This book is to
the las

Hatch and Sumner's Textbook of Paediatric Anaesthesia

Hatch and Sumner's Textbook of Paediatric Anaesthesia

Third edition

Edited by

Robert Bingham FRCA
Consultant Anaesthetist, Great Ormond Street Hospital
for Children NHS Trust, London, UK

Adrian R Lloyd-Thomas FRCA
Consultant Anaesthetist, Great Ormond Street Hospital
for Children NHS Trust, London, UK

Michael RJ Sury FRCA
Consultant Anaesthetist, Great Ormond Street Hospital
for Children NHS Trust, London, UK

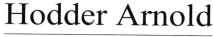
Hodder Arnold
www.hoddereducation.com

First published in Great Britain in 1989 by Baillière Tindall
Second edition published in Great Britain in 2000 by Hodder Arnold
This third edition published in 2008 by
Hodder Arnold, an imprint of Hodder Education, part of Hachette Livre
UK, 338 Euston Road, London NW1 3BH

http://www.hoddereducation.com

Distributed in the United States of America by
Oxford University Press Inc.,
198 Madison Avenue, New York, NY10016
Oxford is a registered trademark of Oxford University Press

*Hachette Livre UK's policy is to use papers that are natural, renewable and
recyclable products and made from wood grown in sustainable forests. The
logging and manufacturing processes are expected to conform to the
environmental regulations of the country of origin.*

Whilst the advice and information in this book are believed to be true
and accurate at the date of going to press, neither the author[s] nor the
publisher can accept any legal responsibility or liability for any errors or
omissions that may be made. In particular (but without limiting the
generality of the preceding disclaimer) every effort has been made to
check drug dosages; however it is still possible that errors have been
missed. Furthermore, dosage schedules are constantly being revised and
new side-effects recognised. For these reasons the reader is strongly
urged to consult the drug companies' printed instructions before
administering any of the drugs recommended in this book.

British Library Cataloguing in Publication Data
A catalogue record for this book is available from the British Library

Library of Congress Cataloging-in-Publication Data
A catalog record for this book is available from the Library of Congress

ISBN-13 978 0 340 912201

1 2 3 4 5 6 7 8 9 10

Commissioning Editor: Gavin Jamieson
Project Editor: Francesca Naish
Production Controller: Andre Sim
Cover Designer: Helen Townson
Indexer: Laurence Errington

Typeset in 10/12, Minion by Charon Tec Ltd (A Macmillan Company),
Chennai, India www.charontec.com
Printed and bound in the UK by MPG Books, Bodmin

What do you think about this book? Or any other Hodder Arnold
title? Please visit our website: **www.hoddereducation.com**

To trainees in paediatric anaesthesia – the future of the specialty.

Contents

Appendices

Contributors

J Mark Ansermino MBBCh FFA(SA) FRCPC
Assistant Professor
Anaesthesiology, Pharmacology
and Therapeutic Department
University of British Columbia
Vancouver, Canada

Brian J Anderson PhD, FANZCA, FJFICM
Associate Professor of Anaesthesiology
University of Auckland
New Zealand

James Bennett MBBS FRCA
Consultant Anaesthetist
Birmingham Children's Hospital
Birmingham, UK

Justus Benrath MD
Professor of Anaesthesia and Intensive Care Medicine
Medical University Vienna
Department of Anaesthesia and Intensive Care Medicine
Waehringer Guertel
Vienna, Austria

Robert Bingham FRCA
Consultant Anaesthetist
Great Ormond Street Hospital for Children NHS Trust
London, UK

Bruno Bissonnette MD
Professor of Anaesthesia
University of Toronto
Director of Neuroanaesthesia
The Hospital for Sick Children
University of Toronto
Ontario, Canada

Ann E Black MB BS, FRCA
Consultant Anaesthetist
Great Ormond Street Hospital for Children NHS Trust
London, UK

Peter D Booker MB, BS, MD, FRCA
Consultant Anaesthetist
Royal Liverpool Children's Hospital,
Eaton Road
Liverpool, UK

Adrian T Bösenberg MBChB (Cape Town),
DA (SA), FFA (SA)
Professor and Second Chair of Anaesthesia
Faculty of Health Sciences
University Cape Town
Observatory, South Africa and
Red Cross War Memorial Children's Hospital
Rondebosch, South Africa

Liam Brennan BSc MBBS FRCA
Consultant Anaesthetist
Addenbrooke's Hospital
Cambridge, UK

Mike Broadhead FRCA
Consultant Anaesthetist
Great Ormond Street Hospital for Children NHS Trust
London, UK

Peter Bromley MBBS FRCA
Consultant Anaesthetist
Birmingham Children's Hospital
Birmingham, UK

Anthony Chisakuta BSc MB ChB MSSc MMedSc
FFARCSI
Consultant Anaesthetist
The Royal Belfast Hospital for Sick Children
Belfast, N. Ireland, UK

Peter Crean MB BCh FRCA FFARCSI
Consultant Anaesthetist
The Royal Belfast Hospital for
Sick Children
Belfast, N. Ireland, UK

Philip M D Cunnington MB, BS, FRCA
Consultant Anaesthetist
Great Ormond Street Hospital for Children NHS Trust
London, UK

John Currie FRCA
Consultant Anaesthetist
Royal Hospital for Sick Children
Glasgow, UK

Andrew John Davidson MBBS, MD, FANZCA
GradDipEpiBiostats
Staff Anaesthetist
Royal Children's Hospital and
Clinical Associate Professor
University of Melbourne
Research Group Leader
Murdoch Children's Research Institute
Melbourne, Australia

David De Beer FRCA
Consultant Anaesthetist
Great Ormond Street Hospital for Children NHS Trust
London, UK

Bruce Emerson FRCA
Consultant Anaesthetist
St Andrew's Centre for Plastic Surgery and Burns
Broomfield Hospital
Chelmsford, UK

Patrick Thomas Farrell MBBS FRCA FANZCA
Director of Anaesthesia
John Hunter Hospital
Newcastle, NSW, Australia

Hilary Glaisyer FRCA
Consultant Anaesthetist
Great Ormond Street Hospital for Children NHS Trust
London, UK

Richard F Howard BSc MB ChB FRCA
Consultant in Anaesthesia and Pain Management
Great Ormond Street Hospital for Children NHS Trust
London, UK

Jane E Herod BSc, FRCA, MBBS
Consultant Anaesthetist
Great Ormond Street Hospital for Children NHS Trust
London, UK

Elizabeth Jackson BSc, MRCP, FRCA, PhD
Consultant Anaesthetist
Great Ormond Street Hospital for Children NHS Trust
London, UK

Ian James MB, ChB, FRCA
Consultant Anaesthetist
Great Ormond Street Hospital for Children NHS Trust
London, UK

Justin John MB BS
Staff Anaesthetist
The Hospital for Sick Children
University of Toronto
Ontario, Canada

Stephan Kettner MD
Professor of Anaesthesia and Intensive Care Medicine
Medical University Vienna
Department of Anaesthesia and Intensive Care Medicine
Waehringer Guertel
Vienna, Austria

Hannu Kokki MD, PhD, Docent
Professor of Anaesthesia
Department of Pharmacology and Toxicology
University of Kuopio and
Department of Anaesthesiology and Intensive Care
Kuopio University Hospital
Kuopio, Finland

Gillian R Lauder FRCA
Consultant Anaesthetist
Bristol Royal Hospital for Children
Bristol, UK

Adrian R Lloyd-Thomas FRCA
Consultant Anaesthetist
Great Ormond Street Hospital for Children NHS Trust
London, UK

Per-Arne Lönnqvist
Consultant Anaesthesiologist
Astrid Lindgrens Children's Hospital/Karolinska
University Hospital and
Associate Professor
Dept of Physiology, Pharmacology and Anaesthesiology
Karolinska Institute, Stockholm, Sweden

Jane Lockie FRCA
Consultant Anaesthetist
University College Hospital NHS Trust
London, UK

Igor Luginbuehl MD
Assistant Professor of Anaesthesia
University of Toronto and
Staff Anaesthetist
The Hospital for Sick Children
University of Toronto
Ontario, Canada

Daniel Lutman FRCA
Consultant Anaesthetist
Children's Acute Transport Service
Great Ormond Street Hospital for Children NHS Trust
London, UK

Anne M Lynn MD
Professor of Anesthesiology and Pediatrics (adjunct)
University of Washington School of Medicine
Attending Anesthesiologist
Children's Hospital and Regional Medical Center
Seattle, USA

Duncan Macrae FRCA
Consultant Anaesthetist and
Director of Paediatric Intensive Care
Royal Brompton Hospital
London, UK

S Mallory FRCA
Consultant Anaesthetist
Great Ormond Street Hospital for Children NHS Trust
London, UK

Peter Marhofer MD
Medical University Vienna
Waehringer Guertel
Vienna, Austria

Rebecca Martin FRCA
Consultant Anaesthetist
St Andrew's Centre for Plastic Surgery and Burns
Broomfield Hospital
Chelmsford, UK

Richard Martin FRCA
Consultant Anaesthetist
Great Ormond Street Hospital for Children NHS Trust
London, UK

Jean-Xavier Mazoit MD PhD
Staff Anaesthesiologist
Département d'Anesthésie-Réanimation Hopital
Bicêtre Assistance Publique Hôpitaux de Paris and
UPRES
'Traumatisme tissulaire et inflammation'
Université Paris-Sud
Le Kremlin-Bicêtre, France

Angus McEwan FRCA
Consultant Anaesthetist
Great Ormond Street Hospital for Children NHS Trust
London, UK

George Meakin FRCA
Consultant Anaesthetist
Royal Manchester Children's Hospital and
Senior Lecturer in Paediatric Anaesthesia
University of Manchester
Manchester, UK

Neil S Morton MBChB, FRCA, FRCPCH
Consultant in Paediatric Anaesthesia and Pain
Management
Royal Hospital for Sick Children
Glasgow, UK

Monty Mythen FRCA, PhD
Professor of Anaesthesia
Portex Anaesthesia, Intensive Therapy and
Respiratory Unit
Institute of Child Health
London, UK

Isabelle Murat MD PhD
Professor of Anaesthesiology
University Paris VI and
Chairman
Service d'Anaesthésie Réanimation
Hôpital Armand Trousseau
Paris, France

Reema Nandi FRCA, MD
Consultant Anaesthetist
Great Ormond Street Hospital for Children NHS Trust
London, UK

Kar-Binh Ong FRCA
Consultant Anaesthetist
Great Ormond Street Hospital for Children NHS Trust
London, UK

Mark J Peters MRCP FRCPCH PhD
Children's Acute Transport Service
Paediatric and Neonatal Intensive Care Units
Great Ormond Street Hospital for Children NHS Trust
London, UK

Sally E Rampersad MB, DCH, FRCA
Assistant Professor of Anesthesiology
University of Washington School of Medicine and
Attending Anesthesiologist
Children's Hospital and Regional Medical Center
Seattle, USA

Derek J Roebuck FRCR, FRANZCR
Consultant Radiologist
Great Ormond Street Hospital for Children NHS Trust
London, UK

Desiré Schabort MD
Department of Anatomy
School of Medicine
University of Pretoria
Pretoria, South Africa

Stephen Scuplak FRCA
Consultant Anaesthetist
Great Ormond Street Hospital for Children NHS Trust
London, UK

Janet Stocks PhD
Professor of Respiratory Physiology
Portex Anaesthesia, Intensive Therapy and
Respiratory Medicine Unit,
Institute of Child Health
London, UK

Peter Stoddart BSc, MB BS, MRCP, FRCA
Consultant Anaesthetist
Bristol Royal Hospital for Children
Bristol, UK

Michael RJ Sury FRCA
Consultant Anaesthetist
Great Ormond Street Hospital for Children NHS Trust
London, UK

Mark Thomas FRCA
Consultant Anaesthetist
Great Ormond Street Hospital for Children NHS Trust
London, UK

Isabeau Walker FRCA
Consultant Anaesthetist
Great Ormond Street Hospital for Children NHS Trust
London, UK

Johan van der Walt MB ChB, FFARCSI, FANZCA
Emeritus Staff Anaesthetist
Women's and Children's Hospital
Adelaide, Australia

Dr Kathy Wilkinson MRCP, FRCA, FRCPCH
Consultant Anaesthetist
Norfolk and Norwich University Hospital
Norwich, UK

Glyn Williams FRCA, MD
Consultant in Anaesthesia and Pain Management
Great Ormond Street Hospital for Children NHS Trust
London, UK

Sally Wilmshurst FRCA
Consultant Anaesthetist
Great Ormond Street Hospital for Children NHS Trust
London, UK

Andrew R Wolf FRCA, PhD
Professor and Consultant in Anaesthesia
University of Bristol
Bristol, UK

Foreword

From the early days of anaesthesia children were given priority for what was a scarce resource. However, formal training was non-existent, and there are few references to the special needs of children in the early literature, although complications, and even deaths, were reported in the leading medical journals from as early as 1847 [1]. The most well known, though not the first, was that of Hannah Greener in 1848. Since those pioneering days many people around the world have striven to make anaesthesia safer both for adults and for children. John Snow presented a paper on asphyxia and the resuscitation of newborn children in 1841 [2], so it seems likely that he took a particular interest in the safe administration of ether and chloroform to children. Indeed, in his famous treatise on chloroform, published posthumously in 1858, he noted that induction and recovery were quicker in children than in adults, a fact that he attributed to the quicker breathing and circulation [3]. He also kept a meticulous record of his cases, writing:

'I have given chloroform in a few cases as early as the ages of eight and ten days, and in a considerable number before the age of two months; and I have at this time, June 30th 1857, memoranda of the cases of 186 infants under a year old to whom I have administered this agent. There have been no ill effects from it either in these cases or in those of children more advanced in life; and it is worthy of remark that none of the accidents from chloroform which have been recorded, have occurred to young children.'

Frederic Hewitt, writing in *The Lancet* in 1910, recognised that children required special consideration. He acknowledged the importance of gaining their confidence and never deceiving them or losing patience with them [4]. He was ahead of his time in documenting the psychological aspects of the approach to children, though his suggestion that relatives should be excluded during induction of anaesthesia would not receive much support today.

It soon became apparent that not only were children physiologically and pharmacologically different from adults, but also the apparatus designed for the administration of anaesthesia to adults was not satisfactory for children. This may partly explain why the simple 'rag and bottle' method survived for so long. Although Magill described a device for insufflation anaesthesia in children [5], Philip Ayre's simple T-piece [6], later modified by Jackson Rees [7], was one of the most important developments in anaesthetic apparatus for children of the first half of the twentieth century. The high cost of inhalational agents used for children together with concerns about environmental pollution have stimulated a resurgence of interest in circle breathing systems as a viable alternative to the T-piece.

Advances in monitoring of basic physiological parameters such as blood pressure and ECG have occurred comparatively recently, and some anaesthetists can still recall the era when patient monitoring relied on little more than a finger on the pulse. Undoubtedly, the most significant monitoring advances have been the development of pulse oximetry and capnography, which are now widely used throughout the world. Availability of drugs for children, however, remains disappointing, with so many unlicensed or off-licence drugs being used that the phrase 'therapeutic orphans' is still sadly appropriate for children. The provision of safe sedation for children for the increasing numbers of diagnostic and therapeutic procedures being performed outside the traditional operating environment remains a particularly challenging problem.

For many years little attention was paid to pain management, and indeed many thought that perception of pain was blunted in infants and young children. The advances in regional analgesia and other methods of pain relief, together with the introduction of interdisciplinary acute pain teams, have been among the most dramatic developments in recent years. Other major advances that have occurred outside the operating environment, including advances in critical care, are too numerous to mention.

The first national organisation for improving the standards of anaesthesia for children and enhancing communication between those who anaesthetised them – the Association of Paediatric Anaesthetists of Great Britain and Ireland – was founded in 1973 and was quickly followed by others in the USA and around the world. The first international peer-review journal devoted to the subject – *Paediatric Anaesthesia* – was published in 1991 and reflected the world-wide recognition of paediatric anaesthesia as a major specialty in its own right. The first article of the first issue of that journal is a fine account of the early history of paediatric anaesthesia written by Jackson Rees [8].

Until the early 1990s most anaesthetists regarded themselves as capable of providing anaesthesia for children. However, following the criticism of occasional paediatric anaesthetic practice in the 1989 National Confidential Enquiry into Perioperative Deaths [9] more children are now treated in specialist centres or general hospitals with a large enough caseload to maintain the skills needed for safe paediatric anaesthetic practice. Formal competency-based training in paediatric anaesthesia is now firmly embedded in the curriculum, but the maintenance of skills required to treat emergency cases by anaesthetists without a regular paediatric commitment remains a challenge.

Many of the pioneers of paediatric anaesthesia were more interested in the practical aspects of the subject than the academic ones, and they passed on their knowledge and skills more by oral teaching and demonstration than by writing. Langton Hewer's book on anaesthesia in children, published in 1923, was the first book to be devoted specifically to the topic in the UK [10] and it was not until after the Second World War that other textbooks devoted to the subject began to appear. In America Digby Leigh and Robert Smith produced textbooks, which became a source of reference around the world [11,12]. However, very few textbooks on the subject existed before the 1970s, with teaching largely in the form of apprenticeships and mostly carried out in specialist centres. Nowadays trainees receive less clinical experience and the need for practically orientated textbooks such as this is increasing both for them and for the continuing education of trained staff.

This textbook addresses both the general and the specialised aspects of paediatric anaesthesia, while maintaining the strong grounding in basic sciences established by its predecessors. While many of the chapters are underpinned by decades of local experience and expertise, the broadly based international authorship of the book as a whole reflects the increasing amount of knowledge that is accepted globally in this modern age of rapid electronic communication.

David J Hatch and Edward Sumner

REFERENCES

1. Gardner J. On ether vapour, its medical and surgical uses. *Lancet* 1847; **1**: 431–4.

2. Snow J. On asphyxia, and the resuscitation of still-born children. *Lond Med Gaz* 1841; **29**: 222–7.

3. Snow J. *On chloroform and other anaesthetics: their action and administration.* Edited by Richardson BW. London: J Churchill, 1858: 49.

4. Hewitt FW. The aesthetics of anaesthetics. *Lancet* 1910; **i**: 625.

5. Magill IW. An expiratory attachment for endotracheal catheters. *Lancet* 1924; **i**: 1320.

6. Ayre P. Endotracheal anesthesia for babies: with special reference to hare-lip and cleft palate operations. *Anesth Analg* 1937; **Nov–Dec**: 330–3.

7. Rees G.J. Anaesthesia in the newborn. *BMJ* 1950; **ii**: 1419–22.

8. Jackson Rees G. An early history of paediatric anaesthesia. *Paediatr Anaesth* 1991; **1**: 3–11.

9. Camplin EA, Devlin HB, Lunn JN. *The Report of the National Confidential Enquiry into Perioperative Deaths 1989.* London: NCEPOD, The Royal College of Surgeons of England, 1990.

10. Hewer CL. *Anaesthesia in children.* London: HK Lewis, 1923.

11. Leigh MD, Belton MK. *Pediatric anesthesia.* New York: Macmillan Co., 1948.

12. Smith RM. *Anesthesia for infants and children.* St Louis, MO: CV Mosby, 1959.

Introduction

In the autumn of 2005 we began the project of this third edition aiming to expand the textbook and retain its respected *Hatch and Sumner* name. We feel privileged to follow the editorial paths mapped out by David and Ted who were our friends, colleagues and teachers. In the 8 years since their second edition paediatric anaesthesia has advanced with fresh knowledge, new challenges and practice to make another edition necessary.

Our particular gratitude goes to our authors who were chosen not only from our own hospital but also more widely in order to capture the opinions of experts from many parts of the globe. Together they have created 50 chapters, each of which can stand alone either as a review of the science or as an essay of current best practice. Their brief was to provide the reader with a concise, pithy account of up-to-date practice supported by scientific evidence where it exists. They were asked not to provide detailed coverage of standard anaesthesia knowledge that can be found elsewhere but to concentrate on material that is extra and special to our paediatric specialty. Details of surgical operations or medical diseases have been limited to those that are relevant and important enough to either the practical or organisational management of children. At the risk of reducing clarity, controversial issues have not been evaded. Our intention was to cover what is both known and unknown so that future debate may be better informed and research is stimulated. References have been included if they were published within the last decade; older references can be found in their bibliographies although some older iconic or historical ones have been included if they were considered sufficiently important to justify their continued quotation. We have marked crucial references that we feel should be known by trainees (these could be used to direct discussion in tutorials). It may be that paper-based textbooks will be outdated and superseded by the electronic format (and we intend to develop this further ourselves) but until that day comes we hope that our book will be used as a quick clinical reference in operating theatres and for browsing in libraries.

Many daylight and nocturnal hours have been taken up by this enterprise and we owe considerable debts to our families and friends for their support, help and, most of all, their patience.

Robert Bingham, Adrian R Lloyd-Thomas
and Michael RJ Sury
August 2007

Abbreviations

5-HT	5-hydroxytryptamine (serotonin)
ABF	aortic blood flow
AChRs	acetylcholine receptors
ACS	acute chest syndrome
ACT	activated coagulation time
ACTH	adrenocorticotrophic hormone
ADH	antidiuretic hormone
ADHD	attention deficit hyperactivity disorder
AE	acute epiglottitis
AEP	auditory-evoked potential
AIDS	acquired immune deficiency syndrome
AIMS	Australian Incident Monitoring Study
ANZCA	Australian and New Zealand College of Anaesthetists
APAGBI	Association of Paediatric Anaesthetists in Great Britain and Ireland
APLS	Advanced Paediatric Life Support
APSF	Australian Patient Safety Foundation
APTT	activated partial thromboplastin time
ARDS	acute respiratory distress syndrome
AS	aortic stenosis
ASA	American Society of Anesthesiology
ASD	atrial septal defect
AVM	arteriovenous malformation
AVSD	atrioventricular canal defect
BBB	blood–brain barrier
BiPAP	bi-level positive pressure ventilation
BIS	Bispectral Index
BMR	basal metabolic rate
BNF	*British National Formulary*
BPA	British Paediatric Association
BPD	bronchopulmonary dysplasia
BSA	body surface area
BT	Blalock–Taussing (shunt)
Cl	clearance
CATS	Children's Acute Transport Service
CBF	cerebral blood flow
CBV	cerebral blood volume
CCAM	congenital cystic adenomatoid malformation
CDH	congenital diaphragmatic hernia
CESP	Confederation of European Specialists in Paediatrics
CFAM	cerebral functioning analysing monitor
CFM	cerebral function monitor
CHAOS	congenital high airway obstruction syndrome
CHARGE	(association) *c*oloboma of the eye, *h*eart defects, *a*tresia of the choanae, *r*etardation of growth and/or development, *g*enital and/or urinary abnormalities, and *e*ar abnormalities and deafness)
CHD	congenital heart disease
CI	cardiac index
CLD	chronic lung disease
CLDI	chronic lung disease of infancy
$CMRO_2$	cerebral metabolic rate for oxygen
CNS	central nervous system
CO	cardiac output
COREC	Central Office for Research Ethics Committees
CPAP	continuous positive airway pressure
CPB	cardiopulmonary bypass
CPP	cerebral perfusion pressure
C_{pss50}	50 per cent depression of electromyograph twitch
CR_{CO_2}	cerebrovascular reactivity to carbon dioxide
CS	cervical spine
CSAa	aortic cross-sectional area
CSF	cerebrospinal fluid
CSW	cerebral salt wasting
CT	computed tomography
CTEV	congenital talipes equinovarus
CV	closing volume
CVA	cerebrovascular accident
CVC	central venous catheter
CVP	central venous pressure
C_w	chest wall compliance
CXR	chest X-ray
DA	ductus arteriosus
DHCA	deep hypothermic circulatory arrest
DLT	double-lumen tubes
EA	emergence agitation
EAR	enclosed afferent reservoir
ECF	extracellular fluid
ECG	electrocardiogram
ECMO	extracorporeal membrane oxygenation
EDHF	endothelial-derived hyperpolarising factor
EEG	electroencephalogram
ELSO	extracorporeal life support organisation
EMG	electromyograph

EMLA	eutectic mixture of local anaesthetics
EMO	Epstein–Macintosh–Oxford (vaporiser)
ENT	ear, nose and throat
EPLS	European Paediatric Life Support
ESRF	end-stage renal failure
EWTD	European Working Time Directive
EXIT	*ex utero* intrapartum treatment
FAST	focused abdominal sonography for trauma
FEV_1	forced expiratory volume in one second
FFP	fresh frozen plasma
FiO_2	inspired oxygen concentration
FOI	fibre-optic intubation
FOT	forced oscillation technique
FRC	functional residual capacity
FTc	corrected flow time
FVC	forced vital capacity
GABA	γ-aminobutyric acid
GCS	Glasgow Coma Scale
GEDV	global end-diastolic volume
GFR	glomerular filtration rate
GOR	gastro-oesophageal reflux
GUCH	'grown-up congenital heart disease'
GVHD	graft-versus-host disease
HAS	human albumin solution
Hb	haemoglobin
HbA	adult haemoglobin
HbF	foetal haemoglobin
HBIR	Hering–Breuer inflation reflex
HDU	high-dependency unit
HFOV	high-frequency oscillatory ventilation
HIV	human immunodeficiency virus
HLHS	hypoplastic left heart syndrome
HME	Heat and moisture exchanger
HOCM	hypertrophic obstructive cardiomyopathy
HPA	human platelet antigen
HPS	hepatopulmonary syndrome
HPV	hypoxic pulmonary vasoconstriction
HRS	hepatorenal syndrome
HRV	heart rate variability
IAP	intra-abdominal pressure
ICC	interventional cardiac catheterisation
ICH GCP	International Conference on Harmonisation Good practice Guideline
ICP	intracranial pressure
ICU	intensive care unit
IFT	isolated forearm technique
ILMA	intubating laryngeal mask airway
iNO	inhaled nitric oxide
INR	international normalised ratio
IPPV	intermittent positive pressure ventilation
ISS	injury severity score
ITBV	intrathoracic blood volume
IUGR	intrauterine growth restriction
IV	intravenous
IVC	inferior vena cava
LA	local anaesthesia/anaesthetic
LAP	left atrial pressure

LIP	lymphocytic interstitial pneumonitis
LMA	laryngeal mask airway
LP	lumbar puncture
LV	Liquid ventilation
LVAD	left-ventricular assist device
LVH	Left-ventricular hypertrophy
LVOT	left-ventricular outflow tract
LVOTO	left-ventricular outflow tract obstruction
M-3-G	morphine-3-glucuronide
M-6-G	morphine-6-glucuronide
MAC	minimum alveolar concentration
MAP	mean arterial pressure
MAPCA	major aortopulmonary collateral artery
MBW	multiple breath inert gas washout
MH	malignant hyperthermia
MHRA	Medicines and Healthcare products Regulatory Agency
MLB	microlaryngoscopy and bronchoscopy
MLR	middle latency response
MMS	masseter muscle spasm
MRI	magnetic resonance imaging
MRV	magnetic resonance venography
MUA	manipulation under anaesthesia
N_2O	nitrous oxide
NACS	Neurologic and Adaptive Capacity Score
NAI	non-accidental injury
NAPQI	*N*-acetyl-*p*-benzoquinone imine
NCA	nurse-controlled analgesia
NCEPOD	National Confidential Enquiry into Perioperative Deaths (UK)
NGT	nasogastric tube
NHMRC	National Health and Medical research Council
NHS	National Health Service
NIBP	automated non-invasive blood pressure
NICU	neonatal intensive care unit
NMDA	*N*-methyl-D-aspartic acid
NO	nitric oxide
NPSA	National Patient Safety Authority
NSAID	non-steroidal anti-inflammatory drug
NSF	National Service Framework
NYHA	New York Heart Association
OCR	oculocardiac reflex
OIB	Oxford Inflating Bellows
OMV	Oxford Miniature Vaporiser
τ_{rs}	expiratory time constant
ORS	oral rehydration solution
OSA	obstructive sleep apnoea
$PaCO_2$	partial pressure of arterial carbon dioxide
PACU	post-anaesthesia care unit
PALS	Paediatric Advanced Life Support
PaO_2	partial pressure of arterial oxygen
PAP	pulmonary arterial pressure
PAPVD	partial anomalous pulmonary venous drainage
PCA	patient-controlled analgesia or postconceptional age
PCO_2	partial pressure of carbon dioxide

PCRA	patient-controlled regional anaesthesia		SIGN	Scottish Intercollegiate Guideline
PDA	patent ductus arteriosus		SIMV	synchronised intermittent mandatory ventilation
$P_{ET}CO_2$	end-tidal carbon dioxide tension		SLV	single lung ventilation
PEEP	positive end-expiratory pressure		SpO_2	peripheral haemoglobin oxygen saturation
PEFR	peak expiratory flow rate		STRS	South Thames Retrieval Service
$P_{ET}CO_2$	end-tidal carbon dioxide partial pressure		SVC	superior vena cava
PFO	Patent foramen ovale		SvO_2	venous oxygen saturation
PIC	paediatric intensive care		SVR	systemic vascular resistance
PICU	paediatric intensive care unit		TAPVD	total anomalous pulmonary venous drainage
PMETB	Postgraduate Medical Education and Training Board		TB	tuberculosis
PN	parenteral nutrition		TBI	traumatic brain injury
POCA	perioperative cardiac arrest		$TcCO_2$	transcutaneous carbon dioxide
PONV	postoperative nausea and vomiting		TCD	transcranial Doppler
POV	postoperative vomiting		TCI	target-controlled infusion
PPH	persistent pulmonary hypertension		TCPC	total cavopulmonary connection
PSA	procedural sedation and analgesia		t_E	expiratory time
PT	prothrombin time		Teq	equilibration half-time
PVD	pulmonary vascular disease		TIVA	total intravenous anaesthesia
PVI	pressure–volume index		TLC	total lung capacity
PVR	pulmonary vascular resistance		TOE	transoesophageal echocardiography
RA	relative analgesia		ToF	tetralogy of Fallot
RAE	Ring–Adair–Elwyn tracheal tube		$Tpeak$	time to peak effect
R_{aw}	airway resistance		TPN	total parenteral nutrition
RCoA	Royal College of Anaesthetists		TT	thrombin time
RCPCH	Royal College of Paediatrics and Child Health		TT	tracheal tube
RCSEng	Royal College of Surgeons of England		UAO	upper airway obstruction
RCT	randomised controlled trial		URTI	upper respiratory tract infection
RDS	respiratory distress syndrome		$\dot{V}/\dot{Q}$	ventilation/perfusion
RED	rigid extraction device		VAE	venous air embolism
REM	rapid eye movement		VATS	video-assisted thoracic surgery
RR	respiratory rate		Vc	volume of distribution in the central compartment
R_{rs}	total respiratory resistance		VC	vital capacity
RSI	rapid sequence induction		VCFS	velocardiofacial syndrome
SA	surface area		V_d	volume of distribution
SaO_2	arterial oxygen saturation		Vf	flow velocity
SCD	sickle cell disease		VLTB	viral laryngotracheobronchitis (croup)
SCPP	spinal cord perfusion pressure		VO_2	oxygen uptake
SEF	spectral edge frequency		VSD	ventricular septal defect
SESAM	Society in Europe for Simulation Applied to Medicine		V_{ss}	volume of distribution at steady state
SGS	subglottic stenosis		WBC	white blood cell
SIDS	sudden infant death syndrome		WHO	World Health Organization

PART I

SCIENTIFIC BASIS OF PAEDIATRIC ANAESTHESIA

1

Normal development

ANDREW J DAVIDSON

KEY LEARNING POINTS

Growth
- Growth charts aid assessment of health and nutrition.
- Formulae are useful to estimate body weight.
- Different parts of a child grow at different rates, leading to significant changes in proportion.
- Breast-feeding is associated with a reduced incidence of a wide range of diseases.

Normal physical development
- Periods of rapid growth occur in infancy and puberty.
- Foetal physiology, such as haemoglobin and pulmonary vascular reactivity, lingers in the early neonatal period.
- Neonates lack a breadth of function in many organ systems.
- Neonatal metabolic rate is significantly higher than in adults.

Normal behavioural and psychological development
- Behavioural development is determined by genes and environment.

- Before surgery, children aged 2–7 years focus on single concepts.
- Cognition and rudimentary concepts of self are evident from early infancy.
- There is evidence that infants have memory.

Child health
- Accidents are the commonest cause of death after the neonatal period.
- Upper respiratory infection is the commonest reason for primary care.
- Behavioural problems are the commonest indication for specialist referral.
- Approximately 5 per cent of children have an anaesthetic each year. The commonest procedure involves ear, nose or throat surgery.

INTRODUCTION

Paediatric anaesthesia is distinct from adult anaesthesia. The pathology, procedures and intercurrent illnesses differ and, most importantly, children in themselves are different. Together with size and proportion, their physiology and behaviour also undergo substantial change with age. Understanding how a child grows and develops is fundamental to paediatric anaesthesia.

This chapter will describe normal growth and summarise normal development. Greater detail of physiological and anatomical development for each organ system can be found in later chapters. Also in this chapter there is detailed discussion on behavioural and psychological development. Finally, the current status of child health in the developed world is described, along with incidence of anaesthesia in children.

GROWTH

Growth is an increase in size while development is an increase in complexity and functional capacity. In a statistical sense, the term *normal* refers to a distribution of values

Table 1.1 Mean weight, length and head circumference

Age	Girls			Boys		
	Weight (kg)	Length (cm)	Head circumference (cm)	Weight (kg)	Length (cm)	Head circumference (cm)
Birth	3	50	35	3	50	35
3 months	6	61	41	6	60	40
6 months	8	66	44	8	66	42
1 year	10	76	46	10	74	45
2 years	13	88	48	12	86	47
4 years	17	103	50	16	102	49
6 years	21	116	52	19	115	51
8 years	25	127	52	24	127	52
10 years	32	137	53	32	139	53
12 years	40	150	54	41	153	54
14 years	51	164	54	50	161	54
17 years	67	176	55	57	164	54

Data adapted from Centres of Disease Control and Prevention (http://www.cdc.gov/growthcharts/) and Paxton *et al.* Paediatric Handbook, 7th edn. Melbourne: Blackwell Publishing, 2003.
Note: formulae for approximate weight (age is in years).
For age <9 years: weight (kg) = (2 × age) + 9.
For age >9 years: weight (kg) = 3 × age.

that have a gaussian or bell-shaped distribution. A gaussian distribution is produced when the magnitude of the dependent variable is determined by a large number of independent, binary and random inputs. In a gaussian (normal) distribution 95 per cent of values will be expected to fall within 2 standard deviations (SDs) of the mean and 99.7 per cent within 3 SDs of the mean.

Many anthropometric measures are normally distributed. In a population of children at a particular age, their height and weight will be normally distributed and an individual child who is far from the mean may be arbitrarily classified as abnormal. Alternatively, the further the child's measure is from the mean, the greater the chance that the measure is determined by pathological factors rather than the random influence of non-pathological determinants.

Centiles are commonly used to describe an individual's dimensions relative to the population. The centile is the percentage of children that have a certain measured quantity at that age. As children grow normally they tend to follow a particular centile. 'Falling down' centiles with age may be an indication of disease. A variety of growth charts have been developed to aid assessment of various aspects of normal growth. Population growth charts have been compiled by the Centres of Disease Control and Prevention and can be accessed and downloaded from http://www.cdc.gov/growthcharts/.

Growth charts may be specific to the population where they were derived. For example, compared with bottle-fed babies, breast-fed babies normally have higher weights for the first 6 months then lower in the second 6 months, and more recent charts are derived from populations including higher proportions of bottle-fed babies. The growth chart

may also be difficult to interpret around puberty because the growth spurt is more closely related to onset and timing of puberty rather than age.

Various formulae have also been derived to give very approximate estimates of normal weight (Table 1.1) [1]; these quick formulae are particularly useful.

The rate of growth for a child is not uniform and there are three periods of rapid growth: *in utero* (most rapid), infancy and puberty. After birth, the newborn initially loses 5–10 per cent body weight in the first 24–48 hours because of loss of body water. Birth weight is usually regained by 10–14 days. Growth is then rapid for the first 6 months, birth weight being doubled by 5–6 months and tripled by 1 year. After 1 year the rate of growth falls off gradually, remaining fairly steady after 2 years, before accelerating again at puberty. Growth rates in weight, length and head circumference follow similar patterns (Table 1.2). On a shorter time-scale, growth is not continuous, occurring in brief spurts and varying from day to day.

Different parts of a child also grow at different rates, leading to significant changes in proportion. At birth the head is relatively large and the trunk is long with short arms and legs. If the symphysis pubis is used to divide the body into upper and lower segments, the ratio of upper to lower body segments is about 1.7 at birth, 1.3 at 3 years and 1.0 by 7 years. The body surface area, relative to mass, is greatest at birth and thus there is an increased risk of hypothermia.

The relative mass of organs also changes with growth. This has implications for pharmacokinetics and drug delivery. In classic pharmacokinetic models, drugs are delivered first to well-perfused organs such as the brain, heart and liver, then redistributed to muscle and lastly to

Table 1.2 Rates of growth

Age	Weight (g/day)	Length	Head circumference
0–3 months	30	3.5 cm/month	2 cm/month
3–6 months	20	2 cm/month	1 cm/month
1 year	12	1.2 cm/month	0.5 cm/month
4–6 years	6	3 cm/year	1 cm/year

poorly perfused fat. In neonates, the proportion of cardiac output supplying skeletal muscle is only half that of adults, and therefore relatively more blood goes to other organ systems, influencing the onset of action of drugs and their redistribution. Although the relative size of organs such as kidney, brain and liver is greater, the blood flow to these organs may not be simply related to size. For example, the liver and kidneys are relatively large in neonates but have lower relative blood flows. Also, the maturity of organ systems may influence how the organs handle the drugs independent of blood flow.

The relative blood flow to the brain is also age dependent. In neonates the brain receives a similar proportion of cardiac output compared with adults despite its relatively greater mass, so neonates have a relatively low brain blood flow. In infants and toddlers, however, the brain receives twice the proportion of the cardiac output compared with adults, and therefore the relative blood flow to the brain is greater. This may explain the rapid onset of intravenous anaesthesia in children of this age.

Nutrition

Children require a healthy diet for normal growth and development. Nutritional and energy requirements vary significantly throughout childhood and are expressed in a variety of ways. The estimated average requirement (EAR) is the average amount needed to achieve a defined physiological endpoint, while the recommended daily intake (RDI) is the amount needed to meet the requirement of most healthy members of the population. The RDI is hence greater than the EAR. Owing to difficulties collecting data, the EAR and RDI for most nutrients are not known with certainty.

In the first year nutritional requirements are relatively high because of rapid growth and high metabolic rate. Expressed relative to body weight, an infant requires three times the energy intake of an adult. The energy RDI rises during infancy before falling in later childhood. The energy RDI at 1–6 months is 2310 kJ/day compared with 3013 kJ/day at 7–12 months, and 4494 kJ/day at 1–3 years. The energy can be provided as either fat or carbohydrate, although there is increasing evidence that infants particularly need long-chain polyunsaturated fatty acids. These are present more in breast milk than formula feeds, which may explain the superior visual and cognitive development in breast-fed

infants. The infant also requires relatively more protein, especially essential amino acids. Breast milk is ideally suited to infant nutrition and is associated with a reduced incidence of a wide range of significant diseases. Although the average infant is born with iron stores sufficient for several months, iron deficiency is not uncommon because of significant variability in storage and adsorption.

Feeding

Feeding patterns are often irregular in the first month of life, but by the first week most infants have settled into some routine. Most healthy infants want six to nine feeds per day. Gastric emptying in infants is very variable and the period between feeds may vary from 2 to 4 hours. Breast-fed infants tend to be satisfied for shorter periods than formula-fed infants. The number of feeds per day declines over the first year and by 12 months most infants will be satisfied with three meals per day.

Breast milk can provide all nutritional needs for the first 4–6 months. The use of breast milk, formula and cows' milk varies widely between cultures. Cows' milk is often gradually introduced from 7 to 8 months, coinciding with cup drinking. Although solids should be introduced at around 6 months there is no definite time for weaning. By 8–9 months lumpy food can be eaten and by 2 years the child should be eating the same food as the rest of the family.

Children begin to show food preferences from 1 year of age. While selection of food may vary from day to day, in general, over a prolonged period, young children tend to select well-balanced diets.

Reflux

Gastro-oesophageal reflux is the involuntary passage of gastric contents into the oesophagus. The difference between physiological reflux and disease may be difficult to define. About 50 per cent of 3- to 4-month-olds will regurgitate or occasionally vomit. There are many causes for reflux disease but it is particularly common in children with neurological impairment. Reflux disease may lead to recurrent aspiration and chest infection, weight loss and anaemia. The risk from reflux related to paediatric anaesthesia is uncertain. Rapid sequence induction is not routinely practised in children with reflux, although it certainly should be if there is any suspicion of oesophageal achalasia.

Failure to thrive

Failure to thrive (FTT) is arbitrarily defined as a child falling below the third centile, or dropping two weight centile tracks. In long-standing FTT, poor weight gain is accompanied by failure of linear growth. Some children defined as failing to thrive, will simply be normal variants, while more than 50 per cent of FTT is caused by poor nutrition and psychosocial factors. It can also be caused by a wide variety of diseases including renal, cardiac, respiratory, gastrointestinal, metabolic, genetic, intrauterine, chronic infectious and neurological.

NORMAL PHYSICAL DEVELOPMENT

Development is the increase in complexity or refinement of function that occurs with age and is determined by genetic and environmental factors. Like growth, there is a normal distribution of ages at which children achieve developmental milestones. Disease can also affect development either directly or indirectly by altering the child's social environment.

Development is often described in terms of transitions. The first major transition is birth. The extrauterine environment is significantly different from life in the womb and many aspects of neonatal development are linked to the transition of birth. The other major transition occurs during adolescence, when a child enters competitive and sexually active adult life. Between birth and adolescence other important transitions are the increased mobility and upright posture attained with walking, and the relative increase in independence when children go to school. Not all development occurs as sudden transitions (e.g. organ systems gradually mature, taking months or years to reach their full capacity and breadth of function). A child's steadily increasing size and mass may also directly influence some aspects of organ development.

Later chapters will discuss development of body systems in greater detail.

Neonatal and infant development

The most dramatic changes in development occur *in utero*. In the embryonic period the organ systems differentiate and by birth the bulk of the maturational process has occurred. After birth, the neonatal period is the time of greatest development. The physiology of a neonate is quantitatively and qualitatively different from adults, there being more difference between a 2-day-old and a 2-year-old, than between a 2-year-old and a 20-year-old. For paediatric anaesthesia, neonates present the greatest challenge and the greatest risk [2,3].

In the neonatal period there are changes in maturity and size, and changes that reflect the recent transition from uterine to extrauterine life. Immature organ systems frequently lack a capacity for wide variation in function, for example, neonates are less able to concentrate urine. The maximum urine concentration is 0.6 osmol/kg for a neonate, compared with 1.2 osmol/kg in adults. Also, despite the fact that the kidneys are relatively large, the renal blood flow and glomerular filtration rate (GFR) are low in the newborn,

limiting their ability to excrete water. When adjusted for size, GFR reaches adult levels by 2–3 years.

CARDIOVASCULAR DEVELOPMENT

The cardiovascular and respiratory systems are those most affected by the transition at birth. At birth the lungs aerate and the umbilical vessels are clamped. The pulmonary vascular resistance (PVR) decreases, increasing flow to the lungs and, as the placenta is no longer perfused, the systemic vascular resistance (SVR) increases. *In utero* the left and right ventricles are of similar size but after birth there is a greater workload on the left ventricle (LV) which responds by rapidly increasing in size. The left-to-right size ratio achieves the adult ratio of 3:1 by 3 months [4]. Ventricular growth results from an increase in the size and number of myocytes up until 7 months; further growth is by size only [5].

Some aspects of the foetal circulation linger through the neonatal period. The neonatal PVR can increase in response to hypoxia, hypercapnia and acidosis, and the foramen ovale may also remain functionally open up to the third month; it may remain probe patent into adulthood. If PVR is increased, right-to-left shunting can occur across the patent foramen ovale resulting in further hypoxia. This is seen clinically when neonates are relatively slow to recover from a period of hypoxia. The PVR decreases over the first few months of life.

Lingering foetal physiology is also present in haemoglobin. In neonates the total haemoglobin concentration is high (135–200 g/L at birth), with a high percentage of foetal haemoglobin (70 per cent). The haemoglobin concentration falls to a nadir of about 90–140 g/L by about 2 months and then rises as more adult haemoglobin is produced. Normally, by 4 months all foetal haemoglobin is replaced by adult haemoglobin.

Cardiac output is relatively high in the neonate and this corresponds to the high oxygen consumption. The resting cardiac output of a neonate is 350 mL/kg/min, at 2 months it is 150 mL/kg/min and it then gradually falls toward adult levels of 75 mL/kg/min. The high resting cardiac output may limit the neonate's ability to further increase cardiac output. Resting heart rate also changes significantly with age. It is between 95 beats/min and 145 beats/min at term and rises to a peak of 110–175 beats/min between 3 months and 6 months, before it gradually declines with age [1]. In contrast, stroke volume, adjusted for size, increases throughout childhood [6]. Normal blood pressure also increases throughout childhood from a mean of between 40 mmHg and 60 mmHg in neonates to 50–90 by 1 year. The total blood volume is relatively high in neonates, averaging at 86 mL/kg while adult values are closer to 70 mL/kg.

The LV also has a higher basal level of contractility in early infancy compared with later childhood, which may be due to increased cardiac sympathetic activity. Over the first 6 months of life there is a gradual decrease in adrenergic tone and an increase in cholinergic tone.

Neonates also have a reduced capacity to accommodate changes in afterload and preload. This is due to the immature intracellular and extracellular structure of the heart. Neonatal myocardium is relatively less compliant than adult myocardium, restricting the capacity to increase stroke volume in response to an increasing preload. Neonates are hence more vulnerable to overfilling.

Although it is commonly thought that heart rate is the major determinant of cardiac output in neonates, neonates do retain the capacity to alter cardiac output significantly with change in stroke volume despite their relatively decreased diastolic function [7].

Compared with older children, neonates are also more sensitive to changes in afterload so that when SVR increases they may have more difficulty maintaining cardiac output. However, the evidence for this is contradictory [8]. The aetiology may be that neonatal myocardium cannot generate the same contractile force as adult myocardium [9].

RESPIRATORY DEVELOPMENT

At birth the lungs are expanded, the amniotic fluid is expelled and regular respiration commences. The triggers for the continuation of normal respiration after birth are unclear, but probably relate to the relative hyperoxic environment outside the womb. The foetus makes some regular breathing-like movements well before birth and this activity is depressed by hypoxia. After birth, neonates may continue to respond to hypoxia with suppression of respiration. Response to carbon dioxide is also slightly reduced in the neonate.

Periodic breathing consists of apnoeic pauses up to 10 seconds long, without bradycardia or cyanosis, and occurs in up to 80 per cent of term neonates. It decreases with age, but may still be present in up to 30 per cent by 10 months [10,11]. Apnoea is the cessation of breathing for more than 15 seconds, or less if associated with bradycardia or cyanosis. Central apnoea is uncommon in term neonates. Newborns may also become apnoeic after stimuli that would usually result in increased respiration in older children, such as upper airway obstruction and stimulation of the carina or areas supplied by the superior laryngeal nerve.

There are also important differences in the anatomy of the neonatal airways, lungs and thorax. In neonates the epiglottis and tongue are relatively large and the larynx higher and more anterior. During quiet respiration the majority of neonates are obligate nasal breathers, while by 6 months most infants can mouth breathe.

The tidal volume of a neonate is 6–10 mL/kg and is similar to adults. The oxygen consumption is relatively higher in neonates (6–8 mL/kg/min in neonates versus 4–6 mL/kg/min in adults) and therefore the minute ventilation is also relatively higher. The functional residual capacity (FRC) of neonates and adults is also similar in proportion to size, but the higher minute volume/FRC ratio results in more rapid oxygen desaturation with apnoea.

The chest wall of the neonate is highly compliant because it is cartilaginous and has less muscle. Compared with the adult the outward recoil of the thorax is considerably less, while the pulmonary elasticity is only slightly less. Accessory muscles are used to maintain FRC and prevent the chest wall collapsing during inspiration. The FRC is also maintained by the use of laryngeal adductors 'breaking' the expiratory airflow. Anaesthesia relaxes these muscles resulting in a significant fall in FRC in neonates and infants [12]. Closing volume is also higher in neonates and therefore hypoxia may more readily occur if FRC falls. By 6 months of age chest wall compliance is closer to adult levels, although anaesthesia-related changes in FRC are still marked in children up to the age of 12 [13]. The neonate is also highly dependent on diaphragmatic breathing, making abdominal excursion more obvious during quiet breathing. The ribs are oriented more horizontally and the diaphragm less domed, restricting the neonate's total lung capacity; this does not reach adult levels until 5 years [14].

Airway resistance is highly dependent on airway diameter. The smaller airways in infants could be expected to produce great resistance; however, this is more than adequately countered by the relatively greater diameters when adjusted for weight [15,16]. Airway resistance is thus relatively lower in neonates, but it is important to note that in neonates small absolute changes in the diameter of airways will have a significantly greater impact on airway resistance.

NEUROLOGICAL DEVELOPMENT

Although the brain is relatively large at birth, there is still significant growth and development during childhood. The brain weighs 335 g at birth and doubles in weight in 6 months. By 1 year it weighs 900 g, at 2 years 1000 g and it achieves the adult weight of 1200–1400 g by 12 years of age.

On a cellular level, neuronal development consists of division, growth, migration, differentiation, increasing connectivity and selective cell death. Neurogenesis and division are complete by 18 weeks' gestation. In the embryo there is an overabundance of neurons and glia and with maturity the excess cells undergo programmed cell death (apoptosis). While the number of neurons decreases, they increase in the complexity of their synapses. The period of increasing dendrite formation, or arborisation, is also known as the growth spurt period and lasts, in humans, from the third trimester up until 2–3 years of age. In an animal model, neurons undergo apoptosis after exposure to some anaesthetic agents [17].

Connectivity is determined by a combination of inherent (or genetic) and environmental influences. Molecular programmes, independent of activity or experience, largely determine the path-finding of axons to target areas of the brain. However, the formation of synapses between specific cells depends at least in part on patterned neural traffic evoked by sensory input. An excess number of synapses are initially formed and then pruned on a 'use it or lose it basis'.

The influence of the environment is both general and specific. Synapse generation can be classified as *experience expectant* where normal wiring occurs as a result of stimuli that any human occupying a normal environment would have, and *experience dependent* where connections are formed and reorganised throughout life as a function of an individual's particular experiences [18]. This theme of combined genetic and environmental influence is central to neurological, behavioural and psychosocial development.

Development also occurs in the myelination of axons. Myelination enables faster nerve conduction leading to more rapid reflexes and more complex cognitive processing. Myelination is rapid in the first 2 years and continues to occur up until 7 years of age.

Neonatal responses to physical stimuli

Behavioural and reflex responses to physical stimuli may be useful in the early identification of abnormal neurological development. There are two well-known methods of evaluating neurological behaviour in neonates and they have been used to describe the normal range. Brazelton [19] used responses to 27 simple tests and the reliability of the scoring is heavily dependent upon observer training. Originally, the normal range of scores for neonates was described in Caucasian infants, who were not exposed to appreciable doses of maternal sedation or analgesia and who had 'good' Apgar scores. Since many infants can be discoordinated for 48 hours after delivery, the behaviour on the third day was taken as the expected mean. The scale has been used in a wide variety of situations and it can be reliable enough to demonstrate differences in behaviour

between Oriental and Caucasian infants (Oriental babies are more calm and habituate to stimulation with light more readily) and between normal infants and those whose mothers are methadone addicts. Prechtl [20] also developed

Table 1.3 Summary of descriptors used for defining sleep states in infants

Brazelton [19]	Prechtl [20]
1. Deep sleep, regular breathing, eyes closed, no spontaneous activity	1. Eyes closed, regular respiration, no movements
2. Light sleep, eyes closed; rapid eye movements, irregular respiration	2. Eyes closed, irregular respiration, small movement
3. Drowsy, eyes may be open or closed, eyelids fluttering	3. Eyes open, no movements
4. Alert, with bright look; seems to focus attention on source of stimulation	4. Eyes open, gross movements
5. Eyes open; considerable motor activity, with thrusting movements of limbs	5. Crying (vocalisation)
6. Crying; characterised by intense crying which is difficult to break through with stimulation	6. Other state e.g. coma

Table 1.4 Standard criteria for natural sleep and wakefulness in neonates [18]: summary of criteria for sleep, awake and drowsy states in normal full-term newborn infants

State	Face	Body	Vocalisation	Respiration
Sleep (eyes closed)				
Quiet sleep	Occasional mouth movements	None	Quiet	Regular
Active sleep	Smiles, grimaces, frowns, bursts of sucking	Moves digits or limbs, slow body writhing, sudden jerks	Brief grunts, whimpers and cries	Irregular
Indeterminate sleep	Mixed and changing	Mixed	Mixed	Mixed
Awake				
Crying	Flushed and grimacing	Vigorous and diffuse	Crying	Mixed
Active awake	Eyes moving	Gross	No crying	Mixed
Quiet awake	In active, eyes bright, can follow slow-moving object	Inactive	Quiet	Mixed
Sleep onset and drowsiness	Eyes glassy, cannot follow slow-moving object	NS	NS	Mixed

Sleep state	EOG	EMG	EEG (frequency or pattern)
Quiet sleep	REM negative	Present	TA, HVS, mixed
Active sleep	REM positive	Minimal	LVI, mixed or rarely HVS
Indeterminate sleep	Mixed	Mixed	Mixed

EEG, electroencephalogram; EMG, electromyograph; EOG, electro-oculography; HVS, high voltage, slow; M, mixed; NS, not significant; LVI, low voltage, irregular; REM, rapid eye movement; TA, tracé alternant.

a detailed method of neurological examination of infants that could be used as a reference to identify abnormalities. Both these authors have emphasised the importance of describing the state of sleep or wakefulness in order to interpret the scores from their scales. They each categorised the conscious state similarly although Prechtl does not have a 'drowsy' category (Table 1.3).

Other methods have also been described but have their problems. The Neurologic and Adaptive Capacity Score (NACS) is a scale of behaviour in newborns and was developed to determine the effects of maternal drugs rather than birth asphyxia [21]. It assesses 20 items and can be completed in only 60–90 seconds. Although it was originally said to have high inter-rater reliability, and has been used in many studies, it is now generally regarded as unreliable [22,23].

Development of wakefulness and sleep

In 1971 Anders, Emde and Parmelee and others formed a committee to recommend standard descriptors of natural sleep in infants for use in sleep research [24]. An earlier committee had standardized a description of sleep in adults [25] but this needed modification, as it was clearly not useful in the developing infant. They defined sleep states based on behavioural and physiological characteristics from polygraphic recordings and these are summarised in Table 1.4. The primary criterion to define sleep is sustained eye closure – transient eye openings of up to one epoch per minute may be ignored depending on other observations – and the three secondary behaviour observations are facial and body movements, and vocalisation. The number, combination and weighting of coded observations can be varied and therefore the descriptions of sleep and wake states have to be specified. Detailed accounts of natural sleep development can be found in textbooks of sleep medicine [26,27] and the following is a brief summary of normal development of patterns of sleep and wakefulness.

Spontaneous foetal movements begin at gestation of 10 weeks and rhythmical cycling of activity and rest periods have been observed from 28 to 32 weeks. In premature neonates differentiation between active and quiet sleep is not possible until about 28 weeks when sleep is mostly active sleep, with eye movements and irregular respiration, or intermediate sleep. With increasing age the proportion of intermediate sleep declines while the proportion of quiet sleep increases [28]. By term the foetus has roughly equal amounts of quiet and active sleep. Interestingly, in experiments with pregnant ewes, uterine windows have been surgically implanted to observe the activity of lambs and their eyes do not open until after birth.

Electroencephalogram (EEG) recording of the foetus is possible, transabdominally, from 12 weeks' gestation and shows continuous low-voltage activity that is unrelated to body movement [29]: sleep or waking states cannot be completely defined by EEG until the foetus is much older, by about 36 weeks.

Up until 24 weeks it is difficult to differentiate an EEG associated with from one without limb movement. After 24–27 weeks bursts of high-voltage slow waves (2–6 seconds) followed by very depressed activity (4–8 seconds) is predominant. This pattern is called discontinuous EEG or 'tracé discontinue' [29–32]. From 26 weeks onwards there is a gradual increase of continuous EEG activity. Active sleep develops during this period and is characterised by continuous mixed frequency EEG. Over the same period 'tracé discontinue' is gradually replaced during quiet sleep by 'tracé alternant'. 'Tracé alternant' consists of 3- to 8-second bursts of high-voltage low-amplitude activity interspersed with low-voltage mixed frequency EEG. During quiet sleep 'tracé alternant' normally completely replaces 'tracé discontinue' by 36 weeks and itself disappears by 2 months of age [28]. Sleep spindles, which are characteristic of non-rapid eye movement (non-REM) sleep, usually appear by the age of 3 months. Non-REM and REM sleep develop from quiet and active sleep respectively.

At the start of normal term labour the foetus goes into quiet sleep. The EEG becomes further depressed with hypoxia. This may be a protective reflex. Awakening occurs with the stimulation and changes in circulation and oxygenation at birth.

At term, neonates sleep for approximately 16 hours per day compared with 12 hours by 3 months, and 10 hours by 1 year. The temporal spacing or architecture of sleep develops from short naps between feeding into more prolonged nocturnal periods. Neonates spend approximately 50 per cent of their sleep in active or REM states compared with 25 per cent of 10-year-olds. Neonates begin their sleep with REM and this starts to change at 3 months with REM tending to occur at the end of the sleep period.

During the first 3 months of life babies may be categorised into three groups according to crying. Approximately 50 per cent have paroxysms of unexplained irritable crying lasting for about 3 hours each day for no more than 3 days per week and this is regarded as normal. Crying for more than 3 hours on more than 3 days per week occurs in about 25 per cent of 'fussy' babies but the seriously fussy 25 per cent have paroxysms of crying over a period of longer than 3 weeks (These babies have 3-month colic).

Sudden infant death syndrome

The cause of sudden infant death syndrome (SIDS) is unknown, and despite the major decline in incidence over the last decade it remains an important cause of death in infants. The incidence is rare in the first month, peaks at 2–3 months of age and then decreases; the peak incidence coincides with maturation of vital reflexes and changes in sleep architecture [33]. The following are risk factors for SIDS: sleeping in the prone position, sleeping on a soft surface, maternal smoking during pregnancy, overheating, late or no prenatal care, young maternal age, preterm birth or low birth weight and male gender. Recommendations to reduce SIDS include: supine sleeping, sleeping on a firm surface with no loose bedding or soft objects within reach, no smoking during pregnancy, sleeping in the same room as the infant but not in the same bed, use of a pacifier at bedtime and avoiding overheating [34].

Development through later childhood

By the end of infancy the transition to extrauterine life is complete and most organ systems have achieved a substantial degree of maturity. Increasing size and moving to an upright posture result in continuing development of some organ systems.

The cardiovascular system develops to accommodate the larger body mass, changing proportions and increased activity. The heart progressively increases its weight and stroke volume throughout childhood, both in absolute terms and when adjusted for body surface area. Heart rate gradually falls with age, while, in order to perfuse increasingly distant peripheries, blood pressure steadily increases (it being more closely related to height and weight than age alone).

There are significant respiratory changes beyond infancy. The surface area available for gas exchange increases owing to septation, folding and lengthening of alveoli. The newborn has about 20–50 million alveoli and, by school age, there are roughly 10 times this number. Throughout childhood the lungs and alveoli continue to grow in size to meet the respiratory demands of a larger body. With age, the compliance of the chest wall falls and the elasticity of the lungs increases. Respiratory rate falls as the chest wall compliance falls. The proportions of the upper airway also change; up until 8 years of age the cricoid cartilage is the narrowest point.

The first primary teeth appear at 6–7 months and the last at 2–3 years of age. The first permanent teeth appear at about 6–7 years and the last primary teeth are lost by 12 years (Table 1.5).

Adolescence

With adolescence comes increasing independence and potential for reproduction. There is acceleration in both general and gender-specific growth, together with sexual and psychological maturation. This transition is regulated by both hormonal changes and social factors.

Table 1.5 Normal development of the teeth

Tooth	Eruption of primary teeth (months)	Eruption of permanent teeth (years)
Central incisor	6–12	6–8
Lateral incisor	9–16	6.5–8.5
Canine	16–23	9–13
First premolar	–	9.5–11.5
Second premolar	–	10–3
First molar	13–19	5.5–7
Second molar	23–33	11–13
Third molar	–	17+

Adolescence occurs between 10 and 20 years of age and may be divided into early, middle and late periods. There is considerable variation in both the onset and progression but it starts with the onset of puberty, which is triggered by the increased sensitivity of the pituitary to gonadotrophin-releasing hormone. The time taken to reach growth maturity varies also between racial groups.

The height growth spurt starts in early adolescence but may not peak until 13–14 years of age in boys and 11–12 years of age in girls. It usually finishes by about 17–18 years of age in boys and 14–15 years of age in girls. The growth spurt begins in the hands and feet, before arms and legs, and then last in the trunk and chest. Weight gain follows several months behind height and this makes an adolescent look gangly.

Total muscle mass increases, particularly in boys. The lean body mass before puberty is about 80 per cent. During adolescence this increases to 90 per cent in boys, but decreases to 75 per cent in girls owing to subcutaneous fat. Heart size and lung capacity double, and blood pressure, haematocrit and blood volume also increase.

Menarche usually occurs 1 year after the onset of the growth spurt but may vary enormously and is determined by genetic factors, disease and weight. Compared with the previous century, it is occurring at younger ages in developed countries.

NORMAL BEHAVIOURAL AND PSYCHOLOGICAL DEVELOPMENT

General factors and theories

For children, hospitalisation and anaesthesia are stressful events [35,36] and their perioperative care is increasingly becoming the domain of the anaesthetist. The anaesthetist must understand how children are likely to behave, the nature of their fears and anxieties, and how to communicate effectively with them. This requires a good understanding of cognitive and social development. From another perspective, a primary role of the anaesthetist is to render an individual unconscious and amnestic. The paediatric anaesthetist should understand how and when memory and consciousness develop.

THE BIO-PSYCHOSOCIAL MODEL OF DEVELOPMENT

Neurological, behavioural, psychological and social aspects of development are all linked. For many years nature versus nurture was the central issue in understanding development but now more complex models give a fuller explanation of normal development. The bio-psychosocial model involves three determinants of development: for example, the gene set inherited by the child determines some aspects of neuronal connectivity. The connectivity is further determined by neuronal use directed by environmental stimuli. Finally, with maturity, environmental factors are altered by the child's own choices. This mix of genes and environment has been well illustrated by twin studies that found inheritance consistently accounts for about half of the variability in intelligence. There can also be interaction between neurological and sociological factors: for example, slow development for biological reasons may lead to parental neglect, furthering developmental delay. Children born into poverty are at greater risk of abnormal development as they are exposed to greater biological risk and have less access to support. Alternatively, a child with neurological injury will develop further with nurture.

Temperament is expressed in terms of emotional, motor and attention reactivity and it tends to remain constant across situations and age [37]. A child's temperament is often called 'easy' or 'difficult' and an easy baby usually becomes an easy adolescent. However, the environment is important; a difficult child may develop normally if the environment is supportive.

Normal behavioural development

No other aspects of development undergo as much change during childhood as behavioural and psychological development. Like other aspects of development, there is a mix of transitional and continuous change. Recognised milestones are often used to track normal development but there is considerable normal variation (Table 1.6).

NEONATAL PERIOD

After birth neonates are exposed to new challenges such as cold and hunger, to which they respond with heightened arousal. Crying is a behaviour adopted to alert the parent to these threats. Six normal behavioural states have been described in neonates: quiet sleep, active sleep, drowsy, alert, fussy and crying. Each state is defined by various behaviour and observations including spontaneous movement, muscle tone and EEG.

The senses also adjust to extrauterine life. A neonate's vision has a fixed focal length of 20–30 cm, poor contrast sensitivity and poor colour vision until about 2–3 months. Acuity at birth is approximately 6/120, by 12 months this has improved to 6/12 and adult acuity is present by 18 months. Maturation of the visual cortex is slower. Neonates are insensitive to noise. The faintest sound audible is four times louder than that for an adult. However, like vision, hearing rapidly improves.

Neonates typically display uncontrolled writhing of limbs and purposeless hand opening and closing. In the first few months there are reflexes such as the grasp reflex, the rooting reflex (touch the side of the cheek near the mouth and the head will turn and mouth open) and the tonic neck reflex (turning the infant's head to the right results in the right arm extending, the left arm flexing and the right knee flexing). Neonates smile spontaneously.

2–6 MONTHS

Gradually writhing is replaced by fidgety movement. The infant also begins to explore their bodies by staring at their hands, vocalising and touching themselves. The infant learns how they can control their environment. Facial expressions increase in diversity and rolling over normally first occurs by 4–6 months of age. The sleep EEG also matures with REM and non-REM sleep development.

6–12 MONTHS

Milestones in this period include sitting (7 months), pincer grasp (9 months), crawling (8 months) and walking (12 months). At this age objects are characteristically picked up, looked at, banged, placed in the mouth and dropped. Non-verbal communication increases with facial expressions and vocal tones; first 'words' soon follow. At this time separation from parents becomes more difficult, while autonomy is also developing (for example, sporadic refusal to eat). After this age an infant is more likely to be distressed by separation prior to anaesthesia.

12–24 MONTHS

Toddlers explore their environment as mobility increases. In language understanding precedes expression. Simple statements are understood, and by 15 months the average

Table 1.6   Average attainment of some developmental milestones

Age	Gross motor	Vision and fine motor	Language	Cognitive and social
2–4 months	Head steady sitting	Follows object 180 degrees, reaches for objects	Squeals with pleasure, smiles	Stares at hand
5–8 months	Sits without support, rolls over	Passes object hand to hand	Monosyllabic babble, understands 'no'	Bangs two cubes
9–12 months	Stands without support, cruises and crawls	Neat pincer grip	First word	
12–16 months	Walks well without help	Stacks two cubes	Three words	Drinks from a cup
16–24 months	Walks up steps	Imitates scribbling	Identifies body parts	Listens to stories with pictures, feeds self
24–36 months	Jumps	Draws line in imitation	Refers to self with 'I'	Helps with dressing
3–4 years	Balances on one foot	Draws a face	Tells a story	Plays with several children

child uses four to six words correctly, increasing to 10–15 words by 18 months and over 100 words by 2 years of age. Consistent labelling of objects indicates the onset of symbolic thought. 'Clinginess' increases and objects may have increased attachment as representative symbols of parents (for example, soft toys or blankets).

PRESCHOOL

Left- or right-handedness is normally apparent by 3 years of age. Bladder and bowel control is normally established but varies greatly within and between cultures. Vocabulary increases to about 2000 words and sentence structure advances. Language development at this stage is closely linked to cognitive and emotional development. Magical thinking is common in this period. Magical thinking includes attributing life-like qualities to inanimate objects (animism), confusion between coincidence and causality, and unrealistic beliefs about powers and wishes. Magical thinking can lead to intense fears and misunderstanding when simple procedures are explained, but can also be used to help distract children.

Preschoolers explore the boundaries of their emotional experiences. This may lead to apparent inconsistencies in behaviour, from stubborn opposition to cheerful compliance, and from bold exploration to clinging dependence. At this time the interaction between a child's environment and their abilities or temperament also becomes increasingly important. Energetic and physically more coordinated children thrive if physical activity is encouraged, while more thoughtful children thrive when quiet play is encouraged. Play is increasingly complex and imaginative, and becomes more cooperative and rule governed. Rules tend to be absolute, reflecting the stage of cognitive development. Similarly, preschoolers are unable to focus on more than one aspect of a situation at a time, making them unable to understand complex explanations or reassurance.

SCHOOL AGE

School places an increasing demand on cognitive, perceptual and language skills. With increasing separation from parents, interaction with others increases and the child develops their own self-evaluation as well as an increasing perception of how others see them.

ADOLESCENCE

Development in adolescence is influenced by gender, subculture and social factors. Important issues are separation from family, increasing self-identity and self-consciousness. Self-consciousness increases significantly with the physical signs of puberty. Adolescents ask questions and analyse issues such as who they are, why do they exist and where are they going in life. In this period idealistic or absolutist ideas may flourish as well as increased religious behaviour. Later, there may be increasing thought about abstract ideas such as injustice and fairness.

Theories of cognitive development

Familiarity with the main theories of cognitive development helps the clinician to appreciate the level of understanding that can be expected in children of various ages.

PIAGET

Piaget's theory remains one of the most influential cognitive theories. A central component is the premise that children are actively constructing knowledge for themselves in response to their experiences. Children generate hypotheses, conduct experiments and draw conclusions. Piaget described children as undergoing assimilation (seeking experience and translating information into understandable forms) and accommodation (adapting their implicit ideas about the world in response to new experience). Children are also constantly seeking equilibrium – trying to balance assimilation and accommodation to form stable understanding. Another central tenet of Piaget's theory is that a child progressively passes through qualitatively different cognitive stages (Table 1.7).

When explaining procedures to a child the anaesthetist should consider the cognitive stage of the child. Infants and toddlers are in the sensorimotor stage and may be easily distracted with objects. In contrast children in the preoperational stage will focus on particular perceptual points. They may not understand that a needle will be painless, even if they are told that the anaesthetic cream has numbed the skin. Similarly a preoperational child may be just as distressed by the attachment of a big syringe to the cannula as

Table 1.7 Piaget's stages of cognitive development

Stage	Age (years)	Key features
Sensorimotor	0–2	Experiment with objects establishing rudimentary concepts of the properties of objects, causality and space
		Object consistency established at about 9 months
Preoperational	2–7	Use symbolic thought and characteristically focus on single aspects of an event or object
		Egocentric behaviour – unable to see another's perspective
Concrete operational	7–12	Can apply logic to concrete objects and events
Formal operational	>12	Abstract and hypothetical reasoning

by the intravenous cannula insertion itself. Explanations to preoperational children should be simple and clear. A concrete operational child will understand more complex explanations, but may have difficulty with abstract ideas such as how anaesthesia differs from normal sleep.

INFORMATION-PROCESSING THEORY

Central to Piaget's theory is the progression through stages. More recent theories have considered cognitive development to be a more continuous phenomenon, without discrete qualitatively different stages. Like Piaget's theory, other information-processing theories also see children as problem solvers and focus on the mental processes.

From infancy children actively pursue goals, encounter obstacles and devise strategies to attain goals. Several mental processes are involved in problem solving, including basic processes such as associating events with each other, recognising objects as familiar, generalising from one instance to another and encoding. Encoding involves representing in memory information that draws attention or is considered important. Children encode features about objects and events, and then remember which features go together. The speed of basic processing increases with age. The rate of increase results from biological maturation and experience. Myelination is one biological process that is correlated with process speed. Processing speed and efficiency also increase with age as children develop strategies for learning and memory. Between 5 and 8 years of age children develop the ability to perform rehearsal – repeating information over and over. Selective attention also is developed by around the age of 7 or 8 years. Lastly, knowledge also increases with age. As knowledge increases a child's ability to recall and encode new material is enhanced by their increased ability to relate it to past experience.

Alternative information processing theories include neural network or connectionist theories, dynamic systems and overlapping wave theories.

CORE KNOWLEDGE AND SOCIOCULTURAL THEORY

The main concept of this theory is that children are born with innate or core knowledge. The content of this innate knowledge is determined by evolutionary or Darwinian forces, and therefore includes vital knowledge such as language and face recognition. In contrast, sociocultural theory emphasises the importance of others teaching children the skills and knowledge of their particular culture.

Theories of emotional and social development

Just as cognitive theories may explain how children understand, theories of social development may help to explain how children behave.

FREUD

Freud describes three personality structures. From birth basic biological drives comprise the *id*. Later, in infancy, the *ego* emerges as the rational aspect of personality. Eventually the ego becomes the 'self', though the id is always strongest. From 3 to 6 years behaviour is also influenced by a sense of right and wrong; this is the *superego*, or conscience. Freud's theory of psychosexual development involves five body-centred or sexual stages. The stages are oral (age 0–1 years), anal (2–3 years), oedipal (3–6 years), latency (6–12 years) and adolescence. At each stage there is potential for conflict and progression to the next stage occurs only after conflict resolution. Similarly, Erickson also proposed that each stage of development was characterised by a crisis or set of issues that had to be resolved or the child would struggle with that issue into maturity (Table 1.8).

BEHAVIOURAL THEORY

Behaviourists such as Watson and Skinner believe that all behaviour is learned from previous responses to the

Table 1.8 Erickson's psychosocial stages

Stage	Age (years)	Features
Basic trust and mistrust	0–1	If the mother is consistent and caring the child will acquire a basic trust, if not the child will continue to have difficulty forming intimate relationships
Autonomy versus shame and doubt	1–3	Increasing cognitive and motor skills increase desire to explore. At the same time parental control is apparent. A child must achieve self-control without loss of self-esteem, therefore gaining a balanced sense of autonomy
Initiative versus guilt	4–6	The child sets itself increasingly demanding goals that may not be achievable. They must be able to set higher standards but not be crushed by guilt when they are not always reached
Industry versus inferiority	6 to puberty	Child must master important cognitive and social skills. Parents and teachers set increasingly difficult tasks. Success can lead to a sense of competence while failure can lead to feelings of inadequacy
Identity versus role confusion	Adolescence to adulthood	Adolescent must identify who they are and what they want or become confused by what roles they should adopt as adults

environment, and less emphasis should be placed on a person's inner experience. This theory explains why children tend to repeat behaviour that has a favourable outcome, and avoid behaviour that is punished or ignored.

COPING MECHANISMS

The perioperative period is a stressful time and children use direct and indirect methods of coping. Young children use direct coping mechanisms such as hiding or attempting to run away, while children between 5 and 9 years may use more sophisticated direct avoidance strategies such as refusing the premedication because it tastes bad. Older children use indirect, internal coping strategies such as reframing an issue to a more favourable perspective (for example, believing the premedication will make them better) or using distraction. However, stress tends to cause children to regress to immature coping mechanisms.

Consciousness

A simple and primary aim of anaesthesia is to produce loss of consciousness but the definition of consciousness is complex. From an internal perspective, consciousness is being aware of our mental processes, our immediate environment and our effect on the environment. Unfortunately, we cannot remember much of what was going on in our minds before 3 or 4 years of age. To analyse consciousness below this age we need to approach it from an external or observer perspective.

Neurophysiologists, psychologists, philosophers and theologians have all tackled the problem of defining consciousness from an external perspective. Despite centuries of discourse we can never be entirely certain that anybody (or anything) else is conscious. In this respect we have not advanced far from the original thoughts of Rene Descartes who, in 1641, believed that the only certainty was that he was thinking – 'cogito, ergo sum'.

Nevertheless, from an external perspective, consciousness requires evidence that the individual sees themselves as a self or unified entity, separate to their environment and others. There should also be evidence of intentionality or thought. When does a child perceive itself as a 'self'? When do they start to think?

EVIDENCE OF THOUGHT

Learning begins in early infancy but there is controversy over the degree of knowledge, thought and reasoning. Core-knowledge theorists argue that children are born with innate knowledge, while others think that at first only learning mechanisms are present. It may be that infants have no true thought but only complex subconscious reflexes.

Yet there is evidence that infants do think. Piaget originally argued that infants had no concept of a hidden object (no sense of object permanence) but if an infant is shown an attractive object, and then suddenly plunged into darkness, the infant will still search for it [38]. Thought is demonstrated also by violation of expectancy. Infants as young as 4 months will stare longer when presented with events that appear impossible given their prior observations. An infant aged 7 months will be surprised at a ball rolling up a slope, and a 3-month-old will be surprised if a box released in mid-air does not fall to the ground.

EVIDENCE FOR SELF

Evidence for 'self' is demonstrated by their differentiation between themselves and their surroundings. From the ages of 2–4 months, infants enthusiastically move a mobile attached to their limbs with a string, but if the string is removed, the mobile is no longer under their control, and they are angry. Evidence for consciousness, is more obvious by 18 months when children will look into a mirror and realise that the image they see is their own. If a red dot is placed on their forehead, they will touch their face rather than their reflection [39]. Almost all 30-month-olds, and over 60 per cent of 20- to 25-month-olds, point to themselves in pictures.

Behaviour and emotions also reflect a strengthening sense of self. Two-year-olds demonstrate self-assertion and opposition to parental requests. Complex emotions such as embarrassment, pride, envy, shame and guilt reflect an enhancement or injury to the child's sense of self; these are self-conscious emotions. Embarrassment and envy are recognisable from 18 to 24 months while pride, shame and guilt appear between 2 and 3 years of age.

Language also demonstrates consciousness. Children begin to use the pronouns 'I' and 'me' just before the age of 2 years, followed soon after by the use of 'you'.

THEORY OF MIND

Theory of mind is the understanding of how the mind influences behaviour. Between the ages of 2 and 5 years children begin to understand that another child has a mind and this means that they recognise the concept of their own mind.

Most 2-year-olds can predict that actions of others will be dictated by the desires of others. By 3 years children understand that beliefs may predict another's action, but they do not understand false beliefs until aged 4 years.

Memory

INFANTILE AMNESIA

When adults are asked, their first memories are usually from when they were 3–4 years old. The lack of memory for anything earlier is known as infantile amnesia, yet despite infantile amnesia there is evidence that infants can form memories.

BEHAVIOUR INFLUENCED BY EXPERIENCE – IMPLICIT MEMORY

DeCasper *et al.* demonstrated that a neonate's behaviour is altered by stories read out loud during the last weeks of pregnancy [40]. Newborns can recognise and therefore remember their mother's voice (although not the father's) [41,42]. By observing behaviour associated with heel pricking, it is also apparent that neonates can learn to associate certain actions with previous nociceptive or painful stimuli [43].

A neonate prefers to look at new rather than familiar images [44,45], yet this memory formation is only short term. Longer-term memory is established in the later part of the first year and, as age increases, an infant's memories exist for longer periods. A 9-month-old child can establish a memory for 4 weeks, a 10-month-old can establish memories for up to 6 months [46] and there is evidence that an 11-month-old infant can form memories for up to 12 months [47,48].

EXPLICIT MEMORY

Although infants can form some implicit memories that are preserved into later years, there is no evidence that these memories can be consciously recalled – there is no evidence for explicit memory. Two examples demonstrate lack of explicit memory. Toddlers, who, as infants had performed auditory localisation tests, were more familiar with the tests compared with those who had not had the tests before, but none of the toddlers had any conscious memory of the tests [49]. An 18-month-old had a fish bone caught in her throat and was distressed when it was removed. Six months later, when she was old enough to talk, she had no recollection of the incident although she recognised the doctor and she refused to eat fish [50].

As language develops, formation of explicit memory becomes more obvious and easier to detect. For example, in a review of children who had presented to the emergency department, Howe *et al.* demonstrated that all the children who were verbal at the time of presentation (from 27 months old), were able to recall the event explicitly 6 months later, whereas non-verbal children could not recall the visit [50].

PAIN MEMORY

Pain pathways, although not fully developed, are intact in neonates and infants [51], and a neonate's behavioural and hormonal response to a nociceptive stimulus is similar to that of an adult [52,53]. The hormonal and haemodynamic response to a nociceptive stimulus has also been demonstrated in an unborn foetus [54,55]. A recent interesting study demonstrated that the stress associated with a later painful stimulus is greatest in babies who had an assisted delivery [56]. This may imply that babies form some memory of a particularly painful birth.

CONSCIOUSNESS MEMORY AND ANAESTHESIA

In summary there is increasing evidence that neonates and infants have some consciousness and memory; however, there are challenges of how anaesthesia effect can be measured and judged to be adequate. Anaesthesia for adults is given in doses to guarantee loss of consciousness and explicit memory. Finding the appropriate dose is more difficult in small children because we have less precise measures of their consciousness or memory.

CHILD HEALTH

The events, diseases and injuries that befall children vary widely between countries and societies. Ninety per cent of children on earth are born into the developing world, where the death rate in children younger than 5 years of age is over 10 times higher than in the developed world. Of approximately 1000 infants who die world-wide every hour, only 30 die in developed countries. In this section I briefly outline the common diseases of childhood in developed countries and typical reasons why children present for anaesthesia. Paediatric anaesthesia in the developing world is covered in Chapter 50.

Diseases of childhood

There are good data on mortality in children. Mortality reports are often complete and well defined, but mortality is only one crude measure of child health. Morbidity is of greater importance but data are less precise.

MORTALITY

In developed countries child mortality has markedly decreased over the last two centuries. In the early nineteenth century almost half the children born in the UK died under the age of 12 years, prompting one physician of the time to comment: 'It is really astonishing, that so little attention should in general be paid to the preservation of infants. What labour and expense are daily bestowed to prop an old tottering carcass for a few years while thousands of those who might be useful in life perish without being regarded!' [57].

The relative causes for mortality have also changed, with a dramatic decline in infectious disease. In Victoria, Australia, in 2004, the overall child death rate (up to 14 years) was 40.3 per 100 000. The rate was highest in the neonatal period with a rate of 453 deaths per 100 000 in children aged less than 1 year, compared with 16.4 per 100 000 in children aged 1–4 years, 9.1 in children aged 5–9 years and 10.8 in those aged 10–14 years [58]. Deaths in infants were most commonly birth related or caused by genetic or congenital conditions, SIDS and infection. The number of children dying from SIDS decreased from 67 in 1991 to 18 in 2004 [57].

In the USA statistics are similar. Infant mortality was roughly 7 per 1000 live births in 2002. In the neonatal period the leading causes of death were prematurity, low birth weight, congenital malformations, chromosomal abnormalities, maternal complications of pregnancy, respiratory causes and sepsis [59]. In the period from 28 days to 1 year the leading causes were SIDS, congenital malformations and chromosomal abnormalities, accidents, diseases of the circulatory system and septicaemia [59]. For children aged 1–19 years, accidents, congenital malformations and cancer remain leading causes for death (Table 1.9). In adolescents 75 per cent of deaths were due to accidents, homicide and suicide, but the single leading cause of death was motor vehicle accidents (40 per cent) [59]. These mortality patterns are also beginning to become apparent in developing nations, for example now in Vietnam the commonest cause of death in post-neonatal children is motorcycle trauma.

MORBIDITY

In developed societies, the morbidity and mortality from infectious disease have also decreased over the last century. The most significant improvement has been a fall in the incidence of tuberculosis, chronic suppuration of the chest, bone and ear, and all forms of streptococcal disease. The decline in these diseases resulted from improvements in hygiene, housing and education. The introduction of chemotherapeutic agents also played a role, though most of the decline had occurred before the introduction of antibiotics or vaccines.

Although the incidence of many diseases is declining, the incidence of some, such as asthma, is increasing. Asthma is now the leading cause for admission to Australian hospitals [60]. In the USA 13 per cent of children have, at some stage, been diagnosed with asthma [61]. There is also evidence that obesity is increasing, with the prevalence of overweight children in the USA rising from 4 per cent in 1963–70, to 15.8 per cent in 1999–2000.

The relative frequency of childhood illness can also be gauged by health-care attendances. The most frequent reasons for attendance of children to primary health-care physicians are for upper respiratory tract infections (URTIs), tonsillitis, asthma, bronchitis and immunisation. In the first 5 years of life children average six to eight URTIs per year, although the majority are viral, mild and last 5–7 days. They occur earlier and more often in children with older siblings and also in those who attend day-care centres [60].

Behavioural problems are also a frequent problem. Over 12 months in one region of Australia, 10 per cent of all children attended specialist paediatricians and of these 35 per cent had consultations for behavioural problems, and 76 per cent of these related to attention deficit hyperactivity disorder (ADHD). Over half of all consultations involved some form of chronic illness [62]. In the USA, it has been estimated that 8 per cent of children (3–17 years) have a learning disability and 6 per cent have ADHD [61].

Limitation of activity is another useful measure of childhood illness. In the USA between 1997 and 2002, 6–7 per cent of children had limitation of activity because of chronic ill health [63]. In children less than 5 years old the most common causes of chronic ill health were speech problems, asthma, learning disability or other developmental problems, while in children over the age of 5 years, the most common were learning disabilities and ADHD.

Finally, normal emotional and social development is vital to reduce health risk. This aspect of child health is more difficult to quantify but may be of increasing importance in developed countries as the gap between rich and poor widens, the environment is degraded and the pace of change in family and social structures increases. In the USA 40 per cent of children in poor families have excellent health compared with 60 per cent in better-off families [61]. Child maltreatment, behaviour and learning problems, youth suicide, eating disorders, substance abuse and early criminal behaviour are all increasing.

IMMUNISATION

Immunisation effectively prevents many infectious diseases and has in the past been responsible for a reduction in morbidity, permanent disability and mortality [64]. Schedules vary but most include immunisation against hepatitis B, diphtheria, tetanus, pertussis, *Haemophilus influenzae* b and poliovirus during infancy. Toddlers and preschool childhood receive boosters and further immunisation against measles, mumps and rubella. Immunisation is also possible for hepatitis A, tuberculosis (BCG), influenza, varicella and several pneumococcal and meningococcal strains.

Immunisation is often associated with mild fever or local inflammation, while anaphylaxis is very rare. There has been debate over whether children should receive immunisation when they are scheduled for anaesthesia. In theory, major surgery may suppress the immune response leading to failure of immunisation, and any fever associated with immunisation may be confused with postoperative wound infection [65]. However, the evidence behind the arguments against immunisation in the perioperative period is weak and the theoretical advantage of withholding immunisation must be weighed against the greater risk of infection resulting from missing immunisation altogether. Immunisation during anaesthesia (for other procedures) may be justified in children with significant needle phobia or a history of poor health-care attendances.

How many children have anaesthetics?

Defining the frequency of anaesthesia in children is important for planning and calculation of risk. Studies in several countries have estimated how often children are anaesthetised. The estimates vary as sedation and anaesthesia

Table 1.9 Leading causes for mortality in children in the USA for 2002. Rates as deaths per 100 000

Rank	Age 1–4 years		Age 5–9 years		Age 10–14 years		Age 15–19 years	
	Cause	Rate	Cause	Rate	Cause	Rate	Cause	Rate
	All causes	**31.2**	**All causes**	**15.2**	**All causes**	**19.5**	**All causes**	**67.8**
1	Accidents	10.5	Accidents	5.9	Accidents	7.3	Accidents	35.0
2	Congenital malformations and chromosomal abnormalities	3.4	Malignancy	2.7	Malignancy	2.5	Assault	9.3
3	Assault	2.7	Congenital malformations and chromosomal abnormalities	1.0	Suicide	1.2	Suicide	7.4
4	Malignancy	2.6	Assault	0.7	Congenital malformations and chromosomal abnormalities	1.0	Malignancy	3.5
5	Disease of the heart	1.1	Disease of the heart	0.5	Assault	1.0	Disease of the heart	2.0
6	Influenza and pneumonia	0.7	Other neoplasms	0.2	Disease of heart	0.8	Congenital malformations and chromosomal abnormalities	1.2
7	Septicaemia	0.5	Septicaemia	0.2	Chronic lower respiratory disease	0.4	Chronic lower respiratory disease	0.5
8	Chronic lower respiratory disease	0.4	Chronic lower respiratory disease	0.2	Cerebrovascular disease	0.3	Influenza and pneumonia	0.4
9	Specific conditions arising in the perinatal period	0.4	Influenza and pneumonia	0.2	Septicaemia	0.3	Diabetes	0.3
10	Other neoplasms	0.4	Cerebrovascular disease	0.2	Influenza and pneumonia	0.3	Cerebrovascular disease	0.3

Data from Centers of Disease Control and Prevention [59].

practice varies. The geographical isolation of the Australian state of Western Australia has enabled an accurate assessment of anaesthesia in children [66]. Over a 12-month period from a population of 456 753 children aged up to 16 years, 28 522 general anaesthetics were administered to a total 24 981 children (5.5 per cent); 90 per cent had only one anaesthetic. The most common procedures were those of ear, nose and throat surgery (28 per cent). There was a bimodal distribution of incidence over age, with peaks at 4 years and 16 years. In all age groups, anaesthesia was more frequent in males than in females, and twice as many male infants had anaesthesia compared with females (7.8 per cent versus 3.2 per cent) [66].

These gender differences were similar in a French study from 1996. Of all children having anaesthesia 11.6 per cent were infant boys and 7.1 per cent were infant girls. Ear, nose and throat procedures were again the most common cause for anaesthesia [67].

In the USA, data from the National Hospital Discharge Survey and the National Survey of Ambulatory Surgery have been used to estimate rates of surgical and non-surgical procedures performed in children. It was estimated that in 1996 24 per cent of children aged less than 1 year had a procedure compared with 9 per cent of 1–4 year olds and 5 per cent of 5–14 year olds [68]. The most frequent procedures were, in descending order, myringotomy with insertion of tubes, tonsillectomy and/or adenoidectomy, dental procedures, reduction of fractures, excision of skin lesion, circumcision and repair of inguinal hernia [68]. Not all children had anaesthesia for these procedures.

REFERENCES

Key references

Brazelton TB. Neonatal behavioural assessment scale. Clinics in developmental medicine no. 50. London: Heinemann, 1973.

DeCasper A, Spence M. Prenatal maternal speech influences newborns perception of speech sounds. *Infant Behav Dev* 1986; **9**: 133–50.

Howe M, Curage M. How can I remember when 'I' wasn't there: long-term retention of traumatic experiences and emergence of the cognitive self. *Conscious Cogn* 1994; **3**: 327–55.

Sims C, Stanley B, Milnes E. The frequency of and indications for general anaesthesia in children in Western Australia 2002–2003. *Anaesth Intensive Care* 2005; **33**(5): 623–8.

Taddio A, Shah V, Gilbert-Macleod C, Katz J. Conditioning and hyperalgesia in newborns exposed to repeated heel lances. *JAMA* 2002; **288**(7): 857–61.

References

1. Shann F. *Drug doses*, 13th edn. Melbourne: Collective, 2005.
2. Murat I, Constant I, Maud'huy H. Perioperative anaesthetic morbidity in children: a database of 24 165 anaesthetics over a 30-month period. *Paediatr Anaesth* 2004; **14**(2): 158–66.
3. Morray JP, Geiduschek JM, Ramamoorthy C *et al*. Anesthesia-related cardiac arrest in children: initial findings of the Pediatric Perioperative Cardiac Arrest (POCA) Registry. *Anesthesiology* 2000; **93**(1): 6–14.
4. Halon DA, Amitai N, Gotsman MS, Lewis BS. Serial echocardiography during the first 3 months of life in normal neonates. *Eur J Cardiol* 1979; **9**(5): 393–404.
5. Huttenbach Y, Ostrowski ML, Thaller D, Kim HS. Cell proliferation in the growing human heart: MIB-1 immunostaining in preterm and term infants at autopsy. *Cardiovasc Pathol* 2001; **10**(3): 119–23.
6. Poutanen T, Jokinen E, Sairanen H, Tikanoja T. Left atrial and left ventricular function in healthy children and young adults assessed by three dimensional echocardiography. *Heart* 2003; **89**(5): 544–9.
7. Gullberg N, Winberg P, Sellden H. Changes in stroke volume cause change in cardiac output in neonates and infants when mean airway pressure is altered. *Acta Anaesthesiol Scand* 1999; **43**(10): 999–1004.
8. van Hare GF, Hawkins JA, Schmidt KG, Rudolph AM. The effects of increasing mean arterial pressure on left ventricular output in newborn lambs. *Circ Res* 1990; **67**(1): 78–83.
9. Anderson PA, Glick KL, Manring A, Crenshaw C Jr. Developmental changes in cardiac contractility in fetal and postnatal sheep: *in vitro* and *in vivo*. *Am J Physiol* 1984; **247**(3 Pt 2): H371–9.
10. Kelly DH, Riordan L, Smith MJ. Apnea and periodic breathing in healthy full-term infants, 12–18 months of age. *Pediatr Pulmonol* 1992; **13**(3): 169–71.
11. Kelly DH, Stellwagen LM, Kaitz E, Shannon DC. Apnea and periodic breathing in normal full-term infants during the first twelve months. *Pediatr Pulmonol* 1985; **1**(4): 215–9.
12. Agostoni, E. Volume–pressure relationships of the thorax and lung in the newborn. *J Appl Physiol* 1959; **14**: 909–13.
13. Dobbinson TL, Nisbet HI, Pelton DA. Functional residual capacity (FRC) and compliance in anaesthetized paralysed children. I. *In vitro* tests with the helium dilution method of measuring FRC. *Can Anaesth Soc J* 1973; **20**(3): 310–21.
14. Thorsteinsson A, Larsson A, Jonmarker C, Werner O. Pressure–volume relations of the respiratory system in healthy children. *Am J Respir Crit Care Med* 1994; **150**(2): 421–30.
15. Motoyama EK. Pulmonary mechanics during early postnatal years. *Pediatr Res* 1977; **11**(3 Pt 2): 220–3.
16. Stocks J, Godfrey S. Specific airway conductance in relation to postconceptional age during infancy. *J Appl Physiol* 1977; **43**(1): 144–54.
17. Jevtovic-Todorovic V, Hartman RE, Izumi Y *et al*. Early exposure to common anesthetic agents causes widespread neurodegeneration in the developing rat brain and persistent learning deficits. *J Neurosci* 2003; **23**(3): 876–82.
18. Greenough WT, Black JE, Wallace CS. Experience and brain development. *Child Dev* 1987; **58**(3): 539–59.
19. Brazelton TB. Neonatal behavioural assessment scale. *Clinics in developmental medicine no. 50*. London: Heinemann, 1973.

20. Prechtl HF. The behavioural states of the newborn infant (a review). *Brain Res* 1974; **76**(2): 185–212.

21. Amiel-Tison C, Barrier G, Shnider SM *et al*. A new neurologic and adaptive capacity scoring system for evaluating obstetric medications in full-term newborns. *Anesthesiology* 1982; **56**(5): 340–50.

22. Halpern SH, Littleford JA, Brockhurst NJ *et al*. The neurologic and adaptive capacity score is not a reliable method of newborn evaluation. *Anesthesiology* 2001; **94**(6): 958–62.

23. Brockhurst NJ, Littleford JA, Halpern SH. The Neurologic and Adaptive Capacity Score: a systematic review of its use in obstetric anesthesia research. *Anesthesiology* 2000; **92**(1): 237–46.

24. Anders T. *A manual of standardized terminology, techniques and criteria for scoring sleep states of sleep and wakefulness in newborn infants*. Los Angeles: UCLA Brain Information Service, 1971.

25. Rechtschaffen A, Kales A. *Techniques and scoring system for sleep stages in human subjects*. Los Angeles: Brain Information Service/Brain Research Institute, 1968.

26. Anders NK, Sadeh A, Appareddy V. Normal sleep in neonates and children. In: Ferber R, Kryger M, eds. *Principals and practice of sleep medicine in the child*. Philadelphia: WB Saunders Co., 1995: 7–18.

27. Shneerson J. *Handbook of sleep medicine*, 1st edn. Oxford: Blackwell Science, 2000.

28. Mirmiran M, Maas YG, Ariagno RL. Development of fetal and neonatal sleep and circadian rhythms. *Sleep Med Rev* 2003; **7**(4): 321–34.

29. Okamoto Y, Kirikae K. Electroencephalographic studies on brain of foetus, of children of premature birth and newborn, together with a note on reactions of foetus brain upon drugs. *Folia Psychiatr Neurol Jpn* 1951; **5**(2): 135–46.

30. Torres F, Anderson C. The normal EEG of the human newborn. *J Clin Neurophysiol* 1985; **2**(2): 89–103.

31. Dreyfus-Brisac C. Ontogenesis of sleep in human prematures after 32 weeks of conceptional age. *Dev Psychobiol* 1970; **3**(2): 91–121.

32. Parmalee A, Akiyama Y, Shultz M. Analysis of electroencephalograms of sleeping infants. *Activ Nerv Suppl* 1969; **11**: 111.

33. Glotzbach SF, Ariagno RL, Harper MH. Sleep and sudden infant death syndrome. In: Ferber R, Kryger M, eds. *Principals and practice of sleep medicine in the child*. Philadelphia: WB Saunders Co., 1995: 7–18.

34. The changing concept of sudden infant death syndrome: diagnostic coding shifts, controversies regarding the sleeping environment, new variables to consider in reducing risk. *Pediatrics* 2005; **116**(5): 1245–55.

35. Caldas JC, Pais-Ribeiro JL, Carneiro SR. General anesthesia, surgery and hospitalization in children and their effects upon cognitive, academic, emotional and sociobehavioral development – a review. *Paediatr Anaesth* 2004; **14**(11): 910–5.

36. Watson AT, Visram A. Children's preoperative anxiety and postoperative behaviour. *Paediatr Anaesth* 2003; **13**(3): 188–204.

37. Rothbart M. Bates J. Temperament. In: Eisenberg N, ed. *Social, emotional, personality development*. New York: Wiley, 1998: 105–76.

38. Hood B, Willatts P. Reaching in the dark to an object's rembered position: evidence of object permanence in 5-month-old infants. *Br J Dev Psychol* 1986; **4**: 57–65.

39. Lewis M, Brooks-Gunn J. *Social cognition and the acquisition of self*. New York: Plenum Press, 1979.

40 DeCasper A, Spence M. Prenatal maternal speech influences newborns perception of speech sounds. *Infant Behav Dev* 1986; **9**: 133–50.

41. DeCasper AJ, Fifer W. Of human bonding: newborns prefer their mothers' voices. *Science* 1980; **208**(4448): 1174–6.

42. DeCasper AJ, Prescott PA. Human newborns' perception of male voices: preference, discrimination, reinforcing value. *Dev Psychobiol*, 1984; **17**(5): 481–91.

43. Taddio A, Shah V, Gilbert-Macleod C, Katz J. Conditioning and hyperalgesia in newborns exposed to repeated heel lances. *JAMA* 2002; **288**(7): 857–61.

44. Fagan JF 3rd. Infants' delayed recognition memory and forgetting. *J Exp Child Psychol* 1973; **16**(3): 424–50.

45. Pascalis O, de Schonen S. Recognition memory in 3- to 4-day-old human neonates. *Neuro Report* 1994; **5**(14): 1721–4.

46. Carver LJ, Bauer PJ. The dawning of a past: the emergence of long-term explicit memory in infancy. *J Exp Psychol Gen* 2001; **130**(4): 726–45.

47. McDonough L, Mandler JM. Very long-term recall in infants: infantile amnesia reconsidered. *Memory* 1994; **2**(4): 339–52.

48. Bauer PJ. What do infants recall of their lives? Memory for specific events by one- to two-year-olds. *Am Psychol* 1996; **51**(1): 29–41.

49. Perris EE, Myers NA, Clifton RK. Long-term memory for a single infancy experience. *Child Dev* 1990; **61**(6): 1796–807.

50. Howe M, Curage M. How can I remember when 'I' wasn't there: long-term retention of traumatic experiences and emergence of the cognitive self. *Conscious Cogn* 1994; **3**: 327–55.

51. Fitzgerald M, Beggs S. The neurobiology of pain: developmental aspects. *Neuroscientist* 2001; **7**(3): 246–57.

52. Owens ME. Pain in infancy: conceptual and methodological issues. *Pain* 1984; **20**(3): 213–30.

53. Owens ME, Todt EH. Pain in infancy: neonatal reaction to a heel lance. *Pain* 1984; **20**(1): 77–86.

54. Teixeira J, Fogliani R, Giannakoulopoulos X, Glover V, Fisk NM. Fetal haemodynamic stress response to invasive procedures. *Lancet* 1996; **347**(9001): 624.

55. Giannakoulopoulos X, Sepulveda W, Kourtis P, Glover V, Fisk NM. Fetal plasma cortisol and beta-endorphin response to intrauterine needling. *Lancet* 1994; **344**(8915): 77–81.

56. Taylor A, Fisk NM, Glover V. Mode of delivery and subsequent stress response. *Lancet* 2000; **355**(9198): 120.

57. Buchan W. *Domestic medicine*. London: W Lewis, 1822: 4.

58. CCOPMM. *Annual report for the year 2004, incorporating the 43rd survey of perinatal deaths in Victoria*. Melbourne: The Consultative Council on Obstetric and Paediatric Mortality and Morbidity, 2005.

59. Anderson R, Smith B. Deaths: leading causes for 2002. *Natl Vital Stat Rep* 2005; **53**: 1–89.

60. Robinson M, Roberton D, eds. *Practical paediatrics,* 5th edn. Edinburgh: Churchill Livingstone, 2003.

61. Dey A, Bloom B. Summary health statistics for US Children: National Health Interview Survey, 2003. *Vital Health Stat* 2005. **10**(223).

62. Hewson PH, Anderson PK, Dinning AH *et al.* A 12-month profile of community paediatric consultations in the Barwon region. *J Paediatr Child Health,* 1999. **35**(1): 16–22.

63. NCHS. *Health, United States, 2004 with chartbook of trends in the health of Americans.* Hyattsville: National Center for Health Statistics, 2004.

64. Department of Health, UK. Immunisation against infectious disease – 'The Green Book'. 2006: http://www.dh.gov.uk/PolicyAndGuidance/HealthAndSocialCareTopics/GreenBook/fs/en

65. Short JA, van der Walt JH, Zoanetti DC. Immunization and anesthesia – an international survey. *Paediatr Anaesth* 2006; **16**(5): 514–22.

66. Sims C, Stanley B, Milnes E. The frequency of and indications for general anaesthesia in children in Western Australia 2002–2003. *Anaesth Intensive Care* 2005; **33**(5): 623–8.

67. Clergue F, Auroy Y, Perquignot F, Jougla E, Lienhart A, Laxenaire MC. French survey of anesthesia in 1996. *Anesthesiology* 1999; **91**(5): 1509–20.

68. Flick R, Moriarty J. Frequency of surgical and nonsurgical procedures performed in children in the United States, 1996. *Anesthesiology* 2005; **103**: A1349.

69. Flick R, Moriarty J. The most frequently performed procedures on children in the United States: 1996. *Anesthesiology* 2005; **103**: A1311.

The respiratory system

JANET STOCKS

KEY LEARNING POINTS

- Most alveolar development occurs during the last trimester of pregnancy and the first 2–3 years. Damage during this period may have life-long effects.
- Infants and young children are vulnerable to respiratory problems resulting from both immunological immaturity and developmental differences in respiratory structure and function. The latter include small airways, increased chest wall compliance, tendency for airway closure within the tidal range, increased oxygen consumption, reduced respiratory reserve and immature regulation of breathing patterns.

- Other risk factors are male gender, preterm birth, intrauterine growth retardation, maternal smoking during pregnancy and concurrent respiratory infections.
- Differences in developmental physiology increase the susceptibility of infants and young children to the potentially adverse ventilatory effects of anaesthesia – anaesthetic agents, intubation and ventilatory support may all result in iatrogenic damage.
- An extensive range of techniques is now available to assess lung function in infants and preschool children, including those receiving intensive care.

INTRODUCTION

The respiratory system presents challenges during anaesthesia and intensive care and the aim of this chapter is to provide a scientific basis for understanding the development of the respiratory system, and the clinical implications of such development, with respect to:

- structure (prenatal and postnatal changes);
- function (with emphasis on why infants and young children are more vulnerable to respiratory disease and failure);
- control of breathing;
- increased vulnerability of children requiring intubation, anaesthesia or ventilatory support.

The broad aim of this chapter is to cover essential knowledge for paediatric anaesthetists. Further detailed reviews of developmental respiratory anatomy and physiology are recommended [1–3] and details of common respiratory diseases of childhood can be found in standard texts [4]. Comprehensive accounts of paediatric lung function tests have been described previously [5,6] and this chapter will discuss their application and interpretation. References will generally be limited to those published during the last 5 years, the bibliographies of which will provide the reader with the wider literature.

STRUCTURE

Foetal growth

During foetal development the lung bud, lined by epithelium, appears as a ventral diverticulum of the foregut at

4 weeks' gestational age. This immediately divides within the surrounding mesenchyme to form the two main bronchi, with the formation of a preliminary capillary network by 5 weeks. During the next 11 weeks there is rapid dichotomous branching, such that by the end of the pseudoglandular phase (about 16 weeks) all the major conducting airways, including the terminal bronchioles, have formed (Fig. 2.1). The pulmonary nerves appear by 5–8 weeks, alongside bronchial smooth muscle, and by birth there are as many as there are in adults. The canalicular period is characterised by development of the respiratory bronchioles, each of which terminate in two or three thin-walled dilatations called terminal sacs or primitive alveoli. During this period there is also rapid proliferation of the pulmonary capillaries and the epithelium becomes thinner, allowing close contact between airspaces and blood flow. While a primitive gas-exchanging surface is established by 22–23 weeks (which is the current limit of viability for preterm infants), this is suboptimal and infants delivered at this stage are unlikely to survive without prenatal administration of corticosteroids, postnatal administration of surfactant and some ventilatory support. From this stage, fibrin, collagen and elastic fibres, which are important for true alveolar development, begin to be laid down and both cuboidal (type II, responsible for surfactant secretion) and thin (type I) epithelial cells line the airspaces. During the alveolar period, further refinement of lung microstructure occurs as tiny secondary septa form on the walls of larger saccules. These out-pouchings grow into the lumen, thereby increasing the gas-exchanging surface area further and forming the walls of the 'true alveoli'. Although true alveoli do not appear until between 30 and

36 weeks, by birth it is thought that about 150 million are present, representing between one-third to one-half of the final adult complement. Development of the pulmonary vasculature coincides with that of the airways and airspaces, and the pulmonary circulation is fully formed by the seventh week of gestation.

Surfactant development has been studied intensively during the past 30 years, ever since the cause of respiratory distress syndrome (RDS) in preterm infants was attributed to surfactant deficiency. Identifiable type II cells appear after about 22 weeks, but surfactant in the airspaces does not increase until after 30 weeks. The lung normally matures functionally after about 35 weeks' gestation; however, it has a remarkable capacity to mature early, stimulated by both maternal corticosteroids and exposure to chorioamnionitis. Indeed, antenatal inflammation is a potent promoter of maturation and increased surfactant [7]. There is considerable individual variability in surfactant production including, on average, a 1- to 2-week delay in boys and white infants, which undoubtedly contributes to gender and ethnic differences in morbidity and mortality in preterm infants [8,9].

The control of lung development is highly complex and known to be influenced by interactions between the pulmonary mesenchyme and epithelium. Fibroblast growth factors play a key role in cell proliferation, migration and differentiation. Together with secretion of lung liquid, foetal breathing movements stretch and distend the foetal lung and both are essential for normal lung development; diminution in either is associated with lung hypoplasia. Morbidity and mortality following preterm delivery are inversely proportional to gestational age, being more likely in infants born

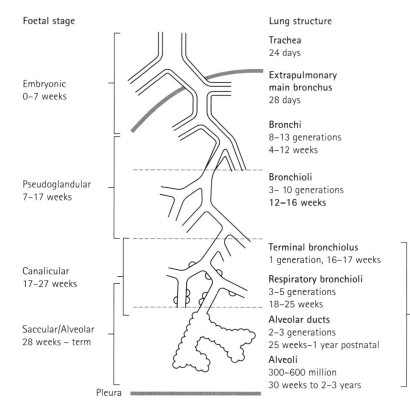

Figure 2.1 Stages of lung development during foetal and early postnatal life. © Janet Stocks.

before 26 weeks, males and those with associated intrauterine growth retardation. Despite increasing survival of extremely preterm infants, the incidence of chronic lung disease of infancy (CLDI) or bronchopulmonary dysplasia (BPD) has not declined [10] and may be associated with long-term changes in cardiorespiratory function [11]. In the past, mechanical ventilation with high peak inspired pressures and oxygen concentrations was predominantly implicated in the pathogenesis of BPD. While these factors may still play a role, 'new BPD' or CLDI can also develop in extremely preterm infants who require minimal ventilatory support at birth. This is generally associated with prenatal infection, pulmonary inflammation, oedema, dysmaturity of alveolarisation and angiogenesis [10,12].

Postnatal growth

Lung growth occurs well into the adolescent years and, in males, continues for several years after somatic growth has ceased, primarily owing to increases in thoracic dimensions. Although lung structure is suited to optimising gas exchange in health, some shortcomings in design become apparent during anaesthesia when, for example, retained secretions can rapidly lead to airway obstruction and atelectasis [13]. Major developmental changes in the anatomy of the airways, lungs and thorax occur during childhood. By adulthood the tracheal diameter has tripled. The majority of postnatal lung growth involves the terminal respiratory unit and the gas-exchanging surface area maintains a close relationship to body mass (about 1 m^2/kg). Rapid alveolarisation continues during the first 2–4 years of life, after which alveolar multiplication slows considerably, with lung growth occurring primarily owing to increasing size of existing components; the alveolar diameter increases from 50–100 μm at birth to around 300 μm in the adult. The final number of alveoli has been estimated to be between 250 and 500 million, this being higher in males and closely correlated with final lung size [14]. As alveolar multiplication occurs, new blood vessels appear within the acinus, so that the alveolar to arterial ratio decreases rapidly to approach adult structure within 2 years of birth.

Bronchial smooth muscle increases up to 1 year of postnatal age. A rapid increase in the relative amount of bronchiolar smooth muscle occurs immediately after birth, which is probably related to adaptation to air breathing. There is excessive bronchial smooth muscle in babies who require ventilatory support during the neonatal period, those with BPD and children with asthma.

FUNCTION

Adaptation to air breathing

Dramatic changes occur during the transition from intrauterine life to air breathing, triggered by removal of placental humeral inhibition, a surge in catecholamines, increased CO_2 levels and temperature, and tactile stimulation of the skin.

These changes include:

- absorption of alveolar liquid;
- rapid aeration and establishment of a resting lung volume;
- twentyfold increase in pulmonary blood flow;
- resetting of chemoreceptors;
- establishment of continuous rhythmic breathing.

The increase in pulmonary blood flow is due to a combination of mechanical expansion of the vessels, removal of hypoxic pulmonary vasoconstriction, a massive release of kinins from lung granulocytes in response to the rise in PaO_2, and dilatation of the pulmonary vascular bed. These changes initially reverse the flow through, and subsequently close, both the ductus arteriosus and the foramen ovale.

In the lung tissue itself there is a rapid rise in compliance and decrease in resistance so that relatively stable values are achieved within the first 12–24 hours after birth. Nevertheless, many other aspects of lung development, including histochemical maturation, development of respiratory reflexes and control of breathing, follow a predestined time course and do not appear to be affected by birth as such.

Approximately 10 per cent of newborns fail to establish adequate respiration immediately after birth and require some form of resuscitation. Over-zealous intervention in this situation, by either inadequate or excessive lung distension, can lead to degradation of surfactant function and iatrogenic RDS [7]. Furthermore, there is growing evidence to suggest that pulmonary function recovers faster and mortality is reduced when room air is used instead of unhumidified cold 100 per cent oxygen [15].

Postnatal development

The main developmental differences in respiratory physiology that contribute to increased vulnerability of infants to respiratory compromise are summarised in Table 2.1.

Following the establishment of regular respiration after birth, the alveolar ventilation, minute ventilation and gas mixing efficiency of a normal neonate become similar to those of an adult in proportion to body size and metabolic rate [16,17]. However, the relatively large surface area to body mass ratio and rapid growth in infants are such that oxygen consumption is much higher (6–8 ml/kg/min in neonates versus 4–6 ml/kg/min in adults) [18].

The epiglottis and tongue are relatively large in neonates and the larynx is higher and more anterior. While this facilitates simultaneous suckling and breathing, these anatomical differences mean that babies rarely breathe through their mouths until 3–6 months of age. Since nasal resistance comprises 50 per cent of total airway resistance, and

Table 2.1 Main developmental differences in respiratory physiology that contribute to increased vulnerability of infants to respiratory compromise

- ↑ Metabolism: rapid growth, large surface area/body weight, ↑ O_2 consumption
- ↓ Resting lung volume (decreased oxygen reserves), ↓ number of alveoli
- Dynamic elevation of FRC – rapid fall in FRC during expiratory pauses or apnoea, and during anaesthesia
- Immature control of breathing: Hering–Breuer inflation reflex active during tidal breathing
- Biphasic response to hypoxaemia during first 6 months of life? Risk of apnoea
- Hypercapnic increase in ventilation mediated primarily through increased tidal volume with respiratory rate decreasing or remaining unchanged
- ↓ Endurance of respiratory muscles
- High chest wall compliance, ↓ elastic recoil, contributes to recession/paradoxical breathing efforts
- ↑ Tendency for peripheral airway closure during tidal breathing
- ↑ Work of breathing
- ↑ Upper airway resistance – preferential nose breathers (nasal resistance comprises approximately 50 per cent total resistance)

FRC, functional residual capacity.

resistance is inversely proportional to the fourth power of the radius, even minor obstruction from nasal secretions, oedema or a nasogastric tube may increase the work of breathing and compromise very young or small infants. The narrowest part of the infant larynx is the non-distensible ring-like cricoid cartilage, and a tracheal tube that is too large can cause temporary subglottic oedema or permanent scarring and stenosis. By 10–12 years of age upper airway anatomy resembles that in the adult. Anatomical dead space appears to be relatively constant through life at approximately 1–2 ml/kg body weight.

The larynx, trachea and bronchi of infants are far more compliant than in older children, making the neonatal airway highly susceptible to distending or compressive forces. Furthermore, activity of the genioglossus and other muscles responsible for maintaining upper airway patency is decreased in infants. In the presence of any upper airway obstruction the generation of increased negative intrathoracic airway pressure required to effect inspiratory flow will cause further narrowing of the compliant extrathoracic airway and may result in audible inspiratory stridor. In contrast, in the presence of any lower airway obstruction, work of breathing is primarily increased during *expiration*. This is because the negative pressure that keeps the intrathoracic airways patent during inspiration is far less during expiration, resulting in airway narrowing. In the presence of marked obstruction, forced expiratory efforts can cause airway closure. Crying will also exacerbate these problems.

Abnormal airway function and respiratory illness are more common in boys than in girls during both infancy and childhood. Similarly, there are marked ethnic differences. Although overall infant mortality rate is higher in black infants, neonatal mortality (especially in low-birth-weight infants) is lower and they are less likely to develop RDS [8,9]. Although some remodelling of the lung may occur during the first year of life, those born with suboptimal function tend to have lower centile function thereafter. This suggests that lung and airway function may be determined for life during foetal and early postnatal development. During the rapid growth period, factors such as prenatal exposure to infection and cigarette smoke, preterm delivery, intrauterine growth retardation, neonatal lung disease and its treatment may all have long-term and irreversible effects [6,19,20]. Following the adolescent growth spurt, the male disadvantage disappears and respiratory and wheezing illnesses become relatively more common and severe in girls.

Mechanics of the respiratory pump

The adequacy of the respiratory pump depends upon the mechanical properties and interactions of the diaphragm, chest wall, the airways and lung parenchyma (Fig. 2.2). Detailed descriptions of these processes have been published elsewhere [3], and only developmental changes will be discussed that are relevant to respiratory disease or anaesthesia.

The diaphragm, which is innervated by the phrenic nerve, is the principal muscle of inspiration and is responsible for around 75 per cent of the inhaled gas volume during quiet breathing in children and adults, the remaining 25 per cent being attributable to ribcage movement. Efficiency of breathing is reduced in the presence of hyperinflation, owing to the flattening of the diaphragm. In adults, the downward sloping ribs allow a significant increase in both the anteroposterior and lateral diameters of the thorax when the diaphragm descends. Some of the reduction in lung volumes caused by anaesthesia has been attributed to cephalad movement of the diaphragm [1]. Infants have a limited ability to increase tidal volume largely because of their cartilaginous, horizontally placed ribcage, and because the diaphragm is more horizontal than in older subjects. Consequently, maximal diaphragmatic activity during severe respiratory disease leads to paradoxical in-drawing of the lower rib cage. Furthermore, the infant diaphragm has a relatively low muscle mass and reduced proportion of high-endurance muscle fibres so that fatigue occurs earlier than in older subjects. The adult rib cage configuration gradually develops during the first

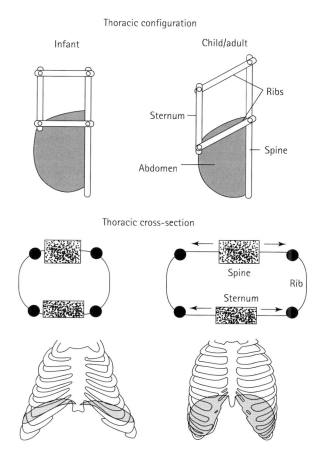

Thoracic configuration

Thoracic cross-section

Figure 2.2 Changes in chest configuration from infancy to early adulthood. In adults, the downward sloping ribs allow a significant increase in both the anteroposterior and lateral diameters of the thorax when the diaphragm descends during inspiration. Infants have a limited ability to increase tidal or minute volume in response to increased ventilatory demands. This is largely because of the horizontally placed ribcage at end-expiration together with limitations imposed by the flaccid (highly compliant) ribcage, © Janet Stocks.

2 years of life. The external intercostal muscles play a vital role in stabilising the ribcage but this is lost or severely diminished during inhalational anaesthesia.

The resting point of outward chest spring and inward lung collapse determines the functional residual capacity (FRC). The FRC is the lung's physiological reserve and acts as a reservoir for gas exchange. Loss of lung elasticity (inward recoil) as with ageing or in emphysema results in an increased FRC, whereas either a loss of outward recoil (high chest wall compliance because of the flaccid ribcage in infancy) or increased lung recoil (e.g. surfactant deficiency), will result in a smaller FRC and reduced oxygen reserves (Fig. 2.3). The high chest wall compliance found in infants also increases the likelihood of ribcage recession, particularly in the presence of lung disease (requirement for more negative intrapleural pressure swings during inspiration), during rapid eye movement (REM) sleep (reduced intercostal muscle tone and chest wall stability) and in those born

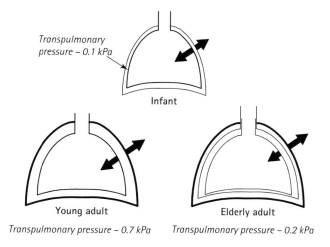

Figure 2.3 Maturational changes in lung and chest wall recoil and transpulmonary pressure at end-expiration. At end-expiration, transpulmonary pressure is less negative in both the infant and the elderly than in the young adult. In the elderly this is caused by emphysematous changes with loss of lung recoil. By contrast, in the infant, lung recoil is similar to an adult's but the extremely compliant thoracic cage results in less outward recoil with which to keep the lungs and airways distended, © Janet Stocks.

prematurely. Many inhalational anaesthetics also reduce intercostal muscle tone thereby contributing to a fall in FRC when compared with the awake state [1]. Recession increases the work of breathing, since much of the inspiratory effort is wasted in distorting the chest wall rather than in effecting gas exchange, and this contributes to respiratory failure. Increased chest wall compliance in early life not only impairs gas exchange and ventilation–perfusion balance, particularly in the dependent parts of the lung but, together with the small absolute size of the airways, renders the infant and young child particularly susceptible to airway obstruction and wheezing disorders [21]. Ossification of the ribcage, sternum and vertebrae begins *in utero* and continues until about 25 years of age, while calcification of costal cartilage continues into old age. There is a progressive decrease in chest wall compliance with ageing, owing to both increased calcification and narrowing of the intervertebral disc spaces. There have been relatively few studies of infant respiratory muscle function, but recent development of less invasive measurement techniques should facilitate future research [22,23]. Both the elastic and resistive components of the work of breathing (i.e. those required to stretch the lung and to generate airflow) may be increased in children with respiratory disease although, beyond the neonatal period, airway disease is far more common than parenchymal disease.

Lung volumes

Passive lung emptying is determined by the product of resistance (R) and compliance (C), commonly known as

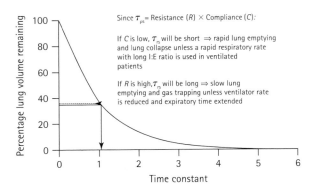

Figure 2.4 Clinical significance of the expiratory time constant (τ_{rs}), which is the time taken for the lung to deflate to 37 per cent of its original volume. After $3\tau_{rs}$ lung emptying is 95 per cent complete. If expiratory time is less than $3\tau_{rs}$, dynamic hyperinflation (auto-positive end-expiratory pressure) will occur. I:E ratio = inspiratory:expiratory ratio, © Janet Stocks.

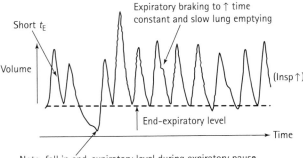

Note fall in end-expiratory level during expiratory pause.

Figure 2.5 Dynamic elevation of functional residual capacity (FRC) in infants. Infants modulate both expiratory time and flow in order to maintain a dynamically elevated FRC above that which would be determined by the outward recoil of the chest wall and inward recoil of the lung. By increasing respiratory rate and shortening expiratory time (t_E), they can breathe in before the passively determined FRC is reached. This is assisted by braking (i.e. slowing) expiratory flows and hence lung emptying by using laryngeal or diaphragmatic muscle activity to increase the expiratory time constant. Note the fall in end-expiratory level when a more prolonged expiration occurs. A similar but more prolonged change can occur during apnoeic spells, and on induction of anaesthesia because of loss of intercostal muscle tone, © Janet Stocks.

the expiratory time constant (τ_{rs}). An expiratory time (t_E) equivalent to $3\tau_{rs}$ is required to allow 95 per cent lung emptying during a passive expiration, whereas lung emptying will be 99 per cent complete if $t_E = 5\tau_{rs}$. Dynamic elevation of lung volume, by *auto-PEEP* (positive end-expiratory pressure), can occur in the presence of a rapid respiratory rate or elevated airway resistance, i.e. whenever $t_E < 3\tau_{rs}$ (Fig. 2.4). The lower the compliance (e.g. in RDS), the higher the elastic recoil and hence the faster the lung emptying and the risk of lung collapse is increased. The higher the resistance (e.g. in asthma or bronchiolitis), the slower the emptying and the risk of hyperinflation is increased. While this may be a useful way of increasing airway calibre and hence flows in patients with severe lung disease [24], breathing at higher lung volumes can increase the work of breathing since ventilation may then occur on the flatter (stiffer) portion of the volume–pressure curve. It may also put the diaphragm and other respiratory muscles at a mechanical disadvantage, thereby increasing risk of respiratory muscle fatigue. Failure to lengthen expiratory time to allow sufficient lung emptying in ventilated patients with airway obstruction can lead to inadvertent and potentially detrimental hyperinflation. For this reason, the use of high-frequency oscillatory ventilation (HFOV) rarely helps patients with airflow obstruction, despite its potential benefits in those with stiff lungs.

During the first months of life, infants partially compensate for their compliant chest wall by dynamically modulating both expiratory timing and flow to elevate the volume of air remaining in their lungs at end-expiration (FRC) (Fig. 2.5). This is mediated through vagal stretch receptors that are exquisitely sensitive to changes in resting lung volume. This is evident from the almost instantaneous change in breathing rate and pattern in response to the application of continuous negative or positive pressure. Infants also use laryngeal and diaphragmatic activity to slow or brake expiratory flow. Grunting is an extreme form

of glottic braking that results from partial closure of the vocal cords during expiration. This increases intra-alveolar pressure and limits alveolar collapse in the presence of high surface tensions such as occur in RDS. Infants frequently expire to a lower level when t_E is prolonged, as can be observed during apnoeic pauses (Fig. 2.5). End-expiratory volume is dynamically elevated until about 6–12 months of age, after which the mechanical characteristics of lung and chest wall determine FRC, as in an adult.

A mean reduction of around 35 per cent in FRC on induction of either barbiturate or inhalational anaesthesia has been documented in infants and young children compared with values in the awake, supine state. The use of a neuromuscular blocking agent does not seem to lead a further reduction [1]. This may be attributed to depression of respiratory drive, loss of intercostal muscle tone, lack of end-expiratory pressure (due to intubation) and possible shifts in intrathoracic blood volume. By contrast, anaesthesia with ketamine is not associated with the reduction in FRC and indeed children anaesthetised with ketamine tend to have an increased FRC [1].

Ventilation

CHEMOSENSITIVITY

During foetal life, arterial oxygen tension in the umbilical vein is approximately 3.3–4.7 kPa and postnatal adaptation of the peripheral chemoreceptors to the higher *ex utero* arterial oxygen tensions requires time. The arterial partial pressure of oxygen (PaO$_2$) ranges from 8.7 to 10.7 kPa in the neonate, compared with 10.7–12.7 kPa in adults. There is currently no consensus regarding optimal blood gases for preterm infants requiring supplemental oxygen [15,25]. The lack of objective criteria to determine which infants actually require supplemental O$_2$ is of increasing concern, since currently this often seems to be based purely on local hospital policy [26]. It is, however, possible to quantify the type (shunt or ventilation/perfusion imbalance) and severity of gas exchange impairment in a graded fashion, simply by making non-invasive paired measurements of inspired oxygen concentration (FiO$_2$) and pulse oximetry (SpO$_2$), and this approach has recently been used in preterm infants to assess precise oxygen requirements at specified time points during early development [27].

Major developmental changes in ventilatory control occur during the first weeks of life. This is a complex area to study, and interpretation of results is highly dependent on behavioural state, the type of technique and stimulus used, and the underlying respiratory mechanics. Functional chemoreceptors are not essential to commence or even to sustain breathing efforts immediately at or after birth and it seems that intense brain activation, which occurs at this time, provides sufficient stimuli. During subsequent days to weeks this 'neurogenic' drive weakens and chemoreceptors become crucial in generating and maintaining normal breathing rhythm. Failure of chemoreceptor development becomes an important cause of breathing dysfunction, particularly during sleep [28]. In addition to the carotid and aortic bodies, similar chemosensitive tissues in the thorax and abdomen are crucial for maintaining oxygen homeostasis [29].

In contrast to older subjects, newborn infants do not demonstrate a sustained increase in ventilation on exposure to hypoxia, but show a 'biphasic response' – the initial transient increase in ventilation on exposure to low oxygen rapidly being replaced by depression. This immature hypoxic ventilatory response persists until at least 6 months of age, but is most marked in the first weeks of life. The ventilatory decline that follows initial hypoxic hyperpnoea has been attributed to immaturity of the peripheral and central chemoreflexes and appears to mimic foetal responses to hypoxia designed to reduce oxygen consumption. Postnatally, however, it may put the infant at risk.

Arousal to hypoxia is an essential protective reflex. Prematurity, intrauterine growth restriction, foetal exposure to maternal smoking during pregnancy and prenatal or perinatal hypoxia have all been associated with a diminished arousal response to a variety of stimuli, including hypoxia in young infants [30,31]. Failure to arouse has been implicated in the sudden infant death syndrome (SIDS). Infants are more likely to arouse during active sleep than in quiet sleep. However, haemoglobin saturation may fall more quickly during an active sleep apnoea because of high oxygen demand.

As in older subjects, hypercapnia produces a rapid, sustained increase in minute ventilation in infants. However, in contrast to adults, during infancy this is primarily caused by an increase in tidal volume with minimal change or even a decrease in respiratory frequency. While hypercapnia stimulates an increase in electromyogram activity of laryngeal abductors at all ages, among infants the diaphragmatic expiratory braking mechanism elevates end-expiratory lung volume, thereby prolonging expiratory time. A weak hypercapnic ventilatory response may predispose to apnoeas in preterm infants.

Effects of anaesthesia on ventilation

Marked age-related differences in respiratory physiology make infants and young children more susceptible to adverse effects of anaesthesia than adults. These effects can often be minimised when spontaneous breathing is maintained by using light planes of anaesthesia supplemented by appropriate regional nerve block. Numerous studies have been undertaken to compare the relative effects of the different inhalational anaesthetics on patterns of respiration in children. Details of these have been summarised in a previous review [1] and are also discussed in Chapter 10. Studies are often difficult to compare due to differences in premedication, induction agent and whether a laryngeal mask or tracheal tube was *in situ*. All currently used inhalational anaesthetic agents, including halothane, isoflurane, enflurane, sevoflurane and desflurane, have a dose-dependent depressant effect on ventilation [1,32–34]. Desflurane induces respiratory depression at concentrations higher than 1 MAC (minimum alveolar concentration), mainly as a result of a decrease in tidal volume and should therefore be used cautiously at high concentrations during spontaneous ventilation [32]. Tidal volume may be reduced from 6 to 10 mL/kg in sleeping or sedated infants to as little as 4 mL/kg in those allowed to breathe spontaneously during halothane anaesthesia. This reduction in tidal volume has been reported to be less marked when using a laryngeal mask than tracheal tube, possibly owing to the lower resistance and hence diminished workload of the former [33,35]. Since nitrous oxide does not produce any significant depression of ventilation, it may be used in combination with other inhalational agents such as isoflurane or halothane to minimise the reduction in tidal volume. There are marked differences on the effects of these different agents on respiratory rate: halothane causes an increase, enflurane a reduction and isoflurane little change. The effects of anaesthesia and intermittent positive pressure ventilation (IPPV) on alveolar–arterial oxygen tension differences do not appear to be clinically significant when oxygen-enriched mixtures are used, but may contribute to postoperative hypoxaemia.

The reduction in minute ventilation on induction of anaesthesia is accompanied by increases in end-tidal carbon dioxide tension (P$_{ET}$CO$_2$) up to 8 kPa, the greatest increases being seen in the youngest infants. Most agents appear to have a similar effect on P$_{ET}$CO$_2$. Non-opioid premedication (midazolam) causes less depression of ventilatory frequency and minute ventilation than opioids, and without any significant difference in P$_{ET}$CO$_2$. While healthy anaesthetised children appear to tolerate increased CO_2 tensions without clinical problems, this may not be the case with children with prior cardiorespiratory difficulties. The depression in ventilatory response to CO_2 has generally been attributed to depression of the respiratory neurons in the medullary centre but may also result from preferential suppression of intercostal muscle activity. Ventilatory depression during anaesthesia is greater in infants, because they depend more on inspiratory intercostal activity to stabilise the compliant thorax. During quiet sleep, ventilatory response to CO_2 appears to depend more on the ribcage than the diaphragm and it has been postulated that this helps preserve the diaphragm in its most efficient configuration. However, the response of the ribcage is not maintained during REM sleep and may also be compromised during inhalational anaesthesia. The contribution of profound depression of the ribcage to ventilation has been demonstrated in children during halothane anaesthesia and may result in paradoxical inward movement of the highly deformable chest wall, leading to a downward spiral of reduced ventilatory efficiency and increasing diaphragmatic fatigue.

Postoperative ventilatory function

The impairment of gas exchange occurring during anaesthesia persists into the postoperative period. Since children are potentially more susceptible to airway closure than adults, routine oxygen saturation monitoring is desirable at least in the immediate recovery period. Preterm infants are more prone to complications after anaesthesia than full-term infants, particularly with respect to life-threatening apnoeic episodes. This may be related to maturational differences in chest wall compliance as well as immaturity of respiratory control. Infants with a preanaesthetic history of idiopathic apnoea are particularly at risk and such infants should not undergo surgical procedures as outpatients. Continuous postoperative monitoring is recommended for 12–48 hours in preterm infants below 60 weeks' postconceptional age (PCA), and non-essential surgery should be delayed until after 44 weeks' PCA.

UPPER AIRWAY AND LUNG RECEPTORS

Upper airway and lung reflexes appear to play a more important role during early life, perhaps reflecting the relative immaturity of the central control of breathing. The laryngeal reflex has the most inhibitory effect on respiration and is inversely related to PCA. Tiny amounts of water or any fluid with low concentrations of chloride that drop into the larynx can induce marked apnoea, especially under anaesthesia. The laryngeal reflex is also reinforced by hypoxia, infection and gastro-oesophageal reflux. Laryngeal irritability during anaesthesia is more pronounced in children than adults and may lead to serious hypoxaemia. Despite its advantages with respect to rapid induction time, isoflurane has been found to be more irritant than halothane, with increased incidence of laryngospasm,

salivation, coughing and breath holding [1]. The reduction in respiratory frequency and occurrence of respiratory pauses in response to trigeminal stimulation of the face and nasal mucosa are more marked during infancy. In contrast to older children and adults, the vagally mediated Hering–Breuer inflation reflex (HBIR), which results in inhibition of inspiration (expiratory pause or apnoea) if the lungs are inflated, remains active over the tidal range in infants during the first year of life. The strength of the HBIR is volume dependent and inversely related to age, such that even relatively small lung inflations can induce marked apnoeic pauses in preterm infants. This is often seen during anaesthesia and ventilatory support [36]. 'Head's paradoxical reflex' is an inspiratory gasp in newborn infants, elicited by distension of the upper airways, and is thought to be vagally mediated and have an important role in initial lung inflation at birth.

PERIODIC BREATHING AND APNOEA

Periodic breathing is commonly seen in otherwise normal preterm infants and occasionally in term neonates. It is characterised by apnoea lasting from 3 to 10 seconds alternating with periods of ventilation lasting 10–15 seconds. Its incidence diminishes with increasing maturity and usually disappears by 40 weeks' PCA (i.e. term equivalent). The cause of periodic breathing is unknown, but may reflect brain-stem immaturity. All anaesthetic techniques are associated with an increased risk of apnoea in preterm infants. The term 'apnoea' has been variously defined as a respiratory pause lasting somewhere between 2 and 20 seconds, making comparison between studies extremely difficult. Given that long respiratory pauses are more likely to be associated with life-threatening changes in cardiovascular, neurological or metabolic function, it is probably more appropriate to categorise respiratory pauses by whether or not these secondary events are present, rather than simply by duration. Since infants have high oxygen consumption and reduced oxygen stores, they may be more vulnerable to brief respiratory pauses than older subjects [37,38]. It should be noted that even normal infants, children and adults exhibit respiratory pauses from time to time, especially during REM sleep. Indeed, the absence of such irregularities may indicate abnormalities of respiratory control.

EFFECTS OF GROWTH ON VENTILATION

During the first months of life the weight-corrected tidal volume remains relatively constant at between 6 and 10 ml/kg [6,39] so that any increase in minute ventilation is achieved primarily through an increased respiratory rate. The tidal breathing pattern is particularly variable at this stage and mainly depends upon age and chest wall maturation. Newborn infants have an 'abdominal breathing' pattern in that inspiration coincides with an outward displacement of the abdomen. This may be accompanied by sternal and intercostal recession, so that ribcage expansion

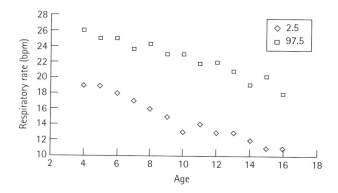

Figure 2.6   Age-related changes in respiratory rate. Data from Wallis *et al.* [41], showing the upper (97.5 centile) and lower (2.5 centile) limits of normal respiratory rate in awake children, derived from 1109 healthy children aged 4–16 years. Adapted with permission from BMJ Publishing Group.

contributes relatively little to overall air exchange. With growth, stiffening of the chest wall and reduction in the relative size of the liver, outward displacement of the chest wall becomes the primary mechanism for lung expansion. Abdominal breathing is rare after 1 year of age.

Elevations in respiratory rate are a sensitive, early, but non-specific indicator of respiratory disease. Although it is generally accepted that respiratory rate is inversely proportional to age throughout childhood, values quoted for the 'normal range' in health vary widely. A study to establish reference ranges in young children below 3 years of age showed that respiratory rate (RR) decreases rapidly after birth and is particularly variable during the first 3 months of life [40]. In this study, mean (SD) RR was 48 (9) breaths per minute (bpm) in awake and 40 (9) bpm in sleeping infants less than 2 months, falling to 27 (4) bpm and 21 (4) bpm in awake and sleeping children by 3 years of age. Data from older children showed that, on average, respiratory rate falls from 22 (range 20–26) bpm in a 4-year-old to 14 (11–18) bpm by 16 years of age, the latter approaching values commonly reported in adults (Fig. 2.6) [41].

CLINICAL APPLICATION AND INTERPRETATION OF LUNG FUNCTION TESTS

An extensive range of techniques is now available to assess lung function in infants and children of all ages [5,6,19,42]. Measurements are also feasible during intensive care, although accuracy may be reduced because of leakage around uncuffed tracheal tubes, interactions between spontaneous and mechanical ventilation, and inherent inaccuracies in many current monitors [43–45].

Lung volumes

Both plethysmographic and gas dilution methods for assessing resting lung volumes have been successfully

adapted for use in sleeping infants and in awake children as young as 3 years of age [6]. The FRC increases from around 100 mL in a newborn infant to 3–4 L in adults. Like most lung volumes, FRC is proportional to height at all ages, but, after puberty, is greater in males than females for any given height. Recently, it has become possible to obtain lung volume measurements in infants over an extended volume range, by passively inflating the lungs towards total lung capacity (TLC) using what has become known as the 'raised volume technique'. Similar measurements are feasible by voluntary effort in 60–80 per cent of children between 3 and 6 years of age [6], and in the majority thereafter [5].

Lung volumes and capacities are influenced by many factors, including muscle strength, elastic properties of the lungs and chest wall, airway properties (including calibre and airway wall compliance) and patient age, cooperation, height and gender. Volumes are some 10 per cent lower in African–Caribbeans when compared with age-matched white children, which is probably related to their lower trunk:leg ratio. The TLC is reached when the force generated by voluntary contraction of the inspiratory muscles equals that determined by the combined elastic inward recoil of the lungs and chest wall. The FRC (i.e. end-expiratory volume) is generally determined when the inward recoil of the lung is equal to the outward recoil of the chest wall (Fig. 2.7), although this is not the case in infants who, as discussed above, compensate for their low elastic equilibrium volume by dynamically elevating their FRC.

Lung volumes and capacities increase rapidly during infancy and childhood. Adult values are achieved by around 18 years in females and 25 years in males. Serial measures of absolute lung volumes, used in combination with forced expiratory manoeuvres, may be used to discriminate between restrictive and obstructive lung disease. A reduction in both vital capacity (VC) and TLC can occur in a wide range of restrictive diseases, including muscle weakness, loss of chest wall elasticity, loss of lung tissue or diminished lung growth. Conversely, in obstructive airway disease, there will a reduction in forced flows and volumes, but TLC will be preserved. An elevated residual volume (RV = volume of air remaining in the lungs after a forced expiration) in relation to total lung capacity (i.e the RV:TLC ratio) may be a valuable indicator of trapped gas secondary to airway obstruction. At residual volume it is not possible to empty any further air from the alveoli because of dynamic airway collapse (airway closure). The point at which dynamic compression of the airways begins is called the closing volume (CV). In healthy children and adults this occurs only at volumes well below the FRC. However, the CV increases with age, smoking, lung disease, anaesthesia and body position (being greater when supine than erect) and may move into the tidal range. This may also occur in healthy infants and young children because of their highly compliant chest wall, but will be exacerbated in the presence of airway disease. Airway collapse increases the work of breathing and leads to ventilation–perfusion mismatch.

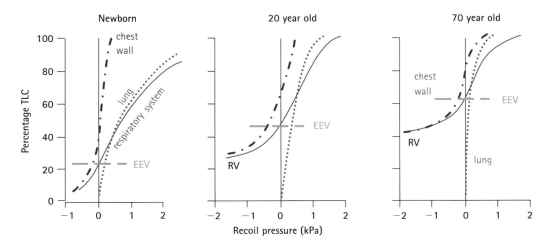

Figure 2.7 Effect of maturational changes in lung and chest wall recoil on lung volumes. Abbreviations: EEV, elastic equilibrium volume; RV, residual volume; TLC, total lung capacity. Note the very low transpulmonary pressure at EEV in infants due to the highly compliant chest wall (see also Fig. 2.3). This yields a small resting lung volume which may predispose to premature airway closure unless functional residual capacity (FRC) is dynamically elevated (see text). In the elderly, loss of lung recoil and stiffening of the chest wall leads to a relative increase in EEV and RV and a reduction in vital capacity, © Janet Stocks.

Auto-PEEP occurs when there is inadequate time for expiration, for example in bronchoconstriction or mucus plugging, so that airway pressure remains positive at end-expiration. The increased work of breathing associated with auto-PEEP can be offloaded by applying continuous positive airway pressure (CPAP) at the trachea or mouth above the auto-PEEP level in order to splint open the connecting airways. Similarly, in mechanically ventilated patients, airway collapse can be prevented by applying positive pressure to the airway throughout the respiratory cycle. Positive end-expiratory pressure or CPAP works by increasing FRC, maintaining alveolar recruitment, facilitating gas exchange and reducing the workload of breathing. The patient requires sufficient PEEP to prevent alveolar de-recruitment, but not so much that alveolar overdistension, dead space ventilation and hypotension occur. The ideal level of PEEP is that which prevents de-recruitment of the majority of alveoli, while causing minimal overdistension. Recruitment manoeuvres are used to reinflate collapsed alveoli before applying a sustained pressure to prevent de-recruitment [46–50]. This is discussed further below with respect to optimising ventilation in relation to the pressure–volume characteristics of the lung.

Lung elasticity

During ventilation, energy is required to overcome impedance of the respiratory system. The reduction in lung volume and compliance, and the increase in resistance occurring during anaesthesia, are likely to result in increased work in breathing. This is usually only clinically significant during spontaneous breathing, but may also lead to under-ventilation when pressure-generating lung ventilators are used. The elasticity of the lung results from

both structural components, including elastic fibres within the lung parenchyma and the geometry of the terminal air-spaces, and the surface tension generated at the air–liquid interface. Surfactant deficiency, fibrosis, oedema and interstitial lung disease all result in 'stiffer' lungs, (i.e. increased elasticity or decreased compliance). Compliance (the reciprocal of elastance) is defined as the change in volume for a given unit change in pressure. Lung compliance (C_L) increases 20- to 30-fold with growth, from around 60 mL/kPa (6 mL/cmH$_2$O) in a neonate to 1.3–1.9 L/kPa in an adult. However, specific compliance (C_L/FRC) remains relatively consistent throughout life in normal lungs, at least until the onset of emphysematous changes in the elderly, when it increases. Dynamic lung compliance can be measured during quiet breathing by relating changes in volume to changes in oesophageal pressure between points of no flow [6]. Among children, however, this technique is generally limited to neonates or ventilated children because of the relatively invasive nature of the oesophageal catheter.

PRESSURE–VOLUME RELATIONSHIPS

The amount of pressure required to inflate the lung at any given moment depends not simply on lung compliance, but on the volume at which lung inflation is initiated and on events immediately preceding such inflation – termed the pressure–volume (PV) history. Interpretation of changes in both lung and total respiratory compliance (combination of lung and chest wall compliance) is often confounded by the failure to take PV history into account. Thus, a sudden change in compliance in an infant with RDS, or as a result of changing PEEP level, is more likely to reflect opening or closure of a number of lung units rather than any intrinsic change in lung elasticity. It is therefore important to standardise such factors if comparisons are

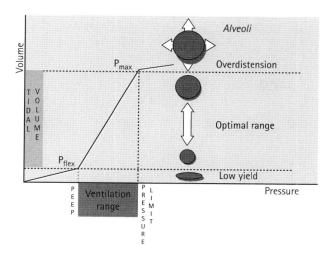

Figure 2.8 Significance of the respiratory pressure–volume curve for optimising ventilation. The pressure–volume (PV) relationships within the lung are such that more pressure is required to effect the same degree of lung inflation at very low and high volumes than in the more compliant central portion. Owing to gravitational changes and effects of disease, some areas of the lung may be over-distended while others remain collapsed (see Fig. 2.9). To minimise lung injury, the lung should be ventilated on the portion of the PV curve between the lower (shown here as P_{flex}) and the upper inflection points (P_{max}). © Janet Stocks.

to be made within or between subjects. More pressure is required to inflate the lungs by a given amount at both high and low lung volumes (Fig. 2.8). If a subject breathes at a fixed, low tidal volume for some time, portions of the lung (particularly in dependent areas) will not be ventilated and may become atelectatic, requiring high pressures to reinflate. Computed tomography techniques have shown that pulmonary densities develop in areas of collapse in the dependent parts of the lung during anaesthesia, which may adversely affect gas exchange. These can probably be attributed to the reductions in both tidal volumes and FRC induced by most inhalational anaesthetic agents [1].

There has been increasing emphasis on the need to optimise both resting lung and tidal volumes in ventilated infants and young children in order to minimise lung injury, although accurate adjustment of these parameters is extremely difficult, using standard ventilator equipment [44,45]. Inflammation caused by lung overdistension is thought to be important in the pathogenesis of bronchopulmonary dysplasia [12,51,52] and preterm infants with variable lung compliance are particularly at risk. Mechanical ventilators that deliver a set pressure rather than volume can cause inadvertent over-distension or *volutrauma* of the more compliant portions of the lung, particularly if there is a sudden change in compliance – as for example immediately after surfactant administration. Volume-targeted neonatal ventilators have been developed as alternatives to traditional pressure-limited ventilators

because they are better able to deliver more consistent and appropriate tidal volumes. It is suggested that these should provide a more effective and safer means of ventilating the newborn infant [53]. Inappropriate equipment and methods of neonatal resuscitation may also greatly increase the risk of lung injury at birth, with long-term impact [7,54].

General anaesthesia promotes atelectasis but this can be reduced by using an alveolar recruitment manoeuvre immediately after induction of anaesthesia [46]. Further paediatric studies are needed to determine the role of recruitment manoeuvres in anaesthesia and intensive care [47,49,55–57]. During ventilatory support, the aim is to maintain ventilation over the central, more compliant portion of the PV curve to achieve maximum ventilation with minimum pressure swings, thereby avoiding lung injury associated with the opposite extremes of over-distension and atelectasis (Fig. 2.8) [50]. Some investigators have suggested that the ratio of compliance over the final 20 per cent portion of the breath in relation to that over the entire breath (the so-called C20/C ratio) can help guide management in this respect, but mechanisms underlying both atelectasis and lung recruitment are generally too heterogeneous for this simplistic approach.

The shape of the PV curve around the lower inflection point depends on many factors, such as non-linear characteristics of lung and chest wall tissue, surfactant redistribution, collapse and reopening of the alveoli and bronchi, and dynamic hyperinflation. Sudden reopening of closed airways is accompanied by short, transient sounds called 'crackles' and it has been recently demonstrated that quantification of airway closure on the basis of subsequent recruitment is feasible by monitoring intratracheal crackle sounds. Since these acoustic signals precede any accompanying changes in resistance, elastance or the shape of the transpulmonary PV curve, this may prove to be a valuable non-invasive clinical monitoring technique in the near future [58].

Chest wall elasticity

The chest wall is also elastic but, in contrast to the lung, tends to 'spring out' at low lung volumes and only demonstrates any measurable inward recoil at high lung volumes. Chest wall compliance (C_w) is rarely measured but total respiratory compliance (C_{rs}, which is $C_w + C_L$) is useful to assess the elastic characteristics of the respiratory system in young infants in whom values approximate to C_L because of their to their very high C_w. Accurate measurements of C_{rs} can only be made during a respiratory pause when there is total relaxation of the respiratory muscles. Changes in volume above FRC are related to pressure changes at the airway opening (tracheal tube or facemask) during a respiratory pause induced by brief airway occlusion. In the absence of any airflow or respiratory effort, these pressure changes are assumed to reflect alveolar, and hence total elastic recoil, pressure. Adults can be trained to perform breath-holding manoeuvres at different lung volumes in order to obtain a static PV curve, and similar measurements can be performed in the ventilated, para-lysed infant. These measurements are rarely possible in children but can be undertaken in spontaneously breathing infants by taking advantage of the Hering–Breuer inflation reflex [6,36].

Airway resistance

Respiratory work has to be done to overcome not only the elastic but also the resistive properties of the lungs and airways. The energy required to overcome the frictional resistance to airflow only accounts for about one-third of total respiratory work during quiet breathing in health, but may rise considerably in the presence of airway disease. Airflow is either laminar (streamlined) or turbulent, and depends on gas density, airway calibre and airflow velocity: the higher the flow, the denser the gas and the wider the airway, the greater the tendency for turbulent flow. Hence flow is generally laminar in peripheral, but turbulent in larger airways (maximal in the trachea). Resistance is directly proportional to the length of the airways, but inversely proportional to the fourth (laminar flow) or fifth (turbulent flow) power of the radius. Hence, halving airway calibre results in a 16- or 32-fold increase in resistance, respectively. Resistance to turbulent (but not laminar) flow is also proportional to gas density and therefore the work of breathing can be reduced in upper or central airway obstruction by breathing Heliox (70 per cent helium, 30 per cent oxygen) [59].

Resistance is defined as change in pressure per unit change in flow expressed as kilopascals/litre/second (kPa/L/s) whereas conductance (G) (its reciprocal) describes the change in flow per unit pressure change. The site of pressure measurement affects which type of resistance is assessed. Airway resistance (R_{aw}) is estimated by measuring change in alveolar pressure using whole-body plethysmography in relation to airflow. A combination of lung tissue and airway resistance is estimated from the transpulmonary pressure difference using oesophageal manometry, and is referred to as 'pulmonary' or 'lung' resistance. Total respiratory resistance (R_{rs}) combines the components of the airways, lung and chest wall and requires estimation of pressure at the airway opening (i.e. mouth or nose).

Resistance falls as lung volume and airway calibre increase with growth. Consequently, specific resistance remains relatively constant throughout life. Specific resistance is resistance × FRC, unlike other variables that are proportional to FRC. Airway resistance falls from around 3 kPa/L/s (30 cmH$_2$O/L per s) in a newborn to around 1 kPa/L/s by 1–2 years and to 0.1–0.2 kPa/L/s in an adult. It is, however, important to appreciate that, during infancy these measurements include nasal resistance, which comprises 50 per cent of R_{aw}. Indeed, despite their small absolute size, the calibre of the conducting airways is relatively large in relation to airflow during the first years of

life, resulting in a very short time constant, or emptying time of the lung, when compared with older subjects. This reflects that all conducting airways are formed well before birth, whereas the majority of alveolarisation occurs postnatally. Following delivery, growth of lung volume outstrips that of the airways (dysanaptic growth) such that there is a gradual lengthening of the expiratory time constant. Nasal breathing must be taken into account when interpreting measurements, since changes in lower airway resistance may be masked, especially if there has been a recent upper respiratory infection. Similarly, since the nose acts as an efficient filter, less aerosolised material (such as a bronchodilator) may reach the lung in an infant than in a mouth-breathing adult [3].

In addition to growth-related increases, airway calibre is determined by the balance between forces tending to narrow the airways and those tending to tether them open.

Forces tending to narrow the airways include:

- obstruction by secretions, mucus or foreign bodies
- thickening of the airway wall (muscle hypertrophy, inflammation or oedema)
- increased bronchial smooth muscle tone (bronchoconstriction due to a range of irritants, cold, hypoxia, hypercapnia and active mediators such as histamine and acetylcholine)
- increased airway wall compliance (floppy airways)
- decreased elastic recoil from both the lung (e.g. emphysematous changes or low lung volumes) and chest wall (in infancy, heavy sedation, anaesthesia or paralysis).

Forces helping to tether the airways open include:

- during inspiration, resistance falls because the airways are tethered open by the negative intrapleural pressures that develop as the thorax expands
- similarly, transpulmonary pressure becomes increasingly negative at higher lung volumes due to the increased lung recoil.

The effect of anaesthetic agents and related drugs on airway smooth muscle tone in children requires further study [1]. Increased smooth muscle tone, reduction in airway calibre owing to accumulation of secretions or oedema and reduction in lung volume will all increase airway resistance.

AIRWAY RESPONSIVENESS

Although the airways are fully innervated at birth and airway responsiveness appears to be similar to that in older children, bronchodilator therapy is rarely effective in wheezy infants during the first 6 months of life. This is probably because of the structural and physiological differences that predispose the infant to wheeze in the absence of any bronchoconstriction. Indeed, while around 30 per cent of infants may wheeze [60], most will not go on to develop asthma. Infants born to mothers who smoke during pregnancy have diminished airway function (increased resistance and low airflows) and a fourfold increased risk of 'transient' wheezing, which is probably caused by impaired prenatal and postnatal airway growth [6,20,60].

ASSESSMENT OF AIRWAY FUNCTION

Measurement of lung resistance by oesophageal manometry was once commonplace in infants, but has generally been replaced by the less invasive assessments of passive respiratory mechanics using one of the occlusion techniques. Respiratory resistance and airway responsiveness can be assessed in awake preschool children using either the interrupter technique (Rint) or plethysmographic assessments of specific airway resistance. The forced oscillation technique (FOT), in which the impedance of the respiratory system (Zrs) is measured by superimposing small amplitude pressure oscillations on the respiratory system and measuring the resultant oscillatory flow has also been adapted for use in both infants and preschool children [6]. Depending on the frequency of the applied pressure wave, the resultant impedance contains different mechanical information and can be adapted to allow partitioning of lung function into airway and tissue parameters or to study airway wall mechanics [61,62].

An alternative method of assessing airway function is to measure rate of airflow using spirometry during forced expiratory manoeuvres: lower flows and forced expired volumes (e.g. forced expired volume in 1 second, FEV_1) are associated with diminished airway calibre. During studies in sleeping infants, voluntary efforts are replaced by rapidly inflating a jacket, which is wrapped around the chest and abdomen to force expiration either at end-tidal inspiration or after passively inflating the lung towards total lung capacity. This is called the raised volume rapid thoraco-abdominal compression technique [63]. Full forced expiratory manoeuvres can also be obtained in intubated children using the forced deflation technique [64,65].

Until recently, attempts to obtain forced expiratory manoeuvres by voluntary effort were generally restricted to children above the age of 5–6 years. It has now been shown that with suitable encouragement (including use of computer incentive games) and adaptation of quality control criteria, such measurements are feasible in 60–80 per cent of 3- to 6-year-olds [6]. However, the rapid lung emptying during early life means that it may not be possible to obtain an FEV_1 in infants and young children, so expired volumes over shorter intervals (e.g. $FEV_{0.75}$ or $FEV_{0.5}$) are used as alternative outcome measures. Detailed discussions of how to perform and interpret these measurements in both infants and children have been published recently [5,6]. Conventional tests such as spirometry measure only the function of the larger conducting airways and as such may be relatively insensitive to early lung disease, which often starts in, or affects, the peripheral (small) airways.

Dependence on these tests may result in misdiagnosis and delay effective therapeutic interventions in diseases such as cystic fibrosis and asthma until after irreversible lung damage has occurred [6,39]. Consequently, there is increasing emphasis on the need for sensitive tests of small airway function such as the multiple breath inert gas washout (MBW) technique. The MBW is a non-invasive, tidal breathing method applicable to subjects of all ages, which provides information on both lung volume and ventilation inhomogeneity as sensitive indicators of early airway disease [6,39,66,67]. Although the calibre of individual airways in the periphery of the lung is tiny, their combined surface area is huge. Indeed, while obstruction of 50 per cent of peripheral airways has dramatic effects on gas exchange, this results in only a 10 per cent rise in resistance, which is why this part of the lung is often referred to as the 'silent zone'. In contrast, even minimal changes in the calibre of the trachea or major bronchi, which represent the narrowest part of the airway tree, can cause dramatic and potentially life-threatening increases in resistance.

Regional distribution of ventilation and lung volumes

Gravitational differences in pleural pressure gradient, together with regional differences in airway resistance and compliance, and hence time constants, means that even in health, neither ventilation nor volumes are evenly distributed. General anaesthesia causes some impairment of gas exchange due both to the reduction in FRC, with subsequent shunting of blood through unventilated areas of the lung, and to alterations in the ventilation–perfusion ratio. Differences exist between children and adults in relation to the distribution of ventilation and pulmonary perfusion. In spontaneously breathing adults, ventilation and perfusion are distributed preferentially to dependent parts of the lungs (Fig. 2.9a), whereas, during IPPV, more ventilation is diverted to non-dependent regions. In spontaneously breathing infants, the distribution of ventilation appears to be similar to that seen during IPPV in adults (Fig. 2.9b). This finding is of importance in children with unilateral lung disease in whom oxygenation improves when the good lung is uppermost, this being the reverse of the situation in adults. It is therefore possible that ventilation–perfusion mismatch may be greater in anaesthetised children during spontaneous breathing than when IPPV is used, although this has yet to be confirmed. The age at which the 'adult pattern' is attained with respect to postural changes in regional ventilation is currently unknown, although it probably occurs by school age. Recent developments in new non-invasive methods of assessing regional ventilation, including electrical impedance tomography [6,66,68], are likely to shed further light on this phenomenon in the near future. Such methods may also prove invaluable for optimising lung volumes and ventilation and minimising lung injury in children requiring ventilatory support [66].

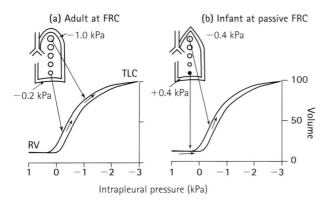

Figure 2.9 Developmental changes in regional ventilation and lung volumes. The pressure–volume (PV) curve of the lung is sigmoid. The lung expands most easily over the central portion (i.e. the curve is steepest at around functional residual capacity [FRC] and the tidal breathing range) but becomes increasingly difficult to inflate at very low and high volumes (i.e. the curve flattens towards total lung capacity [TLC] and residual volume [RV], respectively). Intrapleural pressure is less negative at the base than at the apex of the lung because of the weight of the lung. (a) In the adult, the base of the lung is relatively compressed when breathing at FRC, but expands better (greater unit ventilation) on inspiration than the apex because of its position on the PV curve. In contrast, the apex of the lung has a relatively larger resting volume at FRC than the base of the lung but receives relatively little ventilation for the same pressure change during inspiration (see also Fig. 2.8), © Janet Stocks. (b) In infants intrapleural (transpulmonary) pressures are less negative throughout the lung because of increased chest wall compliance and diminished outward recoil (see Fig. 2.3), such that pressure at the base of the lung may exceed airway pressure at low lung volumes. As a consequence airway closure occurs in this region and no gas enters with small tidal volumes. This situation may also occur during tidal breathing in the elderly or those with emphysema and during anaesthesia because of loss of chest wall recoil and associated reductions in FRC, © Janet Stocks.

Gas exchange and diffusion

The vital process of gas exchange occurs in the terminal respiratory units and, once an adequate air–blood interface has been established, is very similar in infants as in older subjects. During anaesthesia, dead space and resistance of breathing systems are more critical during spontaneous breathing than during IPPV. During IPPV the main effect of using a high-resistance system is to increase lung volume. In respiratory support of infants, flow resistive characteristics of tracheal tubes and connectors are of critical importance and it is also essential to minimise all equipment deadspace [65,69–71]. This is particularly pertinent (and challenging) in the preterm infant, in whom the absolute tidal volume may be as low as 5 mL. Diffusing capacity can be measured relatively routinely in children over 10 years of age but such measurements are difficult in

younger children. Development of reliable, non-invasive methods of assessing the surface area available for gas exchange (alveolar size and number) are essential in order to further our knowledge of disease and therapeutic interventions in the developing lung. Non-invasive lung imaging using hyperpolarised magnetic resonance imaging (MRI) hold some promise [72].

Assessing mechanically ventilated children

Although there is no firm evidence to suggest that pulmonary function testing can guide the clinical management of individual ventilated children, it can provide a valuable educational tool for more rational ventilation of sick children [43,65]. It is possible to assess both baseline respiratory mechanics and lung volumes, and the response to ventilatory strategies or therapeutic interventions in intubated children [1,19,22,62,64,65,67,73–75]. End-tidal CO_2, arterial oxygen tensions and/or saturations and compliance can be readily measured, but it is increasingly realised that additional information such as the lower and upper inflection points on the pressure volume curve, or measurement of intrinsic (auto) PEEP, is required to facilitate optimal mechanical lung support (see above).

Airway pressures measured during manual or mechanical ventilation do not equate to those in the spontaneously breathing patient, in that not only are they positive during inspiration, but they reflect the total force required to expand the lung and thorax and to overcome the resistance of both the intrinsic airways and the tracheal tube. The latter may represent a very significant proportion of total airway resistance especially in young infants [35,43,70,71]. Mechanical properties of the respiratory pump must be considered when using assisted or triggered ventilation modes in children, since instability and inspiratory deformation of the ribcage may make it difficult to detect the negative deflections of airway pressure that are required to indicate intended inspirations.

One of the major challenges in assessing the effects of different types of anaesthesia or ventilatory modes on respiratory mechanics relates to appropriate adaptation of equipment for use in ventilated infants [44,45,69,71,76]. Ultimately, the aim should be to provide continuous on-line monitoring of both tidal and regional lung volumes, and partitioned respiratory mechanics. This will require continuing attempts to minimise apparatus dead space and resistance, increase frequency response and minimise gas sampling flows. In the past, attempts to undertake such measurements have been limited by:

1. The relative invasiveness of these techniques in clinically unstable infants.
2. Insensitivity to changes in respiratory mechanics within individuals due, for example, to the relative magnitude of resistance of the tracheal tube, and marked intrasubject variability.

3. Inaccuracies in displayed values of tidal volume or pressure [44,45].
4. Confounding of results due to interactions between the ventilator and spontaneous breathing activity.
5. Leaks around the tracheal tube [77].

In most patients, a leak can be eliminated by applying gentle cricoid pressure, or by the use of a tube with a cuff. It has been traditionally taught that only uncuffed tracheal tubes should be used in small children. Recent studies suggest that cuffed tubes can be used safely even in small infants, although cuffs reduce the largest size of tube that can be inserted and can therefore potentially increase the resistance to airflow and the work of spontaneous breathing. Nevertheless, in ventilated patients, a properly sized, positioned and inflated modern (low-pressure, high-volume) cuffed tracheal tube offers better control of air leakage, lower rate and better control of flow of anaesthetic gases, and decreased risk of aspiration and infection [78,79].

Further adaptation of non-invasive, sensitive techniques to measure gas exchange, tissue mechanics, ventilation distribution and pulmonary perfusion may provide more pertinent and reliable information in the future [56,61,62,66,73,80,81]. Several new methods are currently being used in specialised research settings, but considerable further work is required before they will find their way into clinical practice.

REFERENCES

Key references

Hatch DJ, Fletcher M. Anaesthesia and the ventilatory system in infants and young children. *Br J Anaesth* 1992; **68**: 398–410.

Keidan I, Fine GF, Kagawa T *et al.* Work of breathing during spontaneous ventilation in anesthetized children: a comparative study among the face mask, laryngeal mask airway and endotracheal tube. *Anesth Analg* 2000; **91**(6): 1381–8.

Marraro GA. Protective lung strategies during artificial ventilation in children. *Paediatr Anaesth* 2005; **15**(8): 630–7.

Saugstad OD. Oxygen for newborns: how much is too much? *J Perinatol* 2005; **25** (suppl 2): S45–9.

Tusman G, Bohm SH, Tempra A *et al.* Effects of recruitment maneuver on atelectasis in anesthetized children. *Anesthesiology* 2003; **98**(1): 14–22.

References

1. Hatch DJ, Fletcher M. Anaesthesia and the ventilatory system in infants and young children. *Br J Anaesth* 1992; **68**: 398–410.
2. Hatch DJ. Respiratory physiology in neonates and infants. *Curr Opin Anaesthesiol* 1995; **8**: 224–9.
3. Stocks J, Hislop AA. Structure and function of the respiratory system: Developmental aspects and their relevance to aerosol therapy. In: Bisgaard H, O'Callaghan C, Smaldone GC, eds. *Drug delivery to the lung: clinical aspects.* New York: Marcel Dekker, Inc., 2002: 47–104.
4. Chernick V, Boat, TF, Wilmott RW. Bush A, eds. *Kendig's disorders of the respiratory tract in children,* 7th edn. Philadelphia: Elsevier, 2006.
5. Castile RG. Pulmonary function testing in children. In: Chernick V, Boat TF, Wilmott RW, Bush A, eds. *Kendig's disorders of the respiratory tract in children.* Philadelphia: WB Saunders Company, 2006: 168–85.
6. Stocks J. Pulmonary function tests in infants and young children. In: Chernick V, Boat TF, Wilmott RW, Bush A, eds. *Kendig's disorders of the respiratory tract in children,* 7th edn. Philadelphia: Elsevier, 2006: 129–67.
7. Jobe AH. Transition/adaptation in the delivery room and less RDS: 'Don't just do something, stand there!'. *J Pediatr* 2005; **147**(3): 284–6.
8. Henderson-Smart DJ, Hutchinson JL, Donoghue DA *et al.* Prenatal predictors of chronic lung disease in very preterm infants. *Arch Dis Child Fetal Neonatal Ed* 2006; **91**(1): F40–5.
9. Morse SB, Wu SS, Ma C *et al.* Racial and gender differences in the viability of extremely low birth weight infants: a population-based study. *Pediatrics* 2006; **117**(1): e106–12.
10. Allen J, Zwerdling R, Ehrenkranz R *et al.* Statement on the care of the child with chronic lung disease of infancy and childhood. *Am J Respir Crit Care Med* 2003; **168**(3): 356–96.
11. Stocks J, Coates AL, Bush A. Lung function in infants and young children with chronic lung disease of infancy: The next steps? *Pediatr Pulmonol* 2007; **42**: 3–9.
12. Kallapur SG, Jobe AH. Contribution of inflammation to lung injury and development. *Arch Dis Child Fetal Neonatal Ed* 2006; **91**(2): F132–5.
13. West JB. How well designed is the human lung? *Am J Respir Crit Care Med* 2006; **173**(6): 583–4.
14. Zeman KL, Bennett WD. Growth of the small airways and alveoli from childhood to the adult lung measured by aerosol-derived airway morphometry. *J Appl Physiol* 2006; **100**: 965–71.
15. Saugstad OD. Oxygen for newborns: how much is too much? *J Perinatol* 2005; **25** (suppl 2): S45–9.
16. Al Hathlol K, Idiong N, Hussain A *et al.* A study of breathing pattern and ventilation in newborn infants and adult subjects. *Acta Paediatr* 2000; **89**(12): 1420–5.
17. Aurora P, Kozlowska WJ, Stocks J. Gas mixing efficiency from birth to adulthood measured by multiple-breath washout. *Respir Physiol Neurobiol* 2005; **148**: 125–39.
18. Schulze A, Abubakar K, Gill G, Way RC, Sinclair JC. Pulmonary oxygen consumption: a hypothesis to explain the increase in oxygen consumption of low birth weight infants with lung disease. *Intensive Care Med* 2001; **27**(10): 1636–42.
19. Stocks J, Lum S. Applications and future directions of infant pulmonary function testing. In: Hammer J, Eber E, eds.

Paediatric pulmonary function testing. Basel: Karger, 2005: 78–93.

20. Stocks J, Dezateux C. The effect of parental smoking on lung function and development during infancy. *Respirology* 2003; **8**(3): 266–85.

21. Greenspan JS, Miller TL, Shaffer TH. The neonatal respiratory pump: a developmental challenge with physiologic limitations. *Neonatal Netw* 2005; **24**(5): 15–22.

22. Manczur TI, Greenough A, Pryor D, Rafferty GF. Assessment of respiratory drive and muscle function in the pediatric intensive care unit and prediction of extubation failure. *Pediatr Crit Care Med* 2000; **1**(2): 124–6.

23. Traeger N, Panitch HB. Tests of respiratory muscle strength in neonates. *Neo Rev* 2004; **5**(5): e208–14.

24. Kosmas EN, Milic-Emili J, Polychronaki A *et al.* Exercise-induced flow limitation, dynamic hyperinflation and exercise capacity in patients with bronchial asthma. *Eur Respir J* 2004; **24**(3): 378–84.

25. Walsh M, Engle W, Laptook A *et al.* Oxygen delivery through nasal cannulae to preterm infants: can practice be improved? *Paediatrics* 2005; **116**(4): 857–61.

26. Walsh MC, Szefler S, Davis J *et al.* Summary Proceedings from the Bronchopulmonary Dysplasia Group. *Paediatrics* 2006; **117**: 52–6.

27. Quine D, Wong CM, Boyle EM *et al.* Non-invasive measurement of reduced ventilation–perfusion ratio and shunt in infants with bronchopulmonary dysplasia: a physiological definition of the disease. *Arch Dis Child Fetal Neonatal* Ed 2006; **91**: F409–14.

28. Cohen G, Katz-Salamon M. Development of chemoreceptor responses in infants. *Respir Physiol Neurobiol* 2005; **149**(1–3): 233–42.

29. Nattie E. Why do we have both peripheral and central chemoreceptors? *J Appl Physiol* 2006; **100**(1): 9–10.

30. Baldwin DN, Pillow JJ, Stocks J, Frey U. Lung-function tests in neonates and infants with chronic lung disease: tidal breathing and respiratory control. *Pediatr Pulmonol* 2006; **41**(5): 391–419.

31. Horne RS, Parslow PM, Harding R. Postnatal development of ventilatory and arousal responses to hypoxia in human infants. *Respir Physiol Neurobiol* 2005; **149**(1–3): 257–71.

32. Behforouz N, Debousset AM, Jamali S, Ecoffey S. Respiratory effects of desflurane anesthesia on spontaneous ventilation in infants and children. *Anesth Analg* 1998; **87**(5): 1052–5.

33. Brown K, Aun C, Stocks J *et al.* A comparison of the respiratory effects of sevoflurane and halothane anaesthesia in infants and young children. *Anesthesiology* 1998; **89**: 86–92.

34. Erb T, Christen P, Kern C, Frei FJ. Similar haemodynamic, respiratory and metabolic changes with the use of sevoflurane or halothane in children breathing spontaneously via a laryngeal mask airway. *Acta Anaesthesiol Scand* 2001; **45**(5): 639–44.

35. Keidan I, Fine GF, Kagawa T, Schneck FX, Motoyama EK. Work of breathing during spontaneous ventilation in anesthetized children: a comparative study among the face mask, laryngeal mask airway and endotracheal tube. *Anesth Analg* 2000; **91**(6): 1381–8.

36. Brown K, Stocks J, Aun C, Rabbette PS. The Hering–Breuer reflex in anesthetized infants: end-inspiratory vs. end-expiratory occlusion technique. *J Appl Physiol* 1998; **84**(4): 1437–46.

37. Katz-Salamon M. Delayed chemoreceptor responses in infants with apnoea. *Arch Dis Child* 2004; **89**(3): 261–6.

38. Martin RJ, Abu-Shaweesh JM. Control of breathing and neonatal apnea. *Biol Neonate* 2005; **87**(4): 288–95.

39. Aurora P, Bush A, Gustafsson P *et al.* Multiple-breath washout as a marker of lung disease in preschool children with cystic fibrosis. *Am J Respir Crit Care Med* 2005; **179**: 249–56.

40. Rusconi F, Castagneto M, Gagliardi L *et al.* Reference values for respiratory rate in the first 3 years of life. *Paediatrics* 1994; **94**: 350–5.

41. Wallis LA, Healy M, Undy MB, Maconochie I. Age related reference ranges for respiration rate and heart rate from 4 to 16 years. *Arch Dis Child* 2005; **90**(11): 1117–21.

42. American Thoracic Society/European Respiratory Society. Pulmonary function testing in preschool children: official statement. *Am J Respir Crit Care Med* 2007; **175**: 1304–45.

43. Stocks J. Infant respiratory function testing: is it worth all the effort? *Paediatr Anaesth* 2004; **14**: 537–40.

44. Castle RA, Dunne CJ, Mok Q *et al.* Accuracy of displayed values of tidal volume in the pediatric intensive care unit. *Crit Care Med* 2002; **30**(11): 2566–74.

45. Dela Cruz RH, Banner MJ, Weldon BC. Intratracheal pressure: a more accurate reflection of pulmonary airway pressure in pediatric patients with respiratory failure. *Pediatr Crit Care Med* 2005; **6**(2): 175–81.

46. Tusman G, Bohm SH, Tempra A *et al.* Effects of recruitment maneuver on atelectasis in anesthetized children. *Anesthesiology* 2003; **98**(1): 14–22.

47. Thorsteinsson A, Werner O, Jonmarker C, Larsson A. Airway closure in anesthetized infants and children: influence of inspiratory pressures and volumes. *Acta Anaesthesiol Scand* 2002; **46**(5): 529–36.

48. Rimensberger PC, Cox PN, Frndova H, Bryan AC. The open lung during small tidal volume ventilation: concepts of recruitment and 'optimal' positive end-expiratory pressure. *Crit Care Med* 1999; **27**(9): 1946–52.

49. Marraro GA. Protective lung strategies during artificial ventilation in children. *Paediatr Anaesth* 2005; **15**(8): 630–7.

50. Halbertsma FJ, van der Hoeven JG. Lung recruitment during mechanical positive pressure ventilation in the PICU: what can be learned from the literature? *Anaesthesia* 2005; **60**(8): 779–90.

51. Carney D, DiRocco J, Nieman G. Dynamic alveolar mechanics and ventilator-induced lung injury. *Crit Care Med* 2005; **33**(3 suppl): S122–8.

52. Christou H, Brodsky D. Lung injury and bronchopulmonary dysplasia in newborn infants. *J Intensive Care Med* 2005; **20**(2): 76–87.

53. McCallion N, Davis PG, Morley CJ. Volume-targeted versus pressure-limited ventilation in the neonate. *Cochrane Database Syst Rev* 2005; (3): CD003666.

54. O'Donnell CP, Davis PG, Morley CJ. Resuscitation of premature infants: what are we doing wrong and can we do better? *Biol Neonate* 2003; **84**(1): 76–82.

55. Tingay DG, Mills JF, Morley CJ *et al.* The deflation limb of the pressure-volume relationship in infants during high-frequency ventilation. *Am J Respir Crit Care Med* 2006; **173**(4): 414–20.

56. Pillow JJ, Sly PD, Hantos Z. Monitoring of lung volume recruitment and derecruitment using oscillatory mechanics during high-frequency oscillatory ventilation in the preterm lamb. *Pediatr Crit Care Med* 2004; **5**(2): 172–80.

57. Keenan WJ. Neonatal resuscitation: what role for volume expansion? *Pediatrics* 2005; **115**(4): 1072–3.

58. Petak F, Habre W, Babik B *et al.* Crackle-sound recording to monitor airway closure and recruitment in ventilated pigs. *Eur Respir J* 2006; **27**(4): 808–816.

59. Nawab US, Touch SM, Irwin-Sherman T *et al.* Heliox attenuates lung inflammation and structural alterations in acute lung injury. *Pediatr Pulmonol* 2005; **40**(6): 524–32.

60. Dezateux C, Stocks J, Wade AM *et al.* Airway function at one year: association with premorbid airway function, wheezing and maternal smoking. *Thorax* 2001; **56**: 680–6.

61. Pillow JJ, Stocks J, Sly PD, Hantos Z. Partitioning of airway and parenchymal mechanics in unsedated newborn infants. *Pediatr Res* 2005; **58**(6): 1210–15

62. Petak F, Babik B, Asztalos T *et al.* Airway and tissue mechanics in anesthetized paralyzed children. *Pediatr Pulmonol* 2003; **35**(3): 169–76.

63. ATS–ERS Consensus Statement, Lum S, Stocks J, Castile R *et al.* Raised volume forced expirations in infants: Recommendations for current practice. *Am J Respir Crit Care Med* 2005; **172**(11): 1463–71.

64. Hammer J, Patel N, Newth CJ. Effect of forced deflation manoeuvres upon measurements of respiratory mechanics in ventilated infants. *Intensive Care Med* 2003; **29**(11): 2004–8.

65. Hammer J, Newth CJ. Pulmonary function testing in the neonatal and paediatric intensive care unit. In: Hammer J, Eber E, eds. *Paediatric pulmonary function testing.* Basel: Karger, 2005: 266–81.

66. Pillow JJ, Frerichs I, Stocks J. Lung function tests in neonates and infants with chronic lung disease: global and regional ventilation inhomogeneity. *Pediatr Pulmonol* 2006; **41**(2): 105–21.

67. Schibler A, Henning R. Positive end-expiratory pressure and ventilation inhomogeneity in mechanically ventilated children. *Pediatr Crit Care Med* 2002; **3**(2): 124–8.

68. Frerichs I, Schiffmann H, Oehler R *et al.* Distribution of lung ventilation in spontaneously breathing neonates lying in different body positions. *Intensive Care Med* 2003; **29**(5): 787–94.

69. Frey U, Stocks J, Coates A, Sly P, Bates J. Standards for infant respiratory function testing: Specifications for equipment used for infant pulmonary function testing. *Eur Respir J* 2000; **16**: 731–40.

70. Manczur T, Greenough A, Nicholson GP, Rafferty GF. Resistance of pediatric and neonatal endotracheal tubes: influence of flow rate, size, and shape. *Crit Care Med* 2000; **28**(5): 1595–8.

71. Miller DM, Adams AP, Light D. Dead space and paediatric anaesthetic equipment: a physical lung model study. *Anaesthesia* 2004; **59**(6): 600–606.

72. Waters B, Owers-Bradley J, Silverman M. Acinar structure in symptom-free adults by Helium-3 magnetic resonance. *Am J Respir Crit Care Med* 2006; **173**(8): 847–51.

73. Habib RH, Pyon KH, Courtney SE. Optimal high-frequency oscillatory ventilation settings by nonlinear lung mechanics analysis. *Am J Respir Crit Care Med* 2002; **166**(7): 950–3.

74. Habib RH, Pyon KH, Courtney SE, Aghai ZH. Spectral characteristics of airway opening and chest wall tidal flows in spontaneously breathing preterm infants. *J Appl Physiol* 2003; **94**(5): 1933–40.

75. Schibler A, Frey U. Role of lung function testing in the management of mechanically ventilated infants. *Arch Dis Child Fetal Neonatal Ed* 2002; **87**(1): F7–10.

76. Leipala JA, Iwasaki S, Milner A, Greenough A. Accuracy of the volume and pressure displays of high frequency oscillators. *Arch Dis Child Fetal Neonatal Ed* 2004; **89**(2): F174–6.

77. Main E, Castle R, Stocks J *et al.* The influence of endotracheal tube leak on the assessment of respiratory function in ventilated children. *Intensive Care Med* 2001; **27**: 1788–97.

78. Fine GF, Borland LM. The future of the cuffed endotracheal tube. *Paediatr Anaesth* 2004; **14**(1): 38–42.

79. Newth CJ, Rachman B, Patel N, Hammer J. The use of cuffed versus uncuffed endotracheal tubes in pediatric intensive care. *J Pediatr* 2004; **144**(3): 333–7.

80. Pillow JJ. High-frequency oscillatory ventilation: mechanisms of gas exchange and lung mechanics. *Crit Care Med* 2005; **33**(3 suppl): S135–S141.

81. Willis BC, Graham AS, Yoon E *et al.* Pressure-rate products and phase angles in children on minimal support ventilation and after extubation. *Intensive Care Med* 2005; **31**(12): 1700–5.

The cardiovascular system

PETER D BOOKER

KEY LEARNING POINTS

- Failure of the pulmonary circulation to undergo successful transition at birth results in persistent pulmonary hypertension of the newborn which is associated with a significant morbidity and mortality.
- Major postnatal morphological changes occur in the heart and great vessels

- There are important developmental changes in cardiac intercellular structure and organisation.
- After birth there is clinically relevant development of the cardiomyocyte, cardiovascular function (and its regulation) and the response to vasoactive drugs.

INTRODUCTION

Significant physiological changes occurring after birth have an effect not only on myocardial performance, but also on the structure, functioning and control of the cardiovascular system as a whole. Our understanding of these developmental processes has advanced substantially in recent years. In this chapter, I have described those aspects of postnatal development that affect the cardiovascular system, giving most emphasis to those changes that have a direct influence on perioperative care.

TRANSITIONAL CIRCULATION [1–4]

During intrauterine life, the placenta serves as the organ for gas exchange, and the lungs receive <10 per cent of right ventricular output. The relatively low pulmonary blood flow, sufficient for normal lung growth and development, results from a combination of a high pulmonary vascular resistance (PVR) in the non-aerated lung and a relatively low systemic vascular resistance (SVR) relating to the placental circulation. The contrasting vascular impedances result in 90 per cent of the right ventricular output shunting across the ductus arteriosus to the descending aorta. It is probable that an oxygen sensor within the mitochondria in the vascular smooth muscle cell senses alterations in partial pressure of arterial oxygen (PaO_2). This creates a signal that modulates redox-sensitive K^+ channels, thereby controlling membrane potential, Ca^{2+} entry and vascular tone. The oxygen tension in the foetal alveoli and arterioles is about 3 kPa, thus hypoxic pulmonary artery vasoconstriction (HPVC) is the principal reason for the resting high vascular tone.

In human foetal lung vessels expression of endothelial nitric oxide (NO) synthase decreases markedly after mid-gestation, and stays low thereafter. Concentrations of endothelin-1 are higher in the third trimester foetus than in the neonate. Activation of endothelin-A (ET_A) receptors causes vasoconstriction, whereas activation of endothelin-B (ET_B) receptors (probably) causes vasodilatation. Hence, the net effect of endothelin-1 is dependent on the balance between the opposing effects of the two types of endothelin receptor activation. Although ET_A-receptor gene expression increases with gestational age in the developing foetus, ET_B-receptor expression is higher in the term foetus and neonate. Other endothelium-derived products – vasodilators (e.g. epoprostenol) and vasoconstrictors (e.g. leukotrienes) – also influence vascular tone. Mechanical compression of the distal non-muscular pulmonary arteries by fluid-filled alveoli, and increased phosphodiesterase (PDE-5) activity also accentuate the high resting tone.

Foetal pulmonary arteries have a thicker muscular layer relative to their external diameter than those in adults and this is one reason for the increased vasoreactivity found in the near-term foetus. The relatively small lumen size also contributes to the high resting PVR. During foetal growth, the number of small pulmonary arteries increases both in absolute terms and per unit volume of lung, a 10-fold increase in vessels per unit of lung in the last trimester allows rapid recruitment of precapillary arteries into the pulmonary circulation after birth. The PVR of the term foetus, however, remains high because of active vasoconstriction.

The imbalance between vasoconstrictor and vasodilator mediators changes abruptly in the postnatal period. The cessation of placental blood flow causes an immediate decrease in pressure in the inferior vena cava and right atrium, and an increase in the SVR; PVR decreases acutely with lung aeration, resulting in an increase in pulmonary blood flow and pulmonary venous return. Consequently, the pressure in the left atrium exceeds that in the right, and shunting through the foramen ovale is minimised. Hence, the direction of blood flow through the heart alters acutely, and the three shunts that permitted much of the blood to bypass the liver and lungs start to close; consequently, the left ventricular stroke volume increases from 1.2 mL/kg to 2.2 mL/kg.

The dramatic postnatal reduction in PVR results not only from a reduction in HPVC, but also from increased local release of vasodilator mediators such as bradykinin, NO, epoprostenol and endothelium-derived hyperpolarising factor (EDHF). This factor induces smooth muscle cell hyperpolarisation by activating K_{ATP} channels. Endothelin-1, acting on endothelin-B receptors, also may have potent vasodilatory effects in the newborn. Simultaneously, within a few minutes after birth, the external diameter of the precapillary non-muscular arteries increases. The rise in oxygen tension causes previously cuboidal endothelial cells to assume a flattened appearance and spread out within the vessel wall, increasing lumen diameter and lowering resistance. The relative paucity of interstitial connective tissue aids this process.

Failure of the pulmonary circulation to undergo this transitional process results in persistent pulmonary hypertension of the newborn, a condition that is associated with a significant morbidity and mortality rate.

POSTNATAL MORPHOLOGICAL CHANGES OCCURRING IN THE HEART AND GREAT VESSELS

In addition to the early physiological adaptations of the neonate to extrauterine life, structural changes in the cardiovascular system occur throughout infancy.

Atrial septum [5]

In the foetus, oxygenated inferior vena caval blood from the placenta flows preferentially across the foramen ovale in the atrial septum to the left atrium, and thereby to the left ventricle (Fig. 3.1). The foramen ovale has a 'flap' valve derived from the septum primum, so that when left atrial pressures (LAPs) become higher than right atrial pressures (RAPs) after birth, the septum closes functionally. Subsequent anatomical closure depends on the septum developing

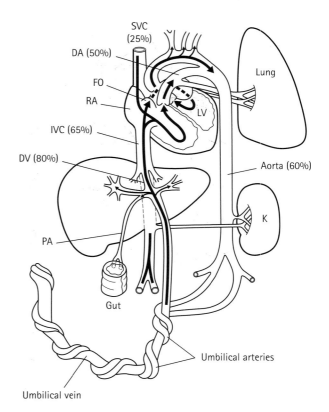

Figure 3.1   Diagram of the foetal circulation. Typical oxygen saturation values are given in parentheses. SVC, superior vena cava; IVC, inferior vena cava; DA, ductus arteriosus; FO, foramen ovale; RA, right atrium; LV, left ventricle; DV, ductus venosus; PV, portal vein; K, kidney.

fibrous bands that seal the previously patent anterosuperior margin. The channel remains patent in 50 per cent of children for up to 5 years, and persists in about 30 per cent of adults and may become functionally significant if, at any time, RAP exceeds LAP.

Ductus arteriosus [6]

At the origin of the left pulmonary artery, the ductus arteriosus forms a direct continuation of the pulmonary trunk with the distal aortic arch and, in the foetus, is similar in size to both (Fig. 3.1). The media of the ductus arteriosus consists of circular smooth muscle fibres. Localized intimal thickenings progressively enlarge from 20 weeks' gestation. During the first 24 hours of postnatal life, active muscular contraction of the ductus occurs and approximation of the opposing surfaces of the intimal cushions occludes its lumen (duct diameter 4.3 mm at 2 h and 2.1 mm at 12 h and closed at 24 h in 90 per cent of term neonates).

Oxygen-induced potassium (K^+) channel inhibition leads to smooth muscle cell depolarisation, opening of voltage-gated L-type calcium channels, influx of Ca^{2+} and vasoconstriction. The proximal mitochondrial electron transport chain serves as the oxygen sensor: mitochondria respond to rises in the partial pressure of O_2 by increasing their production of reactive oxygen species (ROS), and increase inhibits the voltage-gated K^+ channels. The ductus arteriosus in preterm infants may fail to close normally because their ductal smooth muscle cells are relatively deficient in voltage-gated K^+ channels. Following functional closure, the opposing surfaces of the ductal cushions fuse and additional fibrous tissue proliferation, or thrombus, completes the anatomical obliteration of the lumen. With time, the formerly muscular artery becomes a thin fibrous ligament. Complete anatomical closure generally occurs by 4–8 weeks of age. However, 4.5 per cent of healthy term infants aged between 2 and 6 months have a (silent) ductus arteriosus.

Cardiac chambers [7]

Once the foetal circulatory shunts have functionally closed, rather than both ventricles working in parallel to pump oxygenated blood into the descending aorta, the cardiovascular system shifts to the adult 'in series' configuration. The right and left ventricles in the full-term neonate are symmetrical cone-like structures at birth, with both chambers being circular in cross-section. In the first few months of life, the left ventricle (LV) rapidly increases in size in response to the increase in its afterload. In contrast, the right ventricle (RV) gains weight relatively slowly, reflecting its much lower afterload. The adult ratio of about 3:1 for LV:RV weight is attained by 3 months of age. Thereafter, the thickness of both the LV and RV walls increases progressively with increasing age throughout childhood.

The heart in a full-term neonate weighs approximately 20 g. In the first year of life, while body weight doubles, the weight of the heart increases by 80 per cent. Thereafter, up until puberty, the weight of the heart increases in direct proportion to body size, averaging about 0.5 per cent of body weight (Fig. 3.2). Subsequently, the correlation between LV mass and body size progressively decreases because of the increasing variability of haemodynamic workload and increasing effect of gender. Growth of the heart results from an increase in the size (hypertrophy) and number (hyperplasia) of cardiomyocytes. However, hyperplasia plays a relatively minor role in cardiac growth, and only up to about 7 months of age. At birth, both RV and LV myocardial fibres average 8 μm in diameter, whereas in the adult LV fibres are 20 μm and RV fibres 16 μm.

Ductus venosus and umbilical arteries [8]

The umbilical arteries arise from both internal iliac arteries and carry foetal blood to the placenta. Oxygenated blood leaves the placenta via the umbilical vein, traverses the liver in the ductus venosus, and empties into the inferior vena cava (see Fig. 3.1). The umbilical vein remains catheter patent in 64 per cent of neonates during the first 6 days after birth.

During the third trimester, the ductus venosus directs about 20 per cent of umbilical venous blood towards the foramen ovale to maintain preferential streaming to the left atrium. Blood distribution through the foetal ductus venosus is dependent on umbilical venous pressure and active regulation of the lumen diameter. In postnatal life, the flow velocity through the ductus venosus reflects the portocaval pressure gradient and pressure in the right atrium. The ductus venosus closes functionally between day 3 and 7 in about 76 per cent of term neonates, the remainder usually before day 18. The ductus venosus stays open for up to 14 days in healthy preterm neonates. The exact stimulus for closure remains unknown, though prostaglandin E_1 tends to keep the duct open, while thromboxane promotes its closure.

A combination of muscular contraction and fibrous proliferation of the intima obliterates the umbilical vessels within 3–5 weeks after birth. The umbilical vein extending

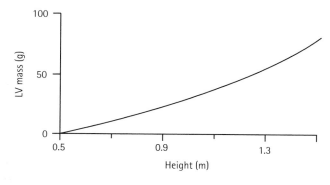

Figure 3.2   Relationship between body size and left ventricular (LV) mass. Data from de Simone et al. [7].

to the liver becomes the ligamentum teres and the ductus venosus becomes the ligamentum venosum. Proximally, the umbilical arteries persist as the hypogastric arteries, and the obliterated distal segments become the lateral umbilical ligaments.

Structure of arterial vessel walls [9]

At birth, the growth and microscopic appearance of the great arteries mirror the symmetry of the left and right ventricles. In the newborn, the walls of the pulmonary trunk and aorta are similar in size and wall thickness, and the elastic fibres of both are long, uniform and parallel. However, by 6 months of age, the pulmonary trunk is thinner than the aorta, and the elastic fibres more loosely arranged. Wall thickness of the aorta and density of elastic fibres both increase with postnatal growth and development. The pulmonary artery achieves adult structure by about 2 years of age. At this time, the wall thickness of the main pulmonary artery is 60 per cent that of the aorta and its elastic tissue is relatively sparse.

DEVELOPMENTAL CHANGES IN CARDIAC INTERCELLULAR STRUCTURE AND ORGANISATION

The myocardium consists of millions of myocytes supported in an extracellular matrix of connective tissue (ECM), the latter determining myocyte shape and alignment, and maintaining structural integrity during individual myocyte contraction and relaxation.

Extracellular matrix [10]

The ECM consists of interstitial collagens, proteoglycans (such as hyaluronic acid), glycoproteins and proteases. It surrounds the cardiomyocytes, fibroblasts and capillaries in a three-dimensional network. The structural proteins of the ECM, which bind to cell surface receptors called *integrins* (see below), maintain cellular alignment and are an important determinant of the passive and active mechanical properties of the myocardium.

Cardiomyocytes occupy about 75 per cent of normal myocardial tissue by volume, but account for only about 35 per cent of total cell numbers. About 90 per cent of the non-myocyte cells in the heart are fibroblasts; the remainder is made up of relatively small numbers of other cell types such as smooth muscle cells. Fibroblasts produce two subtypes of collagen, type I and type III; the latter is more compliant and flexible than the former. During the neonatal period, collagen production increases and collagenous connections between cardiomyocytes develop rapidly; the LV afterload increase results in the production of more type I than type III. Normal adult concentrations are attained by about 5 months of age, as type I collagen production declines relative to type III. This developmental change in collagen quality and quantity during early infancy partly explains the relatively stiff, non-compliant myocardium seen in this age group.

Cell adhesion molecules, such as fibronectin and laminin, are glycoproteins that link myocytes and endothelial cells, and collagen and other matrix proteins. Fibronectin has numerous binding sites for collagen and integrins (see below), and has a homogeneous distribution throughout the extracellular space. Production of fibronectin decreases during the neonatal period. The rate of production of laminin, another glycoprotein that has both collagen- and integrin-binding sites, does not vary with age, though its spatial distribution changes with cardiac development. In the neonate, the distribution of laminin is relatively homogeneous around the cardiomyocyte, whereas in the adult heart it localises to the basement membrane and Z discs, where collagen bundles contact the sarcolemma. The affinity of the neonatal cardiomyocyte for laminin, mediated by integrins, is significantly lower than in the adult (Table 3.1).

Table 3.1 Myocardial intercellular structure: the main differences between neonate and adult and their clinical implications

Structural component	Neonate versus adult	Clinical implications
Collagen	Relatively high total collagen content. Relatively high type I/type III ratio	Myocardial compliance reduced in neonate
Cell adhesion molecules, e.g. laminin	Regular distribution around myocyte in neonate; localised to Z discs in adult	Reduced structural integrity and reduced force transduction in neonate
Integrins	Increased expression of α_1 subunit Affinity of myocyte for laminin reduced	Reduced structural integrity and reduced force transduction in neonate
Gap junctions	Expression of connexion isoforms changes Uniform distribution of gap junctions in neonate; localised to intercalated disc in adults	Reduced intercellular conduction velocity in neonate

Integrins [11]

Integrins are heterodimeric cell membrane receptors (α and β subunits) that bind to cell adhesion molecules, and to components of the cytoskeleton. Integrins are necessary for myofibrillar alignment and for the formation of the rod-shape cell phenotype. Integrins mediate the organised arrangement of the ECM proteins relative to the cytoskeleton and myofibrils, and so optimise transduction of the force developed by the sarcomere into ventricular pressure.

Significant changes in the arrangement of the components of the ECM and integrins occur during cardiac remodelling; furthermore ECM–integrin interactions function in a bidirectional manner across cell membranes. For example, when laminin binds to an integrin receptor, it modulates adenylyl cyclase-mediated signalling within cardiac myocytes, an example of 'outside-in' signalling. In contrast, a signalling event initiated through non-integrin cellular receptors but which modifies integrin function is termed 'inside-out' signalling. For example, sustained adrenoreceptor agonism leads to increased binding of integrin to various ECM proteins and to clustering of integrins within the sarcolemma.

Developmental changes in the expression of isoforms of the integrin α subunits may alter the affinity of ECM proteins for integrins and so affect cardiac contraction. For example, increased affinity for interstitial collagens by myocytes is associated with expression of the α_1 subunit. Increased expression of this isoform occurs when collagen synthesis increases, during the neonatal period and when cardiac hypertrophy occurs in response to pressure overload. The integrin α_1 subunit is usually undetectable in the healthy adult heart.

When physiological or pathological hypertrophy occurs, the cardiomyocyte undergoes a significant change in cell shape. In order to adjust to the change in cell shape, integrins must change their position on the cell surface and their contact with the ECM and cytoskeleton. During the initial physiological adaptation that occurs with the increase in LV afterload in early infancy, expression of fibronectin and its integrin receptor increases in parallel. In contrast, during pathological hypertrophy, there may be disruption of the coordinated connection between fibronectin and its integrin receptor, resulting in myocytes being released from their ECM attachment sites, and the cell being subjected to forces that are detrimental to its survival.

Gap junctions [12]

An array of membrane channels, called 'gap junctions', link the cytoplasm of adjacent cells, thereby allowing myocardial cells to function as a syncytium by providing a low-resistance pathway for the propagation of an electrical impulse. Each of the apposed membranes in a gap junction is composed of a honeycomb-like array of transmembrane channels termed connexons. Connexons from adjacent cells combine to form an intercellular channel that is 1–2 nm in diameter, large enough to permit the diffusion of small molecules from one myocyte to another. Connexons are composed of six identical protein subunits termed connexins. The four connexin isoforms found in the heart can each produce a physiologically distinct gap junction that exhibits different channel conductances and gating mechanisms. Connexin isoforms found in conduction tissue and endocardium are different, and the resultant disparity in conductivity found within the myocardium aids the orderly and sequential spread of activation throughout the heart. The potential difference between connected cells is the main regulator of intercellular communication through gap junctions, though other factors such as intracellular pH can influence the strength of the intercellular link, allowing rapid functional uncoupling of healthy myocytes from damaged ones.

The developmental change in the expression of connexin isoforms results in a gradual decrease in the voltage dependence of the gap junction. The membrane density of gap junctions increases during late gestation, correlating with a developmental increase in conduction velocity. The increase in expression of connexins peaks during early neonatal life. The increase in density of gap junctions accompanies an increase in the proportion of large gap junctions, which have gating properties that are relatively voltage independent. In the neonate, gap junctions have a uniform distribution along the sarcolemma of ventricular myocytes. During postnatal development, as cell size increases, the gap junctions preferentially localise to the end of each cell, a region of specialised sarcolemma known as the intercalated disc. The relatively poor coupling of immature myocytes can be advantageous during a time of cardiac remodelling because it allows healthy immature myocytes to uncouple more easily from damaged ones.

POSTNATAL DEVELOPMENT OF THE CARDIOMYOCYTE

In response to the greater workload taken on by the postnatal LV, the population of myocytes increases during neonatal life more rapidly in the LV than in the RV. However, hyperplasia ceases after the first few months of life, and subsequently hypertrophy becomes the major mechanism through which ventricular mass increases.

During heart development, the cardiomyocyte changes its shape from spherical into the rod-shaped phenotype, and organises its internal structure into a clearly defined arrangement of contractile elements, supporting cytoskeleton, and sarcoplasmic reticulum. As the density of myofibrils in the myocyte increases, they become more orientated to the long axis of the cell, and extend from one side of the cell to the other. In immature cells, the central mass of non-contractile material appears to introduce an internal load against which the myofibrils contract. In the adult cell, by comparison, the myofibrils connect to the Z discs and the intermediate filaments, so that they lie as layers that extend throughout the cell, which is a much more efficient process for transmitting force developed by the cardiomyocyte into ventricular pressure.

Cytoskeleton [13]

The cytoskeleton is a complex meshwork of structural proteins that gives the cell its shape and organisation. The microtubules and desmin filaments connect the Z discs to the myofibrils and the myofibrils to the T-tubules, mitochondria and nuclei. The distribution of desmin is uniform in the late gestational foetus, and only starts to localise to the region of the Z disc postnatally. The expression of actinin, a cytoskeletal protein that is a major component of the Z disc, changes qualitatively and quantitatively during development, resulting in a maturational decrease in the thickness of the Z disc. In addition to the thick and thin filaments, sarcomeres also contain a third filament system composed of titin. This giant filamentous molecule, which links the thick filaments to the Z disc, determines the elasticity of myofibrils. There are two isoforms of titin found in the myocardium, one longer and more compliant than the other, but their relative proportion does not change with development.

The maturational changes in the cytoskeletal organisation and in the isoforms of at least some of the proteins that make up this force-transducing system help explain why the passive properties of the myocardium change with development.

Sarcolemmal ion channels

Significant changes in the expression of many sarcolemmal proteins occur during postnatal development. Although the neonatal myocyte may contain the same membrane proteins that allow trans-sarcolemmal transport of ions in the adult, they are often found in different relative proportions and have a different distribution in the sarcolemma. There are large inter-species differences in the developmental changes affecting the regulation of ionic currents in

the cardiomyocyte, and so much of the experimental data reported in the past is not applicable to the human. It is only recently that the relevant experiments using human material have been performed. There are five potentially clinically important ion channels.

L-TYPE CALCIUM CHANNELS [14,15]

In the adult cardiomyocyte, during each action potential, Ca^{2+} ions enter the cell mainly through voltage-gated L-type calcium channels. Membrane depolarisation to -30 mV opens these channels, and it is this inward Ca^{2+} current (I_{Ca}), which peaks within 2–3 milliseconds, that triggers the release of Ca^{2+} from the sarcoplasmic reticulum (SR) via ryanodine-sensitive Ca^{2+} channels, which are arrayed in close proximity to the L-type calcium channels. The resultant huge increase in local cytosolic Ca^{2+} concentration (from $0.1\,\mu$mol/L to $>100\,\mu$mol/L) activates crossbridge cycling and mechanical force production by the contractile proteins. At the same time, the local increase in Ca^{2+} concentration and change in transmembrane potential act, in concert, to inactivate the L-type calcium channels and to prevent excessive Ca^{2+} influx.

The mean basal I_{Ca} in cells taken from infants (1.2 pA/pF) is about half that seen in cells taken from adults (2.5 pA/pF). β-Adrenoreceptor stimulation increases I_{Ca} via protein kinase A phosphorylation shifting gating behaviour; the maximum I_{Ca} appears similar in all age groups (8.4–9.2 pA/pF), but lower levels of adrenoreceptor stimulation produce less proportional change in I_{Ca} in infant cells compared with those from adults. These developmental differences relate partly to the comparatively high concentration of $G_i\alpha_3$ protein found in infant cells, which acts to inhibit adenylyl cyclase activity. The concentrations of other G_i proteins, such as $G_i\alpha_2$, do not appear to vary significantly with age.

Another factor that contributes to the low basal I_{Ca} in neonatal cardiomyocytes is the reduced number of L-type calcium channels found in their sarcolemma. There is about 33 per cent less mRNA for L-type calcium channels in cardiomyocytes taken from the human neonate compared with the adult (Table 3.2). However, this deficit may be

Table 3.2   Relative density of sarcolemmal ion channels in the cardiomyocyte in the neonate compared with the adult and their clinical implications

Type of channel	Neonate versus adult	Clinical implications
L-type Ca^{2+}	Reduced (33%)	Contributes to lower basal Ca^{2+} current and reduced response to isoprenaline
T-type Ca^{2+}	Increased (10%)	Insignificant
Na^+/Ca^{2+} exchange	Increased (45%)	Contributes to reduction of systolic function
Na^+/K^+ ATPase	Increased (?)	Reduces sensitivity to digoxin
Na^+ entry (all)	No difference (?)	Insignificant
Na^+/H^+ exchanger	Increased (?)	Increases susceptibility to ischaemia–reperfusion injury

(?) Signifies data not confirmed in humans.

compensated somewhat by the relatively slow early repo-larisation of infant cells (produced by a faster inactivating transient outward current), which allows greater time for trans-sarcolemmal Ca^{2+} influx through both the L-type calcium channels and reverse-mode NCX (Na^+/Ca^{2+} exchanger, see below), and Ca^{2+} release from the sarcoplasmic reticulum.

Na^+/Ca^{2+} EXCHANGE [16]

Normal contraction and relaxation of the heart is dependent on tightly regulated intracellular Ca^{2+} homeostasis. In adults, the decrease in intracellular Ca^{2+} concentration that occurs during diastole is caused by take up of Ca^{2+} ions by the sarcoplasmic reticulum (70 per cent), and by transport out of the cell through the NCX channel (30 per cent). The principal cardiomyocyte extrusion mechanism, the NCX, uses the Na^+ electrochemical gradient across the sarcolemma to mediate the electrogenic countertransport of three Na^+ ions for one Ca^{2+} ion. Exchange is bidirectional and capable of moving Ca^{2+} in either direction across the sarcolemma. The highest density of NCX is in the T-tubular membranes. The NCX activity depends primarily on the potential difference and Na^+ gradient across the sarcolemma. Na^+ and Ca^{2+} also exert regulatory functions: exposure of the intracellular surface of the NCX to high concentrations of Na^+ results, after a few seconds, in a new steady-state (reduced) level of NCX activity.

Developmental changes in expression of NCX suggest that it has a more important role in controlling intracellular Ca^{2+} concentration in the immature myocyte than in adult cells. In the adult myocyte, the NCX functions primarily as a mechanism for removing Ca^{2+} from the cell, while in the perinatal heart the NCX also increases Ca^{2+} influx during the action potential. This is because when the transmembrane potential is positive, and/or when intracellular Na^+ concentration is increased, the NCX functions in reverse mode, allowing Ca^{2+} into the cell and expelling Na^+. Concentrations of NCX mRNA and protein are much higher in the human foetus than in the adult and, though they decrease postnatally, NCX protein concentrations in neonatal cardiomyocytes are about 45 per cent higher than in adult cardiomyocytes. Reverse-mode NCX Ca^{2+} entry is promoted by a low intracellular Ca^{2+} concentration and by a high intracellular Na^+ concentration, the latter observation helping to explain the positive force-frequency response.

Experimental studies have demonstrated that chronic β-adrenoreceptor agonism stimulates NCX expression and function, perhaps explaining why upregulation of NCX is normal in the neonatal period. Although a high density of NCX can partly compensate for compromised function of the calcium channels in the sarcoplasmic reticulum (SR), it does so primarily by depleting SR Ca^{2+} stores, hence potentially compromising systolic function. In addition, upregulation of NCX leads to spatial rearrangement of NCX within the sarcolemma and, with closer proximity to the L-type calcium channels, the NCX acts to reduce the

local Ca^{2+} in the microdomains between the T-tubular membrane and sarcolemma, and around the ryanodine receptors. Moreover, NCX operating in reverse mode is less efficient for triggering SR Ca^{2+} release compared with I_{Ca}. Experimental studies indicate that heart rate and intracellular Na^+ concentration are the main factors regulating the predominant direction of Ca^{2+} transport via NCX during an action potential.

Na^+/K^+-ATPASE CHANNEL [17]

This pump uses energy derived from the hydrolysis of adenosine triphosphate (ATP) to exchange three Na^+ ions for two external K^+ ions. This channel is the main regulator of intracellular Na^+ and K^+ concentrations, so influencing membrane potential and excitability. It indirectly affects cytosolic Ca^{2+} by maintaining the Na^+ gradient across the sarcolemma, so influencing NCX function. In addition, these pumps contain receptors for endogenous and therapeutic cardiac glycosides such as digoxin. The α subunit, of which there are three isoforms, is responsible for the catalytic activity and digoxin-binding properties of the enzyme, whereas the β subunit, of which there are four isoforms, is required to fix the enzyme to the sarcolemma. Developmental changes in the relative amount of the protein, its ATPase activity and its isoform expression occur in many different species, but only limited data are available in humans. Studies have demonstrated that Na^+/K^+-ATPase activity in human neonatal erythrocytes is higher than in adults, decreasing over the first 6 months of life. The ratio of α_1 to α_2 subunits also decreases during this period. Extrapolation of this data to cardiomyocytes would help explain why the neonatal myocardium is relatively less sensitive to digoxin than adult myocardium, irrespective of any pharmacokinetic differences.

SODIUM ENTRY CHANNELS [18]

In the steady state, the balance between Na^+ influx and efflux determines the intracellular concentration of Na^+. There are several pathways for Na^+ entry into the cardiomyocyte, but only one extrusion mechanism – the Na^+/K^+-ATPase pump. In addition to the NCX and Na^+/H^+ exchange pumps, other Na^+ entry channels include the Na^+/HCO_3^- cotransporter, an important acid extruding mechanism, and the Na^+/Mg^{2+} exchanger, involved in extruding Mg^{2+} from the cell. In addition, the $Na^+/K^+/2Cl^-$ cotransporter is important in cell volume regulation. Voltage-gated sodium channels are the primary channels responsible for the sudden influx of Na^+ into the cell subsequent to membrane depolarisation.

Na^+/H^+ EXCHANGER [19,20]

Accumulation of protons in the cell during ischaemia activates the Na^+/H^+ exchanger (NHE), which is the major regulatory protein responsible for control of intracellular pH. Activation of the NHE results in influx of one Na^+ ion into the cell in exchange for at least one H^+ ion. Extracellular acidosis inhibits proton extrusion through the NHE. An increase in intracellular Na^+ concentration causes reduced extrusion of Ca^{2+} by the NCX and increased Ca^{2+} influx through reverse-mode Na^+/Ca^{2+} exchange. Displacement of Ca^{2+} from intracellular buffers by H^+ may exacerbate the increase in intracellular Ca^{2+} concentration that results from intracellular acidosis. The NHE activity in myocytes taken from neonatal rats is two to three times that measured in adult rat cardiomyocytes. In human neonates too, it is likely that NHE activity is relatively high, as both α_1-adrenoreceptor agonism and triiodothyronine (T_3) stimulate NHE, and concentrations of norepinephrine and T_3 are relatively high in the neonatal period. High NHE activity helps explain why neonatal cardiomyocytes are relatively susceptible to ischaemia–reperfusion injury, as excess Ca^{2+} accumulating in the cell during periods of ischaemia can cause cell damage.

SARCOPLASMIC RETICULUM [21]

The primary site for Ca^{2+} storage in the cardiomyocyte is the SR. In the adult, the SR is composed of specialised regions with specific functions, notably the longitudinal elements and the junctional components. The longitudinal elements contain a calcium-dependent ATPase (SERCA2a) that removes Ca^{2+} from the cytosol and translocates it into the lumen of the SR. The longitudinal elements of the SR surround the sarcomere from Z disc to Z disc, so allowing for rapid removal of Ca^{2+} bathing the myofibrils. The junctional components of the SR contain the calcium-binding protein calsequestrin, and have large numbers of calcium-releasing channels – ryanodine receptor channels (RyRs) – covering their cytosolic surfaces. The junctional components of the SR are located at the level of the Z disc, in close proximity to the T-tubular system, which are sarcolemmal extensions that extend deep into the cell. The T-tubules that adjoin the junctional component of the SR have a high density of L-type calcium channels. This close structural relationship ensures that the opening of the calcium channels produces an increase in Ca^{2+} concentration in close proximity to the cytosolic surface of the junctional SR. In response to the increase in cytosolic Ca^{2+}, the RyRs allow Ca^{2+} to flow from the SR lumen into the cytosol.

The localisation of specific functions to specific regions of the SR, and the structural relationship between different regions of the SR and the Z disc, occurs only after postnatal maturation. The relative volume of the SR increases during late gestation and postnatally. Hence, although components of the SR are present in early postnatal life, the lack of differentiation and ordered relation with other membrane systems prevent the close coupling of L-type calcium channels and RyRs. The proximity of these proteins is important, as the Ca^{2+} concentration in this region increases more than an order of magnitude greater than in the rest of the cytosol. The relative abundance of NCX offers some compensation for the relative paucity of L-type calcium channels and the poor coupling of the SR and calcium channels. The activation of RyRs by NCX reverse-mode Ca^{2+} influx requires proximity of these two proteins, and (probably) Na^+ channels. While depolarisation favours reverse-mode NCX Ca^{2+} influx, a local increase in intracellular Na^+ concentration markedly enhances this effect.

In addition to the morphological changes in the SR and T-tubular system, the biochemical function of these membrane systems changes with development. Cardiomyocytes from adult hearts contain about 30 per cent more SERCA2a protein than those from neonates. Experimental studies demonstrate that there are relatively few RyRs in immature myocytes, and the increase in RyR expression parallels the increase in L-type calcium current density. Nevertheless, although the rate of release of Ca^{2+} through RyRs increases with age, even in early postnatal life it remains the primary mechanism for transiently increasing Ca^{2+} concentration in the cardiomyocyte in response to an action potential.

Mitochondria [22,23]

The mitochondria of cardiomyocytes increase in size and number during the neonatal period, but show little change thereafter. Mitochondria in immature myocytes are scattered randomly throughout the cytoplasm, and only become organised, to surround each sarcomere, gradually during the postnatal period. The relative volume of the mitochondria within the myocyte, particularly in those from the LV, increases during postnatal development. It is probable that local demand for energy substrates governs mitochondrial ATP production.

In the foetal heart, which functions in a relatively hypoxic environment, glucose and lactate are the main fuel substrates, used by glycolysis and lactate oxidation respectively. Postnatally, metabolism in the heart becomes primarily oxidative, and long-chain fatty acids are the primary substrate for ATP production. The transition to reliance on fatty acids for myocardial energy production begins in the immediate postnatal period, at a time when nutritional intake is composed of high-fat content milk. This metabolic shift allows for a greater amount of ATP production per mole of substrate compared with glycolysis, albeit at a greater oxygen consumption cost. Not surprisingly, therefore, there is a dramatic increase in the expression of genes encoding enzymes in the mitochondrial fatty acid β-oxidation pathway during the first 2 months of postnatal life. Specific mitochondrial membrane-associated and cytoplasmic proteins involved in long-chain fatty acid uptake are also upregulated in the early postnatal period.

Contractile proteins

Myofilaments taken from newborn hearts develop a relatively greater amount of force than do myofilaments from

Table 3.3 Cardiomyocyte contractile and regulatory proteins: the main differences between neonate and adult, and their clinical implications

Protein	Neonate versus adult	Clinical implications
Myosin	Relative proportion of MLC-2 isoforms changes postnatally	Contributes to reduction in myocardial contractility
Actin	Proportion of skeletal α-actin relatively low	Contributes to reduction in myocardial contractility
Troponin C	No difference	None
Troponin I	Relatively high proportion of mTnI isoform	Reduces ventricular relaxation, particularly during
	Relatively high proportion of cTnI phosphorylated	β-adrenergic stimulation
Troponin T	Relatively high proportion of TnT-1	Contributes to relatively poor ventricular relaxation
Tropomyosin	Relatively high proportion of β-tropomysin	Contributes to relatively poor ventricular relaxation

MLC, myosin light chains; mTnI, troponin I isoform seen in slow skeletal muscle; cTnI, cardiac isoform.

adult hearts in the presence of the same Ca^{2+} ion concentration. Developmental changes in the expression of contractile protein isoforms are probably responsible for this difference in sensitivity to Ca^{2+} (Table 3.3).

MYOSIN [24]

Myosin is the protein complex responsible for energy transduction and force development in cardiac muscle. Myosin possesses enzyme activity that promotes ATP hydrolysis, the reaction providing the energy required for muscle contraction. Each myosin molecule is composed of two heavy chains (MHCs), each of which contains an actin-binding site and an ATP hydrolysis site, and four light chains (MLCs).

Human cardiac myocytes express two functionally different forms of MHCs that are encoded by two separate genes; the two isoforms are designated α and β. Throughout life, from neonate to adult, about 95 per cent of total MHC in ventricular myocytes is composed of the β-MHC isoform. α-MHC comprises about 86 per cent of total MHC in atrial myocytes in all age groups studied.

Each pair of MLCs consists of an essential light chain (MLC-1) and a regulatory light chain (MLC-2). The human cardiomyocyte produces two essential MLC isoforms, ALC-1 and VLC-1. The concentration of ALC-1 in ventricular cardiomyocytes taken from the human foetus is high, but it rapidly decreases during early postnatal life. It persists in the atria throughout life, and may be re-expressed in the ventricles of patients with obstructive heart lesions. Ventricular myosin with high amounts of ALC-1 shows a higher detachment rate, rate of force development and Ca^{2+} sensitivity than fibres containing low amounts of ALC-1. Human ventricular cardiomyocytes express two isoforms of MLC-2. Phosphorylation of MLC-2 increases myofibrillar sensitivity to Ca^{2+}, probably owing to a change in crossbridge cycling kinetics. Developmental change in the relative proportion of MLC-2 isoforms contributes to the postnatal changes in myocardial contractility.

ACTIN [25]

The adult human heart expresses two isoforms of α-actin, skeletal and cardiac. The relative amount of skeletal α-actin is low during foetal development, but its concentration increases postnatally and it represents about 50 per cent of total actin by the end of the first decade. Cardiac α-actin is the dominant isoform in the developing foetal heart, accounting for >80 per cent of total actin in both ventricular and atrial cardiomyocytes during early postnatal life. During childhood, the concentration of cardiac α-actin decreases somewhat, such that in adults it comprises about 50 per cent of total actin. In normal adult hearts, the highest concentration of skeletal α-actin is found in the subendocardial region of ventricular muscle (67 per cent), whereas in the subepicardial area only about 28 per cent is skeletal α-actin, the remainder being cardiac α-actin. It is probable that this transmural gradient of skeletal α-actin relates to the transmural gradient in contractility, as a high proportion of skeletal α-actin is required to achieve a high level of contractility.

Regulatory proteins

In the relaxed state, intracellular Ca^{2+} concentration is low, and the thin filament regulatory proteins, tropomyosin (TM) and the troponin complex, block strong actin–myosin interactions to inhibit force generation. The troponin complex consists of three subunits, troponin C (TnC), troponin I (TnI) and troponin T (TnT). Calcium binding to TnC causes conformational changes within the regulatory proteins. The location of TM on the thin filament determines the state of actin–myosin interaction. In the 'blocked state', TM lies on the outer regions of actin and blocks significant actin–myosin interaction in the absence of Ca^{2+}. The 'closed state' follows the binding of a small number of TnC molecules with Ca^{2+}, which causes the inhibitory region of TM to relocate from its binding surface on actin to allow the formation of weakly bound crossbridges on the periphery of the actin molecule. The 'open state' occurs once a sufficient number of TnC molecules bind to Ca^{2+}, which allows TM to move into the inner domains of the actin molecule, thereby freeing actin-binding sites for strong interactions with the myosin ATPase of the thick filament.

TROPONIN C [26]

The myocardium contains only a single isoform of TnC, the smallest of the regulatory proteins. The cardiac isoform has only one functioning low-affinity Ca^{2+}-binding site; attachment of Ca^{2+} to this site removes the troponin I inhibition of actin–myosin interaction. Troponin C also possesses two high-affinity Ca^{2+}-binding domains, which are always occupied, and which are essential for the attachment of TnC to the troponin complex.

TROPONIN I [27]

The isoform expression of troponin I, the regulatory protein that inhibits myofibrillar ATPase activity at diastolic levels of Ca^{2+}, changes with development. A developmental switch in expression from the isoform seen in slow skeletal muscle (mTnI) to the cardiac isoform (cTnI) occurs during the first 9 months of postnatal life; cTnI is the only isoform detectable in the normal adult heart. Both phosphorylated and dephosphorylated forms of cTnI coexist in cardiomyocytes, their relative proportions depending on the level of β_1-adrenergic stimulation. The neonate has a high baseline level of sympathetic activity, so has a relatively high proportion of cTnI in the phosphorylated form. This protein kinase A-mediated phosphorylation results in a reduction in myofilament Ca^{2+} sensitivity, an increase in cross-bridge cycling, a shortening in twitch duration and enhanced relaxation. Similarly, the phosphorylation of cTnI at other specific sites that are substrates for protein kinase C leads to persistent phosphorylation of cTnI, a decrease in tension generation and reduced Ca^{2+} sensitivity. Concentrations of the three protein kinase C isoforms found in human cardiomyocytes, relative to total protein, are relatively high in the newborn but decrease rapidly over the first month of life. Furthermore, protein kinase C activation by noradrenaline (norepinephrine), endothelin or angiotensin II is higher in the neonate than in the adult. These mechanisms, by which phosphorylation of cTnI is increased in the neonate, only partially compensate for the absence of protein kinase A-dependent phosphorylation sites in the mTnI isoform. Hence, β-adrenergic stimulation shortens the twitch duration of an immature cardiomyocyte that contains mTnI much less than that of the adult cardiomyocyte, which contains exclusively cTnI. The presence of this mTnI isoform partly explains the relatively poor ventricular relaxation seen in the neonate.

TROPONIN T [28]

Troponin T is the subunit that binds TM, TnC and TnI, anchoring the troponin complex to the thin filament and aiding in the propagation of Ca^{2+}-induced conformational changes. Foetal myocardium expresses predominantly TnT-1, with very little expression of TnT-2, TnT-3 and TnT-4. During postnatal development, the expression of TnT-1 decreases and TnT-3 increases to become the only cTnT isoform found in the normal adult heart. Myofibrils containing TnT-1 and TnT-2 have a reduced ability to inhibit myosin ATPase activity compared with those containing TnT-3, and show reduced relaxation between contractions.

TROPOMYOSIN [29]

Tropomyosin, a helical coil wrapped around the actin filaments, stabilises the actin filament and facilitates the transmission of conformational changes between the actin monomers that are induced by interaction with TnI and myosin. The human heart expresses three isoforms of tropomyosin; α-TM, β-TM and α-slow TM. α-Slow TM is expressed in the adult myocardium only at low levels. The ratio of α-TM to β-TM increases from about 5:1 in the foetal heart to 60:1 in the adult. The β-TM isoform confers an increased sensitivity to Ca^{2+} and a reduction in myofibril relaxation rate.

DEVELOPMENTAL CHANGES IN THE REGULATION OF CARDIOVASCULAR FUNCTION

Cardiomyocyte hypertrophy can be induced not only by mechanical loading, but also by various hormones, which can induce both morphological and transcriptional changes. Many of these hormones act through G-protein-coupled receptors in the heart, resulting in protein kinase C activation. Protein kinases activate many known trophic triggers, including adrenergic agonists, vasoactive peptides such as endothelin and angiotensin II, growth factors, adrenocorticoids, insulin, growth hormone and triiodothyronine. I have limited my discussion to those hormones that are required for the normal perinatal development of cardiac function.

Triiodothyronine [30,31]

Triiodothyronine, the biologically active thyroid hormone, exerts profound effects on the cardiovascular system. After transport to the myocyte nucleus, T_3 binds to thyroid hormone nuclear receptors, which in turn bind to T_3-responsive genes. Nuclear receptors for T_3 are expressed at increasing levels during late gestation. Triiodothyronine-regulated cardiac-specific genes include those that encode contractile proteins, regulatory proteins, mitochondrial proteins, β_1-adrenoreceptors and ion channel proteins. Triiodothyronine can either activate or repress gene transcription and so has a major controlling influence on the relative proportions of most of the important proteins governing ventricular contractile function. Therapeutic administration of T_3 not only has effects on gene transcription, but also results in acute changes in cardiovascular function. These acute effects do not involve T_3 binding to nuclear receptors.

Phospholamban is a protein that regulates sarcoplasmic reticulum Ca^{2+}-ATPase (SERCA2) activity. Phosphorylation of phospholamban by cAMP-dependent protein kinase prevents its inhibition of SERCA2. This is the primary mechanism by which β-adrenoreceptor agonists exert positive inotropic actions. Calcium/calmodulin-dependent protein kinase phosphorylates phospholamban, so any increase in Ca^{2+} cycling tends to increase SERCA2 activity. In addition to regulating the expression of phospholamban at the transcriptional level, T_3 is able to increase the degree of phospholamban phosphorylation directly.

Triiodothyronine also exerts effects on mitochondrial metabolism. In the mature heart, substantial increases in ATP production follow small increases in cytosolic ADP. In contrast, mitochondrial ATP production in the immature heart increases in response only to large increases in cytosolic ADP. This is because the expression of the protein carrier responsible for mitochondrial ADP/ATP exchange, adenine nucleotide translocator (ANT), is relatively low in the foetal heart. Expression of ANT increases postnatally under the influence of T_3, so increasing the sensitivity of myocytes to small changes in ADP concentrations. Other important mitochondrial constituents regulated by T_3 in the postnatal period include cardiolipin, a phospholipid essential for normal cytochrome oxidase activity, transport proteins involved in NADH production and medium-chain acyl-CoA dehydrogenase, an enzyme required for the β-oxidation of medium-chain fatty acids. Hence, the normal postnatal increase in T_3 is important in establishing the metabolic transition that is necessary for the foetal heart to adapt to its extrauterine environment.

Corticosteroids [32]

Serum concentrations of cortisol and adrenocorticotrophic hormone (ACTH), which are very high after birth, decline postnatally, reaching a nadir by about 2 months of age. These perinatal changes in cortisol secretion affect myocardial structure and function, as cortisol inhibits cardiomyocyte proliferation and induces cell hypertrophy. Myocardial wall thickness increases more in preterm infants given dexamethasone than in controls. These changes may have long-term implications, as premature hypertrophy limits the reserve of the cardiomyocyte for further increase of its size.

Most preterm infants have impaired adrenal function, and they may be deficient in several important steroidogenic enzymes. In addition, immaturity of the hypothalamus or pituitary may be partly responsible for clinically significant adrenal insufficiency. Transient adrenal insufficiency is common in preterm infants in the postnatal period, and this often manifests as cardiovascular dysfunction. Steroid administration to preterm infants with refractory hypotension may result in marked amelioration of their cardiovascular status within 2 hours of starting treatment. This rapid cardiovascular response is secondary to a nongenomic mechanism, though delayed genomic mechanisms may occur in addition. Experimental studies show that high concentrations of hydrocortisone increase the L-type

calcium current in cardiomyocytes, signifying an inotropic effect. It is likely, however, that the antihypotensive effects of hydrocortisone in preterm infants relate more to its effects on the peripheral vasculature as, in preterm neonates, mean arterial pressure is more dependent on vascular tone than myocardial function. Experimental studies show that glucocorticoids downregulate the expression of epoprostenol and endothelial NO synthase, resulting in an increase in basal SVR.

Adrenergic agonists and the autonomic nervous system [33–35]

The interval between each heartbeat fluctuates, due mostly to changes in the autonomic input to the sinoatrial node. Power spectral analysis of this heart rate variability (HRV) can assess the relative contribution of parasympathetic and sympathetic tone in maintaining cardiovascular homeostasis. Vagal tone is the principal contributor to the high-frequency (HF) component of HRV, whereas both vagal and sympathetic tone influence the lower frequencies (LF). The ratio of LF/HF power reflects sympathetic–parasympathetic balance. Preterm infants do not change their LF/HF power ratio with changes in posture, whereas with increasing postnatal age the LF component of the power spectrum increases with head-up tilt. These findings suggest that neural regulation of cardiac function undergoes changes with maturation, becoming more functional with postnatal development. There is normally a progressive decline in the LF/HF power ratio associated with increasing postnatal age, indicating an increase in the parasympathetic contribution to control of resting heart rate with maturation (Fig. 3.3). Nevertheless, even preterm infants have significant vagal tone and increase their heart rate in response to atropine.

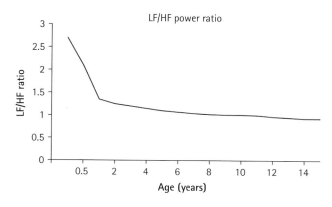

Figure 3.3   Change in parasympathetic/sympathetic nervous system activity with age. The high-frequency (HF) component of the heart rate variability (HRV) spectrum is mediated principally by the vagus. The low-frequency (LF) component of the HRV spectrum is mediated by both the sympathetic and parasympathetic nervous systems. The LF/HF ratio is a sensitive index of autonomic balance.

Baroreceptors buffer acute changes in blood pressure by initiating changes in heart rate and SVR. The responses are mediated by both parasympathetic and sympathetic systems. The postnatal resetting of the arterial baroreceptors, which involves many neural, hormonal and metabolic factors, influences maturational changes in the regulation of vascular tone. Passive head-up tilting in preterm infants results in significant vasoconstriction of the lower limbs and a slight decrease in blood pressure but no change in heart rate. In term infants, however, tachycardia accompanies the decrease in blood pressure and vasoconstriction.

The clinical data demonstrating initial sympathetic dominance in the autonomic control of the heart during infancy, and its gradual transition into sympathetic and parasympathetic codominance in later childhood, correlate well with anatomical findings. Despite cardiac sympathetic dominance, however, neonates demonstrate marked haemodynamic stability following high thoracic spinal anaesthesia. This relative lack of response relates more to low parasympathetic activity than to any deficiency in peripheral adrenoreceptors.

Noradrenaline acts entirely through interaction with G-protein-coupled adrenoreceptors. Activation of a G-protein involves binding of guanosine triphosphate (GTP) to the α-subunit of the G protein. This complex disassociates from the other subunits and associates with an effector molecule such as adenylyl cyclase. Different subtypes of G proteins alter the activity of adenylyl cyclase: G_i proteins inhibit while G_s proteins stimulate. For example, vagal stimulation decreases contractility via cholinergic receptors, which act through G_i proteins. Vagal tone is relatively weak in the neonate and so it is unsurprising that the density of cholinergic receptors in the heart is relatively low in this age group; repeated β_1-adrenoceptor stimulation reduces it further.

Human cardiomyocytes produce many different subtypes of adrenoreceptors, including three types of β-adrenoreceptor and three types of α_1-adrenoreceptor. Thyroid receptor stimulation contributes to a constitutively high level of β_1-adrenoreceptor transcription during late foetal and early postnatal life. Prolonged, excessive β-adrenoreceptor stimulation can lead to cell damage or death and receptor desensitisation is the main mechanism for preventing this from occurring. However, the ability of β-adrenoreceptor agonists to elicit desensitisation is acquired only during postnatal development. Repeated β_1-adrenoreceptor agonist administration to neonatal mammals increases the adenylyl cyclase response to β-adrenoreceptor stimulation, instead of uncoupling receptors from the signalling pathway as occurs in the mature cardiomyocyte. Repeated β-adrenoreceptor agonist administration to neonates decreases cardiac G_i expression and enhances β_1-adrenoreceptor coupling to G_s, a response pattern opposite to that seen in the adult. During mammalian development, changes in the relative expression of specific isoforms of the α subunit of G_s proteins significantly affect β_1-adrenoreceptor/adenylyl cyclase signalling. However, these experimental findings may not apply to the human, as there are many interspecies differences in adrenoreceptor function. Relevant human data are lacking.

DEVELOPMENTAL CHANGES IN CARDIOVASCULAR FUNCTION

The predominant influence on left ventricular systolic function in the first few days after birth is the reduction in preload secondary to ductal closure. Thereafter, the gradual increase in LV afterload and decrease in RV afterload are the major determinants of systolic function. Sequential echocardiographic studies of term neonates have shown that LV stroke volume correlates directly with the lumen size of the ductus arteriosus. Contractility does not change significantly over the first 120 h of extrauterine life.

Systolic function [36,37]

Preterm neonates have slightly lower, though not significantly different, systolic function than term neonates. Studies of preterm infants without a ductus arteriosus have shown significant age- and growth-related changes in LV function in the first 3 months of postnatal life. The left ventricular end-systolic pressure and end-systolic wall stress all increase with growth, although contractility changes little. Hence, despite the significant increase in afterload that occurs normally during the neonatal period, the LV of a preterm infant is able to maintain the same level of contractility.

Although cardiac output in infants alters mainly by changes in heart rate rather than by changes in stroke volume, neonates and infants are able to change stroke volume to a greater extent than is often presumed. Three-dimensional echocardiographic studies show that LV mass, end-diastolic volume, emptying rates and stroke volume index all increase throughout childhood from the neonatal period onwards (Fig. 3.4). However, load-independent measures of contractility suggest that the LV exhibits a higher basal level of contractility in early infancy than in later childhood. This may partly relate to the relatively low afterload experienced by the immature heart, as LV wall stress in neonates

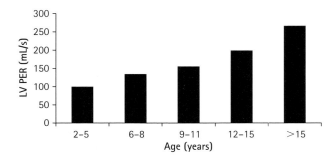

Figure 3.4   Effect of age on left ventricular peak emptying rates in healthy children at rest. LV, left ventricle; PER, peak emptying rate. Data from Poutanen *et al.* [37].

is significantly lower than in children. Another important factor is the level of sympathetic stimulation in early infancy. Serum concentrations of neuropeptide Y, a marker of sympathetic activity, and noradrenaline (due mainly to spill-over from postganglionic sympathetic nerve terminals) are initially high, but decrease with age throughout infancy and childhood. The increase in cholinergic, and decrease in adrenergic, modulation of heart function takes place predominantly over the first 6 months of life.

The high sympathetic tone affecting cardiac function during infancy appears at variance with the relatively low SVR found in the same age group. Term neonates vasoconstrict in response to certain stimuli, showing that they have sufficient adrenoreceptors in the peripheral vasculature to respond normally to sympathetic neurohormonal stimulation. However, induced vasoconstriction is not always accompanied by a significant change in heart rate, suggesting that the regulation of vascular tone and cardiac function are less well coupled in infancy than adulthood.

Diastolic function [37–39]

Diastolic function is dependent on myocardial relaxation and compliance. The neonatal myocardium is less compliant than that of older infants, and improvement of diastolic function is reliant on structural maturation of the myocardium. Diastolic function is difficult to measure, particularly in early infancy, as Doppler-derived indices of LV filling are affected by the interaction of many factors, including heart rate, preload, afterload and contractility. Nevertheless, there is good evidence that diastolic function improves not only in the first few months of postnatal life, but throughout childhood. Early diastolic filling at 1 month of age is significantly lower than in older infants and children. The peak velocity of early diastole, which relates to active ventricular relaxation, increases by about 70 per cent during the first 6 months of age. It then increases more slowly up to the age of 36 months, thereafter showing little change.

Ventricular compliance and heart rate influence late diastolic filling, caused by active atrial contraction. Flow wave velocity increases by 30 per cent over the first month after birth, even after correcting for heart rate. Echocardiographic studies have shown that left atrial volume per unit of body surface area, and the ratio of active/passive emptying of the left atrium both increase throughout childhood and adolescence.

Systemic vascular resistance [40,41]

Systemic vascular resistance is defined as the pressure difference across the systemic vascular bed (mean arterial pressure minus mean right atrial pressure) divided by the cardiac index. Thus, systemic arterial blood pressure is a function of both blood flow and SVR, and is a poor surrogate marker for LV afterload, particularly as cardiac index increases

throughout childhood. The relationship between mean arterial blood pressure and cardiac output is particularly weak in preterm infants, as the lumen size of the ductus arteriosus affects it greatly. A normal blood pressure in a preterm infant does not equate to normal systemic flow, as left-to-right shunting through the duct may result in a relatively high LV output and decreased systemic flow. The normal SVR in a preterm neonate varies between 108 and 383 mmHg/L/min/kg.

Although mean arterial blood pressure increases during the first 5 days after birth in term neonates by about 20 per cent, their SVR does not change significantly because cardiac output also increases by a similar proportion, due principally to an increase in stroke volume. The mean SVR in term neonates is about 244 mmHg/L/min/kg, compared with a mean value of 723 in healthy young adults.

The metabolic rate in infants is twice that of adults, hence tissue oxygen demand is also higher; cardiac output (Q) is commensurately elevated at $4 L/min/m^2$ declining with growth to an adult figure of $2.5–3.0 L/min/m^2$.

Vessel size and wall distensibility determine arterial compliance, which is another important component of myocardial afterload. The systemic vascular bed increases in size in proportion to body size, so arterial compliance is normalised to body surface area. Normalised arterial compliance decreases significantly during the first 20 years of life, with the most rapid rate of decrease occurring in the first 5 years of life. Medial and intimal thickness of the thoracic aorta, and density of the elastic fibres in the media, progressively increase during early childhood.

Pulmonary vascular resistance [4,42]

Pulmonary vascular resistance is defined as the pressure difference across the pulmonary vascular bed (pulmonary artery pressure minus pulmonary venous pressure) divided by the flow rate (cardiac index in the normal adult). In the first few weeks after birth, partially muscular arteries become non-muscular, completely muscularised arteries become partially muscular, and the muscle layer in the more proximal larger vessels becomes thinner. This overall reduction in muscularity increases lumen diameter, and reduces the reactivity of the vessels to vasoconstrictive stimuli. The developmental adaptations in the mechanical properties of the vessel wall are also influenced by an overall increase and compositional change in connective tissue deposition in the media and adventitia. During the neonatal period, PVR indexed to body surface area is normally 3–5 Wood units/m², but by 2 months of age has decreased to equal adult values of 0.8–1.9.

DEVELOPMENTAL CHANGES IN THE RESPONSE TO VASOACTIVE DRUGS

If the patient cannot maintain adequate cardiac function after optimisation of heart rate, rhythm and preload, then

Table 3.4 Age-related differences in the pharmacokinetics of inotropic drugs. Data taken from studies of critically ill patients requiring drug infusions

Drug	<12 months	1–12 years	Adult
Adrenaline (epinephrine)			
CL	–	34	64
V_D	–	–	
Dobutamine			
CL	90	151	90
V_D	–	1.1	0.2
Dopamine			
CL	82	46	50
V_D	1.8	–	1.2
Milrinone			
CL	3.4	6.7	2.5
V_D	0.5	0.5	0.5
Enoximone			
CL	9.7	10.5	3.5
V_D	3.6	10	4
Levosimendan			
CL	3.8	3.6	3.3
V_D	0.43	0.35	0.33
Digoxin			
CL	4.5	13.3	3.1
V_D	–	–	8.5

CL, clearance (mL/min/kg); V_D, volume of distribution at steady state (L/kg).

use of inotropic drugs should be considered. Three main classes of drugs can be used to increase myocardial contractility: β-adrenoreceptor agonists (catecholamines), phosphodiesterase III inhibitors and calcium sensitisers. Each different type of drug has its own advantages and disadvantages, and they are commonly administered concurrently. The rational use of these drugs requires knowledge of their pharmacokinetic and pharmacodynamic properties, which can vary with age and development (Table 3.4). Similar comments are applicable to vasodilators and vasoconstrictors. However, although there are many reasons why the response to vasoactive drugs may vary with age, such variation is usually clinically irrelevant. This is because all acutely acting vasoactive drugs should be given by continuous infusion and the drug infusion rate titrated against response.

Catecholamines

Catecholamines exert their effects by binding with specific adrenergic and dopaminergic receptors. They all increase myocardial oxygen consumption, heart rate and contractility, and exert significant effects on vascular tone. Adverse effects increase in severity and frequency as dosage is increased. Drug distribution, clearance and pharmacodynamic response of critically ill patients to catecholamine infusions vary widely. Individual differences in organ receptor density, organ perfusion, metabolising capacity and protein binding are just a few of the many factors affecting individual response. There is no consistent relationship between plasma catecholamine concentration and target-organ effect, so the infusion rate of the drug should be titrated against the desired effect. An understanding of the relative potency of each drug on arteriolar and venous smooth muscle is important because, in addition to the direct effect on contractility, each has a distinctive ability to modify preload and afterload.

ADRENALINE [43–45]

Adrenaline is an agonist at most adrenergic receptors found in the peripheral vasculature and myocardium. It has slightly more potency at β_1- than β_2-adrenoreceptors, but very little activity at β_3-adrenoreceptors. At low dosages (<0.1 µg/kg/min), its agonist effects on β-adrenoreceptors overshadow its effects on α-adrenoreceptors, whereas the converse tends to occur when the infusion rate exceeds 0.1 µg/kg/min. High doses are reserved for acute cardiopulmonary resuscitation.

Experimental studies have shown that adrenaline infused at rates >0.5 µg/kg/min produces a greater proportional increase in cardiac output (and therefore oxygen delivery) than oxygen demand. At rates <0.1 µg/kg/min adrenaline produces significant increases in heart rate and contractility, with vasodilatation in some regional vascular beds and vasoconstriction in others. At higher doses, peripheral vasoconstriction becomes progressively more prominent, increasing preload and afterload, and blood flow is redistributed away from the skin, mucosa, kidneys, muscle and gut. Adrenaline increases hepatic glucose production and inhibits insulin-induced glucose uptake in skeletal muscle and adipose tissues, leading to a rapid increase in plasma glucose concentration.

The steady-state plasma concentration of adrenaline is linearly related to the infusion rate, though interindividual differences in disposition and clearance result in a 34 per cent coefficient of variation in normalised steady-state concentrations. Endogenous production of adrenaline usually contributes <5 per cent of measured plasma concentrations in patients receiving an adrenaline infusion. The context-sensitive half-time of adrenaline is only a few minutes, owing to active uptake by tissues and organs throughout the body. Hence, infusion rates should be gradually reduced rather than abruptly terminated.

NORADRENALINE

Noradrenaline (norepinephrine) is equipotent to adrenaline at β_1-adrenoreceptors, but has significantly less potency at β_2-adrenoreceptors. However, it has a relatively high affinity for the β_3-adrenoreceptor subtype, and increases glucose uptake and its utilisation in skeletal muscle and adipose tissues in an insulin-independent manner. Noradrenaline produces a greater proportional increase in oxygen demand than in cardiac output. For a given increase in oxygen delivery, oxygen consumption increases by two to three times more with noradrenaline than with other catecholamines.

Its agonist activity at β-adrenoreceptors predominates when infused at rates <0.1 μg/kg/min and cardiac output and heart rate increase in a dose-related manner. At doses >0.1 μg/kg/min, noradrenaline causes widespread arterial and venous smooth muscle vasoconstriction as noradrenaline is a potent agonist at α_1- and α_2-adrenoreceptors. Hence, its use is usually restricted to patients exhibiting marked vasodilatation. The context-sensitive half-time of noradrenaline, like adrenaline, is only a few minutes, owing to active uptake by tissues and organs throughout the body. Hence, infusion rates should be gradually reduced rather than abruptly terminated.

DOPAMINE

Dopamine is an agonist at all adrenoreceptors found in the peripheral vasculature and myocardium, and an agonist at dopaminergic receptors in the peripheral vasculature. There are five subtypes of dopaminergic receptors, categorised into either D_1 or D_2. D_1 receptors are found on vascular smooth muscle in most major organs, renal tubules and the juxtaglomerular apparatus. Their stimulation causes regional vasodilatation and promotion of urinary sodium and water excretion. D_1 receptors are coupled to G_s and G_q proteins, and their activation causes an increase in intracellular concentrations of adenylyl cyclase and cyclic AMP. In contrast, D_2 receptors are coupled to G_i proteins; their activation causes a decrease in intracellular concentrations of adenylyl cyclase and cyclic AMP. D_2 receptors are found on postganglionic sympathetic nerve terminals, glomeruli, renal cortex and renal tubules. Activation of prejunctional D_2 receptors on sympathetic nerve terminals causes inhibition of noradrenaline release and vasodilatation. The distribution and density of the different receptor subtypes varies between different vascular beds.

Dopamine pharmacokinetics varies widely in critically ill patients, due mainly to interpatient variation in sulphoconjugation and renal function. Steady-state plasma dopamine concentrations may vary fourfold among patients receiving the same dose. Moreover, some infused dopamine is converted into noradrenaline, the proportion varying because of polymorphism of the gene controlling dopamine β-hydroxylase. Fortunately, however, intrapatient pharmacokinetics are relatively linear, so that infusion rates can easily be titrated to desired clinical response.

The predominant cardiovascular effects of dopamine at normal therapeutic plasma concentrations relate to its agonist actions at β_1-adrenoreceptors, whereas, at high plasma concentrations, its agonist actions at α-adrenoreceptors become increasingly dominant. In the preterm neonate, these vasoconstrictive effects may be useful in maintaining systemic blood pressure. However, even when the vasoconstrictive effects of dopamine are required in a particular patient, the drug should be started at a low dose and the infusion

rate increased according to response. Patients with pulmonary hypertension should not be given dopamine, as it may increase PVR even when given at low dosage.

ISOPROTERENOL

Isoproterenol, a synthetic catecholamine, is the most potent agonist at all β-adrenoreceptors found in the peripheral vasculature and myocardium. It has pronounced chronotropic and inotropic effects, and its use is reserved for patients with bradyarrhythmias. As it has no significant agonist effects at α-adrenoreceptors, it is a safe agent to use in patients with pulmonary hypertension, but may produce pronounced peripheral vasodilatation. Infusion rates should be started at 0.05 μg/kg/min, and titrated against effect; an excessive tachycardia usually precludes infusion rates >0.1 μg/kg/min.

The steady-state plasma concentration of isoproterenol is linearly related to the infusion rate. Isoproterenol is rapidly metabolised by catechol-o-methyltransferase, primarily in the liver, and excreted into the urine and bile in its free or conjugated form. Isoproterenol may also be excreted unchanged in the urine, or conjugated by hepatic sulphatase and glucuronidase enzymes, before urinary excretion. Extraneuronal tissues, such as myocardium, smooth muscle and fat, which also contain catechol-o-methyltransferase, provide an alternative metabolic pathway.

DOBUTAMINE

Dobutamine, a synthetic catecholamine, is a racemic mixture of two stereoisomers: (−)-dobutamine has only minor agonist activity at β_1- and β_2-adrenoceptors, and is primarily a partial α_1-adrenreceptor agonist, whereas (+)-dobutamine stimulates both β_1- and β_2-adrenoreceptors, and is a competitive antagonist at α_1-adrenoreceptors. At normal therapeutic doses, the vasodilatation produced by α_1-adrenoreceptor antagonism and β_2-adrenoreceptor agonism usually predominates over α_1-adrenoreceptor-mediated vasoconstriction. The racemate is equipotent with dopamine with regard to its inotropic effects, and is safe to use in patients with pulmonary hypertension. Dobutamine 10 μg/kg/min produces a greater proportional increase in cardiac workload (as expressed by rate–pressure product), than in oxygen demand. Dobutamine induces coronary vasodilatation, and does not increase efferent cardiac sympathetic activity.

Dobutamine pharmacokinetics vary widely in critically ill patients, mainly owing to interpatient variation in sulphoconjugation and renal function. However, intrapatient pharmacokinetics are relatively linear, and clinical effects follow a classic dose–response curve. It is conventional to start a dobutamine infusion at a rate of 5 μg/kg/min. Infusion rates above 20 μg/kg/min are associated with an increased incidence of excessive tachycardia, arrhythmias and no further increase in contractility. In common with all catecholamines, it is better to use dobutamine at a moderate dose and add a phosphodiesterase inhibitor or adjuvant drug rather than increase the dose in poorly responding patients.

DOPEXAMINE

Dopexamine, a synthetic catecholamine, is an agonist at β_2-adrenoreceptors in the myocardium and peripheral vasculature, but has only negligible activity at β_1- adrenoreceptors. Dopexamine is also an agonist at D_1- and D_2-dopaminergic receptors in the peripheral vasculature, but unlike dopamine has no demonstrable effects on α-adrenoreceptors. Dopexamine is also an agonist at prejunctional D_2 receptors located at sympathetic neuroeffector junctions in the ventricle; stimulation of these receptors inhibits noradrenaline release from sympathetic nerve terminals. Dopexamine is about one-third as potent as dopamine as a D_1-receptor agonist, and about one-sixth as potent as a D_2-receptor agonist. The predominant D_1-receptor and β_2-adrenoreceptor agonism produced by dopexamine in moderate dosage results in vasodilatation and moderate increases in contractility and heart rate. At infusion rates $<1.5\,\mu g/kg/min$, dopexamine produces a greater proportional increase in cardiac output (and therefore oxygen delivery), compared with myocardial oxygen demand, than any other catecholamine. Dopexamine induces regional vasodilatation, particularly in the splanchnic vascular bed, though comparative studies with dopamine have been unable to show any significant difference between the two drugs when given at equipotent inotropic doses. Infusion rates should be started at $0.5\,\mu g/kg/min$, but not increased above $1\,\mu g/kg/min$ unless a tachycardia is desired.

Phosphodiesterase inhibitors

Catecholamines increase myocardial oxygen requirements proportionately more than they increase mechanical function, thereby depleting myocardial energy reserves. Phosphodiesterase (PDE-III) inhibitors, like catecholamines, increase Ca^{2+} loading of the cytosol and SR and so inevitably increase myocardial oxygen consumption. In addition, however, they cause coronary vasodilatation and increase myocardial oxygen delivery. Furthermore, PDE-III inhibitors decrease afterload, so reducing myocardial oxygen requirements and increasing metabolic efficiency.

There are no clinically significant differences among the three PDE-III inhibitors with regard to their cardiovascular effects. All three drugs require administration of a loading dose to achieve therapeutic plasma concentrations rapidly, though hypotension will occur unless the drug is infused over at least 20 minutes and preload is adequate. Cardiovascular effects in most patients are maximised at the suggested infusion rates. The PDE-III inhibitors have wide therapeutic margins of safety, and appear devoid of obvious adverse effects during short-term infusions.

All three drugs are relatively selective competitive inhibitors of PDE-III, the intracellular enzyme that catalyses

the hydrolysis of cAMP. The resultant increase in the intracellular concentration of cAMP promotes protein phosphorylation through activation of various protein kinases. In myocardial cells, activation of protein kinases increases intracellular Ca^{2+} concentrations following depolarisation, by prolonging the opening time of Ca^{2+} channels in the sarcolemma and SR. In addition, protein kinase-mediated phosphorylation of phospholamban disinhibits the uptake of Ca^{2+} by SR ATPase, so improving diastolic function. In vascular smooth muscle cells, an increase in cAMP concentration causes vasodilatation by several distinct mechanisms: activation of protein kinase G, which stimulates activity of Ca^{2+}-activated potassium channels, so indirectly reducing Ca^{2+} influx; protein kinase inhibition of sarcolemmal Ca^{2+} channels, so directly reducing Ca^{2+} influx; and disinhibition of the uptake of Ca^{2+} by SR ATPase.

Phosphodiesterase III inhibitors possess moderate inotropic and vasodilator properties that are additive to those produced by catecholamines. These inhibitors reduce systemic, coronary and pulmonary vascular resistances, and have beneficial effects on RV function in patients with severe pulmonary hypertension. Platelet activity is regulated by intracellular concentrations of cAMP. The PDE-III-mediated increase in cAMP concentrations results in a concentration-dependent inhibition of platelet activation, adhesion and aggregation.

The published pharmacokinetic data suggest that milrinone has the shortest context-sensitive half-time of the three drugs, though this would seldom be a clinically significant factor in the individual choice of a PDE-III inhibitor used for a short-term infusion. The context-sensitive half-time for all three drugs will be several hours after a 48-hour infusion, so slow weaning from the drug requires only cessation of the infusion.

MILRINONE

Milrinone is excreted primarily via the urine; 80–85 per cent of the drug is cleared unchanged. Most of the remaining drug is metabolised in the liver to the glucuronide, which is excreted in the urine. Drug accumulation can be expected in oliguric patients, and the infusion rate must be reduced accordingly. Pharmacokinetic studies suggest that a loading dose of $75\,\mu g/kg$, infused over 20 minutes, followed by an infusion at 0.5–$0.75\,\mu g/kg/min$, quickly achieves a therapeutic plasma concentration in most infants and children.

INAMRINONE

Inamrinone is eliminated mainly by hepatic acetylation and glucuronidation, though up to 40 per cent of the parent drug is excreted in the urine. Inamrinone acetylation is affected by the acetylator phenotype; plasma clearance in slow acetylators is approximately 45 per cent of that in fast acetylators. Neonates eliminate inamrinone at a slower rate than infants and children. Pharmacokinetic studies suggest that therapeutic concentrations are best achieved by giving a loading dose of 3 mg/kg, infused over 20 minutes, followed by an infusion at 10 μg/kg/min. The infusion rate should be reduced in patients with hepatic or renal dysfunction and in neonates.

ENOXIMONE

Enoximone is primarily metabolised in the liver by oxidation to enoximone sulphoxide. This metabolite is renally excreted, and accumulation will occur in oliguric patients. Enoximone sulphoxide has about one-seventh the potency of the parent drug and can be reduced back to enoximone in the kidney and liver. Hence, reduction of dose is required in patients with severe hepatic or renal dysfunction. Pharmacokinetic studies suggest that a loading dose of 0.5 mg/kg, infused over 20 minutes, should be followed by an infusion at 10 μg/kg/min. There are no significant age-related pharmacokinetic differences among neonates, infants, children and adults. Enoximone has one major disadvantage compared with milrinone and inamrinone; it is incompatible with a large number of drugs commonly used in the paediatric intensive care unit (PICU), and must be given via a dedicated infusion line.

Vasodilators [46]

Vasodilators are drugs that primarily reduce vascular tone, but have no significant direct effect on myocardial contractility. However, a poorly contracting myocardium requires a low afterload to perform optimally. Afterload, the force opposing ventricular ejection, is influenced primarily by wall thickness and vascular impedance. It is quantifiable as the instantaneous wall tension per unit cross-sectional area of the myocardium during systole; this 'wall stress' constantly changes during systole, but is usually assessed echocardiographically only at end-systole. Another variable used frequently as a surrogate for afterload is systemic vascular resistance, which, though relatively easy to measure, does not take into account elastic forces (large vessels distend with each beat) or reflective forces (pressure waves reflected back).

Patients may have relatively normal myocardial contractility, yet may require urgent reduction in afterload. Examples include rebound hypertension following relief of left ventricular outflow tract obstruction, or hypertensive emergencies in children with renal disease. However, many vasodilators reduce both afterload and preload. In patients with hypertrophied, poorly compliant ventricles, such therapy may be detrimental, as the stiff ventricle depends on an elevated preload to generate an adequate stroke volume. Afterload applies to both ventricles. Right ventricular failure may result secondary to pulmonary hypertension. Reduction of RV afterload without causing significant alteration of LV afterload is achieved by giving inhaled NO or epoprostenol, or intravenous sildenafil.

Many different types of vasodilator drugs can be used to reduce LV afterload acutely, including the so-called 'NO donors', adrenoreceptor antagonists, epoprostenol, calcium channel blockers and dopamine agonists. With the notable exception of fenoldopam, a dopamine agonist, all these drugs have significant effects on both systemic and pulmonary vessels. In addition, most direct-acting vasodilators share common adverse effect profiles, including the tendency to inhibit hypoxic pulmonary vasoconstriction, produce reflex tachycardia, increase intracranial pressure in patients with altered intracranial compliance and increase intraocular pressure.

NITRIC OXIDE DONORS [47]

Sodium nitroprusside (SNP) does not liberate NO spontaneously: it requires partial reduction (one-electron transfer) by a reducing agent, such as endogenous NO. The breakdown of the SNP molecule releases NO, which activates guanylyl cyclase in vascular smooth muscle cells. In contrast, glyceryl trinitrate (GTN) induces vasodilatation by directly stimulating guanylyl cyclase, without eliciting a significant increase in vascular endothelial NO formation. The increased activity of guanylyl cyclase, caused either directly or indirectly by both drugs, catalyses the conversion of GTP to cyclic guanosine monophosphate (cGMP), which activates cGMP-dependent protein kinases. These protein kinases mediate vasorelaxation via phosphorylation of several proteins regulating the concentration of intracellular Ca^{2+}, myosin light chain phosphorylation and actin-binding proteins. The vascular responsiveness to GTN and SNP varies between blood vessels of different size because the relative magnitude of the various pathways leading to cGMP-induced vasorelaxation is different in cells from large arteries compared with those from microvessels. An infusion of either drug results in a decrease in both afterload and preload, the latter owing to venodilatation. Glyceryl trinitrate has a more pronounced effect on venous capacitance vessels than SNP.

Tolerance to GTN develops within 24 h of continuous administration; this may be due to reduced enzymatic biotransformation of GTN within the cell by cytochrome P450, or induced endothelial dysfunction. Tolerance may also develop during SNP administration, though the potential for accumulation of the cyanide and thiocyanate metabolites makes prolonged SNP therapy inadvisable. The initial infusion rate for both GTN and SNP is 0.5 μg/kg/min, and the dose thereafter adjusted according to response. Severe hypotension and reflex tachycardia may occur, and both drugs require gradual diminution of dosage to avoid rebound hypertension. The infusion rate of SNP should not exceed 8 μg/kg/min. Close monitoring of thiocyanate and methaemoglobin concentrations and acid–base balance is necessary after 12 h of infusion.

ADRENORECEPTOR ANTAGONISTS [48,49]

Phenoxybenzamine alkylates all types of α-adreno-receptors, so preventing their interaction with agonists.

Phenoxybenzamine, which has a biological half-time of about 28 hours, dilates arterioles in both the systemic and pulmonary vascular beds, and is a venodilator. The recommended dose of phenoxybenzamine is 2 mg/kg, given over 30 minutes, every 24 hours. Phenoxybenzamine produces a long-lasting reduction in afterload that is difficult to reverse; significant hypotension and a reflex tachycardia are prominent in some patients.

β-Adrenoreceptor antagonists have certain advantages over other vasodilators: they reduce heart rate and myocardial oxygen consumption, and do not increase intracranial pressure. However, they have a negative inotropic effect. Drugs that have relative selectivity for β_1-adrenoreceptors, such as atenolol and esmolol, are less likely to induce bronchospasm in susceptible individuals compared with the non-selective antagonists. Esmolol has the advantage of a very short offset time, owing to its rapid metabolism by esterases in the cytosol of red blood cells. The initial infusion rate in infants and children is 100 μg/kg/min.

EPOPROSTENOL [50]

Epoprostenol is a synthetic analogue of prostacyclin, which is an endogenous prostaglandin primarily produced by vascular endothelial cells from arachidonic acid. Prostacyclin has three main actions: it is a powerful vasodilator, and it inhibits platelet aggregation and vascular cell proliferation. The vasodilator activity of prostacyclin is determined by the expression of specific receptors in vascular smooth muscle. Prostacyclin receptors are coupled to adenylyl cyclase, and the resultant increase in cAMP stimulates ATP-sensitive K^+ channels to cause hyperpolarisation of the cell membrane, thus preventing Ca^{2+} influx and so inhibiting smooth muscle contraction. Epoprostenol has a less pronounced effect on the venous capacitance vessels than SNP or GTN and so reduces LV afterload without significantly reducing RV preload.

Epoprostenol is hydrolysed rapidly at neutral pH in blood and is subject to extensive enzymatic degradation. It must be given by continuous infusion as it has a context sensitive half-time of only about 6 minutes. No loading dose is required, as it has a small volume of distribution. The infusion rate should be started at 5 ng/kg/min and adjusted according to response. Crossover studies in adults have shown that similar systemic vasodilatation is produced by SNP 2.3 μg/kg/min, GTN 12.6 μg/kg/min, and epoprostenol 20 ng/kg/min. Epoprostenol and SNP produce comparable decreases in PVR. Epoprostenol is expensive and reserved for chronic treatment of patients with pulmonary hypertension, as it has a low incidence of adverse effects compared with the other vasodilators even when given over long periods.

NICARDIPINE [51,52]

Nicardipine is one of the few calcium channel blockers that can be given by continuous infusion, and has been used successfully in the treatment of hypertensive emergencies in neonates and children. Prospective studies that have compared nicardipine and SNP for treating hypertensive emergencies in adults have shown similar efficacy. Onset and offset times are slightly longer for nicardipine than for SNP. However, there are no published paediatric pharmacokinetic data. Nicardipine should be administered via a central vein at an initial infusion rate of 0.5 μg/kg/min, which can be increased according to response up to a maximum of 3 μg/kg/min.

FENOLDOPAM [53]

This drug is a selective agonist at peripheral dopamine D_{A1} receptors. It has no significant activity at D_{A2} or adrenoreceptors. Most vascular smooth muscle cells contain D_{A1} receptors, though their concentration is highest in renal and splanchnic arteries, and lowest in coronary and cerebral arteries. Activation of D_{A1} receptors, which are coupled to G proteins, increases intracellular cAMP-dependent protein kinase A activity, resulting in reduction of Ca^{2+} influx, and relaxation of the myocyte. In addition, D_{A1} receptors are found in cells in the juxtaglomerular apparatus and renal tubules; their activation causes inhibition of Na^+/K^+ ATPase and Na^+/H^+-exchanger activity via activation of protein kinase A, resulting in an increase in urinary sodium and water excretion.

Fenoldopam has a context-sensitive half-time <10 min even after prolonged infusions. It is poorly lipid soluble and has an apparent volume of distribution of about 0.6 L/kg in adults. There are no published paediatric pharmacokinetic data. Fenoldopam has the disadvantages of displaying tolerance after infusing for >48 hours, increases intraocular pressure and is expensive. The recommended initial infusion rate is 0.5 μg/kg/min.

Vasoconstrictors [54]

It is rare for children to require vasoconstrictor therapy in isolation. Although many hypotensive children are peripherally vasodilated, usually they will respond to restoration of vascular volume and inotropic support. However, a proportion of children with meningococcal septicaemic shock, for example, will require a noradrenaline infusion in addition to large fluid volume infusions and other inotropic drugs, to achieve a normal systemic blood pressure. Some patients may develop severe vasodilatory hypotension without having significant myocardial dysfunction. This hypotension may be refractory to conventional therapeutic regimens such as noradrenaline, but respond to vasopressin, given by constant infusion at a rate of 0.0003–0.002 U/kg/min. This same drug, in higher dose, has been suggested for the treatment of prolonged paediatric cardiac arrest. Other vasoconstrictors in common use include phenylephrine, a specific α_1-adrenoreceptor agonist, which has been used successfully to treat chronic orthostatic intolerance in adolescents. The recommended initial infusion rate of phenylephrine is 1 μg/kg/min. Intermittent injections of phenylephrine 10 μg/kg may help reverse severe oxygen desaturation in children with tetralogy of Fallot.

REFERENCES

Key reference

Lake CL, Booker PD. *Pediatric cardiac anesthesia*, 4th edn. Baltimore, MA: Lippincott, Williams & Wilkins, 2004.

References

1. Kluckow M. Low systemic blood flow and pathophysiology of the preterm transitional circulation. *Early Hum Dev* 2005; **81**: 429–37.
2. Levy M, Maurey C, Chailley-Heu B *et al*. Developmental changes in endothelial vasoactive and angiogenic growth factors in the human perinatal lung. *Pediatr Res* 2005; **57**: 248–53.
3. Lévy M, Maurey C, Dinh-Xuan AT *et al*. Developmental expression of vasoactive and growth factors in human lung. Role in pulmonary vascular resistance adaptation at birth. *Pediatr Res* 2005; **57**: 21R–5R.
4. Wojciak-Stothard B, Haworth SG. Perinatal changes in pulmonary vascular endothelial function. *Pharmacol Ther* 2006; **109**: 78–91.
5. Connuck D, Sun JP, Super DM *et al*. Incidence of patent ductus arteriosus and patent foramen ovale in normal infants. *Am J Cardiol* 2002; **89**: 244–7.
6. Michelakis ED, Rebeyka I, Wu X *et al*. O_2 sensing in the human ductus arteriosus. Regulation of voltage-gated K^+ channels in smooth muscle cells by a mitochondrial redox sensor. *Circ Res* 2002; **91**: 478–86.
7. de Simone G, Devereux RB, Kimball TR *et al*. Interaction between body size and cardiac workload. Influence on left ventricular mass during body growth and adulthood. *Hypertension* 1998; **31**: 1077–82.
8. Kiserud T. The ductus venosus. *Semin Perinatol* 2001; **25**: 11–20.
9. Senzaki H, Akagi M, Hishi T *et al*. Age-associated changes in arterial elastic properties in children. *Eur J Pediatr* 2002; **161**: 547–51.
10. Salih C, McCarthy KP, Ho SY. The fibrous matrix of ventricular myocardium in hypoplastic left heart syndrome: a quantitative and qualitative analysis. *Ann Thorac Surg* 2004; **77**: 36–40.
11. Ross RS. The extracellular connections: the role of integrins in myocardial remodeling. *J Cardiac Fail* 2002; **8**: S326–31.
12. Lo CW. Role of gap junctions in cardiac conduction and development. *Circ Res* 2000; **87**: 346–8.
13. Hein S, Kostin S, Heling A *et al*. The role of the cytoskeleton in heart failure. *Cardiovasc Res* 2000; **45**: 273–8.
14. Tipparaju SM, Kumar R, Wang Y *et al*. Developmental differences in L-type calcium current of human atrial myocytes. *Am J Physiol* 2004; **286**: H1963–9.
15. Wagner MB, Wang Y, Kumar R *et al*. Calcium transients in infant human atrial myocytes. *Pediatr Res* 2005; **57**: 28–34.
16. Reuter H, Pott C, Goldhaber JI, Henderson SA *et al*. Na^+/Ca^{2+} exchange in the regulation of cardiac excitation-contraction coupling. *Cardiovasc Res* 2005; **67**: 198–207.
17. McDonough AA, Velotta JB, Schwinger RHG *et al*. The cardiac sodium pump: structure and function. *Basic Res Cardiol* 2002; **97**: 19–24.
18. Bers DM, Barry WH, Despa S. Intracellular Na^+ regulation in cardiac myocytes. *Cardiovasc Res* 2003; **57**: 897–912.
19. Avkiran M, Haworth RS. Regulatory effects of G protein-coupled receptors on cardiac sarcolemmal Na^+/H^+ exchanger activity: signaling and significance. *Cardiovasc Res* 2003; **57**: 942–52.
20. Li X, Misik AJ, Rieder CV *et al*. Thyroid hormone receptor α_1 regulates expression of the Na^+/H^+ exchanger. *J Biol Chem* 2002; **277**: 28656–62.
21. Frank KF, Bölck B, Erdmann E, Schwinger RHG. Sarcoplasmic reticulum Ca^{2+}-ATPase modulates cardiac contraction and relaxation. *Cardiovasc Res* 2003; **57**: 20–7.
22. Lehman JJ, Kelly DP. Transcriptional activation of energy metabolic switches in the developing and hypertrophied heart. *Clin Exp Pharmacol Physiol* 2002; **29**: 339–45.
23. Marin-Garcia J, Ananthakrishnan R, Goldenthal MJ. Heart mitochondrial DNA and enzyme changes during early human development. *Mol Cell Biochem* 2000; **210**: 47–52.
24. Reiser PJ, Portman MA, Ning X-H, Moravec CS. Human cardiac myosin heavy chain isoforms in fetal and failing adult atria and ventricles. *Am J Physiol* 2001; **280**: H1814–20.
25. Suurmeijer AJH, Clément S, Francesconi A *et al*. α-actin isoform distribution in normal and failing human heart: a morphological, morphometric, and biochemical study. *J Pathol* 2003; **199**: 387–97.
26. Lindhout DA, Sykes BD. Structure and dynamics of the C-domain of human cardiac troponin C in complex with the inhibitory region of human cardiac troponin I. *J Biol Chem* 2003; **278**: 27024–34.
27. Metzger JM, Michele DE, Rust EM *et al*. Sarcomere thin filament regulatory isoforms. *J Biol Chem* 2003; **278**: 13118–23.
28. Gomes AV, Guzman G, Zhao J, Potter JD. Cardiac troponin T isoforms affect the Ca^{2+} sensitivity and inhibition of force development. *J Biol Chem* 2002; **277**: 35341–9.
29. Wolska BM, Wieczorek DF. The role of tropomyosin in the regulation of myocardial contraction and relaxation. *Pflugers Arch* 2003; **446**: 1–8.
30. Dillman WH. Cellular action of thyroid hormone on the heart. *Thyroid* 2002; **12**: 447–52.
31. Klein I, Ojamaa K. Thyroid hormone and the cardiovascular system. *N Engl J Med* 2001; **344**: 501–9.
32. Bolt RJ, van Weissenbruch MM, Lafeber HN *et al*. Development of the hypothalamic–pituitary axis in the fetus and preterm infant. *J Pediatr Endocrinol Metab* 2002; **15**: 759–69.
33. Andriessen P, Janssen BJA, Berendsen RCM *et al*. Cardiovascular autonomic regulation in preterm infants: the effect of atropine. *Pediatr Res* 2004; **56**: 939–46.

34. Chow LTC, Chow SSM, Anderson RH, Gosling JA. Autonomic innervation of the human cardiac conduction system: changes from infancy to senility – an immunohistochemical and histochemical analysis. *Anat Rec* 2001; **264**: 169–82.

35. Ducrocq J, De Broca A, Abdiche M *et al.* Vasomotor reactivity in premature neonates at term. *Biol Neonate* 2002; **82**: 9–16.

36. Barlow AJ, Ward C, Webber S *et al.* Myocardial contractility in premature neonates with and without patent ductus arteriosus. *Pediatr Cardiol* 2004; **25**: 102–7.

37. Poutanen T, Jokinen E, Sairanen H, Tikanoja T. Left atrial and left ventricular function in healthy children and young adults assessed by three-dimensional echocardiography. *Heart* 2003; **89**: 544–9.

38. Harada K, Suzuki T, Tamura M *et al.* Role of age on transmitral flow velocity patterns in assessing left ventricular diastolic function in normal infants and children. *Am J Cardiol* 2003; **76**: 530–2.

39. Schmitz L, Koch H, Bein G, Brockmeier K. Left ventricular diastolic function in infants, children, and adolescents. Reference values and analysis of morphologic and physiologic determinants of echocardiographic Doppler flow signals during growth and maturation. *J Am Coll Cardiol* 1998; **32**: 1441–8.

40. de Simone G, Roman MJ, Daniels SR *et al.* Age-related changes in total arterial capacitance from birth to maturity in a normotensive population. *Hypertension* 1997; **29**: 1213–17.

41. Gentles TL, Colan SD. Wall stress misrepresents afterload in children and young adults with abnormal left ventricular geometry. *J Appl Physiol* 2002; **92**: 1053–7.

42. Archer S, Michelakis E. The mechanism(s) of hypoxic pulmonary vasoconstriction: potassium channels, redox O_2 sensors and controversies. *NewsPhysiol Sci* 2002; **17**: 131–7.

43. Fisher DG, Schwartz PH, Davis AL. Pharmacokinetics of exogenous epinephrine in critically ill children. *Crit Care Med* 1993; **21**: 111–17.

44. Hoffmann C, Leitz MR, Oberdorf-Maass S *et al.* Comparative pharmacology of human β-adrenergic receptor subtypes – characterization of stably transfected receptors in CHO cells. *Naunyn-Schmiedeberg's Arch Pharmacol* 2004; **369**: 151–159.

45. Scheeren TWL, Arndt JO. Different response of oxygen consumption and cardiac output to various endogenous and synthetic catecholamines in awake dogs. *Crit Care Med* 2000; **28**: 3861–8.

46. Patel HP, Mitsnefes M. Advances in the pathogenesis and management of hypertensive crisis. *Curr Opin Pediatr* 2005; **17**: 210–14.

47. Yamamoto T, Bing RJ. Nitric oxide donors. *Proc Soc Exp Biol Med* 2000; **225**: 200–6.

48. Cuneo BF, Zales VR, Blahunka PC, Benson DW Jr. Pharmacodynamics and pharmacokinetics of esmolol, a short-acting beta-blocking agent, in children. *Pediatr Cardiol* 1994; **15**: 296–301.

49. Wiest DB, Garner SS, Uber WE, Sade RM. Esmolol for the management of pediatric hypertension after cardiac operations. *J Thorac Cardiovasc Surg* 1998; **115**: 890–7.

50. Kieler-Jensen N, Houltz E, Rickstein SE. A comparison of prostacyclin and sodium nitroprusside for the treatment of heart failure after cardiac surgery. *J Cardiothorac Vasc Anesth* 1995; **9**: 641–6.

51. Flynn JT, Mottes TA, Brophy PD *et al.* Intravenous nicardipine for treatment of severe hypertension in children. *J Pediatr* 2001; **139**: 38–43.

52. Milou C, Debuche-Benouachkou V, Semama DS *et al.* Intravenous nicardipine as a first-line antihypertensive drug in neonates. *Intensive Care Med* 2000; **26**: 956–8.

53. Murphy MB, Murray C, Shorten GD. Fenoldopam – a selective peripheral dopamine-receptor agonist for the treatment of severe hypertension. *N Engl J Med* 2001; **345**: 1548–57.

54. Tanaka K, Kitahata H, Kawahito S *et al.* Phenylephrine increases pulmonary blood flow in children with tetralogy of Fallot. *Can J Anaesth* 2003; **50**: 926–9.

4

Water, electrolytes and the kidney

ISABEAU WALKER

KEY LEARNING POINTS

- Intravenous fluids should be prescribed with the same care as any other medication. It is always preferable to use the oral route for fluid administration, if possible.
- Administration of electrolyte-free water in the presence of raised antidiuretic hormone (ADH) levels results in a fall in plasma osmolality and sodium. The brain is vulnerable to rapid changes in plasma osmolality, particularly if superimposed on long-standing adaptive changes.
- Iatrogenic hyponatraemia is related to traditional prescribing habits, such as the use of hypotonic intravenous solutions during surgery.
- Intravenous fluids should be prescribed as 'maintenance' to replace insensible and urinary losses and 'replacement' to expand the extracellular fluid (ECF) volume, maintain blood pressure or replace abnormal losses. Replacement fluids must always be given as isotonic fluids.
- Confusion or seizures secondary to acute hyponatraemia is a medical emergency; initial treatment should be with intravenous hypertonic saline.
- Hypernatraemia is frequently multifactorial, and usually caused by excess water loss rather than excess sodium administration. Long-standing hypernatraemia should be corrected slowly over 48 hours. In particular, dehydration in diabetic ketoacidosis has developed over many weeks – it must be corrected slowly to avoid cerebral oedema.

INTRODUCTION

Administration of intravenous fluids is routine in paediatric anaesthesia. However, the rationale for fluid administration is often poorly understood and errors in fluid management can lead to serious morbidity and mortality. The paediatric anaesthetist must give careful consideration to the type and volume of fluids administered in the perioperative period, prescribing intravenous fluids with the same care as any other medication. The first part of this chapter will review basic and developmental physiology of the kidney and fluid compartments and the management of electrolyte abnormalities. The second part will consider the rationale for perioperative fluid management, including maintenance fluids, replacement fluids, the need for glucose and, finally, specific clinical situations in paediatric anaesthetic practice.

RENAL PHYSIOLOGY, DEVELOPMENT OF THE KIDNEY, MATURATION OF RENAL FUNCTION AND ELECTROLYTE DISORDERS

Fluid compartments, osmolality, tonicity and basic renal physiology

In adults, the body consists of 50–60 per cent water, one-third in the extracellular fluid (ECF) compartment and two-thirds in the intracellular fluid (ICF) compartment. The newborn infant has a greater percentage of body water, representing 75 per cent of total body weight; half of this is ECF and half is ICF [1]. After an initial rapid reduction in ECF volume at birth, there is a gradual reduction in body water with age because of alterations in relative proportions of fat and muscle. The adult distribution of body water is reached by the age of 10 years. Blood volume in adults is 8 per cent of total body weight; immediately after birth the blood volume depends on when the umbilical cord is clamped but is normally 80–85 mL/kg; it is 75 mL/kg from 6 weeks to 2 years and 70 mL/kg from 2 years to adulthood.

The cell membrane acts as a semipermeable membrane. Sodium is the predominant extracellular cation, potassium is the predominant intracellular cation, and the distribution of ions is determined by their electrochemical gradients and the activity of transmembrane ion channels. Plasma membrane potential is dependent on the ratio of intracellular to extracellular ions, predominantly sodium and potassium. Small changes in extracellular potassium result in large changes in the electrical properties of cell membranes.

Plasma osmolality is normally 285–295 mosmol/kg and is determined by the principal osmotically active ions, sodium, chloride and bicarbonate, and urea and glucose. The following formula can be used to calculate an approximate plasma osmolality:

$$\text{Plasma osmolality (mosmol/kg)} = 2[Na^+]\ (\text{mmol/L}) + \text{urea (mmol/L)} + \text{glucose (mmol/L)}$$

Intracellular osmolarity is determined by potassium and organic particles. If cells are exposed to hypotonic fluids water moves into them to regain osmotic equilibrium and the cells swell. Water can be extruded from the cells to compensate for the increase in ICF volume, but only if these changes occur slowly. Compensation is achieved by the movement of potassium and organic osmolytes out of the cells. If cells are exposed to hypertonic fluids, water will move out of the cells and the cells will shrink. Adaptation over a period of time is possible by the accumulation of electrolytes and organic osmolytes. The brain is particularly vulnerable to rapid changes in plasma osmolality, especially if superimposed on long-standing adaptive changes.

The function of the kidney is to eliminate waste products of metabolism and to conserve water, essential nutrients and ions to maintain homeostasis, despite wide variations in intake of water and solutes. Individual nephrons consist of a glomerular tuft with afferent and efferent arterioles, a proximal convoluted tubule surrounded by the cells of the juxtaglomerular apparatus, the loop of Henle, which descends towards the renal medulla surrounded by the vessels of the vasa recta, a distal convoluted tubule and the collecting ducts which drain to the renal medulla.

The concentration of solute in glomerular filtrate resembles that in plasma. In the mature kidney, 99 per cent of filtered sodium and water is reabsorbed, principally in the proximal convoluted tubule. Sodium reabsorption is via sodium transporter proteins either in exchange for

hydrogen ions or via co-transporters (glucose, phosphate, amino acid, lactate, chloride, potassium), or via sodium channels in the collecting duct, under the influence of aldosterone which allows 'fine tuning' of sodium reabsorption in exchange for potassium and hydrogen ions. Aldosterone is secreted by the adrenal cortex and is released via the renin–angiotensin system in response to a fall in blood volume or ECF volume. It promotes the reabsorption of sodium (and water) in the collecting duct to expand the ECF volume. Aldosterone secretion is also stimulated by the stress response and by a high potassium intake. Glucocorticoids and thyroid hormone are required for normal tubular reabsorption of sodium.

If the ECF volume is expanded a naturesis will be induced by a combination of increase in plasma volume, cardiac output and increase in glomerular filtration rate (GFR), plus a reduction in tubular reabsorption of sodium. Loss of potassium chloride from the body causes sodium to move into cells to compensate; two osmotically active cations are therefore lost from the ECF (Na^+ and K^+) and the plasma sodium falls. Potassium supplements are therefore an important component of fluid regimens.

Normal plasma sodium is maintained within the range 135–145 mmol/L. The main determinant of plasma sodium concentration is the plasma water content, which is the balance of intake (determined by thirst and behavioural factors) and urinary losses of water, and is independent of sodium excretion. Water excretion is controlled by the action of arginine vasopressin or ADH, which is synthesised in the hypothalamus, stored in the posterior pituitary and activates water channels (aquapores) in the collecting duct such that water reabsorption increases and more concentrated urine is produced. Antidiuretic hormone is released in response to activation of central osmoreceptors by a rise in plasma osmolality. Conversely, if an individual drinks a fluid load, ADH release is suppressed, water reabsorption is reduced and the excess water load is excreted. By 1 year of age, healthy children can vary urine osmolality between 50 mosmol/kg and 1400 mosmol/kg, depending on water intake. Excretion of the urinary solute load can be achieved with a minimal urine output of only 25 mL/kg/day (approximately 1 mL/kg/h) [2]. Specific gravity of urine is used as a bedside test of urinary concentration relative to water. Normal values are between 1.002 and 1.028. Sodium and potassium are the principle cations contributing to urine osmolality.

Antidiuretic hormone is also released in response to hypovolaemia and a variety of other non-osmotic stimuli (see Table 4.2). The effects of hypovolaemia and non-osmotic factors override the effects of osmolality, an appropriate response in evolutionary terms to conserve water in the presence of an acute illness and reduced oral intake. This is not the case if inappropriate intravenous fluids are given.

The tonicity of a solution describes its osmolality relative to plasma; a solution of 0.9 per cent saline has the same osmolality as plasma (isotonic to plasma) and rapidly equilibrates with the ECF compartment. A solution of 5 per cent dextrose is initially isotonic but becomes hypotonic as the glucose is metabolised – the net effect is infusion of a hypotonic solution devoid of electrolytes (100 per cent electrolyte-free water). Similarly, a 0.45 per cent saline solution is hypotonic and contains 50 per cent electrolyte free water (see Table 4.10). If an individual receives electrolyte free water in the presence of non-osmotic release of ADH they will excrete concentrated urine but will be unable to excrete the free water load; plasma osmolality and sodium will fall.

Development of the kidney and renal function

Nephrogenesis begins at 5 weeks' gestation and the first definitive nephrons produce urine from 8 to 10 weeks' gestation. The placenta performs the excretory function of the foetus and the main function of the foetal kidney is the production of amniotic fluid; intrauterine renal impairment may result in oligohydramnios and pulmonary hypoplasia. Nephrogenesis occurs from the juxtamedullary region to the cortical region in a preprogrammed manner – by 35 weeks each kidney contains its full complement of approximately 1 million nephrons. The postnatal increase in weight of the kidney results almost entirely from the increase in complexity, in particular, the length of the tubules. Babies who are premature or small for dates have reduced numbers of nephrons and impaired renal function in infancy. They develop normal renal function by early childhood, but this relative loss of nephrons results in an increased incidence of hypertension, diabetes and related diseases in adult life [3].

At birth there is a dramatic period of adaptation to extrauterine life and the kidney takes over the role of water and electrolyte homeostasis from the placenta. Lactation becomes established after the first 48–96 hours and fluid intake is initially low as the baby takes small amounts of colostrum from the mother. During this time, levels of ADH in the infant are high, water is conserved and urine output is low. This is likely to represent an appropriate evolutionary response to a period of low fluid intake. After the first few days of life there is a brisk diuresis and a period of postnatal weight loss. This occurs because the newborn infant has a relatively expanded ECF compartment. The diuresis is in part due to cardiopulmonary adaptation, triggered by a progressive fall in pulmonary vascular resistance, increase in left atrial filling and the release of atrial natriuretic peptide. Excessive fluids or sodium prior to the postnatal diuresis, particularly in premature infants, is associated with delayed weight loss, an expanded ECF compartment and an increase in complications of prematurity (patent ductus arteriosus, respiratory distress syndrome and necrotising enterocolitis) [4]. The relevance of this to infants who undergo surgery in the first few days of life has not been studied, but it would seem appropriate to avoid fluid overload during this time.

The GFR is low at birth but increases rapidly in the first few months of life under the influence of locally released prostaglandins (which cause renal vasodilatation), and increasing mean arterial pressure. The GFR reaches normal adult indexed values by 2 years of age. Plasma creatinine at birth reflects maternal renal function and falls within the first week of life to reach a steady state by 1 month of life (Table 4.1). The newborn kidney is sensitive to non-steroidal anti-inflammatory drugs (NSAIDs) (prostaglandin synthetase inhibitors), or other causes of renal hypoperfusion in the newborn period, such as anoxia or sepsis, which may result in acute renal failure.

Renal handling of sodium in infants

Renal function in the newborn infant favours retention of sodium, an appropriate adaptation as the sodium intake from breast milk is low but the child is growing rapidly. Sodium wasting in the kidney is minimised by the low mean arterial blood pressure and GFR and very high activity of the renin–angiotensin–aldosterone system (RAAS), which promotes reabsorption of sodium in the collecting duct. There is a further increase in responsiveness of the collecting duct to aldosterone during the first months of life. As a consequence, the newborn infant is unable to handle sodium loading and excessive sodium intake in the first few days of life may result in hypernatraemia. It is customary to use low-sodium-containing intravenous fluids during this time. The ability to develop a natriuresis develops after a few weeks, and results from downregulation of sodium channels and the RAAS [1].

In contrast, the premature neonate is prone to acquired hyponatraemia due to tubular immaturity and limited sodium reabsorption, particularly in the proximal convoluted tubule. The number of sodium transporters is reduced, as is the enzyme responsible for active sodium transport (Na^+/K^+ ATPase). The relatively low sodium content in human breast milk (1–1.5 mmol/kg/day) is sufficient to maintain sodium balance in term babies but premature neonates require sodium supplements in the first weeks of life to prevent hyponatraemia and promote optimal growth [5].

Table 4.1 Normal values glomerular filtration rate (GFR) and plasma creatinine

	Birth	1 week	1 month	6 months	1 year	2 years
GFR (mL/min/1.73 m^2)		20–40	50	80	100	120
Plasma creatinine (μmol/L)	70–90	15–40	15–40	18–40	19–43	20–44

Renal handling of water in infants

The ability to respond to ADH develops during foetal life and is responsible for reduced urine output at the time of birth. After the first few days of life, however, the healthy infant is able to suppress ADH release and excrete a water load (up to 200 mL/kg/day), provided that sodium intake is constant [1]. This is not the case in the postoperative neonate in whom the stress response and high ADH levels result in the inability to excrete excess free water.

Healthy babies produce relatively large amounts of dilute urine with low solute concentration, a situation that is appropriate to their stage of development. The ability to concentrate the urine is determined by the action of ADH, the tonicity of the renal medulla and the countercurrent mechanism. Dilute urine is produced in the newborn infant as a result of reduced expression of aquaporins, short loops of Henle and poorly developed solute concentration gradients in the renal medulla. The requirement for solute excretion is low as, during rapid growth in the first few months of life, waste products of metabolism can be incorporated into new tissues; in fact, growth has been referred to as the 'third kidney' [5]. Production of concentrated urine via the countercurrent mechanism would therefore represent an unnecessary expenditure of energy [5].

In addition, because babies obtain their calories from a liquid diet, a relatively high urine output is required to maintain water balance and the urine is usually isotonic to plasma (300 mosmol/kg). If required, babies can concentrate their urine after the first few months of life to achieve a urinary osmolality of 500–700 mosmol/kg and can obtain adult values of urinary osmolality by 1 year of age (1200–1400 mosmol/kg). However, this means that young babies are prone to dehydration if access to water is restricted; excessively long periods of preoperative starvation should be avoided. The relatively immature renal function in infants may be exposed in the postoperative child who is catabolic and may show signs of early renal impairment.

Disorders of water and electrolyte balance

DISORDERS OF SODIUM BALANCE

Hyponatraemia

Hyponatraemia is defined as a plasma sodium less than 135 mmol/L. The adverse effects of hyponatraemia result from cerebral oedema and depend on the severity and speed with which hyponatraemia develops. Children become symptomatic sooner than adults and over 50 per cent of children with plasma sodium <125 mmol/L will develop hypo-natraemic encephalopathy. Children are thought to be particularly vulnerable as they have a relatively large brain to intracranial volume ratio compared with adults (greater increase in intracranial pressure for any increase in brain volume), and possibly an impaired adaptive ability to extrude water from brain cells in the presence of hyponatraemia. The outcome from symptomatic hyponatraemic

encephalo-pathy is poor in children, possibly related to their susceptibility to airway obstruction and the compounding effects of hypoxia [6].

Although hyponatraemia may be caused by sodium deficiency in the ECF, it usually results from excess water. Children are particularly vulnerable to hypovolaemia from gastrointestinal and third space losses of sodium and water; they will become rapidly hyponatraemic if water is replaced appropriately but the sodium is not.

Causes of hyponatraemia are listed in Table 4.2.

Hospital-acquired hyponatraemia

There have been repeated reports of iatrogenic hyponatraemia in children, with more than 50 reported deaths or cases of serious neurological morbidity in previously healthy children receiving intravenous fluid therapy [6].

Table 4.2 Causes of hyponatraemia [7–9]

Deficit of sodium in the ECF

Extrarenal loss of sodium (urinary $Na^+ < 30$ mmol/L)*	Gastrointestinal losses
	Third space losses
	Bowel obstruction, peritonitis, burns
	Excess sweating
Renal loss of sodium (urinary $Na^+ > 30$ mmol/L)	Diuretics
	Osmotic diuresis (glucose, urea, mannitol)
	Adrenal insufficiency (Addison's disease)
	Diabetic ketoacidosis
	Salt-wasting nephropathy
	Renal tubular abnormalities
	Cerebral salt wasting
	Congestive cardiac failure
	Nephrotic syndrome
	Cirrhosis
	Hypothyroidism
	ECF volume expansion

Excess electrolyte-free water

Hypotonic intravenous fluids*
Polydipsia
Reduced solute intake (dilute infant formula)
Renal failure
Non-osmotic release of ADH*
Hypovolaemia
Postoperative pain, stress, nausea
Drugs (opioids, NSAIDs, carbamazepine, vincristine)
Pulmonary disorders: pneumonia, bronchiolitis, IPPV
CNS disorders: tumours, trauma, haemorrhage

ADH, antidiuretic hormone; CNS, central nervous system; ECF, extracellular fluid; IPPV, intermittent positive pressure ventilation; NSAID, non-steroidal anti-inflammatory drug.
*Hyponatraemia is common if these factors are combined.

Many were undergoing elective surgery (tonsillectomy, fracture setting, appendectomy or orchidopexy). The syndrome has also been described in association with illnesses such as gastroenteritis, bronchiolitis, pneumonia and meningitis. In all cases, children received hypotonic intravenous fluids, often in volumes in excess of 'standard maintenance fluids' described below.

The clinical course was typified by progressive lethargy, headache, and nausea and vomiting, followed by confusion and rapid deterioration with seizures, respiratory arrest and coma. Fatal cerebral oedema occurring during surgery has also been reported [10]. Acute hospital-acquired hyponatraemia has been seen in 10 per cent of children presenting to the accident and emergency department [11], including one fatality from cerebral oedema caused by an acute fall in plasma sodium from 142 mmol/L to 128 mmol/L. Hyponatraemia was seen in 33 per cent of infants presenting to the paediatric intensive care unit (PICU) with bronchiolitis; hyponatraemic encephalopathy was seen in 4 per cent [12]. The vulnerability of children to iatrogenic hyponatraemia may be related to traditional fluid prescriptions, involving the use of hypotonic fluids [13]. A recent systematic review indicated that the odds of developing hyponatraemia using hypotonic intravenous solutions was 17.2 times greater than with isotonic fluids [95 per cent confidence interval [CI] 8.67–34.2] [14], although these conclusions are based on a small number of studies involving very few postoperative patients.

Perioperative iatrogenic hyponatraemia has also been described despite near-isotonic saline infusion, with some fatalities [15]. This is thought to be due to excessive fluid administration in the perioperative period with expansion of the ECF volume, when there are elevated levels of ADH (hypertonic urine). Expansion of the ECF volume leads to a natriuresis but, in the presence of ADH, the associated water load is not excreted and hyponatraemia ensues. This process has been termed 'desalination'.

The incidence of hospital-acquired hyponatraemia can therefore be reduced by avoiding hypotonic fluids in the perioperative period or in a child who is otherwise 'unwell', and avoiding unnecessary ECF volume expansion.

Diagnosis of hyponatraemia (Table 4.3)

A careful history should be taken, including of recent illnesses, medications and weight changes, possible sources of salt losses or excessive water ingestion. Fluid balance and plasma electrolytes should be routinely checked in any child receiving intravenous fluids, and especially if their recovery is not following the expected course. Hypothyroidism and adrenal insufficiency should be excluded. The child should be examined clinically to gain an impression of their ECF volume status (comparison with recent weight, examination of heart rate, blood pressure, capillary refill, skin tissue turgor, assessment of urine output and fluid balance). Additional investigations should include the plasma osmolality (normal value 285 mosmol/kg), urine osmolality (range 200–1400 mosmol/kg) and the urinary sodium concentration ('spot urine') which may be low (<30 mmol/kg), indicating low renal perfusion or suppression of ADH, or high (>30 mmol/kg), indicating normal or increased renal perfusion, or defective tubular function.

Treatment of hyponatraemia

The duration of hyponatraemia and the occurrence of symptoms will determine the correct treatment. Chronic hyponatraemia should be corrected slowly by fluid restriction as rapid changes in plasma sodium carry the risk of cerebral osmotic demyelination syndrome. Hyponatraemia associated with hypovolaemia should be treated with 0.9 per cent saline; in the absence of neurological symptoms,

Table 4.3 Diagnostic features characteristic of different causes of hyponatraemia

	Cause	Clinical signs and symptoms	Plasma osmolality	Urinary osmolality	Urinary sodium	Clinical examples
Sodium loss	Extrarenal sodium loss	Weight loss, dehydration; symptoms suggestive of cause	Low	High	Low	Gastrointestinal losses, peritonitis, burns
	Renal sodium loss	Weight loss, dehydration	Low	Isotonic	High	Osmotic diuretics, cerebral salt wasting
Water excess	Non-osmotic release of ADH	Weight gain or stable; history suggestive of cause	Low	High	High	Perioperative
	Renal failure, diuretics	Weight gain or stable; history suggestive of cause	Low	Isotonic	High	Intrinsic renal disease, nephrotoxins
	Low GFR, polydipsia	Weight gain or stable; history suggestive of cause	Low	Isotonic	Low	Toddler polydipsia, low-solute infant feeds

ADH, antidiuretic hormone; GFR, glomerular filtration rate.

there is no indication for hypertonic saline. However, a child presenting with confusion or seizures secondary to acute hyponatraemia (<48 hours) is at risk of cerebral oedema and requires rapid correction of plasma sodium by the administration of hypertonic saline (3 per cent). The risk of osmotic demyelination syndrome in this situation is thought to be low but rapid correction of plasma sodium should be undertaken after specialist consultation, in a monitored environment with 1- to 2-hourly measurement of plasma sodium. Suggestions include a target rate of correction of 8–12 mmol/L/day [16], or at a rate of 1–2 mmol/L/h for a few hours until the child is alert and seizure free or the plasma sodium is 125–130 mmol/L, whichever occurs first [8,16].

The plasma sodium can be raised by 1 mmol/L by the intravenous infusion of 1 mL/kg 3 per cent sodium chloride solution (assuming total body water is 50 per cent total body weight) [16].

Osmotic demyelination syndrome

Osmotic demyelination syndrome occurs after overcorrection or rapid correction of long-standing hyponatraemia. It leads to irreversible neurological damage (quadriplegia, pseudobulbar palsy and pseudocoma with 'locked-in' state), usually occurring a few days after elevation of the plasma sodium concentration [9,16]. Extensive demyelinating lesions are seen on MRI (magnetic resonance imaging). Patients who are malnourished, have liver disease or are potassium depleted, or whose clinical course is complicated by a hypoxic event are particularly vulnerable. Correction of chronic hyponatraemia such as that associated with Addison's disease should proceed extremely slowly and should not exceed 4 mmol/kg/day, particularly if the patient does not have hyponatraemic symptoms [17].

Hypernatraemia

Hypernatraemia is defined as a plasma sodium >145 mmol/L, while severe hypernatraemia is a plasma sodium >160 mmol/L. There are potent physiological responses to protect against hypernatraemia (ADH and thirst); it is therefore always pathological. Hypernatraemia causes cerebral dehydration. Severe and rapidly developing hypernatraemia may lead to structural changes; cerebral haemorrhage, venous sinus thrombosis, cerebral infarction and diffuse demyelinating lesions have been reported. Children may complain of intense thirst, vomiting, irritability, lethargy, or progress to seizures and coma. Severe hypernatraemia may be associated with hyperglycaemia or rhabdomyolysis. Hypernatraemia has a high mortality rate in hospitalised children (15 per cent), although deaths are often related to the underlying condition [16].

Causes of hypernatraemia (Table 4.4)

Hypernatraemia may occur as a result of excess sodium intake but is more commonly caused by excessive water loss. Examples include large insensible losses with inadequate water intake in premature neonates, or water loss in excess of sodium loss in severe gastroenteritis causing hypernatraemic dehydration [16].

Table 4.4 Causes of hypernatraemia [9]

Excess sodium	Isotonic or hypertonic parenteral fluids
	Hyperosmolar infant feeds
	Salt poisoning
	CNS injury – abnormal thirst
	Sodium-containing drugs (antibiotics, sodium bicarbonate)
Deficit of electrolyte-free water	
Inadequate fluid intake	Restricted access to fluids
	Excessive fluid restriction
	Ineffective breast-feeding
	Neurological impairment
	Reset osmostat (rare)
Excess water loss	
Renal water loss	Central diabetes insipidus
	Nephrogenic diabetes insipidus
	Diuretics
	Hyperglycaemia
	Post-obstructive diuresis
	Diuretic phase of ATN
Insensible water loss	Fever, tachypnoea, dry environment, especially in premature neonates
Gastrointestinal water loss	Gastroenteritis
	Ileostomy/colostomy losses
	Malabsorption

ATN, acute tubular necrosis; CNS, central nervous system.

Diagnosis of hypernatraemia (Table 4.5)

A detailed medical history is required to elicit the cause of hypernatraemia, which is often multifactorial and iatrogenic in the hospital setting. There may be signs of dehydration with weight loss (excess water loss); rarely there is an increase in weight due to expansion of the ECF space associated with excess sodium intake. Plasma osmolality will be high in all cases; urinary sodium and osmolality may be high or low, depending on aetiology.

Hypernatraemic dehydration associated with gastroenteritis may present with circulatory collapse. Diabetes insipidus (DI) (nephrogenic or central) is indicated by polyuria and polydipsia – these children may have normal plasma sodium but will become rapidly hypernatraemic if access to water is restricted. They may be differentiated by the response to the ADH analogue desmopressin which causes concentration of urine in children with central DI, but not nephrogenic DI [16]. Salt poisoning may be differentiated from hypernatraemic dehydration by weight gain rather than weight loss and by comparing the fractional excretions of sodium and water. Fractional excretion of sodium is calculated by comparison of sodium and creatinine concentrations in paired 'spot' urine and plasma samples and is >2 per cent in salt poisoning and <1 per cent in dehydration [18].

Treatment of hypernatraemia

Treatment of hypernatraemia requires correction of the plasma sodium abnormality, the possible circulatory volume

Table 4.5 Diagnostic features characteristic of different causes of hypernatraemia

	Cause	Clinical signs and symptoms	Plasma osmolality	Urinary osmolality	Urinary sodium	Clinical examples
Excess sodium	Excess sodium	Weight gain, oedema or weight stable	High	High	High	Excess sodium administration Salt poisoning
			High	Low	Variable	Reset osmostat
Excess water loss	Renal water loss	Weight loss, clinical dehydration	High	High or isotonic	High	Diuretics, glycosuria, post-obstructive, ATN
			High	Low	Low	Diabetes insipidus
	Insensible water loss	Weight loss, clinical dehydration	High	High	Low	Neonates, fever, tachypnoea, IPPV
	GI loss	Weight loss, clinical dehydration	High	High	Low	Diarrhoea and vomiting

ATN, acute tubular necrosis; GI, gastrointestinal; IPPV, intermittent positive pressure ventilation.

deficit and the underlying cause of the condition. Correction via the oral route is preferable for all patients, but children who are shocked, for example from gastroenteritis, may require initial fluid resuscitation with 0.9 per cent saline 20 mL/kg. Rapid correction of hypernatraemia is reasonable if it has developed acutely, but cerebral oedema may develop if there have been adaptive changes to long-standing hypernatraemia. In these patients it is preferable to correct the plasma sodium over 48 hours and by no more than 0.5 mmol/L per h. The goal of treatment is to achieve a plasma sodium of 145 mmol/L or, in severe hypernatraemia (>170 mmol/L), slow correction to 150 mmol/L over 48–72 hours. If intravenous fluids are used, electrolytes should be assessed 2-hourly initially. Hypotonic fluids will be required, the choice depending on relative losses of sodium and water. If hypernatraemia is caused by sodium and water loss, it is suggested that 0.45 per cent saline in 5 per cent dextrose is used; if primarily caused by water loss, 0.18 per cent saline in 4 per cent dextrose is used [16].

The minimum amount of free water required to correct serum sodium in hypernatraemia may be calculated using the formula [16]:

$$\text{Free water deficit (mL)} = 4\,\text{mL} \times \text{lean body weight (kg)} \times \text{desired change in serum sodium (mmol/L)}$$

DISORDERS OF POTASSIUM BALANCE

Potassium stores in the body are largely intracellular as potassium is the predominant intracellular cation (intracellular potassium approximately 150 mmol/L). Plasma potassium is maintained within narrow limits, around 3.5–5 mmol/L. The electrical properties of cell membranes are dependent on the precise balance between intracellular and extracellular potassium, and minor alterations in extracellular potassium can have significant clinical effects.

Dietary potassium intake is 1–2 mmol/kg/day: 90 per cent of this load is renally excreted and the remainder lost largely through the intestine, but these are slow processes. Minute-to-minute control of plasma potassium is achieved by the movement of potassium across cell membranes via ion channels controlled by insulin, catecholamines, thyroid hormone, parathyroid hormone and acid–base status.

Renal excretion of potassium is determined by the plasma potassium concentration and dietary intake, acid–base status, GFR, distal sodium delivery and the effects of aldosterone, and to a lesser extent ADH. Aldosterone is secreted in response to a rise in plasma potassium or a rise in angiotensin II. Its main action is on the collecting duct to increase potassium excretion in exchange for sodium which is reabsorbed. Potassium excretion also occurs in the distal tubule via Na^+/K^+-ATPase channels, dependent on plasma potassium levels, independent of aldosterone. Adaptation to renal impairment includes an increase in distal tubular Na^+/K^+-ATPase activity. Potassium excretion also depends on distal sodium delivery: if the GFR is increased, potassium excretion is increased and vice versa.

Insulin increases the uptake of potassium by liver, skeletal muscle and fat cells. Catecholamines increase intracellular uptake of potassium via β_2-receptors, independent of insulin. Metabolic acidosis induces exchange of potassium and hydrogen ions across cell membranes to increase plasma potassium [19].

Hyperkalaemia

Hyperkalaemia is defined as plasma potassium greater than 5 mmol/L. The clinical effects of hyperkalaemia depend on the magnitude of the rise in plasma potassium, and the speed with which it develops, as well as associated abnormalities such as acidosis, hyponatraemia and hypocalcaemia. The principal adverse effects of hyperkalaemia are on the heart. Progressive electrocardiogram (ECG) changes are seen with rising potassium, but may not always be present. Typical ECG changes are: peaked T waves (K^+ 6–7 mmol/L), broad P waves, wide QRS complex (K^+ 7–8 mmol/L), sinusoidal QRS (K^+ 8–9 mmol/L), AV dissociation, ventricular fibrillation and asystole (K^+ > 9 mmol/L) [20]. Cardiac arrest may be the presenting feature of hyperkalaemia. Non-cardiac effects of hyperkalaemia include diarrhoea or ileus, abdominal pain, myalgia and flaccid paralysis [19].

Causes of hyperkalaemia are listed in Table 4.6 [19]; it may result from a combination of abnormalities, in paediatric practice most commonly due to low cardiac output leading to metabolic acidosis and acute renal failure.

Table 4.6   Causes of hyperkalaemia [19]

Increased potassium load	
Exogenous	Potassium chloride (drug error)
	Stored blood
Endogenous	Haemolysis
	Exercise
	Catabolic states
	Rhabdomyolysis
	Acute tumour lysis
Decreased renal potassium excretion	
Renal impairment (acute/chronic)	
Distal renal tubular abnormalities	Interstitial nephritis
	Papillary necrosis
	Postrenal transplantation
	Obstructive uropathy
Abnormalities of renin–angiotensin–aldosterone system	
Drugs	Spironolactone
	ACE inhibitor
	NSAIDs
	Tacrolimus
	Ciclosporin
Primary hypoaldosteronism	
Congenital adrenal hypoplasia	
Type IV renal tubular acidosis	
Adrenal insufficiency	Primary
	Infection, e.g. tuberculosis
Sodium channel block	
Drugs	Amiloride
	Trimethoprim
Decrease in distal sodium delivery	Heart failure
	Renal failure
	Salt-wasting nephropathy
Transcellular shift	
	Hyperglycaemia
	Suxamethonium
	Acute haemolysis
	Hyperkalaemic periodic paralysis
	Acute metabolic acidosis
	Extreme prematurity

ACE, angiotensin-converting enzyme; NSAIDs, non-steroidal anti-inflammatory drugs.

Rhabdomyolysis is an unusual cause of hyperkalaemic cardiac arrest, but in children may be the initial presentation of a previously undiagnosed neuromuscular disorder such as Duchennes muscular dystrophy [21], particularly when suxamethonium is used [20]. Suxamethonium may also induce hyperkalaemia in children in other situations, all associated with upregulation of muscle nicotinic acetylcholine receptors, for example upper or lower motor neuron defects, prolonged infusion of muscle relaxants, direct muscle trauma, tumour or inflammation, burns, prolonged immobility or severe infection [20]. The potassium concentration of stored blood increases by 1 mmol/L/day; irradiation of blood to remove competent white cells accelerates potassium rise and such blood should be transfused within 24 hours. Transient hyperkalaemia is common in extremely low-birth-weight infants in the first week of life, despite the absence of potassium intake. This rise is due to transcellular shift of potassium and plasma levels fall with the onset of the postnatal diuresis. The rise in plasma potassium may be attenuated by prophylactic administration of calcium gluconate to maintain ionised calcium within normal limits [22].

Treatment of hyperkalaemia (Table 4.7)

Severe hyperkalaemia is a medical emergency, particularly when plasma potassium exceeds 7.5 mmol/L. Treatment strategies depend on whether the child is symptomatic, and in particular the presence of cardiac arrhythmias. Treatment is aimed at counteracting the effect of potassium on the myocardium, promoting intracellular uptake of potassium

Table 4.7   Treatment of hyperkalaemia

Stabilise cell membranes (cardiac arrhythmias)			
10% calcium gluconate:	0.5 mL/kg (0.1 mmol/kg) slow intravenous injection		
Promote intracellular uptake of potassium			
Salbutamol			
Nebulised salbutamol	Age (years)		Dose (mg)
	<2.5		2.5
	2.5–7.5		5
	>7.5		10
Intravenous salbutamol injection over 5 min	4 μg/kg		
Insulin and dextrose			
Glucose infusion only	20% dextrose 2.5 mL/kg/h (0.5 g/kg/h)		
Insulin infusion (if plasma glucose > 10 mmol/L)	0.05 units/kg/h (initial rate: titrate to plasma glucose)		
Increase potassium excretion			
Calcium resonium	Loading dose: 1 g/kg (oral/rectal)		
	Maintenance: 1 g/kg/day divided doses		

and increasing the excretion of potassium. Therapy should also be aimed at the cause of hyperkalaemia.

Intravenous calcium stabilises plasma membranes and reduces the arrhythmic threshold. Although the randomised evidence to support its use is lacking, intravenous calcium is the immediate treatment of choice in the presence of cardiac arrhythmias [23].

Salbutamol is a β_2 agonist and is effective in reducing plasma potassium within 30 minutes whether administered intravenously, in a nebulised form or as a multidose inhaler. The dose may be repeated if necessary. Insulin (with dextrose) promotes intracellular uptake of potassium and is rapidly effective within 15 minutes. Administration of a dextrose load to a non-diabetic child is probably just as effective, and does not carry the risk of inadvertent hypoglycaemia, although dilute dextrose solutions may induce hyponatraemia. Sodium bicarbonate is useful, particularly in the presence of metabolic acidosis, but may cause hypernatraemia or worsen ionised hypocalcaemia, causing tetany or hypotension. The treatment of choice to promote intracellular uptake of potassium is nebulised salbutamol as it has the least side-effects; combining salbutamol and glucose infusion probably results in a greater fall in plasma potassium [23].

Excretion of potassium is increased by haemofiltration, peritoneal dialysis, haemodialysis or ion-exchange resins such as calcium resonium. Calcium resonium is safe but only reduces plasma potassium levels slowly; it is recommended that dialysis is instituted early in cases of hyperkalaemic cardiac arrest [24].

Hypokalaemia

Hypokalaemia is defined as plasma potassium <3.5 mmol/L. Treatment is seldom an emergency, except when severe. Mild hypokalaemia leads to non-specific clinical symptoms of generalised weakness and lassitude, but increasing severity may lead to muscle necrosis ($K^+ < 2.5$ mmol/L) or ascending paralysis ($K^+ < 2$ mmol/L). Mild-to-moderate hypokalaemia is associated with cardiac arrhythmias in children with underlying heart disease but this is rarely seen in children with a normal myocardial function, even when plasma potassium is <3 mmol/L [25]. The most frequent cause of hypokalaemia (Table 4.8) in children is loss of potassium from the gastrointestinal tract, particularly from an acute diarrhoeal illness when losses may be profound [26]. The other major cause of hypokalaemia is increased urinary loss associated with drugs, principally diuretics. Hypokalaemia due to transcellular shift of potassium is less common.

Treatment of hypokalaemia [24]

Treatment of hypokalaemia is rarely an emergency; if asymptomatic, oral supplements should be used. Intravenous potassium should be given if the child has cardiac arrhythmias or other symptoms; overzealous treatment can result in fatal cardiac arrhythmias from hyperkalaemia. Potassium chloride is highly irritant and must be diluted to a solution of <80 mmol/L (e.g. 40 mmol in 500 mL 0.9 per

Table 4.8 Causes of hypokalaemia [25]

Increased loss of potassium
  Gastrointestinal
    Infectious diarrhoea
    Vomiting
    Stoma losses
    Tumours (Zollinger–Ellison syndrome)
    Malabsorption
  Renal
    Mineralocorticoid excess
      Primary hyperaldosteronism
      Secondary hyperaldosteronism
        Hypovolaemia
      Congenital adrenal hyperplasia
      Renin-secreting tumour
      Cushing's syndrome
        Pituitary
        Adrenal
      Vasculitis
    Renal tubular abnormalities
      Barrter's syndrome
      Gitelman's syndrome
      Liddle's syndrome
    Drugs causing increased renal loss of potassium
      Diuretics
      High-dose steroids
      High-dose penicillin
      Magnesium depletion
        Aminoglycosides
        Amphotericin B
  Other abnormal losses
      Post surgical abdominal drain losses
      Excessive sweating – cystic fibrosis
Transcellular shift of potassium
  Drugs
    β_2 Agonists (salbutamol, adrenaline)
    Caffeine
    Insulin
  Metabolic alkalosis
  'Stress', e.g. asthma attack
  Hypokalaemic periodic paralysis

cent saline) and administered via a central line with ECG monitoring. When using intravenous potassium infusions, 0.08–0.25 mmol/kg/h should be given The plasma potassium should be checked frequently. Higher rates of replacement (2 mmol/kg/h) have been given to children with profound hypokalaemia due to gastroenteritis [26].

DISORDERS OF CALCIUM BALANCE

Calcium is the most abundant mineral in the body; 98 per cent is found in bone, less than 1 per cent in the circulation and the remainder in the intracellular and extracellular compartments. Ionised calcium is biologically active and constitutes 50 per cent of the plasma calcium; the remainder is bound to plasma proteins (40 per cent) or combined with various anions (10 per cent). Total intracellular calcium is similar to extracellular calcium but the ionised form of calcium is 1000 times lower because of active sequestration, extrusion and buffering. Calcium has an important structural role in bone and is pivotal in many biological processes. It is the major intracellular messenger needed for normal cellular function including excitation–contraction coupling in myocardial, smooth and skeletal smooth muscle, enzyme processes and coagulation of blood.

Calcium homeostasis is complex, involving interactions of parathyroid hormone (PTH) and vitamin D (1,25-dihydroxyvitamin D_3, or calcitriol), calcitonin and the calcium-sensing receptor, which in turn affect intestinal absorption of calcium-bone resorption and urinary excretion of calcium and phosphate [27]. Vitamin D is obtained from dietary sources, is also formed in the skin by the action of sunlight, and is activated in the liver and kidney to increase intestinal absorption of calcium and serum calcium levels. Parathyroid hormone is secreted by the parathyroid glands and promotes bone resorption (thus releasing calcium), reduces urinary calcium and increases urinary phosphate excretion, and enhances the activation of vitamin D. Severe hypomagnesaemia (<0.45 mmol/L) impairs the secretion and activity of PTH. Calcium-sensing receptor is found in the parathyroid, kidney and bone and responds to a decrease in ionised extracellular calcium by increasing the secretion of PTH. Calcitonin is released from the thyroid, in response to elevated plasma calcium, to enhance renal excretion of calcium and reduce bone resorption.

Hypercalcaemia

Normal plasma calcium is 2.1–2.6 mmol/L. Hypercalcaemia usually occurs when the influx of calcium from the intestine or bone exceeds urinary excretory capacity for calcium. Symptoms of hypercalcaemia are often non-specific such as failure to thrive, weight loss, abdominal pain, lethargy and vomiting. Hypercalcaemia interferes with the action of ADH in the collecting duct and leads to polyuria and polydipsia; severe dehydration may occur if combined with poor fluid intake due to vomiting. Acute pancreatitis may occur. Long-term effects of hypercalcaemia on the kidney include impaired renal function with secondary hypertension, interstitial nephritis, nephrocalcinosis, hypercalciuria and nephrolithiasis. A hypercalcaemic crisis may be precipitated by acute nausea and vomiting, leading to generalised muscle weakness, confusion or coma. The ECG may show a prolonged QT interval and arrhythmias are common. Fatal intraoperative cardiac arrest has been reported with a plasma calcium >5.6 mmol/L [28]. Recognition of hypercalcaemia in children is often delayed as laboratory investigation of non-specific symptoms is unusual. Causes of hypercalcaemia are listed in Table 4.9.

Treatment of hypercalcaemia

Treatment of hypercalcaemia is only urgent in children who are symptomatic or with plasma calcium >3.2 mmol/L.

Table 4.9   Causes of hypercalcaemia [28]

Hyperparathyroidism
Hypervitaminosis D, A
Idiopathic hypercalcaemia of infancy (Williams' syndrome)
Down syndrome
Malignancy
Skeletal disorders
Immobility
Thiazide diuretics

Rehydration with 0.9 per cent saline is usually sufficient to dilute the plasma calcium and increase urinary calcium excretion. Furosemide may also be given to increase calcium excretion. The underlying cause of hypercalcaemia should be investigated and dietary intake of calcium restricted. Steroids reduce the production of calcitriol and intestinal absorption of calcium; they are useful in vitamin D toxicity and hypercalcaemia associated with malignancy. Bisphosphonates such as pamidronate reduce osteoclast activity and bone resorption. They have been used in the treatment of resistant hypercalcaemia associated with malignancy or hyperparathyroidism but may induce severe hypocalcaemia and febrile reactions and should be used after specialist consultation only [29].

Hypocalcaemia

Hypocalcaemia occurs as a result of inadequate uptake of calcium from the intestine or bone, or abnormal losses or chelation in the plasma. Hypocalcaemia is defined as plasma calcium less than 1.7, 2.0 and 2.2 mmol/L in preterm, term newborns and children, respectively [27]. Plasma calcium is bound to albumin, and this must be taken into account in the diagnosis of hypocalcaemia (for each 10 g/L reduction in plasma albumin, add 0.2 mmol/L to the total plasma calcium concentration). The ionised calcium is a much more useful measure: levels below 1.0 mmol/L are clinically significant and life-threatening complications occur when ionised calcium is less than 0.5 mmol/L [28].

Symptoms of hypocalcaemia relate to the effects on excitable tissues, cardiovascular, respiratory and neurological symptoms being of particular importance. The severity of symptoms depends on the degree of hypocalcaemia and the speed with which it develops. It may be associated with profound hypotension (loss of vascular tone) and impaired cardiac contractility, particularly in children with sepsis and after cardiopulmonary bypass. Citrate-anticoagulated blood or blood products are a common cause of hypocalcaemia, particularly after cardiac surgery. Neonates are particularly sensitive to the cardiovascular effects of ionised hypocalcaemia as the sarcoplasmic reticulum is immature and calcium required for excitation–contraction coupling is obtained from the extracellular fluid. The ECG is not diagnostic – it may be normal or show a prolonged QT and ST interval, T-wave inversion or arrhythmias, including ventricular fibrillation.

Table 4.10 Causes of hypocalcaemia [28]

Sepsis
Massive blood transfusion
Vitamin D deficiency
Hypoparathyroidism
Hypomagnesaemia
Malabsorption
Renal failure
Hepatic impairment
DiGeorge syndrome
Neonatal asphyxia
Acute pancreatitis
Hyperphosphataemia
Calcium-sensing receptor defect

Hypocalcaemia of longer duration may present with paraesthesiae, muscle cramps, carpopedal spasm, muscle weakness, tetany or seizures. It should be considered in the differential diagnosis of an infant presenting with stridor [30]. Vitamin D is a fat-soluble vitamin present in the diet, but only in low quantities in human breast milk. Babies who are exclusively breast-fed and have limited exposure to sunlight may become deficient in vitamin D. Rickets is the bone disease associated with hypocalcaemia, caused by undermineralisation of metaphyseal growth plates. It commonly presents at 2 months to 3 years of age with bowing and flaring of the ends of long bones, rib abnormalities (rachitic rosary, Harrison's groove) and fractures. It may result from dietary deficiency of calcium or vitamin D (as above) or from chromosomal abnormalities interfering with vitamin D metabolism (vitamin D-dependent rickets types I and II). Mineralisation of bones occurs during the last trimester of pregnancy; rickets of prematurity occurs when the dietary intake of minerals is inadequate. DiGeorge anomaly is caused by a deletion in chromosome 22q11. It is associated with thymic aplasia, cardiac abnormalities, cleft palate and hypocalcaemia due to hypoplasia or aplasia of the parathyroid glands [27]. Causes of hypocalcaemia are shown in Table 4.10.

Treatment of hypocalcaemia

Ionised hypocalcaemia associated with hypotension or seizures should be treated with dilute intravenous calcium, preferably via a central line as calcium is highly irritant to the tissues. The ECG should be monitored. Two forms of calcium are available which have a different content of elemental calcium. Either may be given, taking care to ensure the correct dose, depending on which preparation is used [24]: intravenous injection should be over at least 10 minutes and the doses are either 10 per cent calcium gluconate 0.3 mL/kg or 10 per cent calcium chloride 0.1 mL/kg.

Long-term treatment of hypocalcaemia should be directed at the underlying cause. Oral calcium and vitamin D metabolites are usually required.

DISORDERS OF MAGNESIUM BALANCE

Magnesium is the fourth most common cation. Like potassium, magnesium is predominantly intracellular, with extracellular magnesium accounting for <1 per cent of total body content [31]. Magnesium is essential for life and is a cofactor required for numerous enzymatic reactions and cellular energy metabolism, and has an important role in membrane stabilisation, nerve conduction and calcium channel activity.

Magnesium homeostasis depends on the balance of intestinal absorption, renal excretion and movement between stores, principally in bone and muscle. Renal excretion is determined principally by the concentration of magnesium in plasma, regulated by the calcium–magnesium-sensing receptor in the loop of Henle.

Hypomagnesaemia

The main clinical effects of magnesium imbalance result from hypomagnesaemia, which is common in hospitalised patients. The normal plasma magnesium is 0.7–1.0 mmol/L and, although ionised magnesium may be more meaningful clinically, ion-selective electrodes may not offer an accurate measurement [32]. Magnesium deficiency may be caused by increased gastrointestinal or renal losses.

Hypomagnesaemia is commonly associated with other ion deficiencies such as hypocalcaemia, hypokalaemia and metabolic alkalosis, which respond to treatment only after magnesium replacement. Magnesium increases intracellular calcium uptake into the sarcoplasmic reticulum. Deficiency of magnesium results in increased intracellular calcium and increased smooth muscle contraction. Deficiency of magnesium may have a role to play in the development of bronchospasm, neuromuscular hyperexcitability and seizures. Magnesium may have a role in the treatment of asthma, sepsis, acute cerebral ischaemia and other critical illnesses in children.

Hypomagnesaemia causes neuromuscular abnormalities, weakness, carpopedal spasm and seizures. Cardiovascular abnormalities include ECG abnormalities (widened QRS complex, prolongation of PR interval, inverted T wave, U wave) and severe ventricular arrhythmias; magnesium is the treatment of choice for polymorphic (torsade de pointes) ventricular tachycardia. Addition of magnesium to the pump prime of children undergoing cardiopulmonary bypass prevents hypomagnesaemia and hypokalaemia, and reduces the incidence of cardiac junctional arrhythmias [33]. If a child has signs and symptoms of magnesium deficiency, magnesium should be administered, even if plasma magnesium levels fall within the normal range [32].

Treatment of hypomagnesaemia [24]

Magnesium should be administered by slow intravenous injection over at least 10 minutes and suggested doses are given in Table 4.11.

Table 4.11 Magnesium treatment [24]

Septicaemia	0.4 mmol/kg (100 mg/kg) $MgSO_4$ over 30 minutes, single dose, max. 20 mmol (5 g)
Asthma (over 6 years)	0.1–0.16 mmol/kg (25–40 mg/kg) $MgSO_4$ over 20 minutes, single dose, max. 8 mmol (2 g)
Torsade de pointes	0.1–0.2 mmol/kg (25–50 mg/kg) $MgSO_4$, single dose, max. 8 mmol (2 g)

PRESCRIBING INTRAVENOUS FLUIDS IN CHILDREN

When administering intravenous fluids, the anaesthetist must take into account whether the fluid is for maintenance or replacement, the requirements for electrolytes and free water and the ability of the individual to excrete any excess free water. Reference values for commonly used intravenous fluids are shown in Table 4.12.

Maintenance fluids in children: the Holliday–Segar formula

Holliday and Segar proposed a formula to estimate the maintenance need for water in parenteral fluid therapy for children in 1957 and this formula has been in common use to calculate maintenance fluids for children ever since

(Table 4.13). The requirement for water was linked to the caloric expenditure in healthy children. Estimations were made for 'average' energy requirements, insensible losses and urinary losses, with an allowance for the water of oxidation produced during metabolism [34] (Fig. 4.1). They proposed that the daily maintenance electrolyte requirement should be equivalent of the dietary intake of milk-fed infants, that is, sodium chloride 2–3 mmol/kg/day and potassium chloride 1 mmol/kg/day. An ideal, isosmolar solution for maintenance therapy was formulated (4 per cent dextrose, 0.2 per cent saline) to which potassium could be added. The authors also pointed out that caloric expenditure is reduced in hospitalised children and urinary losses may vary according to the clinical situations and the effects of ADH. Holliday stated that 'maintenance' fluid requirements should be restricted postoperatively in the presence of increased ADH secretion and that that volume deficits should be managed separately and replaced with a 20–40 mL/kg bolus of isotonic saline [34,35].

The Holliday–Segar formula has been criticised because it may overestimate fluid requirements, particularly in a catabolic patient after surgery [2]. A minimum amount of water is required daily in order to excrete the waste products of metabolism in the urine and stool, and replace insensible water losses from the respiratory tract and skin. Holliday and Segar may have overestimated insensible water losses and oversimplified water requirements to replace urinary losses. They estimated insensible water losses to be 50 mL/kg/day. However, insensible water loss varies widely

Table 4.12 Sodium content and osmolality of commonly used intravenous fluids

Intravenous fluid	Sodium (mmol/L)	Chloride (mmol/L)	Osmolality (mosm/kg H_2O)	Percentage electrolyte-free water	Osmolality (compared with plasma)	Tonicity (after metabolism of dextrose)
5% dextrose	0	0	252	100	Isosmolar	Hypotonic
10% dextrose	0	0	555	100	Hyperosmolar	Hypotonic
0.18% saline/ 4% dextrose	30	30	282	80	Isosmolar	Hypotonic
0.45% saline/ 2.5% dextrose	77	77	293	50	Isosmolar	Hypotonic
0.45% saline/ 5% dextrose	77	77	432	50	Hyperosmolar	Hypotonic
Compound sodium lactate (Hartmann's solution or lactated Ringer's)*	131	111	278	16	Isosmolar	Isotonic
0.9% saline	154	154	308	0	Isosmolar	Isotonic
5% dextrose/ 0.9% saline	154	154	560	0	Hyperosmolar	Isotonic
4.5% human albumin solution	100–160		275	0	Isosmolar	Isotonic
Succinylated gelatin (e.g. Gelofusine)	154	120	274	0	Isosmolar	Isotonic

*Compound sodium lactate also contains K^+ 5 mmol/L, Ca^{2+} 2 mmol/L, lactate 29 mmol/L.

Table 4.13 The Holliday–Segar formula: the average maintenance requirement for fluid in healthy children [34]

Body weight (kg)	Average maintenance allowance for fluid	
	(mL/day)	(mL/h)
0–10	100 mL/kg	4 mL/kg
10–20	1000 mL + 50 mL/kg for each kg over 10 kg	40 mL + 2 mL/kg for each kg over 10 kg
20–30	1500 mL + 20 mL/kg for each kg over 20 kg	60 mL + 1 mL/kg for each kg over 20 kg

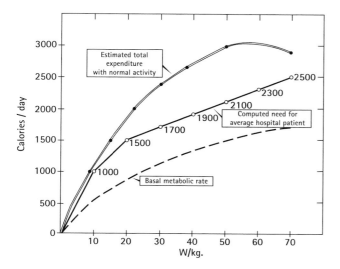

Figure 4.1 Comparison of energy expenditure in basal and ideal state, redrawn from Holliday and Segar [34], with permission from the American Academy of Pediatrics. Weights at the 50th percentile were selected for converting calories at various ages to calories related to weight. The computed line for calories required for the average hospital patient was derived from the following equations:

1. 0–10 kg   100 cal/kg
2. 10–20 kg   1000 cal + 50 cal/kg for each kg over 10 kg
3. ≥20 kg   1500 cal + 20 cal/kg for each kg over 20 kg

depending on the clinical situation: from a maximum of 120 mL/kg/day for the 1 kg premature infant on day 1 of life [1] to 12–27 mL/kg/day for a 1-year-old, or 10 mL/kg/day for the catabolic patient with renal failure [2]. If the urine is maximally concentrated in the presence of ADH, excretion of the urinary solute load can be achieved with a minimal urine output of only 25 mL/kg/day [2], rather than the 'average' urinary loss of 67 mL/kg/day suggested by Holliday and Segar [34].

The maintenance requirement for water can therefore vary from as much as 180 mL/kg/day in the premature infant on day 1 of life, to as little as 50–60 mL/kg/day in a child who is acutely unwell or following surgery. The Holliday–Segar formula should be used as a simple starting

point for maintenance fluid and requires modification in the light of the clinical circumstances.

The Holliday–Segar formula has also been criticised because of the recommendation to use hypotonic infusions, especially in the perioperative period. A small study in adolescents undergoing scoliosis surgery randomised patients to receive either Hartmann's solution or hypotonic dextrose saline intraoperatively and postoperatively. Patients receiving hypotonic fluid had significantly lower plasma sodium at all time points up to 48 hours, including the first postoperative sample [36]. In another study, children undergoing elective minor surgery were randomised to receive either 2.5 per cent dextrose, 0.43 per cent saline or 5 per cent dextrose, 0.33 per cent saline. In both groups there was a fall in plasma sodium, but this was significantly greater in the group receiving more electrolyte-free water [37]. A recent prospective randomised trial of intravenous rehydration in children with gastroenteritis showed that 2.5 per cent dextrose, 0.9 per cent saline was better than 2.5 per cent dextrose, 0.45 per cent saline in protecting against hyponatraemia, but was not associated with hypernatraemia [38]. Numerous case reports suggest that hypotonic fluid is associated with iatrogenic hyponatraemic encephalopathy in the postoperative period [6].

'Replacement' fluids and 'maintenance' fluids

The Holliday–Segar formula describes the requirements for 'maintenance' fluids to replace insensible and urinary losses when oral intake is suspended. Intravenous fluids may also be required as 'replacement' fluids to expand the ECF volume, maintain blood pressure or replace abnormal fluid losses [7]. Such replacement fluids should have the same composition as ECF.

During the intraoperative period, the stress response to surgery causes maximal vasopressin release and urinary losses will be low. Insensible losses (sweating/respiratory water losses) will also be low; therefore the requirement for maintenance water is low. However, anaesthetic agents induce a fall in blood pressure and fluid is also required to replace deficits caused by fasting and ongoing losses associated with surgery. These deficits/losses are from the extracellular compartment and should be replaced by an isotonic solution. Hypotonic solutions would be expected to result in a fall in plasma sodium and should not be used during the intraoperative period; only isotonic solutions should be used during surgery in children, in line with adult practice.

Crystalloid versus colloids for intravascular fluid resuscitation

The debate regarding the relative benefits of crystalloid versus colloid for fluid resuscitation in adult and paediatric practice has continued for many years. Albumin and other colloid solutions are often favoured by anaesthetists as they may lead to greater plasma volume expansion and increase in cardiac output than comparable fluid loading with crystalloids [39], with reduced oedema formation but increased risk for transfusion-related infection if human-derived products are used. The choice between synthetic colloids, that is, gelatins starch solutions, probably has much to do with local tradition and marketing [40]. Questions remain about the side-effects of starch solutions in children, such as pruritis, renal function and bleeding, even with the newer lower-molecular-weight solutions [41].

The Saline versus Albumin Fluid Evaluation ('SAFE') study group conducted a double-blind randomised controlled study of albumin versus saline for fluid resuscitation of nearly 7000 adult patients admitted to intensive care [42]. There was no difference in outcome between each group at 28 days, although subgroup analysis indicated a trend towards increased mortality in the albumin group in patients with traumatic brain injury, and a decreased mortality in patients with sepsis [43]. Another recent randomised controlled trial in adults found no difference in long-term outcome when hypertonic saline was compared with lactated Ringer's solution for prehospital resuscitation in hypotensive patients with traumatic brain injury [44]. The Cochrane Injuries group has revised their previous advice regarding increased mortality in patients receiving albumin but pointed out the lack of survival benefit of colloids and increased expense when compared with crystalloids [45]. Current Advanced Paediatric Life Support (APLS) guidelines for fluid resuscitation in children suggest initial fluid resuscitation with isotonic crystalloid 20 mL/kg (0.9 per cent saline or Hartmann's), subsequent fluid bolus with crystalloid or colloid, but favouring 4.5 per cent albumin in sepsis [24].

Hyperchloraemic acidosis, isotonic saline and balanced salt solutions

Isotonic saline contains non-physiological concentrations of chloride compared with normal plasma (150 mmol/L versus approximately 105 mmol/L). In contrast, Hartmann's solution and lactated Ringer's solution are balanced electrolyte solutions with an electrolyte composition close to that of plasma (sodium 131 mmol/L, potassium 5 mmol/L, calcium 2 mmol/L, lactate 29 mmol/L and chloride 111 mmol/L). Lactate is rapidly metabolised to bicarbonate and is used because the latter is less stable in solution. Fluid resuscitation with isotonic saline may result in a persistent metabolic base deficit due to hyperchloraemia, which may be predicted by Stewart's 'strong ion theory'. Traditional diagnostic descriptions of acid–base abnormalities take into account plasma bicarbonate and hydrogen ion concentrations only. In contrast, Stewart's method of assessing acid–base abnormalities takes three independent variables into account – the measure of carbon dioxide in the blood (PCO_2), concentration of weak acids (plasma albumin and inorganic phosphate) and the 'strong ion difference' (SID), that is, the difference

between the concentration of the strong cations (Na^+, K^+, Ca^+ and Mg^+) and strong anions (chloride, lactate) in plasma, the term 'strong' denoting substances completely ionised in plasma. The normal SID is 40 mmol/L. For electroneutrality, the sum of the strong cations in plasma is equal to the sum of the strong anions and weak acids (phosphate, bicarbonate and albumin) – a reduction in SID, for example caused by hyperchloraemia, is associated with a reduction in bicarbonate and a reduction in plasma pH [46].

Hyperchloraemic acidosis is seen in both adults and children after saline resuscitation [47–50], but not with balanced saline solutions in adults [49,50]. The physiological importance of hyperchloraemia is not clear – hyperchloraemia may be benign but has been associated with abdominal discomfort, reduced urine output, reduced splanchnic perfusion and increased postoperative nausea and vomiting [50]. The main problem with hyperchloraemic acidosis in children is the temptation for overzealous fluid administration to correct a persistent base deficit due to hyperchloraemia in the mistaken assumption that it is caused by tissue hypoperfusion [47,48]. The theoretical problem of balanced salt solutions causing hyperkalaemia (for example, after renal transplantation) is unfounded [51] and it has been suggested that lactated Ringer's solution with or without low-dose dextrose would be the ideal solution to use for perioperative infusion in children [52]. Large-volume infusion of Hartmann's solution (or Ringer's) may be associated with hyponatraemia (sodium concentration only 131 mmol/L) and should be used with caution in patients at risk of raised intracranial pressure. The ideal crystalloid solution for perioperative use should approximate as closely as possible to the electrolyte composition of plasma, with the addition of low-dose dextrose (1–2 per cent) to avoid postoperative hypoglycaemia or fluid that is excessively hypertonic with reference to the veins. The ideal crystalloid solution may be closer to solutions currently used for haemodialysis or haemofiltration replacement fluid, rather than intravenous fluids currently licensed for intravenous replacement.

The need for dextrose in the perioperative period

There has been much discussion in the paediatric literature about the need for dextrose during surgery. Some children are particularly vulnerable to intraoperative hypoglycaemia (neonates, those with sepsis or receiving preoperative dextrose infusions or parenteral nutrition) and should have their blood glucose monitored regularly during surgery [37,53]. However, the majority of children maintain their blood sugar perioperatively as a result of the stress response to starvation and surgery [54], even if they do not receive dextrose during surgery. If there are concerns about intraoperative hypoglycaemia, for example in prolonged surgery in small infants, the use of 1 per cent dextrose added to the electrolyte solution is sufficient to avoid hypoglycaemia and prevent ketosis

[52]. Conversely, fluids containing 4 or 5 per cent dextrose may be associated with hyperglycaemia, which may have deleterious effects [52]. Hypotonic fluids containing dextrose, should never be used during surgery (either 4 per cent dextrose, 0.18 per cent saline or 2–5 per cent dextrose, 0.45 per cent saline) as this fluid is associated with dilutional hyponatraemia and hyperglycaemia. For the majority of children intraoperative fluid should be an isotonic solution with or without low-dose dextrose. A 1 per cent solution of dextrose in Hartmann's is not commercially available in the UK at present.

Perioperative fluid management

Fluids should be prescribed with great care, particularly in the perioperative period, taking into account the potential for significant harm.

Intraoperative fluids

The volume of fluid administered during surgery depends on the clinical situation and the type of surgery. Various regimens for fluid administration have been described [55,56], but generous fluid regimens with large-volume replacement of (estimated) insensible losses in adult practice have been associated with increased postoperative weight gain and postoperative complications [57].

A simple regimen, and the one followed in our unit, is to replace the fasting deficit with Hartmann's solution 10–20 mL/kg with subsequent fluid boluses of 20 mL/kg only if necessary (determined by clinical assessment of the patient, remembering that the blood volume is approximately 80 mL/kg). Assessment includes heart rate, capillary refill and blood pressure, measurement of the base excess and haematocrit, as well as close observation of the surgical field, weighing surgical swabs and measuring suction losses. If significant fluid losses or volume shifts are expected (for example, in cardiothoracic surgery or abdominal tumour resection), clinical monitoring is supplemented by invasive monitoring (central venous pressure, invasive arterial pressure). Initial fluid bolus is given as 20 mL/kg of crystalloid; with significant fluid losses boluses of 20 mL/kg of colloid or blood may be given, depending on the clinical circumstances. Blood transfusion is discussed in Chapter 24.

Children undergoing minor surgery only require a fluid bolus of 10–20 mL/kg, which is equivalent to their fasting deficit. This may improve postoperative recovery, particularly for procedures associated with a high incidence of postoperative nausea and vomiting. Administration of intraoperative fluids and withholding oral fluids for 4–6 hours postoperatively has been shown to reduce vomiting in children undergoing day surgery, particularly those receiving opioids [58]. Intravenous fluid therapy during surgery has been shown to reduce postoperative nausea and vomiting in children after strabismus surgery [59]. A small study in children undergoing tonsillectomy showed that perioperative saline infusion was associated with significantly lower postoperative ADH levels compared with control children who did not receive intraoperative fluids; the difference is presumed to be due to correction of hypovolaemia [60]. However, excessive volumes of fluid should be avoided and intravenous fluids should be continued after minor surgery only if the child is unable to tolerate oral fluids. It is much better to allow the child to control their own water balance postoperatively.

Intravenous fluids after major surgery

When oral intake is precluded or inadequate in the postoperative period, maintenance fluids are required to replace insensible losses and urinary losses, and provide a source of dextrose. In addition, isotonic replacement fluids may be required for ongoing or abnormal losses (such as losses from wound drains or gastrointestinal losses). The Holliday–Segar formula [34,35] is a useful starting point for calculating fluid replacement in paediatric practice but prescriptions should be individually tailored to the clinical situation for each child and the outcomes monitored.

The choice of postoperative maintenance fluid remains controversial, although it is clear that hypotonic fluids may harm some children. In the absence of definitive randomised prospective trials in postoperative patients, most experts favour the use of isotonic fluid for postoperative maintenance [6,61–65], although some favour the use of restricted isotonic fluids [2]. Where there is concern that isotonic fluids may be associated with hypernatraemia and fluid overload it is suggested that hypotonic fluids may be used, restricted to 50 per cent of maintenance to take account of the rise in ADH levels, with isotonic fluids administered for replacement of abnormal losses or as a bolus to maintain blood pressure if required [35,66]. A recent survey of perioperative fluid prescription by anaesthetists caring for children suggests that unrestricted hypotonic dextrose saline solutions continue to be the most widely prescribed fluids for children in the UK, a practice likely to place children at risk from iatrogenic hyponatraemia [13]. A recent systematic review has reiterated the lack of experimental evidence to support the use of hypotonic fluids in children, with greater morbidity if hypotonic solutions are used and a significantly increased risk of developing acute hyponatraemia (odds ratio 17.22, 95 per cent CI 8.67, 34.2) [14].

The Department of Health in Northern Ireland has issued guidance on the use of postoperative fluids in children [67], and the National Patient Safety Agency (NPSA: http://www.npsa.nhs.uk) issued guidance in 2007. The latter referred to all children, except neonates and those in intensive care units and specialist areas such as renal or cardiac units. It recommended that 4 per cent dextrose, 0.18 per cent saline should be withdrawn from use in the UK – except in specialist areas – and that isotonic solutions should be used for maintenance fluids in the perioperative period.

Suggested guidance for postoperative fluid administration after major surgery:

- All children should be weighed before surgery and, if practical, daily thereafter.
- Plasma electrolytes should be measured at the start of intravenous fluid therapy, daily thereafter.
- Postoperative fluids should be prescribed at 60 per cent of maintenance described by the Holliday–Segar formula [34,35], for the first 24 hours.
- Hypovolaemia should be treated by a bolus of 20 mL/kg 0.9 per cent saline, Hartmann's, colloid or blood, depending on the clinical situation.
- Children who are at risk from hyponatraemic encephalopathy, for example those who are hyponatraemic already or after head injury, should receive 0.9 per cent saline as maintenance postoperatively (± 5 per cent dextrose).
- For other children, our current practice is to prescribe 2.5 per cent dextrose, 0.45 per cent saline for maintenance fluid; electrolytes are monitored daily and fluid changed to an isotonic fluid if the plasma sodium falls below 136 mmol/L.
- Continuing abnormal losses should be replaced millilitre for millilitre with the appropriate intravenous fluid – for example, nasogastric losses are replaced with 0.9 per cent saline with potassium (20 mmol K^+ per 500 mL 0.9 per cent saline).
- Potassium should be added to maintenance fluids on the second postoperative day.
- Fluid balance should be assessed daily by clinical examination and the use of fluid balance charts, monitoring all sources of fluid input and output.

The issue of hyperchloraemic acidosis has not been addressed [68].

Special clinical situations in anaesthetic practice

NEONATES

Insensible losses through the skin are particularly high in premature infants as the protective layer of the skin, the stratum corneum, is poorly developed. Evaporative losses in these babies may exceed urinary losses in the first few days of life, especially if the infant is cared for in a cold or draughty environment at low ambient humidity [1]. Allowance is made for additional losses when calculating daily water intake. Antidiuretic hormone levels are high in the first few days of life and maintenance requirement for water is low. Similarly, ADH levels remain elevated after surgery, and it is our practice to restrict fluids to 50–60 per cent of maintenance in the initial 24–48 hours after surgery. For surgery in the first few days of life there is no need

to restrict fluids further on top of the restrictions already in place. Fluid balance and electrolytes should be checked 12-hourly to determine subsequent fluid requirements. The sodium requirements in the first few days of life are low and 10 per cent dextrose or 4 per cent dextrose, 0.18 per cent saline is used initially for maintenance. However, gastrointestinal losses should be replaced with 0.9 per cent saline millilitre for millilitre; only isotonic fluids should be used for correction of hypovolaemia. Colloids (gelatins, albumin, blood, depending on requirements and local preference) may be used to replace third-space losses, which may be significant, for example, following placement of an abdominal wall silo in a neonate with gastroschisis.

FLUID RESUSCITATION: SHOCK

Shock occurs when perfusion is inadequate to metabolic demands of the tissues. Common causes of shock in children presenting for surgery include gastrointestinal losses, peritonitis and haemorrhage, for example caused by intussusception, appendicitis, volvulus, trauma or occasionally pyloric stenosis. The clinical signs of shock in a child include tachycardia, cool peripheries, delayed capillary refill and reduced volume pulses. More worrying signs suggesting decompensated shock are hypotension, mottling and confusion. Immediate management should be according to standard APLS guidelines with assessment of the airway, administration of high-flow oxygen and an isotonic crystalloid fluid bolus of 20 mL/kg. Clinical signs should be reassessed and the fluid bolus repeated if required. The choice of further fluid management depends on the clinical situation, and can be with crystalloid, colloid, blood or 4.5 per cent albumin in sepsis.

DEHYDRATION

Dehydration and shock may occur independently of each other or may coexist. Shock implies an acute reduction in circulating volume and dehydration loss of fluid from all fluid compartments, occurring over a period of time, possibly associated with electrolyte abnormalities. Dehydration may occur due to abnormal renal losses of fluid, such as diabetic ketoacidosis or diabetes insipidus, or result from abnormal gastrointestinal losses such as pyloric stenosis or gastroenteritis. The severity of dehydration may be estimated from clinical signs, although these are not very reliable. Weight is a useful measure of severity of dehydration, although it is unusual to have a recent weight in a child who is acutely unwell, but it is also useful to monitor rehydration therapy. The type of dehydration (and therefore therapy) depends on the relative losses of sodium and water. If water and sodium are lost in equal amounts, isonatraemic dehydration will result – this is the most common form of dehydration. If sodium is lost in excess of water, or excessive electrolyte-free water is given as treatment, hyponatraemic dehydration will occur; if water is lost in excess of sodium, hypernatraemic dehydration occur.

Table 4.14   Clinical signs of dehydration

Degree of dehydration	Mild	Moderate	Severe
Weight loss (%)	5	10	15
Volume of deficit (mL/kg)	50	100	150
Clinical state	Not unwell	Apathetic, unwell	Usually shocked
Pulse	Normal	Tachycardia	Tachycardia
Capillary refill (s)	<2	2–4	>4
Anterior fontanelle	Normal	Normal	Sunken
Tears	Present	Decreased	Absent
Eyes	Normal	Sunken	Deeply sunken
Mucous membrane	Normal	Dry	Parched
Skin	Normal	Reduced turgor	Doughy
Mental state	Normal	Lethargic	Unresponsive
Blood pressure	Normal	Normal	Reduced
Urine specific gravity	>1.020	>1.020	Oliguric or anuric

Table 4.14 illustrates clinical signs as a guide to assess dehydration, although, if losses are rapid and severe, shock may be the presenting sign and in hypernatraemic dehydration the clinical signs may underestimate the fluid deficit [69].

PYLORIC STENOSIS

In pyloric stenosis, the primary fluid lost gastric acid, which contains a high concentration of hydrogen, chloride and sodium ions. Early diagnosis may not be associated with any electrolyte disturbance – continued vomiting results in the classic picture of hypochloraemic and hypokalaemic metabolic alkalosis and dehydration. The plasma sodium may be normal, high or low. Correction of dehydration, acid–base and electrolyte disturbance is important prior to surgery, in particular the metabolic alkalosis as the baby will otherwise be prone to postoperative apnoeas. Mild dehydration may be corrected over 6–12 hours but severe electrolyte disturbances may require correction over 36–72 hours. If the baby is shocked they should receive an initial rapid bolus of 20 mL/kg 0.9 per cent saline. The fluid deficit should be estimated and given in addition to maintenance fluid, the choice of fluid (either 5 per cent dextrose, 0.9 per cent saline or 5 per cent dextrose, 0.45 per cent saline) depending on the initial electrolytes and the duration of dehydration (slow rehydration in hypernatraemic dehydration). Potassium should be added once the baby is passing urine. Fluid balance and electrolytes should be monitored until the target electrolyte balance is achieved: surgery should not be undertaken until the chloride is at least 90 mmol/L and bicarbonate <26 mmol/L.

DIARRHOEAL DEHYDRATION

Diarrhoeal dehydration in children remains one of the leading causes of death in children worldwide. Children with mild-to-moderate dehydration should be treated with oral rehydration solution (ORS) administered in small volumes orally or via a nasogastric tube. Rehydration solutions containing glucose and sodium are particularly effective, as transport of sodium (and water) is coupled with glucose in the small intestine. The standard World Health Organization (WHO) ORS contains sodium 90 mmol/L and glucose 111 mmol/L (osmolarity 311 mosm/L). However, this has been associated with hypernatraemia and reduced osmolarity solutions containing 45–75 mmol/L sodium may be preferable [70]. If the child is severely dehydrated (>10 per cent), they should receive intravenous rehydration with an initial 20 mL/kg bolus of isotonic fluid; the remaining fluid deficit should be replaced over 12–72 hours with 5 per cent dextrose, 0.45 per cent saline (isonatraemic dehydration), 5 per cent dextrose, 0.9 per cent saline (hyponatraemic dehydration) or 4 per cent dextrose, 0.18 per cent saline (hypernatraemic dehydration), ideally with electrolyte monitoring. Rapid rehydration must be avoided in chronic hypernatraemia or hyponatraemia to avoid osmotic demyelination and there is a concern about sodium overload in the treatment of shock in patients with severe malnutrition [71].

DIABETIC KETOACIDOSIS

Diabetic ketoacidosis (DKA) is the leading cause of morbidity and mortality in children with diabetes, with the majority of deaths resulting from cerebral oedema which occurs in 0.3–1 per cent of all episodes of DKA. Diabetic ketoacidosis is associated with hyperglycaemia, hyperosmolality and metabolic acidosis due to ketosis, which in turn lead to osmotic diuresis, severe dehydration and loss of electrolytes. Shock is rare in DKA, although the ECF volume may be significantly contracted.

Therapy in DKA is aimed at restoring circulating volume, replacing sodium and potassium, restoration of the ECF and ICF water deficit, and restoration of GFR to enhance clearance of glucose and ketones [72]. However, it should be remembered that DKA develops slowly over weeks, allowing physiological adaptation to take place, with movement of water from the ICF to the ECF to compensate for the osmotic disequilibrium. It is important that treatment is instituted slowly in order to prevent fluid shifts and the development of cerebral oedema. Risk factors for cerebral oedema are large volumes of hypotonic fluids, rapid changes in blood glucose and severe acidosis and dehydration at presentation. Children with severe DKA should be managed in an intensive care unit with hourly assessment of fluid, glucose and electrolyte balance. An initial fluid bolus of isotonic saline may be required, but should be limited to 7.5–10 mL/kg; fluid management should be conservative with dehydration corrected slowly over 48 hours with isotonic fluid only. Insulin should be given as a continuous infusion avoiding bolus administration [73].

NEUROSURGERY

Neurosurgical patients may suffer from a complex series of abnormalities affecting their sodium balance, which may occur alone or in combination, especially after procedures for hypothalamic–pituitary tumours: syndrome of inappropriate antidiuretic hormone secretion (SIADH), cerebral salt wasting (CSW), or transient or permanent diabetes insipidus (DI). Surgery may also interfere with the central osmoreceptors and thirst.

CENTRAL DIABETES INSIPIDUS

Central DI results from a deficiency in ADH, which may be caused by hypothalamic tumours such as craniopharyngiomas, infiltrative lesions such as Langerhans' cell histiocytosis, or destructive lesions, such as head injury or hypoxic brain injury. It is associated with polyuria with compensatory polydipsia provided that the thirst mechanism is intact, so that plasma osmolality is maintained. The child will develop hypernatraemic dehydration if access to adequate (hypotonic) fluid is restricted. It should be suspected in a neurosurgical patient who develops a urine output >5 mL/kg/h; the urine osmolarity is inappropriately low in the presence of high plasma osmolarity. The treatment of DI is desmopressin, starting with low doses and allowing breakthrough polyuria to obtain a picture of the requirement for desmopressin and avoid water intoxication with excessive doses.

SYNDROME OF INAPPROPRIATE ANTIDIURETIC HORMONE SECRETION AND CEREBRAL SALT WASTING

Syndrome of inappropriate ADH secretion may occur after neurosurgery, head injury, cerebral haemorrhage or meningitis, or in association with drugs such as carbamazepine. It is associated with reduced free-water clearance; the urine osmolarity is inappropriately high in the presence of low plasma osmolarity. The clinical picture is of ECF volume expansion with weight gain.

Cerebral salt wasting occurs under similar circumstances to SIADH and is difficult to differentiate from it;

however, treatments are radically different. Cerebral salt wasting is associated with a natriuresis and diuresis due to a number of potential natriuretic peptides, including atrial natriuretic peptide. As in SIADH, urine osmolarity is inappropriately high in the presence of low plasma osmolarity, but in CSW there is a contraction of the ECF volume with weight loss, elevated urea and haematocrit.

Treatment of hyponatraemia in SIADH is fluid restriction, unless associated with seizures or coma, in which treatment with 3 per cent saline is indicated, as described previously. Conversely, treatment of CSW is expansion of the ECF volume with isotonic saline to replace the deficit of sodium and water, using 3 per cent saline in the presence of severe symptomatic hyponatraemia. If it is not possible to differentiate between CSW and SIADH on clinical grounds, sodium supplements should be given and fluid intake maintained – central venous access may be required to estimate volume status [74].

REFERENCES

1. Modi N. Fluid and electrolyte balance. In: Rennie J, ed. *Roberton's textbook of neonatology*, 4th edn. Edinburgh: Churchill Livingstone; 2005: 333–54.
2. Taylor D, Durwood A. Pouring salt on troubled waters. *Arch Dis Child* 2004; **89**: 411–14.
3. Simeoni U, Zetterstrom. Long-term circulatory and renal consequences of intrauterine growth restriction. *Acta Paediatr* 2005; **94**: 819–24.
4. Hartnoll G, Betreniuex P, Modi N. Randomised controlled trial of postnatal sodium supplementation on body composition in 25–30 weeks gestational age infants. *Arch Dis Child* 2000; **80**: F19–23.
5. Haycock G. Disorders of the kidney and urinary tract. In: Rennie J, ed. *Roberton's textbook of neonatology*, 4th edn. Edinburgh: Churchill Livingstone; 2005: 929–44.
6. Moritz ML, Ayus JC. Preventing neurological complications from dysnatraemias in children. *Paediatr Nephrol* 2005; **20**: 1687–1700.
7. Shafiee MA, Bohn D, Hoorn EJ, Halperin ML. How to select optimal maintenance intravenous fluid therapy. *Q J Med* 2003; **96**: 601–10.
8. Adrogué HJ, Madias NE. Hyponatraemia. *N Engl J Med* 2000; **342**: 1581–4.
9. Reynolds R, Padfield P, Seckl J. Disorders of sodium balance. *BMJ* 2006; **332**: 702–5.
10. Armour A. Dilutional hyponatraemia: a cause of massive fatal intraoperative cerebral oedema in a child undergoing renal transplantation. *J Clin Pathol* 1997; **50**: 444–6.
11. Hoorn EJ, Geary D, Robb M *et al.* Acute hyponatraemia related to intravenous fluid administration in hospitalised children: an observational study. *Pediatrics* 2004; **113**: 1279–84.
12. Hanna S, Tibby SM, Murdoch IA. Incidence of hyponatraemia and hyponatraemic seizures in severe respiratory syncytial virus bronchiolitis. *Acta Paediatr* 2003; **92**: 430–4.

13. Way C, Dhamrait R, Wade I, Walker I. Perioperative fluid therapy in children: a survey of current prescribing practice. *Br J Anaesth* 2006; **97**: 371–9.

14. Choong K, Kho M, Menon K, Bohn D. Hypotonic versus isotonic saline in hospitalised children: a systematic review. *Arch Dis Child* 2006; **91**: 828–35.

15. Steele A, Gowrishankar M, Abrahamson S *et al*. Post-operative hyponatraemia despite near-isotonic saline infusion. A phenomenon of desalination. *Ann Intern Med* 1997; **126**: 20–5.

16. Moritz ML, Ayus JC. Disorders of water metabolism in children: hyponatraemia and hypernatraemia. *Pediatr Rev* 2002; **23**: 371–80.

17. Lin S-H, Hsu Y-J, Chiu J-S *et al*. Osmotic demyelination syndrome: a potentially avoidable disaster. *Q J Med* 2003; **96**: 935–47.

18. Coulthard MG, Haycock GB. Distinguishing between salt poisoning and hypernatraemic dehydration in children. *BMJ* 2003; **325**: 157–60.

19. Evans K, Greenberg A. Hyperkalaemia: a review. *J Intensive Care Med* 2005; **20**: 272–90.

20. Martyn JAJ, Richtsfeld M. Succinylcholine-induced hyperkalaemia in acquired pathologic states. *Anesthesiology* 2006; **104**: 158–69.

21. Girshin M, Mukherjee J, Clowney R, Wasnick J. The postoperative cardiovascular arrest in a 5-year-old male: an initial presentation of Duchenne's muscular dystrophy. *Pediatr Anesth* 2006; **16**: 170–3.

22. Iljima S, Uga N, Kawase Y, Tada H. Prophylactic calcium administration for hyperkalaemia in extremely low birth weight infants. *Am J Perinatol* 2005; **22**: 211–16.

23. Mahony BA, Smith WAD, Lo DS *et al*. Emergency interventions for hyperkalaemia. *Cochrane Database Syst Rev* 2005 Issue 2. Art no CD003235.DOI:1002/14651858. CD003235.pub2.

24. Advanced Life Support Group. Fluid and electrolyte management. In: Mackway-Jones K, Molyneux E, Philips B, Wieteska S, eds. *Advanced paediatric life support – the practical approach*, 4th edn. Oxford: Blackwell, 2005.

25. Gennan FJ. Hypokalaemia. *N Engl J Med* 1998; **339**: 451–9.

26. Welfare W, Sasi P, English M. Challenges in managing profound hypokalaemia. *BMJ* 2002; **324**: 269–70.

27. Umpaichitra V, Bastian W, Castellis S. Hypocalcaemia in children: pathogenesis and management. *Clin Pediatr* 2001; **40**: 305–12.

28. Aguilera I, Vaughan R. Calcium and the anaesthetist. *Anaesthesia* 2000; **55**: 779–90.

29. Shaw NJ, Bishop NJ. Biphosphonate treatment of bone disease. *Arch Dis Child* 2005; **90**: 494–9.

30. Train JJ, Yates R, Sury MJ. Lesson of the week: hypocalcaemic stridor and infantile nutritional rickets. *BMJ* 1995; **310**: 48–9.

31. Weisinger JR, Bellorin-Font E. Magnesium and phosphorus. *Lancet* 1998; **352**: 391–6.

32. Tong GM, Rude RK. Magnesium deficiency in critical illness. *Intensive Care Med* 2005; **20**: 3–17.

33. Dorman BH, Sade RM, Burnette JS *et al*. Magnesium supplementation in the prevention of cardiac arrhythmias in pediatric patients undergoing surgery for congenital heart defects. *Am Heart J* 2000; **139**: 522–8.

34. Holliday MA, Segar WE. The maintenance need for water in parenteral fluid therapy. *Pediatrics* 1957; **19**: 823–32.

35. Holliday MA, Friedman AL, Segar WE, Chesney R, Finberg L. Acute hospital-induced hyponatraemia in children: a physiologic approach. *J Pediatr* 2004; **145**: 584–7.

36. Brazel PW, McPhee IB. Inappropriate secretion of antidiuretic hormone in postoperative scoliosis patients: the role of fluid management. *Spine* 1996; **21**: 724–7.

37. Hongat JM, Murat I, Saint-Maurice C. Evaluation of current paediatric guidelines for fluid therapy using two different dextrose hydrating solutions. *Paediatr Anaesth* 1991; **1**: 95–100.

38. Neville KA, Verge CF, Rosenberg AR *et al*. Isotonic is better than hypotonic saline for intravenous rehydration of children with gastroenteritis: a prospective randomised study. *Arch Dis Child* 2006; **91**: 226–32.

39. Paul M, Dueck M, Herrmann J, Holzki J. A randomised controlled study of fluid management in infants and toddlers during surgery: hydroxyethyl starch 6 per cent (HES 70/0.5) vs. lactated Ringer's solution. *Paediatr Anaesth* 2003; **13**: 603–8.

40. Söderlind M, Salvignol G, Izard P, Lönnqvist PA. Use of albumin, blood transfusion and intraoperative glucose by APA and ADARPEF members: a postal survey. *Paediatr Anaesth* 2002; **11**: 685–9.

41. Bork K. Pruritis precipitated by hydroxyethyl starch: a review. *Br J Dermatol* 2005; **152**: 3–12.

42. Finfer S, Bellomo R, Boyce N *et al*. A comparison of albumin and saline for fluid resuscitation in the intensive care unit. *New Engl J Med* 2004; **350**: 2247–57.

43. Fan E, Stewart TE. Albumin in critical care: SAFE, but worth its salt? *Crit Care* 2004; **8**: 297–9.

44. Cooper DJ, Myles PS, McDermott *et al*. Prehospital hypertonic saline resuscitation of patients with hypotension and severe traumatic brain injury: a randomised controlled trial. *JAMA* 2004; **291**: 1350–7.

45. Roberts I, Alderson P, Bunn F *et al*. Colloids versus crystalloids for fluid resuscitation in critically ill patients. *Cochrane Database Syst Rev* 2004; **4**: CD000567.

46. Fencl V, Jabor A, Kazda A, Figge J. Diagnosis of metabolic acid-base disturbances in critically ill patients. *Am J Respir Crit Care Med* 2000; **162**: 2246–51.

47. Skellet S, Mayer A, Durwood A *et al*. Chasing the base deficit: hyperchloraemic acidosis following 0.9 per cent saline fluid resuscitation. *Arch Dis Child* 2000; **83**: 514–16.

48. Hatherill M, Salie S, Waggie *et al*. Hyperchloraemic acidosis following open cardiac surgery. *Arch Dis Child* 2005; **90**: 1288–92.

49. Scheingraber S, Rehm M, Sehmisch C, Finsterer U. Rapid saline infusion produces hyperchloraemic acidosis in patients undergoing gynecologic surgery. *Anesthesiology* 1999; **90**: 1265–70.

50. Wilkes N, Woolf R, Mutch M *et al*. The effects of balanced versus saline-based hetastarch and crystalloid solution on acid-base and electrolyte status and gastric mucosal perfusion in elderly surgical patients. *Anesth Analg* 2001; **93**: 811–16.

51. O'Malley C, Frumento R, Hardy M *et al*. A randomized, double-blind comparison of lactated Ringer's solution and 0.9 per cent NaCl during renal transplantation. *Anesth Analg* 2005; **100**: 1518–24.

52. Berleur M-P, Dahan A, Murat I, Hazebroucq G. Perioperative infusions in paediatric patients: rationale for using Ringer-lactate solution with low dextrose concentration. *J Clin Pharm Ther* 2003; **28**: 31–40.

53. Larsson LE, Nilsonn LE, Niklasson A *et al*. Influence of fluid regimens on perioperative blood glucose concentrations in neonates. *Br J Anaesth* 1990; **64**: 419–24.

54. Nilsonn K, Larsson LE, Andreasson S, Ekstrom-Jodal B. Blood glucose concentrations during anaesthesia in children. Effects of starvation and perioperative fluid therapy. *Br J Anaesth* 1984; **56**: 375–9.

55. Leelanukrom R, Cunliffe M. Intraoperative fluid and glucose management in children. *Paediatr Anaesth* 2000; **10**: 353–9.

56. Berry FA. Practical aspects of fluid and electrolyte therapy. In: Berry FA, ed. *Anesthetic management of difficult an routine pediatric patients*, 2nd edn. New York: Churchill Livingstone, 1990: 89–120.

57. Brandstrup B, Tønnesen H, Beier-Holgerson R *et al*. Effects of intravenous fluid restriction on postoperative complications: comparison of two perioperative fluid regimens. *Ann Surg* 2003; **238**: 641–8.

58. Kearney R, Mack C, Entwistle L. Withholding oral fluids from children undergoing day surgery reduces vomiting. *Paediatr Anaesth* 1998; **8**: 331–6.

59. Goodarzi M, Matar M, Shafa M *et al*. A prospective randomized blinded study of the effect of intravenous fluid therapy on postoperative nausea and vomiting in children undergoing strabismus surgery. *Paediatr Anaesth* 2006; **16**: 49–53.

60. Judd BA, Haycock GB, Dalton N, Chantler C. Hyponatraemia in premature babies and following surgery in older children. *Acta Paediatr Scand* 1987; **76**: 385–93.

61. Sterns RH, Silver SM. Salt and water: read the package insert. *Q J Med* 2003; **96**: 549–52.

62. Duke T, Molyneux E. Intravenous fluids for seriously ill children: time to reconsider. *Lancet* 2003; **302**: 1320–3.

63. Halberthal M, Halperin M, Bohn D. Acute hyponatraemia in children admitted to hospital: retrospective analysis of factors contributing to its development and resolution. *BMJ* 2001; **322**: 780–2.

64. Bohn D. Problems associated with intravenous fluid administration in children: do we have the right solutions? *Curr Opin Pediatr* 2000; **12**: 217–21.

65. Arieff AI, Ayus JC, Fraser CL. Hyponatraemia and death or permanent neurological damage in healthy children. *BMJ* 1992; **304**: 1218–22.

66. Hatherill M. Rubbing salt in the wound. *Arch Dis Child* 2004; **89**: 414–18.

67. Department of Health, Social Services and Public Safety Northern Ireland. Any child receiving prescribed fluids is at risk of hyponatraemia. http://www.dhsspsni.gov.uk (accessed 5.11.06).

68. Cunliffe M. Four and a fifth and all that. *Br J Anaesth* 2006; **97**: 274–77.

69. Ireland JD. Gastrointestinal disorders. In: Harrison V, ed. *Handbook of paediatrics for developing countries*. Cape Town: Oxford University Press, 2005: 206–23.

70. Hahn S, Kim Y, Garner P. Reduced osmolarity oral rehydration solution for treating dehydration due to diarrhoea in children: a systematic review. *BMJ* 2001; **323**: 81–5.

71. Molyneux E, Maitland K. Intravenous fluids – getting the balance right. *N Engl J Med* 2005; **353**: 941–4.

72. Dunger DB, Sperling MA, Acerini *et al*. ESPE/LWPES consensus statement on diabetic ketoacidosis in children and adolescents. *Arch Dis Child* 2004; **89**: 188–94.

73. Bohn D, Daneman D. Diabetic ketoacidosis and cerebral oedema. *Curr Opin Pediatr* 2002; **14**: 287–91.

74. Albanese A, Hindmarsh P, Stanhope R. Management of hyponatraemia in patients with acute cerebral insults. *Arch Dis Child* 2001; **85**: 246–51.

5

The liver and gastrointestinal tract

PETER BROMLEY, JAMES BENNETT

KEY LEARNING POINTS

Liver

- Coagulation factors are among the key proteins synthesised in the liver.
- The liver has a key role in the maintenance of plasma glucose levels.
- Liver disease varies depending whether it is acute or chronic.
- Acute liver disease typically causes hypoglycaemia, acidosis and raised intracranial pressure.
- Chronic liver disease typically causes portal hypertension.

Gastrointestinal tract

- The gastrointestinal tract has a complex interplay of autonomous function and regulation by hormones, neural input, and local chemical and electrical control.

- Normal digestion and absorption depends on proper motility, input of enzymes and other secretions, and a plethora of different absorptive processes.
- Disturbance of gastrointestinal tract function commonly causes dehydration, and electrolyte and acid–base abnormalities.
- Intestinal failure has many causes and has life-threatening consequences in addition to lack of nutrition, in particular liver disease, sepsis and loss of central venous access.

INTRODUCTION

The liver has many vital functions of which the anaesthetist has to be aware. Liver disease is not common in children, but its effects can so alter the physiology that an understanding of the topic is essential.

The objective of this chapter is to give the anaesthetist an overview of the anatomy and physiology of the liver and gastrointestinal tract relevant to the practice of paediatric anaesthesia, first in the normal healthy state, and then as it may be changed in the diseased condition, including the effects that may manifest as a result of conditions originating elsewhere. Also included are the effects that may appear in other organs and systems secondary to disease of the liver and gastrointestinal tract. The intention is not to replace or replicate the standard texts of anatomy and physiology to which the interested reader is referred for a more detailed account.

THE LIVER

Anatomy

The liver is a large organ, up to 5 per cent of the body weight of the term neonate, which declines towards 2 per cent of the adult weight. Its blood supply is large and is derived from the hepatic artery and the portal vein, together around 25 per cent of the cardiac output. Various factors change the relative proportion that the two supply, but if portal vein blood flow is reduced then hepatic artery blood flow increases to compensate (hepatic arterial buffer response), a finding that holds true even in the presence of cirrhosis [1].

Macroscopically the liver is made up of four lobes, the large right and left lobes and the smaller caudate and quadrate lobes. Functionally the liver comprises eight segments, each with its own branch of hepatic artery, portal vein, hepatic vein and bile duct, but in the human the boundaries of the lobes are not obvious to the observer, and there is quite a bit of variation in how the segments and their respective vessels and ducts are arranged, sometimes to the inconvenience of the surgeon who wishes to divide the liver in a segmental fashion. On a smaller scale the liver lobules are arranged around portal tracts, where the small branches of the artery, portal vein and bile duct run together. Blood passes along sinusoidal vessels from the portal tracts to the tributaries of the hepatic veins. There are usually three large veins, the right, middle and left hepatic veins, which after a short course open into the inferior vena cava. The sinusoids have large fenestrations to allow the liver cells to have access to the flow of plasma. The bile canaliculi are sealed off from the sinusoids by tight junctions between adjacent hepatocytes. The cells are arranged so that those hepatocytes carrying out metabolic processes which are the most oxygen dependent (gluconeogenesis, urea synthesis) are closest to the portal tracts; the cells can be divided into three zones having progressively lower oxygen tension nearer to the venules, where the less energy-dependent processes (glycolysis, liponeogenesis) occur [2].

Microscopically liver parenchyma comprises hepatocyte epithelial cells, stellate cells, Kupffer's cells and pit cells. Most of the functions generally thought of as carried out by the liver are performed by epithelial cells, which contribute about 60 per cent of the liver cells. The Kupffer cells are fixed macrophages; they are part of the reticuloendothelial system and are concerned with immunological functions. Stellate cells have also been known as lipocytes because of the large amount of fat that they store, but they also maintain the matrix of the liver and are much involved in the fibrosis that occurs in cirrhosis. The pit cells are natural killer cells which are important in protection from tumours [3].

The functions of the liver

The liver carries out many functions, which is one of the reasons why it has been so difficult to devise an artificial liver. Only an outline sketch of this enormous topic will be presented here, concentrating on those aspects where derangement of function leads to problems relevant to the anaesthetist. Broadly, liver functions may be classified under the headings below (Table 5.1).

PROTEIN SYNTHESIS

Albumin forms the largest proportion of the liver's protein output. It has a major contribution to plasma oncotic pressure and transports many substances in plasma, including drugs. Its weakly anionic properties make it a buffer for plasma

Table 5.1 Outline of the functions of the liver

Synthesis of proteins	Albumin
	Coagulation factors (except Factor VIII)
	Other 'transport' proteins
	Lipoproteins
Intermediary metabolism	Carbohydrate
	Fats
	Cholesterol and the steroid hormones
Catabolic	Deamination of proteins, formation of urea
	Breakdown of many hormones, formation of bile and bile salts
	Detoxification and excretion
Immunological	

acid–base balance. Despite this, low albumin concentration in itself causes only minor problems, although it may aggravate the troublesome consequences of altered physiology elsewhere, for example increasing the volume of ascites in portal hypertension. Serum albumin concentration is widely used as a measure of liver synthetic capacity, although, as the half-life is long (20 days), it is not very responsive.

Coagulation factors merit important consideration for the anaesthetist who has to care for a child with liver disease undergoing surgery. The liver synthesises all the coagulation factors except the von Willebrand fraction of factor VIII, which originates from vascular endothelium. Factors II, VII, IX and X require vitamin K for their synthesis and so are liable to fall if there is any biliary obstruction because the fat-soluble vitamin K will not be well absorbed unless fat in the gut is properly emulsified by bile salts. Classically, the coagulation cascade was described as having an intrinsic and an extrinsic pathway. It is now widely recognised that this is an over-simplification and that the whole process of clot formation *in vivo* is much more integrated. The traditional intrinsic/extrinsic model remains useful as it does explain the results of the commonly used tests of coagulation, the prothrombin time (PT) and activated partial thromboplastin time (APTT). Prothrombin time particularly is used to track liver synthetic capability. Factor V levels are also used for this purpose and since it has a rapid turnover and does not require vitamin K for its synthesis, it is not so influenced by biliary obstruction. Fibrinogen levels are generally preserved unless there is excessive consumption.

Low levels of clotting factors will eventually lead to coagulopathy. However, there is a considerable margin available in the normal levels of clotting factors before prolongation of the commonly used tests becomes detectable, and still more before bleeding problems become clinically apparent. Patients can therefore have advanced liver disease without significant coagulopathy, particularly if the disease is chronic and secondary to cholestasis, when synthetic function is often preserved until the end-stage.

ROLE OF THE LIVER IN INTERMEDIARY METABOLISM

The liver has a fundamental role in the regulation of many aspects of metabolism.

Carbohydrate and fats

The liver is crucially important in glucose homeostasis. In response to falling blood glucose levels and mediated by glucagon, the liver generates and releases glucose by glycogenolysis. The activity of the enzyme catalysing this reaction, phosphorylase, is also promoted by stimulation of β_2-adrenergic receptors and many other hormones have regulatory effects [4]. Only about one-quarter of the body store of glycogen is in the liver. Most is in muscle but is only available for local use as muscle lacks the glucose-6-phosphatase (present in liver cells) needed to convert glucose-6-phosphate (G6P) into glucose. Glycogen stores may be low in disease states or exhausted after a period of starvation, and gluconeogenesis may occur from protein or fat catabolism. If glucose demand cannot be met from glycogen then ketone bodies are generated in the liver from fatty acids generated by lipolysis. The organs take some time to adapt to utilising ketone bodies and so the predominant initial substrate for gluconeogenesis is protein. Clearly, it is not in the organism's interests to lose too much protein and so later fat is the major substrate. In liver disease serum glucose levels may not be maintained because of reduced insulin breakdown, the excess insulin thereby inhibiting gluconeogenesis.

When glucose levels rise, insulin promotes the uptake of glucose into the liver and muscle, and the formation of glycogen. Fatty acids are synthesised and esterified to triglyceride in the liver, and transported to adipose tissues as very low-density lipoprotein (VLDL).

Cholesterol

The major site of cholesterol synthesis is in the liver, although appreciable amounts can be derived from the diet, which can greatly reduce the amount that the liver synthesises [5]. Cholesterol and its derivatives are ubiquitous in animal cells as structural lipids in cell membranes, and the steroids are all derived from it. Lipids including cholesterol are hydrophobic and are transported in plasma in lipoproteins, the protein components of which (apoproteins) are also made in the liver. There are various types of lipoprotein: chylomicrons, VLDL, low-density lipoprotein (LDL), high-density lipoprotein (HDL), and so on. These lipid–protein complexes vary in the types and proportions of lipid that they transport, and the protein parts regulate the entry and exit of lipids at particular target sites.

The steroid derivatives include glucocorticoids, mineralocorticoids, the sex hormones and vitamin D. It is obvious that disruption of the levels of any of these can have far-reaching effects.

Bile salts are also cholesterol derivatives. These are the sodium or potassium salts of bile acids (chenodeoxycholic and cholic acid) conjugated to glycine or taurine and excreted in bile. They emulsify fats and form micelles in the gut lumen. Failure of emulsification results in fat appearing in the faeces (steatorrhoea), and fat-soluble vitamins A, D, E and K are not absorbed – the earliest consequence of this is coagulopathy. Vitamin K is not stored and cannot be synthesised by humans, although it is synthesised by colonic bacteria and it may be absorbed from there. Neonates do not have a developed colonic flora and haemorrhagic disease of the newborn may result. Bile salts are extensively reabsorbed in the terminal ileum and recirculated, typically many times in a day, both in their original form and altered by gut flora.

Protein catabolism and the urea cycle

The liver is the major site of protein catabolism. The products of protein breakdown, the amino acids, cannot be stored; they must be used directly for protein synthesis, or deaminated by aminotransferases and used to produce glucose (or fed into the glycolytic pathway or citric acid cycle), ketones or fatty acids. The product of deamination, the ammonium ion, is converted into urea. Accumulation of ammonia is toxic and contributes to the raised intracranial pressure and encephalopathy seen in acute liver failure. There are a few rare inborn errors of metabolism that can have the same effect, although a total failure of the urea cycle is incompatible with life.

Drug metabolism

The liver is the major site of drug metabolism. The role of the liver in regulating the processing and disposition of all the substances brought to it from the gut means that it will often have the systems that are needed to alter alien substances (xenobiotics), which may include drugs, administered by the gut or not, and sometimes having little resemblance to any naturally occurring substance. In many cases a general chemical route is followed which transforms the substance into a more polar and water-soluble form that is more readily excreted. These are the phase 1 and phase 2 reactions and are discussed in Chapter 9.

Phase 1 reactions

Phase 1 reactions are the result of electron transfers carried out by the cytochrome P450 enzymes, NADPH and NADPH–cytochrome c reductase, and cause oxidation by electron removal, or sometimes reduction by electron addition. Other types of phase 1 reaction such as hydrolysis of esters and amides, sulphation, dehalogenation, N-dealkylation, O-demethylation, etc., are all achieved by a similar mechanism. Cytochrome P450 (CYP) is a group of iron-containing enzymes bound to endoplasmic reticulum that are involved in many essential biological processes, as well as handling of xenobiotics. There are thousands of CYP variants found across all classes of organism, and they show considerable variation within the same species. The human has at least 57 CYP genes [6], which produce enzymes that can be classified according to the degree of amino acid homogeneity that they show. There are 18 (at least) families of them in humans, and they are named as 'CYP' plus a number, then a letter, then a final number (e.g. CYP2D6, which is the enzyme responsible for the metabolism of codeine). The relevance of this to the practising anaesthetist is that individuals will vary in the alleles in their genome that code for CYP enzymes (7 per cent of Caucasians have no CYP2D6), and this will lead to differences in drug handling. Furthermore, the activity of some of the enzymes can vary with age, and they are also susceptible to induction or inhibition by other drugs or even foodstuffs (e.g. grapefruit juice inhibits CYP3A4, which is responsible for the handling of nearly 50 per cent of all drugs). This all adds to a huge unpredictability in how drug handling might differ in the normal condition, let alone in the disease state. This restricts us to no more than very broad generalisations about how pharmacokinetics and pharmacodynamics may be affected in liver disease.

Phase 2 reactions

Phase 2 reactions are synthetic reactions in which a compound is conjugated with a substrate to form a more polar and water-soluble conjugate, for example a glucuronide, sulphate or acetylated derivative. Glucuronides are formed by the addition of an activated form of glucose (uridine diphosphate glucuronic acid, UDPGA) by the enzyme glucuronyl transferase. Glucuronides are readily excreted in urine or, especially in the case of larger compounds, in bile. Bilirubin is excreted in this way, but in the newborn the activity of glucuronyl transferase is low (but soon rises), and so a significant amount of haemolysis will overload the conjugating capacity of the enzyme and result in the accumulation of unconjugated bilirubin. It will similarly reduce the conjugation of other substances, slowing elimination and resulting in raised levels (e.g. chloramphenicol). The situation can be helped by inducing the enzyme with phenobarbital.

Pharmacokinetics: first–pass metabolism, protein binding and volume of distribution

The rate of clearance of drugs by the liver depends on the amount of a drug presented to it, the hepatic blood flow and the intrinsic ability of the liver to metabolise it. Drugs that have a high intrinsic clearance are subject to a high first-pass metabolism if given by the oral route as more or less all of the absorbed drug has to pass through the liver, and so systemic levels will be much lower for these drugs given orally compared with the parenteral route. For drugs that have a high intrinsic clearance, increasing clearance further, for example by enzyme induction, will have little effect on levels of drug given parenterally, but may decrease levels of orally administered drugs. Conversely, increased intrinsic clearance of a low extraction ratio drug will increase the clearance of the drug regardless of the route by which it is given.

Increasing liver blood flow will also have a different effect depending on route of administration and intrinsic clearance. For a drug that has a low clearance, increasing liver blood flow within the physiological range will not have much effect. For a high-extraction drug given orally, there will similarly be little effect, as most of it is cleared on the first pass anyway; however, more of the parenterally administered drug will be presented to the liver, so its clearance will increase [7].

Protein binding has a potentially large influence on the activity of a drug and its clearance. Protein binding is itself influenced by age and liver disease. For a drug that is highly protein bound, its free fraction, which is the fraction responsible for its biological effect, may be greatly increased by a small fall in protein binding; for example, if protein binding falls from 98 per cent to 96 per cent, the free fraction will double from 2 per cent to 4 per cent. This may double its biological effect, and may also increase the volume of distribution, as high protein binding tends to inhibit the movement of drug out of the plasma space.

Albumin levels are not so much affected by age, with adult levels being attained within the first few months. However, these are reduced in liver disease and in the acute-phase response. α_1-Acid glycoprotein, which is important in the binding of basic drugs, is markedly reduced in the neonate, but rises in the acute-phase response. Enzyme activity tends to be lower in neonates, but then rises in children to higher than adult levels, before falling again towards puberty. Liver disease has a more unpredictable effect. Metabolising ability may be decreased or more normal depending on the enzyme system; oxidation reactions tend to be more affected than glucuronidation, for example. The situation is further complicated by the presence of portosystemic shunts in chronic liver disease, which may allow drugs to escape first-pass metabolism, greatly increasing the bioavailability of high-extraction drugs.

Liver function tests

SYNTHETIC FUNCTION

Coagulation: PT, APTT, fibrinogen. The clotting cascade and the effect of liver disease on it have already been reviewed. Prolongation of the clotting times is an indicator of hepatic epithelial cell dysfunction.

Albumin: this is a less sensitive test as the half-life of albumin is over 20 days, so levels fall slowly.

Pseudocholinesterase activity is sometimes measured as the enzyme is exclusively synthesised in the liver but again the half-life is long.

Liver enzymes: aspartate aminotransferase (AST), alanine aminotransferase (ALT), γ-glutamyltranspeptidase (γGT or GGT), alkaline phosphatase (ALP)

Aspartate aminotransferase is present in liver and muscle. It is found in both cytosol and mitochondria: the cytosolic form is concentrated in the portal areas, whereas the mitochondrial form is evenly distributed. It has a half-life of less than 20 hours.

Alanine aminotransferase is more specific for the liver. It is exclusively cytosolic. Its half-life is over 40 hours. It is said that the fact that AST is (partially at least) a microsomal enzyme means that it will rise fastest in conditions that cause cell death, for example with secondary deposits of tumours or with massive necrosis, whereas conditions that cause the cells to become 'leaky', for example viral hepatitis, will cause a relatively greater rise in ALT. This explanation is not entirely satisfactory as most AST is cytosolic, but it is true that a low (<1) AST:ALT ratio is a feature of hepatitis and that the ratio tends to rise above 1 when cirrhosis becomes established [8].

Both GGT and ALP are membrane bound and do not leak out of the damaged hepatocyte.

γ-glutamyltransferase is a marker of enzyme induction, and both GGT and ALP rise if there is biliary obstruction. Alkaline phosphatase is found in large amounts in bone, although this is a different isoenzyme that can be distinguished if necessary. Both these enzymes are age sensitive, with GGT and ALP being, respectively, up to three and five times the adult levels in the neonate. The levels of ALP fall to two or three times adult level in childhood and then rise again in puberty [9].

These characteristics mean that AST is the most sensitive indicator of liver cell damage (because of its shorter half-life) provided that there is not any doubt that it is of liver origin.

BILIRUBIN

Bilirubin originates in the reticuloendothelial system as a product of haem breakdown. It is sparingly soluble in water and in the blood is tightly bound to albumin. It is taken up in the liver and conjugated with glucuronide by UDP-glucuronyl transferase. In adults mainly diglucuronide is formed but in children relatively more monoglucuronide is formed. Conjugated bilirubin is excreted into the bile; there are tight junctions between hepatocytes and bile canaliculi, which in normal function prevent the reflux of any conjugated bilirubin back into plasma. In the gut conjugated bilirubin may be metabolised into urobilinogen by microbial activity. Some urobilinogen may be reabsorbed, and since it is quite water soluble, some may then be filtered through the glomerulus and appear in the urine.

Further investigations of liver disease, which may include other blood tests, microbiology or histopathology, ultrasound scans, radiology, isotope scans or other more invasive procedures, may be suggested by the putative diagnosis. These investigations are outside the scope of this chapter.

Table 5.2 Causes of acute liver disease in children (the list is not exhaustive)

Infective	Hepatitis viruses, HAV, HBV, 'seronegative' hepatitis, herpesvirus, echovirus, others
Metabolic	Galactosaemia, tyrosinaemia, haemochromatosis, fructose intolerance, Wilson's disease, mitochondrial disease
Autoimmune hepatitis	
Drugs and toxins	Valproate, isoniazid, paracetamol, carbamazepine
Ischaemia	Congenital heart disease, myocarditis, asphyxia, shock

HAV, HBV, hepatitis A and hepatitis B virus, respectively.

Liver disease

The features of liver disease depend on whether the presentation is acute or chronic, and on the precise aetiology. The features of liver disease in general will be reviewed (Table 5.2).

Acute liver failure

Acute (fulminant) liver failure is defined as hepatic necrosis in a previously normal liver leading to hepatic encephalopathy within 8 weeks of disease onset [10].

Acute liver failure in children is not common; it accounts for 10–15 per cent of presentations to specialist units in the UK. The incidence and aetiology vary with age; it is somewhat commoner in infants <1 year old, and these are more likely to have probable viral hepatitis where the agent is not discovered (non-A–G hepatitis), or certain inborn errors of metabolism (e.g. haemochromatosis, galactosaemia). Older children are more likely to have Wilson's disease, autoimmune hepatitis or cystic fibrosis, for example. Across all age ranges a high proportion (>30 per cent) have an indeterminate cause [11].

COAGULOPATHY

Abrupt loss of synthetic function will cause a coagulopathy. Often, however, prolongation of clotting times does not cause a bleeding tendency until the abnormality is marked. Because of this, and because coagulation provides a useful marker of the evolution of the liver problem, coagulopathy is often not corrected until it becomes dangerous, or a decision has been taken to transplant the liver. Both PT and APTT are affected. Fibrinogen levels usually take longer to respond. The platelet count tends to fall.

HYPOGLYCAEMIA

The central role of the liver in carbohydrate metabolism means that hypoglycaemia is common, occurs early and may be severe. Serum lactate levels rise as the liver fails to clear it, and a metabolic acidodis develops.

JAUNDICE

Jaundice may take a while to become apparent, but bilirubin levels will rise inexorably if there is no recovery. A variable fraction of the bilirubin may be conjugated depending on whether any liver cells retain conjugating capacity; usually it will be predominantly conjugated early on. Bilirubin levels rarely climb as high as those seen in chronic conditions, especially those with a biliary cause.

OTHER FINDINGS FROM LABORATORY INVESTIGATIONS

The serum transaminases are often very high initially. Falling levels may indicate recovery, or may be because most of the liver cells are already dead, so recovery must be corroborated by signs of improvement elsewhere (falling glucose requirement, shorter clotting times). The serum ammonia will be high ($>100\,\mu$mol/L).

ENCEPHALOPATHY

Encephalopathy will develop after a while. It is conventionally graded into four stages (Table 5.3) [10].

The progression of encephalopathy can be measured by electroencephalogram (EEG). The cause is not completely understood but raised ammonia levels certainly contribute, and there are features compatible with stimulation of central nervous system γ-aminobutyric acid (GABA) receptors. Sometimes an improvement can be obtained by giving the GABA antagonist flumazenil [12]. Increased levels of nitric oxide and short-chain fatty acids may also be involved [13]. Cerebral oedema usually aggravates the condition in stages III and IV (and may be the cause of death), but will probably not be present in the earlier stages. Some infants with metabolic disease present with convulsions.

CARDIOVASCULAR SYSTEM

Classically, patients develop a high cardiac output with a low or very low systemic vascular resistance from dilated peripheries and arteriovenous shunting [14]. There is often tachycardia. The picture closely resembles septic shock. Bradycardia and severe hypotension are late signs and these patients will suffer high mortality, although recovery or transplantation is still possible. Often the hyperdynamic circulation appears volume loaded (especially after resuscitation) but this may be appropriate. Pulmonary oedema is sometimes seen.

RENAL FUNCTION AND ELECTROLYTE IMBALANCE

Renal impairment is usual but may develop slowly or late. Prerenal failure may result from hypovolaemia due to bleeding or under-resuscitation, or there may be acute tubular necrosis or hepatorenal syndrome (see Chronic liver disease, below). Renal support may be required. Patients are generally too unstable for intermittent haemodialysis. Usually, if the liver function recovers (either the native liver or after successful transplantation) then renal function also recovers, although after liver transplantation nephrotoxicity from immunosuppressant agents may be a problem [15]. Electrolyte imbalance is often seen. There may be hyponatraemia or hypernatraemia, often consequent on the nature of fluids and diuretics administered. There is usually sodium and water retention from increased aldosterone and antidiuretic hormone activity. Potassium levels are usually low for the same reason unless there is haemolysis or renal failure. Hypocalcaemia and hypomagnesaemia are common.

SECONDARY INFECTION

Impaired liver function predisposes to infection. Grampositive bacteria from skin (staphylococci and streptococci) are frequent causes, but sepsis from other organisms, especially fungi, is common. Sepsis should always be considered if there is a sudden deterioration in condition, for example depressed conscious level or hypoglycaemia. Classic signs of infection may not be seen or may be masked by the sepsislike features of acute liver failure. Common foci are lungs or urinary tract, but there may be primary septicaemia or peritonitis [16].

TREATMENT AND CLINICAL COURSE

The liver has an enormous capacity to regenerate. In children the likelihood of spontaneous recovery is not easy to predict but in general is better for metabolic causes, if the biochemical mechanism can be controlled, for example by diet in galactosaemia. Viral hepatitis (except hepatitis A virus, HAV) does not have as good a prognosis, fewer than 50 per cent recovering without transplantation. In most cases, where liver regeneration occurs there will not be any long-term sequelae in the liver, and the effects in other systems will resolve. In patients who die from acute liver failure the cause is generally cerebral oedema or sepsis. Some patients succumb to a bleeding diathesis. The danger is not past the moment there is unequivocal evidence of liver

Table 5.3 Grades of hepatic encephalopathy

Stage I	Mild intellectual impairment, reversed sleep/awake cycle
Stage II	Drowsy, confused, mood swings
Stage III	Very drowsy, delirious, unresponsive to speech, hyperreflexia
Stage IV	Coma, decorticate → decerebrate

recovery; quite a few children die of brain-stem herniation or sepsis with a recovering liver.

The management is generally supportive [17]. The child often requires resuscitation from volume depletion and electrolyte disturbance, which may have occurred from reduced intake or vomiting. Glucose support is often needed, sometimes in large amounts. Vitamin K is usually given although there may not be much response if liver synthetic function is poor. Broad-spectrum antibiotics (including antifungals) should be given. Early transfer to a specialist centre is strongly recommended. Once the child has been resuscitated an improvement in some of the clinical parameters may be seen. It is important to come to a view early regarding the probability of spontaneous recovery, as the outcome from transplantation is better if the child is not in extremis, and once the decision to transplant has been taken there may well be a wait (longer for smaller children) before a suitable organ becomes available.

If there is a need for general anaesthesia then this must be undertaken cautiously. The child should be intubated for airway protection anyway if the grade of encephalopathy merits it. Conscious level may be markedly worsened on emergence from anaesthesia by an enhanced effect and duration of drugs. Moderate hyperventilation might be helpful in the short term to reduce intracranial pressure [18].

Nutritional support is considered important, although there is no consensus about how this should be achieved; a majority of centres use enteral feeding [19].

N-Acetylcysteine (NAC) has a well-established role in the treatment of acute liver failure due to paracetamol poisoning [20]. It is an antioxidant and is effective in mitigating the harmful effects of hepatotoxic substances in laboratory animals if given before the poison. Its use in non-paracetamol-induced liver failure is not so firmly established although it is widely used [21].

Haemorrhage into the gastrointestinal tract is a recognised threat and it is usual to give H_2-receptor blockers (ranitidine) and sucralfate to protect against this.

Chronic liver disease

Chronic liver disease (Table 5.4) generally results in cirrhosis. Mediators released from injured or dying hepatocytes promote fibrosis and regeneration. Activation of the hepatic stellate cell causes collagen production [22], and hepatocytes will tend to regenerate in nodules; these processes distort the liver architecture and cause cirrhosis. The result is much the same regardless of the aetiology of the liver disease. Cirrhosis impedes the flow of blood and bile through the liver, causing portal hypertension and cholestasis. Once the process is initiated it may continue even though the original noxious stimulus is no longer present.

JAUNDICE

Jaundice is a common reason for presentation but in compensated liver disease the child may appear quite well and

Table 5.4 Causes of chronic liver disease in children (the list is not exhaustive)

Biliary	EHBA, choledochal cyst, Alagille's syndrome, familial intrahepatic cholestasis, stones, prolonged parenteral nutrition
Hepatitis	Chronic infection with hepatitis viruses (not HAV), autoimmune, drugs
Metabolic	α_1-Antitrypsin deficiency, galactosaemia, fructosaemia, glycogen storage disease types III and IV, tyrosinaemia, haemochromatosis, Wilson's disease, cystic fibrosis, lipid storage disorders, urea cycle defects
Vascular	Budd–Chiari syndrome, veno-occlusive disease, ischaemia

EHBA, extrahepatic biliary atresia; HAV, hepatitis A virus.

not be jaundiced. Presentation may be because of hepatosplenomegaly, because the skin stigmata of liver disease are noticed, or because blood tests produce abnormal results. Sometimes the disease only comes to light because of bleeding (haematemesis or nosebleeds usually) or because of transformation to acute liver failure, as is common with Wilson's disease. If cirrhosis is established it tends to progress, and in time problems become more numerous and serious.

GROWTH FAILURE AND MALNUTRITION

The child will tend to trail down the growth centiles and show reduced lean mass and fat stores. This may be addressed by dietary advice, but later supplementary enteral feeding by tube will often need to be started. In advanced disease there may be a poor response to this. Vitamin supplements (A, D, E and K) are often given, but rickets is common and may be difficult to treat. Optimal nutrition for liver disease includes protein and carbohydrate provision in excess of normal maintenance amounts but the topic is complex (providing adequate protein without provoking encephalopathy, for example) and treatment should be carried out in a specialist centre [17].

PORTAL HYPERTENSION

Increased resistance to portal vein flow can have several consequences. Collateral circulations will tend to open up, causing umbilical veins to open and visible veins to radiate away from the umbilicus (caput medusae). Oesophageal and gastric varices may form which have the potential to bleed catastrophically. The back-pressure in the splenic vein may cause splenomegaly and hypersplenism leading to a pancytopenia, the thrombocytopenia aspect being potentially troublesome. Partly because of the increased hydrostatic pressure and partly because of reduced plasma oncotic pressure, ascites may form. If severe this can cause diaphragmatic splinting and respiratory difficulties, which can be further worsened by pleural effusion.

COAGULOPATHY

Synthesis of clotting factors is often fairly well preserved until the late stages of cirrhosis, so in quite advanced disease may still only be a slight prolongation of the clotting times. Nevertheless, there may be evidence of problems such as easy bruising and nosebleeds. Coagulation may quickly become significantly impaired if there is an episode of decompensation secondary to sepsis or bleeding, for example. Especially in biliary cirrhosis there may be impairment of the synthesis of anticoagulant proteins (protein C, protein S and antithrombin III) which may outweigh the reduction in levels of clotting factors and so 4 high resistance to portal vein flow, the flow pattern may become biphasic or reverse, and in these conditions portal vein thrombosis may occur and lead to a sudden worsening in condition.

ENCEPHALOPATHY

Encephalopathy is usually mild to start with, and may be difficult to detect in children. Difficulties at school or with sleep patterns may be the only signs. Worsening of encephalopathy can be precipitated by many factors: increased nitrogen load from the gut into the systemic circulation might be responsible and can occur from the formation of intrahepatic shunts or an increase in flow from the portal vein into collateral vessels, as well as from bleeding into the gut. Hypoglycaemia, electrolyte disturbance or sepsis can also lead to acute decompensation.

HEPATOPULMONARY SYNDROME

Hepatopulmonary syndrome (HPS) is seen fairly frequently in children. There is liver disease, arterial hypoxaemia and true intrapulmonary shunting. The hypoxaemia may be multifactorial, but there is ventilation/perfusion ($\dot{V}/\dot{Q}$) mismatch and new vessel formation in the lungs [23]. The shunting is worse in basal parts of the lung, where the blood flow is highest, and so lying the patient flat will divert some blood flow to more normal areas and improve the hypoxaemia. A ($\dot{V}/\dot{Q}$) mismatch will tend to respond to supplemental oxygen whereas true shunt will not, and this can be a useful bedside test of the relative contribution of the two. Other causes of potentially remediable hypoxia (e.g. large vessel shunts) need to be eliminated by cardiological assessment. Intrapulmonary shunting can be demonstrated by radiolabelled aggregated albumin scan or by agitated saline echocardiography, but while this may be useful for classification purposes it rarely alters management. The degree of hypoxaemia is not necessarily related to the severity of the liver disease, but may prove to be the most limiting problem for the patient. There is no specific therapy other than liver transplantation, which will usually reverse the changes, although this may take months. Acute deterioration can sometimes be treated with inspired nitric oxide [24].

PORTOPULMONARY HYPERTENSION

This rare condition is quite distinct from HPS; there may not be any hypoxaemia, and the cardinal feature is pulmonary hypertension. The condition carries a high (>50 per cent) mortality [25,26]. It may resolve after transplantation. In adults treatment has been attempted with long-term (months) intravenous prostacyclin infusions, or with the endothelin antagonist bosentan, with some evidence of efficacy. There are no comparable data for children.

HEPATORENAL SYNDROME

The hepatorenal syndrome (HRS) is a progressive deterioration in renal function (rising creatinine and declining glomerular filtration rate) in the setting of end-stage liver disease. It seems to be less common in children than in adults. The urinary sodium is low (<10 mmol/L) and the urine:plasma creatinine ratio is high (>40). There is oliguria. The mechanism is uncertain, but despite plasma volume being expanded there is renin–angiotensin activation, reduced renal blood flow, and high aldosterone and antidiuretic hormone activity. There is intense renal vasoconstriction and splanchnic vasodilatation. The patient tends to be hyponatraemic. The primary problem is in the circulation of the patient with liver disease, not in the kidneys; indeed, kidneys have been transplanted from patients with end-stage HRS and have functioned satisfactorily. Hepatorenal syndrome is divided into type 1 and type 2. Type 1 is more acute in onset, with a doubling of plasma creatinine in 2 weeks, whereas type 2 has a more insidious onset. The condition carries a high mortality. Volume expansion and dopamine infusions are not helpful. The only definitive treatment remains liver transplantation; if liver function is restored then the kidneys will recover. There may be a role for terlipressin infusion and regular albumin [27].

It should be remembered that other forms of renal failure are frequently found in patients with liver disease, and HRS remains a condition diagnosed by exclusion of other causes.

INFECTIVE COMPLICATIONS

Chronic liver failure predisposes to infection. Bacterial infection with a range of organisms frequently occurs in the respiratory and urinary tracts, and an obstructed biliary system is prone to cholangitis. Portal hypertension makes bacterial translocation from the gut more likely, and indwelling central venous lines are prone to becoming colonised. Spontaneous bacterial peritonitis is a threat and the diagnosis should be suspected in a sick child with ascites. Paracentesis should be carried out to allow antibiotic therapy to be directed against the causative organism.

The jaundiced baby

The jaundiced baby warrants a special mention because, unlike most forms of paediatric liver disease, it is common. Up to half of term babies are jaundiced in the first week, and possibly up to 20 per cent have a bilirubin >200 μmol/L. The characteristic of the so-called physiological jaundice is that bilirubin is unconjugated and that it resolves (or begins to) by 14 days [28]. The danger is that unconjugated bilirubin may diffuse into the central nervous system and cause direct toxic damage in specific areas, for example the basal ganglia (kernicterus), and cause movement disorders, learning disability and deafness. The mechanism is thought to be immaturity of the glucuronyltransferase conjugating enzyme, and possibly poor uptake of bilirubin by hepatocytes, and an increased bilirubin load because of shortened red cell life span. Treatment is not generally undertaken unless the bilirubin level is >300 μmol/L in the term baby or >200 μmol/L in the premature one, who are more vulnerable to the complications.

Jaundice prolonged beyond 14 days should be investigated. Breast-milk jaundice is an unconjugated hyperbilirubinaemia in an exclusively breast-fed baby, which may persist for a month or two. The cause is not known. The bilirubin should fall by 50 per cent within a few days of stopping breast-feeding. Conjugated hyperbilirubinaemia or pale (acholic) stools suggest liver disease. There are a large number of possible causes, most of them rare or very rare.

The neonatal hepatitis syndrome

Neonatal hepatitis syndrome (NHS) is a non-specific disorder that may result from a number of causes. Common features include jaundice, which may be mild at first, but the bilirubin is conjugated. There may be pale stools and dark urine, the baby is prone to hypoglycaemia, there is often hepatomegaly and the baby is often small for gestational age. Serum transaminase levels are generally raised, but there is not usually coagulopathy unless there is vitamin K deficiency.

The possible causes can be divided into broad groups as described in Table 5.5.

The management of these babies is essentially supportive with urgent efforts to establish the diagnosis, as specific treatments may be available, for example antimicrobials, surgical interventions, dietary manipulations, and so on. Nutritional support is important and should include supplementation of the fat-soluble vitamins. Liver transplantation may be necessary for some.

Specific conditions causing chronic liver disease

The management of these children is a specialist task, which is not within the scope of a general text like this; however, a

Table 5.5 Causes of the neonatal hepatitis syndrome (NHS)

Infective	'TORCH' (*Toxoplasma*, rubella, cytomegalovirus, herpes simplex) infections. Cytomegalovirus is the commonest of these to cause NHS
	Varicella
	Paramyxovirus (giant cell hepatitis)
	Enteric virus (echovirus, Coxsackie, adenovirus)
Endocrine	Hypothyroidism
Cholestatic conditions	Biliary atresia, choledochal cyst, Alagille's syndrome, parenteral nutrition
Metabolic	α_1-Antitrypsin deficiency
	Cystic fibrosis
	Galactosaemia
	Tyrosinaemia, etc.
Autoimmune	Neonatal lupus

brief indication of the particular features of the commoner conditions is offered below.

α_1-ANTITRYPSIN DEFICIENCY

α_1-Antitrypsin deficiency commonly presents in the neonatal period. Although many (30 per cent) recover completely, some develop chronic liver disease in childhood. The normal protein (PiM) protects the lung from neutrophil elastase. An abnormal protein (of which there are several types) can fold and be retained in the liver. The commonest in the UK is the PiZZ genotype. Lung problems do not occur in childhood. The only treatment is supportive or liver transplantation [29].

WILSON'S DISEASE

Wilson's disease is an abnormality of copper metabolism, an abnormal copper-handling enzyme in the hepatocyte causes failure of normal copper excretion and transportation, leading to toxic copper deposition in various tissues including in the liver itself. It may present after age 3 years with an acute or chronic liver disease, or with neurological or psychiatric problems. Penicillamine chelates copper and can successfully treat some patients (zinc and pyridoxine are also given); others need transplantation [30].

CYSTIC FIBROSIS

Cystic fibrosis typically causes liver disease in older children. The liver disease itself can cause problems with portal hypertension or decompensation, or the malnutrition and susceptibility to infection resulting from the liver disease can worsen the respiratory problems to the extent that liver transplantation is justified; it is often well tolerated and produces improvement in respiratory function and quality of life, although heart/lung/liver transplantation may be needed for some [17].

AUTOIMMUNE HEPATITIS

Autoimmune hepatitis is the commonest cause of liver disease in older children. Most children (>80 per cent) respond to immunosuppression with prednisolone or azathioprine. There are immunological similarities to sclerosing cholangitis and many patients are now ascribed to 'overlap syndrome' [31].

BILIARY HYPOPLASIA DISORDERS

The biliary hypoplasia disorders are reviewed in Chapter 41.

THE GASTROINTESTINAL TRACT

The gastrointestinal tract is perhaps not accorded as much importance in the minds of many anaesthetists as it deserves. It may be that the physiology and pharmacology of the cardiovascular, respiratory and renal systems have a much more immediate relevance in our daily work, but the gastrointestinal tract has such a great influence on the survival and well-being of the organism that our interest should extend a little beyond the recommended starvation times before anaesthesia.

This account will provide an overview of the functioning of the normal gastrointestinal tract, and at the relevant point briefly describe the features of some of the commoner disorders in children, concentrating on those that most often present to the anaesthetist.

The gastrointestinal tract extends from mouth to anus. There are, of course, huge structural and functional differences between the various parts of the gastrointestinal tract but there are some features that are common to many parts, particularly to do with the regulation of the whole organ system.

Regulation: hormones, nerves and smooth muscle cells

The full details of the regulation of the gastrointestinal tract are not known. All the gastrointestinal tract hormones are peptides, and they may be described as endocrine, paracrine or neurocrine depending on the method by which the peptide reaches its target site. An endocrine is released into the general circulation, and so usually exerts its effects remote from the site of its release. Its effects are not a property of the compound itself but depend on the specificity of its receptor at the target. A paracrine diffuses through the extracellular space and so has its effect close to the point of its release. A neurocrine is released from a nerve ending and diffuses across the very short distance of the synaptic gap, and so is a neurotransmitter. Not all neurotransmitters are peptides.

Two of the gastrointestinal tract hormones (gastrin and secretin) were the first to be discovered. The gastrointestinal tract hormones are released into the portal circulation, pass through the liver and back to the gastrointestinal tract via the systemic circulation. They regulate its movements and secretions, and the growth of various parts. There are five peptides that are recognised as 'full' gastrointestinal tract hormones: gastrin, secretin, cholecystokinin (CCK), gastric inhibitory peptide (GIP) and motilin. Many others are known as candidate hormones because they have not been fully characterised or their actions established.

Gastrin is found in the antrum of the stomach and to a lesser extent in the duodenum. Its release is stimulated by distension and protein, and directly by neural stimulation. It promotes acid secretion and mucosal growth. Acid inhibits the release of gastrin.

Secretin is found in the duodenum. Its release is stimulated by acid, and to a lesser extent by fat. It promotes the secretion of bicarbonate in the bile and pancreatic juice, and is a pancreatic growth factor. It inhibits acid secretion.

Cholecystokinin is found in the duodenum, jejunum and ileum. It is released by protein and fat. It promotes bicarbonate secretion by the pancreas, and the secretion of pancreatic enzymes, and is a pancreatic growth factor. It stimulates gallbladder contraction and delays gastric emptying.

Gastric inhibitory peptide is found in the duodenum and jejunum. It is released by protein, fat and carbohydrate. It enhances the release of insulin and inhibits acid secretion.

Motilin is also found in duodenum and jejunum and its release is principally under neural control. It promotes gastric and intestinal motility.

Most gastrointestinal tract hormones can exist in two or more forms.

Paracrines are are more difficult to study than endocrines because their effects cannot be correlated with changes in blood levels. Somatostatin functions to inhibit gastrin release and gastric acid secretion. Histamine is released by gastrin and promotes acid secretion by parietal cells. It also potentiates the effect of gastrin and acetylcholine (ACh) on acid production; hence the H_2-receptor blockers reduce gastric acid secretion.

Neurocrines known to have a physiological role in the gut are vasoactive intestinal peptide (VIP), gastrin releasing peptide (GRP) and the enkephalins leu-enkephalin and met-enkephalin. Vasoactive intestinal peptide causes the relaxation of gut smooth muscle by promoting the production of nitric oxide, and so may also be important in local vasodilatation. Gastrin-releasing peptide is found in gastric mucosa, is released by vagal activity and promotes gastrin release. The enkephalins act on opiate receptors and cause contraction of the lower oesophageal, pyloric and ileocaecal sphincters, and reduce intestinal secretion. They slow transit time and may be involved in the regulation of peristalsis.

The gastrointestinal tract is under the neural control of the intrinsic and extrinsic autonomic nervous systems. The extrinsic system is the familiar sympathetic/parasympathetic system. The intrinsic system consists of several distinct networks of nerves, such as the myenteric and submucosal plexus. The intrinsic autonomic system uses many neurotransmitter compounds, and acetylcholine, serotonin, VIP and somatostatin have all been found in intrinsic interneurons. Acetylcholine and substance P have been mapped to excitatory neurons, and VIP and NO to inhibitory ones. Both intrinsic and extrinsic systems provide numerous afferent pathways to supply sensation and responsiveness. The contractile tissues of the gastrointestinal tract are (voluntary sphincters aside) smooth muscles. The contractions of smooth muscle can be phasic, lasting a few seconds, or tonic, sustained for much longer. These contractions can occur without any neurohumoral input and are a property of the cells themselves, although the periodicity and strength of contraction can be modulated.

Swallowing

Swallowing is initiated voluntarily, but, once initiated, the process proceeds as a reflex. Relaxation of the upper oesophageal sphincter, peristalsis down the oesophagus and relaxation of the lower oesophageal sphincter (LOS) are coordinated from the brain stem. The LOS is a zone of smooth muscle not discernible anatomically, but for a variable length from a few millimetres to several centimetres the pressure in the lumen is 20–40 mmHg higher than on either side. Resting tone is increased by cholinergic agents and gastrin, and decreased by isoprenaline and prostaglandin E_1. Relaxation is mediated through intrinsic nerves which may use VIP or NO.

Gastro-oesophageal reflux is common in infants less than 6 months old. It is due not so much to low LOS tone but more to transient relaxation, which may be a result of postural problems, gastric distension or liquid diet. Reflux can cause oesophagitis, and be the cause of respiratory problems such as apnoeas, laryngitis, recurrent pneumonitis and asthma. In older children it may frequently complicate cerebral palsy, Down syndrome or head injury [32,33].

Gastric secretion

The important constituents of gastric juice are acid, pepsin, intrinsic factor and mucus. The proximal 80 per cent of the stomach (the fundus and body) contain oxyntic glands at the base of pits in the mucosa. In the glands, parietal cells produce acid and chief cells produce pepsinogen. Mucus-producing cells are found towards the neck of the pits. Parietal cells secrete hydrogen ions by an energy-dependent H^+/K^+ pump. Pure parietal cell secretion can contain up to 150 mmol H^+. Acid secretion is promoted by gastrin and histamine. Both acid secretion and histamine release are triggered by ACh from postganglionic, muscarinic, cholinergic nerves. Pepsinogens are precursor molecules which are cleaved into active pepsin in an acid environment.

Pepsin breaks internal peptide links in protein to begin the digestive process. Mucus is secreted in two forms, soluble and insoluble. Soluble mucus mixes with and lubricates gastric contents. Insoluble mucus forms a protective alkaline layer protecting the stomach between meals. Parietal cells also secrete intrinsic factor, a large mucoprotein that combines with vitamin B_{12} and is essential for the absorption of vitamin B_{12} in the ileum. Gastric secretion is under complex control; it is promoted by the thought of food, gastric distension and the presence of digestive products, as well as neurohumoral influences previously described. It is inhibited by somatostatin, secretin, GIP and nervous reflexes from the duodenum in response to gastric emptying.

Gastric emptying

Emptying is accomplished by muscular contractions of longitudinal, circular and oblique layers of muscle in the stomach wall. Not all contractions are peristaltic; some are retropulsive and enhance mixing in the stomach. The nature and pattern of the contractions depend on the digestive state; liquids are cleared rapidly and solids more slowly. The rate of emptying is slowed by neurohumoral responses triggered by the presence of digestive products in the duodenum, (particularly acid, fatty acids and a hyperosmolar solution), to prevent the digestive capacity from being overwhelmed. Muscular contractions of the various regions of the stomach are coordinated by waves of depolarisation that spread through it. The speed and force of the contraction can be modulated as required, but generally they start slowly and weakly in the proximal part and become faster and stronger towards the pylorus.

Digestion

The assimilation of food takes place primarily in the small intestine. The surface area is greatly increased by folding and the presence of villi, and microvilli on the enterocytes themselves, which form the 'brush border'. There are tight junctions between enterocytes forming a barrier between the gut lumen and the extracellular space adjacent to the enterocytes, bordered by the basolateral membrane. The principal cell types are enterocytes, which carry out the digestive and secretory functions, and goblet cells, which secrete mucus. Digestion partly takes place in the gut lumen where food is broken down by digestive enzymes secreted by salivary glands, stomach and pancreas, and partly by membrane-bound enzymes in the microvilli. Digestive products are taken into the enterocyte by passive diffusion, facilitated diffusion or active transport.

CARBOHYDRATES

In the western diet about half the carbohydrate (CHO) intake is starch, one-third is sucrose and the rest comprises lactose, maltose and others. Starches are broken down by α-amylase in salivary and pancreatic secretions. The yield is a series of different oligosaccharides. These are broken by a series of different membrane-bound disaccharidases (glucoamylase, sucrase, isomaltase, etc.) which yield the basic hexose sugars glucose, galactose and fructose. There is quite a large redundancy in disaccharidase activity so the rate-limiting step is the absorption of the hexoses. Glucose and galactose are transported by an active carrier (SGLT-1), while fructose is absorbed by facilitated diffusion [34]. Inherited defects of carbohydrate absorption are rare; however, acquired lactase deficiency is fairly common. Lactase activity usually declines after infancy in all except those of European ancestry, but lactase activity is lower than that of other disaccharidases and is concentrated near the tips of the villi, which are most vulnerable to damage from inflammation or ischaemia. Insufficiency leads to bloating and, at worst, an osmotic diarrhoea [35].

PROTEINS

Protein digestion starts with pepsin in the stomach. As chyme leaves the stomach CCK and secretin stimulate the release of bicarbonate and enzymes from the pancreas. Pancreatic enzymes are secreted as inactive precursors. Trypsinogen is converted to the active trypsin by enterokinase located on the intestinal brush border. Trypsin then activates other precursor enzymes, including more trypsinogen and chymotrypsinogen; however, the exact mechanism for the activation of some of the other enzymes (elastase, carboxypeptidases, etc.) is more complicated, involving a sequence of several steps. The absorption of the resulting amino acids or small peptides is complex. Some groups of amino acids compete for shared carriers which are energy dependent and require a sodium gradient, while others do not. There are rare inherited disorders of amino acid absorption affecting classes of amino acids that share a transporter, such as Hartnup's disease (neutral amino acids) and cystinuria (basic amino acids).

LIPIDS

There is no significant fat absorption in the stomach. In the duodenum bile is added, containing lecithin and bile salts, which emulsifies fats. Pancreatic lipase, phospholipase A_2 and cholesterol esterase then break down the various dietary lipids. Bile salts, above a critical concentration, form micelles; these are small aggregates of fat with a hydrophilic exterior, which are much smaller than emulsified fat droplets (3–10 nm versus 200–5000 nm). Micelles are not absorbed entire but they allow fats to pass easily through the aqueous 'unstirred' layer next to the microvilli from where the fats can be absorbed, mainly by diffusion. Within the cell lipids can be assembled back into triglycerides in the endoplasmic reticulum. Some glycerol and free fatty acids pass directly into capillaries, but triglycerides, phospholipids, fat-soluble vitamins and cholesterol esters are packaged with apoproteins into chylomicrons, which are exported from the cell by exocytosis into lacteals, then into the circulation via the thoracic duct, and eventually are taken up by the liver. Lipid malabsorption is most often the result of exocrine pancreas insufficiency or cholestasis. Steatorrhoea can lead to failure to thrive, coagulopathy or deficiency of the other fat-soluble vitamins.

The commonest causes of pan-malabsorption are cystic fibrosis [36] or the result of widespread mucosal damage, such as may occur as a result of coeliac disease or the inflammatory bowel diseases [37,38].

Fluid and electrolyte absorption

A huge amount of water goes into the gastrointestinal tract every day: in the adult about 9 L (2 L from diet, 1 L saliva, 2 L gastric juice, 2 L pancreatic juice, 1 L bile and 1 L small intestinal secretions). Only about 100 mL water is normally lost in faeces. Most of the water is reabsorbed because of the movement of ions and solutes from the gut lumen into blood. The osmolarity of gut contents is usually similar to that of plasma until the distal colon, where the osmolarity is 350–400 mosm/L. In the duodenum, the sodium concentration is similar to plasma, and the major anion is chloride. Sodium concentration falls progressively, to 125 mmol/L in the ileum and 35 mmol/L in the colon. Potassium concentration rises from the serum level to 9 mmol/L in the ileum to 90 mmol/L in the colon, where it is actively secreted. Chloride is retained avidly in exchange for bicarbonate. In the event of excessive fluid loss from the colon the major ions lost are therefore potassium and bicarbonate (but not in the case of secretory diarrhoea, when large amounts of chloride can be lost). Fluid losses originating from more proximal parts of the gut will contain proportionally more sodium and chloride.

Sodium is absorbed from the lumen by several mechanisms: by restricted diffusion through water-filled paracellular channels, by cotransport with solutes such as glucose or amino-acids, by exchange for hydrogen ions or by cotransport with chloride. The Na^+/K^+-ATPase pump maintains a low intracellular sodium, so sodium is always absorbed along its concentration gradient. The serosal side of the cell is weakly positively charged compared with the gut lumen, so chloride continually moves out of the lumen, whereas potassium leaks into it. Chloride is also moved into the cell against both electrical and concentration gradients by cotransport with sodium and in exchange for bicarbonate. In the colon chloride can be secreted into the lumen by a cAMP/calcium-dependent mechanism. Usually this is not active but cholera toxin can greatly elevate intracellular cAMP and cause profuse chloride loss (secretory diarrhoea). Water absorption follows an osmotic gradient as solutes and ions are absorbed. The colon is sensitive to aldosterone and the sodium content of faecal water can fall from 30 mmol/L to 2 mmol/L, and the potassium concentration rise from 75 mmol/L to 150 mmol/L.

OTHER IONS

Calcium is taken up in the proximal small intestine. The amount absorbed is increased by vitamin D through an incompletely understood mechanism. Since intracellular free calcium levels have such a profound effect on the workings of the cell, there is a binding mechanism to prevent this. Calcium is secreted from the cell across the basement membrane by an energy-dependent process.

Iron is also principally absorbed in the proximal small bowel. Body iron stores are tightly conserved and so the amount absorbed is usually low compared with the amount ingested. The enterocyte secretes a transferrin, which binds two iron molecules, and the complex is then absorbed by receptor-mediated endocytosis. Some iron is stored intracellularly bound to ferritin. Iron is exported from the cell bound to a different transferrin. If body iron stores are low then more iron receptors are generated on the brush border, and the intracellular storage of iron falls, promoting export into the circulation.

Small bowel motility

The small bowel musculature consists of an inner circular and outer longitudinal layer. The inner circular layer is the thicker. Both layers become thinner more distally. Like the stomach, small and large bowel smooth muscle cells exhibit regular slow-wave depolarisations, on top of which there may be spike potentials, which are required to produce a contraction, but can occur only in the plateau phase of the slow wave. In fasting conditions, periodic strong waves of contraction (the migrating motor complex, MMC) sweep the gut from stomach to rectum, helping to empty the proximal gut and keep bacterial counts there low [39]. Typically, MMCs occur every 90 minutes or so, and take about the same time to travel from stomach to terminal ileum. After feeding, contractions become much more frequent, but not so forceful. Segmentations are seen, which affect only a few centimetres of gut at a time, and which may be peristaltic for just a few centimetres. Movement of contents is generally from proximal to distal, but not as rapid or coordinated as in the MMC. The bowel contractions serve to mix the contents with digestive secretions and to stir the contents, maximising contact with the absorptive brush border. If a bolus is presented to the small bowel, the bowel at that point contracts, and the neighbouring distal segment relaxes, propelling the bolus forwards (the so-called peristaltic reflex). However, in normal conditions this reflex may not be so important. Intrinsic and extrinsic nerve plexus supply the small bowel, the most recognisable series being the myenteric or Auerbach plexus between the muscle layers. Plexal neurons receive input from the central nervous system via sympathetic and parasympathetic trunks, both preganglionic and postganglionic fibres. Many neurotransmitter substances have been identified in addition to noradrenaline and acetylcholine, including somatostatin,

CCK, substance P, enkephalins, neuropeptide Y, and so on. The interplay of endocrine, paracrine and neurogenic input modifies the patterns of motility that are observed.

Large bowel motility

In the large bowel the pattern of muscle arrangement is similar to that in the small bowel but the longitudinal fibres are gathered into three bands, the taenia coli. The large bowel diameter is not constant, but constrictions (haustrations) are seen more or less regularly; these are functional rather than anatomical features, and their position may move. The ileocaecal valve controls the passage of gut contents from the terminal ileum into the caecum. This sphincter relaxes in response to ileal distension or a meal, and closes if the caecum distends. The large bowel shows frequent segmental contractions and occasional (just a few times daily) coordinated peristaltic waves from caecum to rectum (the mass movement). Passage through the colon is slow, usually taking days. Water and electrolytes are absorbed in the colon and, although there is not much homeostatic response to what is presented to it (most is absorbed in any case), the colon does respond to aldosterone by absorbing more sodium in exchange for potassium. The rectum is usually empty or nearly empty; when it distends with faeces, the urge to defecate is felt, but of course the external anal sphincter is under voluntary control and the reflex can be overridden. Colonic motility is greatly influenced by neural and endocrine input, and by state of mind. If the neural networks are disrupted, for example by the congenital absence of ganglia in Hirschprung's disease, then movement of contents is functionally blocked and there is distension of the proximal gut as contents back up. If not relieved by surgical intervention then megacolon can result.

Splanchnic blood flow

Blood flow to the gut is high – generally around 30 per cent of the cardiac output, despite only constituting about 10 per cent of the body mass in the adult. The supply is via coeliac trunk and superior and inferior mesenteric arteries. However, the flow is highly responsive and much of the one-third of the blood volume that is in the organs of the gastrointestinal tract can be diverted elsewhere [40]. Most of this regulation occurs in the smooth muscle walls of the resistance vessels. Multiple systems exert control here, including cardiovascular, endocrine, paracrine, autonomic nervous and digestive systems. At the level of the vascular smooth muscle cell, controls are exerted by a number of complex mechanisms, the final pathway being that vasoconstriction occurs in response to a rise in intracellular calcium, and a fall in intracellular calcium causes relaxation.

Autonomic nervous control is exerted by sympathetic, parasympathetic, primary sensory and enteric nerves. Sympathetic activity causes catecholamine release.

Noradrenaline binding to α_1-adrenergic receptors causes vasoconstriction. However catecholamines also bind to β_2-receptors which cause vasodilatation. This and the action of other vasodilators explain why noradrenaline causes an initial intense vasoconstriction which gradually wears off (autoregulatory escape), and is followed, when catecholamine levels then fall, by a reactive hyperaemia. Parasympathetic nerves tend to cause vasodilatation via their neurotransmitters ACh, VIP and ATP, which act by inducing nitric oxide production. Primary sensory nerves respond to neuropeptides (e.g. substance P) by increasing blood flow through reflexes which may be local, or via ganglia or at spinal level. Enteric nerves form networks through local plexuses projecting to more distant segments of gut, mostly using ACh to cause vasodilatation.

Hormones released into the circulation at distant sites can influence splanchnic blood flow; angiotensin II, vasopressin and catecholamines all tend to cause splanchnic vasoconstriction. Vasodilatory hormones generally originate from the gastrointestinal tract; gastrin, CCK and secretin all enter the circulation in response to a meal and have widespread effects, causing vasodilatation, regulating motility and promoting secretion from pancreas, biliary system and gut epithelium, as well as promoting energy-dependent processes such as absorption of digestive products. The local rise in products of metabolism causes further vasodilatation. Products of inflammatory processes (histamine, bradykinin, prostaglandins, etc.) will also tend to cause local hyperaemia. Somatostatin, released in response to the presence of acid in the gastric antrum, reduces the secretion of gastrin and causes vasoconstriction in the splanchnic circulation, thereby switching off the gastric phase of gastric secretion. Its selective effect on the splanchnic circulation can be used to reduce bleeding from varices, but more often now its synthetic analogue octreotide is used therapeutically for this purpose. Other local effects on the circulation include the myogenic response of the vascular smooth muscle cell, which is the same as that found in many organ systems: an increase in perfusion pressure causes an increase in wall tension, which in turn leads to constriction, reducing the vessel diameter and smoothing out any changes in blood flow. Digestive products in the gut lumen will also increase blood flow locally, independent of hormonal or extrinsic nerve influence. This postprandial hyperaemia is mediated by VIP from enteric nerves.

Pathological disturbances of splanchnic blood flow can have disastrous consequences. Thrombosis in a major vascular supply will result in gut ischaemia and septic shock unless corrected promptly. More commonly, a low-flow state can result in non-occlusive ischaemia. Microthrombi can cause a more localised ischaemia, and in the villi a countercurrent exchange-type mechanism can worsen the situation. Each villus has arterioles projecting into it and venules draining from it; when flow is poor oxygen can diffuse from the arteriole to the venule, leading to a very low oxygen tension in the tip of the villus. Epithelial sloughing at the tips of the villi is an early sign of ischaemia. The breakdown of the epithelial barrier can allow bacterial translocation and diffusion of toxins from the gut lumen into the tissues.

Intestinal failure and the short gut syndrome

The term neonate has a small bowel length of about 250 cm, which grows to about 750 cm in the adult, the most rapid period of growth being in the first year. Significant amounts of small bowel may be lost because of surgical resection for many reasons, among the commonest being gastroschisis, volvulus and necrotising enterocolitis. The result may be osmotic diarrhoea with high water and electrolyte losses, leading initially to dehydration, electrolyte disturbance and acidosis, and later to nutritional failure, sepsis and liver disease from dependence on parenteral nutrition. Intestinal failure may also occur because of motility disorders or mucosal diseases (Hirschprung's, microvillous inclusion disease, etc). Before the advent of parenteral nutrition (PN) in the early 1970s these children did not survive, but long-term PN is associated with life-threatening problems, in particular cholestatic liver disease and loss of central venous access. In the case of short gut, often the loss of inhibitory factors normally secreted by the small bowel leads to rapid gastric emptying and excessive gastric acid secretion. The high output of acidic fluid can badly damage the skin around a stoma or the anus, and a fast transit time limits the amount that can be absorbed. Fortunately, a considerable degree of gut adaptation is possible, and even the colon can acquire the ability to absorb nutrients. However, only terminal ileum can absorb vitamin B_{12} and bile salts – in fact the ileum is the most adaptable part of the bowel. The presence of the ileocaecal valve (ICV) is important as it slows intestinal transit time and prevents bacterial overgrowth of the small bowel; with an intact valve as little as 12 cm of small bowel may eventually be enough to sustain enteral feeding, but probably 25 cm is needed without the ICV [41]. Adaptation in these patients may take many years. With over 40 cm and an intact ICV enteral feeding should usually be possible fairly quickly (<1 year), provided that there is no motility or absorption defect. Complex feeding regimens are needed to cope with the problems of a short gut. Intestinal transplantation is sometimes indicated. Intestinal failure places a huge burden of suffering on patients and their families, and enormous demands on finances and institutions that care for them. Although the specialty is fairly small there is an active international effort aimed at making progress in this field [42].

REFERENCES

Key references

Beath SV. Hepatic function and physiology in the newborn. Semin Neonatol 2003; **8**: 337–46.

Bihari D, Gimson A, Williams R. Cardiovascular, pulmonary and renal complications of fulminant hepatic failure. *Semin Liver Dis* 1986; **6**: 119–128.

Kelly DA. Managing liver failure. *Postgrad Med J* 2002; **78**(925): 660–7.

Krowka MJ. Hepatopulmonary syndrome and portopulmonary hypertension: implications for liver transplantation. *Clin Chest Med* 2005; **26**(4): 587–97.

Lee WS, McKiernan P, Kelly DA. Etiology, outcome and prognostic indicators of childhood fulminant hepatic failure in the UK. *J Pediatr Gastroenterol Nutr* 2005; **40**(5): 575–81.

References

1. Richter S, Mucke I, Menger MD, Vollmar B. Impact of intrinsic blood flow regulation in cirrhosis: maintenance of hepatic artery buffer response. *Am J Physiol – Gastrointest Liver Physiol* 2000; **279**(2): G454–62.

2. Jungermann K, Katz N. Functional hepatocellular heterogeneity. *Hepatology* 1982; **2**(3): 385–95.

3. Nakatani K, Kaneda K, Seki S, Nakajima Y. Pit cells as liver-associated natural killer cells: morphology and function. *Med Electr Microsc* 2004; **37**: 29–36.

4. Exton JH. Mechanisms of hormonal regulation of hepatic glucose metabolism. *Diabetes/Metab Rev* 1987; **3**(1): 163–83.

5. Quintão E, Grundy SM, Ahrens EH Jr. Effects of dietary cholesterol on the regulation of total body cholesterol in man. *J Lipid Res* 1971; **12**(2): 233–47.

6. Nelson D, Zeldin DC, Hoffman SM *et al.* Comparison of cytochrome P450 (CYP) genes from the mouse and human genomes, including nomenclature recommendations for genes, pseudogenes and splice-variants. *Pharmacogenetics* 2004; **14**(1): 1–18.

7. Wilkinson GR, Shand DG. Commentary; a physiological approach to hepatic drug clearance. *Clin Pharm Ther* 1975; **18**(4): 377–90.

8. Williams AL, Hoofnagle JH. Ratio of serum aspartate to alanine aminotransferase in chronic hepatitis. Relationship to cirrhosis. *Gastroenterology* 1988; **95**(3): 734–39.

9. Knight JA, Hammond RE. Gamma-glutamyl transferase and alkaline phosphatase activities compared in the serum of normal children and children with liver disease. *Clin Chem* 1981; **27**(1): 48–51.

10. Trey C, Davidson C. The management of fulminant hepatic failure. *Progr Liver Dis* 1970; **3**: 282–98.

11. Lee WS, McKiernan P, Kelly DA. Etiology, outcome and prognostic indicators of childhood fulminant hepatic failure in the UK. *J Pediatr Gastroenterol Nutr* 2005; **40**(5): 575–81.

12. Bansky G, Meier PJ, Riederer E *et al.* Effects of benzodiazepine receptor antagonist flumazenil in hepatic encephalopathy in humans. *Gastroenterology* 1989; **97**(3): 744–50.

13. Shawcross D, Jalan R. The pathophysiologic basis of hepatic encephalopathy: central role for ammonia and inflammation. *Cell Mol Life Sci* 2005; **62**(19–20): 2295–304.

14. Bihari D, Gimson A, Williams R. Cardiovascular, pulmonary and renal complications of fulminant hepatic failure. *Semin Liver Dis* 1986; **6**: 119–128.

15. Mention K, Lahoche-Manucci A, Bonnevalle M *et al.* Renal function outcome in pediatric liver transplant recipients. *Pediatr Transplant* 2005; **9**(2): 201–7.

16. Rolando N, Harvey F, Brahm J *et al.* Prospective study of bacterial infection in acute liver failure: an analysis of fifty patients. *Hepatology* 1990; **11**(1): 49–53.

17. Kelly DA. Managing liver failure. *Postgrad Med J* 2002; **78**(925): 660–7.

18. Larsen FS, Wendon J. Brain edema in liver failure: basic physiologic principles and management. *Liver Transplant* 2002; **8**(11): 983–9.

19. Suddle A, Foster G, Powell-Tuck J. The nutritional and metabolic management of hepatic failure in European liver units – a surprising lack of consensus ? *Clin Nutr* 2004; **23**(5): 953–4.

20. Keays R, Harrison PM, Wendon JA *et al.* Intravenous acetylcysteine in paracetamol induced fulminant liver failure: a prospective controlled trial. *BMJ* 1991; **303**(6809): 1026–9.

21. Sklar GE, Subramaniam M. Acetylcysteine treatment for non-acetaminophen-induced liver failure. *Ann Pharmacother* 2004; **38**(3): 498–500.

22. Reeves HL, Friedman SL. Activation of hepatic stellate cells – a key issue in liver fibrosis. *Frontiers Biosci* 2002; **7**: d808–26.

23. Lange PA, Stoller JK. The hepatopulmonary syndrome. *Ann Intern Med.* 1995; **122**(7): 521–9.

24. Durand P, Beaujard C, Grosse AL *et al.* Reversal of hypoxaemia by inhaled nitric oxide in children with severe hepatopulmonary syndrome type 1 during and after liver transplantation. *Transplantation* 1998; **65**(3): 437–9.

25. Krowka MJ. Hepatopulmonary syndrome and portopulmonary hypertension: implications for liver transplantation. *Clin Chest Med* 2005; **26**(4): 587–97.

26. Condino AA, Ivy DD, O'Connor JA *et al.* Portopulmonary hypertension in pediatric patients. *J Pediatr* 2005; **147**(1): 20–6.

27. Cardenas A. Hepatorenal syndrome: a dreaded complication of end-stage liver disease. *Am J Gastroenterol* 2005; **100**(2): 460–7.

28. Beath SV. Hepatic function and physiology in the newborn. *Semin Neonatol* 2003; **8**: 337–46.

29. Primhak RA, Tanner MS. Alpha-1 antitrypsin deficiency. *Arch Dis Child* 2001; **85**(1): 2–5.

30. Brewer GJ. Recognition, diagnosis and management of Wilson's disease. *Proc Soc Exp Biol Med* 2000; **223**(1): 23–46.

31. Gregorio GV, Portmann B, Karani J *et al.* Autoimmune hepatitis/sclerosing cholangitis overlap syndrome in childhood: a 16-year prospective study. *Hepatology* 2001; **33**(3): 544–53.

32. Orenstein SR. Gastroesophageal reflux in children. *Pediatr Rev* 1999; **20**(1): 24–8.

33. Cezard JP. Managing gastro-oesophageal reflux in children. *Digestion* 2004; **69**(suppl 1): 3–8.

34. Scheepers A, Joost H-G, Schürmann A. The glucose transporter families SGLT and GLUT: molecular basis of normal and aberrant function. *J Parenter Enteral Nutr* 2004; **28**(5): 364–72.

35. Swagerty DL Jr, Walling AD, Klein RM. Lactose intolerance. *Am Fam Phys* 2002; **65**(9): 1845–58.

36. Durie PR. Pathophysiology of the pancreas in cystic fibrosis. *Neth J Med* 1992; **41**(3): 97–100.

37. Bai JC. Malabsorption syndromes. *Digestion* 1998; **59**(5): 530–46.

38. Farrell RJ, Kelly CP. Celiac sprue. *N Engl J Med* 2002; **346**(3): 180–9.

39. Kellow JE, Borody TJ, Phillips SF *et al.* Human interdigestive motility: variations in patterns from esophagus to colon. *Gastroenterology* 1986; **91**(2): 386–95.

40. Reilly PM, Wilkins KB, Fuh KC *et al.* The mesenteric hemodynamic response to circulatory shock: an overview. *Shock* 2001; **15**(5): 329–43.

41. Goulet O, Baglin-Gobet S, Talbotec C *et al.* Outcome and long-term growth after extensive small bowel resection in the neonatal period: a survey of 87 children. *Eur J Pediatr Surg* 2005; **15**(2): 95–101.

42. Kocoshis SA, Beath SV, Booth IW *et al.* Intestinal failure and small bowel transplantation, including clinical nutrition: working group report of the second world congress of pediatric gastroenterology, hepatology and nutrition. *J Pediatr Gastroenterol Nutr* 2004; **39**(suppl 2): S655–61.

6

The central nervous system

JUSTIN JOHN, IGOR LUGINBUEHL, BRUNO BISSONNETTE

KEY LEARNING POINTS

- The brain weighs about 335 g at term, 900 g by 1 year, reaching adult weight of 1200–1400 g by 12 years.
- The cerebral metabolic rate in children is much higher than in adults.
- Oxygen uptake is 5.8 versus 3.5 ml O_2/100 g/min.
- Glucose usage is 6.8 versus 5.5 mg glucose/100 g/min.
- Cerebral blood flow (CBF) increases with age, peaking at 3–4 years (100–110 mL/100 g/min) then decreasing to adult level by age 9 years (80 mL/100 g/min).
- Even though infants have open fontanelles, an acute increase in intracranial volume causes a rapid increase in intracranial pressure.
- Potent inhalational agents cause a dose-dependent decrease in cerebral vascular resistance and cerebral metabolic rate for oxygen ($CMRO_2$).

- In anaesthetised infants and children there is a direct and logarithmic change in CBF velocity with end-tidal CO_2, suggesting that a much lower arterial partial pressure of CO_2 ($PaCO_2$) is required to produce cerebral vasoconstriction than in adults.
- Isoflurane (<1.5 minimum alveolar concentration, [MAC]) does not change CBF during normocapnia and has minimal effects on cerebrovascular reactivity to carbon dioxide in children
- Desflurane increases CBF significantly at 1 MAC.
- There are developmental changes in the electroencephalogram (EEG). An infant's EEG is much more irregular than an adult's, and it has a different power spectrum.

INTRODUCTION

A significant portion of central nervous system development occurs after birth during the first year of life, resulting in major anatomical, physiological and psychological changes. An awareness of neurological maturation is particularly import when caring for children with neurovascular dysfunction. In patients with neurological pathology the perilesional area is particularly at risk of ischaemia and an understanding of neurophysiology can significantly minimise or prevent neuronal damage. This chapter reviews the concepts needed to understand the anaesthetic management of the child with neurological disease.

NEUROEMBRYOLOGY AND DEVELOPMENT

The central nervous system (CNS) is the first organ system to begin development in the foetus and probably the last to complete. When defects occur in particular stages of CNS development they result in specific neuropathological disorders. Knowledge of the timing and sequencing of major developmental milestones of the CNS helps to understand the various neurological disorders. Human embryological development occurs in stages classified according to both morphology of the embryo and its age. The embryonic period comprises 23 stages. Development of the CNS involves the three major

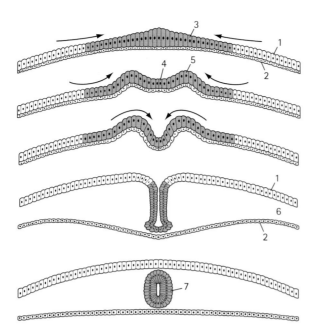

Figure 6.1   Schematic presentation of neurulation (see text for details). The arrows indicate the direction of the cell movement. 1, embryonic ectoderm; 2, embryonic endoderm; 3, neural ectoderm; 4, neural plate with neural groove; 5, neural fold; 6, mesoderm; 7, neural tube.

processes of neurulation, canalisation and retrogressive differentiation.

Neurulation is the process by which the neural plate, derived from the neuroectodermal layer, folds upon itself to make a groove, and in time fuses to form the neural tube (Fig. 6.1). It is divided into early and late periods. Differentiation of the neural tube is part of an extensive process of development, which occurs within the first 60 days following the fertilisation of the ovum. The nervous system does not appear until stage 6, corresponding to the second week of gestation. Differentiation of the cerebral cortex primarily takes place during the third trimester of the gestation period. Gestational age can be estimated from the surface of the developing brain as fissures and sulci develop. The cerebellar primordium begins during stage 13 when the pontine and cervical flexures are forming. Most of early cerebellar development occurs about 4 weeks after fertilisation of the ovum but at this time the cerebellar primordia are not identifiable.

Canalisation is the formation of the caudal neural tube and includes the development of the lower lumbar, sacral and coccygeal segments. Within the neural tube groups of cells, with their corresponding vertebrae, proliferate and produce an excess number of segments. These excess segments degenerate in a process called retrogressive differentiation and the filum terminale and the cauda equina remain. The growth of the spinal column brings the conus medullaris to its adult level.

Defects

Neural tube defects occur during neurulation and can be classified into those involving (1) the brain and spinal cord, (2) only the brain and (3) only the spinal cord. For example, when there is failure of neurulation in early development, total dysraphism occurs within both the brain and spinal cord. If only the brain fails to close, the condition is termed anencephaly. Congenital hydrocephaly is characterised by an increased amount of cerebrospinal fluid (CSF) within the cranial vault and spinal column. Abnormal neuronal migration results in cortical malformations. Schizencephaly (clefts in the cerebral wall), pachygyri (sparse, broad gyri) and polymicrogyria are examples of anomalies strongly associated with migrational disorders. Lissencephaly (smooth brain) is a severe anomaly that may be produced by either migrational anomalies or earlier disruptions in neurogenesis. Partial or complete agenesis of the corpus callosum may be associated with any of the above anomalies. Failure of canalisation results in a spectrum of lesions called spina bifida. This includes a myelocele if the lesion exposes only neural tissue, a myelomeningocele if there is an additional dorsal outpouching of the meninges or a meningocele if the mass contains only meninges.

The ventricular system and cerebrospinal fluid pathway

By the end of stage 12, the posterior neuropore closes and the ventricular system becomes enclosed within the primitive brain, and the spinal cord encloses the central canal. Evaginations of the cerebral hemispheres form the lateral ventricles, the third ventricle and the foramen of Monro. Later, the lateral ventricles become the largest within the ventricular system as a result of expansion of the cerebral hemispheres. Shortly thereafter, a perforation in the roof of the fourth ventricle occurs, thereby creating the foramen of Magendie. The foramina of Luschka, which are lateral apertures of the fourth ventricle, form at approximately 12 weeks of gestational age. The aqueduct of Sylvius narrows as the tectal plate and midbrain tegmentum enlarge. The CSF volume within the lateral, third and fourth ventricles becomes somewhat reduced as the choroid plexus proliferates and the brain substance increases. Normally, the central canal of the spinal cord is obliterated after birth by proliferation of cells within the spinal cord. Thus, the ventricular system terminates at the midline of the dorsal surface of the medulla oblongata that marks the caudal angle of the rhomboid fossa in the floor of the fourth ventricle. In the Arnold–Chiari malformation, which accounts for 40 per cent of congenital hydrocephalus, the embryological development of the caudal cerebellum is disturbed resulting in herniation below the foramen magnum (Fig. 6.2), which may lead to an enlarged central canal progressing to syringomyelia (Morvan's disease).

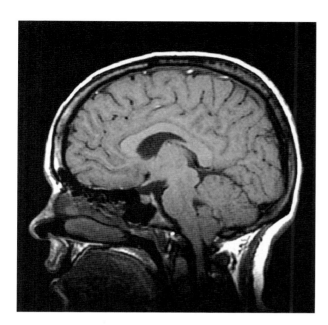

Figure 6.2 Abnormal cerebellar anatomy associated with Arnold–Chiari malformation. Sagittal magnetic resonance imaging (MRI) scan of a 17-year-old patient showing early herniation of the cerebellar tonsils through the foramen magnum and into the cervical spinal canal.

Cerebral vascular development

The cerebral vasculature develops during five distinct periods. In the first period (stages 8 and 9), a system of primordial endothelium-lined channels is present in which neither arteries nor veins are distinguishable. These channels form a plexiform network and ultimately differentiate into arteries and veins. This neovascular system provides the initial circulation to the head with direct communication from the primitive aortic system to the jugular system. The fourth period corresponds to stage 19 wherein there is separation of the arterial and venous systems. The fifth and final period extends beyond birth and is characterised by late histological changes in the vascular walls, transforming them into the adult form. It is believed that most vascular malformations, which seem to be the result of a defect in the structure of the primitive arteriolar–capillary network, occur before the embryo attains a length of 40 mm and prior to arterial wall thickening.

NEUROANATOMY

The following is a review of the important aspects of clinical neuroanatomy. At birth, the calvarium (skull cap) is composed of ossified plates, which cover the dura mater. The plates are separated by fibrous sutures and fontanelles. The posterior and anterior fontanelles close between 2 and 3 months and between 10 and 18 months of age, respectively, and become ossified during adolescence. The dura

mater is relatively non-compliant and unable to accommodate an acute rise in intracranial pressure (ICP), even when the fontanelles are open. An acute increase in intracranial volume will therefore result in a rapid increase in ICP that will compress and displace vital CNS tissue and cause dysfunction. A slow rise in pressure may be accommodated to a limited extent by expansion of the fontanelles and separation of fibrous sutures[1]. The fontanelles tend not to close if there is any chronic process that increases the intracranial volume including tumours, hydrocephalus and haemorrhage. Intracranial pressure may be clinically monitored in the infant by palpation of open fontanelles or by application of skin surface pressure transducers[2,3].

At birth the brain weighs about 335 g, comprising about 10–15 per cent of the total body weight. Rapid brain growth occurs within the first year of life; brain weight doubles by 6 months of age and reaches 900 g by 1 year. By 12 years, the brain achieves its adult weight of 1200–1400 g and accounts for approximately 2 per cent of total body weight. The intracranial space is separated by a special horizontal layer of dura mater, called the tentorium cerebelli, into two major compartments – the supratentorial and infratentorial compartments. Neuropathology is often differentiated according to these compartments.

The supratentorial compartment

This is the largest compartment of the cranial space and includes, within the anterior and middle cranial fossae, the cerebrum and all the structures formed from the diencephalon. The shape of the skull and the tentorium cerebelli determines its volume. The tentorium is tent shaped and forms a roof over the posterior cranial fossa that contains the cerebellum.

The cerebrum, located in the anterior cranial fossa, is separated into two hemispheres by the longitudinal cerebral fissure and falx cerebri. The cerebral hemispheres are further divided into the frontal, temporal and parieto-occipital lobes. This physical division corresponds with division of function. The frontal lobe, located anterior to the central sulcus and lateral fissure, is associated with motor function, speech, cognition and affective behavior. Lesions in specific areas of the frontal lobe can result in contralateral spastic upper motor neuron paralysis and motor aphasia. The parietal lobe, located between the central sulcus and the parieto-occipital fissure, is involved in somatosensory processing. Lesions in this area may result in contralateral paraesthesiae and tactile agnosia. The occipital lobe, located posterior to the parieto-occipital sulcus, contains the visual cortex and lesions in this area may result in homonymous visual field defects (hemianopia) and various other visual abnormalities. The temporal lobe, inferior to the lateral sulcus, is involved in memory and audition; lesions in this area may result in sensory aphasia.

The diencephalon is the most rostral part of the brain stem. It is located in the central portion of the supratentorial compartment and consists predominantly of the thalamus with some epithalamic, subthalamic and hypothalamic regions. The brain stem is continuous with the spinal cord and after passing through the tentorial notch (incisura tentorii) of the tentorium cerebelli it reaches the middle cranial fossa and its anterior surface lies on the body of the sphenoid bone. It is bound posteriorly by the basioccipital bone. Lesions in the diencephalon, depending on the specific location, may result in thalamic dysfunction including decreased thresholds for pain, temperature and tactile stimulation, as well as ballism (involuntary, jerking, proximal limb movements), paralysis agitans (Parkinson's disease) and autonomic nervous system dysfunction (dysregulation of temperature, appetite, thirst and hormone secretion). The diencephalon is susceptible to ischaemia or neoplasms. In particular, the anterior pituitary gland may have benign tumours, which may impinge on the optic chiasm and cause visual field defects.

If a primary lesion or injury involves gross expansion by haemorrhage or oedema, structures near to the tentorium and the falx become sites of secondary injury. This secondary injury is caused by both the pressure and ischaemia from anterior cerebral artery compression. If the pressure continues to rise within the supratentorial compartment, the diencephalon, cerebral peduncles, oculomotor nerves, posterior communicating artery and the uncus of the temporal lobe may eventually herniate through the incisura tentorii (uncal herniation) resulting in contralateral hemiplegia, ipsilateral pupil signs (dilated, irregular, poor reaction to light) and abnormal posturing (Fig. 6.3).

The infratentorial compartment

The infratentorial compartment is located within the posterior cranial fossa and contains the cerebellum, pons and

medulla oblongata, which are protected by the anterior and posterior occipital parts of the skull. The cerebellum is a dorsal expansion of the brain stem with a function that is expressed ipsilaterally and predominantly regulates motor functions. Cerebellar lesions may result in ataxia decreased tendon reflexes, asthenia, intention tremor and nystagmus. The medulla oblongata lies inferior to the pons and contains the nuclei of cranial nerves VII–XII as well as the ascending sensory and descending motor pathways.

Lesions in the infratentorial compartment may result in irreversible, devastating consequences secondary to displacement and compression of vital areas of the brain including the reticular system, cardiac and respiratory control centres, and the cranial nerves. Increasing pressure within the posterior fossa may initially present as relatively subtle neurological symptoms; however, as the pressure continues to rise, herniation of the cerebellar tonsils (postero-inferior prolongations of the cerebellum) through the foramen magnum may occur. This form of herniation is widely known as 'coning' and is often fatal if not treated quickly (Fig. 6.3).

The spinal canal compartment

The spinal cord and CSF are contained within the cylindrical vertebral canal. The spinal cord is a continuation of the brain stem. Following retrogressive differentiation, its caudal tip is located at the intervertebral space of L3 at birth (Fig. 6.4a), but by the age of 8 years the spinal cord reaches its adult level of L1–L2 (normal range T12–L3; Fig. 6.4b). It is important to note that the spinal cord extends below L2 in approximately 1 per cent of the general population, particularly in short-statured individuals. Therefore lumbar puncture (LP) should not be performed above the level of L4. Between L2 and S2 lies a reservoir of CSF located within the subdural space. The spinal compartment is more compliant than the skull and serves to slow down any rise in ICP. If there is high ICP, herniation can be precipitated by an acute decompression of the spinal compartment caused by an LP. Therefore, if increased ICP is suspected, computed tomography (CT) scans may be warranted to assess this risk before performing an LP.

Vascular anatomy

Although in adults the brain comprises only 2 per cent of total body weight it uses 20 per cent of the blood supply. Cerebral blood flow is supplied by an extensive network of arteries originating from paired internal carotid and vertebral arteries. The vertebral arteries join to form a single midline basilar artery that divides again at the junction of the pons and midbrain into paired posterior cerebral and superior cerebellar arteries. The posterior cerebral arteries become interconnected with the vessels originating from the carotid arteries to form the circle of Willis. The

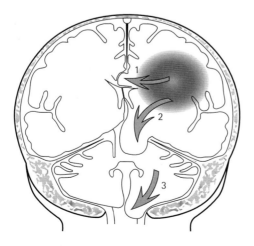

Figure 6.3 The different potential effects of a cerebral space-occupying lesion in the brain: 1, falx herniation; 2, uncus herniation; 3, herniation of the cerebellar tonsils through the foramen magnum.

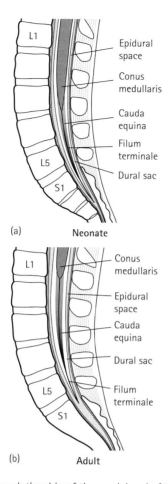

(a)   **Neonate**

Labels in (a): Epidural space, Conus medullaris, Cauda equina, Filum terminale, Dural sac; vertebrae L1, L5, S1

(b)   **Adult**

Labels in (b): Conus medullaris, Epidural space, Cauda equina, Dural sac, Filum terminale; vertebrae L1, L5, S1

Figure 6.4   The relationship of the caudal end of the spinal cord within the vertebral canal in neonates (a) and in adults (b).

communicating arteries are effective anastomoses that reduce the risk of clinical ischaemia if a contributing vessel is occluded.

The vessels of the circle of Willis are prone to the formation of berry aneurysms, which are congenital birth defects related to defective arterial wall formation. Although berry aneurysms are present at birth, they rarely rupture until early to middle adulthood. Arteriovenous malformations (AVMs) are the most frequently occurring cerebrovascular malformations in children. They result in shunting of blood from the arterial to the venous circulation and approximately 50 per cent of patients present with seizures or neurological deficits that result from compression or an ischaemic steal phenomenon; the other 50 per cent present with cerebral haemorrhage. Approximately 90 per cent of AVMs are located in the supratentorial compartment.

Cerebral veins run in the pia and into collecting veins within the subarachnoid layer. They eventually transverse the subdural space and open into venous sinuses that lie between the dura mater and the cranial periosteum. The cerebral venous system is valveless and its walls are thin and without smooth muscle. Although the brain is insensitive to

pain, the cerebral dura mater's nociceptive responsiveness can be demonstrated, particularly around the venous sinuses – this is a potential cause of headache.

The superior sagittal sinus is clinically important because it is superficial and midline, making it vulnerable to damage during surgery for craniosynostosis or craniectomy. It empties into a confluence of sinuses that drains into bilateral transverse sinuses. The occipital sinus, which lies along the foramen magnum, also ends in the confluence of sinuses. The cavernous sinus, which surrounds the sella turcica, joins the superior petrosal sinuses and drains into the transverse sinus. The transverse sinuses then course laterally along the attachment line of the tentorium to the occipital bone and become continuous with the sigmoid sinus located within the posterior cranial fossa finally to form the venous enlargements known as the internal jugular venous bulbs. The sigmoid sinus is separated anteriorly from the mastoid antrum and mastoid air cells by only a thin plate of bone and is therefore vulnerable during mastoid surgery.

SPINAL CORD VASCULAR ANATOMY

The arterial blood supply to the spinal cord primarily arises from a single anterior spinal artery and two posterior spinal arteries, both originating from the vertebral arteries. The anterior spinal artery supplies the ventromedial aspect of the spinal cord which contains the corticospinal tracts and motor neurons. The two posterior spinal arteries form a plexus-like network on the posterior cord surface, and supply the dorsal and lateral aspects of the spinal cord, which contain the sensory tracts responsible for proprioception and light touch[4].

The anterior spinal artery does not supply the whole length of the spinal cord. Supplemental blood flow is also received from radicular arteries originating from spinal branches of the ascending cervical, deep cervical, intercostal, lumbar and sacral arteries (Fig. 6.5). A large anterior radicular artery, called the artery of Adamkiewicz, is responsible for supplying blood to as much as the lower two-thirds of the spinal cord. It arises at a variable level from the aorta but is most commonly located between T9 and L5 on the left side. All the other radicular arteries provide important collateral flow to the thoracic and lumbar spinal cord. Only six to eight of the 62 original radicular vessels persist into adulthood and up to 45 per cent of the general population have fewer than five. Generally, most individuals possess one or two cervical, two to three thoracic, and one or two lumbar radicular arteries. This renders the spinal cord particularly susceptible to ischaemia in the upper thoracic and lumbar areas, especially during trauma or surgery to the aorta or spine.

The venous drainage of the spinal cord consists of two median, two anterolateral veins and two posterolateral longitudinal veins that empty via anterior and posterior radicular veins into the internal vertebral venous plexus, which lies between the dura mater and the vertebral periosteum. All the veins are thin walled and valveless. The internal

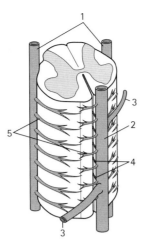

Figure 6.5 Blood supply for the spinal cord is provided by the following vessels: 1, posterior spinal arteries; 2, anterior spinal artery; 3, anterior radicular artery; 4, sulcal branch arteries; 5, pial arterial plexus.

plexus communicates with an external plexus, which then drains via vertebral, intercostal, lumbar and lateral sacral veins into ascending lumbar, azygos or hemiazygos veins. At the cervical levels, the internal plexus connects to a basivertebral vein, which communicates through the foramen magnum with the occipital and basilar sinuses.

NEUROPHYSIOLOGY

The physiology of cerebral metabolism, blood flow and ICP, CSF dynamics and electrophysiology are reviewed in the following sections.

Energetics of cerebral metabolism

The human brain is one of the most complex biological systems. A major aspect of its complexity stems from the myriad of synaptic connections, voltage- and ligand-gated channels and intracellular second messenger systems that mediate interneuronal communications. The energy required to maintain and regulate these systems is significant, as demonstrated by the brain's consumption of more than 20 per cent of the total body ATP. Normally, the main substance used for energy production in the brain is glucose. During aerobic metabolism D-glucose is used to generate high-energy substrates in the citric acid cycle which produces ATP from ADP and inorganic phosphate as well as NADH from NAD^+. Depletion of brain glucose leads to coma and eventually brain death. The brain stores minimal amounts of glycogen compared with muscle and liver tissue (respectively, these store 10 and 100 times as much per unit mass). Consequently, the brain can store only enough glycogen to sustain approximately 3 minutes of normal ATP consumption and further glucose supply is completely dependent on blood flow. In the awake resting state the overall metabolic rate for brain tissue in children (mean age 6 years) is much higher than in adults as demonstrated by the increased demand for oxygen (5.8 versus 3.5 ml O_2/100 g/min of brain tissue) and glucose (6.8 versus 5.5 ml O_2/100 g/min). During stable conditions, the concentration of glucose in the whole brain is approximately 25–35 per cent of the plasma concentration. In the presence of hyperglycaemia, neuronal glucose content increases. This is important because the extent of brain lactic acidosis depends on the amount of glucose present at the time of oxygen deprivation. Cerebral tissue pH will decrease faster if the amount of glucose available to the brain before the ischaemic insult is high. Neonatal mammals have much greater glycogen stores and appear to be more resistant to longer periods of oxygen deprivation.

When neuronal oxygen supply is reduced to a minimum, a cascade of mechanisms is activated that will reduce ATP consumption until cerebral perfusion is re-established. These mechanisms include utilisation of phosphocreatinine stores, production of ATP at low levels through anaerobic glycolysis and abrupt cessation of spontaneous electrophysiological activity, thereby reducing energy demand by up to 60 per cent. Nevertheless, in the absence of oxygen, pyruvate is transformed to lactate to enable NAD^+ regeneration and this process reduces intracellular pH and threatens conductivity and viability.

Cerebral blood flow and cerebral blood volume

An increase in CBF augments cerebral blood volume (CBV) which tends to elevate ICP. Indirect manipulation of ICP is therefore possible by controlling CBF although this may be diminished or abolished by intracranial lesions or diseases. The CBF is dependent on the pressure gradient known as the cerebral perfusion pressure (CPP) and is defined as mean arterial pressure (MAP) minus either ICP or central venous pressure (CVP), whichever is greater.

Global CBF in adults and neonates is similar and is 50 mL/100 g/min and 40–42 mL/100 g/min, respectively. Cerebral blood flow increases in infants to 90 mL/100 g/min by 6 months of age, before it reaches its peak of 100–110 mL/100 g/min at 3–4 years. Thereafter, it slowly decreases to approximately 80 mL/100 g/min by the age of 9 years. Total CBF in infants and small children is therefore more than twice that in adults, and this matches the higher energy requirements of the developing brain [5–8]. The CBF to grey matter is two-thirds higher than that to white matter throughout the entire lifespan [9]. Some areas of the brain show greater metabolic activity than others and, consequently, have a preferential blood flow. Moreover, energy requirements change minute by minute so that the demand-and-supply relationship for oxygen requires vasodilatation and vasoconstriction to increase or decrease regional blood flow. The automaticity of this vasoactivity is known as autoregulation and is mediated by regional tissue adenosine concentrations as a secondary response to changing tissue lactate levels. During periods of increased oxygen consumption, such as during fever and seizure activity, there is an increase in CBF with a corresponding increase in CBV. This may increase ICP. Conversely, factors that decrease $CMRO_2$ will decrease CBF and CBV. For example, during hypothermia, there is a decrease in both $CMRO_2$ and CBF of approximately 7 per cent per degree centigrade temperature reduction [10]. The $CMRO_2$ varies with age. In anaesthetised newborns and infants, $CMRO_2$ is 2.3 mL O_2/100 g/min, whereas in children 3–12 years of age it is 5.2 mL O_2/100 g/min [5,6]. Owing to the energy requirements for the developing brain, $CMRO_2$ in children is substantially greater than in adults.

The CBF is autoregulated to maintain oxygen delivery constant over a wide range of perfusion pressures. Adults can maintain a constant CBF over a range of MAP between 50 and 150 mmHg [11]. Cerebral oedema may occur with acute increases in MAP above 150 mmHg caused by disruption of the blood–brain barrier. Autoregulation thresholds for infants and children are not known fully, but animal studies suggest that neonatal limits may be between 40 and 90 mmHg MAP (Fig. 6.6). While it is not possible to be certain of the effect of hypotension on CBF, induced hypotension in infants appears not to cause overt damage [12]. Once the limits for autoregulation have been exceeded, CBF changes passively with blood pressure. Haemodilution and anticoagulants may increase oxygen delivery by decreasing blood viscosity [13], but this triggers autoregulation and compensatory cerebral vasoconstriction so that CBF remains constant. Focal or global autoregulation is impaired by intracranial trauma, tumour, abscess,

ischaemia hypoxia, vasodilators and high concentrations of volatile anaesthetics [13–15]. Neonates in severe physiological distress may have altered autoregulation [14] as there may be minimal change in CBF in response to varying $PaCO_2$ levels. In preterm infants, because autoregulation can be impaired or ineffective, intraventricular haemorrhage is common and leads to potentially fatal damage [16].

Hypocapnia may be used clinically to reduce CBF. In adults CBF increases change with $PaCO_2$ in the range 2.7–10.7 kPa (20–80 mmHg). The CBF is reduced by 3 per cent with every 0.1 kPa decrease in $PaCO_2$. Past studies have indicated that the immature brain is relatively unresponsive to small changes in $PaCO_2$ but a study in foetal rabbits has demonstrated that CBF can respond to $PaCO_2$ [17]. Transcranial Doppler ultrasound in anaesthetised infants and children has demonstrated a direct and logarithmic change in CBF velocity with end-tidal CO_2 ($PETCO_2$), suggesting that a much lower $PaCO_2$ is required to produce vasoconstrictive effects on the cerebral vasculature than is required in adults [18]. With a steadily decreasing $PaCO_2$, there is an associated increase in CSF pH and periarteriolar pH leading to vasoconstriction. Chronic hyperventilation causes a slow diffusion of bicarbonate ions out of the CSF, normalising CSF pH and CBF within 24 hours [10]. Although the neonatal cerebral vasculature shows little response to hyperventilation [19] a sudden increase in $PaCO_2$ after chronic hyperventilation of more than 24 hours' duration may result in cerebral vasodilatation and increased ICP [20].

Cerebral vascular response to hypoxia has not been well studied in children, but in adults there is no change in CBF until the partial pressure of arterial oxygen (PaO_2) falls below 6.7 kPa (50 mmHg), and thereafter CBF begins to increase exponentially.

Cerebrospinal fluid

Most of the CSF (50–80 per cent), which surrounds the brain and spinal cord, is produced by the choroid plexus (lining the floor of the lateral ventricles and the roof of the third and fourth ventricles) and is thought to be the product of ultrafiltration and active secretion via Na^+/K^+-dependent ATPase pumps. The composition of CSF differs from that of plasma; there is a minimal amount of protein (0.15–0.45 g/L), reduced levels of glucose (2.8–4.4 mmol/L) and potassium (2.6–3.3 mmol/L), and the chloride concentration is slightly higher (119–131 mmol/L). Differences in CSF composition within infant age groups can be found elsewhere [21].

There seems to be a circadian rhythm in CSF production because production may double at night time. Up to 30 per cent of CSF may be formed at sites other than the choroid plexus (such as the ependyma, brain parenchyma and endothelium of cerebral capillaries) [22–24]. The CSF produced by the choroid plexus flows from the lateral ventricles through the interventricular foramen of Monro into the third ventricle, then into the cerebral aqueduct of

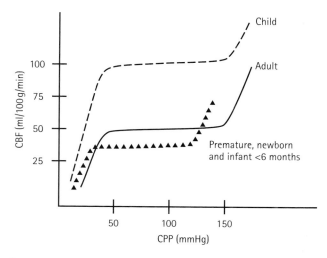

Figure 6.6 The relationship of cerebral blood flow (CBF) to cerebral perfusion pressure (CPP) at different ages. Compared with adults, the CPP range of CBF autoregulation is set at a higher range in children aged 6 months to 12 years and at a lower range in neonates and preterm infants.

Sylvius to the fourth ventricle. It finally leaves the interior of the brain through the two lateral foramina of Luschka and the single medial foramen of Magendie to enter the subarachnoid space. The CSF is absorbed by the arachnoid villi, which project into the superior sagittal sinus to the venous drainage system. Although the exact mechanism of resorption is unknown, the choroid plexus has been suggested as a possible second site of absorption. The mean production rate in children is approximately 0.35 mL/min, which equates to about 500 mL/day [25].

Intracranial pressure is much more dependent on CBF and CBV than the volume of CSF. There is approximately a 1.1 mmHg reduction of ICP for a 35 per cent reduction in CSF production [26]. Therefore, medications causing a reduction in CSF production, such as furosemide and acetazolamide, have minimal effects on ICP. Nevertheless, these drugs may be beneficial in patients who have decreased intracranial compliance. In addition, in this subset of patients, anaesthetic agents who may increase CSF production or decrease CSF absorption should be avoided (e.g. enflurane) [27].

Spinal cord blood flow

Until recently nearly all spinal cord circulation physiology data have been obtained from animal studies. New data from transcranial Doppler ultrasound are useful because it is non-invasive and, in cats, it has been shown that there is a good correlation between directly measured and Doppler inferred blood flow [28]. Animal data suggest that spinal cord blood flow physiology is influenced by the same factors as CBF, albeit the flow itself is lower, matching the lower spinal metabolic rate [29,30]. Adjusting for the lower metabolic rate in the spinal cord, the ratio of demand and supply appears similar to that of the brain. Spinal cord perfusion pressure (SCPP) is the product of MAP − (CSF + extrinsic pressure). This concept is clinically useful because it highlights the influence of not only CSF pressure, but also other potential sources of extrinsic pressure, such as tumours, haematomas or spinal venous congestion. Spinal blood flow is autoregulated within a MAP range of 50–150 mmHg (in adults) [29,30]. Autoregulatory mechanisms may be affected by an MAP exceeding these limits, and also by hypoxia, hypercapnia, trauma or other factors that potentially eliminate vascular reactivity [31,32]. Spinal cord vasculature responds to changes in PaO_2 and $PaCO_2$ much like the cerebral vasculature. In dogs, the spinal cord does not respond to changes in PaO_2 until it falls below 6–6.6 kPa (45–50 mmHg) and at this point blood flow drastically increases (as does CBF) [32]. There may be a linear relationship between spinal cord blood flow and $PaCO_2$ (within a $PaCO_2$ range from 3 to 8 kPa) of approximately 0.3–0.4 mL/100 g/min for every 1 mmHg (0.13 kPa) change in $PaCO_2$ [32]. In contrast, there is a change in CBF of

approximately 1–2 mL/100 g/min for every 1 mmHg change in $PaCO_2$ [33].

Spinal CSF pressure may be affected by epidural anaesthesia. The administration of 10 mL of solution into the epidural space has been noted to cause a transient increase in CSF pressure, but this probably has little effect on SCPP [34].

Intracranial pressure

An uncontrolled increase in ICP is potentially lethal because it can critically reduce CPP. Therefore efforts to control ICP can be crucial. The cranial vault is a confined space containing brain parenchyma (70 per cent of the volume), extracellular fluid (10 per cent), blood (10 per cent) and CSF (10 per cent). For ICP to remain constant, an increase in volume of any one of these components must be compensated by a reduction in another. Once this compensatory mechanism is exhausted the ICP increases. The relationship of ICP to intracranial volume is represented by the intracranial compliance curve. Normal adult ICP is between 8 and 18 mmHg, and the ICP in children typically lies between 2 and 4 mmHg. The ICP in neonates is positive on the day of birth, but then becomes negative [35,36] probably because of salt and water loss. Intracerebral volume also decreases and is matched by a reduction in head size during this period [35]. Negative ICP is a potential risk factor for intraventricular haemorrhage.

Infants can compensate for slow increases in ICP because of their open fontanelles and suture lines. However, acute changes in intracranial volume are not tolerated because the fibrous connective tissue bridging the fontanelles and sutures is relatively difficult to separate. The cranial vault of older children is rigid and the ICP is dependent on intracranial volume. A small change in volume may result in an insignificant increase in ICP in a patient with a normal baseline ICP, but, once the non-compliant point on the intracranial compliance curve is reached, a small volume change causes a greater rise in ICP. The smooth logarithmic nature of the intracranial compliance curve is accounted for by the buffering of intracranial mass, the compliance of cerebral vasculature and pressure-driven CSF absorption [37]. The pressure–volume index (PVI) is a measurement of the compliance that occurs with the injection of an intrathecal volume bolus and is defined as $\delta V/\log10(Pp/Po)$ where δV is the volume of the bolus, Pp is the peak ICP after bolus injection and Po is the baseline ICP [38]. Baseline ICP increases by a factor of 10 with intrathecal administration of approximately 25 mL fluids in adults while in infants the required volume for an equal increase is only 10 ml because of the decreased neural axis volume. This explains why infants and children are more vulnerable to the effects of sudden intracranial haemorrhage.

Using the principles above, the ICP can be controlled by shifting the patient's intracranial compliance curve, changing the slope of the curve or altering the patient's position on the curve.

Electrophysiology

NORMAL ELECTROENCEPHALOGRAM

The electroencephalograms (EEGs) of awake adults are characterised by fast-frequency (8–13Hz, 'alpha'), low-amplitude activity and, when sleep occurs, there is an obvious change to much lower frequency and higher voltage signals [39]. This trend continues as sleep deepens. The lower frequencies are related to thalamic activity in contrast to the irregularity of 'awake' cortical activity [40]. When there is awakening there is a sudden return to fast frequency activity. Natural sleep has another sleep stage in which there is rapid eye movement (REM), irregular breathing and other automatic and autonomic changes, but very low skeletal electromyograph (EMG) activity. This is associated with dreaming and the EEG has 'awake' high-frequency activity.

There are developmental changes in the EEG. An infant's EEG is much more irregular than an adult's [41–43] and it has a different power spectrum. For example, the power in the alpha wave frequency band (8–13 Hz) does not become similar to adults until age 6–8 years [44]. Consequently, any monitor based upon the adult EEG may not be applicable in small infants. For example, Bispectral index (BIS, Aspect Medical Systems, Inc.) can be low in anaesthetised infants even at low anaesthetic doses [45–47] and this may be because the EEG of an anaesthetised infant has a lower amplitude compared with an adult at comparable doses. However, in a clinical study to determine the BIS score at various steady-state sevoflurane concentrations, BIS scores were slightly higher in infants than in older children [48]. Very few normative data have been published on EEG changes during anaesthesia in neonates [49]. Power spectrum have been measured in infants anaesthetised with halothane and the dose was related to EEG power in the occipital channels [50].

INFLUENCE OF SPINAL CORD ACTIVITY

The MAC that prevents movement may not represent the MAC that prevents awakening. Movement, caused by reflex spinal cord responses, may be unrelated to cortical activity. Indeed, this has been demonstrated in rats in which the MAC of decorticate and intact animals is the same [51]. In experiments in a goat model, in which the brain blood supply was isolated from the spinal cord, anaesthetic levels in the spinal cord were more important than those in the brain in preventing both movement, and cortical arousal [52], which suggests that the spinal cord is directly responsible not only for reflex movement, but also for cortical arousal [53]. The sedative effect of spinal anaesthesia is well known in adults and has been described recently in infants [54].

NEUROPHARMACOLOGY

General principles

Animal studies have suggested that the lethal dose of medications is significantly lower in neonates and infants compared with adults [55]. The increased sensitivity noted in neonates to sedatives, hypnotics and opiates is believed to be secondary to brain immaturity (incomplete myelination and blood–brain barrier) and increased permeability to medications, particularly those that are lipid soluble [56]. Minimum alveolar concentration in neonates is significantly lower than in infants between the ages of 1 month and 6 months [57]. The combination of increased dose required (to cause immobility) and appreciable cardiovascular depression results in a narrower safety margin [58]. Dosage must be appropriately calculated and the effects closely monitored.

The effect of anaesthetic agents on cerebral blood flow and intracranial pressure

Depression of the CNS through the use of potent inhalational agents is indicated by dose-dependent decreases in cerebral vascular resistance and $CMRO_2$. Inhalational drugs increase the ratio of CBF to metabolic rate. Commencing with a 0.6 MAC, CBF increases as vascular resistance decreases [59]. The extent of CBF increase is dependent on the specific inhalational agent used. The increase is most pronounced with halothane, less with enflurane and lowest with isoflurane and desflurane [59]. A maximal change in CBF with halothane in children was found at 1.0 MAC [60]. Cerebral blood flow and cerebral autoregulation are less affected by isoflurane than halothane at equivalent MAC doses in cats [61]. The CBF does not change during normocapnia with isoflurane anaesthesia between 0.5 MAC and 1.5 MAC. Isoflurane also has minimal effects on cerebrovascular reactivity to carbon dioxide (CR_{CO_2}) in children [62]. Although isoflurane and halothane differ in their effects on CBF, both equally increase ICP in the animal model, which may be secondary to an increase in CBV [63].

Desflurane allows for rapid emergence and changes in depth of anaesthesia which makes it ideal for neuroanaesthesia [64]. However, it increases CBF significantly in concentrations of 1.0 MAC and 1.5 MAC when compared with 0.5 MAC [64]. Cerebrovascular reactivity to carbon dioxide is preserved during hypocapnia in children anaesthetised with 1.0 MAC, but not 1.5 MAC [65]. The lack of further increase in CBF at higher $PETCO_2$ concentrations was likely to be due to the significant cerebral vasodilatory effect of desflurane, which may have important implications in children with reduced intracranial compliance [65]. Changing propofol anaesthesia to desflurane results in a significant increase in CBF, whereas changing from isoflurane anaesthesia to desflurane does not [66].

Sevoflurane differs from desflurane by not significantly affecting CBF at 0.5, 1.0 and 1.5 MAC in healthy children [67]. In recent studies, autoregulation was preserved with up to 1.5 MAC sevoflurane while CR_{CO_2} was preserved up to 1.0 MAC [68,69].

Nitrous oxide (N_2O) increases CBF when used alone or with other anaesthetic agents such as propofol or sevoflurane. In the presence of nitrous oxide CR_{CO_2} is preserved at 1.0 MAC sevoflurane provided that $PETCO_2$ is less than 5.9 kPa (45 mmHg) [70]. Nitrous oxide does not affect CR_{CO_2} in children receiving propofol anaesthesia and this suggests that a combination of nitrous oxide with propofol anaesthesia would be a suitable choice in children who require preservation of CR_{CO_2} [71].

Under propofol anaesthesia CR_{CO_2} is preserved in children within an $PETCO_2$ range of 3.3–7.2 kPa (25–55 mmHg) [72]. High-dose propofol infusion is associated with lower CBF and MAP in children, which may be secondary to cerebral vasoconstrictive properties of propofol [73]. However, hyperventilation to end-tidal carbon dioxide values below 4.6 kPa (35 mmHg), in the presence of propofol and nitrous oxide, did not result in any further reduction in CBF [71]. Hyperventilation to $PETCO_2$ values below 30 mmHg did not cause a further reduction of CBF in children receiving propofol anaesthesia alone [74].

Opioids have either no or little effect on CBF, $CMRO_2$ and ICP, and therefore preserve CR_{CO_2} and cerebral autoregulation provided that the sympathetic system is not activated [75]. When combined with propofol, remifentanil decreases MAP and heart rate in children without changing CBF [76] and this may be helpful if hypotensive anaesthesia is desired. In children under sevoflurane anaesthesia, fentanyl was found to be more effective than remifentanil at preventing increased CBF during and immediately following direct laryngoscopy and tracheal intubation while providing a more stable haemodynamic profile [77].

Benzodiazepines may decrease CBF and $CMRO_2$ by approximately 25 per cent and thus can reduce ICP [78]. Similarly, barbiturates cause a dose-dependent decrease in CBF and $CMRO_2$ [79]. A major drawback of barbiturates is their potential to reduce significantly myocardial contractility and systemic blood pressure resulting in a reduction in CPP. Thiopental, in non-clinical dosing (as may be used in total circulatory arrest during cardiac surgery), has been reported to produce an isoelectric EEG and a decrease in $CMRO_2$ of 50 per cent [79]. However, barbiturates are more effective in decreasing ICP than benzodiazepines because of their vasoconstricting effect on cerebral vasculature and CBF reduction. Barbiturates preserve both cerebral autoregulation and CR_{CO_2}. Ketamine has little effect on $CMRO_2$ but may increase CBF by up to 60 per cent under normocapnia [80]. It is therefore considered a contraindication in patients with high ICP, although there it had the practical advantage of maintaining blood pressure and a theoretical advantage of cerebral protective effects of N-methyl-D-aspartic acid (NMDA) receptor antagonism.

Apoptosis and potentially damaging effects of anaesthesia agents on the developing brain

Recent concern for the potentially damaging effects of common anaesthetic drugs on the developing infant brain justifies this section. Apoptosis is an active, genetically programmed and energy-dependent process of normal cell death [81] and it is distinct from oncosis, which is a pathological event where several cells are exposed to an overwhelming noxious stimulus (e.g. trauma), resulting in cell death and tissue necrosis. Oncosis is characterised by massive cell swelling and surrounding inflammation whereas apoptosis is a quiet asynchronous process in which a cell dies and is removed by phagocytes. Apoptosis involves activation of a family of proteases known as caspases, which target many structural and functional proteins leading to an orderly sequence of cell death and degradation. It is a feature of normal brain development and results in refinement of neuronal circuitry. In theory, apoptosis could be triggered by blocking synaptic transmission at a critical stage of rapid brain growth.

It is well known that maternal ethanol and anticonvulsants can cause developmental delay and microcephaly and these agents have also been found to cause cortical apoptosis in rat pups. Ethanol is an NMDA receptor antagonist and an γ-aminobutyric acid (GABA) receptor agonist and there is concern that anaesthetics with similar actions could also damage the developing brain [82,83]. Ketamine and nitrous oxide are NMDA antagonists and volatile agents; benzodiazepines and barbiturates are GABA agonists. In rat pups, prolonged exposure to a combination of midazolam, isoflurane and nitrous oxide triggers cerebral neuronal apoptosis and, when they had matured, they showed permanent behavioural dysfunction [84]. Midazolam or N_2O alone did not trigger apoptosis and the doses may be too large and length of exposure too long to be relevant to clinical situation. Nevertheless, even though the clinical significance is uncertain, these findings have attracted much attention [84]. It is possible that lack of surgical stimulation in the rat model, which is usually present during surgical procedures and intensive care, was an important factor since, in the normal developing brain, unused neurons undergo apoptosis. In addition apoptosis may vary across species. Evidence in the monkey model is inconclusive because of the problem of uncertainty of developmental equivalence.

Even if there is a risk of apoptosis, anaesthesia and analgesia should be used for humanitarian reasons [85]. Evidence of brain damage caused by the appropriate clinical use of anaesthesia agents in preterm infants may be hard to find because these patients may have other causes of brain damage, such as intraventricular haemorrhage and meningitis. One method might be to compare the developmental outcome of infants who have had spinal local anaesthesia with those who have had general anaesthesia. Such a trial would involve large numbers of subjects in order to remove the many confounding factors present in this difficult and vulnerable group.

REFERENCES

Key references

Denman WT, Swanson EL, Rosow D et al. Pediatric evaluation of the bispectral index (BIS) monitor and correlation of BIS with end-tidal sevoflurane concentration in infants and children. Anesth Analg 2000; 90(4): 872–7.

Jevtovic-Todorovic V, Hartman RE, Izumi Y et al. Early exposure to common anesthetic agents causes widespread neurodegeneration in the developing rat brain and persistent learning deficits. J Neurosci 2003; 23(3): 876–82.

Karsli C, Luginbuehl I, Bissonnette B. The cerebrovascular response to hypocapnia in children receiving propofol. Anesth Analg 2004; 99(4): 1049–52.

Leon JE, Bissonnette B. Cerebrovascular responses to carbon dioxide in children anaesthetized with halothane and isoflurane. Can J Anaesth 1991; 38(7): 817–25.

Pilato MA, Bissonnette B, Lerman J. Transcranial Doppler: response of cerebral blood-flow velocity to carbon dioxide in anaesthetized children. Can J Anaesth 1991; 38(1): 37–42.

References

1. Lofgren J, Zwetnow NN. Cranial and spinal components of the cerebrospinal fluid pressure–volume curve. Acta Neurol Scand 1973; 49(5): 575–85.
2. Hill A, Volpe JJ. Measurement of intracranial pressure using the Ladd intracranial pressure monitor. J Pediatr 1981; 98(6): 974–6.
3. Hill A. Intracranial pressure measurements in the newborn. Clin Perinatol 1985; 12(1): 161–78.
4. Ross RT. Spinal cord infarction in disease and surgery of the aorta. Can J Neurol Sci 1985; 12(4): 289–95.
5. Kennedy C, Sokoloff L. An adaptation of the nitrous oxide method to the study of the cerebral circulation in children: normal values for cerebral blood flow and cerebral metabolic rate in childhood. J Clin Invest 1957; 36(7): 1130–7.
6. Settergren G, Lindblad BS, Persson B. Cerebral blood flow and exchange of oxygen, glucose ketone bodies, lactate, pyruvate and amino acids in anesthetized children. Acta Paediatr Scand 1980; 69(4): 457–65.
7. Younkin DP, Reivich M, Jaggi J et al. Noninvasive method of estimating human newborn regional cerebral blood flow. J Cereb Blood Flow Metab 1982; 2(4): 415–20.
8. Cross KW, Dear PR, Hathorn MK et al. An estimation of intracranial blood flow in the newborn infant. J Physiol 1979; 289: 329–45.
9. Ogawa A, Sakurai Y, Kayama T, Yoshimoto T. Regional cerebral blood flow with age: changes in rCBF in childhood. Neurol Res 1989; 11(3): 173–6.
10. Rosomoff HL, Holaday DA. Cerebral blood flow and cerebral oxygen consumption during hypothermia. Am J Physiol 1954; 179(1): 85–8.
11. Lassen NA, Christensen MS. Physiology of cerebral blood flow. Br J Anaesth 1976; 48(8): 719–34.
12. McLeod ME, Creighton RE, Humphreys RP. Anaesthesia for cerebral arteriovenous malformations in children. Can Anaesth Soc J 1982; 29(4): 299–306.
13. Rebel A, Ulatowski JA, Kwansa H et al. Cerebrovascular response to decreased hematocrit: effect of cell-free hemoglobin, plasma viscosity, and CO_2. Am J Physiol Heart Circ Physiol 2003; 285(4): H1600–8.
14. Tweed A, Cote J, Lou H et al. Impairment of cerebral blood flow autoregulation in the newborn lamb by hypoxia. Pediatr Res 1986; 20(6): 516–19.
15. Ong BY, Greengrass R, Bose D et al. Acidemia impairs autoregulation of cerebral blood flow in newborn lambs. Can Anaesth Soc J 1986; 33(1): 5–9.
16. Lou HC, Lassen NA, Friis-Hansen B. Impaired autoregulation of cerebral blood flow in the distressed newborn infant. J Pediatr 1979; 94(1): 118–21.
17. Yamashita N, Kamiya K, Nagai H. CO_2 reactivity and autoregulation in fetal brain. Child Nerv Syst 1991; 7(6): 327–31.
18. Pilato MA, Bissonnette B, Lerman J. Transcranial Doppler: response of cerebral blood-flow velocity to carbon dioxide in anaesthetized children. Can J Anaesth 1991; 38(1): 37–42.
19. Leahy FA, Cates D, MacCallum M, Rigatto H. Effect of CO_2 and 100 per cent O_2 on cerebral blood flow in preterm infants. J Appl Physiol 1980; 48(3): 468–72.
20. Muizelaar JP, van der Poel HG, Li ZC et al. Pial arteriolar vessel diameter and CO_2 reactivity during prolonged hyperventilation in the rabbit. J Neurosurg 1988; 69(6): 923–7.
21. Nouffer JM. Referenzzwerte und interpretationen klinisch-chemischer untersuchungen im kindesalter. In: Kraemer R, Schöni MH, eds. Berner datenbuch der Pädiatrie. Berne: Hans Huber Verlag, 2005: 896.
22. Milhorat TH. Failure of choroid plexectomy as treatment for hydrocephalus. Surg Gynecol Obstet 1974; 139(4): 505–8.
23. Hammock MK, Milhorat TH. Recent studies on the formation of cerebrospinal fluid. Dev Med Child Neurol Suppl 1973: 27–34.
24. Pollay M. Formation of cerebrospinal fluid. Relation of studies of isolated choroid plexus to the standing gradient hypothesis. J Neurosurg 1975; 42(6): 665–73.
25. Rubin RC, Henderson ES, Ommaya AK et al. The production of cerebrospinal fluid in man and its modification by acetazolamide. J Neurosurg 1966; 25(4): 430–6.
26. Cutler RW, Page L, Galicich J, Watters GV. Formation and absorption of cerebrospinal fluid in man. Brain 1968; 91(4): 707–20.

27. Artru AA. Concentration-related changes in the rate of CSF formation and resistance to reabsorption of CSF during enflurane and isoflurane anesthesia in dogs receiving nitrous oxide. *J Neurosurg Anesthesiol* 1989; **1**(3): 256–62.

28. Lindsberg PJ, O'Neill JT, Paakkari IA *et al.* Validation of laser-Doppler flowmetry in measurement of spinal cord blood flow. *Am J Physiol* 1989; **257**(2 Pt2): H674–80.

29. Hickey R, Albin MS, Bunegin L, Gelineau J. Autoregulation of spinal cord blood flow: is the cord a microcosm of the brain? *Stroke* 1986; **17**(6): 1183–9.

30. Marcus ML, Heistad DD, Ehrhardt JC, Abboud FM. Regulation of total and regional spinal cord blood flow. *Circ Res* 1977; **41**(1): 128–34.

31. Guha A, Tator CH, Rochon J. Spinal cord blood flow and systemic blood pressure after experimental spinal cord injury in rats. *Stroke* 1989; **20**(3): 372–7.

32. Griffiths IR. Spinal cord blood flow in dogs. 2. The effect of the blood gases. *J Neurol Neurosurg Psychiatry* 1973; **36**(1): 42–9.

33. Joshi S, Ornstein E, Young WL. Cerebral and spinal cord blood flow. In: Cottrell JE, Smith DS, eds. *Anesthesia and neurosurgery*, 4th edn. St Louis, MO: Mosby, 2001: 19–68.

34. Usubiaga JE, Usubiaga LE, Brea LM, Goyena R. Effect of saline injections on epidural and subarachnoid space pressures and relation to postspinal anesthesia headache. *Anesth Analg* 1967; **46**(3): 293–6.

35. Welch K. The intracranial pressure in infants. *J Neurosurg* 1980; **52**(5): 693–9.

36. Raju TN, Vidyasagar D, Papazafiratou C. Intracranial pressure monitoring in the neonatal ICU. *Crit Care Med* 1980; **8**(10): 575–81.

37. Marmarou A, Maset AL, Ward JD *et al.* Contribution of CSF and vascular factors to elevation of ICP in severely head-injured patients. *J Neurosurg* 1987; **66**(6): 883–90.

38. Shapiro HM. Intracranial hypertension: therapeutic and anesthetic considerations. *Anesthesiology* 1975; **43**(4): 445–71.

39. Rechtschaffen A, Kales A. *A Manual of standardized terminology, techniques and scoring system for sleep stages of human subjects.* Los Angeles: Brain Information Service/Brain Research Institute, 1968.

40. Steriade M. Synchronized activities of coupled oscillators in the cerebral cortex and thalamus at different levels of vigilance. *Cereb Cortex* 1997; **7**(6): 583–604.

41. Ellingson RJ, Peters JF. Development of EEG and daytime sleep patterns in normal full-term infant during the first 3 months of life: longitudinal observations. *Electroencephalogr Clin Neurophysiol* 1980; **49**(1–2): 112–24.

42. Matsuura M, Yamamoto K, Fukuzawa H *et al.* Age development and sex differences of various EEG elements in healthy children and adults – quantification by a computerized wave form recognition method. *Electroencephalogr Clin Neurophysiol* 1985; **60**(5): 394–406.

43. Torres F, Anderson C. The normal EEG of the human newborn. *J Clin Neurophysiol* 1985; **2**(2): 89–103.

44. Gibbs FA, Gibbs EL. *Atlas of electroencephalography.* Cambridge, MA: Addison-Wesley Press, 1950.

45. Bannister CF, Brosius KK, Sigl JC *et al.* The effect of bispectral index monitoring on anesthetic use and recovery in children anesthetized with sevoflurane in nitrous oxide. *Anesth Analg* 2001; **92**(4): 877–81.

46. Kawaraguchi Y, Fukumitsu K, Kinouchi K *et al.* Bispectral index (BIS) in infants anesthetized with sevoflurane in nitrous oxide and oxygen. *Masui – Jpn J Anesthesiol* 2003; **52**(4): 389–93.

47. Davidson AJ, Huang GH, Rebmann CS, Ellery C. Performance of entropy and Bispectral Index as measures of anaesthesia effect in children of different ages. *Br J Anaesth* 2005; **95**(5): 674–9.

48. Denman WT, Swanson EL, Rosow D *et al.* Pediatric evaluation of the bispectral index (BIS) monitor and correlation of BIS with end-tidal sevoflurane concentration in infants and children. *Anesth Analg* 2000; **90**(4): 872–7.

49. Davidson AJ. Measuring anaesthesia in children using the EEG. *Paediatr Anaesth* 2006; **16**(4): 374–87.

50. Sugiyama K, Joh S, Hirota Y *et al.* Relationship between changes in power spectra of electroencephalograms and arterial halothane concentration in infants. *Acta Anaesthesiol Scand* 1989; **33**(8): 670–5.

51. Rampil IJ, Mason P, Singh H. Anesthetic potency (MAC) is independent of forebrain structures in the rat. *Anesthesiology* 1993; **78**(4): 707–12.

52. Antognini JF, Carstens E. *In vivo* characterization of clinical anaesthesia and its components. *Br J Anaesth* 2002; **89**(1): 156–66.

53. Antognini JF, Jinks SL, Atherley R *et al.* Spinal anaesthesia indirectly depresses cortical activity associated with electrical stimulation of the reticular formation. *Br J Anaesth* 2003; **91**(2): 233–8.

54. Hermanns H, Stevens MF, Werdehausen R *et al.* Sedation during spinal anaesthesia in infants. *Br J Anaesth* 2006; **97**(3): 380–4.

55. Goldenthal EI. A compilation of LD50 values in newborn and adult animals. *Toxicol Appl Pharmacol* 1971; **18**(1): 185–207.

56. Kupferberg HJ, Way EL. Pharmacologic basis for the increased sensitivity of the newborn rat to morphine. *J Pharmacol Exp Ther* 1963; **141**: 105–12.

57. Lerman J, Robinson S, Willis MM, Gregory GA. Anesthetic requirements for halothane in young children 0–1 month and 1–6 months of age. *Anesthesiology* 1983; **59**(5): 421–4.

58. Cook DR, Brandom BW, Shiu G, Wolfson B. The inspired median effective dose, brain concentration at anesthesia, and cardiovascular index for halothane in young rats. *Anesth Analg* 1981; **60**(4): 182–5.

59. Eger EI. Isoflurane: a review. *Anesthesiology* 1981; **55**(5): 559–76.

60. Paut O, Lazzell VA, Bissonnette B. The effect of low concentrations of halothane on the cerebrovascular circulation in young children. *Anaesthesia* 2000; **55**(6): 528–31.

61. Todd MM, Drummond JC. A comparison of the cerebrovascular and metabolic effects of halothane and isoflurane in the cat. *Anesthesiology* 1984; **60**(4): 276–82.

62. Leon JE, Bissonnette B. Cerebrovascular responses to carbon dioxide in children anaesthetized with halothane and isoflurane. *Can J Anaesth* 1991; **38**(7): 817–25.

63. Scheller MS, Todd MM, Drummond JC, Zornow MH. The intracranial pressure effects of isoflurane and halothane administered following cryogenic brain injury in rabbits. *Anesthesiology* 1987; **67**(4): 507–12.

64. Luginbuehl IA, Fredrickson MJ, Karsli C, Bissonnette B. Cerebral blood flow velocity in children anaesthetized with desflurane. *Paediatr Anaesth* 2003; **13**(6): 496–500.

65. Luginbuehl IA, Karsli C, Bissonnette B. Cerebrovascular reactivity to carbon dioxide is preserved during hypocapnia in children anesthetized with 1.0 MAC, but not with 1.5 MAC desflurane. *Can J Anaesth* 2003; **50**(2): 166–71.

66. Smith JH, Karsli C, Lagace A et al. Cerebral blood flow velocity increases when propofol is changed to desflurane, but not when isoflurane is changed to desflurane in children. *Acta Anaesthesiol Scand* 2005; **49**(1): 23–7.

67. Fairgrieve R, Rowney DA, Karsli C, Bissonnette B. The effect of sevoflurane on cerebral blood flow velocity in children. *Acta Anaesthesiol Scand* 2003; **47**(10): 1226–30.

68. Wong GT, Luginbuehl I, Karsli C, Bissonnette B. The effect of sevoflurane on cerebral autoregulation in young children as assessed by the transient hyperemic response. *Anesth Analg* 2006; **102**(4): 1051–5.

69. Rowney DA, Fairgrieve R, Bissonnette B. Cerebrovascular carbon dioxide reactivity in children anaesthetized with sevoflurane. *Br J Anaesth* 2002; **88**(3): 357–61.

70. Wilson-Smith E, Karsli C, Luginbuehl I, Bissonnette B. Effect of nitrous oxide on cerebrovascular reactivity to carbon dioxide in children during sevoflurane anaesthesia. *Br J Anaesth* 2003; **91**(2): 190–5.

71. Karsli C, Wilson-Smith E, Luginbuehl I, Bissonnette B. The effect of nitrous oxide on cerebrovascular reactivity to carbon dioxide in children during propofol anesthesia. *Anesth Analg* 2003; **97**(3): 694–8.

72. Karsli C, Luginbuehl I, Farrar M, Bissonnette B. Cerebrovascular carbon dioxide reactivity in children anaesthetized with propofol. *Paediatr Anaesth* 2003; **13**(1): 26–31.

73. Karsli C, Luginbuehl I, Farrar M, Bissonnette B. Propofol decreases cerebral blood flow velocity in anesthetized children. *Can J Anaesth* 2002; **49**(8): 830–4.

74. Karsli C, Luginbuehl I, Bissonnette B. The cerebrovascular response to hypocapnia in children receiving propofol. *Anesth Analg* 2004; **99**(4): 1049–52.

75. Jobes DR, Kennell EM, Bush GL et al. Cerebral blood flow and metabolism during morphine – nitrous oxide anesthesia in man. *Anesthesiology* 1977; **47**(1): 16–8.

76. Lagace A, Karsli C, Luginbuehl I, Bissonnette B. The effect of remifentanil on cerebral blood flow velocity in children anesthetized with propofol. *Paediatr Anaesth* 2004; **14**(10): 861–5.

77. Abdallah C, Karsli C, Bissonnette B. Fentanyl is more effective than remifentanil at preventing increases in cerebral blood flow velocity during intubation in children. *Can J Anaesth* 2002; **49**(10): 1070–5.

78. Nugent M, Artru AA, Michenfelder JD. Cerebral metabolic, vascular and protective effects of midazolam maleate: comparison to diazepam. *Anesthesiology* 1982; **56**(3): 172–6.

79. Michenfelder JD. The interdependency of cerebral functional and metabolic effects following massive doses of thiopental in the dog. *Anesthesiology* 1974; **41**(3): 231–6.

80. Takeshita H, Okuda Y, Sari A. The effects of ketamine on cerebral circulation and metabolism in man. *Anesthesiology* 1972; **36**(1): 69–75.

81. Kam PC, Ferch NI. Apoptosis: mechanisms and clinical implications. *Anaesthesia* 2000; **55**(11): 1081–93.

82. Olney JW, Young C, Wozniak DF et al. Do pediatric drugs cause developing neurons to commit suicide? *Trends Pharmacol Sci* 2004; **25**(3): 135–9.

83. Olney JW, Young C, Wozniak DF et al. Anesthesia-induced developmental neuroapoptosis. Does it happen in humans? *Anesthesiology* 2004; **101**(2): 273–5.

84. Jevtovic-Todorovic V, Hartman RE, Izumi Y et al. Early exposure to common anesthetic agents causes widespread neurodegeneration in the developing rat brain and persistent learning deficits. *J Neurosci* 2003; **23**(3): 876–82.

85. Anand KJ, Soriano SG. Anesthetic agents and the immature brain: are these toxic or therapeutic? *Anesthesiology* 2004; **101**(2): 527–30.

Haematology

REEMA NANDI, RICHARD MARTIN

KEY LEARNING POINTS

- There are important differences in the characteristics of blood in neonates, infants and children, which must be considered in an anaesthetic evaluation.
- Anaemia is the commonest blood disorder in neonates and children; it is often age related and multifactorial in origin.
- Sickle cell disease is a severe, multisystem disorder characterised by endothelial dysfunction.

- The value of preoperative transfusion in sickle cell disease is uncertain. Each child should be considered separately.
- Management of coagulation disturbance requires consideration of the clinical circumstances alongside the results of coagulation testing.

INTRODUCTION

This chapter provides a brief overview of haematological conditions that affect the anaesthetic management of paediatric patients.

In children the blood can be affected by many factors, including environment, diet and illness, so that 'abnormalities' are relatively common. The child's bone marrow is more reactive and small stimuli can cause significant changes in the peripheral blood film; for example, infection may result in mild or moderate degrees of anaemia and elevations of the platelet count. It is essential to assess haematological parameters against age-appropriate range, as these may be different from adults. In addition, important differences exist in the characteristics of blood in neonates and children that must be considered in the anaesthetic evaluation of the paediatric patient.

HAEMATOPOIESIS

Haematopoiesis, is the production of cells of all the haematopoietic lineages and takes place primarily in the bone marrow in children and adults. It begins in the yolk sac during the third week of gestation. By 6–8 weeks' gestation the liver becomes the primary site of haematopoesis, and at 11 weeks it begins in the bone marrow, although the foetal liver remains the principal site of production until the end of the third trimester.

Erythropoiesis in the newborn

Production of new red blood cells and the rate of haemoglobin (Hb) synthesis declines sharply after birth and remains low for the first 2 weeks of life. Erythropoiesis begins to increase after the first 2 weeks but the rise in haemoglobin is not apparent until many weeks later. At 3 months of age a healthy infant should generate 2 mL packed red cells per day. By comparison, during the first 2 months of life maximal red cell production in preterm neonates is approximately 1 mL/day. Neonatal red cells, particularly from preterm babies, have a reduced life span of 35–50 days compared with 60–70 days for term infants and 120 days for healthy adults. This may be because differences in neonatal red cell metabolism increase susceptibility to oxidant-induced injury.

HAEMOGLOBIN

Haemoglobin is a tetramer of two pairs of usually unlike globin polypeptide chains, each associated with a haem group. There are developmental changes in globin type: there are embryonic, foetal and adult haemoglobins. The first globin chain produced is ε-globin, followed almost immediately by α- and γ-globin. Foetal haemoglobin (HbF) ($\alpha_2\gamma_2$) is synthesised from 4–5 weeks' gestation and is the predominant haemoglobin until after birth. Adult haemoglobin (HbA) ($\alpha_2\beta_2$) is produced from 6–8 weeks' gestation but remains at low levels (10–15 per cent) until 30–32 weeks. After this, the rate of HbA production increases concurrently with a fall in HbF production, resulting in an average HbF level at birth of 70–80 per cent, an HbA level of 25–30 per cent, small amounts of HbA_2 and sometimes a trace of Hb Barts (β_4). Normal adult haemoglobin contains three different types of haemoglobin: HbA ($\alpha_2\beta_2$) making up 95–98 per cent of total Hb; HbA_2 ($\alpha_2\delta_2$) making up 1.5–3.2 per cent of total haemoglobin; and HbF making up 0.5–0.8 per cent.

After birth and over the first year of life the level of HbF declines to <2 per cent. In term neonates there is little change in HbF level in the first 15 days but thereafter it declines. However, in preterm babies the HbF level may not change for 6 weeks, before HbA production starts to increase. This delay in HbA production can delay the diagnosis of β-globin disorders in neonates. α-Globin chains are essential for the production of both HbF and HbA and α-thalassaemia major causes severe anaemia from early in foetal life.

In term babies the haemoglobin, haematocrit and red cell indices fall slowly over the first few weeks of life, reaching a mean haemoglobin of 13–14 g/dL at 4 weeks of age and 9.5–11 g/dL at 7–9 weeks of age. In otherwise well premature infants, there is a steeper fall in haemoglobin reaching a mean of 6.5–9 g/dL at 4–8 weeks' postnatal age [1]. Erythropoiesis is suppressed, so the reticulocyte count and numbers of nucleated red cells also fall rapidly after birth. The reticulocyte count starts to rise in term babies at 7–8 weeks of age, reaching 35–200 $\times$ 10^9/L (1–1.8 per cent) at 2 months of age and in preterm babies at 6–8 weeks of age.

Normal blood volume at birth varies with gestational age and the timing of umbilical cord clamping. In healthy term infants average blood volume is 80 mL/kg with a range of 50–100 mL/kg. The blood volume is higher in preterm infants, with an average of 106 mL/kg and range of 85–143 mL/kg. Stores of iron and folic acid are lower in preterm babies and moreover utilisation is more rapid leading to deficiency after 2–4 months, if recommended daily intakes are not maintained. Even term neonates with normal haemoglobin concentration at birth may have depleted their iron stores by the time they have doubled their birth weight.

MEGAKARYOCYTES AND PLATELETS IN THE FOETUS AND NEWBORN

Platelets first appear in the fetal circulation at 5–6 weeks' gestation. Fetal megakaryocytes are smaller and more immature than those in adult marrow, with a reduced formation of pro-platelets; these differences may contribute to the frequent occurrence of thrombocytopenia in sick neonates.

Platelet counts at birth in term and preterm neonates are within the normal adult range [2]. *In vitro* studies of neonatal platelets have identified impaired function, but this is not clinically significant. There is no bleeding tendency in neonates with normal platelet counts and coagulation tests and the bleeding time is normal in term and preterm infants (<135 seconds) [3].

WHITE BLOOD CELLS IN THE FOETUS AND NEWBORN

All types of leukocytes found in adult blood are also found in the foetus and at full term. Monocytes circulate from 4 to 5 weeks' gestation and eosinophils and basophils from 14 to 16 weeks' gestation, each cell type being present in low numbers and increasing slowly to the normal values at term. The neutrophil storage pool (a reserve ready for mobilisation in response to infection) is reduced in the newborn, particularly in preterm infants and in those with intrauterine growth restriction (IUGR) or exposure to maternal hypertension [4]. This may explain the frequency of bacterial infection in such infants.

The neutrophil and monocyte counts vary over the first few days of life even in healthy babies. For the first 12 hours they increase then fall to a nadir at 4 days. Normal values for neutrophils at birth are also affected by other factors including antenatal and perinatal history. The neutrophil count is higher in capillary samples and after vigorous crying; it is lower in neonates with IUGR, those born to mothers with hypertension or diabetes, and in neonates of African origin [5].

RED CELL DISORDERS

Anaemia

Anaemia is the commonest haematological abnormality in newborns and children, and causes vary with age and are

Table 7.1   Causes of anaemia in neonates, infants and childhood

	Neonatal	Infancy	Childhood
Blood loss	Occult bleeding (fetomaternal, fetoplacental, twin to twin) Obstetric accidents Internal bleeding Iatrogenic	Hiatus hernia	Hiatus hernia Epistaxis
Increased destruction	Rhesus incompatibility ABO incompatibility Spherocytosis G6PD deficiency	Sickle cell Thalassaemia Spherocytosis	Sickle cell Thalassaemia Spherocytosis
Decreased production	Infection	Infection Nutritional deficiency Bone marrow depression	Chronic infection Chronic disease
Bleeding disorder	Haemorrhagic disease of the newborn	Haemophilia Christmas disease	Haemophilia Christmas disease
Anaemia of prematurity	Impaired red cell production and reduced red cell lifespan		

G6PD, glucose-6-phosphate dehydrogenase.

often multifactorial. Anaemia is one of the main factors (together with cardiopulmonary function and the position of the haemoglobin–oxygen dissociation curve) influencing tissue oxygenation. In neonates, the two most important factors determining the position of the haemoglobin–oxygen dissociation curve are the HbF and 2,3-diphosphoglycerate (2,3-DPG) concentrations within red blood cells: a high HbF and low 2,3-DPG both cause the curve to be shifted to the left. This is found after birth and is more marked in preterm babies with higher HbF concentrations. Over the first few months of life 2,3-DPG levels rise and HbF levels fall so the haemoglobin–oxygen dissociation curve gradually shifts to the right. This increase in tissue oxygen delivery counteracts the effects of the falling haemoglobin over the first months of life.

The common causes of anaemia in the newborn, infants and children are shown in Table 7.1.

NEONATAL ANAEMIA

Very preterm infants – <26 weeks' post-conceptional age (PCA) – often need prolonged inpatient care; anaemia is universal and often severe. Blood loss is the commonest cause – often from frequent blood sampling. In addition, the anaemia of prematurity is exacerbated by reduced red cell lifespan and low erythropoietin production. Blood transfusion remains the only treatment for nearly all cases of neonatal anaemia. Erythropoietin has been shown to be of limited practical value and its use is confined to prevention or reduction of the late anaemia of prematurity [6].

In term infants, blood loss is often occult. It can occur before or around delivery due to feto-maternal haemorrhage or twin-to-twin transfusion. It may occur as a result

of bleeding from a ruptured cord or abnormal placenta, or there may be internal bleeding, for example intracranial haemorrhage, particularly if the delivery is traumatic.

ANAEMIA IN INFANTS AND CHILDREN

Nutritional deficiencies are the commonest anaemias in childhood, and iron deficiency is the most frequent.

Although severe anaemia can usually be suspected in children during a careful preoperative assessment, mild degrees can be missed without laboratory testing [7]. When anaemia is defined as a haemoglobin concentration of less than 10 g/dL, the incidence appears to be about 0.5 per cent [8]. The prevalence may be higher in patients of a lower socioeconomic group [9]. It has been proposed that routine preoperative haemoglobin testing is indicated only for infants less than 1 year of age, children at risk of sickle cell disease who have never been tested and children with systemic disease [10,11].

APLASTIC ANAEMIAS

These can be inherited or acquired. Fanconi's anaemia is an autosomal recessive condition and the most common of the inherited types. It is a progressive and fatal condition developing after about 5 years of age. Bone marrow transplantation is the main treatment. The literature is limited in this rare condition [12]. Acquired aplastic anaemias can occur at any age. They can be caused by drugs (e.g. chloramphenicol) or following viral infections (e.g. hepatitis A, B or C) but sometimes there is no obvious precipitating cause. Bone marrow transplantation is the current treatment.

ANAESTHESIA ISSUES

In all cases of anaemia standard preoperative evaluation should include an assessment of cardiopulmonary reserve. Adequate blood and blood products should be available and drugs that may exacerbate bone marrow suppression (e.g. chloramphenicol or sulphonamides) should be avoided. Nitrous oxide should be avoided for long procedures (longer than 6 hours) as it may cause bone marrow suppression.

Haemolytic anaemias

Most of the haemolytic disorders that cause clinical problems in childhood are inherited. Haemolysis is defined by an increased rate of red cell destruction with a shortening of the normal lifespan of the cell from 120 days to as little as a few days in severe haemolysis. Haemolysis is usually associated with raised blood unconjugated bilirubin.

RED CELL MEMBRANE DISORDERS

Hereditary spherocytosis

Hereditary spherocytosis (HS) is the commonest hereditary haemolytic anaemia in north Europeans. It caused by a variety of different genetic defects in the red cell skeletal proteins. It affects 1 in 5000 people and is autosomal dominant. There are mutations in genes that encode the red cell membrane proteins essential for maintaining normal cellular integrity. In severe disease a splenectomy will remove the site of red cell destruction, thereby returning the haemoglobin to normal and the red cell lifespan to near normal.

Hereditary elliptocytosis

This common disorder is usually inherited as an autosomal dominant trait and is often diagnosed as an incidental finding. Rare homozygous variants with chronic severe haemolysis may require splenectomy.

ANAESTHETIC ISSUES

There is little in the literature about anaesthetic management of these disorders. Transfusion to bring the haemoglobin to an appropriate level for the surgery and the condition of the child is the main anaesthetic consideration.

Red cell enzyme defects

Genotypic and phenotypic variations have been reported for almost every red blood cell enzyme. The most common red cell enzymopathies that may cause anaemia are glucose-6-phosphate dehydrogenase deficiency (G6PD) and pyruvate kinase (PK) deficiency.

GLUCOSE-6-PHOSPHATE DEHYDROGENASE DEFICIENCY

Glucose-6-phosphate dehydrogenase deficiency is the most common abnormality of red cell enzymes and, indeed, is the most common human genetic disorder with a worldwide distribution. Glucose-6-phosphate dehydrogenase maintains red cell glutathione in its reduced state, thereby protecting red cell membranes from oxidant damage. Drugs (Table 7.2), chemicals or an intercurrent infection can induce oxidation and haemolysis occurs as a result of oxidative cell membrane damage. Deficiency may confer some resistance to malaria because infected red cells cannot detoxify parasite oxidant metabolites so both cell and parasite die prematurely.

There are many variants of G6PD deficiency. The vast majority of individuals are asymptomatic, although some have moderately severe anaemia and jaundice. A severe variant is associated with a complete absence of enzyme in all red cells. After oxidant exposure, haemoglobin forms intracellular inclusions called Heinz bodies which attach to the red cell membrane and trigger haemolysis. In newborns with G6PD deficiency, stress from delivery, infection or antibiotics can precipitate haemolysis and the diagnosis should be considered in all neonates with haemolytic jaundice and kernicterus. Many areas with susceptible populations (e.g. Hawaii) have introduced newborn screening. Jaundice is particularly common in premature infants with G6PD deficiency.

Favism is a severe form of G6PD deficiency that occurs after ingestion of fava beans. It can result in acute, life-threatening haemolysis which requires blood transfusion. Most cases, however, resolve spontaneously and will not recur if the patient avoids fava beans.

Treatment for patients with G6PD deficiency involves supportive care for acute events and counselling with a list of proscribed drugs.

Anaesthetists must be careful not to administer or prescribe mediations to which these patients may be susceptible (Table 7.2).

PYRUVATE KINASE DEFICIENCY

Pyruvate kinase deficiency is the commonest cause of non-spherocytic haemolysis in northern Europe. Inheritance is autosomal recessive and it results in chronic haemolysis with varying grades of severity in different individuals. Medication is not implicated in this condition. Neonatal jaundice occurs and infection can also precipitate more severe haemolysis. Splenomegaly is usually present.

Pyruvate kinase deficiency causes a rise in 2,3-DPG levels and thus a shift to the right in the oxygen dissociation curve with a consequent improvement in oxygen availability. Thus, patients with PK deficiency can tolerate very low haemoglobin levels and should not be transfused unless clinically unwell or failing to thrive. In severely affected children who require intermittent transfusions, usually

Table 7.2 Drugs that precipitate haemolysis in glucose-6-phosphate dehydrogenase (G6PD)-deficient patients. Deficiency of G6PD has a spectrum of severity; drugs may be considered as those likely to precipitate haemolysis in all affected patients and those that may cause haemolysis in some

Group	Drugs likely to cause haemolysis in most G6PD-deficient patients	Drugs with possible risk of haemolysis in some G6PD-deficient patients
Analgesics	Prilocaine	Aspirin* (acetylsalicylic acid)
Antimalarials	Primaquine, pamaquine, pentaquine	Chloroquine, quinidine, quinine (acceptable risk in acute malaria)
Nitrofurans	Nitrofurantoin, furaltadone	
Quinolones	Ciprofloxacin, moxofloxacin, nalidixic acid, norfloxacin, ofloxacin	
Sulphonamides	Sulfapyridine, sulfisoxazole, sulfadiazine, co-trimoxazole	
Sulphones	Dapsone	
Miscellaneous	Chloramphenicol, menadiol sodium phosphate (water-soluble vitamin K analogue), methylene blue	

*Asprin not recommended for use in children.

because they are decompensated by infections, splenectomy should be considered.

Haemoglobinopathies

Haemoglobinopathies are disorders in haemoglobin structure and synthesis, caused by molecular defects affecting a particular globin chain. Structural abnormalities in haemoglobin result in alterations in oxygen transport, haemoglobin stability or physical changes in the haemoglobin molecule (e.g. sickle cell disease). Haemoglobinopathies resulting from the production of abnormal α- or β-globin chains are called thalassaemias.

SICKLE CELL DISEASE

Sickle cell disease (SCD) is a congenital haemoglobinopathy caused by a structural abnormality in the β-globin chains of haemoglobin. The sickle cell diseases are inherited in an autosomal, co-dominant way, with the homozygous expression of the abnormal gene (SS) producing SCD. The spectrum of sickling disorders is widened by the combination of HbS with other haemoglobinopathies such as thalassaemia and HbC (a different β-globin mutation), HbD and HbE. Sickle cell disease is characterised by deformed red blood cells, acute episodic attacks of pain and pulmonary compromise, widespread organ damage and shortened life expectancy. The perioperative period is hazardous for these patients.

The molecular defect in HbS results from the substitution of valine for glutamic acid in the sixth position of the β-globin chain. This substitution leads to a change in the electrostatic charge of HbS when oxygen is released, turning it into an insoluble polymer and transforming the red

blood cell from a deformable, biconcave disc into a rigid, sickle-cell shape. This structural change is exacerbated in the presence of hypoxia, acidosis and hypertonicity.

Heterozygous expression of the SS gene results in sickle cell trait (AS); less than 50 per cent of haemoglobin is S type, red cell indices are normal and no adverse clinical sequelae occur unless there is severe hypoxia. Generally, no special precautions are required for anaesthesia or other medical interventions. Although sickle trait is almost completely benign, splenic infarction at high altitude has been reported [13].

World-wide there are approximately 4 million people with SCD, of whom 60 000 are in North America. There were estimated to be 12 000 patients with SCD in the UK in 2003 with approximately 70–75 per cent of patients in the London region [14]. Neonatal screening and early diagnosis are essential as mortality from SCD is nearly 20 per cent by 3 years of age without treatment [15]. Sickle cell disease can be diagnosed in the newborn using haemoglobin electrophoresis of umbilical cord blood. DNA analysis of foetal tissue from chorionic villous sampling or amniocentesis allows antenatal diagnosis of SCD. Sickle solubility testing using sodium metabisulphite (Sickledex test) is a simple and quick investigation to confirm the presence of HbS although electrophoresis is necessary to distinguish the genotype. The Sickledex test is not reliable in early infancy when there are low levels of HbS and high levels of HbF which has normal solubility.

CLINICAL MANIFESTATIONS OF SCD

Cickle cell disease is a multisystem disorder (Table 7.3) and patients tend to have a haemoglobin level of 6–9 g/dL and reticulocyte counts of 5–15 per cent, but the combination of a hyperdynamic circulation and the low oxygen affinity of

Table 7.3 The features of sickle cell disease (SCD)

Crises	Acute infarction	Clinical features
Painful	Abdominal	Pallor, icterus
Haemolytic	Pulmonary	Hepatomegaly,
Aplastic	Neurological	splenomegaly
Hepatic	Dactylitis	Chronic leg ulcers
Megaloblastic	Aseptic necrosis	Renal involvement –
	Femoral and	haematuria, inability
	humeral heads	to concentrate urine
		Infections –
		pneumococcal
		septicaemia,
		salmonella
		osteomyelitis

HbS maintains adequate tissue oxygen delivery. Haemolytic crises are rare. Aplastic crises can cause massive suppression of normal erythropoiesis and are usually precipitated by infection [16].

Acute splenic sequestration can occur in the first 5 years of life and may require repeated transfusion and splenectomy. More commonly, splenic infarctions occur resulting in functional hyposplenism usually by the age of 7 years. These patients are at increased risk of infections such as osteomyelitis and splenic abscesses [17] and are particularly susceptible to organisms such as *Streptococcus pneumoniae*, *Neisseria meningitides* and *Haemophilus influenzae* type b.

Recurrent acute pain is common, arising from ischaemia and infarction in the marrow or cortical bone, while abdominal pain can be caused by bowel dysfunction, organ infarction or referred pain from the ribs. Dactylitis – painful swelling of the small bones of the hands and feet – affects up to 50 per cent of SS children by the age of 2. On average, patients experience 0.8 episodes of pain per patient year, although 1 per cent have more than six episodes per year [18]. Precipitants for acute pain crises include intercurrent infection, dehydration, cold, hypoxia and stress. However, 57 per cent of episodes have no identifiable precipitant [19].

ACUTE CHEST SYNDROME

Acute chest syndrome (ACS) is defined as the onset of a new lobar infiltration on chest X-ray, excluding atelectasis, accompanied by fever greater than 38.5°C, respiratory distress or chest pain [20]. It is a leading cause of morbidity and mortality in patients with SCD, with multifactorial aetiology, including infection, infarction, pulmonary sequestration and fat embolism. Data on more than 3750 SCD patients were collected in the Cooperative Study of SCD to look at the features of ACS [21]. The study found that children with SCD, aged between 2 and 4 years, presented with fever and cough and a negative physical examination, and rarely had pain. In contrast, adults were often febrile and complained of shortness of breath, chills and severe pain. Upper lobe lung disease was more common in children but adults had multilobar and lower lobe disease. The incidence of ACS in the postoperative child has been found to be as high as 10.2 per cent [22]. Risk factors include an age of 2–4 years, sickle disease and a persistently raised white cell count [23]. Multiple episodes of ACS in childhood are likely to result in pulmonary fibrosis.

OTHER EFFECTS OF SCD

Cardiac signs reflecting a hyperdynamic circulation, in keeping with chronic anaemia, are typical in SCD patients. Cardiomegaly is a frequent finding and congestive heart failure may occur in some children.

Cerebrovascular accidents (CVAs) are a severe complication of SCD; 5 per cent of children with SCD experience overt CVAs [24] and 17 per cent may have changes on magnetic resonance imaging (MRI) suggestive of infarction or ischaemia with no history of stroke [25]. Children at risk of stroke can be identified using transcranial Doppler (TCD) and, if transfused to maintain an HbS level of less than 30 per cent, the risk of stroke is reduced by 92 per cent [26]. Children with SCD are also at increased risk of intracerebral and subarachnoid haemorrhages. Cerebral endarteritis rather than aneurysms seems to be an important cause of these cerebral events [27].

The kidney is at risk of vaso-occlusion and the incidence of renal parenchymal scarring is high. Priapism is reported by 30 per cent of male SCD patients with attacks starting as young as 8 years [28] and occurring from 1 to 52 times a year. It can occur in the postoperative period and treatment includes hydration, alkalinisation, exchange transfusions and intercavernous injections of α-adrenergic agent.

PATHOPHYSIOLOGY OF SCD

The central pathological event of SCD has been thought to be an irreversible sickling of red blood cells, as a result of the insolubility of deoxygenated HbS, producing clumping of red blood cells and vaso-occlusion. There is now increasing evidence of endothelial dysfunction in SCD suggesting that the endothelium itself may be the immediate origin of symptoms in many acute episodes [29,30]. For example, sickle cell neurological pathology may arise from cerebral arterial damage rather than venous sickling [31]. Arterial damage may be a primary rather than a secondary feature of SCD. Powars *et al.* demonstrated in 1998 that progressive pulmonary vascular damage preceded episodes of ACS and pulmonary infarction [32]. Haemoglobin S is extremely unstable and this may the cause of extensive vascular damage rather than its insolubility. Instability of the globin in HbS accelerates molecular breakdown and there is extensive oxidant damage to the cell membrane, disruption of the phospholipid bilayer and impairment of function. This leads to increased adherence to the vascular endothelium, producing endothelial damage and dysfunction. This is supported by the presence of biochemical markers of endothelial damage in SCD and suggests that the disease should be considered as a chronic inflammatory disorder [33].

RISK FACTORS FOR SICKLE CRISES

Low HbF concentration and leukocytosis are associated with increased risk of early death, ACS and painful episodes [34]. Patients with low steady-state haemoglobin are more likely to suffer early death and stroke but are less likely to have ACS and pain. Both avascular necrosis and sickle retinopathy are associated with a higher steady-state haemoglobin. Other known disease modifiers are the β-globin cluster haplotype and α-thalassaemia [35]. Miller *et al.* tested many putative risk factors in the Cooperative Study for Sickle Cell Disease infant cohort. Infants with SS or sickle-β^0-thalassaemia (Sβ^0) who had a haemoglobin concentration below 7 g/dL in steady state during the second year of life, those with an increased white blood cell count and those who had dactylitis before 1 year of age were at significantly increased risk of an adverse outcome [34].

ANAESTHESIA AND SCD

From 1978 to 1988, the Cooperative Study of Sickle Cell Disease observed 3765 patients with a mean follow-up of 5.3 ± 2.0 years [36]. A total of 1079 surgical procedures were conducted on 717 patients (77 per cent sickle cell anaemia [SS], 14 per cent sickle haemoglobin C disease [SC], 5.7 per cent Sβ^0 thalassaemia, 3 per cent Sβ^0 + thalassaemia). Of these 69 per cent had a single procedure, 21 per cent had two procedures, and the remaining 11 per cent had more than two procedures during the study follow-up. The most frequent operations were cholecystectomy or splenectomy (24 per cent of all surgery, $n = 258$). Of these, 93 per cent received blood transfusion, and there was no association between preoperative HbA level and complication rates (except a reduction in pain crises). Overall mortality rate within 30 days of a surgical procedure was 1.1 per cent (12 deaths after 1079 surgical procedures). Three deaths were considered to be related to the surgical procedure and/or anaesthesia (0.3 per cent). No deaths were reported in patients younger than 14 years of age. Sickle cell disease-related postoperative complications were more frequent in SCD patients who received regional compared with general anaesthesia. There were more non-SCD-related postoperative complications in both SCD and sickle trait patients who received regional anaesthesia than in those who received general anaesthesia. Perioperative transfusion was associated with a lower rate of SCD-related postoperative complications for SCD patients undergoing low-risk procedures, with crude rates of 12.9 per cent without transfusion compared with 4.8 per cent with transfusion.

Elective surgery carries a significant risk of sickle-related complications in the postoperative period to patients with SCD. Perioperative management includes pre-emptive blood transfusion, aggressive hydration, and the avoidance of hypoxia, hypothermia and acidosis.

There are no studies to identify which SCD patients are most at risk of perioperative complications, although it has been found that children under 2 years with dactylitis, severe anaemia with a Hb < 7 and leukocytosis in the absence of infection are likely to develop severe SCD later in life [34].

Preoperative assessment should involve a careful systematic review, with particular attention to possible end-organ damage. Respiratory disease from previous episodes of ACS may result in reduced lung volumes, intrapulmonary shunting, pulmonary infarction and pulmonary hypertension. Cardiomegaly may be seen on chest X-ray (CXR) and diastolic dysfunction seen on echocardiography. Neurological examination is needed to establish any pre-existing deficit from previous CVAs. There may be renal impairment resulting in decreased ability to concentrate urine in the kidney. There may be hepatic dysfunction as a result of vaso-occlusive damage, post-transfusion hepatitis or cirrhosis.

Hypoxia must be avoided in patients with SCD; perioperative and postoperative pulse oximetry (SpO$_2$) monitoring is essential. Premedication and opioid analgesia are not contraindicated, although they should be used with caution. Dehydration is poorly tolerated owing to impaired urine-concentrating ability. An SCD patient should be early on the operating list and intravenous fluid should be considered during periods of fasting. Postoperative fluids should be continued until an adequate oral intake has been established. However, there are no published studies evaluating the effect of aggressive hydration in reducing the incidence of postoperative SCD complications.

BLOOD TRANSFUSION IN SCD

Preparation of patients for elective surgery has involved partial exchange or top-up transfusion to raise the HbA level. This practice, largely based on anecdotal evidence, was thought to reduce the frequency of postoperative sickle-related complications. A systematic review of the literature relating to preoperative transfusion practice in SCD was carried out in 2002 for the Cochrane Collaboration by Riddington and Williamson [37]. This revealed that few large rigorous studies have been carried out in this area and the only study that met the strict Cochrane criteria for inclusion was that of Vichinsky *et al.* in 1995 from the Preoperative Transfusion in Sickle Cell Disease Study Group [38]. These authors concluded that a conservative transfusion regimen was as effective as an aggressive exchange regimen in preventing perioperative complications in patients with SCD, and the conservative approach resulted in only half as many transfusion-associated complications. This has halved the exposure to allogeneic blood, with a concomitant reduction in red cell alloimmunisation.

Griffin and Buchanan [39] reported 57 surgical procedures in children not prepared by preoperative transfusion. Complications occurred in 26 per cent, rising to more than 50 per cent after thoracotomy, laparotomy or adenotonsillectomy. Most complications, however, were minor, and the only case of chest syndrome following adenotonsillectomy was in a girl with pre-existing lung disease. The authors concluded that the benefits of routine preoperative transfusion were open to question [40]. More recently, Buchanan and coworkers [41] reported on 28 SCD children having 38 minor procedures, 35 without preoperative transfusion. Postoperative complications involving transient fever or pain occurred in five patients. No postoperative chest syndrome occurred. Neumayr et al. [42] concluded that routine transfusion was not needed for minor surgery, but that patients having abdominal surgery seemed to benefit.

Experience in parts of the world where routine preoperative transfusion is not practised, but where meticulous care is taken with other aspects of perioperative support, suggests that the frequency of complications is low. In a study of 284 procedures in Jamaica, mainly in adults, Homi et al. [43] reported that two-thirds of patients underwent surgery without any transfusion, and that complications were actually less frequent in untransfused patients (13 per cent versus 28 per cent).

The use of chronic transfusion programmes has a more established role in SCD in the prevention of CVAs, as previously discussed [26,27], and is also required in the treatment of aplastic anaemia, sequestration in the spleen and the prevention of painful crises. The dangers of blood transfusion in SCD, including red cell alloimmunisation and postoperative infections, have been recognised for some time. Alloimmunisation, the development of antibodies to non-ABO blood groups, has a high incidence in SCD, with new alloantibodies developing in 7 per cent of patients during perioperative transfusion regimens [38]. Alloantibodies can complicate future cross-matching and transfusion reactions have been associated with stroke, pain crises and acute respiratory failure. Alloimmunisation to human leukocyte antigen and human platelet antigen, which may cause problems with kidney or bone marrow transplantation, has also been observed in multitransfused sickle patients. There is also evidence that perioperative transfusion increases the risk of developing postoperative infection. This so-called immunomodulatory effect of transfusion has been attributed to donor leukocytes [44]. It is unclear whether the provision of leukodepleted blood will result in a measurable reduction of postoperative infections and hospital length of stay.

Therefore, there is no clear answer to the best protocol for preoperative transfusion in SCD. When considering the need for preoperative transfusion, a multidisciplinary approach should be taken with consultation of paediatrician, haematologist, anaesthetist and surgeon as well as the child's family. Each patient must be considered individually, taking into account the patient's past medical history, risk factors for complications and the surgical procedure. (Suggested guidelines are given in the addendum on page 124.)

Although it is recommended to avoid perioperative hypothermia, there is no published evidence to link it with SCD complications [45]. Similarly, there is no evidence of harm in particular specialised circumstances (e.g. during cardiac or neurosurgery). Common sense suggests that, as with all surgical patients, normothermia should be maintained if possible. Other intraoperative practice is related to the surgical procedure and discussed in other chapters.

MANAGEMENT OF POSTOPERATIVE PAIN

Patients with SCD may have high perioperative analgesic requirements and pain management can be challenging. A recent retrospective study showed that children with SCD self-administered more than double the amount of morphine, reported more intense pain, used more non-opioid analgesia and remained hospitalised for more than twice as long as non-SCD children undergoing the same surgical procedure [46]. The pro-inflammatory nature of SCD might exacerbate acute postoperative pain. In addition, chronic pain is likely to contribute to postoperative hyperalgesia. If central neural sensitisation is an important factor the addition of an N-methyl-D-aspartate (NMDA) antagonist or epidural analgesia may be helpful in managing postoperative pain in SCD. There may be some tolerance to opioids in this group as a result of repeated exposure in the management of painful crises. However, care should be taken in the use of high doses of morphine as there is evidence to suggest that the plasma concentration of morphine and its metabolite morphine-6-glucuronide correlates with the risk of developing ACS [47].

Thalassaemia

Thalassaemias are a large and heterogeneous group of red cell disorders resulting from impaired or absent synthesis of globin chains [48]. In general, abnormalities of the α-globin chain (α-thalassaemia) present in the foetal/neonatal period, while abnormalities of the β-globin gene (β-thalassaemias) present later in infancy or childhood.

α-THALASSAEMIAS

The α-thalassaemias result from the deletion of one or more of the four α-globin genes on chromosome 16. Deletion of one or two genes results in α-thalassaemia trait which may cause only mild anaemia. Deletion of three α-globin chains causes HbH disease and deletion of all four genes causes α-thalassaemia major, which is incompatible with life. Several cases of α-thalassaemia major are seen in the UK each year. The α-thalassaemia genes are particularly common in Asia, but mild genotypes are also common in Africa, where they may modify the clinical severity of sickle cell disease.

β-THALASSAEMIAS

The β-thalassaemias are most common in the Indian sub-continent, Mediterranean and Middle East countries and to a lesser extent in Africa. β-Thalassaemia major occurs when the child inherits an abnormal β-globin gene from each parent resulting in two abnormal β-globin genes. The child is unable to make any HbA ($\alpha_2\beta_2$). They remain well up to 6–12 months of age as they are able to make HbF ($\alpha_2\gamma_2$). After this, with the decrease in HbF production, the child presents with progressive anaemia. Untreated, the child develops severe anaemia with growth retardation, hepatosplenomegaly (extramedullary haematopoiesis) failure to thrive and skeletal abnormalities caused by marrow hyperplasia. The skull X-ray has typical 'hair-on-end' appearance due to medullary expansion. Children with β-thalassaemia major require regular transfusions of red cells to maintain adequate haemoglobin levels, promote normal growth and development, and suppress the erythroid hyperplasia and skeletal manifestations. The child should receive red cells that have been fully phenotyped. The main problem with regular transfusions is iron loading, which is treated with an iron chelator. Iron loading results in tissue damage to endocrine glands (parathyroids, pancreas), failure to progress through puberty, skin discoloration, heart failure and dysrythmias. Cardiac iron loading causes death in inadequately chelated patients, often before the end of the second decade. Bone marrow transplantation is potentially curative in β-thalassaemia major and should be undertaken in young children before there has been significant transfusion iron overload [49].

The literature is sparse on the clinical anaesthetic management of these conditions [50]. Thalassaemia minor does not generally cause any anaesthetic problems. In thalassaemia major a careful preoperative examination is required. The cardiovascular implications of severe anaemia must be considered. In addition, medullary bone hyperplasia can result in increased blood loss in bony surgery and can even make tracheal intubation difficult if the maxilla or mandible is involved [51]. Organ dysfunction associated with iron overload and susceptibility to infection must also be considered.

SECONDARY ANAEMIA

The normal bone marrow produces 10^{11} red cells daily and is readily affected by many disease processes. Children often develop anaemia as a consequence of intercurrent illness. Even a transient infection may cause a significant fall in haemoglobin, but this will recover rapidly when the infection clears. More chronic illnesses such as rheumatoid arthritis and other connective tissue disorders are often complicated by 'the anaemia of chronic disease' which is partly caused by inflammatory cytokines and reduced erythropoietin production. Patients may become iron deficient because of poor diet or blood loss from the gut (possibly due to non-steroidal anti-inflammatory drugs [NSAIDs]). Rheumatoid arthritis is particularly complex because the patients may also develop marrow hypoplasia due to some drugs (e.g. gold therapy). Patients with connective tissue disorders such as systemic lupus erythematosus (SLE) can develop autoimmune haemolysis. Other important diseases associated with anaemia are acute and chronic renal failure, and some endocrine disorders, particularly hypothyroidism. Blood dyscrasias may arise as a result of medication.

WHITE BLOOD CELLS

Haematological malignancy

Children with white cell disorders who require anaesthesia generally have haematological malignancies. The most common childhood conditions within this group are acute lymphoblastic leukaemia, acute myeloid leukaemia and non-Hodgkin's lymphoma.

ACUTE LYMPHOBLASTIC LEUKAEMIA

This is the most common cancer occurring in children. It normally appears between the ages of 2 and 5 years. Prior to the 1970s survivors were rare but currently the survival rate is around 85 per cent. The disease is characterised by rapid proliferation of abnormal lymphoblasts within the bone marrow, destruction of other normal cells, causing marrow failure, and infiltration of liver, spleen, lymph nodes, brain and testes. Children commonly present with signs of anaemia and acute infection in association with hepatosplenomegaly, lymphadenopathy, petechiae and bruising; they have anaemia, thrombocytopenia and neutropenia.

ACUTE MYELOID LEUKAEMIA

Acute myeloid leukaemia is characterised by proliferation of cancerous cells within the bone marrow that under normal conditions would develop into neutrophils, basophils, eosinophils or monocytes. These escape into the circulation and are distributed to distant sites where they proliferate and form malignant infiltration. Symptoms and signs are similar to lymphoblastic leukaemia. Acute myeloid leukaemia is more common in adults than children. At present, more than half of children with this disorder survive but many will suffer relapse or morbidity and mortality caused by the treatment. One such complication is the cardiotoxicity that can affect those who are treated with anthracyclines as part of their chemotherapy; some have required cardiac transplantation.

NON-HODGKIN'S LYMPHOMA

The most common site affected in non-Hodgkin's lymphoma is the mediastinum and this is usually the result of the high-grade T-cell disease. Other types include the high-grade B-cell lymphoblastic form that tends to cause abdominal masses and the anaplastic large cell variety that affects peripheral lymph nodes, skin, lungs, and the maxillary and mandibular bones. A subgroup, Burkitt's lymphoma, originates from the B-lymphocyte line. It is most common in central Africa and is associated with the Epstein–Barr virus. The abnormal cells grow and spread quickly to infiltrate lymph nodes throughout the body and can cause gross swelling of the neck and mandible. Overall most patients with non-Hodgkin's lymphoma are curable. The best outcome is seen in those with B-cell non-Hodgkin's lymphoma who can expect a cure rate above 90 per cent. The prognosis of those with the T-cell form depends on the extent of the disease process but there is still around an 80 per cent cure rate.

ANAESTHESIA FOR CHILDREN WITH HAEMATOLOGICAL MALIGNANCY

Children require anaesthesia for either diagnostic or therapeutic interventions. Diagnostic procedures include imaging, such as angiography, MRI and computed tomography (CT), and direct haematological testing in the form of lumbar puncture, bone marrow aspirate and bone marrow trephine. Therapeutic interventions most commonly involve the insertion or removal of long-term indwelling central venous catheters for the administration of chemotherapy and lumbar puncture for administration of intrathecal chemotherapy. Surgery is also undertaken to biopsy, de-bulk or excise malignant tissue (see also Chapter 32).

The preoperative preparation of children with haematological malignancy can be challenging. In addition to the direct effects of the disease process itself, these children often present with sepsis. Each patient should have a full blood count and clotting screen performed as a minimum requirement. Serum biochemistry, including liver function tests, should be performed as indicated. These tests will commonly reveal anaemia, thrombocytopenia and coagulopathy. Less commonly neutropenia or hyperleukocytosis may be discovered. Guidelines for the use of blood products to correct anaemia, coagulopathy and thrombocytopenia are contentious as there is a lack of research to build an evidence base in children. It is accepted that the trigger for transfusion of any kind cannot be based upon absolute test values alone. Any decision must also take into consideration the clinical condition of the child, whether the condition is improving or deteriorating and whether the deficit is acute or chronic in nature.

In the absence of symptoms or additional cardiorespiratory disease, a haemoglobin level of 7 g/dL or above is generally well tolerated. If blood loss is acute and ongoing, if there are signs or symptoms of physiological compromise or if levels drop below 7 g/dL then transfusion should be considered [52,53]. Hyperleukocytosis, which is defined as a peripheral white cell count greater than 100×10^9/L,

causes signs and symptoms of hyperviscosity. These include arterial thrombosis with ischaemic infarction, haemorrhage, dyspnoea and hypoxia. In patients with this condition, transfusion of red blood cells may further increase blood viscosity and the risk of thrombosis, and should be avoided unless vital.

Transfusion-related graft-versus-host disease (GVHD) is caused when there is disparity in histocompatibility between donor T lymphocytes present in the transfused red cells and the recipient. Gamma irradiation of blood is used to eliminate donor T lymphocytes completely. White cell filtration, now performed routinely on donated blood, does not completely remove all white blood cells. It is recommended that children who have undergone bone marrow transplantation are at risk and should receive irradiated red cells. This should continue until they have finished preventive treatment for GVHD which usually lasts for 6 months post-transplantation. Children with acute leukaemia and non-Hodgkin's lymphoma are not at risk of transfusion-related GVHD and do not routinely need irradiated products [54]. Leukocyte-depleted blood is indicated to prevent graft rejection in patients with aplastic anaemia who may receive a haematopoietic cell transplantation and also in patients who have experienced febrile non-haemolytic transfusion reactions [55]. Specialist advice should be sought (further details can be found in Chapter 24).

Thrombocytopenia

Thrombocytopenia can lead to primary haemostatic failure and haemorrhage. This is of particular concern if there is need for lumbar puncture, central venous cannulation, regional anaesthesia or surgery. Current recommendations suggest that it is safe to perform lumbar puncture or central venous cannulation with a platelet count $>40 \times 10^9$/L. A count $>50 \times 10^9$/L is deemed safe for the insertion of epidurals but, for surgery in critical areas such as the brain or eyes, a count $>100 \times 10^9$/L is recommended [56]. The figure for epidural insertion is contentious and some anaesthetic sources still recommend the more conservative figure of 80×10^9/L.

COAGULOPATHY

For most invasive procedures, coagulopathies should be corrected. For single clotting factor deficiencies, the appropriate factor should be used unless there is no virus-safe fractionated product available to treat it (this applies to factor V deficiency at present). In the presence of a generalised coagulopathy, fresh frozen plasma (FFP) should be given. For cases where there is hypofibrinogenaemia, FFP is initially given. Where the fibrinogen level remains low despite FFP, cryoprecipitate may be indicated, but this a pooled blood product and exposes patients to multiple donors.

It is recommended that the results of any treatment be monitored by repeating coagulation tests after transfusion [57].

NEUTROPENIA

When the neutrophil count is less than 1×10^9/L the risk of infection is increased; below 0.5×10^9/L the risk increases even further. Given that anaesthesia can have an inhibitory effect on immune function in healthy individuals, surgical and diagnostic interventions requiring anaesthesia should be avoided in the presence of neutropenia if possible.

CONDUCT OF ANAESTHESIA AND THE USE OF CENTRAL VENOUS CATHETERS

Although the majority of procedures can be performed using standard anaesthetic techniques, there are circumstances that require special consideration. Anaesthetic techniques for short and day-case procedures, management of the child with a tumour encroaching upon the upper airway and the management of an anterior mediastinal mass are discussed in Chapters 44, 21 and 39, respectively.

Long-term central venous catheters (CVCs) are usually necessary because chemotherapy and other treatment damage peripheral veins. The use of CVCs for intravenous induction of anaesthesia is, therefore, appropriate. Insertion of additional peripheral access should be avoided if possible to conserve peripheral venous sites that may be needed in the future, for example if the CVC becomes infected it will need to be removed and sepsis will need intravenous antibiotics via a peripheral line. A CVC must always be accessed using sterile techniques to prevent contamination and subsequent infection. Our approach is to use sterile surgical gloves and, using the sterile packaging of these gloves as a sterile field, to clean the end of the catheter with an alcohol swab. The residual fluid from the catheter that usually contains heparin is aspirated and discarded. Finally, and most importantly, the catheter must be flushed adequately (20 mL 0.9 per cent saline) after use to ensure that no anaesthetic drugs are left in the line. There are numerous reports of residual anaesthetic drugs being flushed into the patient on return to the ward. The CVC dead space should be filled with heparinised saline later.

RECTAL MEDICATION

It is generally accepted that the rectal route should be avoided in immunocompromised patients due to the risk of bacteraemia associated with breaches in the rectal mucosa, however small. Bacteraemia under these circumstances could lead to significant morbidity or even death from septicaemia. Oncologists may prefer to avoid the use of paracetamol by any route as it may suppress pyrexia, thereby masking an early sign of bacteraemia.

COAGULATION

Coagulation disorders fall into two general categories: primary or secondary haemostatic disorders. Primary haemostasis is the process leading to the formation of the primary haemostatic plug. When endothelial damage occurs, collagen matrix is exposed leading to the adherence of platelets due to activity of von Willebrand's factor (vWF) and a platelet-binding molecule. Platelets are in turn activated and release their contents, which causes further platelet aggregation and the formation a haemostatic plug with a complex of platelet-binding receptor, fibrinogen and vWF. Any congenital or acquired defect of blood vessel function, platelets or vWF will manifest as a primary haemostatic disorder and primary haemostatic failure is the commonest form of coagulopathy [58].

Blood vessel abnormalities

These can be congenital or acquired and manifest as easy bruising, purpura and spontaneous bleeding of the mucosa. Bleeding time, prothrombin time (PT), activated partial thromboplastin time (APTT) and platelet count are usually normal. Inherited causes include hereditary haemorrhagic telangiectasia, Ehlers–Danlos and Marfan's syndromes, osteogenesis imperfecta and pseudoxanthoma elasticum. Acquired causes include vitamin C deficiency, steroids, cryoglobulinaemia, vasculitis and amyloidosis. Management of bleeding resulting from vessel abnormality includes the use of direct compression, desmopressin (DDAVP), tranexamic acid and aprotinin [59].

Platelet function disorders

Congenital dysfunction can be caused by Glanzmann's thrombasthenia, platelet storage pool or metabolic disorders. Glanzmann's thrombasthenia is caused by a defect of the complex platelet-binding receptor that is essential for platelet aggregation. Storage pool disorders include Wiskott–Aldrich, Hermansky–Pudlak and Chédiak–Higashi syndromes, thrombocytopenia absent radius (TAR) and May–Hegglin anomaly. Also, there are α-granule storage defects such as Gray platelet syndrome and α or δ storage pool defects. Many of these above are also associated with thrombocytopenia. Metabolic disorders include thromboxane A_2 receptor defect, cyclo-oxygenase and thromboxane synthetase deficiency. These have a clinical effect similar to that of aspirin.

Acquired disorders may be caused by uraemia, liver failure and the use of certain drugs such as aspirin, other NSAIDs and furosemide.

Management of bleeding resulting from platelet dysfunction requires withdrawal of precipitant drugs and the use of procoagulants such as DDAVP and antifibrinolytics. Cryoprecipitate (for vWF) and platelets are administered.

The treatment of bleeding caused by rare disorders of platelet function and blood vessels is best directed by expert haematological opinion.

Thrombocytopenia

Congenital thrombocytopenia usually does not present with spontaneous bleeding unless the platelet count is very low. All of these conditions are rare and include Wiskott–Aldrich syndrome, Bernard–Soulier syndrome and Chédiak–Higashi syndrome. Children with Wiskott–Aldrich syndrome also have immunodeficiency, and platelet function and lifespan are reduced. Treatment in the short term includes platelet transfusion and splenectomy and, ultimately, bone marrow transplantation. Bernard–Soulier syndrome manifests as thrombocytopenia, a reduction in platelet function and a prolonged bleeding time; binding of platelets, extravascular colloid matrix and vWF is the underlying dysfunction and treatment is with platelet transfusion. Chédiak–Higashi syndrome presents with partial occulocutaneous albinism, peripheral neuropathy, platelet storage dysfunction, pancytopenia, hepatosplenomegaly and lymphadenopathy. Syndromes without the risks of spontaneous bleeding include pseudo-von Willebrand's disease, Montreal platelet syndrome, Gray platelet syndrome, May–Hegglin anomaly, Paris–Trousseau syndrome and Alport's syndrome (with all of its variants). Alport's syndrome presents with deafness, cataracts, haematuria and renal failure, and its variants include Epstein's and Fechtner's syndromes. Children with these conditions having dental surgery, major surgery or following trauma need platelet transfusions.

Acquired thrombocytopenias are caused by decreased production or increased destruction of platelets. Decreased production can be the result of leukaemia, cytotoxic drugs, marrow infiltration and aplastic anaemia. Increased destruction of platelets is either immune or non-immune mediated. Immune causes of thrombocytopenia include autoimmune or idiopathic thrombocytopenia and pregnancy-related thrombocytopenia. Idiopathic thrombocytopenic purpura (ITP) can be acute or chronic and usually affects children aged between 2 and 5 years following a viral illness. The primary disorder is caused by an inappropriate immune response to the child's own platelets leading to immune complex formation and increased destruction. When the platelet count falls below 50×10^9/L the risk of spontaneous bleeding is appreciable. Acute ITP is treated with steroids, immunoglobulin and, if these fail, more immunotherapy. Chronic ITP is treated with splenectomy. Thrombocytopenia related to pregnancy can be caused by immune complex formation by the mother after inoculation with platelets from the foetus or by autoimmune complexes already formed within the mother. Either of these situations can result in these complexes passing to the foetus via the placenta, resulting in platelet destruction. Intrauterine platelet transfusion may be required or simply immunotherapy for the mother. When the mother produces immune complexes without inoculation the risk of

thrombocytopenia include splenomegaly, disseminated intravascular coagulopathy and thrombotic thrombocytopenia purpura.

SECONDARY HAEMOSTATIC DISORDERS

Inherited disorders of secondary haemostasis include haemophilia A and B, deficiencies of fibrinogen, prothrombin, factors VII, X, XI, XII and XIII, and prekallikrein and kininogen disorders. Acquired defects include vitamin K deficiency, haemorrhagic disease of the newborn, liver disease and drug therapy.

Haemophilia

Haemophilia A (factor VIII deficiency) is an X-linked genetic abnormality; it is the second most common congenital coagulation defect and occurs in 1 in 5000 male births. Haemophilia B (factor IX deficiency) is six times less common. Both disorders vary in presentation depending on the severity of the deficiency. Those suffering from these disorders can be asymptomatic unless exposed to severe trauma and surgery or, at the other extreme, can have spontaneous bleeding into the joints. Clotting screening will reveal a raised APTT alone with normal thrombin time (TT) and PT for both disorders. Both conditions are treated by administration of purified factor concentrate with therapy directed by factor assay. Factor VIII has a half-life of 12 hours and factor IX has a half-life of 18–24 hours. As a result, replacement therapy is given twice daily for factor VIII and once a day for factor IX once steady state is attained. Minimum serum levels of these factors to ensure effective haemostasis are 25–30 U/dL for factor VIII and 20–25 U/dL for factor IX. For major surgery, levels are kept above 100 U/dL for both factor VIII and factor IX. Many patients develop resistance and antibodies to factor concentrates. Under these circumstances endogenous factor levels can be boosted with desmopressin, and activated factors further down the cascade can be administered; other measures include immunosuppressants, immunoglobulin or plasma exchange therapy.

Other congenital disorders

Fibrinogen deficiency will lead to significant and often spontaneous bleeding and blood tests will reveal raised PT, TT and APTT. Fibrinogen levels can be normal where the defect is caused by abnormality of the fibrinogen molecule. Treatment is by replacement with fibrinogen concentrate or cryoprecipitate. Blood tests on patients with factor V deficiency will show raised PT and APTT with normal TT. Treatment is with FFP as there is no pure factor treatment available. Factor VII deficiency presents with an isolated abnormal PT. In factor X deficiency, both PT and APTT are raised with normal TT and, for factor XI, XII, prekallikrein and kininogen deficiencies, PT and TT are normal with raised APTT only. Patients with factor XIII deficiency have normal PT, TT and APTT. Concentrated factor therapy is available for factor VII, X, XI and XIII deficiencies. Concentrated factor therapy for factor XI deficiency should be used with caution as thrombosis can occur if levels exceed 100 U/dl. Antifibrinolytic agents can be used as an alternative for minor procedures. Factor XII, prekallikrein and kininogen deficiencies do not result in an increased risk of bleeding.

ACQUIRED DISORDERS

Vitamin K deficiency and haemolytic disease of the newborn affects factors II, VII, IX and X. Both are treated with vitamin K replacement. Liver disease causes a similar defect in addition to deficiency of many of the other procoagulant factors. Treatment includes administration of both vitamin K and FFP (see Chapter 24).

Management of patients on anticoagulant drugs

These include warfarin, heparin and low-molecular-weight heparin (LMWH). Treatment of coagulopathy associated with warfarin and heparin requires the administration of vitamin K and protamine respectively. Fresh frozen plasma can also be used for more rapid reversal of warfarin; LMWH affects factors IIa and IXa. The use of protamine mainly reverses the effect on factor IIa with a lesser effect on factor IXa activity. Furthermore, anticoagulant activity can return 3 hours after protamine administration.

Preoperative management of patients on anticoagulant therapy is similar to adult practice. Warfarin therapy should be stopped 3–4 days prior to surgery and the international normalised ratio (INR) monitored. An INR of less than 1.5 is safe for surgery. When anticoagulation must be continued, conversion to heparin may be indicated and this allows the anticoagulant effects to be reversed easily with protamine.

The use of regional anaesthesia and removal of indwelling catheters should be avoided when a coagulopathy is detected. With warfarin therapy, regional anaesthesia and catheter removal are safe when the INR is less than 1.5. During standard heparin therapy, blood tests should be normal and heparin should not be given less than 1 hour after an epidural catheter is inserted; an epidural catheter should not be removed less than 2–4 hours after the last dose of heparin. Lastly, for LMWH, epidural or spinal needle insertion should take place 10–12 hours after the last dose for twice-daily regimens and 24 hours for once-daily therapy; any catheter removal similarly should occur 12–24 hours after the last dose and the next dose should not be given within the following 2 hours [60].

HAEMOSTATIC AGENTS

Desmopressin increases endothelial release of factor VIII and vWF. It is used to treat mild haemophilia A, von Willebrand's disease and conditions leading to platelet dysfunction such as uraemia and liver disease.

Tranexamic acid competitively inhibits plasminogen activation and at high doses inhibits plasmin. As an antifibrinolytic it inhibits the breakdown of clots in small vessels.

Aprotinin inhibits plasmin, trypsin, chymotrypsin, kallikrein, thrombin and activated protein C. It is not clear how aprotinin works; it does not inhibit clot dissolution in small vessels but does suppress D-dimer formation. It is generally used during cardiac surgery. Hypersensitivity reactions can occur with aprotinin and generally occur in patients with a history of prior exposure to the drug. It is estimated that the risk of reaction on first exposure is around 0.5 per cent, with the risk following a second exposure in less than 200 days being 4–5 per cent. This drops to 1–2 per cent after 200 days. Immunoglobulin E (IgE) and immunoglobulin G (IgG) antibodies to the drug are often present [61]. The increased mortality in adults receiving aprotinin for cardiac surgery is leading to a review of indications for treatment (see Chapter 40).

Recombinant activated factor VII (rFVIIa) has been found to be effective in the management of refractory haemophilia since its introduction in 1996. It has been used, unlicensed, in many other haemorrhagic conditions since but there is little good evidence of its safety and efficacy in children. This subject has been recently reviewed [62].

PROTHROMBOTIC CONDITIONS AND ANTICOAGULATION

Intravascular thrombosis is fortunately rare in children but it does occur [63]. The most common association is with indwelling central venous catheters. It is particularly likely in combination with malignancy, trauma, congenital cardiac disease (particularly in the presence of prosthetic material) and SLE, and is most likely in infants and adolescents. Congenital prothrombotic conditions such as deficiencies of antithrombin, protein C, protein S or activated protein C resistance/factor V Leiden do not seem to result in thromboembolism in childhood. The risk in these conditions begins in adolescence.

If anticoagulant therapy is required, the standard drug is unfractionated heparin (100 U/kg for initiation of anticoagulation). Since heparin acts by catalysis of antithrombin, levels of which are low in neonates (particularly if they are premature), heparin resistance may be encountered in this age group. Low-molecular-weight heparins are attractive for longer-term treatment as they involve less monitoring, which is clearly desirable in children. For most routine surgical care, however, physical methods such as TED (thromboembolic deterrent) stockings or intermittent compression boots are sufficient and should be used in longer operations, particularly in adolescents.

REFERENCES

Key references

Firth PG, Head CA. Sickle cell disease and anaesthesia. *Anaesthesiology* 2004; **101**(3): 766–85.

Hackmann T, Steward DJ, Sheps SB. Anemia in pediatric day-surgery patients: prevalence and detection. *Anaesthesiology* 1991; **75**(1): 27–31.

Miller ST, Sleeper LA, Pegelow CH *et al.* Prediction of adverse outcomes in children with sickle cell disease. *N Engl J Med* 2000; **342**(2): 83–9.

Monagle P, Chan A, Chalmers E, Michelson A. Antithrombotic therapy in children. *Chest* 2004; **126**: 645S–87S.

Roy WL, Lerman J, McIntyre BG. Is preoperative haemoglobin testing justified in children undergoing minor elective surgery? *Can J Anesth* 1991; **38**(6): 700–3.

Vichinsky EP, Haberkern CM, Neumayr L *et al.* A comparison of conservative and aggressive transfusion regimens in the perioperative management of sickle cell disease. The Preoperative Transfusion in Sickle Cell Disease Study Group. *N Engl J Med* 1995; **333**(4): 206–13.

References

1. Oski FA. The erythrocyte and its disorders. In: Nathan A, Oski FA, eds. *Haematology of infancy and childhood.* Philadelphia: WB Saunders, 1993: 18.
2. Roberts IA, Murray NA. Neonatal thrombocytopenia: new insights into pathogenesis and implications for clinical management. *Curr Opin Pediatr* 2001; **13**(1): 16–21.
3. Stuart MJ, Graeber JE. Normal haemostasis in the fetus and newborn: vessels and platelets. In: Polin RA, Fox WM, eds. *Fetal and neonatal physiology.* Philadelphia: WB Saunders, 1998: 1834–48.
4. Christensen RD, Calhoun DA, Rimsza LM. A practical approach to evaluating and treating neutropenia in the neonatal intensive care unit. *Clin Perinatol* 2000; **27**(3): 577–601.
5. Kush ML, Gortner L, Harman CR, Baschat AA. Sustained haematological consequences in the first week of neonatal life secondary to placental dysfunction. *Early Hum Dev* 2006; **82**(1): 67–72.
6. Ohls RK, Dai A. Long-acting erythropoietin: clinical studies and potential uses in neonates. *Clin Perinatol* 2004; **31**(1): 77–89.
7. Hackmann T, Steward DJ, Sheps SB. Anemia in pediatric day-surgery patients: prevalence and detection. *Anesthesiology* 1991; **75**(1): 27–31.
8. Roy WL, Lerman J, McIntyre BG. Is preoperative haemoglobin testing justified in children undergoing minor elective surgery? *Can J Anaesth* 1991; **38**(6): 700–3.
9. O'Connor ME, Drasner K. Preoperative laboratory testing of children undergoing elective surgery. *Anesth Analg* 1990; **70**(2): 176–80.
10. Patel RI, DeWitt L, Hannallah RS. Preoperative laboratory testing in children undergoing elective surgery: analysis of current practice. *J Clin Anesth* 1997; **9**(7): 569–75.
11. Patel RI, Hannallah RS. Laboratory tests in children undergoing ambulatory surgery: a review of clinical practice and scientific studies. *Ambul Surg* 2000; **8**(4): 165–9.
12. Jacob R, Venkatesan T. Anaesthesia and Fanconi anaemia: a case report and review of literature. *Paediatr Anaesth* 2006; **16**(9): 981–5.
13. Sheikha A. Splenic syndrome in patients at high altitude with unrecognized sickle cell trait: splenectomy is often unnecessary. *Can J Surg* 2005; **48**(5): 377–81.
14. Davies SC, Gilmore A. The role of hydroxyurea in the management of sickle cell disease. *Blood Rev* 2003; **17**(2): 99–109.
15. Rogers DW, Clarke JM, Cupidore L *et al.* Early deaths in Jamaican children with sickle cell disease. *BMJ* 1978; **1**(6126): 1515–16.
16. Lawrenz DR. Sickle cell disease: a review and update of current therapy. *J Oral Maxillofac Surg* 1999; **57**(2): 171–178.
17. Cavenagh JD, Joseph AE, Dilly S, Bevan DH. Splenic sepsis in sickle cell disease. *Br J Haematol* 1994; **86**(1): 187–9.
18. Platt OS, Brambilla DJ, Rosse WF *et al.* Mortality in sickle cell disease. Life expectancy and risk factors for early death. *N Engl J Med* 1994; **330**(23): 1639–44.
19. Vijay V, Cavenagh JD, Yate P. The anaesthetist's role in acute sickle cell crisis. *Br J Anaesth* 1998; **80**(6): 820–8.
20. Vichinsky EP, Neumayr LD, Earles AN *et al.* Causes and outcomes of the acute chest syndrome in sickle cell disease. National Acute Chest Syndrome Study Group. *N Engl J Med* 2000; **342**(25): 1855–65.
21. Vichinsky EP, Styles LA, Colangelo LH *et al.* Acute chest syndrome in sickle cell disease: clinical presentation and course. Cooperative Study of Sickle Cell Disease. *Blood* 1997; **89**(5): 1787–92.
22. Delatte SJ, Hebra A, Tagge EP *et al.* Acute chest syndrome in the postoperative sickle cell patient. *J Pediatr Surg* 1999; **34**(1): 188–91.
23. Castro O, Brambilla DJ, Thorington B *et al.* The acute chest syndrome in sickle cell disease: incidence and risk factors. The Cooperative Study of Sickle Cell Disease. *Blood* 1994; **84**(2): 643–49.
24. Ohene-Frempong K, Weiner SJ, Sleeper LA *et al.* Cerebrovascular accidents in sickle cell disease: rates and risk factors. *Blood* 1998; **91**(1): 288–94.
25. Moser FG, Miller ST, Bello JA *et al.* The spectrum of brain MR abnormalities in sickle-cell disease: a report from the Cooperative Study of Sickle Cell Disease. *AJNR Am J Neuroradiol* 1996; **17**(5): 965–72.
26. Adams RJ, McKie VC, Hsu L *et al.* Prevention of a first stroke by transfusions in children with sickle cell anemia and abnormal results on transcranial Doppler ultrasonography. *N Engl J Med* 1998; **339**(1): 5–11.
27. Mehta SH, Adams RJ. Treatment and prevention of stroke in children with sickle cell disease. *Curr Treat Options Neurol* 2006; **8**(6): 503–12.

28. Fowler JE Jr, Koshy M, Strub M, Chinn SK. Priapism associated with the sickle cell haemoglobinopathies: prevalence, natural history and sequelae. *J Urol* 1991; **145**(1): 65–8.

29. Hebbel RP, Osarogiagbon R, Kaul D. The endothelial biology of sickle cell disease: inflammation and a chronic vasculopathy. *Microcirculation* 2004; **11**(2): 129–51.

30. Solovey A, Lin Y, Browne P *et al.* Circulating activated endothelial cells in sickle cell anemia. *N Engl J Med* 1997; **337**(22): 1584–90.

31. Stockman JA, Nigro MA, Mishkin MM, Oski FA. Occlusion of large cerebral vessels in sickle-cell anemia. *N Engl J Med* 1972; **287**(17): 846–9.

32. Powars D, Weidman JA, Odom-Maryon T *et al.* Sickle cell chronic lung disease: prior morbidity and the risk of pulmonary failure. *Medicine (Baltimore)* 1988; **67**(1): 66–76.

33. Platt OS. Sickle cell anemia as an inflammatory disease. *J Clin Invest* 2000; **106**(3): 337–8.

34. Miller ST, Sleeper LA, Pegelow CH *et al.* Prediction of adverse outcomes in children with sickle cell disease. *N Engl J Med* 2000; **342**(2): 83–9.

35. Quinn CT, Miller ST. Risk factors and prediction of outcomes in children and adolescents who have sickle cell anemia. *Haematol Oncol Clin North Am* 2004; **18**(6): 1339–54, ix.

36. Koshy M, Weiner SJ, Miller ST *et al.* Surgery and anaesthesia in sickle cell disease. Cooperative Study of Sickle Cell Diseases. *Blood* 1995; **86**(10): 3676–84.

37. Riddington C, Williamson L. Preoperative blood transfusions for sickle cell disease. *Cochrane Database Syst Rev* 2001; (3): CD003149.

38. Vichinsky EP, Haberkern CM, Neumayr L *et al.* A comparison of conservative and aggressive transfusion regimens in the perioperative management of sickle cell disease. The Preoperative Transfusion in Sickle Cell Disease Study Group. *N Engl J Med* 1995; **333**(4): 206–13.

39. Griffin TC, Buchanan GR. Elective surgery in children with sickle cell disease without preoperative blood transfusion. *J Pediatr Surg* 1993; **28**(5): 681–5.

40. Buchanan GR, Rogers ZR. Conservative versus aggressive transfusion regimens in sickle cell disease. *N Engl J Med* 1995; **333**(24): 1641–2.

41. Fu T, Corrigan NJ, Quinn CT *et al.* Minor elective surgical procedures using general anesthesia in children with sickle cell anemia without pre-operative blood transfusion. *Pediatr Blood Cancer* 2005; **45**(1): 43–7.

42. Neumayr L, Koshy M, Haberkern C *et al.* Surgery in patients with hemoglobin SC disease. Preoperative Transfusion in Sickle Cell Disease Study Group. *Am J Hematol* 1998; **57**(2): 101–8.

43. Homi J, Reynolds J, Skinner A *et al.* General anaesthesia in sickle-cell disease. *BMJ* 1979; **1**(6178): 1599–601.

44. Vamvakas EC, Blajchman MA. Deleterious clinical effects of transfusion-associated immunomodulation: fact or fiction? *Blood* 2001; **97**(5): 1180–95.

45. Firth PG, Head CA. Sickle cell disease and anesthesia. *Anesthesiology* 2004; **101**(3): 766–85.

46. Crawford MW, Galton S, Naser B. Postoperative morphine consumption in children with sickle-cell disease. *Paediatr Anaesth* 2006; **16**(2): 152–7.

47. Kopecky EA, Jacobson S, Joshi P, Koren G. Systemic exposure to morphine and the risk of acute chest syndrome in sickle cell disease. *Clin Pharmacol Ther* 2004; **75**(3): 140–6.

48. Weatherall DJ. The thalassaemias. *BMJ* 1997; **314**(7095): 1675–8.

49. Kitoh T, Tanaka S, Ono K *et al.* Anaesthetic management of a patient with β-thalassaemia intermedia undergoing splenectomy: a case report. *J Anaesth* 2005; **19**(3): 252–6.

50. Olive M, Mora A, Ballve M *et al.* [Thalassemic syndromes and anaesthesia.] *Rev Esp Anestesiol Reanim* 1992; **39**(3): 166–9.

51. Mak PH, Ooi RG. Submental intubation in a patient with β-thalassaemia major undergoing elective maxillary and mandibular osteotomies. *Br J Anaesth* 2002; **88**(2): 288–91.

52. Gibson BE, Todd A, Roberts I *et al.* Transfusion guidelines for neonates and older children. *Br J Haematol* 2004; **124**(4): 433–53.

53. Murphy MF, Wallington TB, Kelsey P *et al.* Guidelines for the clinical use of red cell transfusions. *Br J Haematol* 2001; **113**(1): 24–31.

54. Guidelines on gamma irradiation of blood components for the prevention of transfusion-associated graft-versus-host disease. BCSH Blood Transfusion Task Force. *Transfus Med* 1996; **6**(3): 261–71.

55. Guidelines on the clinical use of leucocyte-depleted blood components. British Committee for Standards in Haematology, Blood Transfusion Task Force. *Transfus Med* 1998; **8**(1): 59–71.

56. Guidelines for the use of platelet transfusions. *Br J Haematol* 2003; **122**(1): 10–23.

57. O'Shaughnessy DF, Atterbury C, Bolton MP *et al.* Guidelines for the use of fresh-frozen plasma, cryoprecipitate and cryosupernatant. *Br J Haematol* 2004; **126**(1): 11–28.

58. Smith OP, Hann IM. Primary haemostatic defects. In: *Essential paediatric haematology*. London: Martin Dunitz Ltd, 2002: 105–18.

59. Hayward CP. Diagnosis and management of mild bleeding disorders. *Hematology Am Soc Hematol Educ Program* 2005: 423–8.

60. Horlocker TT, Wedel DJ, Benzon H *et al.* Regional anaesthesia in the anticoagulated patient: defining the risks (the second ASRA Consensus Conference on Neuraxial Anaesthesia and Anticoagulation). *Reg Anaesth Pain Med* 2003; **28**(3): 172–97.

61. Mahdy AM, Webster NR. Perioperative systemic haemostatic agents. *Br J Anaesth* 2004; **93**(6): 842–58.

62. Matthew P, Young G. Recombinant Factor VIIa in paediatric bleeding disorders – a 2006 review. *Haemophilia* 2006; **12**: 457–72

63. Monagle P, Chan A, Chalmers E, Michelson A. Antithrombotic therapy in children. *Chest* 2004; **126**: 645S–87S.

ADDENDUM

Guidelines for the management of sickle cell disease

Suggested transfusion policy for general anaesthesia at Great Ormond Street Hospital (GOSH). (*This transfusion policy has been agreed locally by the haematologists and anaesthetists at GOSH and referring paediatricians.*)

TRANSFUSION RECOMMENDATIONS FOR ELECTIVE SURGERY

Patients with a history of severe sickle-related problems, such as chest crisis, central nervous system (CNS) disease or frequent painful crises, or with severe obstructive sleep apnoea or patients undergoing major surgery have been found to be at greater risk of serious perioperative complications. However, aggressive transfusion regimens or emergency transfusions with blood of inappropriate red cell phenotype are associated with a higher incidence of transfusion-related complications. A four-tiered approach is recommended, tailored to suit the individual case.

Group 1 Children with no special risk factors, who are currently well, having short procedures with minimal risk of perioperative complications, e.g. insertion of grommets:
– top-up transfusion to haemoglobin (Hb) > 7 g/dL only, irrespective of HbS level.

Group 2 Children with no special risk factors, having intermediate risk surgery, e.g. body surface surgery such as herniorraphy, or tonsillectomy in older children >5 years with mild-to-moderate obstructive sleep apnoea:
– top-up transfusion to Hb 9–11 g/dL, irrespective of HbS level;
– total Hb should not exceed 12 g/dL.

Group 3 Children who have had a chest crisis or suffer frequent painful crises, or children undergoing major surgery, e.g. intra-abdominal surgery (including laparoscopic surgery), or tonsillectomy in children <5 years. Plan exchange transfusion or sequential top-up transfusions to achieve:
– HbS level <30 per cent and Hb 9–11 g/dL;
– total Hb should not exceed 12 g/dL.

Group 4 Children with a history of stroke (usually on a regular transfusion programme), or undergoing high-risk major surgery, e.g. thoracic or neurosurgery. Plan exchange transfusion or sequential top-up transfusions to achieve:
– HbS level <20 per cent and Hb 9–11 g/dL;
– total Hb should not exceed 12 g/dL.

EMERGENCY SURGERY

Children requiring emergency surgery should be treated similarly if time allows. If this is not possible, blood should be crossmatched and standing by. All cases must be discussed with the haematologists at presentation.

CHILDREN UNDERGOING MAGNETIC RESONANCE IMAGING (MRI) BRAIN SCAN FOR SUSPECTED CEREBROVASCULAR DISEASE

Treat as for group 2 patients, i.e. top-up transfusion to Hb 9–11 g/dL (but less than Hb 12 g/dL).

USE OF SURGICAL TOURNIQUETS

Tourniquets for surgery may be used in children with sickle cell trait after careful exsanguination of the limb. However, the safety of tourniquets in non-transfused children with sickle cell disease has yet to be established and should be considered carefully on an individual basis.

SICKLE CELL SCREENING

Current policy is to screen all at-risk children. The results should be obtained before surgery and the parents informed. Sickle screening is unreliable in babies under 3 months of age, particularly if they have been transfused. A high level of HbF will be protective and these children are unlikely to present a problem during anaesthesia. Hb electrophoresis is required for reliable detection of haemoglobinopathies.

Suggested perioperative management

GENERAL RECOMMENDATIONS

Sickle cell disease is a chronic debilitating disease associated with significant perioperative morbidity and mortality. Meticulous perioperative care is required. Families are generally well informed about the condition and appreciate being involved in decisions about care.

Elective surgery
Children with SCD presenting for elective surgery should be discussed with the anaesthetists and haematologists preoperatively. A plan for preoperative transfusion will be formulated depending on the child's condition and the nature of the intended surgery. Preparation for surgery may take at least 3 weeks as above.

Admission
Children should be admitted the day before surgery. They require blood of the appropriate phenotype to be crossmatched which may take up to 6 h.

Scheduling operation
Children should be scheduled early on the operating list to ensure that they are not cancelled.

Precipitating factors
Care should be taken at all times to avoid factors that may precipitate a sickle crisis. These include dehydration, hypoxia, acidosis, hypothermia and pain. The majority of crises occur postoperatively.

8

The effects of prematurity

PETER CREAN, ANTHONY CHISAKUTA

KEY LEARNING POINTS

- The incidence of respiratory distress is inversely related to gestational age and it affects over 90 per cent of infants born at 26 weeks' gestation.
- Oxygen toxicity and barotrauma should be avoided by using minimum inspired oxygen and inspiratory pressures compatible with maintaining oxygen saturations between 89 and 95 per cent or arterial oxygen partial pressures of between 6 and 10 kPa.

- Apnoea occurs in over 80 per cent of babies born at less than 30 weeks' gestation but is a presenting sign of infections and other problems.
- Intraventricular haemorrhage occurs in one-third of babies born at 32 weeks' gestation.
- Necrotising enterocolitis is the commonest surgical emergency in the neonatal period affecting 3–5 per cent of low-birth-weight infants.

INTRODUCTION

There are no accurate recent world-wide data, but estimations of the proportion of births that are preterm ranges from 5–10 per cent in developed countries to 25 per cent in the developing world [1]. The factors that contribute to preterm birth vary. World-wide, the main aetiological factor is infection, and malaria and HIV are most common. In developed countries, induced delivery is responsible for almost half of the births between 28 weeks and 35 weeks; maternal hypertension and pre-eclampsia are the main pathologies. Other factors include multiple pregnancy, intrauterine growth restriction, maternal stress, diabetes, malnutrition and heavy physical work.

LEVELS OF PREMATURITY

Preterm birth is the delivery of a baby before 37 completed weeks of gestation. The degree of prematurity can be defined by gestation age at birth or, alternatively, by birth weight (Table 8.1). Although some concordance exists between gestational age and birth weight, they are not interchangeable. In 2003–04, 7 per cent of all deliveries in England were premature, with 0.5 per cent occurring before 28 weeks, 0.9 per cent between 28 weeks and 31 weeks, and the rest after 32 weeks' gestation [2]. These broad categories of gestational age are based on risk of death and perinatal complications. Most serious problems associated with prematurity occur in the 1.5 per cent of

Table 8.1 Levels of prematurity

Defined by gestational age at birth	Severely premature 24–30 weeks	Moderately premature 30–36 weeks	Borderline premature 36–37 weeks
Defined by birth weight	Extremely low birth weight (ELBW) 500–1000 g	Very low birth weight (VLBW) 1000–1500 g	Low birth weight (LBW) 1500–2500 g

infants born before 32 weeks, and particularly the 0.5 per cent born before 28 weeks. The outcomes for preterm infants born at or after 32 weeks of gestation are similar to those of term infants.

Postconceptional age (PCA) is a term used widely, and is the gestational age at birth plus the postnatal age in weeks.

RESUSCITATION OF THE NEWBORN

Resuscitation of the newborn specifically refers to procedures at or immediately after the delivery of a newly born infant [3,4]. The transition from dependence on placental gas exchange in a liquid-filled intrauterine environment to spontaneous breathing of air presents a major physiological challenge to the infant lasting, normally, from minutes to hours after birth. Ten per cent of all newborns require resuscitation at birth [3]. According to the World Health Organization (WHO), more than 5 million neonatal deaths occur world-wide each year. It has been estimated that birth asphyxia accounts for 19 per cent of deaths, suggesting that the outcome might be improved for some 1 million infants per year through implementation of simple resuscitative techniques. In most cases, the outcome of birth is predictable so that unexpected emergency resuscitation is unusual. Careful assessment of maternal and foetal factors, including the mode of delivery and obstetric care, will predict the majority of newborns who require resuscitation.

Physiological changes at birth

An understanding of the physiological changes that take place in the transition from intrauterine to extrauterine life is important to the conduct of resuscitation of the newborn, and the following is a brief account. The lungs change from fluid filled to air filled, the pulmonary blood flow increases, and the intra- and extracardiac shunts (foramen ovale and ductus arteriosus) reverse their direction and subsequently close. Breathing, which is intermittent in the foetus, becomes continuous after birth and is probably triggered by numerous mechanisms such as the removal of placental humoral inhibition, and the beginning of temperature difference, tactile stimulation, catecholamine surges and rising carbon dioxide concentrations. *In utero* the foetus is entirely dependent upon its mother for glucose but, with the rise in plasma concentrations of adrenaline, noradrenaline and glucagon, and the decline in

insulin during delivery, the newborn's glucose supply becomes dependent on its own stored glycogen and fatty acids. Newborns have a high surface area to mass ratio and lose heat quickly. If positive pressure ventilation is necessary the fluid-filled alveoli require higher ventilation pressures to expand them than those used in rescue breathing during infancy.

Apgar scores

The newborn baby's initial cry and subsequent efforts at breathing must be assessed carefully to ensure that they result in adequate and sustained oxygenation of the lungs. Gasping without additional breathing is inadequate. Abnormal or absent ventilatory patterns will require immediate intervention. The initial assessment of the neonate is based on respiratory activity, colour and heart rate, and these three parameters have been shown to be more accurate in the assessment of the newborn than the total APGAR score [5] (Table 8.2). The status of a newborn can be classified into one of three groups (Table 8.3).

Meconium

The majority of newborns cry within a few minutes of birth and require little more than careful drying and then wrapping in a warm towel to prevent heat loss. If the baby does not cry, he or she should be gently stimulated by more vigorous drying with a towel [3]. More vigorous stimulation is contraindicated and can be potentially dangerous. Of those who do not cry, most only need their airway cleared and bag-and-mask ventilation. Meconium aspiration leads to dangerous respiratory failure and every effort should be made to prevent it. If babies are born through thick meconium and are unresponsive (or 'not vigorous') at birth, the oropharynx and larynx should be inspected (by laryngoscopy) and cleared of meconium. Meconium in the trachea must be removed by a suction catheter. If tracheal intubation is necessary, as much meconium must be removed as possible before positive pressure ventilation begins although ventilation will have to be initiated if there is hypoxic bradycardia. Fortunately, few of these babies need tracheal intubation, circulatory access or drug administration. Intervention in a vigorous baby born through thick meconium should be limited to superficial suction of the mouth and external nares.

Table 8.2 Apgar scoring

	Sign	0 point	1 point	2 points
A	Activity (muscle tone)	Limp	Limbs flexed	Active movement
P	Pulse (beats/min)	Absent	<100	>100
G	Grimace (response to smell or foot slap)	Absent	Grimace	Cough or sneeze Cry and withdrawal of foot
A	Appearance (colour)	Blue	Body pink Extremities blue	Pink all over
R	Respiration (breathing)	Absent	Irregular Weak cry	Good strong cry

The total score is the sum of the scores for the five signs.

Table 8.3 Status and intervention at birth

	Group 1	Group 2	Group 3
Respiratory activity	Vigorous, effective	Inadequate or apnoeic	Inadequate or apnoeic
Colour	Centrally pink	Central cyanosis	Pale or white owing to poor cardiac output and peripheral vasoconstriction
Heart rate	>100 beats/min	>100 beats/min	<100 beats/min or no detectable heart rate
Intervention	Nil (fit and healthy baby)	May respond to tactile stimulation and/or facial oxygen but often need basic life support	Sometimes improve with initial basic life support, but normally require immediate intubation and positive pressure ventilation, progressing to chest compressions and full advanced life support

RESPIRATORY SYSTEM

Respiratory distress syndrome

Respiratory distress syndrome (RDS) of prematurity is a major cause of morbidity and mortality in preterm infants. The incidence is inversely related to gestational age and it affects over 90 per cent of infants born at 26 weeks' gestation. Primarily, RDS is caused by immaturity of the lungs, and in particular the pulmonary surfactant-producing systems. Surfactant, produced by type II pneumocytes, is a complex mixture of phospholipids and proteins that reduce alveolar surface tension and prevent alveolar collapse at end-expiration. As most surfactant is produced after 30–32 weeks' gestation, preterm infants born prior to this will probably develop RDS. In addition to prematurity, several other risk factors for RDS have been identified and these include male gender, Caucasian race, delivery by caesarean section, perinatal asphyxia, maternal diabetes, hypothermia and multiple pregnancy. Deficiency of surfactant leads to reduced lung volumes, decreased lung compliance and ventilation/perfusion abnormalities.

Preterm infants with RDS present immediately or within 4 h of birth. There is worsening respiratory distress with tachypnoea (rate > 60 breaths per minute), thoracic recession,

expiratory grunting, cyanosis and diminished breath sounds. First-line medical treatment includes oxygen delivered via head-box, and ascending to continuous positive airway pressure (via nasal prong or tracheal tube), and then to mechanical ventilation (conventional or high-frequency oscillation) and administration of exogenous surfactant via a tracheal tube. In infants at risk of developing RDS, surfactant replacement is most effective when given at the time of delivery. It is better as prophylaxis rather than 'rescue' treatment. Surfactant therapy reduces mortality by 40 per cent and reduces the rate of pneumothorax by up to 60 per cent [6,7].

During anaesthesia, positive end-expiratory pressure reduces pulmonary collapse and ventilation/perfusion mismatch. The potential problems of oxygen toxicity and barotrauma should be avoided by using minimum oxygen and inspiratory pressures compatible with maintaining oxygen saturations between 89 and 95 per cent or a partial pressure of oxygen in the arterial blood (PaO_2) of between 6 and 10 kPa (45–75 mmHg).

Chronic lung disease

Chronic lung disease (CLD) of prematurity or bronchopulmonary dysplasia (BPD) was first described by Northway and colleagues in 1967 as lung injury in preterm infants resulting from oxygen and mechanical ventilation [6]. Chronic lung disease is usually defined as a need for ventilatory support or supplemental oxygen at a PCA of more than 36 weeks and is associated with several risk factors [8] (Table 8.4). Advances in neonatal care over the past decades have increased survival and, now, CLD is common. The overall incidence of CLD in preterm infants who required ventilation at birth is reported to be 20 per cent, and if the birth weight was <1500 g it can be 15–50 per cent. The main contributing factors include mechanical ventilation (especially if peak inflating pressures are greater than 35 cmH$_2$O), prolonged exposure to high oxygen concentrations, infection, and pulmonary oedema resulting from a patent ductus arteriosus (PDA) or excess fluid administration [8].

Northway *et al.* reported the mortality rate of patients with CLD to be between 30 and 40 per cent [9]. The main causes of death include respiratory failure, systemic infections and cor pulmonale [10]. If infants with CLD survive the neonatal period, they are more likely to develop frequent respiratory infections during the first 2 years of life. An increased incidence of bronchial hyperactivity has been found in severe cases with remission occurring at around 8 years of age. Neurological development is affected in about 40 per cent of patients with CLD; motor and auditory abnormalities, and long-term disability, are reported in 16 per cent.

Medical treatment

POSTNATAL CORTICOSTEROIDS

Meta-analyses suggest a beneficial effect of steroids, given between 7 days and 14 days of age, in terms of reduction in the combined incidence of CLD and death [10]. However, there are concerns of both short-term (hypertension, hyperglycaemia and septic episodes) and long-term side effects (neurodevelopmental impairment and impaired growth). There is also concern about adverse neurological effects of the sulphite moiety of dexamethasone. Sulphite-free dexamethasone is readily available. If a ventilated infant is not improving after 7–14 days (and he or she weighs less than 2000 g) dexamethasone may be helpful (0.25 mg/kg every 12 hours IV) [11]. This dose is halved after 3 days and stopped after 6 days although, if there is a clinical response,

Table 8.4   Risk factors for chronic lung disease

- Level of prematurity
- Small for gestational age
- Severity of respiratory distress syndrome
- Duration of mechanical ventilation
- Duration of oxygen administration
- Patent ductus arteriosus
- Maternal chorioamnionitis
- Postnatal sepsis

the dose may be reduced earlier. Prophylactic inhaled steroids are not effective [12].

BRONCHODILATORS

Bronchodilators (β_2 agonists or anticholinergics) are used in acute wheezing episodes of infants with CLD [12].

DIURETICS

Several randomised trials in preterm infants with CLD have demonstrated short- to medium-term improvements in pulmonary function with both furosemide and thiazide diuretics. Diuretics reduce airway resistance and increase lung compliance, allowing a reduction in oxygen and ventilator requirements [13]. Babies should be monitored for electrolyte disturbance.

OXYGEN THERAPY

Supplementary low-flow oxygen therapy may be required and can be delivered via either twin nasal cannulae or a single feeding catheter inserted into one nostril. Oxygen saturation must be monitored and maintained above 92 per cent to ensure weight gain [14].

Apnoea of prematurity

There are various definitions of apnoea. It may be regarded as a pause in breathing together with bradycardia or cyanosis. It must be differentiated from periodic breathing, which is common in preterm infants. Periodic breathing has an irregular rhythm with bursts of respiratory activity separated with apnoeic pauses lasting at least 3 s. There is an inverse relationship between the frequency of apnoea and gestational age. Apnoea occurs in over 80 per cent of babies born at less than 30 weeks' gestation, 50 per cent in those born at 30–31 weeks, 14 per cent at 32–33 weeks and 7 per cent at 34–35 weeks [15].

Apnoea is classified according to the presence of upper airway obstruction. There are three types: central, obstructive and mixed. Central apnoea is characterised by total cessation of inspiratory effort without any evidence of obstruction. In pure obstructive apnoea, the infant tries to breathe against an obstructed upper airway, resulting in chest wall motion without airflow throughout the entire apnoea. Using an ultrafine fibreoptic scope, the usual site of obstruction has been shown to be at the larynx but it may also occur in the pharynx [16]. Mixed apnoea consists of obstructed respiratory efforts, usually following central pauses, and it accounts for more than half of all long apnoiec episodes. Purely obstructive apnoea is the least common type.

Mechanisms of apnoea are specific for each type of apnoea. Mechanoreceptors of the lung and upper airways, chemoreceptors and inputs from the cerebral cortex provide signals into the respiratory centre, which is responsible for the involuntary control of breathing and thereby maintaining rhythmic ventilation [17]. Delayed maturation of any of these sites could potentially result in central apnoea. Obstructive apnoea has multiple causes including reduced airway muscle tone, asynchrony of the airway muscles and diaphragm, and pathology in either the upper airway or the central nervous system. In mixed apnoea, narrowing of the airway due to loss of muscle tone occurs about 1 second into a central apnoea and then, when breathing begins, airway obstruction can persist to produce a mixed apnoea.

Apnoea may also be the presenting sign of other diseases, or pathophysiological states frequently affecting preterm infants (Fig. 8.1) [17]. It is therefore essential to investigate apnoeas appropriately when they appear unexpectedly. An infection screen (including lumbar puncture and urinalysis), serum glucose and calcium, haemoglobin level, chest X-ray, cranial ultrasound scan, arterial blood gas and viral screen should all be considered. If apnoeas persist despite treatment, an EEG should be obtained to exclude a convulsive disorder.

Treatment of apnoea of prematurity depends on the severity. Many episodes of apnoea are self-limiting and no action needs to be taken. Apnoea or bradycardia can be stopped by applying a gentle stimulus – flicking the foot may be sufficient to restore breathing. If stimulation fails, the infant should be ventilated by bag and mask.

Methylxanthines such as caffeine, aminophylline and theophylline have been standard treatments of apnoea [17], and they have been shown to increase minute ventilation, improve carbon dioxide sensitivity, decrease hypoxic depression of breathing and enhance diaphragmatic activity. These effects are mediated by an increase in respiratory neural output but their precise pharmacological actions are unknown. The likely major mechanisms of action are from phosphodiesterase inhibition and the competitive antagonism of adenosine (adenosine acts as an inhibitory neuroregulator in the central nervous system) [17]. A recent Cochrane Review concluded that caffeine treatment was associated with a significant reduction of symptomatic apnoeas in preterm infants [18]. Treatment is usually 5 mg/kg each day starting 24 h after an initial loading dose of 20 mg/kg (either oral or intravenous preparations); neonates over 44 weeks PCA may require 10 mg/kg twice daily [19].

If an infant continues to have frequent apnoeas, despite treatment with methylxanthines, continuous positive airway pressure (CPAP) needs to be considered [20]. This reduces the incidence of mixed or obstructive apnoea but has no effect on central apnoea. Continuous positive airway pressure appears to splint the upper airway and decrease the risk of pharyngeal or laryngeal obstruction. It probably also increases functional residual capacity (FRC) and so improves oxygenation. For severe or refractory apnoea, tracheal intubation and mechanical ventilation may be needed. The lowest possible oxygen concentration and ventilator pressures should be used to allow for spontaneous ventilatory efforts and to minimise the risk of barotrauma.

Neonates with apnoeic spells do not breathe adequately during anaesthesia and must be ventilated from induction until the end of the surgery [21].

Subglottic stenosis

Subglottic stenosis (SGS) is a rare cause of upper airway obstruction in infants [22]. The reported incidence varies from 0.6 per cent to 2.6 per cent of intubated neonates, and can be either acquired or congenital. In over 95 per cent of cases, SGS develops in low-birth-weight, preterm infants following prolonged tracheal intubation; they usually also have chronic lung disease. Many units have used Cole tracheal tubes in the past because they are wider, except for the narrow tracheal section, and therefore less likely to kink and easier to secure. However, there is a shoulder at the point where the tube narrows that may press against the larynx and this has been blamed for causing tracheal damage. The current risk factors for acquired SGS are summarised in Table 8.5 [23,24].

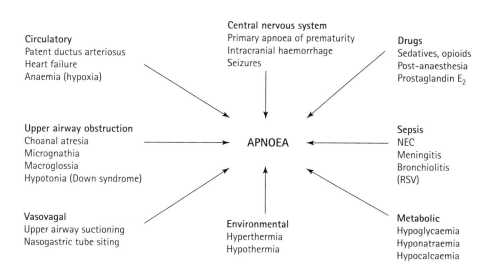

Figure 8.1 Causes of apnoea in the neonatal period.
NEC, necrotising enterocolitis; RSV, respiratory syncytial virus.

Circulatory
Patent ductus arteriosus
Heart failure
Anaemia (hypoxia)

Central nervous system
Primary apnoea of prematurity
Intracranial haemorrhage
Seizures

Drugs
Sedatives, opioids
Post-anaesthesia
Prostaglandin E_2

Upper airway obstruction
Choanal atresia
Micrognathia
Macroglossia
Hypotonia (Down syndrome)

APNOEA

Sepsis
NEC
Meningitis
Bronchiolitis
(RSV)

Vasovagal
Upper airway suctioning
Nasogastric tube siting

Environmental
Hyperthermia
Hypothermia

Metabolic
Hypoglycaemia
Hyponatraemia
Hypocalcaemia

Table 8.5   Risk factors associated with acquired subglottic stenosis

- Low birth weight
- Low gestational age
- Long intubation period (>14 days)
- Traumatic intubation
- Multiple intubations
- Post-extubation stridor
- Large-sized tracheal tube in relation to gestational age
- Respiratory tract infection within 14 days of intubation

Congenital SGS is a narrowed and sometimes elliptically shaped cricoid cartilage or an under-riding of the first tracheal cartilage [22]. The severity of the stenosis is graded using Cotton's classification system [23]. A grade I stenosis occurs when there is 0–50 per cent reduction in lumen cross-section; grade II is between 51 and 70 per cent, grade III from 71 per cent to 99 per cent and grade IV complete obliteration.

The management of SGS will depend upon its severity and evolution. Neonates with a mild degree of stenosis are managed conservatively and, with growth, the condition can improve [22]. With more severe forms, urgent tracheostomy may be required. Moderate oedematous SGS may be treated by splitting the cricoid cartilage and resting the trachea with a period of intubation. More severe long-standing stenosis is likely to require laryngotracheal reconstruction surgery or cricotracheal resection.

CARDIOVASCULAR SYSTEM

Changes at birth

With the first breaths of air, pulmonary blood flow increases. Clamping of the umbilical cord reduces right atrial pressure and, with increased pulmonary blood flow, left atrial pressure rises and causes a functional closure of the foramen ovale. The pulmonary vascular resistance falls as the blood oxygen tension rises, and right-to-left shunting through the ductus arteriosus (DA) ceases. Physiological closure of the DA is normally achieved by 10–15 h after delivery. Permanent closure, by obliteration of the duct lumen, may take several weeks. During this period the duct may reopen if there is hypoxia, acidosis, cardiac failure or severe surgical stress. A Patent DA (PDA) is, in itself, a cause of cardiac failure and is a common problem in the preterm infant. Patency *in utero* is maintained by prostaglandins (particularly PGE_2) released by the placenta.

Patent ductus arteriosus

The DA closes in the same time-scale in well preterm babies as it does in term-born babies; it closes in over 90 per cent of infants by 60 h of age [25]. Small preterm infants often have a PDA noted 5 days after birth especially if they have not received surfactant. This supports the view that the problem is not caused by an abnormality of the DA but rather results from stimuli such as acidosis, hypoxia, surgical stress and high circulating PGE_2 levels. Prematurity and RDS are the two major associated factors.

The incidence of PDA is estimated to be approximately 45 per cent of infants weighing less than 1750 g at birth and 80 per cent of infants less than 1200 g [26]. A PDA should be suspected in a preterm neonate with RDS who is either failing to improve or deteriorates between 5 and 10 days of age, and has bounding pulses (and precordium) and a continuous pulmonary murmur [27]. Other signs include progressive cardiomegaly and worsening lung shadowing on X-ray. Patent DA sometimes presents as apnoea or necrotising enterocolitis. Echocardiography is more sensitive and specific than the clinical signs. Echocardiographic features include volume overloading of the left heart, and visualisation of the ductus itself.

First-line treatment involves optimising oxygen delivery by treating anaemia, oxygen supplementation, fluid restriction and diuretic therapy. However, there are theoretical reasons and clinical evidence to suggest that furosemide may promote ductal patency by its effect on renal prostaglandin synthesis. If first-line treatment proves ineffective, the PDA will need to be closed by either indometacin or surgery. Indometacin inhibits prostaglandin synthetase and has been used for many years in neonatology: it successfully closes 90 per cent of PDAs. An effective regimen is 0.2 mg/kg IV. followed by two doses of 0.1 mg/kg at 12-hourly intervals. The side-effects include oliguria, hyponatraemia, gastrointestinal bleeding and transient reduction in blood flow to organs such as the brain and intestine.

If surgery is undertaken it is likely that the baby is hypovolaemic because they have been treated with fluid restriction and diuretic therapy. Meticulous assessment and monitoring is important and volume loading should be considered.

Myocardial function

Just before birth the combined ventricular output of the fetal heart is high, being in the order of 500 mL/kg/min. The left ventricle (LV) contributes one-third of this combined output. After birth the outputs from the left and right ventricles are the same at 300–400 mL/kg/min. Therefore the LV output increases by about 200 per cent and consequently myocardial performance is close to maximum. Over the next few months cardiac output decreases to 150–200 mL/kg/min and this is associated with the fall in oxygen consumption. There is greater functional myocardial reserve with maturation [28].

Neonatal cardiac output is very sensitive to changes in heart rate and this is due probably to reduced myocardial compliance which limits the ability to increase the stroke volume. Vagal stimulation initially causes a reduction in stroke volume and ventricular output with only a small decrease in heart rate, then, when bradycardia develops, cardiac output falls profoundly [29].

Parasympathetic tone predominates in the neonate and bradycardia is easily induced either by manoeuvres that increase vagal discharge or by hypoxia itself. Volume loading will increase stroke volume (but only over a limited range) [30] – overfilling causes a rapid decline in stroke volume. Optimum right-sided atrial filling pressures are as low as 3–6 mmHg [30].

Mean resting blood pressure is age dependent and ranges from 33 mmHg in a preterm infant of 23 weeks' gestation to 55 mmHg in a term newborn. The increase in pressure is caused by resetting of the carotid baroreceptor reflex, which gradually becomes insensitive to acute rises in arterial pressure, resulting in an increased basal blood pressure.

Persistent pulmonary hypertension

Although the transition from foetal to adult circulation is usually smooth, occasionally this may be delayed or reversed, with serious consequences. The pulmonary vasculature is extremely labile in the neonate because of an abundance of arteriolar smooth muscle, which extends more peripherally than in later life. The pulmonary vasculature constricts in response to hypoxia, hypercapnia, acidosis and other noxious stimuli. This leads to pulmonary hypertension with right-to-left shunting of venous blood across both the PDA and the foramen ovale. The shunting worsens the systemic hypoxaemia which further exacerbates pulmonary vasoconstriction and right-to-left shunting. There is metabolic acidosis and myocardial contractility is impaired.

Persistent pulmonary hypertension (PPH) may be idiopathic or associated with premature closure of the DA, severe intrapartum asphyxia, pneumonia, meconium aspiration, prematurity and lung hypoplasia (for example, in diaphragmatic hernia). Treatment is directed at reducing pulmonary vascular resistance by reversing hypoxia with raised levels of inspired oxygen, inducing a respiratory alkalosis with hyperventilation and intravenous vasodilators. Vasodilator drugs (tolazoline, magnesium sulphate, prostacyclin and sodium nitroprusside) are given in the hope that their effect will be more marked on the pulmonary circulation; however, systemic hypotension is a common and sometimes serious side-effect with these agents. Treatment may ameliorate pulmonary hypertension in some infants, but in many it does not. Extracorporeal membrane oxygenation (ECMO) therapy is life saving for some infants with pulmonary hypertension; however, it is costly, invasive, and associated with important morbidities.

Inhaled nitric oxide (iNO) is a selective pulmonary vasodilator that has become the first-line treatment [31]. Nitric oxide diffuses rapidly across the alveolar–capillary membrane into the smooth muscle of pulmonary vessels to activate guanylyl cyclase, the enzyme that converts guanosine triphosphate (GTP) to guanosine cyclic monophosphate (cGMP). Increased intracellular concentrations of cGMP relax vascular smooth muscles. The physiological effects of cGMP are limited to its area of synthesis by its hydrolysis to GMP by cyclic nucleotide phosphodiesterases (PDEs) or by its removal from the cell. Of the 11 PDE isozymes, PDE5 is the most active in the smooth muscle and possesses a high affinity for cGMP and is selectively inhibited by compounds such as sildenafil and verdenafil. When given to severely hypoxic babies with PPH in concentrations of up to 20 parts per million (p.p.m.), iNO rapidly improves arterial oxygen tension without causing systemic hypotension, and it decreases the need for ECMO therapy. Inhaled NO also has bronchodilatatory, anti-inflammatory and vascular cell antiproliferative effects in the lungs [31,32].

The efficacy of iNO is dependent on its delivery to the target resistance vessels within the lung. High-frequency oscillatory ventilation (HFOV) is a ventilatory strategy that provides adequate gas exchange using very small tidal volumes given at very fast respiratory rates, while maintaining relatively high mean airway pressures. This allows ventilation with relatively high mean lung volumes while minimising the risk of volutrauma and atelectrauma [33]. Christou et al. showed that, when iNO was used in combination with HFOV for PPHN, there was a significant improvement in oxygenation and a reduced need for ECMO [34].

CENTRAL NERVOUS SYSTEM

The brain of the term newborn weighs 330–350 g, which is one-quarter of the weight of an adult brain, and accounts for about 10 per cent of the total birth weight. About 25 per cent of the adult number of brain cells are present at birth. Myelination within the cerebral hemispheres occurs well after birth and progresses over decades.

Pain pathways

There is now overwhelming evidence to show that all the neurophysiological components required for pain perception are present by mid-gestation [35]. Incomplete myelination does not imply lack of function, but merely a slower conduction time, which is offset by shorter interneurone distances in infants. The neural pathways for pain in the newborn infant can be traced from the sensory receptors in the skin to the sensory areas in the cerebral cortex. Cutaneous sensory receptors appear in the perioral area of the human foetus by the seventh week of gestation and spread to all cutaneous and mucous surfaces by the twentieth week. The spread of cutaneous receptors is preceded by the development of synapses between sensory fibres and interneurons in the dorsal horn of the spinal cord.

Nociceptive nerve tracts in the spinal cord and central nervous system undergo complete myelination during the second and third trimester of gestation. Pain pathways to the brain stem and thalamus are completely myelinated by 30 weeks [36].

Cerebral blood flow

Control of cerebral blood flow (CBF) involves the complex interaction of metabolic, chemical and neural factors which produce their effects by direct action on the cerebral vessels. In adults, CBF is constant over a range of mean arterial pressure from 50 mmHg to 150 mmHg. The limits of autoregulation are unknown in newborns but, since systemic blood pressure is lower, they should also be lower. Autoregulation is intact even in premature infants who are mildly asphyxiated or who have respiratory distress. Carbon dioxide has a marked relaxant effect on their cerebral vascular tone.

Moderate hypercapnia increases and moderate hypocapnia decreases CBF. In preterm infants with arterial partial pressure of CO_2 ($PaCO_2$) less than 2.7 kPa (20 mmHg), further reductions in CBF may produce cerebral ischaemia and associated neurodevelopmental deficit. Chronic severe hypercapnia elevates CBF but cerebral oxidative metabolism is unaltered. Acute rises in $PaCO_2$ may depress cerebral metabolism. Hypercapnia may also reduce autoregulation because of vasodilatation, which may add to the risk of brain haemorrhage.

A decrease in arterial oxygen content produces cerebral vasodilatation and increases CBF, thereby maintaining cerebral oxygen delivery constant (CBF × arterial oxygen content). The arterial oxygen content is dependent not only on PaO_2 but also on haemoglobin-carrying capacity.

Intraventricular haemorrhage

Intraventricular haemorrhage (IVH) is a common problem in extremely low-birth-weight (ELBW) babies. Although the incidence has decreased in recent years it still occurs in one-third of babies born at 32 weeks' (or less) gestation. The magnitude of this problem relates to an increase in the absolute number of surviving preterm infants.

The most common site of origin of IVH is the subependymal germinal matrix. This region is highly cellular, gelatinous in texture, richly vascularised and lies immediately ventrolateral to the lateral ventricles. It serves initially as the source of cerebral neuronal precursor cells and then later, by the third trimester, glial cell precursors. The many thin-walled vessels in the matrix are a prime site for haemorrhage. In 80 per cent of patients with IVH the blood enters the lateral ventricles and spreads throughout the ventricular system. The outcome depends on the degree of parenchymal injury; complications include hydrocephalus and neurodevelopmental disability. Intraventricular haemorrhage becomes less common after

34 weeks' gestation [37] when the subependymal germinal matrix gradually involutes and disappears. If CBF autoregulation is impaired, for example with severe asphyxia or cranial trauma or hypercapnia, an acute increase in blood pressure, provoked by a noxious stimulus, could increase CBF and provoke bleeding from the germinal matrix.

During anaesthesia abrupt fluctuations in cerebral arterial and venous pressures, should be avoided. Rapid fluid administration may provoke IVH but hypotension is also potentially damaging. Fluid administration should balance fluid losses; both should be monitored carefully. Airway manipulations, including awake tracheal intubation, have been shown to increase blood pressure and anterior fontanelle pressure. Awake intubation should rarely be required in these infants; intubation conditions are better with adequate anaesthesia and muscle relaxation.

Retinopathy of prematurity

Retinopathy of prematurity (ROP) is an important cause of childhood blindness. The mild form is common but the severe form (requires treatment) occurs in 1.8 per cent of preterm infants screened in the UK [38]. Severe ROP is mostly confined to babies with a birth weight under 1000 g and gestational age of less than 32 weeks. Vascularisation of the retina proceeds centrifugally from the optic disc from about 16 weeks' gestation so that retina is fully vascularised by term. Retinopathy is caused by abnormal growth of retinal vessels. Although oxygen therapy has been identified as a major cause of ROP, the safe limits of duration and concentration are unknown. Meticulous monitoring of oxygenation and minimisation of oxygen therapy have largely eliminated the risk of blinding ROP for the more mature preterm infants.

Treatment is usually by laser therapy and, less frequently, cryotherapy. Many ROP babies have multiple medical problems of prematurity and, during anaesthesia, the lowest inspired oxygen concentration should be used to avoid oxygen desaturations less than 89 per cent. It is possible to conduct treatment in the neonatal intensive care unit under ketamine so that tracheal intubation is avoided.

INFECTION

About 10–20 per cent of neonates in developed countries are treated for suspected sepsis [39]. Serious bacterial infections occur in 1–4 per 1000 live births in developed world compared with 2–21 per 1000 in developing countries, where it remains a major cause of neonatal death. In preterm infants, the incidence of infection and sepsis is 3- to 10-fold more than in normal full-term infants.

Neonates are relatively immunocompromised particularly when they are premature and are therefore prone to infections, often with unusual organisms. This is attributed to reduced cellular and tissue immunity. *In utero*, maternal immunoglobulin G (IgG) is transferred to the foetus across the placenta from 14 weeks' gestation. The process starts slowly but accelerates at around 22 weeks so that after 30 weeks large amounts of IgG are transported. Immunoglobulins M (IgM), A (IgA), D (IgD) and E (IgE) are not transported and if these are found in cord blood they have been synthesised by the foetus. Newborn IgM levels are low and this increases susceptibility to infection by Gram-negative bacteria. Other risk factors for neonatal sepsis include prolonged rupture of the amniotic membranes before delivery, chorioamnionitis, maternal urinary tract infection and invasive intensive care procedures such as tracheal intubation and vascular catheterisation [39].

Neonatal sepsis may be early or late (Table 8.6). Early onset sepsis manifests within 48 h of birth, and the causative organisms are almost always maternal group B streptococci and *Escherichia coli*. Late-onset sepsis is caused by either common organisms from the environment or unusual maternal flora. In developed countries, infections with coagulase-negative staphylococci are commonest, but other causes include Gram-positive coccid (enterococci) and Gram-negative bacilli and fungi [39]. In developing countries, Gram-negative bacilli are the major cause. Candida septicaemia, from either *albicans* or non-*albicans* species of *Candida*, is a particular problem in infants born before 28 weeks. Symptoms and signs of infection are often subtle and non-specific and are summarised in Table 8.6. There should be a very low threshold for suspecting sepsis and initiating empirical antibiotic therapy.

Bacteriological tests and other investigations may be helpful, and these include maternal cultures (blood and high vaginal swab), neonatal blood cultures, and neonatal chest X-ray, lumbar puncture, viral serology and polymerase chain reaction analysis (to detect herpes simplex virus and enteroviruses).

JAUNDICE

Hyperbilirubinaemia in preterm infants is more common, more severe and more protracted than in term infants. It is caused by a combination factors. Bilirubin load is increased because of decreased red cell survival and there may be delayed maturation of bilirubin uptake and conjugation by the liver [40]. If enteral feeding is delayed, and this is common in sick premature newborns, bacterial colonisation is slow resulting in enhancement of bilirubin enterohepatic circulation – this also happens if there is an ileus or bowel obstruction. Unconjugated bilirubin is neurotoxic especially to the basal ganglia, brain-stem auditory pathways and oculomotor nuclei. This can lead to kernicterus which is a condition characterised by opisthotonus and convulsions in the short term, followed by permanent learning disability, choreoathetosis and high-tone deafness. The anatomical preference for bilirubin deposition and vulnerability to toxicity has not been fully explained, but may be a consequence of increased blood flow and metabolic activity in these areas. Damage may also be exacerbated by hypoxia, acidosis, hypercapnia, hypothermia, a low level of serum albumin and disruption of the blood–brain barrier.

Preterm infants tend to sustain neurological damage at lower bilirubin levels than the term infant. P-glycoprotein is a plasma membrane efflux pump found in brain capillary endothelial cells and is considered responsible for limiting the entry of lipophilic substrates into the central nervous system [41]. Expression of P-glycoprotein is related to gestational maturity, and thus may be an important age-related factor.

Monitoring and treating high bilirubin level are important. Specific treatment for hyperbilirubinaemia includes phototherapy and exchange transfusion.

NUTRITION AND HYPOGLYCAEMIA

Infants of less than 34 weeks' gestation seldom have an adequate suck reflex, so that feeding has to be intragastric, transpyloric or intravenous. Nasogastric or orogastric feeding is the most common method. It is important to appreciate that a significant quantity of fat is adsorbed into the polymer of the feeding tube. Transpyloric feeding has been widely used, but is associated with a higher mortality rate [42] probably because infants who need it are very sick. Short-term parenteral nutrition, accompanied by gradually increasing enteral feeding, is often necessary.

Feeding newborns who are less than 1500 g should start early to prevent hypoglycaemia. A common schedule for increasing gastric feed volumes is to give, on the first four successive days, 60, 90, 120 and 150 mL/kg/24 h and to

Table 8.6 Clinical features of neonatal sepsis

Early onset	Late onset
Unexplained birth asphyxia	Bradycardia and apnoea
Respiratory distress	Poor feeding/vomiting/increasing gastric aspirate/abdominal distension
Poor circulatory status (low blood pressure, cold peripheries)	Irritability
Unexplained hypoglycaemia	Convulsions
Unexplained low white cell count	Increasing jaundice
Rash (consider *Listeria*)	Increasing respiratory distress and ventilatory requirements
Hepatosplenomegaly	Unexplained rapid changes in white cells and/or platelets
Jaundice	Signs of local inflammation

make further daily increments to 180 mL/kg/24 h by day 10 and 200 mL/kg/24 h by day 14. Most infants weighing more than 1500 g tolerate 3-hourly feeds, while smaller infants need feeding every 1–2 h. Most hospitals favour gravity feeding (over 10–20 min) rather than using a syringe pump. Necrotising enterocolitis (NEC) should be considered in infants who develop increasing abdominal distension, constipation, loose or bloody stools; enteral feeding should be stopped immediately.

In infants who receive either minimal or no enteral nutrition, the immediate aim of intravenous infusion is to meet the infant's water and electrolyte requirements and to prevent hypoglycaemia. In the first week of life preterm infants often have a greater fall in blood glucose concentration than term infants [43]. Levels of gluconeogenic substrates are higher and glucose-6-phosphatase (the final enzyme of glycogenolysis and gluconeogenesis) activity may be lower. Since the blood sugar level denoting neonatal hypoglycaemia is not clearly defined, pragmatic 'operational thresholds' (blood glucose concentrations at which clinical interventions such as increased feeds should be considered) have been proposed. Such thresholds provide a margin of safety to help achieve 'normoglycaemia'. If there are signs of hypoglycaemia (tremor, irritability, jitteriness, apnoea, hypotonia, abnormal cry, tachypnoea, pallor, feeding difficulties, fits and a reduced level of consciousness), blood glucose concentrations should be raised above 2.5 mmol/L. In hyperinsulinism, an operational threshold of 3.5 mmol/L is appropriate, because there are low levels of alternate fuels. For other 'at-risk' infants who are healthy and without clinical signs, there should be intervention if blood glucose is consistently below 2.0 mmol/L. Intravenous glucose infusions are often required and should provide a least the same amount of glucose as the endogenous hepatic glucose output. This requires at least 6 mg/kg/min glucose, equating to at least 90 mL 10 per cent glucose/kg/day. With such fluid regimens, hypoglycaemia is now rare [43,44].

The diet of preterm neonates should be able to provide energy intake of 120 kcal/kg/day. High intake is required for long-term ventilated infants with chronic lung disease, whose energy requirements are increased by 25–30 per cent. Table 8.7 lists the recommended nutritional requirements for preterm neonates. Fluid intake should in general be restricted to 120–150 mL/kg/day because this is associated with reduced risk of PDA, NEC and death.

TEMPERATURE HOMEOSTASIS

Preterm infants are the most vulnerable of patients to hypothermia because of their thin skin, large surface area and inability to shiver. Normal neonates have some protection from thermogenic brown fat located around the major blood vessels in the neck and thorax. Activated by sympathetic stimulation, mitochondria uncouple oxidative phosphorylation to produce heat rather than ATP. Hypothermia soon after birth is a major risk factor for poor outcome [45] and a simple effective measure is to place the torso in a polythene bag as soon as possible [46,47]. Later, potentially deleterious effects of hypothermia include the reduction of coagulation, cardiac output and drug clearance. Conversely, hypothermia itself may be useful in organ preservation if oxygen delivery is marginal, for example cooling the head for encephalopathy [48]. Management of body temperature is discussed in Chapters 20 and 32. Thermogenesis from brown fat metabolism is suppressed by anaesthesia [49].

HAEMATOLOGY

Normal values at birth for haemoglobin, haematocrit, white blood cells and platelets for preterm babies are shown in Table 8.8.

A preterm neonate should be considered anaemic if the haemoglobin is less than 14 g/dL [50]. The cause of anaemia depends upon when it occurs. During the first 2 weeks of life, it is probably caused by haemorrhage or haemolysis. Blood tests may result in significant blood loss and they are related to immaturity and illness. After the second week there may be 'anaemia of prematurity' and this is maximal by 4–6 weeks when haemoglobin levels reach 6.5–9 g/dL. The severity is related mainly to low erythropoietin concentration, functional immaturity of bone marrow and reduced erythrocyte lifespan [51]. Anaemia of prematurity is always normocytic, normochromic with low reticulocyte count and normal iron levels. Anaemia after the second month is caused by nutritional deficiency of iron, folate or vitamin E. The need for red cell transfusion can be reduced by a combination of limiting blood tests, using iron and folate dietary

Table 8.7 Nutritional requirements for preterm infants (amount per kg per day)

Protein	2.7–3.5 g
Carbohydrate	5–17 g
Lipids	1–3 g
Sodium	3–5 mmol
Chloride	3–5 mmol
Potassium	1–2 mmol
Calcium	1.5–2.2 mmol
Phosphorus	1.5–2.2 mmol
Magnesium	0.3–0.4 mmol

Table 8.8 Normal haematological values at birth in preterm babies

	24–25 weeks	30–31 weeks
Haemoglobin (g/dL)	19.4 ± 1.5	19.1 ± 2.1
Haematocrit	0.63 ± 0.04	0.60 ± 0.08
White cells ($\times 10^9$/L)	3.95	4.44
Platelets ($\times 10^9$/L)	150–450	150–450

supplementation, and erythropoietin [52]. Donated blood can transmit cytomegalovirus infection carried in white blood cells and therefore only leukodepleted packed cells should be used.

Polycythaemia is defined as a central venous haematocrit of >0.65 and it causes very high blood viscosity [53]. It is associated with lethargy, hypotonia, hyperbilirubinaemia and hypoglycaemia, and may also be a contributory factor in neonatal seizures, stroke, NEC, and vascular occlusion of the renal, portal and cerebral veins. Before surgery, the haematocrit should be reduced to 0.55 by partial exchange with crystalloid but this may be associated with intraoperative hypotension if insufficient fluid is not given [21].

The white blood cell count of a normal preterm infant is shown in Table 8.8. The neutrophil count gradually rises in the first and second trimester to reach over 2×10^9/L by term; the count is slightly lower in preterm neonates. The neutrophil 'storage pool' in preterm infants is less than at term and is much lower than in adults. This may explain the frequency of bacterial infections in preterm infants.

By 5–6 weeks of conception, platelets appear in the fetal circulation [50]. During the second trimester, the platelet count rises to normal adult values ($175–250 \times 10^9$/L). Thus, even in the most preterm neonate, a platelet count of less than 150×10^9/L is abnormal. The principal cytokine that regulates platelet production is thrombopoietin and its production is reduced in the newborn, and more so in preterms. Thrombocytopenia is common in neonatal sepsis.

NECROTISING ENTEROCOLITIS

Necrotising enterocolitis [54] is the commonest surgical emergency in the neonatal period affecting 0.5 per cent of all live births and 3–5 per cent of low-birth-weight infants (1500–2500 g). It is characterised by a variable degree of intestinal necrosis, which may or may not be complicated by perforation and fulminant sepsis. The main risk factors include prematurity, enteral feeding and sepsis. The mean PCA of NEC infants is 30–32 weeks and most cases have a low birth weight (<1500 g). The premature gut may be more susceptible to the stresses of hypoxia, ischaemia and mucosal damage of hyperosmolar feeds. Also, hyperosmolar feeds and the bacterial fermentation of carbohydrates can produce large quantities of hydrogen that becomes intramural (pneumatosis intestinalis). Neonates that are breast-fed are 3–10 times less likely to develop NEC than those given formula feeds. Breast milk contains immunoglobulins (IgA and IgG) and white cells that may prevent NEC.

The clinical presentation includes abdominal distension, vomiting and bloody stools. There may be local abdominal tenderness or a mass. There is usually bacteraemia and elevated circulating proinflammatory cytokines. Abdominal X-rays may show distended loops of bowel, intramural gas, free air in the peritoneal cavity and portal venous gas. In more severe cases, there are features of overwhelming sepsis

including respiratory failure, hypotension, thrombocytopenia, coagulopathy and electrolyte disturbance.

Initial management is prompt cessation of enteral feeding and starting nasogastric tube drainage, intravenous antibiotics and systemic support. Total parenteral nutrition (TPN) is often needed. Broad-spectrum antibiotics should cover infection with enterococci, staphylococci and coliforms. Approximately 50 per cent of cases will require surgery. The aim is to remove necrotic bowel quickly but infants need to be stabilised beforehand if they are to survive [21]. Peritoneal drainage is an intermediate conservative measure prior to definitive surgery. Focal disease should be completely resected, whereas extensive disease is best managed with drainage by a proximal stoma and resection of only the worst affected bowel. Extensive bowel resection risks leaving inadequate bowel function so that future survival will be dependent upon lifelong TPN or transplantation.

Anaesthesia in these infants is a major challenge – of all the 'small infant' surgical procedures, laparotomy for NEC is the most difficult. Central venous and arterial catheters are often inserted in intensive care before surgery. Anaesthesia may be induced and maintained with fentanyl combined with a non-depolarising muscle relaxant. During surgery the common difficulties are blood loss and replacement, low cardiac output and maintenance of body temperature. Bleeding and fluid losses arising from bowel oedema and inflammation may require the infusion of large volumes of blood products and other fluids to maintain intravascular volume. Coagulopathy is also common and requires fresh frozen plasma and platelets to control bleeding. Inotropic support is usually necessary in sick infants and should, at least, be made ready before induction.

Occasionally, infection with neuraminidase-producing organisms can damage red cell proteins exposing the T-cryptoantigen (see Chapter 24). Adult but not neonatal plasma usually contains anti-T IgM antibody that is potentially haemolytic. A red cell transfusion should be safe if it contains minimal plasma but other blood products including platelets should be avoided if possible because of the risks of haemolysis. If available, low titre anti-T plasma products are preferred. If there is clinically significant haemolysis exchange transfusion may be necessary.

THE FORMER PRETERM INFANT

Repair of an inguinal hernia is the most common surgical procedure carried out in premature babies. This condition usually occurs in infants born before a gestational age of 32 weeks and a birth weight of less than 1250 g. Surgery is usually performed when the infant has been weaned from ventilation, is growing and is stable, and often this corresponds to when they are ready for discharge home.

Infants born prematurely have more complications after anaesthesia and surgery than term infants, and the most serious of these is apnoea. Most investigators report that

20–30 per cent of otherwise healthy preterm infants undergoing inguinal hernia repair under general anaesthesia have at least one apnoeic episode in the postoperative period; the highest report incidence has been 81 per cent. However, these differences probably result from the definition of apnoea and the variation in either the duration or method of monitoring. Apnoea related to anaesthesia usually occurs within the first 12 postoperative hours. Malviya and colleagues continued monitoring for either a minimum of 24 h or at least 12 apnoea-free hours [55] and in all their infants apnoea occurred within 12 h. Therefore it is generally accepted that apnoea monitoring should be continued for at least 12 h after anaesthesia, or after the last apnoea. Post-anaesthesia apnoeas are usually central but are often mixed with an obstructive element [56]. Obstructive apnoea more often causes desaturation than central apnoea. A combined analysis of eight prospective studies found that the following risk factors were important [57]:

- The incidence of apnoea is inversely related to PCA and becomes less frequent when PCA is more than 43 weeks. Apnoea can occur as late as 55–60 weeks.
- Small-for-gestational-age infants are less likely to develop apnoea. These infants undergo significant intrauterine stress which can induce accelerated maturation and may in some way offer protection against postoperative apnoea.
- Anaemic infants (haematocrit <30 per cent) with a PCA more than 44 weeks are more at risk of postoperative apnoea.
- All anaesthetic agents, including ketamine, are associated with apnoea.

The methylxanthines [58] aminophylline and caffeine have been used for many years to treat apnoea. They are probably effective by multiple actions: they increase respiratory drive and stimulate the diaphragm, have positive inotropic and chronotropic cardiac effects, cause a mild diuresis and increase heat production through utilisation of brown fat. Caffeine, in a dose of 10 mg/kg, given immediately after induction of general anaesthesia reduces apnoea.

Spinal, caudal or combined spinal/caudal blocks have become popular in the management of inguinal hernia repair. Regional techniques, without sedation, may reduce the incidence of postoperative respiratory complications, but the evidence is conflicting. However, regional techniques are technically difficult in awake infants, so that there is a significant failure rate. Spinal techniques have a short duration of action and may be too short for difficult or bilateral repairs. Clonidine, added to a caudal block, may also provoke apnoea.

The newest and shortest-acting volatile agents, sevoflurane and desflurane, appear to produce similar post-operative respiratory problems in infants who have had a caudal block [59]. Desflurane has the advantage of faster recovery than sevoflurane. It has been suggested that the most reliable standard technique for high-risk infants could be light general anaesthesia with either sevoflurane or desflurane, controlled ventilation and a caudal block.

Former preterm infants must be carefully observed following anaesthesia and surgery, irrespective of the anaesthetic technique. Former preterm infants less than a PCA of 60 weeks should not be discharged home the same day. However, the age at which anaesthetic risk becomes minimised is unknown and factors such as growth, development and coexisting medical problems should be considered. Ideally, surgery should be delayed in anaemic infants until the haematocrit is at least 30 per cent.

FOETAL SURGERY

Surgery in a foetus is controversial. It has had poor results in the past but interest is being renewed. The following is a brief account of the important principles and more details can be found elsewhere [60]. Defects that have the potential for foetal correction include repair of meningomyelocele, diaphragmatic hernia and urethral valves. Foetal surgery should, in principle, be undertaken before 30 weeks' gestation in order for the infant to benefit from minimisation of the damage caused by the deformity and to allow maximal time for healing and growth before birth. Surgery can be open, via a hysterotomy, or by minimal access fetoscopy. All procedures require the uterus to be relaxed and this is achieved best by high-dose inhalational anaesthetic agents, especially for open procedures; under these conditions sufficient anaesthetic crosses the placenta to anaesthetise the foetus. Opioids administered to the mother also cross the placenta and, if necessary, supplementary opioid and a muscle relaxant can be given directly to the foetus during open surgery. High doses of isoflurane may decrease placental blood flow and foetal cardiac output, causing a decrease in foetal oxygenation. Safe obstetric anaesthesia and tocolysis are obviously crucial to the foetus. Foetal blood loss during surgery of 10 mL will need transfusion.

Congenital high airway obstruction syndrome (CHAOS) can be managed by *ex utero* intrapartum treatment (EXIT) [61]. In this procedure the infant's head is delivered by caesarean section near to term and the trachea is intubated, by whatever means necessary, while the umbilical placental blood flow is still intact. When the airway is secure, the infant is delivered and treated appropriately.

REFERENCES

Key references

Cote CJ, Zaslavsky A, Downes JJ et al. Postoperative apnea in former preterm infants after inguinal herniorrhaphy: a combined analysis. *Anesthesiology* 1995; **82**: 809–22.

Imai Y, Slutsky AS. High-frequency oscillatory ventilation and ventilator-induced injury. *Crit Care Med* 2005; **33**(3 Suppl): S129–34.

Richmond S (ed.). *Newborn life support – resuscitation at birth*, 2nd edn. London: Resuscitation Council (UK), 2006.

Shaw NJ, Kotecha S. Management of infants with chronic lung disease of prematurity in the United Kingdom. *Early Hum Dev* 2005; **81**: 165–70.

Yeung S, Davies EG. Infection in the fetus and neonate. *Medicine* 2005; **33**(4): 91–7.

References

1. Steer P. The epidemiology of preterm labour. *BJOG* 2005 March; **112**(suppl 1): 1–3.

2. Government Statistical Service for the Department of Health. *NHS maternity statistics, England: 2003–04*. London: Department of Health, 2005.

3. Richmond S, Resuscitation Council. *Newborn life support – resuscitation at birth*, 2nd edn. London: Resuscitation Council (UK), 2006.

4. American Heart Association (AHA 2005). Guidelines for cardiopulmonary resuscitation (CPR) and emergency cardiovascular care (ECC) of pediatric and neonatal patients: pediatric basic life support. *Pediatrics* 2006; **117**(5): e989–1004.

5. Finster M, Wood M. The Apgar score has survived the test of time. *Anesthesiology* 2005; **102**(4): 855–7.

6. Northway WH Jr, Rosan RC, Porter DY. Pulmonary disease following respiratory therapy of hyaline membrane disease: bronchopulmonary dysplasia. *N Engl J Med* 1967; **276**(7): 357–68.

7. Soll RF, Morley CJ. Prophylactic versus selective use of surfactant in preventing morbidity and mortality in preterm infants. *Cochrane Database Syst Rev* 2001; **2**: CD000510.

8. Bancalari E, Claure N, Sosenko IR. Bronchopulmonary dysplasia: changes in pathogenesis, epidemiology and definition. *Semin Neonatol* 2003; **8**(1): 63–71.

9. Northway WH Jr, Moss RB, Carlisle KB *et al.* Late pulmonary sequelae of bronchopulmonary dysplasia. *N Engl J Med* 1990; **323**(26): 1793–9.

10. Halliday HL, Ehrenkranz RA, Doyle LW. Moderately early (7–14 days) postnatal corticosteroids for preventing chronic lung disease in preterm infants. *Cochrane Database Syst Rev* 2003; **1**: CD001144.

11. Shaw NJ, Kotecha S. Management of infants with chronic lung disease of prematurity in the United Kingdom. *Early Hum Dev* 2005; **81**(2): 165–70.

12. Beresford MW, Primhak R, Subhedar NV, Shaw NJ. Randomised double blind placebo controlled trial of inhaled fluticasone propionate in infants with chronic lung disease. *Arch Dis Child Fetal Neonatal Ed* 2002; **87**(1): F62–3.

13. Brion LP, Primhak RA, Ambrosio-Perez I. Diuretics acting on the distal renal tubule for preterm infants with (or developing) chronic lung disease. *Cochrane Database Syst Rev* 2002; **1**: CD001817.

14. Groothuis JR, Rosenberg AA. Home oxygen promotes weight gain in infants with bronchopulmonary dysplasia. *Am J Dis Child* 1987; **141**(9): 992–5.

15. Barrington K, Finer N. The natural history of the appearance of apnea of prematurity. *Pediatr Res* 1991; **29**(4 Pt 1): 372–5.

16. Martin RJ, Abu-Shaweesh JM, Baird TM. Apnoea of prematurity. *Paediatr Respir Rev* 2004; **5**(suppl A): S377–82.

17. Hannam S. Apnoea and bradycardia. In: Rennie JM, ed. *Roberton's textbook of neonatology*, 4th edn. Edinburgh: Elsevier/Churchill Livingstone, 2005.

18. Steer PA, Henderson-Smart DJ. Caffeine versus theophylline for apnea in preterm infants. *Cochrane Database Syst Rev* 2000; **2**: CD000273.

19. Paediatric Formulary Committee 2004–2005. *British national formulary for children*. London: BMJ Publishing Group Ltd, 2005: 186.

20. Miller MJ, Carlo WA, Martin RJ. Continuous positive airway pressure selectively reduces obstructive apnea in preterm infants. *J Pediatr* 1985; **106**(1): 91–4.

21. Gregory GA. Anaesthesia for premature infants. In: Gregory GA, ed. *Pediatric anesthesia*, 4th edn. Philadelphia: Churchill Livingstone, 2002: 353–63.

22. Bath AP, Panarese A, Thevasagayam M, Bull PD. Paediatric subglottic stenosis. *Clin Otolaryngol Allied Sci* 1999; **24**(2): 117–21.

23. Myer CM III, O'Connor DM, Cotton RT. Proposed grading system for subglottic stenosis based on endotracheal tube sizes. *Ann Otol Rhinol Laryngol* 1994; **103**(4 Pt 1): 319–23.

24. Sherman JM, Lowitt S, Stephenson C, Ironson G. Factors influencing acquired subgottic stenosis in infants. *J Pediatr* 1986; **109**(2): 322–7.

25. Evans NJ, Archer LN. Postnatal circulatory adaptation in healthy term and preterm neonates. *Arch Dis Child* 1990; **65**(1 Spec No): 24–6.

26. Moore P, Brook MM, Heyman MA. Patent ductus arteriosus. In: Allen HD, Gutgesell HP, Clark EB, Driscoll DJ, eds. *Moss and Adam's heart disease in infants, children and adolescents including the fetus and young adults*, 6th edn. Philadelphia: Lippincott, Williams & Wilkins, 2001: 652–69.

27. Evans N. Patent ductus arteriosus in the neonate. *Curr Paediatr* 2005; **15**: 381–9.

28. Klopfenstein HS, Rudolph AM. Postnatal changes in the circulation and responses to volume loading in sheep. *Circ Res* 1978; **42**(6): 839–45.

29. Rudolph AM, Heymann MA. Cardiac output in the fetal lamb: the effects of spontaneous and induced changes of heart rate on right and left ventricular output. *Am J Obstet Gynecol* 1976; **124**(2): 183–92.

30. Thornburg KL, Morton MJ. Filling and arterial pressures as determinants of RV stroke volume in the sheep fetus. *Am J Physiol* 1983; **244**(5): H656–63.

31. Ichinose F, Roberts JD, Jr, Zapol WM. Inhaled nitric oxide: a selective pulmonary vasodilator: current uses and therapeutic potential. *Circulation* 2004; **109**(25): 3106–11.

32. Hintz SR, Suttner DM, Sheehan AM, Rhine WD, van Meurs KP. Decreased use of neonatal extracorporeal membrane oxygenation (ECMO): how new treatment modalities have affected ECMO utilization. *Pediatrics* 2000; **106**(6): 1339–43.

33. Imai Y, Slutsky AS. High-frequency oscillatory ventilation and ventilator-induced lung injury. *Crit Care Med* 2005; **33**(3 suppl): S129–34.

34. Christou H, van Marter LJ, Wessel DL *et al*. Inhaled nitric oxide reduces the need for extracorporeal membrane oxygenation in infants with persistent pulmonary hypertension of the newborn. *Crit Care Med* 2000; **28**(11): 3722–7.

35. Fitzgerald M. Development of pain mechanisms. *Br Med Bull* 1991; **47**(3): 667–75.

36. Anand KJ, Hickey PR. Pain and its effects in the human neonate and fetus. *N Engl J Med* 1987; **317**(21): 1321–9.

37. Levene M. The sequelae of periventricular haemorrhage. *Curr Paediatr* 2005; **15**: 375–80.

38. Haines L, Fielder AR, Scrivener R, Wilkinson AR. Retinopathy of prematurity in the UK I: the organisation of services for screening and treatment. *Eye* 2002; **16**(1): 33–8.

39. Yeung S, Davies EG. Infection in the fetus and neonate. *Medicine* 2005; **33**(4): 91–7.

40. Watchko JF, Maisels MJ. Jaundice in low birthweight infants: pathobiology and outcome. *Arch Dis Child Fetal Neonatal Ed* 2003; **88**(6): F455–8.

41. Watchko JF, Daood MJ, Biniwale M. Understanding neonatal hyperbilirubinaemia in the era of genomics. *Semin Neonatol* 2002; **7**(2): 143–52.

42. McGuire W, McEwan P. Transpyloric versus gastric tube feeding for preterm infants. *Cochrane Database Syst Rev* 2002; **3**: CD003487.

43. Hawdon JM, Ward Platt MP, Aynsley-Green A. Patterns of metabolic adaptation for preterm and term infants in the first neonatal week. *Arch Dis Child* 1992; **67**(4 Spec No): 357–65.

44. Deshpande S, Ward PM. The investigation and management of neonatal hypoglycaemia. *Semin Fetal Neonatal Med* 2005; **10**(4): 351–61.

45. Costeloe K, Hennessy E, Gibson AT *et al*. The EPICure study: outcomes to discharge from hospital for infants born at the threshold of viability. *Pediatrics* 2000; **106**: 659–71.

46. Smith CL, Quine D, McCrosson F *et al*. Changes in body temperature after birth in preterm infants stabilized in polythene bags. *Arch Dis Child Fetal Neonatal Ed* 2005; **90**: F444.

47. McCall EM, Alderdice FA, Halliday HL *et al*. Interventions to prevent hypothermia at birth in preterm and/or low birthweight babies. *Cochrane Database Syst Rev* 2005; **1**: CD004210.

48. Gluckman PD, Wyatt JS, Azzopardi D *et al*. Selective head cooling with mild systemic hypothermia after neonatal encephalopathy: multicentre randomised trial. *Lancet* 2005; **365**: 663–70.

49. Lindahl SGE, Grigsby EJ, Meyer DM, Beynen FMK. Thermogenetic response to mild hypothermia in anaesthetized infants and children. *Paediatr Anaesth* 1992; **2**: 23–9.

50. Hann IM. The normal blood picture in neonates. In: Hann IM, Gibson BES, Letsky EA, eds. *Fetal and neonatal haematology*. London: Baillière Tindall, 1991: 29–50.

51. Oski FA. The erythrocyte and its disorders. In: Nathan A, Oski FA, eds. *Haematology of infancy and childhood*. Philadelphia: WB Saunders, 1993: 18–43.

52. Garcia MG, Hutson AD, Christensen RD. Effect of recombinant erythropoietin on 'late' transfusions in the neonatal intensive care unit: a meta-analysis. *J Perinatol* 2002; **22**(2): 108–11.

53. Werner EJ. Neonatal polycythemia and hyperviscosity. *Clin Perinatol* 1995; **22**(3): 693–710.

54. Pierro A. The surgical management of necrotising enterocolitis. *Early Hum Dev* 2005; **81**(1): 79–85.

55. Malviya S, Swartz J, Lerman J. Are all preterm infants younger than 60 weeks postconceptual age at risk for postanaesthetic apnea? *Anesthesiology* 1993; **78**: 1076–81.

56. Kurth CD, LeBard SE. Association of postoperative apnea, airway obstruction, and hypoxemia in former premature infants. *Anesthesiology* 1991; **75**: 22–6.

57. Cote CJ, Zaslavsky A, Downes JJ *et al*. Postoperative apnea in former preterm infants after inguinal herniorrhaphy. A combined analysis. *Anesthesiology* 1995; **82**(4): 809–22.

58. Craven PD, Badawi N, Henderson-Smart DJ, O'Brien M. Regional (spinal, epidural, caudal) versus general anaesthesia in preterm infants undergoing inguinal herniorrhaphy in early infancy. *Cochrane Database Syst Rev* 2003; **3**: CD003669.

59. Sale SM, Read JA, Stoddart PA, Wolf AR. Prospective comparison of sevoflurane and desflurane in formerly premature infants undergoing inguinal herniotomy. *Br J Anaesth* 2006; **96**(6): 774–8.

60. Myers LB, Cohen D, Galinkin J *et al*. Anaesthesia for fetal surgery. *Paediatr Anaesth* 2002; **12**(7): 569–78.

61. Lim FY, Crombleholme TM, Hedrick HL *et al*. Congenital high airway obstruction syndrome: natural history and management. *J Pediatr Surg* 2003; **38**(6): 940–5.

9

Pharmacology: general principles

BRIAN J ANDERSON

KEY LEARNING POINTS

- Most elimination pathways are immature at birth but mature within the first year of life.
- Age-related changes in body composition alter drug disposition during infancy.
- There is considerable pharmacokinetic variability between and within subjects. Size and age are prominent covariates.
- There are few pharmacodynamic data in human infants.

- There is a non-linear relationship between clearance and size. Allometry disentangles size from age, allowing comparison between paediatric and adult data.
- When estimating drug clerance, a per kilogram model under-predicts and a surface area model over-predicts (both get worse as age decreases).

INTRODUCTION

Children are 'therapeutic orphans' because there are insufficient well-conducted pharmacokinetic (PK) and pharmacodynamic (PD) studies. In their stead there is extrapolation from adult or animal data. Neonates, infants and children are different from adults. Paediatric responses to drugs are determined by a large number of factors, which may change independently during development. Growth and developmental aspects account for major changes in infants and small children whereas body size accounts for most of the pharmacokinetic differences between older children and adults. The pharmacodynamic factors that may influence response in early life remain poorly defined.

PHARMACOKINETICS

Absorption

The majority of drugs used in anaesthesia are administered either intravenously or through the lungs. Drugs given via other extravascular routes (e.g. oral, rectal, intramuscular or transdermal routes) must overcome chemical, physical, mechanical and biological barriers to reach the systemic circulation.

The principal enteral site of absorption is the small intestine but the rate at which drug leaves the stomach is the major determinant of speed of absorption. Drug absorption rates are slowest in neonates and young infants because gastric emptying and intestinal motor motility are delayed and may not mature until 6–8 months. Intragastric pH is elevated (>4) in neonates increasing the bioavailability of acid-labile compounds (e.g. benzylpenicillin) and decreasing the bioavailability of weak acids (e.g. phenobarbital). The infant gut is more permeable to large molecule drugs than that of older children. Other effects of the immature gut are either uncertain or not characterised. Immature conjugation and transport of bile salts into the intestinal lumen may affect lipophilic drug blood concentrations. Also, splanchnic blood flow changes in the first few weeks of life may alter concentration gradients across the intestinal mucosa and consequent absorption. The role of altered intestinal microflora in neonates and its effect on drugs (e.g. digoxin inactivation) are uncertain.

The larger relative skin surface area, increased cutaneous perfusion and thinner stratum corneum in neonates increase absorption of topically applied drugs (e.g. corticosteroids or local anaesthetic creams). Skin applications of alcohol and iodine can both be toxic. Neonates have a tendency to form methaemoglobin because they have reduced levels of methaemoglobin reductase and foetal haemoglobin is more readily oxidised. Lidocaine–prilocaine cream can oxidise haemoglobin and this, combined with increased absorption in neonates, has resulted in reluctance to use it in this age group. These fears are unfounded if the cream is used for single dose [1].

Reduced skeletal muscle bulk, blood flow and inefficient contractions in neonates should decrease intramuscular absorption but this is not necessarily the case, partly because of size (see Size models on page 148) and the higher density of skeletal muscle capillaries.

Rectal administration is associated with erratic and variable absorption. Age, formulation, rectal contents and contractions (with consequent expulsion), and the depth of rectal insertion all affect absorption and bioavailability. Rectal drugs may evade first-pass hepatic extraction because not all rectal venous blood passes to the portal system. Age influences the relative bioavailability of rectal paracetamol, but probably not because of first-pass metabolism.

Pulmonary absorption is generally more rapid in infants and children than in adults. Developmental changes of both the lung architecture and mechanics play a role. The more rapid wash-in of inhalational anaesthetics results from higher alveolar ventilation and lower tissue/blood solubility. With the greater fraction of the cardiac output distributed to the vessel-rich tissue group, an anaesthetic reaches its target quicker. Solubility has considerable effect on the uptake of inhalational agents because it determines volume of distribution. The solubilities in blood of halothane and isoflurane are 18 per cent less in neonates than in adults and the tissue solubilities in the vessel-rich tissue group are approximately 50 per cent less. This may be due to the greater water content and decreased protein and lipid concentration in neonatal tissues. These factors do not have an appreciable effect on less soluble agents such as nitrous oxide and sevoflurane but do explain the more rapid uptake and cardiac depression of the more soluble halothane in infants than in children (induction bradycardia is more common in infants). Congenital heat disease can alter pulmonary uptake; right-to-left shunting delays uptake although left-to-right shunting has little effect.

Distribution

BODY COMPOSITION

The volumes of distribution of drugs change dramatically over the first few years of life because of major changes in body composition and proportion. Total body water constitutes 80 per cent of the body weight in the preterm neonate and 75 per cent in term neonates. This decreases to approximately 60 per cent at 5 months and remains relatively constant from this age onwards [2]. The major component contributing to this reduction is the decrease in extracellular fluid (ECF). The ECF constitutes 45 per cent of the body weight at birth and 26 per cent at one year; there is a further reduction during childhood until adulthood where it contributes 18 per cent. Polar drugs such as aminoglycosides and neuromuscular blocking drugs distribute rapidly into the ECF but enter cells more slowly. The initial dose of such drugs is usually higher in the infant compared with older children because of an increased ECF volume. This may explain, in part, why infants require 3–4 mg/kg suxamethonium compared with 2 mg/kg in children and 1 mg/kg in adults to provide equal intubation conditions and duration of action.

Fat contributes 3 per cent of body weight in a 1.5 kg premature neonate, 12 per cent in a term neonate and 24 per cent by 4–5 months of age. 'Baby fat' is lost when the infant starts walking and protein mass increases from 20 per cent in the term neonate to 50 per cent in the adult.

PLASMA PROTEINS

Acidic drugs (e.g. barbiturates) tend to bind mainly to albumin while basic drugs (e.g. diazepam and amide local anaesthetics) bind to globulins, lipoproteins and glycoproteins. In general, plasma protein binding of many drugs is less in neonates than in adults, but the clinical impact is minor for most drugs because reduced clearance in this age group has a greater effect. Protein binding is important for a drug that is more than 95 per cent protein bound and has a narrow therapeutic index [3].

α_1-Acid glycoprotein

α_1-Acid glycoprotein (AAG) concentrations increase after surgical stress. They are reduced in neonates and although variable they tend to reach adult levels by 6 months [4]. Mean preoperative AAG concentrations of 0.38 (SD 0.16) g/L increase to 0.76 (SD 0.18) g/L in infants by day 4 after surgery and remain steady until day 7 [5]. This can cause an increase in total plasma concentration of drugs such as bupivacaine that have low-to-intermediate hepatic extraction. The unbound drug concentration, however, should not change because clearance is by intrinsic hepatic metabolising capacity. Any increase in unbound concentrations observed during long-term epidural is attributable to reduced hepatic clearance rather than AAG concentration.

Albumin

Premature infants have lower plasma albumin concentrations than at other ages and foetal albumin has reduced affinity for drugs. Increased concentrations of free fatty acids and unconjugated bilirubin compete with acidic drugs for binding sites. Neonates also have a tendency to acidosis that alters ionisation and binding properties of plasma proteins. Serum albumin concentrations reach those of adults by 5 months and binding capacity matures by 1 year.

Tissue binding

Maturational changes in tissue binding affect drug distribution. Myocardial digoxin concentrations in infants are sixfold higher than those in adults at similar blood concentrations. The concentration of digoxin in erythrocytes, and perhaps in other tissues, increases gradually and this may explain why infants have a greater apparent volume of distribution and need surprisingly large therapeutic doses.

P-glycoprotein

Most drugs cross membranes as a result of passive diffusion along concentration gradients dependent on factors such as molecular size, ionisation, tissue binding and lipophicity. However, P-glycoprotein, a member of the ATP-binding cassette family of transporters, is capable of producing a biological barrier to membrane passage. This glycoprotein is an efflux transporter that can extrude selected toxins and xenobiotics from cells at diverse sites that include the blood–brain barrier (BBB), hepatocytes, renal tubular cells and erythrocytes. The level of expression of P-glycoprotein appears to be low in neonatal rats and may explain increased brain/plasma phenobarbital ratios in neonates. However, pore density and blood flow distribution differences may also explain this observation.

BLOOD–BRAIN BARRIER

The BBB is a lipid membrane interface between the endothelial cells of the brain blood vessels and the ECF of the brain, and acts as a barrier to water-soluble drugs. Brain uptake of drugs is dependent on lipid solubility and blood flow. It was postulated that BBB permeability to water-soluble drugs, such as morphine, changes with maturation because neonates less than 4 days of age can develop respiratory depression following small doses of intramuscular morphine (0.05 mg/kg) [6]. Respiratory depression in neonates following intramuscular pethidine 0.5 mg/kg is similar to adults [6] and this may be because pethidine, unlike morphine, is lipid soluble and therefore crosses immature or mature BBB equally [6]. Fentanyl is also lipid soluble and causes similar respiratory depression in infants and adults at equal plasma concentrations. However, any increased neonatal respiratory depression after morphine could be due to pharmacokinetic factors. The volume of distribution of morphine is reduced in term neonates [7] and initial concentrations of morphine may then be higher in neonates than in adults. Further, respiratory depression was found to be the same in children from 2 to 570 days of age at the same plasma morphine concentrations [8]. Any developmental differences in BBB transporter activity remain speculative.

Drug metabolism

The main routes by which drugs and their metabolites leave the body are the hepatobiliary system, the kidneys and the lungs. The liver is the primary organ for clearance of most drugs. Non-polar, lipid-soluble drugs are converted to more polar and water-soluble compounds. Water-soluble drugs are excreted unchanged in the kidneys by glomerular filtration and renal tubular secretion. Many of these processes are immature in the neonate but mature within the first year of life; developmental changes are predicted by age and not size or weight.

HEPATIC ELIMINATION

The placenta has enzymatic capacity to clear drugs (conjugation and cytochrome enzymes) and therefore interpretation of foetal hepatic maturation is difficult. Placental transfer of drugs is dependent on the concentration gradient, membrane thickness and drug diffusion constant. Drug transfer can be graded as *limited* (propofol, muscle relaxants, amide local anaesthetics, alfentanil), *high* (thiopental) and *in excess* (ketamine).

Neonates have varying levels of hepatic enzymes, but there is a paucity of data regarding mechanisms for the onset of either extrauterine expression or the specific mechanisms that determine temporal switches [9,10]. Enzyme systems appear to mature and approximate to adult levels within the first year of life but there are exceptions. Isoniazid acetylation, for example, matures by 4 years of age [11].

Phase 1 reactions

Phase 1 metabolic processes involve oxidative, reductive or hydrolytic reactions that are commonly catalysed by mixed function oxidase systems. The activity of the cytochrome P450 group measured in hepatic microsomes obtained from term neonates approaches half of the activity found in adults [12]. It has been claimed, although the evidence is poor, that the specific *in vitro* activity for many of these enzymes approaches adult levels after correction for differences in liver mass. The pathways develop at different rates and are dependent on growth hormone and other mediators. Enzyme systems develop within different hepatic zones and their maturity may take months after birth.

The cytochrome CYP type of the P450 enzyme group is the major system for oxidation of drugs (Table 9.1). There are distinct patterns associated with isoform-specific developmental expression of CYPs. Some appear to be switched on by birth, while in others birth is necessary but not sufficient. CYP2E1 activity surges after birth, CYP2D6 becomes detectable soon after, the CYP3A4 and CYP2C family appear during the first week, and CYP1A2 is the last to appear [13]. Neonates are dependent on the immature CYP3A4 for levobupivacaine clearance and CYP1A2 for ropivacaine clearance, dictating reduced epidural infusion rates in this age group [14,15].

Table 9.1 Examples of some drugs that use cytochrome P450 for metabolism

Cytochrome P450	Substrate
CYP1A2	Ondansetron, paracetamol, caffeine
CYP2C9	Ibuprofen, diclofenac, warfarin
CYP2C19	Phenytoin, diazepam
CYP2D6	Codeine, tramadol, lidocaine, ondansetron
CYP2E1	Alcohol, isoflurane, halothane, sevoflurane, paracetamol, theophylline
CYP3A4	Codeine, midazolam

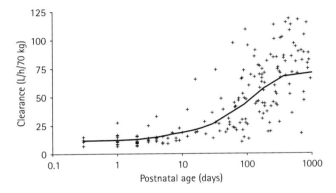

Figure 9.1 Maturation of morphine clearance with age. Total body morphine clearance is 80 per cent that of 'adult' values by 6 months [7]. Redrawn by permission of Oxford University Press.

Phase 2 reactions

Knowledge of maturation of phase II enzymes remains incomplete [10]. Some phase II pathways are mature at birth (sulphate conjugation), while others are not (acetylation, glycination, glucuronidation). The individual isoforms of glucuronosyl transferase (UGT) mature at different rates. Morphine is largely metabolised by uridine 5'-diphosphate UGT2B7 to morphine-3-glucuronide and morphine-6-glucuronide. *In vitro* studies using liver microsomes from foetuses aged 15–27 weeks indicated that morphine glucuronidation is approximately 10–20 per cent of that measured in adult microsomes [16]. Morphine glucuronidation has been demonstrated in premature infants as young as 24 weeks. Clearance increases after birth with maturation half-time at approximately 3 months [7] (Fig. 9.1).

Neonates can use sulphate conjugation as an alternative route for morphine or paracetamol before glucuronidation develops; the sulphate pathway is the dominant metabolic route for paracetamol in infancy. The toxic metabolite of paracetamol, *N*-acetyl-*p*-benzoquinone imine (NAPQI), is formed by CYP2E1, -1A2 and -3A4 and binds to intracellular hepatic macromolecules to produce cell necrosis and damage. CYP2E1 activity surges after birth, but data suggest that infants less than 90 days old have decreased clearance of

CYP2E1 substrates compared with older infants, children and adults. CYP3A4 appears during the first week, whereas CYP1A2 is the last to appear. The lower activity of cytochrome P450 in neonates may contribute to the low occurrence of paracetamol-induced hepatotoxicity.

Another potential advantage of immature drug clearance in preterm infants is the prolonged apnoea prevention effect of a single dose of theophylline. N_7-Methylation of theophylline (a prodrug) produces caffeine and this enzyme is well developed in the neonate. However, oxidative demethylation (CYP1A2), which is responsible for caffeine metabolism, is deficient and develops after a few months. Caffeine is cleared slowly by the immature kidney.

RENAL ELIMINATION

Drugs and their metabolites are excreted by the kidneys by the two processes of glomerular filtration and tubular secretion. The glomerular filtration rate (GFR) is approximately 2–4 mL/min per 1.73 m^2 in term neonates and, sized to surface area, reaches adult values at 5–6 months. Proximal tubular secretion reaches adult capacity by age 7 months. Aminoglycosides are almost exclusively cleared by renal elimination and maintenance dose is predicted by post-conceptional age (PCA) because it predicts the time course of development of renal function. Penicillin is actively secreted by the *p*-aminohippurate pathway, which is immature in neonates and results in an increased elimination half-life for penicillin and related compounds. At birth the urine is slightly acidic (pH 6–6.5) and this decreases the elimination of weak acids.

EXTRAHEPATIC ELIMINATION

Many drugs are metabolised at extrahepatic sites. Remifentanil (and atracurium to some extent) is rapidly broken down by a non-specific esterase in tissue and erythrocytes. Clearance is increased in younger children but this may be attributable to size and not age. The rate constant of hydrolysis by plasma esterases of propacetamol to paracetamol has also been found to be related to size and not age [17]. Ester local anaesthetics are metabolised by plasma pseudocholinesterase, which is reduced in neonates (the *in vitro* plasma half-life of 2-chloroprocaine in umbilical cord blood is twice that in maternal blood, but there are no *in vivo* studies examining the effects of age). The duration of suxamethonium activity is related to rapid redistribution of drug from its site of action in most individuals, although polymorphism reduces pseudocholinesterase activity and prolongs the action of suxamethonium in some individuals.

POLYMORPHISM

An important cause of pharmacokinetic variability is genetic polymorphism. CYP2D6 cytochrome enzymes metabolise a variety of important drugs such as β-adrenoreceptor blockers, antidepressants, neuroleptic agents and opioids.

Deficiency in this system is inherited as an autosomal recessive trait and the consequences may occur in homozygous individuals. For example, some are deficient in the metabolism of codeine to morphine.

Another example is the O-demethylation of tramadol in the liver (CYP2D6] to O-desmethyltramadol and this metabolite has a μ-opioid affinity approximately 200 times greater than tramadol; CYP2D6 isoenzyme activity is therefore very important for tramadol's analgesic effect. N-Acetyltransferase metabolism of caffeine or isoniazid is also polymorphic but because it is immature at birth the acetylation phenotype cannot be determined with certainty in infants.

PHARMACODYNAMICS

The boundary between PK and PD processes is often ill-defined and it seems to require a link to describe the movement of a drug from the plasma to its biophase target. Drugs may exert their effects at non-specific membrane sites, by interference with transport mechanisms, by enzyme inhibition or induction, or by activation or inhibition of receptors. It is postulated that the PD factors that alter the drug–receptor interaction, such as the number, affinity and type of receptors or the availability of natural ligands, are different in children. Pharmacodynamics may be further complicated by the development of functional tolerance and the additive, synergistic or antagonistic effect of drug metabolites or isomers.

Ontogeny of drug action

There are few data describing age-related changes in the number of receptors, their affinity and type of receptors or the availability of natural ligands.

In the newborn rat opioid receptors are not fully developed and the μ and κ receptors are expressed earlier than δ. The relevance of these findings to humans is uncertain because the clinical sensitivity to morphine is more likely attributable to PK rather than to PD differences. Neonates have an increased sensitivity to the effects of neuromuscular blocking drugs [18]. The reasons for this are unknown but it is consistent with the observation that the release of acetylcholine from the infant rat phrenic nerve increases threefold by maturity [19].

γ-aminobutyric acid (GABA$_A$) is an important neurotransmitter at most inhibitory synapses in the human central nervous system and the GABA$_A$ receptor complex is the site of action for benzodiazepines, barbiturates and numerous anaesthetic agents. At birth the cerebellum contains only one-third of the number of GABA$_A$ receptors found in an adult and the receptor subunits themselves have reduced binding affinity for benzodiazepines [20]. Major changes in receptor binding and subunit expression occur during postnatal development [21]. The

GABA$_A$-receptor complex, identified by positron emission tomography, is more prevalent at 2 years and the values then decrease exponentially to 50 per cent of peak values by 17 years [21]. These changes are consistent with age-related concentration effects of inhalational anaesthetics and possibly contribute to different midazolam doses required for sedation at different ages [22].

In spinal anaesthesia amide local anaesthetic agents induce shorter block durations in infants than in adults and larger weight-scaled doses are required to achieve similar dermatome levels. This may be caused, in part, by myelination, spacing of nodes of Ranvier and length of nerve exposed, as well as size factors (see Chapter 14).

Ciclosporin induces greater immunosuppression in infants than older children and adults that is possibly related to the T-lymphocyte response in the infant [23]. Bronchodilators have reduced effect in infants less than 1 year of age because of immaturity of bronchial smooth muscle.

Pharmacogenomic differences also have an impact on PD. Candidate genes involved in pain perception, and pain processing such as opioid receptors, transporters and other targets of pharmacotherapy are under investigation. For example, decreased analgesic potency of morphine and morphine-6-glucuronide has been found in carriers of the single nucleotide polymorphism A118G of the μ-opioid receptor gene. Genetic differences may explain why some patients need higher opioid doses and suffer more adverse effects [24].

Dose–response

EFFICACY – THE SIGMOID E$_{MAX}$ MODEL

The relationship between drug concentration and the magnitude of effect may be described by a sigmoid curve of variable slope according to the equation

$$\text{Effect} = E_0 + \frac{(E_{max} \times C_e^N)}{(EC_{50}^N + C_e^N)}$$

where E_0 is the baseline response, E_{max} is the maximum effect, C_e is the concentration in the effect compartment, EC_{50} is the concentration producing 50 per cent E_{max} and N is the Hill coefficient defining the steepness of the middle part of the concentration–response curve (Fig. 9.2). At low concentrations this non-linear relationship may approach linearity.

Efficacy is the E_{max}. The EC_{50} can be considered to be a measure of potency relative to another drug provided that N and E_{max} for the two drugs are the same. The potency of μ-opioid receptor agonists has been compared in this manner by using the electroencephalogram (EEG) spectral edge frequency (SEF), and the steady-state serum concentration that reduced SEF by half (i.e. EC_{50}) was 6.9 ng/mL

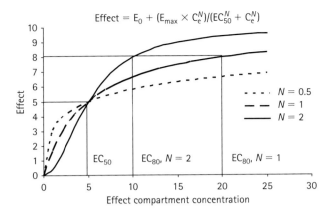

$$\text{Effect} = E_0 + (E_{max} \times C_e^N)/(EC_{50}^N + C_e^N)$$

Figure 9.2 The sigmoid E_{max} (maximum effect) model for three drugs, each with a different Hill coefficient. The EC_{50} (concentration producing 50 per cent E_{max}) and efficacy are the same but the EC_{80} (concentration producing 80 per cent E_{max}) is different for each drug. A higher concentration of the drug with the lower Hill coefficient will be required if an effect of 80 per cent of maximal effect is desired.

for fentanyl, compared with 520 ng/mL for alfentanil [25]. Unfortunately, SEF is not a reliable measure in neonates and so PD differences remain unknown.

QUANTAL EFFECT

The potency of anaesthetic vapours may be expressed by minimum alveolar concentration (MAC) at which 50 per cent of subjects move (or not) in response to a standard surgical stimulus. MAC is similar to an EC_{50} but is an expression of a quantal response rather than magnitude of effect. There are two methods of estimating MAC. Responses can be recorded over the clinical dose range in a large number of subjects and logistic regression is then used to estimate the relationship between dose and quantal effect. The MAC can then be interpolated. Because sufficient numbers of subjects may not be available for this method an alternative called the 'up-and-down' method was described by Dixon [26,27]. This estimates only the MAC and no other quantal effect at any other concentration can be estimated. The method studies only one concentration in each subject and, after the first subject, the concentration studied in the next is either increased if the previous subject did not respond or decreased if they did (Fig. 9.3). Sample sizes less than $n = 6$ can be used and the study can be repeated in batches to determine variability of the MAC estimate.

The dose required to produce a toxic effect in 50 per cent of subjects is called the median toxic dose (TD_{50}). If death is the outcome of interest then the term median lethal dose (LD_{50}) is used. The ratio TD_{50}/ED_{50} is the therapeutic index (ED_{50} = effective dose that produces desired effect in 50 per cent of a population). The margins of safety, expressed as LD_{50}/ED_{50}, have been established for the opioids in adult animals (e.g. morphine = 71, fentanyl = 277, alfentanil = 1080).

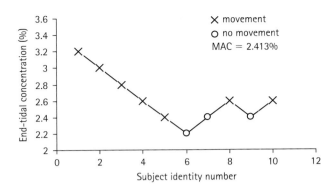

Figure 9.3 The 'up-and-down' method that Dixon used to estimate minimum alveolar concentration (MAC). The nominal sample size is six subjects and is the number of tests after and including the first pair of tests that have opposite results. A statistical table can be checked to determine the maximum likelihood estimate (k), which for this series is -0.935. The final test level (xf) was 2.6 per cent. An end-tidal concentration spacing (σ) of 0.2 per cent was used. MAC = $xf + k\sigma$ = 2.41 per cent [28].

The time-course of drug effect

IMMEDIATE EFFECTS

If the time-course of a drug effect follows its concentration, the concentration half-life matches the effect half-life. This occurs only when the effect site concentration is lower than the EC_{50}. Many drugs, however, have a short concentration half-life but a long duration of effect. This is common for drugs that act on enzymes and the shape of the E_{max} model can predict this.

DELAYED EFFECTS

Observed effects may not be directly related to serum concentration. There may be a delay due to transfer of the drug to effect site (curare), a lag time (furosemide), physiological response (antipyresis), active metabolite (morphine-6-glucoronide) or synthesis of physiological substances (warfarin).

Delayed effect model

A delayed effect can be demonstrated by a plot of plasma concentration against effect which shows a counter-clockwise hysteresis loop. Hull *et al.* [29] and Sheiner *et al.* [30] introduced the effect compartment concept for muscle relaxants. The effect compartment concentration is not the same as the blood concentration and cannot be measured: it is virtual, and calculated, and used to describe the concentration–effect relationship. A single first-order parameter (Teq or $T_{1/2}ke0$) describes the equilibration half-time between the central and effect compartments. The Teq for morphine to equilibrate between plasma and brain in adults is reported as 17 minutes [31] and, because the delay is size dependent (see Size models on page 48), the Teq is expected to be 8 minutes in a term neonate and 10 minutes in a 1-year-old infant.

Physiological substance turnover model

Many drug actions are mediated through the synthesis or elimination of a physiological substance [32]. The concentration at the site of drug effect either stimulates or inhibits the rate of production or elimination of the physiological substance. Warfarin, for example, inhibits the recycling of vitamin K epoxide to the active form of vitamin K, and the change in blood potassium with β agonists is better explained by Na^+/K^+-ATPase activity than by an effect compartment model. Enzyme or protein turnover explains the mechanism of action for many drugs.

Cumulative effects

Many antineoplastic drugs have an effect that is a consequence of cumulative exposure. The extent of binding of a drug to DNA is proportional to drug concentration but is irreversible so that the response is related to cumulative exposure to the drug and can be estimated from the area under the 'concentration versus time' curve.

COMPARTMENT MODELLING (See also Chapter 11)

Compartment models

INSTANTANEOUS INPUT

Mathematical models can be used to describe, and predict, the drug concentration–time relationship. Models may comprise one, two or more compartments (sometimes called mammillary models). A single compartment (Fig. 9.4) is often insufficient to characterise the time–concentration profile. In a two-compartment model (Fig. 9.5) transfer of drug between the central and peripheral compartment is relatively fast compared with the rate of elimination. A plot of the natural log of drug concentration after a bolus dose has two distinct slopes (rate constants, α and β). Consequently the time–concentration profile is described by a poly-exponential function

$$C(t) = Ae^{-\alpha t} + Be^{-\beta t}$$

However, these parameters have little connection with underlying physiology and a better alternative is to have three compartments and rate constants (k_{10}, k_{12} and k_{21}). Another common method is to use two compartment volumes (V_1, V_2) and two clearances (CL and Q: CL is the clearance from the central compartment and Q is the intercompartment clearance). The volume of distribution at steady state (V_{ss}) is the sum of V_1 and V_2.

DOSING BY INFUSION

Anaesthetic drugs are often administered by prolonged infusion and clearance is a very important concept when considering infusion rate. A steady-state plasma concentration

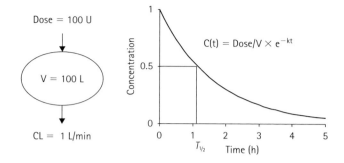

Figure 9.4   A one-compartment model with instantaneous input and first-order elimination, together with time–concentration graph.

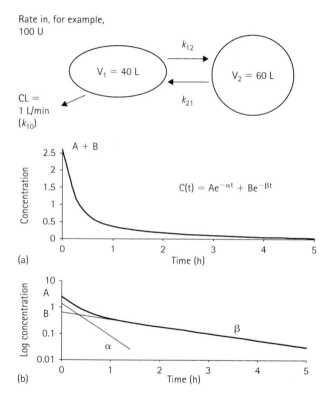

Figure 9.5   A two-compartment, instantaneous input, first-order elimination model together with graphs of (a) plasma concentration against time and (b) log plasma concentration against time – this allows estimation of distributive (α) and terminal elimination (β) rate constants.

is dependent on both the infusion rate and the clearance (rate in = rate out = clearance × steady-state concentration). Whenever the elimination of a drug is related to its concentration the clearance is termed first order and if the elimination is fixed, clearance is said to be zero order. Similar terms can also be applied to input so that drugs given by constant intravenous infusion have zero-order input and, when rate of absorption is determined by gastric emptying or by a controlled-release drug formulation, rate is independent of amount of drug remaining in the gut and is therefore zero order also. The absorption of drugs given extravascularly is first order.

Clearance is often higher in children than in adults (see Size models on page 148) and, consequently, the steady-state concentration achieved is lower for the same infusion rate. It may not be possible to predict the time course of concentration from adult data because of different clearances and volumes of distribution.

Half-life

ELIMINATION HALF-LIFE

Elimination half-life ($T_{1/2}$) is the time required to change the concentration of drug in a compartment by one-half. It is related to the elimination rate constant (k), which represents the slope of the exponential decay curve. Many drugs have multicompartment pharmacokinetics. In a two-compartment model there is an initial distribution (α) half-life and a terminal elimination (β) half-life. Half-life may guide dosing when duration of action of a drug is related to its plasma concentration. Also, it may not be applicable in disease states where V and CL change independently of each other (e.g. digoxin) or in situations where effect continues after drug elimination (e.g. phenoxybenzamine or organophosphates).

CONTEXT-SENSITIVE HALF-TIME

Elimination half-life may not fully characterise the decrease in plasma concentration after an infusion ceases. This is because there is accumulation and distribution to other compartments so that the elimination from the plasma depends on the length of time of the infusion. Therefore, a more useful concept is the context-sensitive half-time and this is the time required for the plasma drug concentration to decline by 50 per cent after terminating an infusion of a specified duration [33]. In a one-compartment model the context-sensitive half-time is the same as the elimination half-life. However, most drugs in anaesthesia conform to multiple compartment models and the context-sensitive half-times are markedly different from their elimination half-lives, for example the half-time of a propofol infusion varies from 12 minutes at 1 hour to 38 minutes at 8 hours, and after a fentanyl infusion the half-time is 1 hour at 24 minutes and 8 hours at 280 minutes. An exception is remifentanil with its half-time constant at 2.5 minutes – this drug is modelled by single-compartment kinetics. Since peripheral compartments are relatively large in children compared with adults drugs tend to remain in the body longer for any given plasma concentration. For example, the context-sensitive half-time of propofol in children is longer [34]. Nevertheless, the context-sensitive half-time describes plasma concentration and may not predict recovery because of PD differences.

Target concentration approach to dosing

A dose can be calculated from the target concentration and pharmacokinetic factors provided that there is a predicable relationship between concentration and effect.

LOADING DOSE

A loading dose raises concentration in the plasma to target concentration promptly and may be desirable in anaesthesia when rapid effect is required. In a one-compartment model the volume of distribution is the proportionality factor that relates dose to target concentration (TC) and loading dose (LD) = V × TC. But this may not be applicable to many anaesthetic drugs with a PK profile described by multiple compartments. If so only using V_1 to calculate loading dose will result in a low plasma concentration but using V_{ss} could mean that the higher loading dose results in excess concentration with undesirable effects (in which case slowing the rate of administration is important during the distributive phase).

TARGET EFFECT DOSE

The time to peak effect (T_{peak}) is dependent on clearance and the effect site equilibration half-time (T_{eq}). At submaximal dose, T_{peak} is independent of dose. At supramaximal doses maximal effect will occur earlier than T_{peak} and persist for longer duration because of the shape of the sigmoid E_{max} model. The T_{peak} concept has been used to calculate optimal initial bolus doses [35], because both V_1 and V_{ss} poorly reflect the required dose-scaling factor. A new parameter, the volume of distribution at the time of peak effect site concentration (V_{pe}) is used and is calculated by:

$$V_{pe} = \frac{V_1}{\left(\dfrac{C_{peak}}{C_0} \right)}$$

C_0 is the theoretical plasma concentration at $t = 0$, and C_{peak} is the predicted effect site concentration at the time of peak effect (Table 9.2). Loading dose can then be calculated as:

$$LD = C_{peak} \times V_{pe}.$$

Table 9.2 Volumes of distribution estimates for opioids in a 70-kg person

	Alfentanil	Fentanyl	Morphine
V_c	2.2	12.7	8.5
V_{ss}	22	339	132
V_{pe}	5.8	79	120

Data adapted from Wada *et al.* [34].
V_c, volume of distribution in the central compartment; V_{ss}, volume of distribution at steady state; V_{pe}, peak effect site concentration. Estimates of V_c and V_{ss} may scale linearly for children beyond infancy.

MAINTENANCE DOSE

Clearance is the most important parameter when defining a rational steady-state dosage regimen. At steady state (ss):

$$\text{Dosing rate}_{ss} = \text{Rate of elimination}_{ss} = CL \times TC.$$

When a drug is given intermittently:

$$\text{Maintenance dose} = \text{Dosing rate} \times \text{Dosing interval.}$$

When a drug is given by constant infusion:

$$\text{Infusion rate}_{ss} = \text{Dosing rate}_{ss}.$$

Once the target concentration of a drug is defined, the infusion rate and clearance should be equivalent but, because many anaesthetic drugs continue to distribute slowly to peripheral compartments, a true steady state may never be achieved.

PRINCIPLES OF THE TARGET–CONTROLLED INFUSION

Propofol is a drug commonly described using a three-compartment model. Redistribution of drug from the central to peripheral compartments does not allow a target concentration of $3\,\mu g/mL$ to be maintained by a constant infusion rate. A simple manual infusion regimen consisting of a 1 mg/kg bolus followed by an infusion of 10 mg/kg/h (0–10 minutes), 8 mg/kg/h (10–20 minutes) and 6 mg/kg/h thereafter was suggested (the '10–8–6 rule') for adults to maintain this steady-state target concentration [36]. This rule was found to be unsuitable in children and alternative rules have been calculated [34]. Computerised pumps, known as target-controlled infusion (TCI) systems can deliver a drug at a rate that achieves and maintains the desired target concentration. The infusion rate changes occur every 10 seconds to maintain a steady-state concentration that can then be altered according to the desired effect. The concentration achieved will vary between individuals because of unexplained PK variability. This subject is discussed in greater detail in Chapter 11.

Interpatient variability

There is considerable variability of both PK and PD parameters. For example, one study found a three- to fivefold variation in the plasma fentanyl concentration that can block a defined response to stimulus in adults [37]. There can also be within-individual variability which may be related to tolerance. Renal and hepatic dysfunction cause further PK variability.

Typical values for population PK parameter variability are 50 per cent for compliance with medication regimens, 30 per cent for absorption, 10 per cent for tissue distribution, 50 per cent for metabolic elimination and 20 per cent for renal elimination [38]. The use of concentration rather than dose allows separation of PK and PD variability, and the PK component has been estimated to be 50 per cent or greater. The variability caused by changes in perfusion of target tissue ranges from 5 per cent to 60 per cent. Receptor sensitivity variability (5–50 per cent) and efficacy variability (30 per cent) also exist. The observed response may not be a direct consequence of drug–receptor binding, but rather through intermediate physiological mechanisms (e.g. antipyretics, angiotensin-converting enzyme inhibitors) and a typical value for this variability is 30 per cent [38].

It is possible to ignore variability for some drugs by giving large doses (e.g. muscle relaxants) but the duration of effect will vary and unwanted side effects will occur.

POPULATION PHARMACOKINETICS

It is desirable to gather measurements of serum concentration or effect in sufficient subjects at set time-points for the purpose of predicting the concentration or effect in an individual. The variation in measurement will be dependent on many potential factors (such as age and weight) and the simplest approach is to minimise these factors. Attempts to predict often become unstuck because a factor accounting for variability between subjects is missing. A useful approach is to develop a model in which all the important causes of variation are included and then to estimate the effect magnitude of each factor. Modelling is a complex statistical process but can identify the major causes of variation. Several approaches are used.

Naive pooled data approach

Data are pooled together as if all doses and all observations pertain to a single subject. No information is available on individual profiles or parameters. It is possible to calculate the standard errors for the structural parameters ('fixed effects') but measures of individual variability cannot be determined. This approach may be satisfactory if data are extensive for each individual and there is only minor interindividual variability, but may result in misrepresentation if data are few.

Standard two–stage approach

Individual profiles are analysed and the individual structural parameters are then treated as variables and combined to achieve summary measures (e.g. arithmetic means). The imprecision in the estimate of an individual's structural parameter is also ignored. If the estimates are not based on a similar number of measurements for each individual, or if the response in one individual is much more variable than another, some form of weighting is required.

Mixed effects models

These provide a means to study sources of variability among a sample of subjects who are representative of the population in whom the drug will be used clinically. The main advantage is that sparse data from a large number of individuals can be used, which is especially valuable in paediatric studies. Interpretation of truncated individual data or missing data (a common occurrence in paediatric PK studies) is also possible with this type of analysis. Models are 'mixed' because they describe the data using a mixture of fixed and random effects.

Explanatory covariates (e.g. age, size, renal function, gender and temperature) can also be introduced that explain part of the interindividual variability. Kataria *et al.* investigated the covariates age, weight and gender on propofol pharmacokinetics, using the mixed effect model, and found that weight-adjusted volumes and clearances significantly improved pharmacokinetic accuracy [17].

SIZE MODELS

'The only principle of drug dosage which survives is that the dose must be adjusted to the individual patient.' [39]

Size is a commonly used to determine dose in children. The normal variation of weight with age (from 3rd centile to 97th centile) is considerable, being least at 1 year (+25 per cent to −20 per cent at 10 kg) and reaching a maximum at about 13 years (+45 per cent to −26 per cent at 40 kg) [40] and it is now recognised that there is a non-linear relationship between weight and drug elimination.

Empirical size models for young children have led to the idea that there is an enhanced capacity of children to metabolise drugs because of their proportionally larger livers and kidneys than their adult counterparts [41]. This idea arises because clearance, expressed per kilogram of body weight, is larger in children than adults.

Dawson, in 1940 [39], reviewed evidence that smaller species are generally more tolerant of drug treatment than larger species and concluded that adjustment of drug dose using a body weight exponent of less than 1 was justified. Body surface area (BSA) was subsequently proposed in 1950 to be a more satisfactory index of drug requirements than body weight or age, particularly during infancy and childhood [42]. A third size model using an exponent of weight ($W^{3/4}$) has also been proposed [43]. The latter, which may be termed the 'allometric ¾-power model' has been found useful in normalising a large number of physiological and pharmacokinetic variables. The linear per kilogram, per surface area and allometric ¾-power models are but three of numerous approaches developed to predict drug effect from body size.

The allometric model

Most body size relationships take the form:

$$Y = aW^b$$

where Y is the biological characteristic to be predicted, W is the body mass and a and b are empirically derived constants. Power relations such as these have been used in such diverse fields as palaeontology, animal morphology, physiology, ecology and animal behaviour. Peters [44] has demonstrated that this simple relationship is a robust and powerful scientific theory when applied to the ecological implications of body size. These theories are realistic because they are built empirically using actual observations and they lend themselves to testing because they are quantitative [44].

In all species studied, including humans, the log of basal metabolic rate (BMR) plotted against the log of body weight produces a straight line with a slope of ¾ [44–47]. This exponential function is the same for homeotherms, poikilotherms and unicellular organisms [44]. Mass- and temperature-compensated resting metabolic rates of microbes, ectotherms, endotherms (including those in hibernation) and plants in temperatures ranging from 0°C to 40°C are similar [48].

Explanations for this phenomenon vary. Kleiber [49] has concluded that the concentration of 'active protoplasm' declines with size and this argument is supported by the finding that smaller species have higher concentrations per cell of RNA, respiratory coenzymes and enzymes ('active protoplasm'). These concentrations rise by a ¾-power function of weight ($W^{3/4}$) in each case [44]. McMahon [50] offers a different structural explanation in that animals cannot remain isometric with increasing size, as loads would increase more than the ability of the skeleton to withstand such loads. Consequently, animals become stockier as size increases. The cross-sectional area of an animal's girth (and generally its limb muscles) increases as a ¾-power function of weight. The maximum power that a muscle can produce depends on cross-sectional area. If metabolic rate of an organism is proportional to power production of its muscles, then metabolic rate rises with muscle cross-sectional area and $W^{3/4}$.

West and colleagues [51] have used fractal geometric concepts to explain this phenomenon. They analysed organisms in terms of the geometry and physics of a network of linear tubes required to transport resources and wastes through the body. Such a system, they reasoned, must have three key attributes: the network must reach all parts of a three-dimensional body; a minimum amount of energy should be required to transport the materials in a fluid medium; and the terminal branches of the networks should all be the same size (because cells in most species are roughly similar sizes). The ¾-power law for metabolic rates was derived from a general model that describes how essential materials are transported through space-filled fractal networks of branching tubes [51].

This allometric ¾-power model may be used to scale metabolic processes such as drug clearance (CL) as follows:

$$CL_i = CL_{std} \times \left(\frac{W_i}{W_{std}} \right)^{3/4}$$

where CL_i is the clearance in the individual of weight W_i and CL_{std} is the clearance in a standardised individual with weight W_{std} [43].

When applied to physiological volumes (V), the power parameter is 1:

$$V_i = V_{std} \times \left(\frac{W_i}{W_{std}} \right)^1 .$$

This index has been demonstrated for blood volume, vital capacity and tidal volume [47,51,52]. The volume of distribution in the central compartment (V_c), volume of distribution by area (V_{beta}) and volume of distribution at steady state (V_{ss}) also show direct proportionality to body weight.

Time-related indices (T) such as heart rate, respiratory rate or drug half-times have a power of ¼:

$$T_i = T_{std} \times \left(\frac{W_i}{W_{std}} \right)^{1/4} .$$

The pharmacokinetic time-scale originated from the concept of physiological time. Most mammals have the same number of heartbeats and breaths in their lifespan and the difference between small and large animals is that smaller animals have faster physiological processes and consequently a shorter lifespan. This power function of ¼ can also be derived mathematically for pharmacokinetic half-times based on more soundly based allometric theory:

$$T_{1/2} = \ln(2) \times \frac{V}{CL} \propto \ln(2) \times \frac{W^1}{W^{3/4}} = \ln(2) \times W^{1/4} .$$

The surface area model

The original surface area model proposed by Du Bois and Du Bois [53] was predicted from nine adults of diverse body shape. These nine individuals included a tall thin adult man, a fat adult woman and a 36-year-old 'cretin' with the 'physical development of a boy of 8 years'. The youngest individual from this group was 12 years old. It is still common practice to use the Du Bois and Du Bois formula to predict surface area from weight (W) and height (H):

$$BSA = W(kg)^{0.425} \times H(cm)^{0.725} \times 0.007184.$$

This formula belongs to the same class of allometric models that include those using weight alone. Nomograms determined from this formula are often used. Surface area can also be estimated from an allometric model with a power parameter of ⅔ [43]. This 'allometric ⅔ power model' assumes that adults and children are geometrically similar. However, infants are not morphologically similar to adults – infants have short stumpy legs, relatively big heads and large body trunks and consequently the surface area formula is inaccurate in children. It underestimates the measured surface area in children who have a predicted surface area of less than 1.3 m² (an average 12-year-old).

When estimating drug clearance, a per kilogram model under-predicts and a surface area model over-predicts, and both get worse as size decreases. Estimation is improved by scaling. The ratio of calculated paediatric BSA (from ⅔ power of body weight) to adult BSA can be applied to adult clearance to estimate paediatric clearance. Clearance estimations scaled to adult BSA of 1.9 m² (rather than the standard 1.73 m²) match those of the allometric ¾ power model except at body weights below 7 kg.

The allometric surface area model does not fit known observations [49,51,54]. The body area of animals rises more slowly than the surface law would suggest, as larger animals are stockier. Also, the surface area model refers to an animal's skin area and does not include other surfaces used in energy exchange such as gut villi or respiratory alveoli; they might be important even though they are distant to the external skin surface. The mass of empirical evidence suggests that the appropriate power factor is significantly different from 0.67 and is actually 0.75.

Surface area has been claimed to be linearly related to ECF volume [55]. This is unexpected because volumes are associated with a weight exponent of 1 and not ⅔. However, the original data [55] were noted to have a non-linear relationship to weight and the surface area model was the only alternative model to the per kilogram model that was tested. Reanalysis of these original data demonstrates that the goodness of fit is improved if an exponent of ¾ is used [56]. This leads to the suggestion that ECF changes may reflect a metabolic process. Water turnover rate, for example, appears to scale with a weight exponent close to ¾ [57]. When clearance is calculated using the allometric surface area model and compared with the ¾-power model, the two models are in close agreement for body weight above 20 kg.

The linear per kilogram model

The linear per kilogram model is the poorest model when used for interspecies scaling of metabolic processes such as total body clearance, but remains the most commonly used in humans. In humans, under-prediction of clearance of more than 10 per cent occurs at body weights less than 47 kg when compared with the allometric ¾-power model. This discrepancy increases as size decreases and approaches 50 per cent for a human neonate of 3.5 kg. Because clearance is reduced in this age group for developmental reasons, use of the linear per kilogram model may get close to the right answer but for the wrong reason.

Scaling for size

Figure 9.6 shows clearance changes with weight for a hypothetical drug using the three different models. Age-related clearance increases throughout infancy and reaches adult rates at approximately 1 year using an allometric ¾-power model. The linear per kilogram model shows an increased clearance compared with adults at approximately 1 year

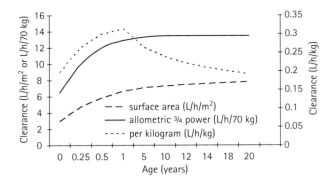

Figure 9.6 Three models of age-related clearance for a hypothetical drug. Each model shows an increase in clearance over the first year of life due to maturation of metabolic pathways. Clearance derived from the per kilogram model decreases after 1 year to reach adult levels in adolescence – this is not evident with the allometric ¾-power and surface area models (from Anderson and Meakin [56], with permission).

Table 9.3 Paediatric maintenance doses of drugs expressed as a percentage of adult dose using an allometric ¾-power model. The neonatal estimate based on size has been reduced further by 50 per cent to account for age-related maturational changes of clearance

Age	Approximate weight (kg)	Percentage of adult dose	Fraction of adult dose
Term	3.2	5	¹⁄₂₀
2 months	4.5	13	¹⁄₈
4 months	6.5	17	
12 months	10	23	¼
18 months	11	25	
5 years	18	36	
7 years	23	43	
10 years	30	53	½
11 years	36	61	
12 years	40	66	
14 years	45	72	¾
16 years	54	82	
Adult	70	100	1

(10 kg). This increased clearance in infants has been interpreted to mean that children have an enhanced capacity to metabolise drugs. It is more likely that the increased clearance seen in 1-year-old children is an artefact of the linear per kilogram model. Drug dosage rules for children, based on allometry, have been described that use percentage of an adult dose to calculate an appropriate child's dose (Table 9.3).

The allometric ¼-power family of models (¼ for times, ¾ for clearance, 1 for volumes) forms a better basis for size scaling than either the surface area or linear per kilogram models. After allometric scaling deviations from predictions are noticeable and their cause can then be sought. The prime

example of such a deviation is the reduced clearance in neonates, attributable to immaturity of hepatic and renal clearance systems.

REFERENCES

Key references

Anderson BJ, Meakin GH. Scaling for size: some implications for paediatric anaesthesia dosing. *Paediatr Anaesth* 2002; **12**(3): 205–19.

Dixon WJ. Staircase bioassay: the up-and-down method. *Neurosci Biobehav Rev* 1991; **15**(1): 47–50.

Kearns GL, Abdel-Rahman SM, Alander SW, Blowey DL, Leeder JS, Kauffman RE. Developmental pharmacology – drug disposition, action, and therapy in infants and children. *N Engl J Med* 2003; **349**(12): 1157–67.

Sheiner LB, Stanski DR, Vozch S, Miller RD, Ham J. Simultaneous modeling of pharmacokinetics and pharmacodynamics: application to D-tubocurarine. *Clin Pharmacol Ther* 1979; **25**: 358–71.

Way WL, Costley EC, Way EL. Respiratory sensitivity of the newborn infant to meperidine and morphine. *Clin Pharmacol Ther* 1965; **6**: 454–61.

References

1. Taddio A, Stevens B, Craig K *et al.* Efficacy and safety of lidocaine–prilocaine cream for pain during circumcision. *N Engl J Med* 1997; **336**(17): 1197–201.

2. Friis-Hansen B. Body water compartments in children: changes during growth and related changes in body composition. *Pediatrics* 1961; **28**: 169–81.

3. Benet LZ, Hoener BA. Changes in plasma protein binding have little clinical relevance. *Clin Pharmacol Ther* 2002; **71**(3): 115–21.

4. Luz G, Wieser C, Innerhofer P, Frischhut B, Ulmer H, Benzer A. Free and total bupivacaine plasma concentrations after continuous epidural anaesthesia in infants and children. *Paediatr Anaesth* 1998; **8**(6): 473–8.

5. Booker PD, Taylor C, Saba G. Perioperative changes in alpha 1-acid glycoprotein concentrations in infants undergoing major surgery. *Br J Anaesth* 1996; **76**(3): 365–8.

6. Way WL, Costley EC, Way EL. Respiratory sensitivity of the newborn infant to meperidine and morphine. *Clin Pharmacol Ther* 1965; **6**: 454–61.

7. Bouwmeester NJ, Anderson BJ, Tibboel D, Holford NH. Developmental pharmacokinetics of morphine and its metabolites in neonates, infants and young children. *Br J Anaesth* 2004; **92**(2): 208–17.

8. Lynn AM, Nespeca MK, Opheim KE, Slattery JT. Respiratory effects of intravenous morphine infusions in neonates, infants, and children after cardiac surgery. *Anesth Analg* 1993; **77**(4): 695–701.

9. Hines RN, McCarver DG. The ontogeny of human drug-metabolizing enzymes: phase I oxidative enzymes. *J Pharmacol Exp Ther* 2002; **300**(2): 355–60.

10. McCarver DG, Hines RN. The ontogeny of human drug-metabolizing enzymes: phase II conjugation enzymes and regulatory mechanisms. *J Pharmacol Exp Ther* 2002; **300**(2): 361–6.

11. Pariente-Khayat A, Rey E, Gendrel D *et al*. Isoniazid acetylation metabolic ratio during maturation in children. *Clin Pharmacol Ther* 1997; **62**(4): 377–83.

12. Aranda JV, MacLeod SM, Renton KW, Eade NR. Hepatic microsomal drug oxidation and electron transport in newborn infants. *J Pediatr* 1974; **85**(4): 534–42.

13. Kearns GL, Abdel-Rahman SM, Alander SW, Blowey DL, Leeder JS, Kauffman RE. Developmental pharmacology – drug disposition, action, and therapy in infants and children. *N Engl J Med* 2003; **349**(12): 1157–67.

14. Berde C. Convulsions associated with pediatric regional anesthesia. *Anesth Analg* 1992; **75**: 164–6.

15. Anderson BJ, Hansen TG. Getting the best from paediatric pharmacokinetic data. *Paediatr Anaesth* 2004; **14**(9): 713–5.

16. Pacifici GM, Franchi M, Giuliani L, Rane A. Development of the glucuronyltransferase and sulphotransferase towards 2-naphthol in human fetus. *Dev Pharmacol Ther* 1989; **14**(2): 108–14.

17. Kataria BK, Ved SA, Nicodemus HF *et al*. The pharmacokinetics of propofol in children using three different data analysis methods. *Anesthesiology* 1994; **80**: 104–22.

18. Fisher DM, O'Keeffe C, Stanski DR, Cronnelly R, Miller RD, Gregory GA. Pharmacokinetics and pharmacodynamics of D-tubocurarine in infants, children, and adults. *Anesthesiology* 1982; **57**(3): 203–8.

19. Wareham AC, Morton RH, Meakin GH. Low quantal content of the endplate potential reduces safety factor for neuromuscular transmission in the diaphragm of the newborn rat. *Br J Anaesth* 1994; **72**(2): 205–9.

20. Brooks-Kayal AR, Pritchett DB. Developmental changes in human gamma-aminobutyric acid A receptor subunit composition. *Ann Neurol* 1993; **34**(5): 687–93.

21. Chugani DC, Muzik O, Juhasz C, Janisse JJ, Ager J, Chugani HT. Postnatal maturation of human GABA A receptors measured with positron emission tomography. *Ann Neurol* 2001; **49**(5): 618–26.

22. Marshall J, Rodarte A, Blumer J, Khoo KC, Akbari B, Kearns G. Pediatric pharmacodynamics of midazolam oral syrup. Pediatric Pharmacology Research Unit Network. *J Clin Pharmacol* 2000; **40**(6): 578–89.

23. Marshall JD, Kearns GL. Developmental pharmacodynamics of cyclosporine. *Clin Pharmacol Ther* 1999; **66**(1): 66–75.

24. Lotsch J, Skarke C, Liefhold J, Geisslinger G. Genetic predictors of the clinical response to opioid analgesics: clinical utility and future perspectives. *Clin Pharmacokinet* 2004; **43**(14): 983–1013.

25. Scott JC, Ponganis KV, Stanski DR. EEG quantitation of narcotic effect: the comparative pharmacodynamics of fentanyl and alfentanil. *Anesthesiology* 1985; **62**(3): 234–41.

26. Dixon WJ. Efficient analysis of experimental observations. *Annu Rev Pharmacol Toxicol* 1980; **20**: 441–62.

27. Dixon WJ. Staircase bioassay: the up-and-down method. *Neurosci Biobehav Rev* 1991; **15**(1): 47–50.

28. Lerman J, Sikich N, Kleinman S, Yentis S. The pharmacology of sevoflurane in infants and children. *Anesthesiology* 1994; **80**(4): 814–824.

29. Hull CJ, van Beem HB, McLeod K, Sibbald A, Watson MJ. A pharmacodynamic model for pancuronium. *Br J Anaesth* 1978; **50**(11): 1113–23.

30. Sheiner LB, Stanski DR, Vozeh S, Miller RD, Ham J. Simultaneous modeling of pharmacokinetics and pharmacodynamics: application to D-tubocurarine. *Clin Pharmacol Ther* 1979; **25**: 358–71.

31. Inturrisi CE, Colburn WA. Application of pharmacokinetic-pharmacodynamic modeling to analgesia. In: Foley KM, Inturrisi CE, eds. *Advances in pain research and therapy. Opioid analgesics in the management of clinical pain.* New York: Raven Press, 1986: 441–52.

32. Holford NHG. Parametric models of the time course of drug action. In: van Boxtel CJ, Holford NHG, Danhof M, eds. *The in vivo study of drug action.* Amsterdam: Elsevier, 1992: 61–9.

33. Hughes MA, Glass PS, Jacobs JR. Context-sensitive half-time in multicompartment pharmacokinetic models for intravenous anesthetic drugs. *Anesthesiology* 1992; **76**(3): 334–41.

34. McFarlan CS, Anderson BJ, Short TG. The use of propofol infusions in paediatric anaesthesia: a practical guide. *Paediatr Anaesth* 1999; **9**: 209–16.

35. Wada DR, Drover DR, Lemmens HJ. Determination of the distribution volume that can be used to calculate the intravenous loading dose. *Clin Pharmacokinet* 1998; **35**(1): 1–7.

36. Roberts FL, Dixon J, Lewis GT, Tackley RM, Prys Roberts C. Induction and maintenance of propofol anaesthesia. A manual infusion scheme. *Anaesthesia* 1988; **43**(suppl): 14–17.

37. Gourlay GK, Kowalski SR, Plummer JL, Cousins MJ, Armstrong PJ. Fentanyl blood concentration-analgesic response relationship in the treatment of postoperative pain. *Anesth Analg* 1988; **67**(4): 329–37.

38. Holford NHG, Peck CC. Population pharmacodynamics and drug development. In: Boxtel CJ, Holford NHG, Danhof M, eds. *The in vivo study of drug action.* New York: Elsevier Science Publishers, 1992: 401–14.

39. Dawson WT. Relations between age and weight and dosages of drugs. *Ann Intern Med* 1940; **13**: 1594–613.

40. Lack JA, Stuart Taylor ME. Calculation of drug dosage and body surface area of children. *Br J Anaesth* 1997; **78**(5): 601–5.

41. Tenenbein M. Why young children are resistant to acetaminophen poisoning. *J Pediatr* 2000; **137**(6): 891–2.

42. Crawford JD, Terry ME, Rourke GM. Simplification of drug dosage calculation by application of the surface area principle. *Pediatrics* 1950; **5**: 783–90.

43. Holford NHG. A size standard for pharmacokinetics. *Clin Pharmacokinet* 1996; **30**: 329–332.

44. Peters HP. Physiological correlates of size. In: Beck E, Birks HJB, Conner EF, eds. *The ecological implications of body size.* Cambridge: Cambridge University Press, 1983: 48–53.

45. Brody S, Proctor RC, Ashworth US. Basal metabolism, endogenous nitrogen, creatinine, and sulphur excretions as functions of body weight. *Univ Mo Agric Exp Sta Res Bull* 1934; **220**: 1–40.

46. Kleiber M. Body size and metabolism. *Hilgardia* 1932; **6**: 315–33.

47. Stahl WR. Scaling of respiratory variables in mammals. *J Appl Physiol* 1967; **22**: 453–600.

48. Gillooly JF, Brown JH, West GB, Savage VM, Charnov EL. Effects of size and temperature on metabolic rate. *Science* 2001; **293**: 2248–51.

49. Kleiber M. *The fire of life: an introduction to animal energetics.* New York: Wiley, 1961.

50. McMahon TA. Scaling physiological time. Lectures on mathematics in the life sciences 1980; **13**: 131–3.

51. West G, Brown J, Enquist B. A general model for the origin of allometric scaling laws in biology. *Science* 1997; **276**: 122–6.

52. Prothero JW. Scaling of blood parameters in animals. *Comp Biochem Physiol* 1980; **A67**: 649–57.

53. Du Bois D, Du Bois EF. Clinical calorimetry: tenth paper. A formula to estimate the approximate surface area if height and weight be known. *Arch Intern Med* 1916; **17**: 863–71.

54. West GB, Brown JH, Enquist BJ. The fourth dimension of life: fractal geometry and allometric scaling of organisms. *Science* 1999; **284**(5420): 1677–9.

55. Friis-Hansen B. The extracellular fluid volume in infants and children. *Acta Paediatr* 1954; **43**: 444–58.

56. Anderson BJ, Meakin GH. Scaling for size: some implications for paediatric anaesthesia dosing. *Paediatr Anaesth* 2002; **12**(3): 205–19.

57. Calder WA, Braun EJ. Scaling of osmotic regulation in mammals and birds. *Am J Physiol* 1983; **244**(5): R601–6.

Inhalational agents

ISABELLE MURAT

KEY LEARNING POINTS

- Sevoflurane and desflurane have a lower blood–gas partition coefficient than the older agents halothane and isoflurane – uptake and elimination are more rapid.
- Minimum alveolar concentration (MAC) of volatile agents decreases with increasing age from infancy to adulthood.
- New volatile agents have minimal toxicity but all volatile agents may trigger malignant hyperthermia.
- Isoflurane, desflurane and sevoflurane share the same safe cardiovascular profile when compared with halothane and are associated with fewer and less severe arrhythmias and less severe myocardial effects.
- Volatile anaesthetic agents depress both central ventilatory drive and respiratory muscles.

- Sevoflurane is probably the best volatile agent when cerebrovascular dynamics are to be maintained.
- Clinical or electrical seizures have been reported during induction and maintenance of anaesthesia with sevoflurane.
- Recovery is more rapid after desflurane or sevoflurane than after halothane, but discharge times are not different after short procedures.
- Emergence agitation is an early and transient phenomenon, observed after sevoflurane anaesthesia but also after other volatile agents.

INTRODUCTION

Inhalational anaesthetics are used extensively in paediatric anaesthesia. Four agents are still available, among them the relatively new anaesthetics sevoflurane and desflurane. Because of its safe cardiovascular profile, sevoflurane has progressively replaced halothane for mask induction in children. Halothane serves as a reference to characterise the properties of the new halogenated agents. Because of its low cost and safe cardiovascular profile, isoflurane is still administered by some as a maintenance agent in children; however, its slower elimination rate compared with that of desflurane and sevoflurane makes it less manageable than the other two agents. Sevoflurane and desflurane have now been used for 15 years, so their pharmacodynamic properties and their

desirable and undesirable effects on organ systems are well known. Since it is too irritating for mask induction, desflurane has not had a major impact in paediatric anaesthesia. In contrast, sevoflurane has become the volatile agent of reference in children as it is both well tolerated for induction and a useful agent for maintenance. Its safety profile has justified its use with a large therapeutic range.

PHYSICAL CHARACTERISTICS

Halothane is a polyhalogenated alkane, isoflurane and desflurane are methyl ethyl ethers and sevoflurane is a methyl isopropyl ether [1]. Physical characteristics of currently used inhalational agents are described in Table 10.1.

Table 10.1   Physical properties of the four currently used halogenated agents

	Halothane	Isoflurane	Sevoflurane	Desflurane
Molecular weight	197.4	184.5	200.1	168
Boiling point (°C)	50.2	48.5	58.6	22.8
Pungency	±	+++	0	++++
Metabolised (%)	15–25	0.2–1	5	0.02
Solubility				
$\lambda_{b/g}$ adults	2.4	1.4	0.66	0.45
$\lambda_{b/g}$ neonates	2.1	1.2	0.66	–
$\lambda_{fat/b}$ adults	57	50	52	29

$\lambda_{b/g}$, blood–gas partition coefficient; $\lambda_{fat/b}$, fat–blood partition coefficient.

Desflurane administration requires a specially designed vaporiser as its vapour pressure exceeds the boiling point (22.8°C) at 1 atmosphere. Both desflurane and sevoflurane have a lower blood–gas partition coefficient than the older agents halothane and isoflurane (Table 10.1). Desflurane has the lowest blood–gas solubility and is comparable to that of nitrous oxide (N_2O) (0.45 versus 0.46). Sevoflurane has a blood–gas partition coefficient of 0.66, allowing for a more rapid uptake and elimination than isoflurane and halothane. The blood–gas partition coefficients of sevoflurane are not different among preterm infants, full-term infants and adults, whereas those of both halothane and isoflurane are decreased in neonates compared with adults [2]. Both desflurane and sevoflurane are stable at ambient temperature. Halothane and sevoflurane are non-irritating for the airways, whereas desflurane and isoflurane are airway irritants.

Uptake and elimination

Uptake (or wash-in) of volatile agents is described as the increase of inspired over alveolar fraction (F_I/F_A) over time of any given volatile agent (Fig. 10.1). Increase in alveolar concentration mainly depends on alveolar ventilation, on cardiac output and on blood–gas and blood–tissue solubilities. Some of these factors are operator dependent such as inspired concentration and alveolar ventilation under controlled ventilation, while others are agent dependent such as blood–gas and blood–tissue solubilities.

The rate of rise of alveolar to inspired partial pressure (F_A/F_I) is higher in infants than in older children and adults (Fig. 10.2). This was first demonstrated for halothane by Salanitre and Rackow [3] in 1969 and modelled later by Brandom *et al.* [4]. Accordingly, for the same inspired fraction of halothane, cerebral (Fig. 10.3a) and heart (Fig. 10.3b) concentrations of halothane are higher in infants than in adults [4]. Subsequent studies found a similar age-related relationship for isoflurane [5]. The three main factors responsible for such higher uptake in infants compared with adults are:

1. The higher alveolar ventilation/functional residual capacity ratio in infants compared with adults. This ratio is approximately 5:1 in neonates compared with

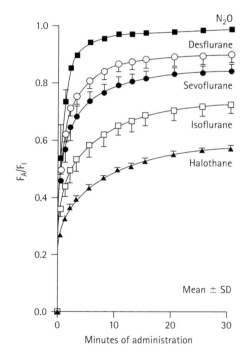

Figure 10.1   Uptake of inhalational agents in adults. The order of wash-in varies inversely with the solubility of these agents in blood. F_A/F_I, ratio of alveolar to inspired partial pressure.

1.5:1 in adults owing to the higher metabolic rate in infants compared with adults.
2. The higher proportion of the vessel-rich group of tissues (brain, heart, kidney, splanchnic organs and endocrine glands) in infants compared with adults (Table 10.2).
3. The lower blood–gas and tissue–gas partition coefficients in neonates compared with adults (except for sevoflurane) [2]. Right-to-left shunting decreases the rate of rise of F_A/F_I ratio whereas left-to-right shunting has minimal effect [6].

Uptake of desflurane and sevoflurane is more rapid than that of isoflurane and halothane. The F_A/F_I ratio is close to 0.9 at 20 minutes for desflurane and to 0.85 for sevoflurane. Unlike the more soluble agents such as halothane or isoflurane, uptake and elimination kinetics of both sevoflurane

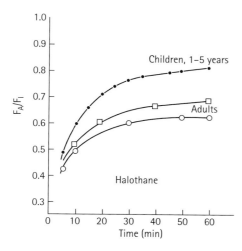

Figure 10.2 Rate of rise of alveolar to inspired partial pressure (F_A/F_I) of halothane in children (closed circles) and adults (open circles and squares). For the same inspired concentration, uptake of halothane is greater and more rapid in infants compared with adults. Source: Salanitre and Rackow [3].

Table 10.2 Tissue volume

Age group	Volume (% of total body volume)		
	Vessel-rich group	Muscle group	Fat group
Newborn	22.0	38.7	13.2
1 year	17.3	38.7	25.4
4 years	16.6	40.7	23.4
8 years	13.2	44.8	21.4
Adult	10.2	50.0	22.3

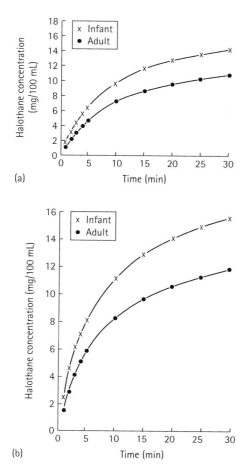

Figure 10.3 (a) Predicted concentration of halothane in the brain in infants and adults. (b) Predicted concentration of halothane in the heart in infants and adults. For the same inspired concentration, brain and heart concentrations are greater in infants compared with adults. Source: Brandom *et al.* [4].

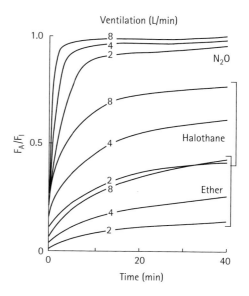

Figure 10.4 Effect of alveolar ventilation on the rate of rise of the alveolar concentration (F_A) relative to the inspired concentration (F_I) of soluble (ether), intermediate (halothane) and insoluble (N_2O) anaesthetics. The wash-in of a more soluble anaesthetic is affected by changes in ventilation to a greater extent than is the wash-in of a less soluble anaesthetic.

and desflurane are minimally different in infants, children and adults owing to their low blood–gas solubility.

Uptake of volatile agents depends on alveolar ventilation. The wash-in of a soluble anaesthetic is affected by changes in ventilation to a greater extent than is the wash-in of a less soluble anaesthetic (Fig. 10.4). Thus, during anaesthesia, uptake of volatile agents varies greatly with the mode of ventilation (i.e. spontaneous versus controlled ventilation). During spontaneous ventilation, respiratory depression limits the depth of anaesthesia, thus protecting against excessive circulatory depression. This is a negative feedback effect. However, if ventilation is controlled, this protective mechanism is bypassed. The F_A/F_I ratio increases relentlessly as cardiac output decreases. There is a positive feedback effect as any decrease in cardiac output will further limit removal of the anaesthetic from the lung. This may explain why most of the cardiac arrests observed in infants during halothane anaesthesia occurred after initiating manually controlled ventilation [7].

Elimination (wash-out) of volatile agents follows an exponential decay that is the reverse of the wash-in curve. Factors affecting elimination are similar to those involved in wash-in: mainly blood–gas and tissue–gas solubilities and alveolar ventilation. The order of wash-out of anaesthetics parallels their blood–gas solubilities, with desflurane being the most rapid followed by sevoflurane, isoflurane and halothane, in that order. The rate of recovery depends on the duration of anaesthesia; the longer the exposure to anaesthetic agents, the longer the recovery time. However, elimination of insoluble agents is less dependent on duration of exposure and is more predictable than that of soluble agents [8]. Thus, recovery after desflurane and sevoflurane is more rapid than after halothane or isoflurane in children. The expected benefit is more important after prolonged anaesthesia than after short exposure. Indeed, applying the concept of context-sensitive half-time to inhaled anaesthetics, Bailey demonstrated that the 80 per cent decrement times of sevoflurane and desflurane are small (<8 min) and do not increase significantly with duration of anaesthesia, whereas it increases significantly after 60 minutes of isoflurane anaesthesia [8]. The 90 per cent decrement time of desflurane increased slightly from 5 minutes after 30 minutes of anaesthesia to 14 minutes after 6 hours of anaesthesia. It remained significantly less than the 90 per cent decrement times of sevoflurane and isoflurane which reached values of 65 minutes and 86 minutes after 6 hours of anaesthesia (Fig. 10.5).

Minimum alveolar concentration

Minimum alveolar concentration is defined as the minimum alveolar (or end-tidal or end-expiratory) anaesthetic concentration at which 50 per cent of patients do not move in response to a stimulus. The classic stimulus used to determine MAC in humans is surgical incision. In this chapter, MAC will refer to MAC for surgical incision unless otherwise indicated. The MAC has also been determined in response to other stimuli such as tracheal intubation (MAC_{INT}), laryngeal mask airway (LMA) insertion (MAC_{LMA}), tracheal extubation (MAC_{EXT}) and awake responsiveness (MAC_{AWAKE}). The MAC that blocks haemodynamic response to painful stimuli is described as MAC_{BAR} (blockage of response to adrenergic stimuli). The MAC of inhalational agents is additive [9].

The MAC of volatile agents varies with age (Table 10.3 and Fig. 10.6). Highest MAC values are observed in infants aged 1–6 months and then MAC decreases with increasing age [10]. The inverse relationship between age and MAC was demonstrated to be identical for all volatile agents [11]. The MAC of sevoflurane measured in infants less than 1 month of age is similar to that of infants aged 1–6 months, whereas MAC values of other volatile agents are decreased in neonates compared with older infants [10,12]. The MAC of isoflurane is lower in preterm infants compared with full-term infants [12] (Fig. 10.7). No data are available in this age group for other volatile agents.

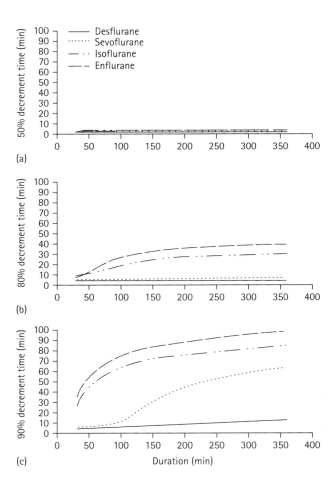

Figure 10.5 (a) The 50 per cent decrement time (context-sensitive half-time) of desflurane, sevoflurane, isoflurane and enflurane as a function of duration of anaesthetic administration. (b) The 80 per cent decrement time of desflurane, sevoflurane, isoflurane and enflurane as a function of duration of anaesthetic administration. (c) The 90 per cent decrement time of desflurane, sevoflurane, isoflurane and enflurane as a function of duration of anaesthetic administration. The 90 per cent decrement time of sevoflurane increases for anaesthesia lasting more than about 80 minutes whereas that of desflurane increases very slightly. Source: Bailey [8].

The MAC of N_2O is 105 per cent in adults. Although the MAC of N_2O has never been measured in children, it has been speculated that the same inverse relationship between age and MAC values exists, suggesting that MAC values for N_2O are higher in infants and children compared with adults [11,13] (Fig. 10.8).

The addition of 60 per cent N_2O decreases the MAC of desflurane by only 24 per cent, compared with 60 per cent for halothane and 40 per cent for isoflurane and sevoflurane [14–17]. The MAC for tracheal intubation is 40–50 per cent higher than the MAC for surgical incision, but the MAC for laryngeal mask insertion is similar to the MAC for surgical incision [18]. The MAC_{EXT} value is approximately 10–25 per cent less than the MAC for skin incision for isoflurane, desflurane and sevoflurane [19,20]; MAC_{AWAKE} corresponds to 0.3 MAC for sevoflurane [21].

Table 10.3   Minimum alveolar concentration (MAC vol%) in 100 per cent O$_2$ of currently used halogenated agents

Age (vol %)	Halothane (vol%)	Isoflurane (vol%)	Sevoflurane (vol%)	Desflurane (vol%)
0–1 months	0.87	1.60	3.3	9.16
1–6 months	1.20	1.87	3.2	9.42
6–12 months	–	1.80	2.5	9.92
1–3 years	0.97	1.60	2.6	8.72
3–5 years	0.91	–	2.5	8.62
5–12 years	0.87	–	2.5	7.98
Adult 25 years	0.73	1.28	2.6	7.25
Adult 40 years	0.74	1.16	2.05	6

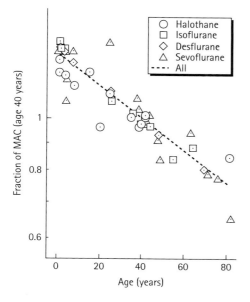

Figure 10.6   Fraction of minimum alveolar concentration (MAC) at age 40 years for halothane, isoflurane, desflurane and sevoflurane. The MAC decreases by 6.7 per cent with each increasing decade of life, whatever the inhalational agent. Conversely, MAC increases with decreasing age to a similar extent for all volatile agents. Source: Eger [13].

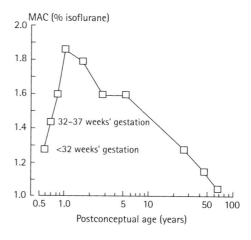

Figure 10.7   Effect of age on the minimum alveolar concentration (MAC) of isoflurane. Postconceptual age is the sum of gestational and postnatal ages. Source: LeDez and Lerman [12].

The MAC, MAC$_{INT}$ and MAC$_{BAR}$ of volatile agents are decreased by the concomitant use of synthetic opioids such as fentanyl or remifentanil, or the use of α_2 agonists such as clonidine, whereas MAC$_{AWAKE}$ is minimally affected (Table 10.4).

Metabolism and toxicity

Studies in humans and animals indicate that desflurane resists biodegradation more than isoflurane, isoflurane more than sevoflurane and sevoflurane more than halothane.

Desflurane undergoes minimal metabolism (less than 0.02 per cent of the delivered dose). Total metabolism of

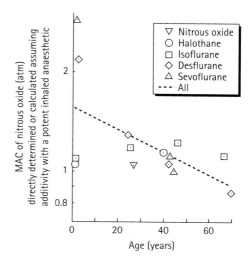

Figure 10.8   Fraction of minimum alveolar concentration (MAC) at age 40 years for N$_2$O. The MAC of nitrous oxide was directly determined or calculated assuming additivity with a potent inhaled anesthetic. Source: Eger [13].

Table 10.4 Effects of adjunctive therapies on minimum alveolar concentration for tracheal intubation (MAC_{INT}) of sevoflurane in children

Adjunct	MAC sevoflurane (%)
MAC_{INT} in oxygen	2.66–3.2
MAC_{INT} in 60% N_2O	1.57
MAC_{INT} in oral clonidine (4 μg/kg)	1.9
MAC_{INT} in oral clonidine (4 μg/kg) and 60% N_2O	1.4

sevoflurane represents 5 per cent of inhaled dose, compared with 75 per cent for methoxyflurane, 41–46 per cent for halothane and 0.2–1 per cent for isoflurane [22]. Sevoflurane is rapidly metabolised into inorganic fluorides and hexafluoroisopropanol, the latter being rapidly conjugated and excreted by the kidneys. Although plasma fluoride concentrations measured may exceed 50 μmol/L (which is the potential nephrotoxic threshold for methoxyflurane), no renal toxicity has been reported after sevoflurane anaesthesia in adults and children, even in those with pre-existing renal insufficiency [23]. Two hypotheses have been proposed to explain the lack of renal toxicity of sevoflurane compared with methoxyflurane: (1) a more rapid elimination of inorganic fluoride with sevoflurane than that observed after methoxyflurane anaesthesia; and (2) differences in intrarenal metabolism; indeed sevoflurane is mainly metabolised in the liver by cytochrome P450 CYP 2E1, whereas methoxyflurane is metabolised in the liver and also in renal tubules by CYP 31 and CYP 2E124. The activity of CYP 2E1 is low during the neonatal period, increasing during the first hour after birth and then gradually increasing during the first year of life to reach adult values in children aged 1–10 years [25]. In children less than 48 months of age, sevoflurane metabolism parallels postnatal development of CYP 2E1 [26].

Sevoflurane is unique among volatile agents as its biodegradation does not produce trifluoroacetic acid (TFA) which has been involved in the occurrence of immune-based hepatitis, mainly described after halothane anaesthesia [27].

Desflurane is not degraded by moist soda lime even at high temperatures. However, desflurane degradation by desiccated soda lime may produce carbon monoxide. Sevoflurane is degraded by soda lime into several compounds. Among them, compound A (olefin) exhibits renal toxicity in rats when exposed to concentration greater than 40 p.p.m. Production of compound A depends on several factors including quantity of inhaled sevoflurane, temperature, type of absorber (soda lime or Baralyme) and fresh gas flow [28]. The production of compound A reaches a maximum after 2–3 hours of anaesthesia and then decreases slowly. No toxicity has been observed in humans during prolonged exposure at low fresh gas flow (1 L/min) [29]. In children, maximal concentration of compound A was less than 15 p.p.m. (mean 5.4 p.p.m.) when fresh gas

flow was set at 2 L/min [30]. The replacement of soda lime by absorbers using strong non-alkali metal bases such as $Ca(OH)_2$ (e.g. Amsorb) causes a large reduction in the production of compound A [31].

EFFECTS ON VITAL SYSTEMS

Cardiovascular system

Isoflurane, desflurane and sevoflurane share the same safe cardiovascular profile when compared with halothane. In terms of cardiovascular safety, the revolution started with isoflurane and minimal further improvement may be attributed to sevoflurane and desflurane. Volatile anaesthetics affect the cardiovascular system either directly (by depressing myocardial contractility or the conduction system or by decreasing systemic vascular resistance) or indirectly (by altering the balance of parasympathetic and sympathetic nervous systems and neurohumoral reflex responses). The cardiovascular responses to inhalational agents are further complicated by maturational changes in the cardiovascular system and its responsiveness to these anaesthetics [32].

In children, halothane and isoflurane decrease arterial pressure to a similar extent with increasing alveolar concentration, but myocardial contractility is much better preserved with isoflurane compared with halothane [33]. Indeed, under halothane anaesthesia, the decrease of arterial pressure mainly reflects the decrease in myocardial function, whereas, under isoflurane anaesthesia, the decrease in arterial pressure is mainly the consequence of the decrease in systemic vascular resistance. Thus, the decrease in blood pressure observed during halothane induction reflects cardiovascular depression, which is more significant in young infants compared with older children [34]. Interestingly, continuous auscultation of heart sounds has recently been demonstrated to be a useful tool for monitoring halothane-induced cardiovascular depression in anaesthetised children [35]. Thus, the continuous use of a precordial stethoscope could be recommended during halothane induction. Most critical cardiovascular incidents are observed when switching from spontaneous ventilation to manually controlled ventilation. Thus, halothane inspiratory concentration has to be reduced when controlled ventilation is initiated. In addition to their direct effects on myocardial function, halothane and isoflurane affect heart rate in an opposite ways. There is a dose-dependent increase in heart rate with isoflurane and a dose-dependent decrease in heart rate with halothane. As cardiac output depends on heart rate, the resulting effect is much better preservation of cardiac output under isoflurane anaesthesia than with halothane anaesthesia in children, especially infants. Indeed, halothane prolongs atrioventricular conduction time much more in infant animals than in adult animals [36]. Atropine increases heart rate and cardiac output during halothane anaesthesia in children, but does not improve myocardial contractility [37,38]. Finally, halothane sensitises the myocardium to catecholamines, thus favouring dysrhythmias particularly during hypercarbia. Indeed halothane decreases the threshold for ventricular extrasystoles during epinephrine administration [39].

Cardiovascular effects of sevoflurane are close to those of isoflurane. Sevoflurane has much fewer undesirable cardio-vascular effects than halothane. It does not sensitise the myocardium to exogenous or endogenous catecholamines [40], and thus promotes less dysrhythmia than halothane especially during ear, nose and throat (ENT) surgery, dental surgery or during endoscopies [41]. Sevoflurane does not modify atrioventricular conduction times. Therefore, the incidence of bradycardia is much lower with sevoflurane than with halothane, especially in infants. Finally, sevoflurane depresses myocardial contractility to a lesser extent than halothane in infants and children [42,43] (Fig. 10.9). The latter is of greatest importance during induction and in children with compromised cardiovascular function [44]. Sevoflurane, and both halothane and isoflurane, markedly depress barore-flex control on heart rate in infants and children [45]. On recovery, baroreflex control on heart rate is more rapidly restored after sevoflurane anaesthesia than after isoflurane anaesthesia, reflecting the more rapid elimination of sevoflu-rane compared with isoflurane in adult patients [46].

Desflurane shares the safe cardiovascular profile of isoflu-rane and sevoflurane. Its haemodynamic effects are very similar to those of isoflurane. The dose-dependent decrease in mean arterial pressure is related to a dose-dependent decrease in systemic vascular resistance. Cardiac output is maintained up to 1.5 MAC because myocardial contractility is only moderately depressed; heart rate increases with increasing desflurane concentration. This dose-dependent increase in heart rate may be of concern in some adult patients with impaired cardiac function but not in most chil-dren. Rapid changes of desflurane alveolar concentration are associated with a transient increase in heart rate and blood pressure [47]. However, this response is easily blunted by the concomitant use of opioids such as fentanyl.

Respiratory system

Volatile anaesthetic agents affect both central ventilatory drive and the activity of respiratory muscles. Volatile agents decrease alveolar ventilation in a dose-dependent fashion, mainly by decreasing tidal volume [48]. During sponta-neous breathing the arterial partial pressure of carbon dioxide ($PaCO_2$) increases with increasing depth of anaes-thesia. All volatile agents markedly decrease ventilatory response to CO_2 [49]. The effects of hypnotics (volatile agents or propofol) and opiates are at least additive on ven-tilatory drive. In addition to their central effects, anaesthetics depress pharyngeal and laryngeal tone and upper airway muscle tone, thus favouring upper airway obstruction [50]. Application of continuous positive airway pressure (CPAP)

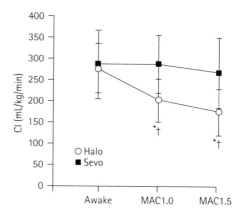

Figure 10.9 Cardiac index (CI) measured by transthoracic echocardiography in infants who received sevoflurane (Sevo) or halothane (Halo). Minimum alveolar concentration (MAC) 1.0 and MAC 1.5 are minimal alveolar concentrations of both agents adjusted for age. Data are mean ± SD. *$P < 0.05$ versus awake; †$P < 0.05$ HALO versus SEVO. Source: Wodey et al. [42].

helps to maintain the airway patency during spontaneous breathing [51], reduces thoraco-abdominal asynchrony [52] and decreases the incidence of atelectasis in depend-ent lung regions [53].

The respiratory effects of sevoflurane are close to those of halothane [54,55]. Sevoflurane produces a dose-dependent decrease in tidal volume identical to that of halothane. Respiratory rate increases up to 1 MAC sevoflu-rane and then decreases at 1.5 MAC. As a result, respiratory depression assessed by changes in end-tidal CO_2 is slightly more significant at deep levels of anaesthesia (1.5 MAC) with sevoflurane than with halothane. Halothane, isoflu-rane and sevoflurane are potent bronchodilators [56].

Halothane and sevoflurane are minimally irritating for the airway and are therefore appropriate for mask induc-tion. Isoflurane and especially desflurane are inappropriate for mask induction because of their pungency. In the only four published paediatric trials on mask induction using desflurane [15,16,57,58] respiratory complications (breath-holding, laryngospasm, coughing, secretions and hypox-aemia) were reported in more than 50 per cent of children and, thus, desflurane is now considered to be contraindicated for mask induction in children. This high incidence of res-piratory complications is partly related to its effects on sites located in the upper airways and the lungs that respond with sympathetic activation during rapid increase in des-flurane concentration independent of systemic anaesthetic changes. In addition, unlike other volatile agents, desflu-rane lacks the ability to cause an early decrease in respira-tory resistance after tracheal intubation (it has been found to cause significant increase in respiratory resistance in smokers) [59]. Although these respiratory effects may be of concern for patients with bronchial hyper-reactivity, main-tenance of anaesthesia with desflurane is not associated with an increased risk of respiratory complications during emergence in paediatric patients [20].

Central nervous system

All inhalational agents have significant cerebrovascular and cerebral metabolic effects.

Halothane is a cerebral vasodilator even in low dose (0.5 MAC) and it increases cerebral blood flow (CBF) in a dose-dependent fashion. In a study in children, CBF increased between 0.5 and 1.0 MAC but not over 1.5 MAC. During the decreasing phase, CBF decreased significantly from 1.5 to 1.0 MAC but no further decrease was observed between 1.0 and 0.5 MAC. This was called a hysteresis phenomenon on the cerebral vasculature, which could be important in children with raised intracranial pressure (ICP) [60]. Halothane decreases cerebral metabolic rate of oxygen ($CMRO_2$), whereas the $CBF/CMRO_2$ ratio is increased and maintained above normal values with prolonged administration. Cerebrovascular reactivity to carbon dioxide is preserved at 0.5 and 1.0 MAC halothane in children, but the vasoconstrictive effect of hypocapnia is weaker at 1.0 MAC halothane compared with 0.5 MAC [61]. For these reasons, halothane should be avoided in patients with known or suspected reduced intracranial compliance until the dura is opened.

Isoflurane affects CBF and cerebral autoregulation less than halothane at equivalent MAC. Isoflurane has minimal effect on the cerebrovascular reactivity to CO_2 in children [61].

Sevoflurane is similar to isoflurane with respect to its effects on CBF, $CMRO_2$ and ICP in adults [62]. In children, sevoflurane decreases cerebral vascular resistance and oxygen consumption, but does not change total cerebral flow and cortical flow at 1 MAC [63]. Cerebral blood flow autoregulation is intact at 1 MAC sevoflurane [64].

Desflurane increases CBF and decreases $CMRO_2$. In children, desflurane increases CBF velocity in a dose-dependent manner and maintains CO_2 reactivity at 1 MAC [65].

Together, these data suggest that sevoflurane is probably the best volatile agent when cerebrovascular dynamics are to be maintained. The effects of N_2O are controversial. When used in combination with other volatile agents or intravenous anaesthetic agents, N_2O increases CBF compared with an air–oxygen mixture [66]. Although N_2O is commonly used in neuroanaesthesia, it would seem prudent to avoid it in patients with raised ICP.

Changes in electroencephalogram (EEG) vary according to the depth of anaesthesia. Compared with awake, loss of consciousness induced by hypnotic agents is accompanied by EEG changes that are close to those seen in normal sleep. With anaesthesia and sedation, beta-type rapid oscillations increase in amplitude. Deeper anaesthesia is associated with global slowing of dominant oscillations, producing theta, then delta-type waveforms, which become regular, before disappearing into an isoelectric tracing of very deep anaesthesia (burst suppression). No clinical or electrical seizure activity has been attributed to the use of halothane, isoflurane or desflurane in children. Conversely, clinical or electrical seizures have been reported during induction and maintenance of anaesthesia with sevoflurane in both children and adults [67,68]. No clinical sequelae have been described to date. A recent review analysed the incidence and prevention of epileptiform activity during sevoflurane anaesthesia [69]. In epileptic patients, sevoflurane has a stronger epileptogenic property than isoflurane, but N_2O or hyperventilation may counteract this side-effect [70]. The mechanism of the epileptogenic effect of sevoflurane is thus far unknown. The hypothesis that it resembles that of enflurane (biphasic and dose-dependent activation of N-methyl-D-aspartate [NMDA] neuronal receptors) is supported by similarity in molecular structure, but remains to be proven. Practical recommendations to limit and/or avoid electrical epileptiform activity may include combination with other agents to decrease the required concentration of sevoflurane (benzodiazepines, N_2O and opioids), and limitation of inspired sevoflurane concentration in order to maintain an alveolar concentration inferior or equal to 1.5 MAC [69].

The Bispectral Index (BIS, Aspect Medical Systems, Inc.) is becoming the gold standard for assessing depth of anaesthesia in adult patients [71]. Indeed, BIS values are highly correlated with the concentration of hypnotic drugs such as propofol or sevoflurane. The BIS is derived from a large database of EEG traces obtained in adults under various conditions of anaesthesia. The BIS values are much higher at given MAC values of halothane compared with sevoflurane [72]. This is not surprising as EEG traces obtained with halothane are different from those integrated in the BIS database (i.e. propofol and more recent volatile agents). The BIS values describe a paradoxical profile during inhalational induction with sevoflurane in children and are not correlated with clinical events or with the clinically assessed depth of anaesthesia [73]. The typical BIS value during rapid inhalational induction with sevoflurane shows an early and abrupt drop after loss of consciousness followed by re-ascension of BIS values with deepening anaesthesia. The nadir of the BIS (lowest BIS value) is usually observed 120–180 seconds after the beginning of induction with 7 per cent sevoflurane (with N_2O) and probably reflects very low EEG frequencies observed around the second minute of induction [73]. The subsequent increase in BIS reflects the shift of EEG rhythms towards faster frequencies. The BIS monitor also displays paradoxical high values during seizure activity [74]. This is of special concern in children anaesthetised with high concentrations of sevoflurane. Indeed, despite the existing controversy regarding the true incidence of epileptiform activity during sevoflurane anaesthesia, it is becoming clear that epileptiform EEG tracings may be observed at very deep levels of sevoflurane anaesthesia [75]. Periodic epileptiform discharges are usually observed before the appearance of burst suppression [67,68].

Renal and hepatic functions

Issues of renal impairment related to metabolism of volatile agents have already been discussed. Basically, the three modern inhalational agents (isoflurane, desflurane and sevoflurane) may affect renal function by changes in renal perfusion pressure. No data specific to paediatric patients are available.

Similarly, the effects of volatile agents on hepatic function have been studied extensively in adult patients and animals. Halothane, isoflurane and desflurane have all been associated with acute postoperative liver dysfunction or failure. In paediatric patients, halothane and sevoflurane produced a slight postanaesthetic increase in α-glutathione S-transaminase (α-GST), which peaked at 1–2 hours after surgery and then returned to normal by 6 hours [76]. Although few case reports implicate sevoflurane as a potential hepatotoxin, the exact mechanism is still uncertain and the direct relationship is very low [77,78].

Malignant hyperthermia

All volatile agents can trigger malignant hyperthermia (MH) episodes in MH-susceptible patients. According to the data of the North American Malignant Hyperthermia Registry, the new volatile agents, sevoflurane and desflurane, may be less potent triggers of malignant hyperthermia than halothane [79].

CLINICAL USE

Induction techniques

Isoflurane and desflurane are not appropriate for mask induction owing to their high pungency. Sevoflurane has replaced halothane for induction of anaesthesia in most developed countries. The main advantage of sevoflurane over halothane is its remarkable cardiovascular safety which has already contributed to decrease the incidence of severe cardiovascular critical incidents during induction of anaesthesia. Indeed, in the 1980s, relative or absolute halothane overdose was reported to be one of the main factors of cardiac arrest or severe bradycardia in infants and young children [80–82]. In the first report of the Paediatric Perioperative Cardiac Arrest (POCA) registry surveying the incidence and causes of cardiac arrests between 1994 and 1997, 33 per cent of anaesthesia-related cardiac arrests occurred in previously healthy ASA (American Society of Anesthesiology Physical Status) 1 and 2 patients, and 64 per cent of them were medication-related errors [7]. Among the latter, 50 per cent of arrests were caused by halothane cardiovascular depression. The second report surveyed the period ranging from 2000 to 2003 in which halothane had been replaced by sevoflurane in most centres [83]. In this second series, the authors reported a marked reduction of medication-related cardiac arrests (from 37 per cent to 12 per cent) mainly due to a near-disappearance of cardiovascular depression by volatile agents.

The safe cardiovascular profile of sevoflurane has changed the practice of mask induction in children. With halothane, a stepwise incremental induction technique was recommended in order to limit the cardiovascular depression, and close monitoring of heart rate and heart sounds was mandatory [35]. Soon after sevoflurane was introduced into clinical practice, it became evident that high concentrations of sevoflurane were tolerated, allowing for rapid induction with very few respiratory and cardiovascular undesirable effects [84,85]. When using 7 or 8 per cent sevoflurane, loss of consciousness is achieved in about 40–45 seconds, and tracheal intubation can be performed without addition of neuromuscular blocking agents in less than 5 minutes in most patients [86–88]. Addition of N_2O reduces time to loss of consciousness and the incidence of agitation during the early induction period [87].

Two techniques have been proposed to perform mask induction in children: the classic technique at tidal volume and the vital capacity technique. The tidal volume technique allows the child to breathe spontaneously. With increasing depth of anaesthesia, tidal volume decreases, respiratory rate increases and minute ventilation decreases in a dose-dependent fashion [89]. Usually, ventilation should be assisted prior to tracheal intubation or LMA insertion. The vital capacity technique involves pre-filling the anaesthesia breathing system with 8 per cent sevoflurane and the patient makes a forced expiration followed by a forced inspiration through the pre-filled circuit. The technique is feasible only in cooperative children and does not offer great advantage over the tidal volume technique [90]. Indeed, forced hyperventilation is followed most of the time by a transient apnoea that should be expected – intervention is usually unnecessary. The tidal volume technique with spontaneous ventilation is the preferred technique for difficult airway management in paediatric anaesthesia [91].

Transient agitation, described as the occurrence of non-purposeful movements requiring restraint during induction, is not uncommon during induction with sevoflurane in children, whatever the induction technique [73,87,88]. Agitation usually occurs after loss of consciousness. Agitation is concomitant with the rapid increase in EEG delta activity and decrease in BIS values, but both clinical and EEG events are transient, whatever the premedication used (Fig. 10.10) [73]. Transient increase in heart rate and arterial pressure is commonly observed at the same time [87,92].

Although the cardiovascular tolerance of high sevoflurane concentrations (7–8 per cent) is usually excellent, recent studies suggest that lower concentrations may be indicated in order to minimise respiratory complications and to avoid too deep a level of anaesthesia. In a study comparing 2, 4, 6 and 8 per cent sevoflurane for inhalational induction in children, Hsu and colleagues [93] found that the incidence of airway reflex response was the highest in the 8 per cent group, and they suggest limiting inspired sevoflurane concentration to 6 per cent. Many studies have

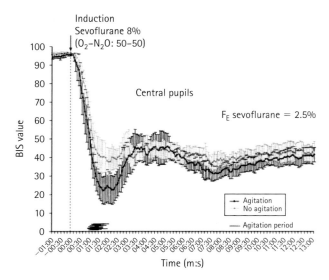

Figure 10.10 Mean values of Bispectral index (BIS) as a function of time, measured during sevoflurane induction (8 per cent sevoflurane in nitrous oxide 50 per cent and oxygen 50 per cent) in children that demonstrated agitation and those that demonstrated no agitation (mean and 95 per cent confidence interval). Intubation was performed when pupils were in central position and then sevoflurane expired concentration (F_E) was maintained at approximately 2.5 per cent. Source: Constant *et al.* [73].

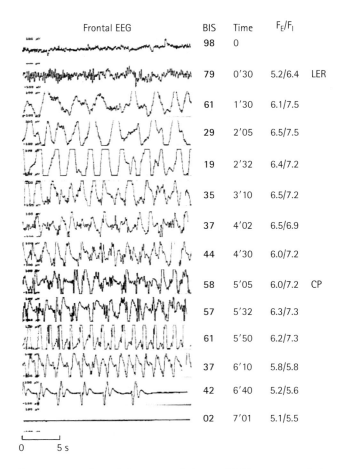

Figure 10.11 Frontal electroencephalogram (EEG) traces recorded in a 5-year-old child during sevoflurane induction (8 per cent sevoflurane in nitrous oxide 50 per cent and oxygen 50 per cent). Epileptiform signs occur around the fourth minute of induction with some spike waves, simple or multiple, followed by periodic discharge (rhythmic polyspikes), leading to periods of epileptiform discharges just before occurrence of burst suppression. The corresponding Bispectral Index (BIS), time and ratio of expired to inspired (F_E/F_I) sevoflurane are noted. The loss of eye lash reflex (LER) and the centralisation of the pupils (CP) are indicated. Source: Constant *et al.* [69].

demonstrated that electrical epileptiform activity is commonly observed during sevoflurane induction, especially when a high concentration (7 or 8 per cent), hyperventilation and vital capacity technique are used (Fig. 10.11) [67,68,73,94]. Thus, recent studies suggest that inspired sevoflurane concentration should not exceed 6 per cent and this concentration should not be maintained for more than 4 minutes in order to avoid too deep a level of anaesthesia. Other options should be considered to limit the inspired concentration of sevoflurane such as coinduction with N_2O and opiates or muscle relaxants if they are required for the surgical procedure. Monitoring EEG changes during anaesthesia will probably become the standard in the near future to optimise the depth of anaesthesia [71]. The BIS monitor may help the anaesthetist avoid too light a level of anaesthesia and its risk of awareness, and to avoid too deep an anaesthesia, which may promote undesirable cardiovascular effects in compromised patients. It may also help to limit potential anaesthesia-induced brain damage in the youngest patients [71,95]. The prerequisite to correctly interpret BIS changes is to be aware of the specific effects of anaesthetic agents on EEG and to know specific EEG changes associated with anaesthesia stages [69]. As already discussed, BIS values show a paradoxical profile during sevoflurane inhalational induction in children and are not correlated with clinical events or with the clinically assessed depth of anaesthesia [73].

Maintenance of anaesthesia

All volatile agents are appropriate for maintenance of anaesthesia whatever the induction technique used (mask or intravenous induction). The choice of inhalational agent for maintenance may depend on expected pharmacodynamic profile, the availability of anaesthesia machines capable of functioning with minimal gas flow and the cost.

As already indicated, isoflurane, desflurane and sevoflurane share the same safe cardiovascular profile and should be preferred to halothane in children with cardiovascular compromise [44,96]. If rapid emergence is a concern, desflurane allows for more rapid recovery than sevoflurane, and sevoflurane is faster than isoflurane and halothane, especially for long procedures [97–99].

All volatile agents potentiate the actions of non-depolarising muscle relaxants. The potentiation of action of non-depolarising muscle relaxants follows the order isoflurane ≈ desflurane ≈ sevoflurane > halothane > N_2O/opiate technique [100].

Desflurane and sevoflurane are more expensive than isoflurane and much more so than halothane. To minimise the extra costs during maintenance, the use of modern anaesthesia machine is mandatory. When fresh gas flow is reduced to 1 L/min or less, the cost of anaesthesia maintenance is very low even when costly inhalational agents are used. One should keep in mind that the total cost of anaesthesia only represents about 7 per cent of the total costs of most planned surgery [101].

Recovery from anaesthesia

Different endpoints are used to describe recovery from anaesthesia such as extubation time, eyes opening on verbal command, and discharge time from recovery room or from hospital. Extubation time and time to eyes opening are more rapid after desflurane or sevoflurane maintenance anaesthesia than after halothane anaesthesia, but late endpoints such as discharge times are not different in most studies after short procedures [85,88,102]. Desflurane allows for more rapid early recovery than sevoflurane or isoflurane in infants [98,99]. The interest in new volatile agents is more evident after long surgical procedures than after short anaesthesia as the context-sensitive half-life of these agent is much shorter than that of halothane and isoflurane [8]. Tracheal extubation can be performed either in a deeply anaesthetised child or in a fully awake child. No differences in terms of respiratory complications have been reported between the two extubation techniques during halothane anaesthesia in children [103]. Extubation in a deeply anaesthetised children has also been reported after anaesthesia maintenance with isoflurane, sevoflurane and desflurane [104,105]. The author's opinion favours the fully awake technique without painful stimulation during emergence in order to decrease the risk of laryngospasm at extubation [106].

Emergence agitation

Emergence agitation (EA) after general anaesthesia is not a new phenomenon, having been first reported 40 years ago. However, this old concern has re-emerged with the introduction of the new inhalational anaesthetics (sevoflurane, desflurane). Emergence agitation has been described as a disturbance in a child's awareness of and attention to their environment with disorientation and perceptual alterations, including hypersensitivity to stimuli and hyperactive motor behaviour in the immediate post-anaesthesia period. A scale has been recently established for quantifying the degree of agitation [107]. Although generally self-limiting, EA can be severe and may result in physical harm to the child and in particular to the site of surgery or any attached catheters or equipment. Emergence agitation in children often requires treatment with additional analgesics or sedatives, which may prolong stay in the recovery ward and increase the workload for the nurses. Finally this behaviour is often clinically indistinguishable from pain and discomfort in preschool-aged children. It may be associated with paranoid delusion.

It is important to minimise contributory factors and to manage agitation appropriately when it occurs. Several studies have found risk factors such as the anaesthetics (sevoflurane and desflurane), preschool age, ENT surgery and postoperative pain. Depending on these previous factors and the definition of agitation, this phenomenon may occur in up to 50 per cent of children anaesthetised with sevoflurane or desflurane [97,108–111].

Several investigators have argued that pain during impaired consciousness contributes to EA in some children; however, no clear relationship has been established. The administration of ketorolac, oxycodone, fentanyl, clonidine, dexmedetomidine or ketamine has been shown to reduce the agitation associated with sevoflurane or desflurane in young children, suggesting a possible relationship between pain and EA. However, Weldon et al. showed that after sevoflurane the incidence of EA was still high (26 per cent) even in pain-free children with caudal anaesthesia [112]. Furthermore, in children recovering from magnetic resonance imaging (MRI) examination, Cravero et al. [113] demonstrated that EA was increased with sevoflurane; there was no obvious pain.

A high level of preoperative anxiety has been suggested to be associated with more EA. Kain et al. [114] demonstrated that in children anaesthetised with sevoflurane without any premedication, the odds of having marked symptoms of EA and development of negative postoperative behavioural increase with the level of preoperative anxiety.

There are conflicting data on the effect of midazolam premedication. Some studies suggest a beneficial effect of midazolam in decreasing preoperative anxiety and in slowing the emergence of children from sevoflurane anaesthesia [115]. Another study demonstrated that children who received midazolam more frequently experienced EA after halothane or isoflurane anaesthesia (30–40 per cent) [116]. Midazolam may induce a gap in the child's memory, recovering abruptly in a strange place with multiple uncomfortable stimuli, resulting in a dreadful fright. These conflicting findings suggest that a randomised double-blind evaluation of midazolam is needed in children anaesthetised with sevoflurane or desflurane.

Avoidance of verbal or physical stimulation until the child is fully awake is desirable, but often impossible in a busy operating room schedule. This may explain why rates of EA were lower in some phase 3 trials than in typical clinical practice [85]. Changing to a different volatile agent (e.g. isoflurane) after sevoflurane induction is used by some anaesthetists, but its effectiveness and safety are not supported by scientific data. Furthermore, this combination was recently demonstrated to be a significant risk factor for EA [108].

Thus, EA is an early and transient phenomenon, observed after sevoflurane anaesthesia but also after other volatile agents, specifically in young children (<5 years). Underlying mechanisms are unknown. Its incidence may be reduced by appropriate pain therapy, analgesic and sedative agents. The long-term consequences of such a phenomenon seem to be minimal as no increased incidence of maladaptive postoperative behaviour change or sleep disturbances has been found in children undergoing anaesthesia with sevoflurane compared with halothane [117].

REFERENCES

Key references

Dubois MC, Piat V, Constant I et al. Comparison of three techniques for induction of anaesthesia with sevoflurane in children. Paediatr Anaesth 1999; 9: 19–23.

Eger EI. New inhaled anaesthetics. Anesthesiology 1994; 80: 906–22.

LeDez KM, Lerman J. The minimum alveolar concentration (MAC) of isoflurane in preterm neonates. Anesthesiology 1987; 67: 301–7.

Mapleson WW. Effect of age on MAC in humans: a meta-analysis. Br J Anaesth 1996; 76: 179–85.

References

1. Eger EI. New inhaled anaesthetics. Anesthesiology 1994; 80: 906–22.
2. Malviya S, Lerman J. The blood/gas solubilities of sevoflurane, isoflurane, halothane, and serum constituent concentrations in neonates and adults. Anesthesiology 1990; 72: 793–6.
3. Salanitre E, Rackow H. The pulmonary exchange of nitrous oxide and halothane in infants and children. Anesthesiology 1969; 30: 388–94.
4. Brandom BW, Brandom RB, Cook DR. Uptake and distribution of halothane in infants: in vivo measurements and computer simulations. Anesth Analg 1983; 62: 404–10.
5. Gallagher TM, Black GW. Uptake of volatile anaesthetics in children. Anaesthesia 1985; 40: 1073–7.
6. Tanner GE, Angers DG, Barash PG et al. Effect of left-to-right, mixed left-to-right, and right-to-left shunts on inhalational anaesthetic induction in children: a computer model. Anesth Analg 1985; 64: 101–7.
7. Morray J, Geiduschek J, Ramamoorthy C et al. Anesthesia-related cardiac arrest in children: Initial findings of the POCA registry. Anesthesiology 2000; 93: 6–14.
8. Bailey JM. Context-sensitive half-times and other decrement times of inhaled anesthetics. Anesth Analg 1997; 85: 681–6.
9. Difazio CA, Brown RE, Ball CG et al. Additive effects of anesthetics and theories of anesthesia. Anesthesiology 1972; 36: 57–63.

10. Lerman J, Robinson S, Willis MM, Gregory GA. Anesthetic requirements for halothane in young children 0–1 month and 1–6 months of age. Anesthesiology 1983; 59: 421–4.
11. Mapleson WW. Effect of age on MAC in humans: a meta-analysis. Br J Anaesth 1996; 76: 179–85.
12. LeDez KM, Lerman J. The minimum alveolar concentration (MAC) of isoflurane in preterm neonates. Anesthesiology 1987; 67: 301–7.
13. Eger EI. Age, minimum alveolar anesthetic concentration, and minimum alveolar anesthetic concentration-awake. Anesth Analg 2001; 93: 947–53.
14. Murray DJ, Mehta MP, Forbes RB, Dull DL. Additive contribution of nitrous oxide to halothane MAC in infants and children. Anesth Analg 1990; 71: 120–4.
15. Zwass MS, Fisher DM, Welborn LG et al. Induction and maintenance characteristics of anaesthesia with desflurane and nitrous oxide in infants and children. Anesthesiology 1992; 76: 373–8.
16. Fisher DM, Zwass MS. MAC of desflurane in 60 per cent nitrous oxide in infants and children. Anesthesiology 1992; 76: 354–6.
17. Lerman J, Sikich N, Kleinman S, Yentis S. The pharmacology of sevoflurane in infants and children. Anesthesiology 1994; 80: 814–24.
18. Inomata S, Watanabe S, Taguchi M, Okada M. End-tidal sevoflurane concentration for tracheal intubation and minimum alveolar concentration in paediatric patients. Anesthesiology 1994; 80: 93–6.
19. Inomata S, Suwa T, Toyooka H, Suto Y. End-tidal sevoflurane concentration for tracheal extubation and skin incision in children. Anesth Analg 1998; 87: 1263–7.
20. Cranfield KA, Bromley LM. Minimum alveolar concentration of desflurane for tracheal extubation in deeply anaesthetized, unpremedicated children. Br J Anaesth 1997; 78: 370–1.
21. Kihara S, Inomata S, Yaguchi Y et al. The awakening concentration of sevoflurane in children. Anesth Analg 2000; 91: 305–8.
22. Kharasch ED, Karol MD, Lanni C, Sawchuk R. Clinical sevoflurane metabolism and disposition. I. Sevoflurane and metabolite pharmacokinetics. Anesthesiology 1995; 82: 1369–78.
23. Ebert TJ, Frink-EJ J, Kharasch ED. Absence of biochemical evidence for renal and hepatic dysfunction after 8 h of 1.25 minimum alveolar concentration sevoflurane anaesthesia in volunteers. Anesthesiology 1998; 88: 601–10.
24. Kharasch ED, Hankins DC, Thummel KE. Human kidney methoxyflurane and sevoflurane metabolism. Intrarenal fluoride production as a possible mechanism of methoxyflurane nephrotoxicity. Anesthesiology 1995; 82: 689–99.
25. Vieira I, Sonnier M, Cresteil T. Developmental expression of CYP2E1 in the human liver. Hypermethylation control of gene expression during the neonatal period. Eur J Biochem 1996; 238: 476–83.
26. Lejus C, Le Roux C, Legendre E et al. Fluoride excretion in children after sevoflurane anaesthesia. Br J Anaesth 2002; 89: 693–6.

27. Njoku D, Laster MJ, Gong DH *et al.* Biotransformation of halothane, enflurane, isoflurane, and desflurane to trifluoroacetylated liver proteins: association between protein acylation and hepatic injury. *Anesth Analg* 1997; **84**: 173–8.

28. Stabernack C, Laster M, Dudziak R, Eger EI. Absorbents differ enormously in their capacity to produce compound A and carbon monoxide. *Anesth Analg* 2000; **90**: 1428–35.

29. Bito H, Ikeda K. Closed-circuit anaesthesia with sevoflurane in humans. Effects on renal and hepatic function and concentrations of breakdown products with soda lime in the circuit. *Anesthesiology* 1994; **80**: 71–6.

30. Frink-EJ J, Green-WB J, Brown EA *et al.* Compound A concentrations during sevoflurane anaesthesia in children. *Anesthesiology* 1996; **84**: 566–71.

31. Kharasch ED, Powers KM, Artru AA. Comparison of Amsorb, sodalime, and Baralyme degradation of volatile anesthetics and formation of carbon monoxide and compound a in swine *in vivo*. *Anesthesiology* 2002; **96**: 173–82.

32. Baum VC, Palmisano BW. The immature heart and anesthesia. *Anesthesiology* 1997; **87**: 1529–48.

33. Wolf WJ, Neal MB, Peterson MD. The hemodynamic and cardiovascular effects of isoflurane and halothane anesthesia in children. *Anesthesiology* 1986; **64**: 328–33.

34. Friesen R, Wurl J, Charlton G. Haemodynamic depression by halothane is age-related in paediatric patients. *Paediatr Anaesth* 2000; **10**: 267–72.

35. Manecke GR Jr, Nemirov MA, Bicker AA *et al.* The effect of halothane on the amplitude and frequency characteristics of heart sounds in children. *Anesth Analg* 1999; **88**: 263–7.

36. Palmisano B, Mehner R, Stowe D *et al.* Direct myocardial effects of halothane and isoflurane. Comparison between adult and infant rabbits. *Anesthesiology* 1994; **81**: 718–29.

37. Barash PG, Glanz S, Katz JD *et al.* Ventricular function in children during halothane anesthesia: an echocardiographic evaluation. *Anesthesiology* 1978; **49**: 79–85.

38. McAuliffe G, Bissonnette B, Cavalle-Garrido T, Boutin C. Heart rate and cardiac output after atropine in anaesthetised infants and children. *Can J Anaesth* 1997; **44**: 154–9.

39. Karl HW, Swedlow DB, Lee KW, Downes JJ. Epinephrine–halothane interactions in children. *Anesthesiology* 1983; **58**: 142–5.

40. Navarro R, Weiskopf RB, Moore MA *et al.* Humans anesthetized with sevoflurane or isoflurane have similar arrhythmic response to epinephrine. *Anesthesiology* 1994; **80**: 545–9.

41. Blayney M, Malins A, Cooper GM. Cardiac dysrhythmias in children during outpatient general anaesthesia for dentistry: a prospective randomized trial. *Lancet* 1999; **354**: 1864–6.

42. Wodey E, Pladys P, Copin C *et al.* Comparative hemodynamic depression of sevoflurane versus halothane in infants. *Anesthesiology* 1997; **87**: 795–800.

43. Holzman RS, van-der VM, Kaus SJ *et al.* Sevoflurane depresses myocardial contractility less than halothane during induction of anesthesia in children. *Anesthesiology* 1996; **85**: 1260–7.

44. Russell IA, Miller Hance WC, Gregory G *et al.* The safety and efficacy of sevoflurane anesthesia in infants and children with congenital heart disease. *Anesth Analg* 2001; **92**: 1152–8.

45. Constant I, Laude D, Hentzgen E, Murat I. Does halothane really preserve cardiac baroreflex better than sevoflurane? A noninvasive study of spontaneous baroreflex in children anesthetized with sevoflurane versus halothane. *Anesth Analg* 2004; **99**: 360–9.

46. Tanaka M, Nishikawa T. Sevoflurane speeds recovery of baroreflex control of heart rate after minor surgical procedures compared with isoflurane. *Anesth Analg* 1999; **89**: 284–9.

47. Weiskopf RB, Moore MA, Eger EI *et al.* Rapid increase in desflurane concentration is associated with greater transient cardiovascular stimulation than with rapid increase in isoflurane concentration in humans. *Anesthesiology* 1994; **80**: 1035–45.

48. Murat I, Chaussain M, Hamza J, Saint-Maurice C. The respiratory effects of isoflurane, enflurane and halothane in spontaneously breathing children. *Anaesthesia* 1987; **42**: 711–8.

49. Murat I, Chaussain M, Saint-Maurice C. Ventilatory responses to carbon dioxide in children during nitrous oxide-halothane anaesthesia. *Br J Anaesth* 1985; **57**: 1197–203.

50. Ochiai R, Guthrie RD, Motoyama EK. Differential sensitivity to halothane anesthesia of the genioglossus, intercostals, and diaphragm in kittens. *Anesth Analg* 1992; **74**: 338–44.

51. Keidan I, Fine GF, Kagawa T *et al.* Work of breathing during spontaneous ventilation in anesthetized children: a comparative study among the face mask, laryngeal mask airway and endotracheal tube. *Anesth Analg* 2000; **91**: 1381–8.

52. Reber A, Bobbia SA, Hammer J, Frei FJ. Effect of airway opening manoeuvres on thoraco-abdominal asynchrony in anaesthetized children. *Eur Respir J* 2001; **17**: 1239–43.

53. Serafini G, Cornara G, Cavalloro F *et al.* Pulmonary atelectasis during paediatric anaesthesia: CT scan evaluation and effect of positive endexpiratory pressure (PEEP). *Paediatr Anaesth* 1999; **9**: 225–8.

54. Erb T, Christen P, Kern C, Frei F. Similar haemodynamic, respiratory and metabolic changes with the use of sevoflurane or halothane in children breathing spontaneously via a laryngeal mask airway. *Acta Anaesth Scand* 2001; **45**: 639–44.

55. Brown K, Aun C, Stocks J *et al.* A comparison of the respiratory effects of sevoflurane and halothane in infants and young children. *Anesthesiology* 1998; **89**: 86–92.

56. Rooke GA, Choi JH, Bishop MJ. The effect of isoflurane, halothane, sevoflurane, and thiopental/nitrous oxide on respiratory system resistance after tracheal intubation. *Anesthesiology* 1997; **86**: 1294–9.

57. Taylor RH, Lerman J. Minimum alveolar concentration of desflurane and hemodynamic responses in neonates, infants, and children. *Anesthesiology* 1991; **75**: 975–9.

58. Taylor RH, Lerman J. Induction, maintenance and recovery characteristics of desflurane in infants and children. *Can J Anaesth* 1992; **39**: 6–13.

59. Goff MJ, Arain SR, Ficke DJ *et al.* Absence of bronchodilation during desflurane anesthesia: a comparison to sevoflurane and thiopental. *Anesthesiology* 2000; **93**: 404–8.

60. Paut O, Bissonnette B. Effect of halothane on the cerebral circulation in young children: a hysteresis phenomenon. *Anaesthesia* 2001; **56**: 360–5.

61. Leon JE, Bissonnette B. Cerebrovascular responses to carbon dioxide in children anaesthetized with halothane and isoflurane. *Can J Anaesth* 1991; **38**: 817–25.

62. Artru AA, Lam AM, Johnson JO, Sperry RJ. Intracranial pressure, middle cerebral artery flow velocity, and plasma inorganic fluoride concentrations in neurosurgical patients receiving sevoflurane or isoflurane. *Anesth Analg* 1997; **85**: 587–92.

63. Monkhoff M, Schwarz U, Gerber A *et al.* The effects of sevoflurane and halothane anesthesia on cerebral blood flow velocity in children. *Anesth Analg* 2001; **92**: 891–6.

64. Rowney DA, Fairgrieve R, Bissonnette B. Cerebrovascular carbon dioxide reactivity in children anaesthetized with sevoflurane. *Br J Anaesth* 2002; **88**: 357–61.

65. Luginbuehl IA, Fredrickson MJ, Karsli C, Bissonnette B. Cerebral blood flow velocity in children anaesthetized with desflurane. *Paediatr Anaesth* 2003; **13**: 496–500.

66. Karsli C, Luginbuehl IA, Bissonnette B. The effect of nitrous oxide on cerebral blood flow velocity in children anesthetised with desflurane. *Anaesthesia* 2003; **58**: 24–7.

67. Vakkuri A, Yli-Hankala A, Sarkela M *et al.* Sevoflurane mask induction of anaesthesia is associated with epileptiform EEG in children. *Acta Anaesth Scand* 2001; **45**: 805–11.

68. Yli-Hankala A, Vakkuri A, Sarkela M *et al.* Epileptiform electroencephalogram during mask induction of anesthesia with sevoflurane. *Anesthesiology* 1999; **91**: 1596–603.

69. Constant I, Seeman R, Murat I. Sevoflurane and epileptiform EEG changes. *Paediatr Anaesth* 2005; **15**: 266–74.

70. Iijima T, Nakamura Z, Iwao Y, Sankawa H. The epileptogenic properties of the volatile anesthetics sevoflurane and isoflurane in patients with epilepsy. *Anesth Analg* 2000; **91**: 989–95.

71. Murat I, Constant I. Bispectral index in paediatrics: fashion or a new tool? *Paediatr Anaesth* 2005; **15**: 177–80.

72. Edwards JJ, Soto RG, Thrush DM, Bedford RF. Bispectral index scale is higher for halothane than sevoflurane during intraoperative anesthesia. *Anesthesiology* 2003; **99**: 1453–5.

73. Constant I, Leport Y, Richard P *et al.* Agitation and changes of Bispectral Index and electroencephalographic-derived variables during sevoflurane induction in children: clonidine premedication reduces agitation compared with midazolam. *Br J Anaesth* 2004; **92**: 504–11.

74. Chinzei M, Sawamura S, Hayashida M *et al.* Change in bispectral index during epileptiform electrical activity under sevoflurane anesthesia in a patient with epilepsy. *Anesth Analg* 2004; **98**: 1734–6, table.

75. Iijima T, Nakamura Z, Iwao Y, Sankawa H. The epileptogenic properties of the volatile anesthetics sevoflurane and isoflurane in patients with epilepsy. *Anesth Analg* 2000; **91**: 989–95.

76. Taivainen T, Tiainen P, Meretoja OA *et al.* Comparison of the effects of sevoflurane and halothane on the quality of anaesthesia and serum glutathione transferase alpha and fluoride in paediatric patients. *Br J Anaesth* 1994; **73**: 590–5.

77. Bruun LS, Elkjaer S, Bitsch-Larsen D, Andersen O. Hepatic failure in a child after acetaminophen and sevoflurane exposure. *Anesth Analg* 2001; **92**: 1446–8.

78. Reich A, Everding AS, Bulla M *et al.* Hepatitis after sevoflurane exposure in an infant suffering from primary hyperoxaluria type 1. *Anesth Analg* 2004; **99**: 370–2.

79. Wappler F, Fiege M. Is desflurane a 'weak' trigger of malignant hyperthermia? *Anesth Analg* 2003; **97**: 295.

80. Keenan RL, Boyan C. Cardiac arrest due to anesthesia. A study of incidence and causes. *JAMA* 1985; **253**: 2373–7.

81. Keenan RL, Shapiro JH, Kane FR, Simpson PM. Bradycardia during anesthesia in infants. An epidemiologic study. *Anesthesiology* 1994; **80**: 976–82.

82. Olsson GL, Hallen B. Cardiac arrest during anaesthesia. A computer-aided study in 250,543 anaesthetics. *Acta Anaesth Scand* 1988; **32**: 653–64.

83. Morray JP. Unexpected cardiac arrest in pediatric anesthesia: causes and prevention. *ASA Refresher Course* 2004; **309**: 1–5.

84. Baum V, Yemen T, Baum L. Immediate 8 per cent sevoflurane induction in children: a comparison with incremental sevoflurane and incremental halothane. *Anesth Analg* 1997; **85**: 313–6.

85. Lerman J, Davis PJ, Welborn LG *et al.* Induction, recovery, and safety characteristics of sevoflurane in children undergoing ambulatory surgery. A comparison with halothane. *Anesthesiology* 1996; **84**: 1332–40.

86. Politis GD, Frankland MJ, James RL *et al.* Factors associated with successful tracheal intubation of children with sevoflurane and no muscle relaxant. *Anesth Analg* 2002; **95**: 615–20.

87. Dubois MC, Piat V, Constant I *et al.* Comparison of three techniques for induction of anaesthesia with sevoflurane in children. *Paediatr Anaesth* 1999; **9**: 19–23.

88. Piat V, Dubois MC, Johanet S, Murat I. Induction and recovery characteristics and hemodynamic responses to sevoflurane and halothane in children. *Anesth Analg* 1994; **79**: 840–4.

89. Walpole R, Olday J, Haetzman M *et al.* A comparison of the respiratory effects of high concentrations of halothane and sevoflurane. *Paediatr Anaesth* 2001; **11**: 157–60.

90. Agnor R, Sikich N, Lerman J. Single-breath vital capacity rapid inhalation induction in children. *Anesthesiology* 1998; **89**: 379–84.

91. Brooks P, Ree R, Rosen D, Ansermino M. Canadian paediatric anaesthesiologists prefer inhalational anaesthesia to manage difficult airways. *Can J Anaesth* 2005; **52**: 285–90.

92. Kern C, Erb T, Frei F. Haemodynamic responses to sevoflurane compared with halothane during inhalational induction in children. *Paediatr Anaesth* 1997; **7**: 439–44.

93. Hsu YW, Pan MH, Huang CJ *et al.* Comparison of inhalation induction with 2 per cent, 4 per cent, 6 per cent, and 8 per cent sevoflurane in nitrous oxide for paediatric patients. *Acta Anaesth Sin* 2000; **38**: 73–8.

94. Vakkuri A, Lindgren L, Kortila K, Yli-Hankala A. Transient hyperdynamic response associated with controlled hypocapneic hyperventilation during sevoflurane nitrous oxide mask induction in adults. *Anesth Analg* 1999; **88**: 1384–8.

95. Davidson AJ, Huang GH, Czarnecki C *et al.* Awareness during anesthesia in children: a prospective cohort study. *Anesth Analg* 2005; **100**: 653–61.

96. Rivenes SM, Lewin MB, Stayer SA *et al.* Cardiovascular effects of sevoflurane, isoflurane, halothane, and fentanyl-midazolam in children with congenital heart disease: an echocardiographic study of myocardial contractility and hemodynamics. *Anesthesiology* 2001; **94**: 223–9.

97. Welborn LG, Hannallah RS, Norden JM *et al.* Comparison of emergence and recovery characteristics of sevoflurane, desflurane, and halothane in pediatric ambulatory patients. *Anesth Analg* 1996; **83**: 917–20.

98. Wolf AR, Lawson RA, Dryden CM, Davies FW. Recovery after desflurane anaesthesia in the infant: comparison with isoflurane. *Br J Anaesth* 1996; **76**: 362–4.

99. O'Brien K, Robinson DN, Morton NS. Induction and emergence in infants less than 60 weeks post-conceptual age: comparison of thiopental, halothane, sevoflurane and desflurane. *Br J Anaesth* 1998; **80**: 456–9.

100. Brandom BW, Fine GF. Neuromuscular blocking drugs in pediatric anesthesia. *Anesth Clin North Am* 2002; **20**: 45–58.

101. Macario A, Vitez TS, Dunn B, McDonald T. Where are the costs in periofative care? Analysis of hospital costs and charges for inpatient surgical care. *Anesthesiology* 1995; **83**: 1138–44.

102. Sury MR, Black A, Hemington L *et al.* A comparison of the recovery characteristics of sevoflurane and halothane in children. *Anaesthesia* 1996; **51**: 543–6.

103. Patel RI, Hannallah RS, Norden J *et al.* Emergence airway complications in children: a comparison of tracheal extubation in awake and deeply anesthetized patients. *Anesth Analg* 1991; **73**: 266–70.

104. Valley RD, Ramza JT, Calhoun P *et al.* Tracheal extubation of deeply anesthetized pediatric patients: a comparison of isoflurane and sevoflurane. *Anesth Analg* 1999; **88**: 742–5.

105. Valley RD, Freid EB, Bailey AG *et al.* Tracheal extubation of deeply anesthetized pediatric patients: a comparison of desflurane and sevoflurane. *Anesth Analg* 2003; **96**: 1320–4, table.

106. Tsui BC, Wagner A, Cave D *et al.* The incidence of laryngospasm with a 'no touch' extubation technique after tonsillectomy and adenoidectomy. *Anesth Analg* 2004; **98**: 327–9.

107. Sikich N, Lerman J. Development and psychometric evaluation of the pediatric anesthesia emergence delirium scale. *Anesthesiology* 2004; **100**: 1138–45.

108. Voepel-Lewis T, Malviya S, Tait A. A prospective cohort study of emergence agitation in the pediatric postanesthesia care unit. *Anesth Analg* 2003; **96**: 1625–30.

109. Cravero JP, Beach M, Dodge CP, Whalen K. Emergence characteristics of sevoflurane compared to halothane in pediatric patients undergoing bilateral pressure equalization tube insertion. *J Clin Anesth* 2000; **12**: 397–401.

110. Davis P, Greenberg J, Gendelman M, Fertal KM. Recovery characteristics of sevoflurane and halothane in preschool-aged children undergoing bilateral myringotomy and pressure equalization tube insertion. *Anesth Analg* 1999; **88**: 34–8.

111. Beskow A, Westrin P. Sevoflurane causes more postoperative agitation in children than does halothane. *Acta Anaesth Scand* 1999; **43**: 536–41.

112. Weldon BC, Bell M, Craddock T. The effect of caudal analgesia on emergence agitation in children after sevoflurane versus halothane anesthesia. *Anesth Analg* 2004; **98**: 321–6.

113. Cravero J, Surgenor S, Whalen K. Emergence agitation in paediatric patients after sevoflurane and no surgery: a comparison with halothane. *Paediatr Anaesth* 2000; **10**: 419–24.

114. Kain ZN, Caldwell-Andrews AA, Maranets I *et al.* Preoperative anxiety and emergence delirium and postoperative maladaptive behaviours. *Anesth Analg* 2004; **99**: 1648–54.

115. Lapin S, Auden S, Goldsmith L, Reynolds A. Effects of sevoflurane anaesthesia on recovery in children: a comparison with halothane. *Paediatr Anaesth* 1999; **9**: 299–304.

116. Cole J, Murray D, McAllister J, Hirshberg G. Emergence behaviour in children: defining the incidence of excitement and agitation following anaesthesia. *Paediatr Anaesth* 2002; **12**: 442–7.

117. Kain ZN, Caldwell-Andrews AA, Weinberg ME *et al.* Sevoflurane versus halothane: postoperative maladaptive behavioural changes: a randomized, controlled trial. *Anesthesiology* 2005; **102**: 720–6.

11

Intravenous induction agents and total intravenous anaesthesia

NEIL S MORTON

KEY LEARNING POINTS

- Healthy young children often need a relatively high induction dose and maintenance infusion rate of intravenous agent per unit of body weight because of higher central compartment volume and clearance.
- Titration to clinical endpoints rather than strict dosing by formula is advisable to allow for wide interindividual variation in pharmacokinetics.
- Three-compartment pharmacological modelling using paediatric parameters is very helpful in understanding drug dosing requirements for total intravenous anaesthesia (TIVA).

- The concept of context-sensitive half-time (CSHT) is crucial to the safe clinical use of intravenous anaesthetics and opioids.
- Target-controlled infusions of propofol in children are possible using enabled infusion devices with validated paediatric datasets such as Paedfusor.
- Whenever propofol is used for TIVA, care should be taken to use 'propofol-sparing' techniques with regional blockade and/or opioids to minimise the risk of toxicity.

INTRODUCTION

The range of paediatric patients is very broad from the tiny preterm infant with immature organ function to the teenager who is (in pharmacological terms) an adult. Organ function matures during the first year of life but differences from adults in regional blood flow, body composition, enzyme activity, integrity of the blood–brain barrier and development of the central nervous system (CNS) mean that extrapolations from adult dosing are inaccurate. Healthy young children often need a relatively high induction dose of intravenous agent per unit of body weight and for total intravenous anaesthesia (TIVA) maintenance infusion rates often need to be higher than the weight-corrected

dose for adults. In contrast, the immature neonate, the critically ill child or those with major organ failure may need considerably reduced doses of intravenous anaesthetic agents and care is particularly needed in children receiving vasodilator medication and with certain forms of congenital heart disease. Allergic reactions to intravenous agents or their solubilising vehicles can occur unexpectedly but some can be prevented by a careful preoperative history (e.g. allergy to egg protein and propofol emulsion). In some medical conditions certain intravenous agents are specifically contraindicated, such as barbiturates in porphyria, but, in contrast, intravenous anaesthesia without volatile anaesthetic agents may be the technique of choice in the child susceptible to malignant hyperthermia. Drugs with sedative properties all potentiate each other's sedating and CNS depressant effects and this can be used to allow a reduction in the dose of each individual agent and possibly, therefore, reduce adverse effects of each. Titration to clinical endpoints rather than strict dosing by formula is advisable to allow for wide interindividual variation in pharmacokinetics (i.e. what the body does to the drug) and pharmacodynamics (i.e. what the drug does to the body). Electronic monitoring may be useful but has not yet been well validated in paediatrics.

BASIC DEVELOPMENTAL PHARMACOLOGY OF INTRAVENOUS INDUCTION AGENTS

Basic pharmacokinetic principles [1]

SINGLE-COMPARTMENT MODEL (FOR NOMENCLATURE USED IN FORMULAE SEE ALSO TABLE 11.6)

When a dose of an intravenous agent is injected or infused into a patient, the body can be considered as a single compartment and the uptake, distribution, metabolism and elimination of the drug can be extrapolated from measurements of the drug and its metabolites in the plasma and urine over time, knowledge of the body composition, knowledge of the solubility of the drug itself in tissues and plasma, and other properties such as the propensity for the drug to bind to plasma proteins and lipids (Table 11.1). In a *single-compartment model* it is assumed that the drug rapidly and evenly distributes throughout the body. This is a big assumption to make when one considers that the drug is being delivered into the venous side of the systemic circulation, has to pass through the pulmonary circulation and then via the systemic arterial circuit to the major organs and other tissues all of which have variable blood flow, metabolic enzyme activity and composition in terms of proportions of fat and water. In children it is even more complex because regional blood flow varies during development as does body composition and body proportions. The apparent volume into which a drug distributes (V_d) therefore varies between individual children, within the same individual at different stages of development and is quite different for different drugs. A drug that is very lipid soluble will seem to have a very large *volume of distribution*, as will one that is heavily bound to plasma proteins. A good visual analogy is to think of fluid vanishing by soaking into a sponge.

Elimination of an intravenous anaesthetic drug from the body is usually by metabolism in the liver and by excretion via the kidneys of the drug and its metabolites. Thus, maturation of liver and renal function is extremely important in affecting elimination of these agents in early life and dysfunction of these organs in illness can have a major adverse effect on drug elimination. A measure of elimination of a drug is the *clearance* (Cl), which is the volume of blood from which the drug is eliminated per unit of time.

Table 11.1 Physical characteristics of intravenous agents

Drug	Percentage ionised at pH 7.4	Percentage plasma protein binding	Lipid solubility
Ketamine	55	47	60
Midazolam	<5	96	34
Propofol	99	98	5000
Thiopental	39	78	600

The time required to achieve a 50 per cent reduction in the drug concentration is known as the elimination half-life ($t_{1/2}$). For our simple single-compartment model, the $t_{1/2}$ is proportional to V_d/Cl and so prolongation of the elimination of a drug can reflect either an increase in the volume of distribution or a reduction in clearance or both. An example might be in the immature neonate where a reduction in hepatic metabolism and renal excretion due to poorly developed organ function leads to slow elimination of the drug, prolongation of its effects and accumulation after repeated dosing or during a continuous infusion.

Simply starting a fixed infusion rate infusion in a single-compartment model will take five half-lives to reach a steady-state concentration. To more rapidly reach steady state in a one-compartment model, a bolus dose could be used to fill the volume of distribution and then a constant rate of infusion can be calculated that will maintain the plasma concentration.

TWO-COMPARTMENT MODEL

We know that once a drug is injected intravenously it distributes rapidly from plasma into tissues and that the drug is then eliminated. This two-phase process of rapid redistribution and slower elimination is mathematically best represented by two exponential curves. The *distribution half-life* and the *elimination half-life* can then be calculated. There are limits on how useful this information is for clinical practice because individuals vary so widely in terms of drug kinetics and dynamics, and processes of uptake, distribution, metabolism and excretion overlap in time and are not discrete, step-wise events in an orderly sequence. Two-compartment models are useful for describing the kinetics of drugs that are highly ionised.

THREE-COMPARTMENT MODEL

For intravenous anaesthetic agents, particularly when considering repeated dosing or delivery by a continuous infusion, it is helpful for practising clinicians to consider a three-compartment model (Fig. 11.1). For intravenous agents, the drug is delivered and eliminated from a central compartment but also distributes to and redistributes from two peripheral compartments, one representing well-perfused organs and tissues (fast compartment, V_1) and the

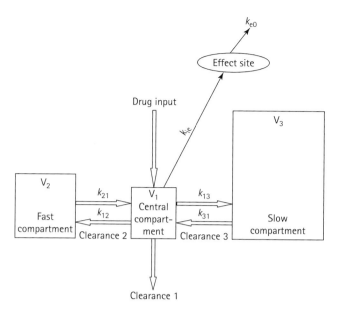

Figure 11.1 Three-compartment pharmacokinetic model with the addition of an effect site.

other representing more poorly perfused tissues such as fat (slow compartment, V_3). The transfer of the drug between the central compartment (V_1) and the two peripheral compartments (V_2 and V_3) and elimination of the drug from the central compartment are described by a series of rate constants (k_{12}, k_{21}, k_{13}, k_{31}, k_{10}). The clinician is interested in the effect of the intravenous anaesthetic agent on the brain and so a fourth rate constant also describes the movement from the central compartment to the effect site in the brain (k_{e0}). This compartment does not have a volume in terms of the model and does not remove a significant amount of drug but time is required for equilibration so there is a time lag before changes in plasma concentration are reflected in the effect site. There is therefore a delay or lag in onset and in offset of effects when an infusion rate is increased or decreased or stopped.

It is useful to think of the compartments as containers filling up with fluid with the central compartment connecting to the peripheral compartments and effect site by pipes of different diameters, and a drainage tap to represent elimination. The anatomy is similar to a water-filled radiator heating system (with a leak) rather than the human body but the clinical applicability of this simple arrangement is extremely helpful in understanding the behaviour of the main intravenous agents that we currently use. The volume of the compartments can be visualised relative to each other for a given drug and patient. The height of the columns of fluid (which represent concentration of drug) illustrates the gradient down which drug moves between the central and peripheral compartments, and this can be animated over time to show filling and emptying of compartments relative to each other. The diameter of the interconnecting pipes between the central and peripheral

compartments represents the inter-compartment clearances, and size of the drainage channel represents elimination. This hydraulic analogy is used in the TIVA Trainer simulation program [2].

FIXED INFUSION RATE AND A THREE-COMPARTMENT MODEL

When a fixed infusion rate is started, the plasma concentration will increase quite rapidly but almost immediately, distribution to the fast compartment starts as does elimination. For most intravenous anaesthetic drugs and opioids used for TIVA, distribution contributes more to removal of drug from plasma than elimination. The notable exception is remifentanil where extremely rapid esterase clearance dominates. As the infusion continues, distribution into the second compartment slows as the concentration gradient between the two compartments lessens but distribution to the slow compartment continues along with elimination. The net effect is that plasma concentration continues to increase but more slowly. As plasma concentration increases, excretion becomes relatively more important. Eventually, a steady state is reached with no net movement between compartments and the concentration is the same in each compartment. Infusion rate equals elimination rate. It can take many hours to achieve this steady state, for example it is approximately 24 hours for propofol.

BOLUS AND VARIABLE RATE INFUSION IN A THREE-COMPARTMENT MODEL

This is the basis for target-controlled infusion (TCI) techniques whether these are designed for maintenance and titration of a target plasma concentration or effect site concentration. A bolus dose can fill the initial volume of distribution, but then a changing rate of infusion is needed to maintain a constant effect site concentration until a steady state is reached. The infusion rate must vary because it has to match the changes in the contribution of distribution and excretion as the infusion continues. Modelling using computer software can be performed for all the intravenous agents and for populations of children of different ages, stages of development and states of health. The relevant studies have not all been done, however, and the models that have been developed are not always well validated in children.

Experience in adult practice has shown the clinical usefulness of delivering intravenous agents based on a robust and well-evaluated population pharmacokinetic model as the starting point, and then using clinical and electronic monitoring to titrate drug to the desired effect for an individual patient. The duration of clinical effects of an intravenous anaesthetic agent is very poorly predicted from the redistribution half-life or the elimination half-life calculated from pharmacokinetic and dynamic modelling. It is a far more clinically relevant exercise to try to relate the change in effect site concentration and its surrogate measure, the plasma concentration, to the pattern of drug delivery (namely single bolus dose, repeated bolus doses, continuous infusion or bolus plus continuous infusion) and to the duration of the infusion.

As drug is delivered into the central compartment it continuously distributes into the peripheral compartments, to the effect site and is being continuously eliminated. If the infusion into the central compartment is stopped then elimination will continue to drain the central compartment and drug will continue for some time to distribute to the peripheral compartments along concentration gradients from the central compartment. Equilibrium may be reached but drug will now start to move back from the peripheral compartments into the central compartment, maintaining the central compartment drug level for a period. Eventually, the central compartment concentration will fall. For most agents, the longer an infusion has been running, the more drug has distributed into the peripheral compartments and the larger the reservoir of drug to be redistributed and eliminated once the infusion stops. The half-time of the decline in drug concentration is therefore related to the duration of the infusion. This is the CSHT where the context is the duration of the infusion. For an individual drug and in a given patient a graph of CSHTs can be drawn by plotting the observed half-time against the duration of the infusion (Figs 11.2 and 11.3). If an infusion carries on long enough, eventually the peripheral compartments reach an equilibrium with the central compartment and the infusion rate will be similar to the elimination rate and a steady state will be achieved. The CSHT graph will then become parallel to the time axis. The infusion therefore becomes context *in*sensitive. This pattern is observed for nearly all intravenous anaesthetics but the half-time of remifentanil becomes context insensitive almost immediately because its elimination is by esterase metabolism. The capacity of the esterase systems is enormous and so elimination is at the same rate regardless of how long the drug has been infused.

For very lipid-soluble drugs such as fentanyl and propofol, V3 is large compared with V1. Intercompartmental clearance between V_1 and V_3 is given by the equation $V_1.k_{13} = V_3.k_{31}$ which implies that, if V_1 is much smaller than V_3, rapid distribution from V_1 to V_3 is associated with very slow redistribution from V_3 to V_1. This is indeed seen with propofol and fentanyl, which have slow offset of effects after prolonged infusion. Propofol has a CSHT that varies between around 3 minutes for a short-duration infusion and 18 minutes after a 12-hour infusion (Fig. 11.3). This is because excretion is quite rapid compared with the rate of redistribution from V_3. For alfentanil, the concentration of the unionised form is 100 times greater than that of fentanyl (alfentanil $pK_a = 6.4$, fentanyl $pK_a = 8.5$). Alfentanil therefore has a more rapid onset time and shorter $t_{1/2} k_{e0}$, a smaller V_1, lower volume of distribution at steady state and lower clearance than fentanyl. However, fentanyl does have a shorter CSHT than alfentanil after a short-duration infusion lasting less than 2 hours but, for

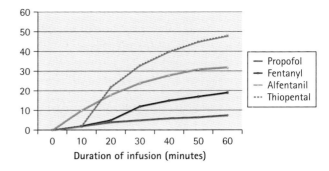

Figure 11.2 Context-sensitive half-times (CSHT) in minutes after short-duration infusions.

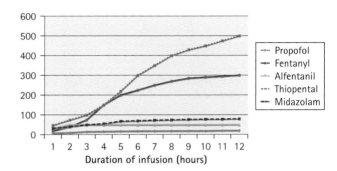

Figure 11.3 Context-sensitive half-times (CSHT) in minutes after long-duration infusions.

longer duration infusions, alfentanil reaches a maximum CSHT after about 90 min whereas for fentanyl the CSHT is still increasing after 12 hours (Fig. 11.2). This is because fentanyl has a huge V_3 and redistribution back to V_1 maintains the plasma concentration when the infusion stops.

Developmental pharmacokinetics and pharmacogenomics

During development there are marked changes in regional blood flow, body composition, protein binding, body proportions, gene expression and enzyme activity that affect drug distribution and elimination (see also Chapter 1).

REGIONAL BLOOD FLOW

The cardiac output corrected for body size is most readily expressed as cardiac output indexed to the body surface area. In neonates, the cardiac index is much lower than in older children (2.6 versus 4.0 L/min/m^2). The pattern of distribution of the cardiac output to different organs varies with development. For vital organs it is important to note that, although their mass constitutes a higher proportion of the body weight in early life, the proportion of the cardiac output distributed to the brain and liver is similar in neonates and adults. A notable exception is the relative hypoperfusion of the neonatal kidneys and skeletal muscle. Renal and hepatic blood flows achieve adult levels by about 1 year of age. Cerebral blood flow values per unit volume of brain are higher in early life than in adulthood and this may explain more rapid onset times of most intravenous agents in children.

BODY COMPOSITION

Body water and fat content and its distribution varies during development and gender differences in body fat content become particularly evident from age 8 years to 20 years. Total body water constitutes up to 80 per cent of a preterm neonate and around 75 per cent of a full-term neonate, with a gradual reduction to the adult proportion of 60 per cent by age 1 year. The total body water is distributed between intracellular and extracellular fluid compartments and the proportions of these change during development as cells multiply and the child grows. Body fat content is about 12 per cent of body weight at birth and rapidly increases to 25 per cent at age 6 months and 30 per cent by age 1 year. There is then a gradual reduction until age 8 years when girls start to have a higher proportion of fat than boys, which is induced by hormonal changes at puberty. The increasing prevalence and severity of childhood obesity are problematic and it may be safer to base drug dosing on lean body mass in such children. Some pharmacokinetic models incorporate corrections for lean body mass or ideal body weight or may have a maximum allowable weight limit (2,3).

PROTEIN BINDING

In the neonate the main drug-binding plasma proteins, albumin and α_1-acid glycoprotein, may be at relatively low levels and a rapid injection of a highly protein-bound drug such as thiopental could have faster clinical effects as there is more free active drug than expected. Neonatal albumin may be structurally different from adult albumin. Drugs may also be displaced by circulating bilirubin in neonates. Changes in plasma protein binding have relatively insignificant effects on drug pharmacokinetics when compared with the effects of hepatic metabolism and renal elimination.

METABOLISM AND EXCRETION

The main site for metabolism of the intravenous anaesthetic drugs is the liver and its function is conversion of these lipid-soluble agents into more water-soluble compounds ready for renal excretion. The most important hepatic microsomal enzyme system is the cytochrome P450 complex and these enzymes undergo varying rates of maturation. Some, such as CYP3A4 (involved in metabolism of midazolam and alfentanil), have low levels of activity in the neonate but reach adult levels by age 6–12 months and have levels above those of adults between the ages of 1 and 4 years. There can be competition between concurrently administered drugs for the same enzyme complex. Other enzyme systems involved in conjugation of drugs by sulphation or glucuronidation mature at different rates and patterns and time courses are extremely variable. Esterase systems may not be fully mature but those involved in clearance of remifentanil do seem to be active even *in utero* as transplacental remifentanil is cleared in the foetus. The kidney is an important route for elimination of water-soluble drugs and water-soluble metabolites of lipophilic drugs by glomerular filtration and tubular excretion. The glomerular filtration rate of the neonate is only 10 per cent of that of the adult but increases rapidly in the first year of life to the proportional adult value. This is a reflection of increase in systemic arterial blood pressure, reduced renal vascular resistance, a relative increase in the distribution of renal blood flow to the outer cortex and the development and growth of more glomeruli. Tubular secretion is also poorly developed in the neonate and matures during the first 6 months of early life, which is of relevance to propofol elimination.

Pathophysiology and pharmacokinetics

Neonates and ill children are prone to pathophysiological changes which can affect drug distribution, elimination and clinical effects.

The circulatory changes occurring at birth and in early postnatal life can be important, when using intravenous agents in patients with the potential for right-to-left intracardiac shunting. If systemic vascular resistance falls suddenly, right-to-left shunt will increase with consequent hypoxia and poor perfusion of liver and kidneys.

Hypotension and hypovolaemia can result in either preferential distribution to the brain of a given intravenous agent or, if autoregulation is impaired, very slow delivery to the brain. Sequestration of drug in the vessel-poor tissues may lead to prolonged recovery once perfusion improves and this depot effect can be quite marked. Low hepatic and renal blood flow can result in reduced elimination and this can occur in hypovolaemia or in low cardiac output states.

Hypoxia causes reduction in glomerular and tubular functions of the kidney because of renal arteriolar constriction.

Acidosis can lead to an increase in the unionised proportion of intravenous agents such as thiopental and this alters its distribution, increases its potency and exacerbates its myocardial depressant effects. An increase in arterial carbon dioxide partial pressure ($PaCO_2$) increases cerebral blood flow and this will affect distribution and uptake into the brain of the intravenous anaesthetic agents.

Hypothermia can reduce hepatic metabolism of certain drugs such as fentanyl and esterase clearance of remifentanil.

PROPERTIES AND DOSES OF INDIVIDUAL DRUGS IN PAEDIATRICS [4]

Propofol

Propofol has been used in paediatric anaesthesia for almost 20 years and its introduction corresponded with the advent of reliable topical anaesthesia of the skin for painless venous cannulation and the widespread adoption of the laryngeal mask airway. More recently, its popularity has declined somewhat with the advent of sevoflurane for inhalational induction. However, with the availability of cheaper generic preparations, alternative formulations to reduce injection pain and lipid load and increasing interest in day-case surgery and TIVA in paediatrics, its continued use is assured for some considerable time.

Propofol is a phenol and is insoluble in water so it is formulated as an emulsion with lipids such as 10 per cent soya bean oil, 2.25 per cent glycerol and 1.2 per cent egg phosphatides. It is available in a concentration of either 10 mg/mL or 20 mg/mL and is buffered to a pH of 6–8.5. Its pK_a is 11 and so it is 90 per cent unionised at pH 7.4. It is 98 per cent plasma protein bound. It rapidly diffuses into brain tissue because it is very lipophilic. Induction of anaesthesia is therefore rapid, within one circulation time. It is also redistributed very rapidly, with its pharmaco-kinetics best described by a three-compartment model. Hepatic metabolism is mainly by conjugation to inactive glucuronides. The clearance of propofol is related to hepatic blood flow and, in young children below age 5 years, propofol clearance is markedly higher. The central compartment volume is much larger in children than in adults by some 30–80 per cent. Thus a scaled-down adult dose of propofol based on body weight will tend to produce a lower peak plasma concentration of propofol and use of scaled-down adult infusion rates will result in relative under-delivery of propofol to children. In contrast, in younger infants and neonates, propofol clearance will be decreased because of immaturity of the hepatic glucuronidation enzyme systems. For single induction doses, however, termination of clinical effects is mainly due to rapid redistribution of drug and so recovery rates after a single dose are similar for all age groups [5].

Injection pain is more troublesome in children, particularly when small veins on the dorsum of the hand are used but pain can be significantly ameliorated by adding lidocaine at a dose of 0.2 mg/kg (1 mL of 1 per cent lidocaine per 10 mL of propofol solution) [6] or preinjecting alfentanil, 15–20 μg/kg [7]. Some of the newer formulations of propofol containing medium-chain triglycerides cause less injection pain [8].

The induction dose of propofol does vary with age (Fig. 11.5a) with young children below age 5 years requiring a relatively high dose [9–12] (Table 11.2). Sedative premedication allows a significant reduction in the induction dose of 30–50 per cent. The relatively large central compartment volume and increased clearance mean that a higher maintenance infusion rate is needed when based on body weight in children whether manual infusion schemes or target-controlled infusion techniques are used (Fig. 11.4a). Recovery after propofol induction is rapid and of excellent quality [7,13–27].

Propofol induction causes a 10–20 per cent decrease in mean systemic arterial pressure because of a reduction in systemic vascular resistance caused by direct relaxation of vascular smooth muscle. This is somewhat more than that seen after an equipotent dose of thiopental. Raised pulmonary vascular tone is reduced by propofol although normal pulmonary vascular resistance is not affected. Heart rate tends to decrease after propofol as a result of depression of baroreceptor reflexes and this is more common in younger children less than age 2 years. The QT interval may be prolonged although a recent study suggests that this is less significant than that caused by sevoflurane, and that neither agent is likely to lead to the malignant arrhythmia torsade de pointes in healthy children [28–31]. Propofol infusion anaesthesia may be associated with a higher incidence of oculocardiac reflexes in children undergoing strabismus surgery when compared with isoflurane anaesthesia [23] and so prophylactic glycopyrrolate or atropine may be useful.

The respiratory effects of propofol in children include respiratory depression, apnoea, and depression of pharyngeal and laryngeal reactive reflexes. Apnoea may occur in up to 50 per cent of children after induction and the ventilatory response to carbon dioxide is depressed, with decreased minute ventilation and carbon dioxide retention. Respiratory mechanics are not significantly altered. Placement of the laryngeal mask airway is facilitated by propofol induction [32] and tracheal intubation can be accomplished without the use of muscle relaxants and with more effective suppression of the haemodynamic response to intubation than is seen with thiopental. Intubating conditions and stress response suppression are improved by alfentanil or remifentanil [33–36].

Propofol produces dose-dependent depression of the central nervous system with significant reduction in cerebral blood flow, cerebral oxygen consumption and intracranial pressure. It should be used cautiously where there is reduced intracranial compliance because of the potential for reduced systemic arterial pressure and thus cerebral perfusion pressure.

Excitatory movements may occur during induction and recovery but these are not usually associated with epileptic activity on the electroencephalogram (EEG) in healthy children. However, at low dose the activity of an epileptiform focus in the brain may increase. Propofol at higher doses suppresses epileptiform activity.

The antiemetic properties of propofol are useful after paediatric day-case surgery and as part of the technique for procedures that carry a higher risk of emesis such as strabismus surgery and ear, nose and throat (ENT) surgery [17,21,23–26,37–40].

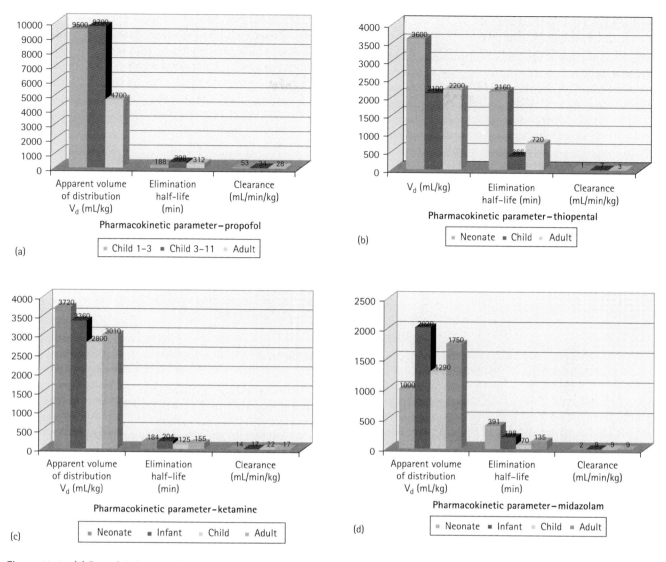

Figure 11.4 (a) Propofol pharmacokinetics. The apparent volume of distribution of propofol in the child is twice that of adults. The clearance of propofol in young children is twice that of adults and elimination is much more rapid. (b) Thiopental pharmacokinetics. The apparent volume of distribution in the neonate is 50 per cent larger than in the adult but elimination is much prolonged in the neonate, with a very low clearance value reflected in very long elimination half-life. In contrast, in the child, clearance rate is more than twice that of the adult and so elimination is more rapid. (c) Ketamine pharmacokinetics. The pharmacokinetic parameters are relatively similar across the ages but neonates and infants have lower clearance of ketamine and thus longer elimination. (d) Midazolam pharmacokinetics. Clearance of midazolam in the neonate is very much reduced due to hepatic enzyme immaturity and elimination half-life is considerably prolonged.

Table 11.2 Induction doses in healthy unpremedicated children

Drug	Induction dose (mg/kg)
Etomidate	0.3
Ketamine	1–2
Midazolam	0.1–0.5
Propofol	3–5
Thiopental	5–7

Notes: premedication or concurrent administration of opioids may reduce the required induction dose by 30–50 per cent. These doses should be reduced in the critically ill, in the child who is hypovolaemic and in the very young infant.

Propofol does not suppress T-cell function or adrenal steroid production, and does not produce tolerance on repeated dosing. The emulsion formulation does support bacterial growth and care is needed when infusion techniques are used. Incidences of anaphylaxis, anaphylactoid reactions and histamine release are comparable to those seen in other intravenous agents. Propofol is not recommended in those with an allergy to soya and should not be used for prolonged sedation in critically ill children under the age of 17 years as it can lead to a syndrome of metabolic acidosis, myocardial depression, rhabdomyolysis, hyperlipidaemia, hepatomegaly and death (propofol infusion syndrome) [41–50].

Thiopental (thiopentone)

Thiopental is a highly lipophilic barbiturate, which rapidly induces anaesthesia within one circulation time (see Tables 11.1 and 11.2). The pharmacokinetics are best described by a three-compartment model. Recovery after a single dose is due to rapid redistribution to vessel-rich tissues and is similar at all ages. Elimination by hepatic metabolism is capacity limited and so neonates with immature hepatic enzyme systems have significantly reduced clearance of the drug (Fig. 11.5b). Repeated doses or continuous infusions in all age groups result in accumulation, as the capacity of the hepatic enzyme system is saturated readily and very prolonged recovery then occurs because elimination occurs at a constant rate whatever the plasma concentration (see Figs 11.2 and 11.3). Clinical effects are even more prolonged as thiopental is metabolised to an active metabolite pentobarbital.

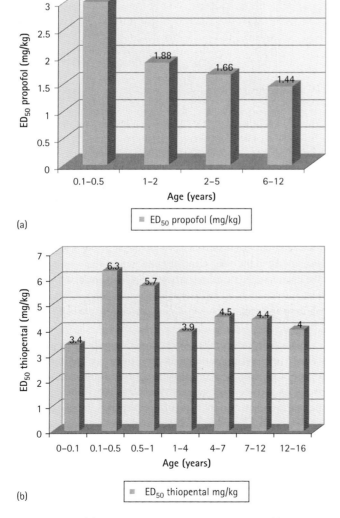

(a)

(b)

Figure 11.5 (a) Age and induction dose of propofol; (b) age and induction dose of thiopental (ED_{50}): the dose required to induce anaesthesia in 50 per cent of healthy, unpremedicated children.

The induction dose of thiopental varies with age with infants requiring relatively high doses to produce anaesthesia and neonates requiring relatively small doses (Fig. 11.5b; Table 11.2). Thiopental does not usually cause intravenous injection pain when a 2.5 per cent solution is used.

Recovery after thiopentone induction is somewhat slower than after propofol with detectable impairment of psychomotor skills for 4 hours. For anaesthesia lasting more than half an hour, the effects of the maintenance agent mask the differences between thiopental and propofol on recovery.

Thiopental does not decrease vascular smooth muscle tone so mean systemic arterial pressure is better maintained than with propofol. It does, however, cause direct myocardial depression and inhibition of CNS sympathetic outflow.

Thiopental is occasionally given by continuous infusion for management of intractable epilepsy or cerebral protection but it takes a long time for its effects to wear off (see Figs 11.2 and 11.3).

Ketamine

Ketamine produces a 'dissociative' state, profound analgesia and amnesia and acts primarily as an N-methyl-D-aspartate (NMDA) antagonist [51]. It is water soluble but as almost half the drug is unionised at normal pH it rapidly crosses the blood–brain barrier. A single injection intravenously of 2 mg/kg (see Tables 11.1 and 11.2) produces 10–20 minutes of dissociation and 30–60 minutes of analgesia. The pharmacokinetics of ketamine are similar in children and adults, although children have slightly higher clearance of ketamine because of their higher hepatic blood flow and neonates have reduced clearance because of reduced hepatic enzyme activity (see Fig. 11.4c). Ketamine has an active metabolite, norketamine, which has one-third the potency of ketamine. This is then further metabolised to water-soluble products which undergo renal excretion. The standard formulation of ketamine is a racemic mixture of equal proportions of $R(-)$ and $S(+)$ enantiomers, with the latter having at least twice the analgesic potency of the former [52–54].

Induction takes more than one circulation time and can be difficult to judge as typically the child's eyes stay open, with unfocused staring and sometimes nystagmus. Involuntary muscle movements may occur and muscle tone tends to increase. Ketamine has sympathomimetic actions with resultant increases in heart rate and systemic arterial pressure. In sick babies blood pressure is better maintained than with fentanyl or isoflurane but care is required as fall in blood pressure and cardiac output can be seen in the critically ill. Ketamine may exacerbate pulmonary hypertension in susceptible children but it is a bronchodilator by multiple mechanisms and is occasionally used to manage severe refractory asthma in the intensive care setting. It inhibits neurogenically mediated bronchoconstriction and that caused by direct stimulation, particularly in the neonate.

Salivary and bronchial secretions are increased by ketamine and glycopyrrolate prophylaxis is extremely helpful. Ketamine does not affect functional residual capacity in spontaneously breathing children and increases intrinsic positive end-expiratory pressure (PEEP), which helps maintain oxygenation and prevents collapse of dependent areas of the lungs. Ketamine significantly reduces the ventilatory response to CO_2 and, although slow administration clinically ameliorates this, the CO_2 response curve is still right shifted even after slow infusion. The respiratory depressant effect correlates with peak plasma concentration and episodes of apnoea tend to occur early after a rapid injection. Ketamine administration may be associated with laryngospasm (usually due to excessive secretions).

Midazolam

The role of the benzodiazepine midazolam is primarily as an anxiolytic and amnestic sedative for premedication, procedural sedation and in intensive care, but it has a secondary role to prevent the psychomotor effects of ketamine. As an anaesthetic induction agent it is not very satisfactory as the onset of action is very slow and recovery can be prolonged [55] (see Tables 11.1 and 11.2). It can be used by slow titration to produce conscious sedation for dentistry [56–59]. It can also be used as a co-induction agent to allow use of lower doses of the principal induction drug and to add anxiolytic and amnestic properties. Midazolam is water soluble at acidic pH below 4 but at pH 7.4 the ring structure closes and it becomes lipophilic (see Table 11.1). The pharmacokinetics are described by a three-compartment model. Midazolam has a hepatic extraction ratio of 50 per cent, so metabolic clearance depends on both hepatic blood flow and enzyme activity; it is noteworthy that the clearance in neonates is much lower than in children and adults (see Fig. 11.4d). Induction of sedation and anaesthesia in healthy children is quite slow and is most safely accomplished by

administration of increments of 0.05–0.1 mg/kg but total doses up to 0.6 mg/kg may be needed. Rapid injection of midazolam can cause hypotension because of reductions in both systemic vascular resistance and cardiac index, and this is most noticeable in critically ill children, children with hypovolaemia and in neonates. To maintain sedation, a continuous infusion of 0.1–0.3 mg/kg/h is used but there are very wide variations in requirements. The effects of midazolam are reversed by the specific benzodiazepine antagonist flumazenil [4,14,60].

Etomidate

The use of etomidate in paediatric anaesthesia is very limited as it causes suppression of adrenal steroid production, particularly after an infusion. Injection pain can be ameliorated with lidocaine or by preinjection of a short-acting opioid. A newer formulation, which contains both medium- and long-chain triglycerides, causes less injection pain. The induction dose is up to 0.3 mg/kg and is accompanied by very stable haemodynamics during and after induction of anaesthesia [61,62] and bronchodilatation. Involuntary movements may occur. Etomidate should not be administered by infusion for maintenance of anaesthesia or for sedation of the critically ill due to steroid suppression.

Opioids

The pharmacology of the opioids is detailed in Chapter 12. The relevant pharmacokinetic parameters for remifentanil, alfentanil and sufentanil are summarised in Table 11.3 [3]. The differences in CSHTs are illustrated in Table 11.4 and Figs 11.2 and 11.3. It is important to emphasise that remifentanil is, in effect, context insensitive while fentanyl has a short CSHT when given by infusion for a short time although this dramatically lengthens after longer-duration infusion. Alfentanil's CSHT becomes constant after approximately

Table 11.3 Pharmacokinetic parameters for short-acting opioids [3]*

	Remifentanil [77,78]	Alfentanil [79]	Sufentanil [80]
V_1	$5.1 - 0.0201(age - 40) + 0.072(LBM - 55)$	Male: 0.111 × weight Female: 1.15 × 0.111 × weight	0.164 × weight
V_2	$9.82 - 0.0811(age - 40) + 0.108(LBM - 55)$	12.0	0.359 × weight
V_3	5.42	10.5	1.263 × weight
k_{10}	$2.6 - 0.0162(age - 40) + 0.0191(LBM - 55)/V1$	$0.356/V_1$	0.089
k_{12}	$2.05 - 0.0301(age - 40)/V_1$	0.104	0.35
k_{21}	$2.05 - 0.0301(age - 40)/V_2$	0.067	0.16
k_{13}	$0.076 - 0.00113(age - 40)/V_1$	0.017	0.077
k_{31}	$0.076 - 0.00113(age - 40)/5.42$	0.0126	0.01
k_{e0}	$0.595 - 0.007(age - 40)$	0.77	0.12

* Adapted with kind permission from Michel Struys.
LBM, lean body mass.

Table 11.4 Context-sensitive half-times of opioids in children

	Infusion duration (minutes)				
	10	100	200	300	600
Remifentanil	3–6	3–6	3–6	3–6	3–6
Alfentanil	10	45	55	58	60
Sufentanil		20	25	35	60
Fentanyl	12	30	100	200	

90 minutes of infusion. The CSHT graphs in Figs 11.2 and 11.3 have been derived from models of healthy adults and are markedly altered by illness and immaturity. Clearance of fentanyl, alfentanil and sufentanil is reduced in neonates and young infants because of immaturity of hepatic enzyme systems or limited capacity of these systems whereas clearance of remifentanil is relatively age independent because the esterases are present and active in early life.

TOTAL INTRAVENOUS ANAESTHESIA [3,22,63–67]

Indications

The main uses of TIVA techniques in paediatrics are:

- in the patient susceptible to malignant hyperthermia where volatile agents are to be avoided
- in those children with a high risk of postoperative nausea and vomiting
- in children undergoing short painful procedures where rapid recovery is needed
- in those undergoing frequent repeated anaesthesia
- in those undergoing major surgery, including cardiac surgery, as an option to control the perioperative stress response
- in neurosurgery to assist with control of intracranial pressure and for cerebral metabolic protection.

Total intravenous anaesthesia has also become popular in some centres for airway procedures. Total intravenous sedation and anaesthesia are used in paediatric intensive care but, in this population, propofol is specifically contraindicated (propofol infusion syndrome) [41–50].

Drugs and techniques

The most commonly used drugs for TIVA in children are propofol, remifentanil, alfentanil and sufentanil. Ketamine techniques are occasionally also used. Drug delivery can be via manual infusion schemes based on body weight and time with titration to effect or using pharmacokinetic model-driven infusion devices with software developed for paediatrics. Recently, computer-controlled infusion

devices that have paediatric software packages built in have become more widely available, although often these are usable down to age 3 years or in children weighing more than 15 kg. The pharmacokinetic parameters used to drive these devices are derived from studies of relatively few healthy children but the performance of some paediatric models can be better than those used commonly in adults. For propofol, programmes that allow for age-, weight- and gender-related changes in central compartment volume, clearance and distribution have been developed and perform well in healthy children. There are considerable gaps in knowledge for some drugs, for ill children and for young children, infants and neonates, so caution is needed in these groups. The clinical anaesthetist still needs to use skill, knowledge and experience to titrate the intravenous agents to effect to avoid awareness, pain and adverse effects of these potent agents.

Pharmacokinetic and pharmacodynamic interactions [68,69]

Propofol administration can affect its own distribution and elimination by altering regional blood flow. Both fentanyl and alfentanil increase the volume of V1 and clearance of propofol while propofol and midazolam inhibit the metabolism of alfentanil by competing for the same cytochrome P450 enzyme isoform, CYP3A4. In addition to these pharmacokinetic interactions, there are important synergistic pharmacodynamic interactions between agents, which suppress central nervous system activity. During TIVA techniques in children, concurrent administration of opioids has a significant 'propofol-sparing' effect while providing analgesia and stress control [69]. It is particularly important to take advantage of this synergism to avoid excessive propofol and lipid load, particularly considering concerns about propofol infusion syndrome. Remifentanil provides the most effective propofol-sparing effect but fast recovery means alternative techniques of analgesia must be well established before remifentanil is discontinued. Fentanyl, alfentanil and sufentanil are effective and local and regional analgesia techniques also allow significant propofol dose reduction once the block becomes established. Nitrous oxide and low doses of volatile agents act synergistically with propofol and opioids, although this does not quite fit with the concept of pollution-free TIVA.

Manual infusion schemes (Table 11.5)

PROPOFOL

A simple scheme was devised by Roberts *et al.* [70] to maintain a plasma concentration of propofol in healthy adults of 3 μg/mL. A bolus dose of 1 mg/kg is followed by a continuous infusion of 10 mg/kg/h for 10 minutes, then 8 mg/kg/h for 10 minutes then 6 mg/kg/h thereafter. When this '10, 8, 6' regimen is modelled and checked using the

Table 11.5   Manual infusion schemes

	Loading dose	Maintenance infusion	Notes	References
Propofol	1 mg/kg	10 mg/kg/h for 10 minutes, 8 mg/kg/h for 10 minutes, 6 mg/kg/h thereafter	Adult regimen to achieve plasma concentration of 3 μg/mL. Underdelivers to children and achieves lower plasma concentration of 2 μg/mL	70
Propofol	1 mg/kg	13 mg/kg/h for 10 minutes, 11 mg/kg/h for 10 minutes, 9 mg/kg/h thereafter	Paediatric regimen with concurrent alfentanil infusion	71
Alfentanil	10–50 μg/kg	1–5 μg/kg/min	Results in plasma concentration of 50–200 ng/mL	81
Remifentanil	0.5 μg/kg/min for 3 minutes	0.25 μg/kg/min	Produces blood concentrations of 6–9 ng/mL	3
Remifentanil	0.5–1.0 μg/kg over 1 minute	0.1–0.5 μg/kg/min	Produces blood concentrations of 5–10 ng/mL	3
Sufentanil	0.1–0.5 μg/kg	0.005–0.01 μg/kg/min	Results in plasma concentration of 0.2 ng/mL for sedation and analgesia	3, 82
Sufentanil	1–5 μg/kg	0.01–0.05 μg/kg/min	Results in plasma concentrations of 0.6–3.0 ng/mL for anaesthesia	3, 82
Fentanyl	1–10 μg/kg	0.1–0.2 μg/kg/min		81
Ketamine	1–2 mg/kg	5–40 μg/kg/min		81
Midazolam	0.05–0.1 mg/kg	0.1–0.3 mg/kg/h		81

Marsh model [64] for an adult patient, the estimated plasma concentration is just over 3 μg/mL and stays reasonably stable, so it does work quite well. However, if the same regimen is modelled using the Paedfusor pharmacokinetic dataset for a child aged 1 year and weighing 10 kg, the plasma concentration achieved is around 2 μg/mL and tends to fall further over time. Thus, this scheme underdelivers propofol. This is because of the larger central compartment and increased clearance in children compared with adults. When the Paedfusor is used to calculate what would be needed to achieve a plasma concentration of 3 μg/mL, a 50 per cent larger bolus dose (1.5 mg/kg) and infusion rates of approximately '18,15,12' are needed to maintain a plasma target concentration of 3 μg/mL. In addition, it takes some 15 minutes for the effect site concentration to reach 3 μg/mL. Browne *et al.* [71] adapted this regimen for children receiving concurrent alfentanil infusions and found the effective dose in 95 per cent of patients (ED_{95}) infusion rates were much higher than the Roberts regimen, as expected from the known pharmacokinetics in children (larger central compartment volume and larger clearance). The infusion regimen could be simplified to '13,11,9' as opposed to '10,8,6' which illustrates the propofol-sparing effect of alfentanil, as without it considerably more propofol would have been needed as noted above (i.e. 18,15,12). These examples illustrate the complexity of the calculations needed to allow for variations in pharmacokinetics, pharmacodynamics and drug interactions and this has been the motivation to develop computer-controlled infusion devices (see below).

OPIOIDS

Simple manual infusion schemes can be used for the opioids fentanyl, alfentanil, remifentanil and sufentanil. The properties of these agents are detailed in Chapter 12. The manual infusion schemes for these opioids in children are summarised in Table 11.5. Transitioning to maintenance analgesia after infusions of these agents is a significant issue and it is important to ensure that either adequate regional or local anaesthesia techniques are established or that adequate doses of systemic analgesia are given well before the infusion is discontinued. Transitioning is somewhat smoother after sufentanil than after alfentanil or remifentanil in children. The problem of acute tolerance to ultra-short-acting opioids has been noted after use of remifentanil in paediatric scoliosis surgery [72].

KETAMINE

Ketamine can be used in a simple basic manual scheme as a loading dose of 1 mg/kg and a maintenance infusion of 0.1 mg/kg/h with additional boluses of 1–2 mg/kg and increase in maintenance rate to 0.2 mg/kg/h.

MIDAZOLAM

Slow bolus dosing of up to 0.1 mg/kg followed by an infusion rate of 0.1 mg/kg/h provide baseline sedation with adjustments and additional bolus doses often needed. Caution is required with bolus dosing in neonates and infants and in the

Table 11.6 Nomenclature for target-controlled infusion (TCI) systems

Term	Meaning	Units
TCI	Target-controlled infusion	
Vc or V_1	Central compartment volume	L
V_2	Fast compartment volume (vessel-rich group) $= V_1 \times k_{12}/k_{21}$	L
V_3	Slow compartment volume (vessel-poor group) $= V_3 \times k_{13}/k_{31}$	L
Cl_1	Elimination clearance $= V_1 \times k_{10}$	L/hour
Cl_2	Clearance between V_1 and $V_2 = V_2 \times k_{21}$	L/hour
Cl_3	Clearance between V_1 and $V_3 = V_3 \times k_{31}$	L/hour
Cp	Blood concentration	
Ce	Effect site concentration	
T	Target concentration	
CALC	Concentration calculated by TCI software	
MEAS	Concentration measured	
k_{10}	Elimination rate constant	per minute
k_{e0}	Rate constant for equilibration between blood and effect site	per minute
k_{12}, k_{21}	Rate constants for movement between V1 and V2	per minute
k_{13}, k_{31}	Rate constants for movement between V1 and V3	per minute

Table 11.7 Paedfusor pharmacokinetic dataset for propofol [64,73,74,83]

Age (years)	Paedfusor dataset
1–12	$V_1 = 0.4584 \times$ weight; $V_2 = V_1 \times k_{12}/k_{21}$; $V_3 = V_1 \times k_{13}/k_{31}$ $*k_{10} = 0.1527 \times$ weight$^{-0.3}$ $k_{12} = 0.114$; $k_{21} = 0.055$ $k_{13} = 0.0419$; $k_{31} = 0.0033$ $k_{e0} = 0.26$
13	$V_1 = 0.400 \times$ weight $k_{10} = 0.0678$ (other constants as above)
14	$V_1 = 0.342 \times$ weight $k_{10} = 0.0792$ (other constants as above)
15	$V_1 = 0.284 \times$ weight $k_{10} = 0.0954$ (other constants as above)
16	$V_1 = 0.22857 \times$ weight $k_{10} = 0.119$ (other constants as above)

*Note: the k_{10} value in the age group 1–12 years is a negative power function of weight, which reflects the increasing clearance values in younger children.

Table 11.8 Comparison between Paedfusor [64,73,74,83] and Kataria [75] models for propofol in children

	'Paedfusor'	Kataria
V_1	$0.458 \times$ weight	$0.41 \times$ weight
V_2	$0.95 \times$ weight	$0.78 \times$ weight $+ 3.1 \times$ age
V_3	$5.82 \times$ weight	$6.9 \times$ weight
k_{10}	$0.1527 \times$ weight$^{-0.3}$	0.085
k_{12}	0.114	0.188
k_{21}	0.055	0.102
k_{13}	0.0419	0.063
k_{31}	0.0033	0.0038
k_{e0}	0.26*	n/a*

*This is the value for adults but Munoz et al. [76] have recently studied these two models to define a more accurate k_{e0} for children age 3–11 years and the values are 0.91 for Paedfusor and 0.41 for Kataria.

critically ill as hypotension may occur and the depth of sedation achieved with midazolam is tremendously variable.

Target-controlled infusion

A TCI [3] is one controlled by a computer which performs rapid sequential calculations every 8–10 seconds to determine the infusion rate required to produce a user-defined drug concentration in the central compartment (which includes the blood) or at the site of action of the drug. Thus, TCI may be blood targeted or effect-site targeted. The standard nomenclature for TCI systems is listed in Table 11.6. Modern TCI systems are computer-controlled syringe drivers capable of infusion rates up to 1200 mL/h with a precision of 0.1 mL/h. They incorporate a user interface and display and a range of safety alarms, monitoring functions and warning systems. For most programmes, the user has to choose a drug and its concentration from a menu and select a pharmacokinetic model. The range of models suitable for paediatrics is quite limited and some models are not suitable for all age groups. Others may be suitable but are not well validated in younger children. Neonatal and infant models are rarely available.

Table 11.9   Target-controlled infusion based on calculated plasma concentration targeting compared with calculated effect-site concentration targeting (both at 5 μg/mL) for a healthy 1 year old, weight 10 kg using the Paedfusor pharmacokinetic dataset

	Plasma concentration targeting	Effect-site concentration targeting	Notes
Loading dose (mg/kg)	1.7	5.7*	*Potential for haemodynamic changes due to high peak plasma concentration from larger bolus dose
Maximum plasma target reached (μg/mL)	5	12*	*Potential for haemodynamic changes due to high peak plasma concentration from larger bolus dose
Total propofol infused after 60 minutes (mg/kg)	23.2	23.3	Virtually the same total dose of propofol in the first 60 minutes
Time to achieve effect site target of 5 μg/mL (minutes)	17.5	4.5**	**Very much shorter time to achieve effect-site target

Experience with the various models may be usefully gained with simulation programs that can run on personal computers such as TIVA Trainer, Rugloop, Stelpump and Stanpump. The TIVA Trainer version 8.5 [2] now allows uploading of new models via a central website and server and contains details and simulations of paediatric models for propofol and neonatal and paediatric models for sufentanil, in addition to a wide range of adult models for propofol, alfentanil, remifentanil, fentanyl, ketamine and midazolam. The simulation shows graphs of plasma and effect-site concentrations against time, infusion rates, volumes, compartment sizes and many other features. Animations are available which vividly illustrate the differences between the behaviour of different drugs and infusion regimens in tables, graphs and hydraulic models.

ACCURACY OF TCI MODELS

The models within TCI systems are derived from studies of small numbers of healthy patients and are only a guide to drug administration to an individual patient. It has already been noted for manual infusions that simply scaling down drug doses and infusion rates by body weight for children leads, in general, to underdelivery of drug and this then risks inadequate levels of anaesthesia and analgesia with all the attendant risks of awareness, excessive stress response to surgery, laryngeal spasm, patient movement and pain. The same applies to TCI systems and so measures to assess the accuracy of TCI systems are needed when paediatric models are proposed [3]. Usually, this is done by using a given dataset and taking accurately timed blood samples to measure drug concentrations in the blood. The accuracy of TCI propofol was assessed by Marsh et al. [63,64] in children and the model was found to perform well in a small prospective series of healthy children. In a subsequent study of children undergoing cardiac surgery the model performed significantly better than the adult model does in adults [73,74]. It has been incorporated into a modified version of the commercial Diprifusor device and is known as the Paedfusor [74], which has been evaluated clinically and

performs well (Table 11.7) [22,63–65]. Another paediatric propofol model that has been reasonably well validated is that of Kataria et al. [75]. As in adult practice, there are differences between paediatric models and care must be taken to learn about these differences before using the TCI systems clinically. One notable difference is that the Paedfusor model makes an allowance for the steady increase in elimination clearance in younger children, particularly those weighing less than 30 kg (Table 11.8). The lower age and weight limits for each model also differ with age 1 year and 5 kg for the Paedfusor system, and 3 years and 15 kg for the Kataria system. In the Paedfusor program, the adult value for k_{e0} of 0.26 is used but there is no value for this parameter in the Kataria model (Table 11.8). Thus, effect-site targeting is possible with the Paedfusor (Table 11.9) but may not be particularly accurate. Munoz et al. have therefore tried to define a more accurate k_{e0} for children in an ingenious study using auditory evoked responses and both the Paedfusor and Kataria models [76]. This revealed that the time to peak effect after a bolus dose was longer in children than adults and the median k_{e0} values for the Paedfusor and Kataria models for children age 3–11 years were 0.91/minute and 0.41/minute. This should allow more accurate effect-site targeting using propofol in the future.

REFERENCES

Key references

Absalom A, Kenny GNC. 'Paedfusor' pharmacokinetic data set. Br J Anaesth 2005; **95**(1): 110.

Aun CS, Short TG, O'Meara ME, Leung DH, Rowbottom YM, Oh TE. Recovery after propofol infusion anaesthesia in children: comparison with propofol, thiopentone or halothane induction followed by halothane maintenance. Br J Anaesth 1994; **72**(5): 554–8.

Morton NS. Total intravenous anaesthesia (TIVA) in paediatrics: advantages and disadvantages. Paediatr Anaesth 1998; **8**(3): 189–94.

SIGN. Safe sedation of children undergoing diagnostic and therapeutic procedures. Edinburgh: Scottish Intercollegiate Guidelines Network, 2004.

Westrin P. The induction dose of propofol in infants 1–6 months of age and in children 10–16 years of age. *Anesthesiology* 1991; **74**(3): 455–8.

References

1. Hill SA. Pharmacokinetics of drug infusions. *Continuing Educ Anaesth Crit Care Pain* 2004; **4**(3): 76–80.
2. Engbers F, Sutcliffe N, Kenny GNC. *TIVA trainer*, 8.5 edn, 2006. http://www.eurosiva.org/TivaTrainer/tivatrainer_main.htm
3. Absalom A, Struys MMRF. *An overview of TCI and TIVA*. Ghent: Academia Press, 2005.
4. Paediatric Formulary Committee. *British national formulary for children*. London: BMJ Publishing Group Ltd, 2007.
5. Patel DK, Keeling PA, Newman GB, Radford P. Induction dose of propofol in children. *Anaesthesia* 1988; **43**(11): 949–52.
6. Morton NS. Abolition of injection pain due to propofol in children. *Anaesthesia* 1990; **45**(1): 70.
7. Hiller A, Saarnivaara L. Injection pain, cardiovascular changes and recovery following induction of anaesthesia with propofol in combination with alfentanil or lignocaine in children. *Acta Anaesth Scand* 1992; **36**(6): 564–8.
8. Nyman Y, von Hofsten K, Georgiadi A *et al.* Propofol injection pain in children: a prospective randomized double-blind trial of a new propofol formulation versus propofol with added lidocaine. *Br J Anaesth* 2005; **95**(2): 222–5.
9. Aun CS, Short SM, Leung DH, Oh TE. Induction dose–response of propofol in unpremedicated children. *Br J Anaesth* 1992; **68**(1): 64–7.
10. Westrin P. The induction dose of propofol in infants 1–6 months of age and in children 10–16 years of age. *Anesthesiology* 1991; **74**(3): 455–8.
11. Valtonen M, Iisalo E, Kanto J, Tikkanen J. Comparison between propofol and thiopentone for induction of anaesthesia in children. *Anaesthesia* 1988; **43**(8): 696–9.
12. Hannallah RS, Baker SB, Casey W *et al.* Propofol: effective dose and induction characteristics in unpremedicated children. *Anesthesiology* 1991; **74**(2): 217–19.
13. Glaisyer HR, Sury MRJ. Recovery after anesthesia for short pediatric oncology procedures: propofol and remifentanil compared with propofol, nitrous oxide, and sevoflurane. *Anesth Analg* 2005; **100**(4): 959–63.
14. Jones RD, Visram AR, Chan MM *et al.* A comparison of three induction agents in paediatric anaesthesia – cardiovascular effects and recovery. *Anaesth Intensive Care* 1994; **22**(5): 545–55.
15. Keidan I, Berkenstadt H, Sidi A, Perel A. Propofol/remifentanil versus propofol alone for bone marrow aspiration in paediatric haemato-oncological patients. *Paediatr Anaesth* 2001; **11**(3): 297–301.
16. Santawat U, Lertakyamanee J, Svasdi-Xuto O. Recovery after total intravenous anesthesia (TIVA) using propofol and inhalation anesthesia (IA) using halothane in day case surgery. *J Med Assoc Thai* 1999; **82**(8): 770–7.
17. Grundmann U, Uth M, Eichner A *et al.* Total intravenous anaesthesia with propofol and remifentanil in paediatric patients: a comparison with a desflurane–nitrous oxide inhalation anaesthesia. *Acta Anaesth Scand* 1998; **42**(7): 845–50.
18. McDowall RH, Scher CS, Barst SM. Total intravenous anesthesia for children undergoing brief diagnostic or therapeutic procedures. *J Clin Anesth* 1995; **7**(4): 273–80.
19. Aun CS, Short TG, O'Meara ME *et al.* Recovery after propofol infusion anaesthesia in children: comparison with propofol, thiopentone or halothane induction followed by halothane maintenance. *Br J Anaesth* 1994; **72**(5): 554–8.
20. Short TG, Aun CS, Tan P *et al.* A prospective evaluation of pharmacokinetic model controlled infusion of propofol in paediatric patients. *Br J Anaesth* 1994; **72**(3): 302–6.
21. Hannallah RS, Britton JT, Schafer PG *et al.* Propofol anaesthesia in paediatric ambulatory patients: a comparison with thiopentone and halothane. *Can J Anaesth* 1994; **41**(1): 12–8.
22. Doyle E, McFadzean W, Morton NS. IV anaesthesia with propofol using a target-controlled infusion system: comparison with inhalation anaesthesia for general surgical procedures in children. *Br J Anaesth* 1993; **70**(5): 542–5.
23. Snellen FT, Vanacker B, van Aken H. Propofol-nitrous oxide versus thiopental sodium-isoflurane-nitrous oxide for strabismus surgery in children. *J Clin Anaesth* 1993; **5**(1): 37–41.
24. Runcie CJ, Mackenzie SJ, Arthur DS, Morton NS. Comparison of recovery from anaesthesia induced in children with either propofol or thiopentone. *Br J Anaesth* 1993; **70**(2): 192–5.
25. Larsson S, Asgeirsson B, Magnusson J. Propofol-fentanyl anesthesia compared to thiopental-halothane with special reference to recovery and vomiting after pediatric strabismus surgery. *Acta Anaesth Scand* 1992; **36**(2): 182–6.
26. Borgeat A, Popovic V, Meier D, Schwander D. Comparison of propofol and thiopental/halothane for short-duration ENT surgical procedures in children. *Anesth Analg* 1990; **71**(5): 511–5.
27. Valtonen M. Anaesthesia for computerised tomography of the brain in children: a comparison of propofol and thiopentone. *Acta Anaesth Scand* 1989; **33**(2): 170–3.
28. Saarnivaara L, Hiller A, Oikkonen M. QT interval, heart rate and arterial pressures using propofol, thiopentone or methohexitone for induction of anaesthesia in children. *Acta Anaesth Scand* 1993; **37**(4): 419–23.
29. Paventi S, Santevecchi A, Ranieri R. Effects of sevoflurane versus propofol on QT interval. *Minerva Anestesiol* 2001; **67**(9): 637–40.
30. Curry TB, Gaver R, White RD. Acquired long QT syndrome and elective anesthesia in children. *Paediatr Anaesth* 2006; **16**(4): 471–8.
31. Whyte SD, Booker PD, Buckley DG. The effects of propofol and sevoflurane on the QT interval and transmural dispersion of repolarization in children. *Anesth Analg* 2005; **100**(1): 71–7.

32. Allsop E, Innes P, Jackson M, Cunliffe M. Dose of propofol required to insert the laryngeal mask airway in children. *Paediatr Anaesth* 1995; **5**: 47–51.

33. Crawford MW, Hayes J, Tan JM. Dose–response of remifentanil for tracheal intubation in infants. *Anesth Analg* 2005; **100**(6): 1599–604.

34. Batra YK, Al Qattan AR, Ali SS *et al.* Assessment of tracheal intubating conditions in children using remifentanil and propofol without muscle relaxant. *Paediatr Anaesth* 2004; **14**(6): 452–6.

35. Blair JM, Hill DA, Wilson CM, Fee JPH. Assessment of tracheal intubation in children after induction with propofol and different doses of remifentanil. *Anaesthesia* 2004; **59**(1): 27–33.

36. Klemola UM, Hiller A. Tracheal intubation after induction of anesthesia in children with propofol – remifentanil or propofol-rocuronium. *Can J Anaesth* 2000; **47**(9): 854–9.

37. Standl T, Wilhelm S, von Knobelsdorff G, Schulte am Esch J. Propofol reduces emesis after sufentanil supplemented anaesthesia in paediatric squint surgery. *Acta Anaesth Scand* 1996; **40**(6): 729–33.

38. Habre W, Sims C. Propofol anaesthesia and vomiting after myringoplasty in children. *Anaesthesia* 1997; **52**(6): 544–6.

39. Tsui BCH, Wagner A, Usher AG *et al.* Combined propofol and remifentanil intravenous anesthesia for pediatric patients undergoing magnetic resonance imaging. *Paediatr Anaesth* 2005; **15**(5): 397–401.

40. Weir PM, Munro HM, Reynolds PI *et al.* Propofol infusion and the incidence of emesis in pediatric outpatient strabismus surgery. *Anesth Analg* 1993; **76**: 760–4.

41. Bray RJ. Propofol infusion syndrome in children. *Paediatr Anaesth* 1998; **8**(6): 491–9.

42. Bray RJ. Propofol-infusion syndrome in children. *Lancet.* 1999; **353**(9169): 2074–5.

43. Hatch DJ. Propofol-infusion syndrome in children. *Lancet.* 1999; **353**(9159): 1117–8.

44. Murdoch SD, Cohen AT. Propofol-infusion syndrome in children. *Lancet.* 1999; **353**(9169): 2074–5.

45. Kelly DF. Propofol-infusion syndrome. *J Neurosurg* 2001; **95**(6): 925–6.

46. Wolf A, Weir P, Segar P *et al.* Impaired fatty acid oxidation in propofol infusion syndrome. *Lancet* 2001; **357**(9256): 606–7.

47. Short TG, Young Y. Toxicity of intravenous anaesthetics. *Best Pract Res Clin Anaesthesiol* 2003; **17**(1): 77–89.

48. Vasile B, Rasulo F, Candiani A, Latronico N. The pathophysiology of propofol infusion syndrome: a simple name for a complex syndrome. *Intensive Care Med* 2003; **29**(9): 1417–25.

49. Riker RR, Fraser GL. Adverse events associated with sedatives, analgesics, and other drugs that provide patient comfort in the intensive care unit. *Pharmacotherapy* 2005; **25**(5 Pt 2): 8S–18S.

50. Tobias JD. Sedation and analgesia in the pediatric intensive care unit. *Pediatr Ann* 2005; **34**(8): 636–45.

51. Krauss B, Green SM. Procedural sedation and analgesia in children. *Lancet* 2006; **367**: 766–80.

52. White M, deGraaf P, Renshof B *et al.* Pharmacokinetics of S(+) ketamine derived from target controlled infusion. *Br J Anaesth* 2006; **96**(3): 330–4.

53. Becke K, Albrecht S, Schmitz B *et al.* Intraoperative low-dose S-ketamine has no preventive effects on postoperative pain and morphine consumption after major urological surgery in children. *Paediatr Anaesth* 2005; **15**(6): 484–90.

54. Lin C, Durieux ME. Ketamine and kids: an update. *Paediatr Anaesth* 2005; **15**(2): 91–7.

55. Salonem M, Kanto J, Iisalo E, Himberg JJ. Midazolam as an induction agent in children. *Anesth Analg* 1987; **66**: 625–8.

56. SDCEP. *Conscious sedation in dentistry.* Dundee: Scottish Dental Clinical Effectiveness Programme, 2006.

57. SIGN. *Safe sedation of children undergoing diagnostic and therapeutic procedures.* Edinburgh: Scottish Intercollegiate Guidelines Network, 2004.

58. Averley PA, Girdler NM, Bond S *et al.* A randomised controlled trial of paediatric conscious sedation for dental treatment using intravenous midazolam combined with inhaled nitrous oxide or nitrous oxide/sevoflurane. *Anaesthesia* 2004; **59**(9): 844–52.

59. Robb ND, Hosey MT, Leitch JA. Intravenous conscious sedation in patients under 16 years of age. Fact or fiction? *Br Dental J* 2003; **194**(9): 469–71.

60. Jones RDM, Lawson AD, Andrew LJ *et al.* Antagonism of the hypnotic effect of midazolam in children. *Br J Anaesth* 1991; **66**: 660–6.

61. Sarkar M, Laussen PC, Zurakowski D *et al.* Hemodynamic responses to etomidate on induction of anesthesia in pediatric patients. *Anesth Analg* 2005; **101**(3): 645–50.

62. Schechter WS, Kim C, Martinez M *et al.* Anaesthetic induction in a child with end-stage cardiomyopathy. *Can J Anaesth* 1995; **42**(5 Pt 1): 404–8.

63. Marsh BJ, Morton NS, White M, Kenny GN. A computer controlled infusion of propofol for induction and maintenance of anaesthesia in children. *Can J Anaesth* 1990; **37**(4 Pt 2): S97.

64. Marsh B, White M, Morton N, Kenny GN. Pharmacokinetic model driven infusion of propofol in children. *Br J Anaesth* 1991; **67**(1): 41–8.

65. Varveris DA, Morton NS. Target controlled infusion of propofol for induction and maintenance of anaesthesia using the paedfusor: an open pilot study. *Paediatr Anaesth* 2002; **12**(7): 589–93.

66. Morton NS. Total intravenous anaesthesia (TIVA) in paediatrics: advantages and disadvantages. *Paediatr Anaesth* 1998; **8**(3): 189–94.

67. Eyres R. Update on TIVA. *Paediatr Anaesth* 2004; **14**(5): 374–9.

68. Vuyk J. Pharmacokinetic and pharmacodynamic interactions between opioids and propofol. *J Clin Anesth* 1997; **9**: 23–6.

69. Drover DR, Litalien C, Wellis V *et al.* Determination of the pharmacodynamic interaction of propofol and remifentanil during esophagogastro-duodenoscopy in children. *Anesthesiology* 2004; **100**(6): 1382–6.

70. Roberts FL, Dixon J, Lewis GT *et al*. Induction and maintenance of propofol anaesthesia. A manual infusion scheme. *Anaesthesia* 1988; **43**(suppl): 14–17.

71. Browne BL, Prys-Roberts C, Wolf AR. Propofol and alfentanil in children: infusion technique and dose requirement for total i.v. anaesthesia. *Br J Anaesth* 1992; **69**(6): 570–6.

72. Crawford MW, Hickey C, Zaarour C *et al*. Development of acute opioid tolerance during infusion of remifentanil for pediatric scoliosis surgery. *Anesth Analg* 2006; **102**(6): 1662–7.

73. Amutike D, Lal A, Absalom A, Kenny GNC. Accuracy of the Paedfusor: A new propofol target-controlled infusion system for children. *Br J Anaesth* 2001; **87**: 175P–6P.

74. Absalom A, Amutike D, Lal A *et al*. Accuracy of the 'Paedfusor' in children undergoing cardiac surgery or catheterization. *Br J Anaesth* 2003; **91**: 507–13.

75. Kataria BK, Ved SA, Nicodemus HF *et al*. The pharmacokinetics of propofol in children using three different data analysis approaches. *Anesthesiology* 1994; **80**: 104–22.

76. Munoz HR, Cortinez LI, Ibacache ME, Altermatt FR. Estimation of the plasma effect site equilibration rate constant (k_{e0}) of propofol in children using the time to peak effect: comparison with adults. *Anesthesiology* 2004; **101**(6): 1269–74.

77. Minto CF, Schnider TW, Egan TD *et al*. Influence of age and gender on the pharmacokinetics and pharmacodynamics of remifentanil. I. Model development. *Anesthesiology* 1997; **86**: 10–23.

78. Minto CF, Schnider TW, Shafer SL. Pharmacokinetics and pharmacodynamics of remifentanil. II. Model application. *Anesthesiology* 1997; **86**: 24–33.

79. Maitre PO, Vozeh S, Heykants J *et al*. Population pharmacokinetics of alfentanil: the average dose-plasma concentration relationship and interindividual variability in patients. *Anesthesiology* 1987; **66**: 3–12.

80. Bovill JG, Sebel PS, C.L. B *et al*. The pharmacokinetics of sufentanil in surgical patients. *Anesthesiology* 1984; **61**: 502–6.

81. Shann F. *Drug doses*, 13th edn. Melbourne: Royal Children's Hospital, 2005.

82. Glass PSA, Shafer SL, Reves JG. Intravenous drug delivery systems. In: Miller RD, ed. *Anesthesia*, 5th edn. New York: Churchill-Livingstone; 2000, 377–411.

83. Absalom A, Kenny GNC. 'Paedfusor' pharmacokinetic data set. *Br J Anaesth* 2005; **95**(1): 110.

12

Opioids

D GLYN WILLIAMS

KEY LEARNING POINTS

- Genetic constitution may alter the physiological response to opioids.
- Neonatal opioid pharmacology and pharmacokinetics are influenced by the immaturity of physiological systems.
- Interindividual variation means that a dose–response cannot be predicted by gestational age.
- Intercurrent illness will affect opioid metabolism.
- Clinical use of opioids in the very young requires titration to effect.

INTRODUCTION

Preparations of the opium poppy *Papaver somniferum* have been used for hundreds of years, as sedatives and for the treatment of pain and diarrhoea. In the early nineteenth century Sertürner isolated a crystalline sample of the main constituent alkaloid and named it after Morpheus, the God of Dreams. Morphine was subsequently shown to be the main analgesic constituent of opium.

Despite advances in the range and techniques of analgesia, opioids, in particular morphine, remain one of the most powerful and widely used analgesic interventions. Opioid analgesia is extensively used in children of all ages and is considered safe in even the most premature of neonates provided that accepted dosing regimens are used, accompanied by appropriate monitoring and staff education.

Clinically, however, opioid action is often variable and unpredictable in the neonate and infant. Organ development is likely to be important in the regulation of opioid analgesia and significant changes occur both before and after

birth that affect opioid analgesic mechanisms. Research in this area is continually increasing our knowledge and will hopefully lead to more effective and safer use of these drugs in the future.

OPIOID ACTION

The analgesic properties of the opioids depend upon their molecular structural and stereochemical properties. This underpins the theory that they produce their effects by interacting with specific receptors. The first opioid receptors were described in 1973 [1,2] and endogenous opioid ligands were identified shortly afterwards [3].

Subsequent research defined three 'classic' types of opioid receptor: μ, κ and δ. These are located on neuronal cells in the brain, spinal cord, myenteric plexus, peripheral nociceptors and many other cell types, including lymphocytes, monocytes, skeletal and cardiac muscle. Genes for these receptors have also been cloned [4]. More recently, cDNA encoding an 'orphan' receptor, ORL_1 (opioid receptor-like), has been identified which has a high degree of homology to the opioid receptors and has been classified as an opioid receptor on structural grounds [5]. Pharmacological and genetic studies have attempted to further subdivide the opioid receptors into subgroups but have proved inconclusive [6].

The μ-opioid receptor has been shown to play a central role in opioid analgesia. Morphine, a μ-opioid receptor agonist, has reduced effect in mu-opioid receptor 'knock-out' mice – as do κ- and δ-opioid receptor agonists [7,8]. κ-Opioid receptor agonists have no effect in κ-opioid receptor 'knock-out' mice whereas the analgesic effects of morphine remain intact [9].

Opioid agonist binding and subsequent receptor activation initiate a cascade of events. The opioid receptors are G-protein-coupled receptors and their signals are transduced through interaction with guanine nucleotide-binding proteins. The resultant common cellular actions, include inhibition of adenylyl cyclase, activation of potassium conductance, inhibition of calcium conductance and direct inhibition of transmitter release. Depending on the site, opioids inhibit the release of excitatory and/or inhibitory transmitters. This can have numerous and complicated effects, which produce the wide range of observed physiological responses.

Opioids act at multiple sites to produce analgesia.

Spinal

Abundant opioid receptors are found in the superficial layers of the dorsal horn, the major site of termination of fine-diameter A- and C-fibres, and fewer are found in the deeper layers. Opioid receptors are mainly associated with C-fibre terminals (both pre- and post-synaptically) and act by reducing release of primary afferent transmitters.

Supraspinal

Opioids reduce nociceptive input to the brain by altering ascending and descending control systems. Opioid receptors are widely distributed throughout the central nervous system (CNS) with high concentrations found in the thalamus, the periaqueductal grey matter, the limbic system and the caudate–putamen.

Peripheral

Increasingly opioid receptors are being found outside the CNS, particularly in painful inflammatory conditions. During the inflammatory process opioid receptors are 'transported' from the dorsal root ganglia to the peripheral sensory nerve endings, where they interact with endogenous opioid peptides, carried by immune cells, to elicit a local analgesic effect.

DEVELOPMENT AND OPIOID EFFICACY

Clinically, it is appreciated that opioids have variable and unpredictable effects in neonates and infants, over and above the variation of drug efficacy at all ages. During development from foetus to infancy and beyond, maturation occurs in all organ systems affecting both opioid handling (pharmacokinetics) and effects (pharmacodynamics). These changes do not occur uniformly in all children because they depend on many factors. For example, the drug doses required in a term neonate at birth may be different from those in a term neonate at 2 weeks and are different again from those in a preterm neonate.

Variation in opioid efficacy during development has been mainly studied in the laboratory because of the ethical issues and technical difficulties of research in young children. A wide range of species, behavioural tests, age ranges, doses and routes of administration have been used and, consequently, results have been variable making it difficult to draw firm conclusions and extrapolate the findings to humans. On the whole, current literature suggests that opioids, mainly morphine, produce a dose-related antinociception in rats at all ages. In studies of the response to mechanical stimulation there is an increased sensitivity to morphine in the younger animals whether given by the epidural or parenteral routes [10,11]. In studies of noxious thermal stimulation, however, the reverse is true, with a greater antinociception effect seen in the older animals [11,12]. This suggests that nociceptive development is important in opioid efficacy.

Early studies showed that opioid-based perioperative analgesia resulted in clinical benefits in the neonate [13,14]. The lack of an objective measure for pain has made the comparison of different opioids and potencies across age groups impossible. Nevertheless, studies show that, like adults, there is no simple relationship between serum morphine concentrations and analgesic efficacy [15,16]. One study showed that younger children (4–8 years) had higher postoperative requirements of morphine after major surgery than older children (9–15 years) [17].

A study in neonates and infants found that age was the most important factor affecting morphine requirements [18]. Following non-cardiac surgery, younger neonates were found to have significantly lower morphine requirements than older neonates. It was also found that morphine plasma concentrations were not correlated with analgesia or respiratory depression.

Several factors may contribute to the developmental variation in opioid efficacy (Fig. 12.1).

Nociceptive development

Nociceptive development involves many changes in the structure and function of primary afferent synapses, neuro-transmitter/receptor expression and function and

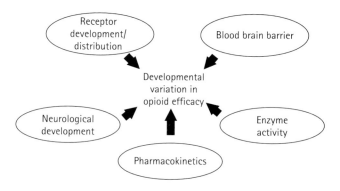

Figure 12.1 Factors affecting developmental variation in opioid efficacy.

excitatory and inhibitory modulation from higher brain centres [19,20]. The changing morphine sensitivity seen in the postnatal period may be part of a general reorganisation in the pattern of central synaptic connectivity that occurs throughout the sensory nervous system.

Receptor development

Laboratory studies show that opioid receptor expression and binding undergo considerable postnatal reorganisation [21,22]. In newborn rats μ-opioid receptor binding is diffusely distributed throughout the dorsal horn of the spinal cord. The density of binding sites increases until day 7 of life, thereafter falling to adult levels by day 21 [22]. The distribution also gradually changes over the first postnatal weeks to achieve the adult pattern of densely packed μ-opioid receptor-binding sites in the superficial dorsal horn and little in the deeper layers.

In the dorsal root ganglion there is a greater proportion of cells expressing the μ-opioid receptor in the first week of life compared with day 21 [21]. Also, in the first postnatal week, the μ-opioid receptor is expressed in cell bodies across the whole diameter range, including non-nociceptive Aβ mechanoreceptors and proprioreceptors as well as nociceptors. By 3 weeks, however, expression is restricted to small- and medium-diameter cells [23]. This suggests that opioid action in the newborn could affect both low threshold and nociceptive neurons and thus be less selective than in the adult. Opioid receptor development at supraspinal level has been less extensively studied but the evidence suggests that developmental regulation in distribution and expression is seen [24].

The μ-opioid receptors in young animals have been shown to be biologically functional despite their altered distribution [11]. The proportion of small Aδ and C nociceptive cells sensitive to μ-opioid receptor agonists is not different between the adult and neonate. In contrast a higher proportion of Aβ cells have μ-opioid receptors in the neonate compared with the adult. This may explain in part the behavioural differences in the sensitivity of morphine with postnatal age.

Pharmacokinetics

Following birth there are changes in the pharmacokinetics of all drugs, due to maturation of organ and enzyme systems, changes in body composition and the withdrawal of maternal hormones (Table 12.1).

Studies of the pharmacokinetics of opioids in neonates and infants have mainly involved morphine. There is much variability between these studies as a result of small numbers of patients, differences in study design, indications for opioid treatment, analytical procedures and pharmacokinetic assumptions and calculations. There is considerable interindividual variability and this contributes to the wide range of morphine serum concentrations observed during constant infusions [25].

Meta-analysis has found that the volume of distribution of morphine is the same irrespective of age [26]. Clearance of morphine matures with postconceptual age and reaches adult levels by 2–12 months of life [25,27]. This enables calculation of an infusion rate of 20 μg/kg/h which matches plasma clearance and which will maintain a steady plasma concentration [28].

A similar pharmacokinetic pattern is also seen with fentanyl. (Table 12.2). The elimination half-life of fentanyl increases with decreasing age [26]. Newer synthetic opioids (fentanyl, alfentanil and remifentanil) are frequently given by infusion during anaesthesia and intensive care. In a three-compartment model, a drug distributes from the central to peripheral compartments and is redistributed back to the central compartment after the infusion stops. The half-time of the decline in drug plasma concentration is therefore related to the duration of the infusion as well as the rate of elimination and this is termed the context-sensitive half-time (CSHT). Remifentanil can be considered context insensitive, whereas the half-times of alfentanil and fentanyl are related to infusion duration (see below).

Table 12.1 Pharmacokinetics of morphine in neonates, infants and children: mean half-life and clearance ($\pm$ SD) [26], clearance for neonates after cardiac surgery presented as a mean and range from Lynn *et al* [31].

	Half–life (hours)	Clearance (mL/kg/min)
Preterm neonates	9.0 (3.4)	2.2 (0.7)
Term neonates	6.5 (2.8)	8.1 (3.2)
After cardiac surgery		5.5 (3.4–13.8)*
Critically ill		2.1
Infants and children	2.0 (1.8)	23.6 (8.5)

From Kart *et al.* [26].
*From Lynn *et al.* [31].

Table 12.2   Age-related clearances of morphine and fentanyl standardised to a 70-kg person: mean clearance (±SD)

Age	Morphine CL allometric ¾ (L/h per 70 kg)	Age	Fentanyl CL allometric ¾ (L/h per 70 kg)
Neonate (<1 week)	13.1 (8.7)	Neonate (<1 month)	31.5 (5.2)
Neonate (1 week–2 months)	18.4 (7.9)		
Infant (2–6 months)	48.8 (15.6)	Infant (1 month)	41.1 (3.2)
Infant (6 months–2.5 years)	51 (13–68)	Child (1–5 years)	34.1 (12.3)
Adult	63 (4)	Adult	43.0 (7.3)

From Tibboel et al. [29].

Protein binding

Protein binding is decreased in the preterm and term neonate compared with adults, although the degree of protein binding for morphine is low in both populations and has a minor effect on the discrepancy in free morphine concentrations [29]. There is a delayed redistribution phase in younger animals leading to higher initial plasma and brain concentrations after single doses [30]. Clinical circumstances such as concurrent illness and type of surgery can all affect morphine pharmacokinetics [29]. Infants undergoing cardiac surgery showed consistently lower morphine clearance compared with their age-matched peers having non-cardiac surgery [31].

Enzyme activity

Drug metabolism occurs via several enzyme systems – mainly in the liver but also in many other organs. The maturation and activity of these systems, and indeed individual enzymes, is not consistent during development. Therefore, the efficacy of a drug during development will depend on the maturation pattern of the particular enzyme or system involved. Hence there is no consistent pattern of enzyme activity on the metabolism of opioids during development. The contrasting development of the metabolism of morphine and codeine is a good example.

Morphine is mainly metabolised by glucuronidation to morphine-3-glucuronide (M-3-G) and morphine-6-glucuronide (M-6-G). The glucuronidation pathway is present but immature at birth and continues to develop after the neonatal period [32,33]. Term neonates, infants and young children are capable of metabolising morphine to M-3-G and M-6-G [34]; however, preterm infants show a reduced metabolic capacity correlated with decreased gestational age and decreased birth weight, but with large interindividual variations [35,36].

Morphine-6-glucuronide is an active and potent metabolite with analgesic properties, whereas M-3-G has no analgesic properties. In experimental models M-3-G has been shown to be a CNS stimulant, and can displace morphine from the μ receptor. In adults the normal ratio of M-3-G to M-6-G is 10:1 whereas in neonates, especially prematures of low birth weight, the ratio approximates to 4:1, though with large interindividual variability [37]. Thus there is relatively more M-6-G present at younger ages and potentially more analgesia. This may be used to explain the longer duration of a single dose of morphine in a neonate [38].

In contrast, the efficacy of codeine may be decreased in neonates and infants as a result of diminished enzyme activity. Codeine analgesia is due almost entirely to its conversion to morphine, a reaction catalysed by the cytochrome P450 enzyme CYP2D6. At birth the activity of this enzyme is low and it increases slowly during early life. In pre-school years the activity is still only 25–50 per cent of adult levels [39]. Laboratory studies have shown that in young rats, where the enzyme activity is low, there is little or no analgesia from a dose of codeine. In contrast, in older animals, CYP2D6 activity is higher and analgesic effect is present [40].

Blood–brain barrier

Developmental differences in the structure and function of the blood–brain barrier (BBB) could have an important effect on the amount of opioid present in the CNS and thus on efficacy. Animal studies suggest that at birth the BBB is intact and that function is unaffected by age [41,42]. The amount of opioid binding in the spinal cord is also unaffected by age [10]. However, removal of morphine from the cerebrospinal fluid (CSF) depends on an active transport system located in the BBB involving P-glycoprotein. Downregulation of this system leads to increased analgesic effect [43]. Little is known about the effect of development on the activity of this transport system, though decreased activity is seen in old age [44].

PHARMACOGENETICS

In addition to developmental factors, the variability in efficacy may also be caused by common factors including intercurrent illness, concurrent drug therapy and psychosocial interactions. The importance of genetic variation in the efficacy of all drugs is being increasingly recognised.

Proteins are involved in every stage of the pharmacological journey of a drug through the body. Genes coding for these proteins show genetic variation and could thus influence efficacy. Furthermore there is genetic variability in how individuals perceive and respond to pain [45]. In animal models, within- and between-strain differences in the efficacy of morphine have been related to altered function of the μ and κ receptors. Genetic variation of these receptor types is one explanation for the difference in function [46,47].

Several mutations of the μ-opioid receptor have been described; their effect on opioid efficacy is unknown but they may influence opioid-regulated behaviours or drug addiction [48]. Opioid receptors have polymorphic regions which might influence expression and function of binding sites. The A118G polymorphism of the μ-opioid receptor has been shown to decrease pupillary constriction by M-6-G and carriers of this polymorphism have a decreased analgesic effect with M-6-G [49,50].

The extent to which an individual metabolises a drug is, in part, genetically determined. During evolution living organisms have developed xenobiotic metabolising enzymes in response to the differing 'foreign' chemicals. Over time genetic changes have led to differences between and within populations in the metabolic abilities of these enzyme systems. In humans the cytochrome P450 enzymes, for example, account for the phase 1 metabolism of most drugs; there are a number of sequence variations in the cytochrome P450 genes, resulting in functionally different phenotypes. Cytochrome enzyme CYP2D6, which converts codeine to morphine, has over 50 different genetic variants, leading to a large interindividual variation in morphine production after codeine administration. Animal and human experiments show that individuals who are unable to produce morphine from codeine will have no analgesic benefit from codeine [51,52].

PHYSIOLOGICAL EFFECTS OF OPIOIDS

Opioids have a wide range of effects on a number of different organ systems (Table 12.3), affording not only clinically desired analgesic effects but also adverse effects.

All opioids cause dose-dependent depression of ventilation primarily by reducing the sensitivity of the brain stem to hypercapnia and hypoxia. They also interfere with the rhythm of breathing regulated by centres in the medulla. Initially, respiratory rate is affected but at higher doses tidal volume is also decreased. Opioids shift the carbon dioxide response curve to the right and reduce its slope; this effect is worsened by the co-administration of a sedative [53]. In neonates and infants respiratory depression has been shown to occur at plasma concentrations as low as 20 ng/mL [54].

The risk of opioid respiratory depression is increased in neonates, in patients who are haemodynamically unstable

Table 12.3 Physiological effects of opioids

1. Central nervous system
   - Analgesia
   - Sedation
   - Dysphoria and euphoria
   - Nausea and vomiting
   - Miosis
   - Seizures
   - Pruritis
   - Psychomimetic behaviours, excitation
2. Respiratory system
   - Antitussive
   - Respiratory depression
      ↓ respiratory rate
      ↓ tidal volume
      ↓ ventilatory response to carbon dioxide
3. Cardiovascular system
   - Minimal effects on cardiac output
   - Heart rate
      bradycardia seen on most occasions
   - Vasodilatation, venodilatation
      morphine >> other opioids ?histamine effect
4. Gastrointestinal system
   - ↓ Intestinal motility and peristalsis
   - ↑ Sphincter tone
      sphincter of Oddi
      Ileocolic
5. Urinary system
   - ↑ Tone
      uterus
      bladder
      detrusor muscles of the bladder
6. Musculoskeletal system
   - ↑ Chest wall rigidity

and in those who have reduced conscious level, disordered ventilation, a tendency to apnoea or a known airway problem. Increasing sedation, miosis and decreasing tidal volume all predict impending respiratory depression. Measurement of sedation is increasingly being recognised as an important method of monitoring children receiving parenteral or spinal opioids.

Nausea and vomiting are commonly reported following the use of opioids. It is thought to result from stimulation of the chemoreceptor trigger zone in the brain stem; however, the pathogenesis of nausea and vomiting is complex and other CNS centres are also involved. Many antiemetics with differing modes of action have been shown to have some efficacy in the treatment and/or prevention of opioid-induced vomiting but no single antiemetic has a high therapeutic index. In children nausea and vomiting have been reported following the use of all opioids. The studies, however, are usually perioperative and, consequently, other factors may be important; codeine may have a low rate compared with morphine [55,56]. Morphine, fentanyl and tramadol have been reported to show an equal risk. Pethidine may have a lower risk because of its anti-muscarinic effects but this has not been proven.

Opioids tend to have little effect on the cardiovascular system. They can cause vasodilatation and venous pooling but this is usually not clinically appreciable unless there are other associated medical problems such as, hypovolaemia or cardiovascular insufficiency. These effects are seen predominately with morphine and are mostly caused by histamine release. In neonates receiving intensive care morphine could be a factor contributing to hypotension; high doses have a greater effect than normal doses [29]. Provision of analgesia may result in hypotension, as pain is often accompanied by increased cardiac sympathetic activity.

Opioids depress the cough reflex by a direct effect on the cough centre in the medulla. They inhibit intestinal smooth muscle activity which decreases peristalsis and increases tone at the pyloric and anal sphincter and the ileocaecal valve. Consequently, they are often used in preparatory remedies for coughs and diarrhoea. Spasm at the sphincter of Oddi occurs with all pure μ-opioid receptor agonists, though there is still much debate as to whether individual opioids have more or less effect in this respect.

SPINAL OPIOIDS

Spinal (epidural or intrathecal) opioid administration was introduced into clinical practice in the hope that it would produce intense spinal analgesia without the systemic side-effects In adults and children it is effective but is associated with adverse effects. There is now strong evidence that not all opioids administered by the epidural or intrathecal route produce analgesia by acting only at the spinal level [57].

Lipid solubility has been shown to be the most important factor affecting the site of action of spinally administered opioids. After epidural administration the more lipid-soluble drugs (fentanyl, alfentanil and sufentanil) remain in the epidural space for longer than the more hydrophilic drugs (morphine and diamorphine) [58,59]. The CSF concentrations of hydrophilic opioids are much higher than those of lipophilic opioids whereas, in simultaneous plasma samples, the reverse is true [57].

When administered into the intrathecal space lipophilic opioids are much more rapidly cleared from the aqueous CSF into the tissues [60] and thus undergo limited rostral spread. In the spinal cord the concentration of hydrophilic opioids is much higher in the grey matter (the site of opioid receptor binding) than that of the lipophilic opioids [60].

These findings suggest that the spinal bioavailability of lipophilic opioids is low and that they work more by redistribution into plasma. Clinical studies in adults confirm this. Continuous epidural infusion of fentanyl has been shown to produce analgesia by uptake into plasma and redistribution to CNS opioid receptors [61]. In contrast, an epidural bolus of fentanyl will produce some spinally mediated analgesia as the larger mass of drug in the epidural space will allow a small fraction to reach the CSF, thereby giving a short-lived spinally mediated effect. When titrated to an equal analgesic effect the doses of epidural and systemic lipophilic opioids are equivalent, whereas much lower doses of hydrophilic opioids are needed. Following intrathecal administration all opioids have some spinally mediated analgesic effect, but the lipophilic drugs result in higher plasma concentrations and equianalgesic doses of the hydrophilic opioids are much lower [57].

This work has not been repeated in children and the dosing regimens are similar to those used in adults. The pharmacology of spinally administered opioids in younger children has not been extensively studied and thus practice varies (age and choice of opioid) between centres [62].

Adverse effects such as pruritis, nausea and vomiting and urinary retention are seen but their incidence at different ages and for the different opioids needs to be clarified.

OPIOIDS IN CLINICAL USE

Morphine

Despite the wide variety of opioids available for clinical use morphine remains the most widely used, and studied, in children. It can be administered by a variety of routes and, using accepted dosing regimens, has been shown to be safe and effective in children of all ages.

No concentration–response relationship for morphine in children has been described. The effectiveness of intravenous morphine in infants has been studied in children using validated pain assessment tools. After major surgery, continuous morphine doses of 10–40 μg/kg/h have been shown to be effective in alleviating pain in children aged 0–14 years [63,64]. Intravenous morphine at continuous doses of 10–30 μg/kg/h has also been shown to decrease pain in premature neonates requiring artificial ventilation [65]. Owing to the large interindividual variations in the developmental pharmacology of morphine it is often titrated to effect, usually an initial intravenous dose of 0.1–0.2 mg/kg. For term and preterm neonates these doses should be reduced in relation to size and maturity. Initial doses of 0.025 mg/kg have been recommended [66]. A lower dose may be wise in critically ill patients or those receiving supplementary analgesics.

Intravenous access and administration are preferred. In a study comparing infusion and bolus administration there was no advantage in infants but in children aged over 1 year a continuous infusion was found to be superior [63]. More sophisticated methods of intravenous morphine delivery such as patient- and nurse-controlled analgesia (PCA and NCA, respectively,) allow greater flexibility. They can be more effective and, although they have been associated with higher opioid consumption, they have similar or increased rates of side-effects [67,68].

Intramuscular injection is considered unacceptable in the non-anaesthetised child and has been shown to be less effective [69]. The subcutaneous route may have similar efficacy to the intravenous route provided that there is good skin perfusion [70]. Again, this route is acceptable only if there is an indwelling subcutaneous cannula.

Morphine can be administered orally, rectally, transtracheally and into intra-articular, epidural and subarachnoid spaces. When administered orally the bioavailability is low and the effect is variable. Nevertheless oral morphine is effective in many situations and can be titrated to effect. Lower doses are recommended in the term and preterm neonate. Absorption via the rectal route is unreliable and there is the potential for delayed respiratory depression. Parenteral morphine is also associated with histamine release, though this is rarely associated with hypotension in children.

Diamorphine

Diamorphine (diacetylmorphine or heroin) is a semisynthetic opioid. It is the 3,6-diacetyl derivative of morphine. It is more lipid soluble than morphine and crosses the BBB far more rapidly and consequently has a faster onset of action. It is considered to be a prodrug because it is active after deacetylation to 6-monoacetylmorphine and morphine. It is licensed in the UK but not widely available in other countries; it is stigmatised by its association with recreational drug addiction.

Despite this problem it has been used effectively and safely in children of all ages via several routes. In adults diamorphine has a better side-effect profile than morphine when given via the epidural or intrathecal route. Recently diamorphine has been used in children via the intranasal route to treat pain in the emergency setting because it is effective and has a fast onset of action [71].

Fentanyl

Fentanyl is a synthetic opioid acting on the μ-opioid receptor and is 50–100 times more potent than morphine. It has few direct cardiovascular effects [72] and is the preferred opioid for critically ill patients with haemodynamic instability; it has been used successfully in neonates with bronchopulmonary dysplasia, pulmonary hypertension, diaphragmatic hernia and those on extracorporeal membrane oxygenation (ECMO) [29]. Fentanyl has a high lipid solubility compared with other opioids and a molecular conformation that enables efficient penetration of the BBB. Consequently, it has a fast onset and short duration of action.

Like morphine, there are age-dependent effects on its pharmacology. Protein binding is greater than for morphine, with increased protein binding in the preterm neonate compared with the term neonate (77 per cent versus 70 per cent)

[73]. The clearance and half-life in preterm neonates are extremely variable and prolonged compared with term neonates and more respiratory depression is seen [74]. Term neonates also have a longer clearance and half-life than older children. Older children (>3 months) have a higher clearance than adults and therefore have a shorter elimination half-life [75]. Fentanyl clearance is dependent on hepatic function and blood flow; thus factors that affect either of these, such as development, mechanical obstruction and disease, will alter clearance. Also, like morphine, the pharmacokinetics are altered during cardiac surgery [76]. In critically ill children on continuous infusions there is marked variability (up to 10-fold) in the elimination half-life and infusion rates needed to achieve similar levels of sedation [77].

Fentanyl metabolism is related to the cytochrome P450 enzyme CYP3A4. All of the metabolites are inactive and only a small amount is renally eliminated unchanged. The CYP3A4 enzyme shows genetic variability and fast and slow metabolisers of fentanyl have been identified. Concurrent administration of medicines metabolised by this enzyme, for example paracetamol, may alter fentanyl metabolism.

Termination of action of fentanyl is by a combination of redistribution and hepatic clearance. At low doses the high lipid solubility allows for this to occur rapidly and also enables the fast onset and short duration of action. High-dose fentanyl accumulates in muscle, fat and other lipid-rich tissue and recirculates more slowly. The context-sensitive half-life after an infusion of 1 hour is approximately 20 minutes but after 8 hours it is 270 minutes [78].

The usual initial bolus dose of intravenous fentanyl is 1–3 μg/kg. Starting doses in term and preterm neonates should be lower. In preterm infants it has been shown to reduce significantly surgical stress responses and improve postoperative outcome [13]. Continuous operative and postoperative infusions of fentanyl are commonly used in paediatric patients of all ages and it has also been used to provide PCA and NCA.

Fentanyl is rapidly absorbed through the oral mucosa, which bypasses the liver and uptake continues for sometime after consumption. This route is effective for premedication, procedural pain, chronic pain and exacerbations of acute pain. Transdermal fentanyl is also increasingly being used with some success in children. It provides continuous low-dose drug administration over a prolonged period. Variations in patch design from different pharmaceutical companies mean that they are not interchangeable (see http://www.mhra.gov.uk).

Alfentanil

Alfentanil is derived from fentanyl and has a rapid onset, a brief duration of action, a smaller volume of distribution, lower lipid solubility and about one-quarter the potency of fentanyl. It is more rapidly eliminated and thus has a shorter duration of action. Studies in adults and children show that the pharmacokinetics are independent of dose [79]. The volume of distribution is smaller in neonates than older children. Clearance is similar at all ages apart from neonates where it is decreased, leading to a prolonged half-life in this age group [80]. Protein binding also increases with age, being 65 per cent in the preterm, 79 per cent in term neonates and 90 per cent in adults [73]. As with fentanyl, hepatic function and blood flow have a marked effect on clearance and any impairment will prolong the clinical effects of alfentanil. Renal failure has little effect on elimination.

The pharmacology of this drug suggests that it has the potential for rapid control of analgesia and rapid awakening from anaesthesia. It has been used for tracheal intubation combined with propofol and high doses have been used in cardiac surgery. High doses also show an increase in context-sensitive half-life.

Sufentanil

Sufentanil, another synthetic opioid, is 5–10 times more potent than fentanyl. Elimination is unaffected by renal failure but dependent on hepatic blood flow. Pharmacokinetic studies in children undergoing cardiac surgery found age-dependent changes; neonates have a larger volume of distribution, slower clearance and a longer and more variable half-life [81]. Protein binding also increases with age.

Bradycardia and asystole have been reported after intravenous bolus and a concurrent vagolytic agent is advised. There are also reports of its use via the intranasal route as premedication [82].

Remifentanil

Remifentanil is a selective μ-opioid receptor agonist that is chemically similar to the fentanyl family, but it is unique in that its metabolism is independent of hepatic and renal function. An ester linkage allows rapid metabolism to a carboxylic acid metabolite by blood and tissue esterases. It is highly lipid soluble, has a higher potency than alfentanil and a duration of action of only a few minutes.

It is usually given as a continuous intravenous infusion (loading dose 0.5–1 μg/kg; maintenance dose 0.1–0.5 μ/kg/min). Unlike the other opioids there is no increase in the context-sensitive half-life irrespective of the dose used or the length of infusion [66]. The elimination half-life is constant across all ages. Other pharmacokinetic data show a deceased clearance with increasing age and a smaller volume of distribution in children than in adults [83].

This favourable pharmacokinetic profile suggests that remifentanil is superior to other opioids in terms of recovery profile and can be used effectively in even the youngest of children. It seems to be haemodynamically stable in neonates and may be considered safe to use in the critically ill patient. It is, however, a profound respiratory depressant

and there is evidence of rapid development of tolerance [84]. Bradycardia has been reported following bolus doses, especially after larger doses and a vagolytic agent may be required. It is being increasingly used in paediatric anaesthesia as part of a balanced anaesthetic technique; infusion rates of 0.25 μg/kg/min appear to be safe and effective in neonates [85].

Codeine

Codeine is a naturally occurring opium alkaloid that is less potent than morphine and considered sufficient for mild-to-moderate pain. It is reputed to have a low incidence of side-effects, which has made it popular for infants and in situations where airway management or neurological assessment is critical.

Codeine can be given by the oral, rectal and intramuscular routes. The intravenous route is not recommended because of reports of profound hypotension, probably due to histamine release. In children it has been used for both acute and chronic pain and as a cough suppressant and antidiarrhoea remedy.

Experimental evidence suggests that codeine is a prodrug for morphine. The analgesic effect of codeine is almost wholly due to its conversion to morphine though, interestingly, the side-effect profile may not be dependent on this conversion [52]. The conversion of codeine to morphine is catalysed by the cytochrome P450 enzyme CYP2D6 which, because of genetic and developmental regulation, leads to large variability in effect. Meta-analysis has estimated that the number needed to treat (NNT) for codeine is 18. This compares with an NNT of 5.0 for paracetamol, although when it is given in combination with paracetamol the NNT is 3.1 [86]. There are few studies of analgesic efficacy of codeine in children, but the efficacy may be low and unpredictable [55].

Tramadol

Tramadol is a weak opioid that is being increasingly used in children. It is described as a unique opioid, in that it binds to μ-opioid receptors but also blocks serotonin and noradrenaline reuptake. Its analgesic effect is not completely abolished by naloxone and this suggests that reuptake inhibition is important. It has been shown to have good analgesic efficacy in adults and a low incidence of respiratory depression and sedation.

Tramadol is also catalysed by the CYP2D6 enzyme, but, unlike codeine, it does have significant analgesic efficacy in its own right. One of its metabolites, M1, also has analgesic effects and thus variable CYP2D6 activity may affect tramadol efficacy.

Tramadol can be given orally, rectally and intravenously and as an additive to local anaesthetic agents for caudal epidural analgesia [87]. It has low incidence of respiratory depression and constipation, and has a nausea and vomiting rate similar to that of other opioids. Few pharmacokinetic data are available in young children. One study showed that the clearance was low in the preterm infants but had increased to 84 per cent of mature values by 44 weeks post-conception [88]. Efficacy in children is uncertain. As a sole agent it seems to be less effective than more potent opioids but as part of a multimodal analgesic technique it has been shown to be effective [89,90].

Pethidine

Pethidine is another synthetic opioid that exerts its analgesic effects as a μ-opioid receptor agonist but, in addition, it also has antimuscarinic and local anaesthetic effects. It is considered a strong opioid and has historically been regarded as an equivalent opioid to morphine. It has been used in children of all ages and by many routes of administration. The usual dose is 1–2 mg/kg.

As with other opioids the pharmacokinetics of pethidine vary considerably in neonates and infants [91]. The half-life in children and adults is approximately 3 hours but in neonates the half-life ranges from 3 to 59 hours. Animal data suggest that the infant respiratory system is less sensitive to pethidine than morphine but this has not been repeated in humans. Pethidine must be used with care when clearance is reduced (e.g. renal failure, neonates) because one of its metabolites, norpethidine, is neurotoxic.

The use of pethidine for acute pain has declined in general because its perceived advantages over morphine have not been proven. As in adult practice it remains popular as part of a sedative technique for painful procedures [92]. In some centres it is also the opioid of choice for pancreatitis caused by biliary spasm, although the antispasmodic effects of pethidine postulated have not been shown *in vivo*.

OPIOID AGONIST–ANTAGONISTS

Buprenorphine and nalbuphine have the perceived advantage of demonstrating good analgesia with a ceiling effect on respiratory depression. They should be used as a sole agent, however, as they may reverse the μ-opioid receptor-mediated analgesic effects of the more potent opioids.

This family of drugs has been used with some success in children, though little is known about the pharmacokinetics, in the younger age groups. Nalbuphine is reported to have a shorter elimination half-life in children than adults [93]. As well as the oral route buprenorphine has also been given with some success via the nasal and transdermal routes in children and it has a role in treating opioid-dependent adolescents.

OPIOID ANTAGONISTS

Naloxone has been used safely in children of all ages, including neonates, for the treatment of opioid side-effects. It is rapidly distributed, metabolised and excreted with a half-life of around 1 hour in adults and children. In neonates the half-life has been reported as being between 70 minutes and 3 hours [94].

The half-life of naloxone is shorter than that of many of the opioids commonly used and thus repeated doses or infusions may be necessary to avoid renarcotisation. Naloxone is a μ-opioid receptor antagonist but it has a lower affinity for the μ-receptor than morphine and other opioids and thus it may have an even shorter clinically relevant half-life [66]. It has also been found to antagonise at the κ-opioid receptor.

More recently, opioid antagonists have been studied in both adults and children for the prevention or antagonism of the opioid non-respiratory adverse effects. Low-dose naloxone decreases pruritis, nausea and vomiting and urinary retention, though variable success has been claimed [95,96].

Studies in adults have shown that low doses of naloxone have an opioid-sparing effect and can prevent acute morphine tolerance; similar work in children has not shown this [97]. This unexpected effect may be explained by the molecular mechanism of action. It has been postulated that opioids bind at low concentrations with stimulatory or antanalgesic G-protein-coupled receptor complexes. Low-dose naloxone may block opioid action at the stimulatory receptor complexes but leave the agonist effects at inhibitory receptor complexes thus preventing adverse effects and enhancing analgesia. Larger doses of opioid antagonist, however, would also block the inhibitory receptor complexes [98–100]. Studies where low-dose naloxone was administered by continuous infusion showed better results than those where it was administered by intermittent bolus [66].

REFERENCES

Key references

Berde CB, Jaksic T, Lynn AM *et al*. Anesthesia and analgesia during and after surgery in neonates. *Clin Ther* 2005; **27**(6): 900–21.

Crain SM, Shen KF. Antagonists of excitatory opioid receptor functions enhance morphine's analgesic potency and attenuate opioid tolerance/dependence liability. *Pain* 2000; **84**(2–3): 121–31.

Hughes J, Smith TW, Kosterlitz HW *et al*. Identification of two related pentapeptides from the brain with potent opiate agonist activity. *Nature* 1975; **258**(5536): 577–80.

Mogil JS. The genetic mediation of individual differences in sensitivity to pain and its inhibition. *Proc Natl Acad Sci USA* 1999; **96**(14): 7744–51.

Nandi R, Beacham D, Middleton J *et al*. The functional expression of mu opioid receptors on sensory neurons is developmentally regulated; morphine analgesia is less selective in the neonate. *Pain* 2004; **111**(1–2): 38–50.

References

1. Pert CB, Snyder SH. Properties of opiate-receptor binding in rat brain. *Proc Natl Acad Sci USA* 1973; **70**(8): 2243–7.
2. Terenius L. Characteristics of the 'receptor' for narcotic analgesics in synaptic plasma membrane fraction from rat brain. *Acta Pharmacol Toxicol (Copenh)* 1973; **33**(5): 377–84.
3. Hughes J, Smith TW, Kosterlitz HW *et al.* Identification of two related pentapeptides from the brain with potent opiate agonist activity. *Nature* 1975; **258**(5536): 577–80.
4. Kieffer BL, Befort K, Gaveriaux-Ruff C, Hirth CG. The delta-opioid receptor: isolation of a cDNA by expression cloning and pharmacological characterization. *Proc Natl Acad Sci USA* 1992; **89**(24): 12048–52.
5. Mollereau C, Parmentier M, Mailleux P *et al.* ORL1, a novel member of the opioid receptor family. Cloning, functional expression and localization. *FEBS Lett* 1994; **341**(1): 33–8.
6. Raynor K, Kong H, Chen Y *et al.* Pharmacological characterization of the cloned kappa-, delta-, and mu-opioid receptors. *Mol Pharmacol* 1994; **45**(2): 330–4.
7. Matthes HW, Maldonado R, Simonin F *et al.* Loss of morphine-induced analgesia, reward effect and withdrawal symptoms in mice lacking the mu-opioid-receptor gene. *Nature* 1996; **383**(6603): 819–23.
8. Sora I, Li XF, Funada M *et al.* Visceral chemical nociception in mice lacking mu-opioid receptors: effects of morphine, SNC80 and U-50,488. *Eur J Pharmacol* 1999; **366**(2–3): R3–5.
9. Simonin F, Valverde O, Smadja C *et al.* Disruption of the kappa-opioid receptor gene in mice enhances sensitivity to chemical visceral pain, impairs pharmacological actions of the selective kappa-agonist U-50,488H and attenuates morphine withdrawal. *EMBO J* 1998; **17**(4): 886–97.
10. Marsh D, Dickenson A, Hatch D, Fitzgerald M. Epidural opioid analgesia in infant rats I: mechanical and heat responses. *Pain* 1999; **82**(1): 23–32.
11. Nandi R, Beacham D, Middleton J *et al.* The functional expression of mu opioid receptors on sensory neurons is developmentally regulated; morphine analgesia is less selective in the neonate. *Pain* 2004; **111**(1–2): 38–50.
12. Giordano J, Barr GA. Morphine- and ketocyclazocine-induced analgesia in the developing rat: differences due to type of noxious stimulus and body topography. *Brain Res* 1987; **429**(2): 247–53.
13. Anand KJ, Sippell WG, Aynsley-Green A. Randomised trial of fentanyl anaesthesia in preterm babies undergoing surgery: effects on the stress response. *Lancet* 1987; **i**(8524): 62–6.
14. Anand KJ, Hickey PR. Halothane-morphine compared with high-dose sufentanil for anesthesia and postoperative analgesia in neonatal cardiac surgery. *N Engl J Med* 1992; **326**(1): 1–9.
15. Scott CS, Riggs KW, Ling EW *et al.* Morphine pharmacokinetics and pain assessment in premature newborns. *J Pediatr* 1999; **135**(4): 423–9.
16. Lynn AM, Opheim KE, Tyler DC. Morphine infusion after pediatric cardiac surgery. *Crit Care Med* 1984; **12**(10): 863–6.
17. Hansen, TG, Henneberg SW, Hole P. Age-related postoperative morphine requirements in children following major surgery – an assessment using patient-controlled analgesia (PCA). *Eur J Pediatr Surg* 1996; **6**(1): 29–31.
18. Bouwmeester NJ, Hop WC, van Dijk M *et al.* Postoperative pain in the neonate: age-related differences in morphine requirements and metabolism. *Intensive Care Med* 2003; **29**(11): 2009–15.
19. Fitzgerald M, Beggs S. The neurobiology of pain: developmental aspects. *Neuroscientist* 2001; **7**(3): 246–57.
20. Pattinson D, Fitzgerald M. The neurobiology of infant pain: development of excitatory and inhibitory neurotransmission in the spinal dorsal horn. *Reg Anesth Pain Med* 2004; **29**(1): 36–44.
21. Beland B, Fitzgerald M. Mu- and delta-opioid receptors are downregulated in the largest diameter primary sensory neurons during postnatal development in rats. *Pain* 2001; **90**(1–2): 143–50.
22. Rahman W, Dashwood MR, Fitzgerald M *et al.* Postnatal development of multiple opioid receptors in the spinal cord and development of spinal morphine analgesia. *Brain Res Dev Brain Res* 1998; **108**(1–2): 239–54.
23. Nandi R, Fitzgerald M. Opioid analgesia in the newborn. *Eur J Pain* 2005; **9**(2): 105–8.
24. Tsang D, Ng SC, Ho KP. Development of methionine-enkephalin and naloxone binding sites in regions of rat brain. *Brain Res* 1982; **255**(4): 637–44.
25. van Lingen RA, Simons SH, Anderson BJ, Tibboel D. The effects of analgesia in the vulnerable infant during the perinatal period. *Clin Perinatol* 2002; **29**(3): 511–34.
26. Kart T, Christrup LL, Rasmussen M. Recommended use of morphine in neonates, infants and children based on a literature review: Part 1 – Pharmacokinetics. *Paediatr Anaesth* 1997; **7**(1): 5–11.
27. Lynn AM, Slattery JT. Morphine pharmacokinetics in early infancy. *Anesthesiology* 1987; **66**(2): 136–9.
28. Bray R J, Beeton C, Hinton W, Seviour JA. Plasma morphine levels produced by continuous infusion in children. *Anaesthesia* 1986 **41**; 7: 654–8
29. Tibboel, D, Anand KJ, van den Anker JN. The pharmacological treatment of neonatal pain. *Semin Fetal Neonatal Med* 2005; **10**(2): 195–205.
30. Windh RT, Kuhn CM. Increased sensitivity to mu opiate antinociception in the neonatal rat despite weaker receptor-guanyl nucleotide binding protein coupling. *J Pharmacol Exp Ther* 1995; **273**(3): 1353–60.
31. Lynn AM, Nespeca MK, Opheim KE, Slattery JT. Respiratory effects of intravenous morphine infusions in neonates, infants, and children after cardiac surgery. *Anesth Analg* 1993; **77**(4): 695–701.
32. McRorie TI, Lynn AM, Nespeca MK *et al.* The maturation of morphine clearance and metabolism. *Am J Dis Child* 1992; **146**(8): 972–6.

33. Choonara IA, McKay P, Hain R, Rane A. Morphine metabolism in children. *Br J Clin Pharmacol* 1989; **28**(5): 599–604.

34. Choonara I, Lawrence A, Michalkiewicz A *et al*. Morphine metabolism in neonates and infants. *Br J Clin Pharmacol* 1992; **34**(5): 434–7.

35. Hartley R, Green M, Quinn MW *et al*. Development of morphine glucuronidation in premature neonates. *Biol Neonate* 1994; **66**(1): 1–9.

36. Bhat R, Abu-Harb M, Chari G, Gulati A. Morphine metabolism in acutely ill preterm newborn infants. *J Pediatr* 1992; **120**(5): 795–9.

37. Faura CC, Collins SL, Moore RA, McQuay H. J.Systematic review of factors affecting the ratios of morphine and its major metabolites. *Pain* 1998; **74**(1): 43–53.

38. Kart T, Christrup LL, Rasmussen M. Recommended use of morphine in neonates, infants and children based on a literature review: Part 2 – Clinical use. *Paediatr Anaesth* 1997; **7**(2): 93–101.

39. Jacqz-Aigrain E, Cresteil T. Cytochrome P450-dependent metabolism of dextromethorphan: fetal and adult studies. *Dev Pharmacol Ther* 1992; **18**(3–4): 161–8.

40. Williams DG, Dickenson A, Fitzgerald M, Howard RF. Developmental regulation of codeine analgesia in the rat. *Anesthesiology* 2004; **100**(1): 92–7.

41. Butt AM, Jones HC, Abbott NJ. Electrical resistance across the blood–brain barrier in anaesthetized rats: a developmental study. *J Physiol* 1990; **429**: 47–62.

42. Murphey LJ, Olsen GD. Diffusion of morphine-6-beta-D-glucuronide into the neonatal guinea pig brain during drug-induced respiratory depression. *J Pharmacol Exp Ther* 1994; **271**(1): 118–24.

43. King M, Su W, Chang A *et al*. Transport of opioids from the brain to the periphery by P-glycoprotein: peripheral actions of central drugs. *Nat Neurosci* 2001; **4**(3): 268–74.

44. Toornvliet R, van Berckel BN, Luurtsema G *et al*. Effect of age on functional P-glycoprotein in the blood-brain barrier measured by use of (R)-[(11)C]verapamil and positron emission tomography. *Clin Pharmacol Ther* 2006; **79**(6): 540–8.

45. Mogil JS. The genetic mediation of individual differences in sensitivity to pain and its inhibition. *Proc Natl Acad Sci USA* 1999; **96**(14): 7744–51.

46. Mogil JS, Wilson SG, Bon K *et al*. Heritability of nociception I: responses of 11 inbred mouse strains on 12 measures of nociception. *Pain* 1999; **80**(1–2): 67–82.

47. Mogil JS, Wilson SG, Bon K *et al*. Heritability of nociception II. 'Types' of nociception revealed by genetic correlation analysis. *Pain* 1999; **80**(1–2): 83–93.

48. Befort, K, Filliol D, Decaillot FM *et al*. A single nucleotide polymorphic mutation in the human mu-opioid receptor severely impairs receptor signaling. *J Biol Chem* 2001; **276**(5): 3130–7.

49. Lotsch J, Skarke C, Grosch S *et al*. The polymorphism A118G of the human mu-opioid receptor gene decreases the pupil constrictory effect of morphine-6-glucuronide but not that of morphine. *Pharmacogenetics* 2002; **12**(1): 3–9.

50. Lotsch J, Zimmermann M, Darimont J *et al*. Does the A118G polymorphism at the mu-opioid receptor gene protect against morphine-6-glucuronide toxicity? *Anesthesiology* 2002; **97**(4): 814–9.

51. Cleary J, Mikus G, Somogyi A, Bochner F. The influence of pharmacogenetics on opioid analgesia: studies with codeine and oxycodone in the Sprague-Dawley/Dark Agouti rat model. *J Pharmacol Exp Ther* 1994; **271**(3): 1528–34.

52. Eckhardt K, Li S, Ammon S *et al*. Same incidence of adverse drug events after codeine administration irrespective of the genetically determined differences in morphine formation. *Pain* 1998; **76**(1–2): 27–33.

53. Yaster M, Nichols DG, Deshpande JK, Wetzel RC. Midazolam–fentanyl intravenous sedation in children: case report of respiratory arrest. *Pediatrics* 1990; **86**(3): 463–7.

54. Lynn A, Nespeca MK, Bratton SL *et al*. Clearance of morphine in postoperative infants during intravenous infusion: the influence of age and surgery. *Anesth Analg* 1998; **86**(5): 958–63.

55. Williams DG, Patel A, Howard RF. Pharmacogenetics of codeine metabolism in an urban population of children and its implications for analgesic reliability. *Br J Anaesth* 2002; **89**(6): 839–45.

56. Semple D, Russell S, Doyle E, Aldridge LM. Comparison of morphine sulphate and codeine phosphate in children undergoing adenotonsillectomy. *Paediatr Anaesth* 1999; **9**(2): 135–8.

57. Bernards CM. Recent insights into the pharmacokinetics of spinal opioids and the relevance to opioid selection. *Curr Opin Anaesthesiol* 2004; **17**(5): 441–7.

58. Bernards CM, Shen DD, Sterling ES *et al*. Epidural, cerebrospinal fluid, and plasma pharmacokinetics of epidural opioids (part I): differences among opioids. *Anesthesiology* 2003; **99**(2): 455–65.

59. Bernards CM, Shen DD, Sterling ES *et al*. Epidural, cerebrospinal fluid, and plasma pharmacokinetics of epidural opioids (part II): effect of epinephrine. *Anesthesiology* 2003; **99**(2): 466–75.

60. Ummenhofer WC, Arends RH, Shen DD, Bernards CM. Comparative spinal distribution and clearance kinetics of intrathecally administered morphine, fentanyl, alfentanil, and sufentanil. *Anesthesiology* 2000; **92**(3): 739–53.

61. Ginosar Y, Riley ET, Angst MS. The site of action of epidural fentanyl in humans: the difference between infusion and bolus administration. *Anesth Analg* 2003; **97**(5): 1428–38.

62. Williams DG, Howard RF. Epidural analgesia in children. A survey of current opinions and practices amongst UK paediatric anaesthetists. *Paediatr Anaesth* 2003; **13**(9): 769–76.

63. van Dijk M, Bouwmeester NJ, Duivenvoorden HJ *et al*. Efficacy of continuous versus intermittent morphine administration after major surgery in 0- to 3-year-old infants; a double-blind randomized controlled trial. *Pain* 2002; **98**(3): 305–13.

64. Farrington EA, McGuinness GA, Johnson GF *et al*. Continuous intravenous morphine infusion in postoperative newborn infants. *Am J Perinatol* 1993; **10**(1): 84–7.

65. Anand KJ, Barton BA, McIntosh N *et al*. Analgesia and sedation in preterm neonates who require ventilatory

support: results from the NOPAIN trial. Neonatal Outcome and Prolonged Analgesia in Neonates. *Arch Pediatr Adolesc Med* 1999; **153**(4): 331–8.

66. Berde CB, Jaksic T, Lynn AM *et al.* Anesthesia and analgesia during and after surgery in neonates. *Clin Ther* 2005; **27**(6): 900–21.

67. Bray RJ, Woodhams AM, Vallis CJ, Kelly PJ. Morphine consumption and respiratory depression in children receiving postoperative analgesia from continuous morphine infusion or patient controlled analgesia. *Paediatr Anaesth* 1996; **6**(2): 129–34.

68. Bray RJ, Woodhams AM, Vallis CJ *et al.* A double-blind comparison of morphine infusion and patient controlled analgesia in children. *Paediatr Anaesth* 1996; **6**(2): 121–7.

69. Hendrickson M, Myre L, Johnson DG *et al.* Postoperative analgesia in children: a prospective study in intermittent intramuscular injection versus continuous intravenous infusion of morphine. *J Pediatr Surg* 1990; **25**(2): 185–90 (discussion 190–1).

70. Doyle E, Morton NS, McNicol LR. Comparison of patient-controlled analgesia in children by i.v. and s.c. routes of administration. *Br J Anaesth* 1994; **72**(5): 533–6.

71. Kendall JM, Reeves BC, Latter VS. Multicentre randomised controlled trial of nasal diamorphine for analgesia in children and teenagers with clinical fractures. *BMJ* 2001; **322**(7281): 261–5.

72. Hickey PR, Hansen DD, Wessel DL *et al.* Blunting of stress responses in the pulmonary circulation of infants by fentanyl. *Anesth Analg* 1985; **64**(12): 1137–42.

73. Wilson AS, Stiller RL, Davis PJ *et al.* Fentanyl and alfentanil plasma protein binding in preterm and term neonates. *Anesth Analg* 1997; **84**(2): 315–8.

74. Santeiro ML, Christie J, Stromquist C *et al.* Pharmacokinetics of continuous infusion fentanyl in newborns. *J Perinatol* 1997; **17**(2): 135–9.

75. Ginsberg B, Howell S, Glass PS *et al.* Pharmacokinetic model-driven infusion of fentanyl in children. *Anesthesiology* 1996; **85**(6): 1268–75.

76. Koren G, Goresky G, Crean P *et al.* Unexpected alterations in fentanyl pharmacokinetics in children undergoing cardiac surgery: age related or disease related? *Dev Pharmacol Ther* 1986; **9**(3): 183–91.

77. Katz R, Kelly HW. Pharmacokinetics of continuous infusions of fentanyl in critically ill children. *Crit Care Med* 1993; **21**(7): 995–1000.

78. Hughes MA, Glass PS, Jacobs JR. Context-sensitive half-time in multicompartment pharmacokinetic models for intravenous anesthetic drugs. *Anesthesiology* 1992; **76**(3): 334–41.

79. Meistelman C, Saint-Maurice C, LePaul M *et al.* Comparison of alfentanil pharmacokinetics in children and adults. *Anesthesiology* 1987; **66**(1): 13–6.

80. Marlow N, Weindling AM, van Peer A, Heykants J. Alfentanil pharmacokinetics in preterm infants. *Arch Dis Child* 1990; **65**(4 Spec No): 349–51.

81. Greeley WJ, de Bruijn NP. Changes in sufentanil pharmacokinetics within the neonatal period. *Anesth Analg* 1988; **67**(1): 86–90.

82. Zedie N, Amory DW, Wagner BK, O'Hara DA. Comparison of intranasal midazolam and sufentanil premedication in pediatric outpatients. *Clin Pharmacol Ther* 1996; **59**(3): 341–8.

83. Ross AK, Davis PJ, Dear GD. Pharmacokinetics of remifentanil in anesthetized pediatric patients undergoing elective surgery or diagnostic procedures. *Anesth Analg* 2001; **93**(6): 1393–401.

84. Vinik HR, Kissin I. Rapid development of tolerance to analgesia during remifentanil infusion in humans. *Anesth Analg* 1998; **86**(6): 1307–11.

85. Davis PJ, Galinkin J, McGowan FX *et al.* A randomized multicenter study of remifentanil compared with halothane in neonates and infants undergoing pyloromyotomy. I. Emergence and recovery profiles. *Anesth Analg,* 2001; **93**(6): 1380–6.

86. Moore A, Collins S, Carroll D, McQuay H. Paracetamol with and without codeine in acute pain: a quantitative systematic review. *Pain* 1997; **70**(2–3): 193–201.

87. Prakash S, Tyagi R, Gogia AR *et al.* Efficacy of three doses of tramadol with bupivacaine for caudal analgesia in paediatric inguinal herniotomy. *Br J Anaesth* 2006; **97**(3): 385–8.

88. Allegaert K, Anderson BJ, Verbesselt R *et al.* Tramadol disposition in the very young: an attempt to assess *in vivo* cytochrome P-450 2D6 activity. *Br J Anaesth* 2005; **95**(2): 231–9.

89. Engelhardt T, Steel E, Johnston G, Veitch DY. Tramadol for pain relief in children undergoing tonsillectomy: a comparison with morphine. *Paediatr Anaesth* 2003; **13**(3): 249–52.

90. Ozer Z, Gorur K, Altunkan AA *et al.* Efficacy of tramadol versus meperidine for pain relief and safe recovery after adenotonsillectomy. *Eur J Anaesthesiol* 2003; **20**(11): 920–4.

91. Pokela ML, Olkkola KT, Koivisto M, Ryhanen P. Pharmacokinetics and pharmacodynamics of intravenous meperidine in neonates and infants. *Clin Pharmacol Ther* 1992; **52**(4): 342–9.

92. Martinez D, Wilson S. Children sedated for dental care: a pilot study of the 24-hour postsedation period. *Pediatr Dent* 2006; **28**(3): 260–4.

93. Jaillon P, Gardin ME, Lecocq B *et al.* Pharmacokinetics of nalbuphine in infants, young healthy volunteers, and elderly patients. *Clin Pharmacol Ther* 1989; **46**(2): 226–33.

94. Stile IL, Fort M, Wurzburger RJ *et al.* The pharmacokinetics of naloxone in the premature newborn. *Dev Pharmacol Ther* 1987; **10**(6): 454–9.

95. Gan TJ, Ginsberg B, Glass PS *et al.* Opioid-sparing effects of a low-dose infusion of naloxone in patient-administered morphine sulfate. *Anesthesiology* 1997; **87**(5): 1075–81.

96. Cepeda MS, Africano JM, Manrique AM *et al.* The combination of low dose of naloxone and morphine in PCA does not decrease opioid requirements in the postoperative period. *Pain* 2002; **96**(1–2): 73–9.

97. Maxwell LG, Kaufmann SC, Bitzer S *et al*. The effects of a small-dose naloxone infusion on opioid-induced side effects and analgesia in children and adolescents treated with intravenous patient-controlled analgesia: a double-blind, prospective, randomized, controlled study. *Anesth Analg* 2005; **100**(4): 953–8.

98. Crain SM, Shen KF. Antagonists of excitatory opioid receptor functions enhance morphine's analgesic potency and attenuate opioid tolerance/dependence liability. *Pain* 2000; **84**(2–3): 121–31.

99. Crain SM, Shen KF. Ultra-low concentrations of naloxone selectively antagonize excitatory effects of morphine on sensory neurons, thereby increasing its antinociceptive potency and attenuating tolerance/dependence during chronic cotreatment. *Proc Natl Acad Sci USA* 1995; **92**(23): 10540–4.

100. Crain SM, Shen KF. Modulatory effects of Gs-coupled excitatory opioid receptor functions on opioid analgesia, tolerance, and dependence. *Neurochem Res* 1996; **21**(11): 1347–51.

13

Non-opioid analgesics

HANNU KOKKI

KEY LEARNING POINTS

- Non-opioid analgesia alone can be effective for the treatment of mild and moderate pain.
- Mild and moderate pain is a common outcome in children with surgery and 80 per cent of children need analgesia for 2–3 days after common operations such as adenoidectomy and herniotomy. Pain after tonsillectomy may last over $1\frac{1}{2}$ weeks.

- For severe pain, non-opioids should be used to enhance analgesia and to reduce the dose and adverse effects of opioids.
- The safety of repeated doses of non-steroidal anti-inflammatory drugs (NSAIDs) in newborns has not been established, but evidence suggests that they are safe in most children over 3 months old.

INTRODUCTION

Pain has negative physical and psychological consequences in a growing body and mind. Recent evidence shows that the incidence and magnitude of troubled behaviour are negligible in children after surgery if they have proactive treatment with non-opioid analgesics as an adjunct to opioids [1].

Pain is a common symptom after surgery, and most children need analgesia even after minor procedures. After myringotomy, half of the children have significant pain [2]. After herniotomy or adenoidectomy analgesics are needed for at least for 2–3 days and after more extended surgery, such as tonsillectomy, abdominal, thoracic, urological, or orthopaedic procedures almost all children have considerable pain beyond the first postoperative week [3–6].

The management of postoperative pain in infants and children has improved significantly over recent years and much information is available for safe and effective use of paracetamol and non-steroidal anti-inflammatory drugs

(NSAID)s in infants and children [7,8]. Nevertheless acute pain is still undertreated because of organisational issues [9].

Analgesia should be adjusted for each patient and situation so that the prescriber should weigh efficacy against possible harm. Children dislike suppositories and they hate intramuscular injections and therefore oral and intravenous formulations should be used more widely [8]. Drug formulations have been refined for use in children.

Surgery causes tissue inflammation associated with pain. Non-steroidal anti-inflammatory drugs block the synthesis of prostaglandins by inhibiting cyclo-oxygenase (COX) types 1 and 2 and thereby reduce the production of mediators of inflammation. They not only reduce peripheral nociception by decreasing local inflammation but also modulate the central response to pain by inhibition of prostaglandin synthesis in the spinal cord [10–12].

Non-opioid drugs are highly effective in the management of mild and moderate pain, particularly in somatic pain conditions. Their efficacy alone is insufficient for severe pain particularly of visceral origin [8] but they can be used for background analgesia together with opioid and regional techniques. Paracetamol is frequently used, but its anti-inflammatory efficacy is weak. Non-steroidal anti-inflammatory drugs such as ibuprofen are especially useful for pain associated with inflammation. Differences in anti-inflammatory activity and analgesic efficacy between different NSAIDs are small, but there may be variation between individuals. In general the main differences between different NSAIDs are in the incidence and type of adverse effects. Safety of NSAIDs in infants has not been established and paracetamol is generally the preferred non-opioid analgesic in this age group [7].

Non-opioid drugs are more effective in prevention rather than in the relief of established pain. It can take 1–2 hours before the maximal analgesic effect is achieved [8] and therefore it is important that they are given regularly whenever pain is likely [1,13]. Pre-emptive treatment does not extend the length of the analgesic effect [14].

MECHANISMS OF ACTION

Non-steroidal anti-inflammatory drugs

The NSAIDs are a group of unrelated organic acids that have analgesic, anti-inflammatory, antiplatelet and antipyretic actions. Their analgesic effect mainly arises from inhibition of prostaglandin (PG) synthesis [15]. After an injury or trauma, arachidonic acid (AA) is released from glycerol-based phospholipids in cell membranes by the action of phospholipase A_2. It is subsequently metabolised into biologically active eicosanoids by three major enzyme systems: COX enzymes convert AA to thromboxane, PGs and prostacyclins; 5-lipoxygenases convert AA to leukotrienes and hydroxyeicosatetraenoic acids; and epoxygenases convert AA to hydroxyeicosatetraenoic and cis-epoxyeicosatrienoic acids.

The COX enzymes catalyse a stepwise conversion of AA into PGG_2, and further by peroxidase activity to PGH_2, which is a common precursor for the synthesis of other PGs. These are various (PGD_2, PGE_2 and $PGF_2\alpha$) of, which PGE_2 is an important mediator in inflammatory pain sensitisation [11,12].

Peripheral sensitisation is produced by the action of PGE_2 and other inflammatory mediators that activate corresponding nerve fibres and nociceptors. PGE_2 binds to G-proteins on sensory neurons and, by activating sodium channels, increases neuronal excitability [11,12,16]. In the spinal cord PGE_2 facilitates the transmission of nociceptive input through the dorsal horn by sensitising both presynaptic receptors of primary afferent neurons and post-synaptic receptors on spinal cord neurones [11,12,16].

Non-steroidal anti-inflammatory drugs are COX inhibitors and prevent the biosynthesis of prostaglandins and thromboxanes from AA. There are two forms of COX inhibitors: COX-1 is the constitutive form of the enzyme and COX-2 is induced by inflammation. Theoretically, inhibition of COX-2 is responsible for the analgesic, anti-inflammatory and antipyretic properties of NSAIDs, whereas inhibition of COX-1 is thought to produce other toxic effects such as those in the gastrointestinal tract. This theory is too simple, because there is evidence for COX-1 inhibition modulating acute nociception, and COX-2 is also expressed constitutively, and maintains homeostasis and organ development [16].

After injury and trauma the time course of PGE_2 production is consistent with an early increase in COX-1 activity followed by increased production 2–3 hours later consistent with COX-2 expression [16]. Therefore COX-1 inhibition is needed for early effective pain relief. COX-2 inhibition has only a weak or nil effect 2–4 hours after injury but pronounced analgesia later [17,18]. Non-steroidal anti-inflammatory drugs that inhibit both COX-1 and COX-2 are ideal.

Non-steroidal anti-inflammatory drugs may act centrally, although slowly, by prevention of PGE_2 generation at the spinal cord [19,20]. However, some have a rapid central action, suggesting that other mechanisms may be involved. Non-steroidal anti-inflammatory drugs do not affect opioid receptors [21]. Cytokines and growth factors also induce or upregulate COX enzymes both peripherally in injured tissue and in the central nervous system.

Paracetamol

The mechanism of action of paracetamol is less well characterised than that of other NSAIDs [22]. Paracetamol has analgesic and antipyretic properties but weak anti-inflammatory activity. Its mechanism of analgesic action is uncertain, but it may be due to inhibition of prostaglandin synthesis both centrally and peripherally.

Paracetamol decreases PG concentrations and decreases swelling and suppresses inflammation after trauma. These effects are similar to COX-2 inhibitors. Inhibition of PG synthesis by paracetamol is weak in damaged cells and strong in intact cells but only when AA concentrations are low [23]. In animal models PGE_2 generation can be inhibited by paracetamol [24,25]. Paracetamol readily penetrates the blood–brain barrier so that cerebrospinal fluid concentrations become similar or above those in plasma quickly. The central nervous system concentrations may be sufficient for inhibition of PGE_2 [26]. Large doses of paracetamol cause COX inhibitor-like adverse effects on gastrointestinal mucosa and renal and platelet funtion [27].

Other mechanisms of action have been suggested. Paracetamol may have a principal central action causing activation of descending inhibitory seroton in ergic pathways [28]. Paracetamol may also reduce hyperalgesia mediated by substance P, and reduce nitric oxide generation involved in spinal hyperalgesia [22].

CLINICAL EFFECTS OF SPECIFIC DRUGS

Paracetamol

Paracetamol, a *p*-aminophenol derivative, is the only agent that has been extensively evaluated in children. Since three decades ago, when it was realised that aspirin could produce Reye's syndrome [29], paracetamol has been the most widely used analgesic to treat mild and moderate pain in children [7].

The supposed analgesic concentration of paracetamol is 10–20 mg/L. In order to achieve and maintain these concentrations the first enteral dose in a child should be 35–45 mg/kg and the cumulative daily dose up to 100 mg/kg [30] – at these doses paracetamol is as effective as NSAIDs. Unfortunately, it is not known how long these doses may be used and, for safety reasons, doses should be lower after the first 2 or 3 days (Table 13.1). Higher doses do not improve analgesia and may produce hepatic failure. In infants and neonates the same single dose may be used but the dose frequency should be less so that the cumulative daily dose does not exceed 75 mg/kg in infants and 60 mg/kg in neonates. Paracetamol is absorbed rapidly and almost completely when administered by mouth. Suppositories are not the ideal formulation because there is wide variation in bioavailability [22] and absorption is erratic, delayed and sometimes insignificant.

Until recently intravenous paracetamol was available as the prodrug propacetamol. This was unstable and therefore available as a powder; it has become obsolete. Now, a stable intravenous formulation of paracetamol is widely available and it is unlikely that the altered chemical structure and formulation would alter either pharmacodynamic efficacy or safety. The first intravenous dose of paracetamol should be 15–30 mg/kg infused over 15 minutes, followed by 15 mg/kg every 6–12 hours – the cumulative daily dose should not exceed 60 mg/kg. Intravenous paracetamol is inactivated by prolonged contact with air(i.e. 30 minutes) and hence the infusion times are recommended as 15 minutes.

Paracetamol, in recommended doses, is generally well tolerated and safe; however, there are reported adverse effects. It may produce gastric inflammation and nephropathy, and it can also inhibit platelet function [27]. Bronchospasm and allergic reactions have also been described [31].

Overdose of paracetamol causes dangerous hepatotoxicity. The therapeutic index is narrow as doses that are only 5- to 10-fold higher than the therapeutic dose may cause severe hepatocellular necrosis [32]. For short postoperative use up to 100 mg/kg/day is regarded as safe.

Ibuprofen

There is evidence of safe use of ibuprofen in children and it is available in both parenteral and enteral formulations. For mild and moderate pain, the recommended dose is 10 mg/kg and this may be repeated every 6–8 hours because the elimination half-life is 1.5–3 hours. The maximum daily dose is 40 mg/kg. At these low doses the risk of gastrointestinal bleeding, renal failure, or anaphylaxis in children is similar to paracetamol [33]. Whether the efficacy and adverse effects are dose dependent has not been established. Ibuprofen can be used to trigger closure of patent ductus arteriosus in preterm infants; it has recently been licensed for this purpose.

Flurbiprofen

Bioavailabilities of oral and rectal administration of flurbiprofen are equivalent and the elimination half-lives ranges from 2 hours to 4 hours. It is available in some countries as an intravenous preparation, which is a practical formulation during surgery. The lowest effective dose for acute pain management seems to be 1 mg/kg intravenously [34]. Flurbiprofen drops may be used for eye surgery.

Table 13.1 Paracetamol in postoperative pain treatment in children (doses should be reduced by one-third after 48–72 hours)

Age group	Loading dose (mg/kg)	Maintenance dose (mg/kg)	Dose interval (hours)	Daily maximum dose (mg/kg)
Enteral				
Preterm infants	20	20	12	40
Neonates and infants <3 months	20–30	15–20	8–12	60
Infants and children >3 months	20–40	15–20	6–8	90
Intavenously*				
Preterm infants	15	15	12	30
Neonates and infants <3 months	15	15	8–12	60
Infants and children >3 months	15–30	15	4–6	60

*Intravenous infusion should be given within 30 minutes of opening container.

Ketoprofen

There are substantial pharmacokinetic, efficacy and tolerability data of ketoprofen in children older than 3 months. The dose is 1–2 mg/kg at every 6–8 hours to a maximum of 5 mg/kg/day. Its elimination half-life in plasma is about 1.5–4 hours. Ketoprofen is available in both parenteral and enteral forms. Dose-finding studies indicate that it has a rapid effect at a low dose of 0.3 mg/kg and analgesia is enhanced by increasing doses up to 3 mg/kg without any increase in adverse effects [35]. It can be given also as a continuous infusion of 0.1–0.2 mg/kg/h after a loading dose of 1 mg/kg; within 24 hours no accumulation has been reported [36]. Ketoprofen readily crosses the blood–brain barrier (BBB) so that cerebrospinal fluid and plasma (unbound) concentrations become similar quickly [37].This may explain its prompt analgesic action [16]. The safety of ketoprofen in neonates has not been established.

Naproxen

Naproxen is available in enteral form only (tablets and suspension). Of all the propionic acid derivatives described here, naproxen has the longest elimination half-life of 12–15 hours. The commonly used daily dose is 10–15 mg/kg after an initial loading dose of 10 mg/kg, and the dose interval is 12 hours. Safe paediatric dosage has not been well established. An oral suspension allows accurate dosing against weight [38]. Because of its long action, it may be useful in replacing parenteral NSAIDs when intavenous access is unnecessary.

Diclofenac

Diclofenac is a phenylacetic acid derivative and may be given by mouth or rectum or as a continuous or intermittent intravenous infusion. The maximum period recommended for parenteral use is 2–3 days. In children 1–12 years old the dose for acute pain management is up to 3 mg/kg daily in divided doses. Diclofenac drops (0.1 per cent) may be useful following eye surgery, laser treatment and trauma [39].

Ketorolac

Ketorolac is a pyrrolizine carboxylic acid derivative and available in injectable form and tablets. The literature on NSAIDs in children is weighted in favour of ketorolac because it is the only parenteral NSAID available in the USA. Nevertheless, in adults, the propionic acid derivatives and diclofenac may have more favourable profiles than ketorolac [40]. Indeed, in adults, ketorolac has the highest incidence of adverse effects and, consequently, many centres have restricted its use in

children [41]. A small series of surgical neonates have been given ketorolac [41] but this drug cannot be recommended for children less than 2 years old. The safety and efficacy of single parenteral doses have been established in children older than 2 years but there are limited data for multiple doses. The elimination half-life of ketorolac after a single dose is 6 hours. In a dose titration study 0.2 mg/kg of ketorolac did not provide sufficient analgesia but a dose of 0.5 mg/kg was as effective as morphine (0.1 mg/kg); there was no improvement in analgesic efficacy with doses of 0.75, 1 and 1.5 mg/kg [42,43]. In children intravenous ketorolac should be used at a dose of 0.5 mg/kg (maximum of 15 mg) every 6–8 hours to a maximum daily dose of 90 mg. The maximum duration of treatment is 48 hours [42]. Ketorolac may also be administered as an intravenous infusion of 0.1–0.15 mg/kg/h. In ophthalmology, preservative-free ketorolac solution may be used topically in children aged over 3 years for 2–3 days to relief inflammation, pain and photophobia [44].

Indometacin

Indometacin is an indole acetic acid derivative. Twenty years ago it was used for postoperative pain management in children. Maunuksela *et al.* [45] showed that it was useful as an infusion in children aged 1–16 years undergoing general or orthopaedic surgery, and rectal indometacin had a significant opioid-sparing effect after appendectomy [46]. In neonates, it is used to close patent ductus arteriosus. Three intravenous doses of 0.2 mg/kg are given spaced by 12–24 hours. If the ductus re-opens, a second course of one to three doses may be given. The terminal half-life in neonates has been reported to be between 12 and 28 hours. Indometacin has also been tried for prevention of intraventricular haemorrhage in preterm infants but, because it causes a significant reduction of cerebral blood volume, oxidised cytochrome oxidase concentration and cerebral blood flow velocity, there are conflicting results for efficacy and safety [47]. In vulnerable neonates indometacin can cause significant ischaemia-related adverse effects on renal, mesenteric and cerebral circulations. In older children, rapid BBB penetration may explain both a highly effective analgesic action and the common CNS adverse effects such as tinnitus, dizziness, headache and agitation [48].

PHARMACOKINETICS AND EFFICACY

In general, children may require higher doses of drugs (per kilogram) than adults because of their higher metabolic rates; however, with NSAIDs these differences are not appreciable and similar doses should be used [49]. In infants, similar single doses are also safe because the volume of distribution is larger, but dose frequency should be less because elimination and clearance are lower.

In awake children, with intact gastrointestinal function, the rate and extent of oral absorption of NSAIDs are similar to those after intramuscular and rectal administration. Both during and immediately after surgery, intravenous administration is the most appropriate route and, later, in cooperative children the drugs should be administered by mouth. Intramuscular administration is almost never necessary in awake children. Postoperative pain disturbs sleep [50] and therefore all children should have effective pain relief for the first night after surgery. Compounds with longer half-life or extended-release preparations should be preferred.

Perioperative factors change pharmacokinetics. The absorption of swallowed drugs may be delayed during immediate postoperative period; for example, the lag time of absorption of paracetamol is 5 minutes before compared with 45 minutes after anaesthesia [51,52]. Relaxation of the sphincters and contraction of the rectum can expel suppositories [53]. Changes in local blood flow distribution may significantly delay absorption of subcutaneous and intramuscular drugs.

Few studies have compared the efficacy of different doses of NSAIDs or paracetamol. It has been suggested that a single dose of 1 mg/kg diclofenac provides similar analgesic efficacy to 1 mg/kg flurbiprofen, 10 mg/kg ibuprofen, 1 mg/kg ketoprofen or 0.5 mg/kg ketorolac [8]. Differences in anti-inflammatory and analgesic activity between different NSAIDs are small, but there may be variation between them in individual patient tolerance and response. The main differences between NSAIDs are in the pharmacokinetics and in the incidence and type of adverse effects. There seems to be significant differences, for example, in the rate and extent of BBB permeation of paracetamol and different NSAIDs [26,37,48].

A rapid intravenous bolus of any NSAID may cause bradycardia [54] and therefore they should be given slowly (>5 minutes) or as a continuous infusion.

DRUG SELECTION

Infants less than 3 months old

Paracetamol is the most commonly prescribed drug in infants and neonates to treat pain after surgery. Oral administration is effective and reliable and now that there is a parenteral formulation available precise dosing and prediction of plasma concentrations are possible. Rectal absorption is unreliable [55].

Evidence of efficacy and toxicity of NSAIDs is limited. Indometacin and ibuprofen are commonly used to close patent ductus arteriosus [47,56]. Similar doses may be useful for analgesia but there are few data. Physiological effects of inhibition of prostaglandin synthesis include alterations in cerebral blood flow and decreased renal function [56]. Neonates may also develop severe gastrointestinal adverse effects such as haemorrhage, perforation and necrotising enterocolitis after exposure to NSAIDs.

Prostaglandins are important for the normal development of the central nervous, cardiovascular and renal systems and theoretically NSAIDs may be adversely affect organogenesis either *in utero* or during the neonatal period.

Older children

In addition to paracetamol, one NSAID may be used; the combination may perform better than paracetamol alone [8,22]. Ibuprofen, flurbiprofen, ketoprofen, naproxen or diclofenac can be considered because evidence supports their efficacy and safety [8] (Table 13.2). Paracetamol, diclofenac and ketoprofen are recommended for intravenous administration. Ketorolac is commonly used in some countries but the side-effect profile in adults is discouraging. Indometacin causes a high incidence of headaches, dizziness and gastrointestinal disturbances in children [45].

Table 13.2 Non-steroidal anti-inflammatory drugs (NSAIDs) in postoperative pain treatment in children 3 months old and older

Drug	Loading dose (mg/kg)	Maintenance dose (mg/kg)	Dose interval (hours)	Daily maximum dose (mg/kg)
Diclofenac	2	1	6–8	3
Flubiprofen	1	1	8–12	3
Ibuprofen	10	10	6–8	40
Ketoprofen*	2	1	6–8	5
Ketorolac†	0.5	0.25	6–8	2
Naproxen	10	5	8–12	15

*Ketoprofen continuous infusion: loading dose 1 mg/kg in 15 minutes, followed by infusion 0.1–0.2 mg/kg/h

†Do not use for longer than 48 hours, and avoid in surgery associated with an increased risk of bleeding.

Minor day-case surgery

Non-steroidal anti-inflammatory drugs and paracetamol are of particular value following day-case surgery because of their lack of sedative and emetic effects. At home, for mild-to-moderate pain, it is sensible to administer NSAIDs regularly for the initial 2 or 3 days [1]. Opioid rescue analgesia will be needed for moderate-to-severe pain.

Proactive analgesia may reduce the incidence of postsurgery distress and behaviour troubles [1,13] and therefore simple non-opioid analgesia should be administered regularly after any procedure where pain is likely [8].

Counselling families is important to ensure that they understand that pain is common and that they can give effective and safe analgesia. There should be emphasis on prevention of pain by early and repeated dosing [57–59]. Preparatory information improves appropriate expectations [60] and, during the hospital admission for children, verbal information should be reinforced with written instructions – these are improved by pictures and cartoons for children [61]. The quality of pain management is also improved by giving clear instructions to staff [3,4]. Parents should be given a contact telephone number for support if analgesic efficacy is insufficient or if adverse effects occur.

Tonsillectomy

Tonsillectomy causes considerable pain that is worst on the third to the fifth postoperative days, and may last longer than 7 days [6,62]. Many children find swallowing and speaking painful and sleeping is disturbed [6]. Pain is unnecessary and increases utilisation of health services [62]. Non-steroidal anti-inflammatory drugs are commonly used for tonsillectomy and there is good evidence that they are effective [63,64]. They minimise the problem of opioid-related nausea and vomiting. Respiratory depression is also avoided and this is especially useful for children with obstructive sleep apnoea [65–67].

Non-steroidal anti-inflammatory drugs inhibit platelet aggregation and prolong bleeding time and may therefore increase operative and postoperative bleeding. The risk of this causing appreciable bleeding is small [68,69]. Further, the risk depends on the drug. In comparison with aspirin, NSAIDs and paracetamol cause reversible platelet dysfunction [27]. The effect on platelets is modest with paracetamol and NSAIDs with short elimination half-lives (such as diclofenac, ibuprofen and ketoprofen), while with compounds with longer elimination half-lives (ketorolac), platelet dysfunction is still present 24 hours after a single dose of 0.4 mg/kg. Ketorolac should probably be avoided.

Contraindications

The use of any NSAID is generally contraindicated in patients in whom sensitivity reactions have been precipitated by NSAIDs, such as asthma, angio-oedema, bronchospasm, rhinitis or urticaria. They should be use with caution, if at all, in children with impaired renal function, hypovolaemia or hypotension, coagulation defects, thrombocytopenia or active bleeding from any cause.

ADVERSE EFFECTS

There is a need for surveillance and reporting of adverse drug reactions in paediatrics because most NSAIDs are not extensively tested in children. Not only are pharmacokinetics and dynamics different in children but also the illnesses and adverse drug reactions can be age related (Tables 13.3 and 13.4). The benefits and risks should be considered for every patient.

Non-steroidal anti-inflammatory drugs cause two types of adverse effects: the predictable (relating to the inhibition of the prostaglandin system) and the idiosyncratic [70]. Idiosyncratic reactions are predominantly of the skin (rash), gut (abdominal discomfort, nausea, diarrhoea) and lung (exacerbation of asthma). They can also cause operative and gastrointestinal bleeding [7,8,22].

Severe adverse effects related to NSAIDs are very rare in children. Aspirin is associated with Reye's syndrome and is not recommended for analgesia [70]. Deaths have been reported due to exacerbation of asthma, and acute liver and renal failure.

Platelet function

By inhibiting the biosynthesis of thromboxane A_2, NSAIDs and paracetamol may prevent platelet aggregation [27]. Single doses cause lengthening of bleeding time and this usually becomes normal within 24 hours [71]. Significant bleeding has been reported with ketorolac during tonsillectomy [72,73] but other NSAIDs and paracetamol have been found to have a negligible effect. However, the risk of bleeding must be appreciated and drugs should be used with caution when there is a haemorrhagic disease [63] or if any bleeding is hazardous – if necessary, non-opioids could be administered after surgery when haemostasis is secure.

Gastrointestinal effects

In adults, gastric mucosal damage resulting in ulceration and bleeding can occur with any NSAID with prolonged use. In children severe gastric adverse effects are rare [38,74]; gastrointestinal bleeding has been reported but the most commonly reported reactions are abdominal pain, nausea, vomiting and diarrhoea [8,41].

Renal effects

The risk of renal damage is increased in patients with dehydration, hypovolaemia and hypotension [75].

Table 13.3 Adverse effects at hospital reported by 943 children aged 1–7 years undergoing day-case adenoidectomy with or without ketoprofen [88, 89]*

Symptom	Ketoprofen (n = 824)	Placebo (n = 119)
Nausea, retching, vomiting	128 (16%)	28 (24%)
Somnolence	45 (5%)	4 (3%)
Difficulty passing urine	15 (2%)	2 (2%)
Pain at the infusion site	9 (1%)	4 (3%)
Abdominal pain	6 (<1%)	
Bleeding	4 (<1%)	
Eyelid oedema	1 (<1%)	1 (<1%)
Shivering	1 (<1%)	
Agitation	1 (<1%)	
Dry mouth	1 (<1%)	
Flushing	1 (<1%)	
Dizziness		1 (<1%)
Fever		1 (<1%)

Table 13.4 Adverse effects reported by 951 children aged 1–12 years undergoing adenoidectomy/tosillectomy with ketoprofen for postoperative pain treatment [90]

Symptom	Ketoprofen (n = 951)
Somnolence	331 (35%)
Fever	193 (20%)
Nausea, retching, vomiting	96 (10%)
Abdominal pain	92 (10%)
Pain at the infusion site	81 (9%)
Dizziness	79 (8%)
Headache	72 (8%)
Minor bleeding	57 (6%)
Constipation	52 (5%)
Diarrhoea	44 (5%)
Sweating	31 (3%)
Significant bleeding	11 (1%)
Difficult in passing urine	6 (<1%)
Skin rash	3 (<1%)
Disturbed sleep	1 (<1%)
Dry mouth	1 (<1%)
Abdominal rumbling	1 (<1%)

Prostaglandin-dependent effects of NSAIDs on the renal perfusion and function are usually reversible [76]. In adults, NSAIDs with intermediate or long half-lives (>4 hours) are more dangerous for renal perfusion and function than short-acting drugs [77]. Reactions involving renal integrity are very rare. However, severe reactions including nephritis and renal papillary necrosis may occur, and papillary necrosis has been reported with prolonged use of excessive doses of NSAIDs and paracetamol [78].

Asthma

Non-steroidal anti-inflammatory drugs (and rarely paracetamol) can precipitate or aggravate asthma [31]. Fortunately, the risk is small and therefore the majority of children with well-controlled asthma can benefit from non-opioid analgesia [79,80]. It is unwise to administer NSAIDs to children who are unstable or uncontrolled asthmatics who have any history of a previous reaction to a NSAID.

Hepatic effects

Paracetamol overdose is a common cause of fulminant hepatic failure in adults and children. Hepatic damage is caused by the toxic metabolite N-acetyl-p-benzoquinone imine (NAPQI), which binds to intracellular hepatic macromolecules to produce cell necrosis and damage [32]. The toxicity of paracetamol is closely linked to its metabolism. There are three pathways for paracetamol metabolism: conjugation with sulphate, conjugation with glucuronide or metabolism by the cytochrome P450 oxidase enzyme system. At therapeutic doses, about 90 per cent of the administered dose is detoxified by the two conjugation reactions. Only a small percentage of paracetamol undergoes oxidative CYP450-dependent (mostly CYP1A2 and CYP2E1) metabolism to the toxic, electrophilic metabolite NAPQI. This metabolite is detoxified by glutathione. The NAPQI that is not detoxified may bind to hepatocytes and produce cellular necrosis. Usually, a relatively small amount of NAPQI is formed [81]. Hepatic glutathione depletion is the critical trigger for hepatotoxicity of paracetamol. At high paracetamol doses the sulfation and glucuronidation pathways become saturated. As a result the amount and rate of formation of NAPQI by CYP450-mediated paracetamol metabolism are greatly increased. At high paracetamol doses, the liver becomes completely depleted of glutathione, and the reactive electrophile NAPQI then covalently binds to hepatocytes, and hepatotoxicity ensues [81].

Hepatic failure can be caused by a large, single dose of >150 mg/kg per or multiple doses adding up to 100 mg/kg/day [82]. The risk of hepatotoxicity is also increased if the child is aged under 2 years and has repeated vomiting, diarrhoea or poor fluid intake for more that 24 hours. Fever and malnourishment are other risk factors [83]. Children with a family history of hepatic toxicity to paracetamol and those with impairment of glucuronidation (e.g. Gilbert's syndrome) have an increased risk of developing a toxic reaction. Some drugs, such as carbamazepine, ethanol and rifampin, may affect paracetamol elimination or NAPQI detoxification [82].

Early symptoms are nausea and vomiting which should settle within 24 hours of ingestion but, if not, hepatic failure occurs, usually associated with right subcostal pain and tenderness. Liver damage is maximal 3–4 days after ingestion and may lead to encephalopathy, haemorrhage, hypoglycaemia, cerebral oedema and death [32]. Rarely, renal tubular necrosis can occur.

Intervention to sustain hepatic glutathione is an effective treatment for paracetamol overdose. The main factors for poor outcome are delayed presentation, and/or delay in establishing treatment. All overdosed children should be treated with N-acetyl-L-cysteine which replenishes glutathione stores [81]. If paracetamol was ingested within the previous hour, absorption may be reduced by activated charcoal administered via a nasogastric tube. After a loading dose of N-acetyl-L-cysteine the plasma paracetamol concentrations should be measured. Plasma concentration above the therapeutic level treatment line should be regarded as carrying a serious risk of liver damage. Further N-acetyl-L-cysteine may be necessary [32].

Young children are more resistant to paracetamol hepatotoxicity than adults because their detoxification predominantly involves sulphation rather than glucuronidation and this probably reduces the formation of NAPQI. Glutathione is synthesised more readily by infants, but fasting enhances hepatotoxicity because it depletes glutathione stores [84]. Treated children seem to recover better than adults [85].

Skin effects

Dermatological reactions may be minor (rash and urticaria) or severe (Lyell's syndrome and Stevens–Johnson syndrome). Minor reactions occur in 0.3 per cent of children (similar rate as in adults) and they may be more common in atopic and asthmatic children. Hypersensitivity to NSAIDs can manifest as facial angio-oedema and this is more common in adults.

Central nervous system effects

Adults can develop dizziness, anxiety, fear, agitation, labile emotions, depersonalisation, paranoia and hallucinations with NSAIDs. There are fewer problems in children but tinnitus, dizziness, headache and agitation have been reported [85–87].

REFERENCES

Key references

Cardwell M, Siviter G, Smith A. Non-steroidal anti-inflammatory drugs and perioperative bleeding in paediatric tonsillectomy. *Cochrane Database Syst* Rev 2005; **2**: CD003591.

Korpela R, Korvenoja P, Meretoja OA. Morphine-sparing effect of acetaminophen in pediatric day-case surgery. *Anesthesiology* 1999; **91**: 442–7.

Reye RDK, Morgan G, Baral J. Encephalopathy and fatty degeneration of the viscera: a disease entity in childhood. *Lancet* 1963; **ii**: 749–52.

Short JA, Barr CA, Palmer CD *et al*. Use of diclofenac in children with asthma. *Anaesthesia* 2000; **55**: 334–7.

van Overmeire B, Allegaert K, Casaer A *et al*. Prophylactic ibuprofen in premature infants: a multicentre, randomised, double-blind, placebo-controlled trial. *Lancet* 2004; **364**: 1945–9.

References

1. Tuomilehto H, Kokki H, Ahonen R, Nuutinen, J. Postoperative behavioral changes in children after adenoidectomy. *Arch Otolaryngol Head Neck Surg* 2002; **128**: 1159–64.
2. Bolton P, Bridge HS, Montgomery CJ, Merrick PM. The analgesic efficacy of preoperative high dose (40 mg × kg^{-1}) oral acetaminophen after bilateral myringotomy and tube insertion in children. *Paediatr Anaesth* 2002; **12**: 29–35.
3. Finley GA, McGrath PJ, Forward SP *et al*. Parent's management of children's pain following 'minor' surgery. *Pain* 1996; **64**: 83–7.
4. Nikanne E, Kokki H, Tuovinen K. Postoperative pain after adenoidectomy in children. *Br J Anaesth* 1999; **82**: 886–9.
5. Kokki H, Heikkinen M, Ahonen R. Recovery after paediatric daycase herniotomy performed under spinal anaesthesia. *Paediatr Anaesth* 2000; **10**: 413–17.
6. Salonen A, Kokki H, Nuutinen J. The effect of ketoprofen on recovery after tonsillectomy in children: a 3-week follow-up study. *Int J Pediatr Otorhinolaryngol* 2002; **62**: 143–50.
7. Litalien C, Jacqz-Aigrain E. Risks and benefits of nonsteroidal anti-inflammatory drugs in children: a comparison with paracetamol. *Paediatr Drugs* 2001; **3**: 817–58.
8. Kokki H. Nonsteroidal anti-inflammatory drugs for postoperative pain: a focus on children. *Paediatr Drugs* 2003; **5**: 103–23.
9. Karling M, Renstrom M, Ljungman G. Acute and postoperative pain in children: a Swedish nationwide survey. *Acta Paediatr* 2002; **91**: 660–6.
10. Vane JR, Botting RM. The mechanism of action of aspirin. *Thromb Res* 2003; **110**: 255–8.
11. Harvey RJ, Deprner UB, Wassle H. GlyR alpha3: an essential target for spinal PGE2-mediated inflammatory pain sensitization. *Science* 2004; **304**: 884–7.
12. Reinhold H, Ahmadi S. Depner UB. Spinal inflammatory hyperalgesia is mediated by prostaglandin E receptors of the EP2 subtype. *J Clin Invest* 2005; **115**: 673–9.
13. Peters JW, Koot HM, de Boer JB *et al*. Major surgery within the first 3 months of life and subsequent biobehavioral pain responses to immunization at later age: a case comparison study. *Pediatrics* 2003; **111**: 129–35.
14. Ochroch EA, Mardini IA, Gottschalk A. What is the role of NSAIDs in pre-emptive analgesia? *Drugs* 2003; **63**: 2709–23.

15. Vane JR. The inhibition of prostaglandin synthesis as a mechanism of action for aspirin-like drugs. *Nat New Biol* 1971; **231**: 232–5.

16. Simmons DL, Botting RM, Hla T. Cyclooxygenase isozymes: the biology of prostaglandin synthesis and inhibition. *Pharmacol Rev* 2004; **56**: 387–437.

17. Nikanne E, Kokki H, Salo J, Linna JP. Celecoxib and ketoprofen in pain management during tonsillectomy: a placebo-controlled clinical trial. *Otolaryngol Head Neck Surg* 2005; **132**: 287–94.

18. Aho M, Kokki H, Nikanne E. Nimesulide versus ibuprofen for postoperative tonsillectomy pain: a double blind, randomised, and active comparator-controlled clinical trial. *Clin Drug Invest* 2003; **23**: 651–60.

19. Björkman R. Central antinociceptive effects of non-steroidal anti-inflammatory drugs and paracetamol. Experimental studies in the rat. *Acta Anaesthesiol Scand Suppl* 1995; **39**: 1–44.

20. Ossipov MH, Jerussi TP, Ren K et al. Differential effects of spinal (R)-ketoprofen and (S)-ketoprofen against signs of neuropathic pain and tonic nociception: evidence for a novel mechanism of action of (R)-ketoprofen against tactile allodynia. *Pain* 2000; **87**: 193–9.

21. Vane JR, Botting RM. Overview-mechanism of action of anti-inflammatory drugs. In: Vane JR, Botting JH, Botting RM, eds. *Improved non-steroid anti-inflammatory drugs.* Cox-2 enzyme inhibitors. Dordrecht/London: Kluwer Academic Publishers/William Harvey Press, 1996: 1–27.

22. Anderson BJ. Comparing the efficacy of NSAIDs and paracetamol in children. *Paediatr Anaesth* 2004; **14**: 201–17.

23. Boutaud O, Aronoff DM, Richardson JH et al. Determinants of the cellular specificity of acetaminophen as an inhibitor of prostaglandin H(2) synthases. *Proc Natl Acad Sci USA* 2002; **99**: 7130–5.

24. Graham GG, Scott KF. Mechanism of action of paracetamol. *Am J Ther* 2005; **12**: 46–55.

25. Muth-Selbach US, Tegeder I, Brune K, Geisslinger G. Acetaminophen inhibits spinal prostaglandin E_2 release after peripheral noxious stimulation. *Anesthesiology* 1999; **91**: 231–9.

26. Kumpulainen E, Kokki H, Halonen T et al. Paracetamol (acetaminophen) penetrates readily into the cerebrospinal fluid of children after intravenous administration. *Pediatrics* 2007; **119**: 766–71.

27. Munsterhjelm E, Munsterhjelm NM, Niemi TT et al. Dose-dependent inhibition of platelet function by acetaminophen in healthy volunteers. *Anesthesiology* 2005; **103**: 712–17.

28. Pickering G, Loriot MA, Libert F et al. Analgesic effect of acetaminophen in humans: first evidence of a central serotonergic mechanism. *Clin Pharmacol Ther* 2006; **79**: 371–8.

29. Reye RDK, Morgan G, Baral J. Encephalopathy and fatty degeneration of the viscera: a disease entity in childhood. *Lancet* 1963; **ii**: 749–52.

30. Korpela R, Korvenoja P, Meretoja OA. Morphine-sparing effect of acetaminophen in pediatric day-case surgery. *Anesthesiology* 1999; **91**: 442–7.

31. Eneli I, Sadri K, Camargo C Jr, Barr RG. Acetaminophen and the risk of asthma: the epidemiologic and pathophysiologic evidence. *Chest* 2005; **127**: 604–12.

32. James LP, Mayeux PR, Hinson JA. Acetaminophen-induced hepatotoxicity. *Drug Metab Dispos* 2003; **31**: 1499–506.

33. Perrott DA, Piira T, Goodenough B, Champion GD. Efficacy and safety of acetaminophen vs ibuprofen for treating children's pain or fever: a meta-analysis. *Arch Pediatr Adolesc Med* 2004; **158**: 521–6.

34. Mikawa K, Nishina K Maekawa N et al. Dose-response of flurbiprofen on postoperative pain and emesis after paediatric strabismus surgery. *Can J Anaesth* 1997; **44**: 95–8.

35. Kokki H, Nikanne E, Tuovinen K. IV intraoperative ketoprofen in small children during adenoidectomy: a dose finding study. *Br J Anaesth* 1998; **81**: 870–4.

36. Kokki H, Karvinen M, Jekunen A. Pharmacokinetics of a 24-hour ketoprofen infusion in children. *Acta Anaesth Scand* 2002; **46**: 194–8.

37. Mannila A, Kokki H, Heikkinen M et al. Cerebrospinal fluid distribution of ketoprofen after intravenous administration in young children. *Clin Pharmacokinet* 2006; **45**: 737–43.

38. Wells TG, Mortensen ME, Dietrich A et al. Comparison of the pharmacokinetics of naproxen tablets and suspension in children. *J Clin Pharmacol* 1994; **34**: 30–3.

39. Morton NS, Benham SW, Lawson RA, McNicol LR. Diclofenac vs oxybuprocaine eyedrops for analgesia in paediatric strabismus surgery. *Paediatr Anaesth* 1997; **7**: 221–6.

40. Forrest JB, Heitlinger EL, Revell S. Ketorolac for postoperative pain management in children. *Drug Safety* 1997; **16**: 309–29.

41. Gupta A, Daggett C, Drant S et al. Prospective randomized trial of ketorolac after congenital heart surgery. *J Cardiothorac Vasc Anesth* 2004; **18**: 454–7.

42. Maunuksela, EL, Kokki H, Bullingham, RE. Comparison of intravenous ketorolac with morphine for postoperative pain in children. *Clin Pharmacol Ther* 1992; **52**: 436–43.

43. Purday JP, Reichert CC, Merrick PM. Comparative effects of three doses of intravenous ketorolac or morphine on emesis and analgesia for restorative dental surgery in children. *Can J Anaesth* 1996; **43**: 221–5.

44. Bridge HS, Montgomery CJ, Kennedy RA, Merrick PM. Analgesic efficacy of ketorolac 0.5 per cent ophthalmic solution (Accular) in paediatric strabismus surgery. *Paediatr Anaesth* 2000; **10**: 521–6.

45. Maunuksela EL, Olkkola KT, Korpela R. Does prophylactic intravenous infusion of indomethacin improve the management of postoperative pain in children? *Can J Anaesth* 1998; **35**: 123–7.

46. Sims C, Johnson CM, Bergesio R. et al. Rectal indomethacin for analgesia after appendicectomy in children. *Anaesth Intensive Care* 1994; **22**: 272–5.

47. Thomas RL, Parker GC, van Overmeire B, Aranda JV. A meta-analysis of ibuprofen versus indomethacin for closure of patent ductus arteriosus. *Eur J Pediatr* 2005; **164**: 135–40.

48. Mannila A, Kumpulainen E, Lehtonen M et al. Plasma and cerebrospinal fluid concentrations of indomethacin in

children after intravenous administration. *J Clin Pharmacol* 2007; **47**; 94–100.

49. Dsida RM, Wheeler M, Birmingham PK *et al.* Age-stratified pharmacokinetics of ketorolac tromethamine in pediatric surgical patients. *Anesth Analg* 2002; **94**: 266–70.

50. Kain ZN, Mayes LC, Caldwell-Andrews AA *et al.* Sleeping characteristics of children undergoing outpatient elective surgery. *Anesthesiology* 2002; **97**: 1093–101.

51. Anderson BJ, Holford NH, Woollard GA *et al.* Perioperative pharmacodynamics of acetaminophen analgesia in children. *Anesthesiology* 1999; **90**: 411–21.

52. Römsing J, Ostergaard D, Senderovitz T *et al.* Pharmacokinetics of oral diclofenac and acetaminophen in children after surgery. *Paediatr Anaesth* 2001; **11**: 205–13.

53. Kearns GL, Abdel-Rahman SM, Alander SW *et al.* Developmental pharmacology – drug disposition, action, and therapy in infants and children. *N Engl J Med* 2003; **349**: 1157–67.

54. Foster PN, Williams JG. Bradycardia following intravenous ketorolac in children. *Eur J Anaesthesiol* 1997; **14**: 307–9.

55. Anderson BJ, Monteleone J, Holford NHG. Variability of concentrations after rectal paracetamol. *Paediatr Anaesth* 1998; **8**: 274.

56. van Overmeire B, Allegaert K, Casaer A *et al.* Prophylactic ibuprofen in premature infants: a multicentre, randomised, double-blind, placebo-controlled trial. *Lancet* 2004; **364**: 1945–9.

57. Kokinsky E, Thornberg E, Ostlund AL, Larsson LE. Postoperative comfort in paediatric outpatient surgery. *Paediatr Anaesth* 1999; **9**: 243–51.

58. Munro HM, Malviya S, Lauder GR *et al.* Pain relief in children following outpatient surgery. *J Clin Anesth* 1999; **11**: 187–91.

59. Wolf AR. Tears at bedtime: a pitfall of extending paediatric day-case surgery without extending analgesia. *Br J Anaesth* 1999; **82**: 319–20.

60. Spafford PA von B, Hicks CL. Expected and reported pain in children undergoing ear piercing: a randomized trial of preparation by parents. *Behav Res Ther* 2002; **40**: 253–66.

61. Hämeen-Anttila K, Kemppainen K, Enlund H *et al.* Do pictograms improve children's understanding of medicine leaflet information? *Patient Educ Couns* 2004; **55**: 371–8.

62. Church JJ. Day case tonsillectomy in children. *Ambul Surg* 1999; **7**: 17–19.

63. Römsing J, Walther-Larsen S. Peri-operative use of nonsteroidal anti-inflammatory drugs in children: analgesic efficacy and bleeding. *Anaesthesia* 1997; **52**: 673–83.

64. Kokki H, Salonen A. Comparison of pre- and postoperative administration of ketoprofen for analgesia after tonsillectomy in children. *Paediatr Anaesth* 2002; **12**: 162–7.

65. Bone ME, Fell D. A comparison of rectal diclofenac with intramuscular papaveretum or placebo for pain relief following tonsillectomy. *Anaesthesia* 1988; **43**: 277–80.

66. Hamunen K, Maunuksela EL. Ketorolac does not depress ventilation in children. *Paediatr Anaesth* 1996; **6**: 79.

67. Moren J, Francois T, Blanloeil Y, Pinaud M. The effects of a nonsteroidal anti-inflammatory drug (ketoprofen) on morphine respiratory depression: a double-blind, randomized study in volunteers. *Anesth Analg* 1997; **85**: 400–5.

68. Moiniche S, Romsing J, Dahl JB, Tramer MR. Nonsteroidal antiinflammatory drugs and the risk of operative site bleeding after tonsillectomy: a quantitative systematic review. *Anesth Analg* 2003; **96**(1): 68–77.

69. Cardwell M, Siviter G, Smith A. Non-steroidal anti-inflammatory drugs and perioperative bleeding in paediatric tonsillectomy. *Cochrane Database Syst Rev* 2005; **2**: CD003591.

70. Royal College of Anaesthetists. *Clinical guidelines for the use of non-steroidal anti-inflammatory drugs in the perioperative period*. London: Royal College of Anaesthetists, 1998.

71. Niemi TT, Taxell C, Rosenberg PH. Comparison of the effect of intravenous ketoprofen, ketorolac and diclofenac on platelet function in volunteers. *Acta Anaesthesiol Scand* 1997; **41**: 1353–8.

72. Rusy LM, Houck CS, Sullivan LJ *et al.* A double-blind evaluation of ketorolac tromethamine versus acetaminophen in pediatric tonsillectomy: analgesia and bleeding. *Anesth Analg* 1995; **80**: 226–9.

73. Splinter WM, Rhine EJ, Roberts DW *et al.* Preoperative ketorolac increases bleeding after tonsillectomy in children. *Can J Anaesth* 1996; **43**: 560–3.

74. Russell RI. Non-steroidal anti-inflammatory drugs and gastrointestinal damage-problems and solutions. *Postgrad Med J* 2001; **77**: 82–8.

75. Gadiyar V, Gallagher TM, Crean PM, Taylor RH. The effect of a combination of rectal diclofenac and caudal bupivacaine on postoperative analgesia in children. *Anaesthesia* 1995; **50**: 820–2.

76. Cuzzolin L, Dal Cere M, Fanos V. NSAID-induced nephrotoxicity from the fetus to the child. *Drug Safety* 2001; **24**: 9–18.

77. Sturmer T, Erb A, Keller F. *et al.* Determinants of impaired renal function with use of nonsteroidal anti-inflammatory drugs: the importance of half-life and other medications. *Am J Med* 2001; **111**: 521–37.

78. Rocha GM, Michea LF, Peters EM *et al.* Direct toxicity of nonsteroidal antiinflammatory drugs for renal medullary cells. *Proc Natl Acad Sci USA* 2001; **9**: 5317–22.

79. Short JA, Barr CA, Palmer CD *et al.* Use of diclofenac in children with asthma. *Anaesthesia* 2000; **55**: 334–7.

80. Lesko SM, Louik C, Vezina RM, Mitchell AA. Asthma morbidity after the short-term use of ibuprofen in children. *Pediatrics* 2002; **109**: E20.

81. American Academy of Pediatrics. Committee on Drugs. Acetaminophen toxicity in children. *Pediatrics* 2001; **108**: 1020–4.

82. Rumack BH. Acetaminophen overdose in young children. Treatment and effects of alcohol and other additional ingestants in 417 cases. *Am J Dis Child* 1984; **138**: 428–33.

83. Russell FM, Shann F, Curtis N, Mulholland K. Evidence on the use of paracetamol in febrile children. *Bull World Health Org* 2003; **81**: 367–72.

84. Peterson RG, Rumack BH. Age as a variable in acetaminophen overdose. *Arch Intern Medical* 1981; **141**: 390–3.
85. Cranswick N, Coghlan D. Paracetamol efficacy and safety in children: the first 40 years. *Am J Ther* 2000; **7**: 135–41.
86. Clunie M, Crone LA, Klassen L *et al.* Psychiatric side effects of indomethacin in parturients. *Can J Anaesth* 2003; **50**: 586–8.
87. Tharumaratnam D, Bashford S, Khan SA. Indomethacin induced psychosis. *Postgrad Med J* 2000; **76**: 736–7.
88. Nikanne E. *Ketoprofen for postoperative pain after day-case adenoidectomy in small children.* Kuopio University Publications D. Medical Sciences 1999; 173.
89. Tuomilehto H. *Pain management and outcome in children after adenoidectomy: a special reference to different administration routes of ketoprofen.* Kuopio University Publications D. Medical Sciences 2002; 269.
90. Salonen A. Ketoprofen in tonsillectomy and adenoidectomy with special reference to the effects on surgical time, postoperative pain, adverse events and recovery after surgery. Kuopio University Publications D. Medical Sciences 2002; 283.

14

Local anaesthetics and their adjuncts

JEAN-XAVIER MAZOIT, PER-ARNE LÖNNQVIST

KEY LEARNING POINTS

- Local anaesthetics (LAs) are bound to plasma proteins, particularly α_1- acid glycoprotein (AAG). Neonates and young infants have low levels of AAG and thus similar doses of LAs will result in higher free plasma levels.
- Cardiac conduction blockade by LAs is markedly stereospecific unlike protein binding or neural blockade. Consequently, the $S(-)$-enantiomers, levobupivacaine and ropivacaine, have similar efficacy and lower cardiac toxicity.
- Cardiac toxicity of LAs is rate dependent – infants and small children may be a greater risk because of their higher heart rates.
- Plasma levels of LAs may be unexpectedly high after three or four half-lives during epidural infusions, especially in infants and young children.
- LA adjuncts (clonidine, ketamine) have been shown to enhance the efficacy of single-shot epidural blockade.

INTRODUCTION

This chapter will explore the pharmacology of local anaesthetic agents with the emphasis on clinical relevance. The differences in pharmacokinetics, pharmacodynamics, clinical activity and toxicity between adults and children will be explored. The pharmacology of adjuvant drugs commonly used in paediatric anaesthesia will be discussed.

PHYSICOCHEMICAL PROPERTIES OF LOCAL ANAESTHETICS

Local anaesthetics (LAs) are weak bases with molecular masses ranging from 270 Da to 320 Da (Table 14.1). Their formula contains an aromatic ring (hydrophobic part of the molecule), an intermediate chain and a hydrophilic residue with a tertiary amine. The intermediate chain is either an ester or an amide function. Only amide local anaesthetics will be considered in this chapter. The extent of substitution of the hydrophilic residue affects hydrophobicity, pK_a and steric bulk. All LAs have a pK_a between 7.6 (mepivacaine) and 8.1 (bupivacaine and ropivacaine). At the physiological pH of 7.40, 60–85 per cent of the molecules are ionised and largely diffuse in the water compartments of the body (Table 14.2). Local anaesthetics are also soluble in lipids and cell membranes. The capacity to cross membranes is measured by the partition coefficient between lipid or organic solvent and water. In comparison with lidocaine, bupivacaine is 10 times more soluble in membranes while ropivacaine is only twice as soluble.

With the exception of lidocaine, all amide LAs possess an asymmetrical carbon. Although the physicochemical properties (pK_a, partition coefficient) of the isomers are

Table 14.1 Physicochemical properties of amide local anaesthetics

Agent	Molecular mass* (Da)	pK_a	Partition coefficient[†]	Protein binding (%)	Onset of action	Duration of action	Potency[‡]
Amides							
Lidocaine	234	7.9	2.9	65	Short	1½ –2 hours	1
Prilocaine	220	7.9	0.9	55	Short	1½–2 hours	1
Mepivacaine	246	7.6	0.8	75	Short	2–3 hours	1
Bupivacaine	288	8.1	27.5	95	Intermediate	3–3½ hours	4
Levobupivacaine	288	8.1	27.5	95	Intermediate	3–3½ hours	4
Etidocaine	276	7.7	141	95	Short	3–4 hours	4
Ropivacaine	274	8.1	6.1	94	Intermediate	2½–3 hours	3.3

*Free base.
[†] *n*-Heptane/buffer partition coefficient at pH 7.40.
[‡] Potency is relative to lidocaine.
Etidocaine is no longer marketed in most countries and is not recommended because of high toxicity.
From: Denson and Mazoit [1].

Table 14.2 Fraction of local anaesthetic molecules in ionised form at normal pH in plasma and tissue

Drug	Plasma (pH 7.40)	Tissue (pH 7.10)
Lidocaine	76	86
Prilocaine	76	86
Mepivacaine	61	76
Bupivacaine	83	91
Etidocaine	66	80
Ropivacaine	83	91

From: Denson and Mazoit [1].

identical, the differences in the molecular conformation lead to different affinities of the enantiomers to biological effectors (channels, receptors, proteins). Ropivacaine is the $S(-)$ enantiomer of the N-propyl-2′,6′-pipecoloxylidide and levobupivacaine is the $S(-)$ enantiomer of bupivacaine (N-butyl-2′,6′-pipecoloxylidide).

Local anaesthetics are marketed as hydrochloride salts in water at a pH of 4–5 in order to have a perfect solubility [2]. It is important to remember that increasing the pH of the solution, for example by adding bicarbonate, may precipitate the salt. Currently, plain solutions are free from any preservative; only solutions with adrenaline contain metabisulphite.

PHARMACOKINETICS

Anaesthetists and pharmacologists have a different vision of pharmacokinetics (Table 14.3). Whereas pharmacologists are interested in the 'true' parameters approaching physiology, i.e. volumes and clearances, anaesthetists are interested in 'practical' parameters, i.e. concentrations, time to reach peak concentrations and half-live, especially context sensitive half-live. We will focus on both aspects [3].

Binding to blood components

Like most weak bases, amide LAs are bound to serum proteins. A small amount is also bound to red cells which may be of clinical relevance especially in newborn and young infants.

BINDING TO RED BLOOD CELLS

Amide LAs bind to red cells [4]. Only 20–30 per cent of the total amount in blood is bound to erythrocytes. Despite their relatively low binding capacity, the buffering capacity of erythrocytes can become important at very high (toxic) concentrations, or when serum protein concentration is markedly decreased. In neonates whose haematocrit often exceeds 50 per cent the buffering capacity of red cells may be clinically relevant.

BINDING TO SERUM PROTEINS

In serum, LAs bind to α_1-acid glycoprotein (AAG) and to human serum albumin (HSA) [5]. The stereospecificity of this binding is insignificant from a clinical point of view.

Despite its low concentration in serum (less than 1 g/L in adults), AAG is the major protein that binds LAs because AAG possess a very high affinity for weak bases such as LAs or phenylpiperidines (fentanyl, sufentanil, alfentanil). The AAG concentration is very low at birth (less than 30 per cent of the concentration measured in adults) [6] and this is why the free fraction of LAs is much higher in neonates and young infants. The AAG concentration progressively increases to reach adult levels by the end of the first year. α_1-Acid glycoprotein is an acute phase protein and its concentration rapidly increases in the postoperative period and all inflammatory states [7,8]. This increase in AAG concentration decreases the free fraction of LA, which may guard against toxicity; however, because there is a concomitant

Table 14.3 Bupivacaine and ropivacaine pharmacokinetics after different routes in infants and children compared with adults

	fu	V_{ss}* (L)	CLT/f (mL/min/kg)	CLU/f (mL/min/kg)	$T_{1/2}$* (h)
Bupivacaine					
Intravenous, adults	0.05	0.85–1.3	4.5–8.1	≈100	1.8
Epidural, adults			4–5.6		5.1–10.6
Infants, caudal single shot	0.16 (0.05–0.35)	3.9	7.1		
Children (5–10 years)		2.7	10		
Infants, epidural prolonged	(0.06–0.24)*		5.5–7.5*	36–73	
	(0.03–0.18)†		3.5–4†	36–73	
Ropivacaine					
Intravenous, adults	0.05	0.5–0.6	4.2–5.3	≈100	1.7
Epidural, adults			4.0–5.7	≈70	2.9–5.4
Caudal single shot					
Neonates	0.07			50–58	
Infants	0.05–0.10	2.1	5.2		
Children	5.2 (1.3–7.3)	2.4	7.4	151	
Epidural prolonged					
Neonates		2.4	4.26		
Infants		2.4	6.15		
Children	0.04		8.5	220	

fu, free fraction; V_{ss}, volume of distribution at steady-state; CL/f, total body clearance over bioavailability (T, total fraction; U, unbound fraction); $T_{1/2}$, terminal half-life. For adults, a mean body weight of 75 kg has been assumed.

*Apparent value, $T_{1/2}$ and volumes measured after non-intravenous injections are overestimated because of a flip-flop effect (see text).

†,† After 3 h infusion and 48 h infusion, respectively. CLT decreases with time because protein binding increases. For references see Mazoit and Dalens [3].

fall in hepatic clearance due to the decreased free fraction, the net effect is unchanged.

Human serum albumin also binds LAs, but with a very low affinity. It is only because HSA is the most abundant protein in serum that its binding capacity becomes significant. In neonates, HSA concentration is similar to that measured in adults. In pathological states AAG concentration increases when HSA decreases, with the exception of nephrotic syndrome.

Several pathological conditions could lead to a decrease in protein binding, but only acidosis has proved to be of clinical relevance.

Absorption

ABSORPTION AFTER TOPICAL ANAESTHESIA

After topical anaesthesia for upper airway procedures, rapid absorption may lead to toxic concentrations, particularly in children less than 4 years old. Topical spray (lidocaine 3–5 mg/kg) should be delivered using a metered nozzle giving 10 mg in each puff [9] or measured doses of either 1 per cent or 4 per cent via an atomising spray.

EMLA (eutectic mixture of local anaesthetics) cream containing an equal amount of lidocaine and prilocaine is not absorbed in significant amount with the exception of premature babies [10]. In neonates and infants prilocaine may induce methaemoglobinaemia [11]. The efficacy of the cream has been questioned in premature babies because of a high skin blood flow at this age (see Chapter 8).

ABSORPTION AFTER CENTRAL AND PERIPHERAL NERVE BLOCKS

Amide LAs are usually considered as having a bioavailability of 1 (metabolism is exclusively hepatic). Since they are liposoluble they bind to the tissues and undergo delayed absorption; the extent of the delay depends upon local conditions. For example, after ilio-inguino–ilio-hypogastric block, absorption occurs faster than after caudal injection. From adult studies we may extrapolate that the speed of absorption decreases from head to foot for peripheral blocks, and from the thoracic to the caudal part of the epidural space (with the possible exception of children not yet walking).

Spinal anaesthesia necessitates high dosage in infants; furthermore, the block duration is brief. Some authors have attributed this to the large volume and rapid turnover of cerebrospinal fluid (CSF) in neonates and infants, in comparison with older children and adults. In fact, the pharmacokinetics of LAs in the CSF is unknown, particularly in the paediatric age group. At the cephalic level, neonates and infants have a lower CSF volume and turnover than children and adults [12]. Extrapolation from animal studies looking at the pharmacokinetics of intrathecal opioids and human studies of epidural LAs suggest that the dural surface area is the determinant of clearance of both spinal and epidural drugs [13]. Dural surface area is related to body surface area not weight, hence LA clearance from CSF is higher in younger patients.

Anton Burm and his collaborators performed a series of elegant studies in adults. Using a double injection technique with stable isotopes, they showed that LAs injected in the epidural space were trapped locally [14]. Three hours after injection, only 70 per cent of a dose of lidocaine and 50 per cent of a dose of bupivacaine were absorbed into the bloodstream, a phenomenon also observed with ropivacaine. This slow absorption process occurs after almost all extravascular injections and is an important safety feature. Lidocaine and bupivacaine concentrations peak about 30 minutes after a caudal or lumbar injection in infants and adults. The time to maximum peak concentration (T_{max}) of ropivacaine is much longer in infants than in children and also longer in children than in adults (Table 14.3). In a study done in patients aged 1–8 years, ropivacaine T_{max} was inversely related to age, from 115 minutes in children aged 1–2 years to 30 minutes in children aged 5–8 years [15]. This correlation is less apparent with levobupivacaine [16].

Adrenaline decreases the peak concentration of LA, even ropivacaine which has intrinsic mild vasoconstrictive properties [17]. Adrenaline also increases the duration of postoperative analgesia after caudal anaesthesia. The usual concentration in clinical practice is 5 mg/L (1/200 000), which has proved to be optimal in adults. It has been suggested this concentration of adrenaline might decrease the spinal cord blood flow in infants, possibly leading to neurological deficits [18] so 1/400 000 adrenaline, which is also effective, may be preferable in this age group.

Distribution

The volume of distribution of local anaesthetics at steady-state (V_{SS}) is slightly below 1 L/kg. Because absorption is delayed after non-intravenous (IV) injection, a 'flip-flop' effect occurs and calculated volumes are markedly overestimated (see Table 14.3). The terminal half-lives are also increased compared with the 'true' value obtained after IV injection. Only the total body clearance is accurately measured after extravascular administration, provided that sampling is performed over a prolonged period.

Local anaesthetics largely distribute in tissue in their ionised form (see Table 14.2). The volume of distribution is probably larger in neonates and infants than in adults. If this hypothesis is true, distribution in a large volume may prevent high serum concentrations after single administration, but not after several reinjections. The volume of distribution of ropivacaine is smaller than that of bupivacaine in adults; this probably also applies in paediatric patients. When dosing is similar, ropivacaine C_{max} (C_{max} is the observed maximum concentration) is sometimes higher than bupivacaine C_{max} despite a delayed T_{max} usually observed with ropivacaine (Table 14.4).

Elimination

METABOLISM

All amide LAs are metabolised in the liver by the cytochrome P450 enzyme group. Bupivacaine is predominantly metabolised into pipecoloxylidide (PPX) by the CYP3A4 [19]. Ropivacaine is mainly metabolised into 3'- and 4'-hydroxy-ropivacaine by the CYP1A2 and to a minor extent to PPX by the CYP3A4 [20]. These enzymes are not fully mature at birth and there are important differences in their developmental expression [21].

Before birth and during the first 3–6 months of life, CYP3A4 is deficient, but parts of its biotransformation activities are achieved by the CYP3A7. In contrast, CYP1A2 is deficient during the first year of life and it is not fully functional before the age of 4 years.

CLEARANCE

Lidocaine has a relatively high hepatic extraction ratio (0.65–0.75) and is considered flow limited rather than rate limited for its elimination. Therefore, any fall in the patient's cardiac output may decrease lidocaine hepatic clearance. The ensuing increase in plasma concentrations may reach toxic levels. Conversely, bupivacaine and ropivacaine have a relatively low hepatic extraction ratio (0.30–0.35) and are considered rate limited for their elimination. Therefore, intrinsic hepatic clearance and free fraction are the major determinants of total clearance. In the postoperative period, protein binding increases due to the increase in AAG concentration in serum. A parallel decrease in clearance is observed [8], but this only leads to a resetting in total serum concentration and the unbound concentration remains constant.

Bupivacaine clearance is low at birth and slightly increases during the first 6–9 months of life [6]. Ropivacaine clearance is also low in neonates and infants and increases during the first 2–6 years of life [15,22–24]. In clinical use even in younger patients, all studies have reported ropivacaine concentrations below toxic levels. After 3 hours of bupivacaine infusion via the lumbar epidural route, Meunier and co-workers found a clearance of 5.5 mL/min/kg in 1-month-old infants, rising to 7.3 mL/min/kg in infants of 6 months [8].

After a single-shot caudal injection of 0.2 per cent ropivacaine, Hansen et al. found a clearance of 5.7 mL/min/kg in infants less than 3 months old and of 6.5 mL/min/kg in infants older than 3 months [22]. These values are similar to the values of 4.3 (infants) and 6.2 mL/min/kg (children) reported by McCann and coworkers [25]. The increase in CL with age is seen with both bupivacaine and ropivacaine but appears to be more marked with ropivacaine. Lönnqvist and coworkers reported that ropivacaine clearance measured after caudal epidural administration increased during the ages 1–8 years: 6.4 mL/min/kg in the 1- to 2-year-old age group, 7.1 mL/min/kg in the 3- to 4-year-old age group and 8.8 mL/min/kg in the 5- to 8-year-old age groups [15].

Table 14.4 Absorption of bupivacaine versus ropivacaine after single-shot administration (venous concentrations)

	Dose	C_{max}	C_{umax}	T_{max}
Bupivacaine				
Adults (epidural)				
	100 mg 0.5%*	0.53		21
Children (caudal)				
1–6 months	2.5 mg/kg 0.5%	0.6–1.9		28
5.5 years	2.5 mg/kg 0.25%	0.96–1.64		29
Children (lumbar or thoracic epidural)				
3–36 months	3.75 mg/kg 0.5%*	1.35		20
1 month–1 year	1.875 mg/kg 0.25%*	0.55–1.10		20
Children (ilioinguinal block)				
10–15 kg	0.25 mL/kg 0.5%	0.43–4.0		18
15–30 kg	–	0.35–1.34		16
Ropivacaine				
Adults (epidural)				
	150 mg 0.75%	1.09		25
Children (caudal)				
0–3 months	2 mg/kg 0.2%	0.42–1.58	10–143	
3–12 months	–	0.41–1.28	7–67	
1–7 years	2 mg/kg 0.2%	0.49–1.05		65
Children (lumbar epidural)				
3–11 months	1.7 mg/kg 0.2%	0.55–0.72		60
12–48 months	–	0.54–0.75		60
Children (ilioinguinal block)				
1–2 years	3 mg/kg 0.5%	0.68–1.84		45
3–4 years	–	0.90–4.77		52
5–12 years	–	0.64–4.77		45

*With adrenaline.
C_{umax} is the maximum observed free concentration after single injection; C_{max} is the maximum observed concentration after a single-shot injection; T_{max} is the time to C_{max}.

A similar observation was made by Bösenberg *et al.* who infused ropivacaine in neonates and infants for postoperative pain relief [24]. In neonates ropivacaine intrinsic clearance was five to six times lower than in the older patients aged 1 year.

After several hours (or days) of administration, total clearance of bupivacaine and of ropivacaine decreases because of the rise in AAG plasma concentration. During the postoperative period, inflammation results in an increase in protein binding, and therefore a decrease in total body clearance. The same studies as above have shown that bupivacaine or ropivacaine total concentration increases during the first 36–48 hours of infusion, whereas the free concentration rapidly reaches near steady-state. The intrinsic hepatic clearance remains constant and, more importantly, the free drug concentration (which is the toxic moiety) rapidly reaches a plateau. Bösenberg *et al.* measured the main metabolites of ropivacaine in urine: pipecoloxylidide (CYP3A4 and CYP-3A7) and 3-hydroxy-ropivacaine (CYP-1A2) [24]. The concentration of 3-hydroxy-ropivacaine in urine increases from birth to the age of 6 months.

Concentrations observed after single-shot or prolonged administration

The concentrations observed after administration by different routes are summarised in Table 14.4.

Concentrations leading to toxicity are largely unknown. In data derived from experimental studies and investigations in adult volunteers, ropivacaine and levobupivacaine are less toxic than racemic bupivacaine. It appears that the threshold of toxicity is about 0.3 mg/L of unbound bupivacaine and 0.6 mg/L of unbound ropivacaine or levobupivacaine in adults. Neonates and infants seem to be more prone to develop toxicity because of reduced serum binding, lower clearance and an increased susceptibility to cardiac effects of LAs (see below). Moreover, because of large interindividual variations in concentrations (the distribution of concentrations is log-normally distributed), some individuals are at greater risk of toxicity. In neonates and infants less than 3 months of age, the free drug concentration may be at the upper limit despite total concentrations far below the threshold of toxicity [6,8,24,26,27]. In these patients clinical manifestations of toxicity may be subtle but will be present on close observation [26].

After single-shot administration, bupivacaine T_{max} is in the region of 25–30 minutes, whatever the route. This is not the case with ropivacaine which has a delayed T_{max}, that is more marked in younger patients. The C_{max} observed with ropivacaine, however, is not lower than with bupivacaine. To date, very few studies have been published with levobupivacaine. From adult studies, we may expect that the kinetics of levobupivacaine will be similar to that of the racemic mixture. In particular, the observed higher intrinsic hepatic clearance of racemic bupivacaine compared with ropivacaine in neonates may offer an advantage if confirmed by further studies.

There have been numerous studies of kinetics during prolonged epidural administration of local anaesthetics for postoperative pain relief. All these investigations assumed that the intrinsic unbound clearance was unaffected during the whole period of administration. Indeed, despite some doubt regarding a possible time-dependent clearance, the clearance of the unbound forms of bupivacaine and ropivacaine appear to be relatively constant in adults and infants. Because of the rise in plasma proteins, the total plasma concentrations of bupivacaine and ropivacaine tend to increase postoperatively over 2–4 days. Concomitantly, the free fraction decreases in a parallel manner and the unbound concentration reaches a steady level 12–18 hours after the initiation of infusion. However, saturation of the buffering properties of the different compartments (epidural fat, fluid compartments, etc.) occurs and after three to four half-lives the steady-state concentration may be higher than the toxic threshold, especially in the younger patients.

PHARMACODYNAMICS

Action on ionic channels

Local anaesthetics block the propagation of impulse along nerve fibres due to the inactivation of voltage-gated sodium channels which initiate the action potential. They are blocked by different toxins like tetrodotoxin (TTX) at the outer side of the cell and by LAs at the cytosolic side of the phospholipid membrane [28]. More precisely, LAs cross the membrane as a free base (unionised), they become ionised and diffuse in the cytoplasm to block the Na^+ channel pore mechanically by binding to a specific amino acid. Local anaesthetics bind differently to the sodium channel depending of the state of the channel. A basal block (tonic block) may be augmented by a phasic block also called frequency-dependent or rate-dependent block. When the frequency of stimulation increases, the molecule cannot unbind from the channel and the intensity of the block increases. Local anaesthetics also block potassium and calcium channels at concentrations slightly higher than those required to block sodium channels. Unlike the central nervous system (CNS) and heart, peripheral nerves express only a small number of potassium channels. Voltage-gated potassium channels initiate repolarisation. Some of these

channels – including the hERG (human *ether-à-go-go related gene*) channel – are responsible for genetically induced arrhythmias such as the long-QT, short-QT or Brugada's syndromes and are blocked by LAs at concentrations just above those blocking sodium channels [29,30]. Both sodium and potassium channel blocks are stereospecific, usually the S-enantiomers causing less blockade than the R-enantiomers. Local anaesthetics bind to neuronal L-type calcium channels [31]. However, the role of L-type calcium channel block in the cardiotoxic effect of long-lasting LAs is unclear. Bupivacaine also binds to the myocardial ryanodine receptor, but the inhibitory effect is significant only at concentrations well above those encountered in clinical practice [32].

Action on nerve conduction

Nerve fibres are classified as myelinated and non-myelinated fibres. In the non-myelinated fibres, the action potential propagates continuously. After the initial depolarisation, the sodium channel is unresponsive to stimulation (the refractory period), thus preventing backward impulse propagation. Like sodium channels, potassium channels are evenly distributed along the fibres. The conduction velocity is low in these small fibres. Myelin is an insulating material and this layer is interrupted regularly by the nodes of Ranvier. Sodium channels are concentrated in these small areas, where they are anchored with a concentration of about 200 000 channels/cm² [33,34]. Potassium channels are distributed along the myelin sheet with a higher concentration in the juxtaparanodal region. The sudden depolarisation of the node induces an electrical field, which extends to two to three nodes. The action potential then 'jumps' rapidly from one node to the other. Because the distance between nodes is much higher in heavily myelinated fibres (there are 3–4 nodes/cm in Aα-fibres compared with 20–30 nodes/cm in Aδ-fibres) the conduction velocity is faster in the fibres involved in motor function and fine sensitivity than in fibres involved in pain. As the electrical field extends over several nodes fibres need to be 'bathed' with LAs for a distance that is greater than the field [35]. This induces a progressive extinction of the signal called decremental conduction. Fortunately, the block is reinforced by the phasic block induced by the high frequency of firing of nerves. Small, Aδ, lightly myelinated fibres are blocked with a lesser amount of drug than heavily myelinated fibres. This phenomenon, called differential nerve block, is explained by the difference in internode distance between fibres. It is not known to what extent the older explanation for these differences – a concentration gradient across the myelin sheet – contributes to this phenomenon.

Developmental aspects of myelinisation and effect of LAs according to age

Myelinisation begins during the third trimester of pregnancy and is incomplete at birth. After birth, myelinisation is rapid and is almost complete at 3–4 years. A last step corresponding to the process of motor and intellectual maturation continues until adolescence. In rats, peripheral neurological maturation is almost complete at the age of 3 weeks [33,34] while nodes of Ranvier are fully mature at the age of 2–3 weeks. The internode distance in mature rats is unchanged from that at 2 weeks of age. In infants and in children, low concentration solutions are used for most procedures. A prolonged motor block is observed with concentrations of bupivacaine or ropivacaine higher that 2–3 mg/L. Benzon and coworkers, using rabbit vagus nerve [36], found that similar LA concentrations led to more intense motor blockade in younger animals. Kohane and coworkers compared the effect of various concentrations and doses of bupivacaine and ropivacaine in a rat model [37]. They were able to show that the dose of either drug inducing a block of similar duration was identical in rats aged 2 weeks and those aged 10 weeks, despite an eightfold difference in body weight. Thus, infants and children require large volumes of low-concentration solutions to achieve blocks of similar intensity and duration to adults. Together with the kinetic factors already discussed, this may explain why spinal anaesthesia duration is so short in neonates and infants.

Action on the central nervous system

Like all inhibitors of sodium channels, LAs possess anticonvulsive effects at low dosage. For example, lidocaine is still used in children with intractable epilepsy [38]; however, the therapeutic ratio is low. At higher doses LAs induce convulsions and even coma. Long-acting LAs also provoke cardiac arrhythmias, which arise at similar concentrations to those leading to convulsions.

Action on the cardiovascular system

With the exception of the nodal conduction, which depends on calcium channels, electrical conduction in the heart is dependent on sodium channels. This is why lidocaine is the chief class Ib antiarrhythmic agent. Indeed, LAs prolong the effective refractory period, but the balance between the increase in effective refractory period and the decrease in the ventricular conduction velocity is unfavourable. Long-lasting local anaesthetics, such as bupivacaine, profoundly decrease the ventricular conduction velocity [39]. This phenomenon is markedly amplified by the addition of a phasic block when heart rate increases [40]. In animal studies, the intensity of the block is the same in neonates and in adults at similar heart rate (Fig. 14.1) [42]. However, because neonates and infants have a higher heart rate than adults, they are more sensitive to the block induced by LAs than adults. Contractility is also impaired by LAs. However, a study on isolated rabbit heart demonstrated that the concentration needed to halve maximum contractile force (EC_{50}) required 10 times the dose of

bupivacaine leading to EC_{50} for ventricular conduction impairment [41]. Contrary to the effect observed on conduction, the effect on contractility was markedly age dependent: newborn rabbits were three times more sensitive to bupivacaine than adult animals. At higher heart rates contractility was even further depressed in the newborn rabbit.

In addition to the effect of sympathetic blockade induced by central block, LAs have direct vasoactive properties and may be vasoconstrictor or vasodilator. Ropivacaine possesses mild vasoconstrictor properties [42], which have been implicated in ischaemia after penile block [43]. However, a direct relationship between ropivacaine and this report seems doubtful as the addition of adrenaline to ropivacaine amplifies the vasoconstrictive effect [17].

Stereospecificity

Mepivacaine, prilocaine, bupivacaine and ropivacaine possess an asymmetrical carbon. Because binding to proteins such as serum proteins, hepatic enzymes or ionic channels may be asymmetrical, different properties of the enantiomers are expected. Table 14.5 summarises our knowledge on the enantioselectivity of pharmacokinetics and of pharmacodynamics. In brief, pharmacokinetics is very little affected, e.g. serum protein binding of bupivacaine differs between the $S(-)$- and the $R(+)$-enantiomers only at concentrations 100 times higher than those encountered in clinical practice. Nerve blockade shows little stereoselectivity [44]. This is why levobupivacaine achieves similar blocking properties to its racemic counterpart. In the heart, conduction is markedly enantioselective (Fig. 14.2), whereas stereoselectivity of contractility appears to be unimportant [45].

Local anaesthetics as anti-inflammatory drugs and antinociceptive agent

Apart from their action on ionic channels, LAs possess anti-inflammatory properties. Local anaesthetics inhibit platelet aggregation *in vitro* and *in vivo* [46]. They decrease leukocyte priming and the production of free radicals [47–49]; consequently lidocaine has been proposed as treatment for adult respiratory distress syndrome. Moreover, systemically administered lidocaine has been shown to have antinociceptive effect particularly on neuropathic pain [50]. Interestingly, by limiting the neuropathic inflammatory processes, LAs can prevent and even treat complex regional pain syndrome in adults and in children [51,52].

TOXICITY OF LOCAL ANAESTHETICS

Toxicity at the site of injection

At the site of injection, the minimum concentration necessary for nerve blockade is 300–1500 μmol/L for lidocaine

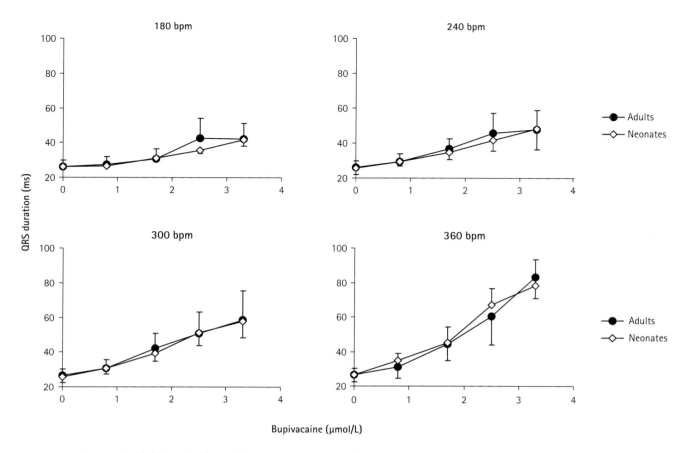

Figure 14.1   Increase in QRS duration (ventricular conduction velocity) in neonatal or adult isolated rabbits hearts as a function of heart rate (from 180 to 360 beats/minute) and dose of bupivacaine. The intensity of the block is similar in the two groups. However, because neonates and infants have a higher heart rate than adults, they are at higher risk of arrhythmias. From Simon *et al.* [41].

Table 14.5   Stereospecificity of the effect

Site	Stereospecificity
Protein binding	Mild
Pharmacokinetics	Mild
Sodium channel (patch)	
Axonal	Mild
Cardiac muscle	Major
Ventricular conduction	
(isolated heart preparation)	Major
Contractility	
(Papillary muscle, V_{max})	Moderate
(Isolated cardiac muscle)	Mild
Whole animal	Mild

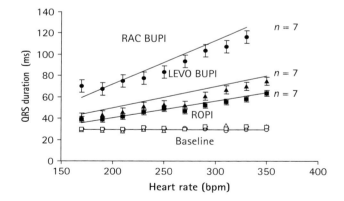

Figure 14.2   Stereospecificity of the effect of local anaesthetics (LAs) on ventricular conduction velocity. The QRS duration was measured in isolated rabbit heart paced at fixed rates. The same amount (5 μmol/L) of racemic bupivacaine, levobupivacaine or ropivacaine was infused. A phasic block was superimposed to the basal tonic block. This phasic block is lower with the *S*-enantiomers than with the racemic drug. From Mazoit *et al.* [40].

and 100–500 μmol/L for bupivacaine. At these concentrations lidocaine may be toxic for nerve structures, leading rarely to cauda equina syndromes or frequently to transient neurological symptoms after spinal anaesthesia [53]. Local anaesthetics are also toxic to muscles and bupivacaine is the agent most implicated. Muscle toxicity has been related to a disorder of the calcium homeostasis [54,55] and is not stereospecific. This perturbation of calcium

homeostasis is caused by the effect of LAs on mitochondrial functions [56]. Care should be taken in certain circumstances such as regional anaesthesia for eye surgery (the oculomotor muscles are particularly sensitive), in children with myopathies (bupivacaine is an *in vitro* model of Duchenne's myopathy) and perhaps in children with mitochondrial cytopathy. It is important to differentiate between central blocks, which have proven efficacy and safety in these circumstances, and peripheral blocks where the injection may be directly into muscles [57].

Systemic toxicity

After local or regional anaesthesia, a rapid rise in blood concentrations may lead to neurological or cardiac toxicity. Neurological toxicity is not rare: a large survey done in adult patients showed that the incidence is about one case in over 1000 patients [58]. Infants are more prone to toxicity than adults because of low protein binding and reduced intrinsic clearance. Since regional anaesthesia is most often practised together with general anaesthesia in paediatrics, care should be paid to this potential complication. The treatment of convulsions includes the maintenance of the airway with oxygen administration and effective ventilation. In intractable convulsions, anticonvulsants such as midazolam, thiopental and propofol are required.

Cardiac toxicity is not as frequent, but arrhythmias may be life threatening. Cardiotoxicity may occur simultaneously with CNS complications. Again, infants are more susceptible than older children or adults and, in addition to pharmacokinetic factors, the rapid heart rate of infants is a major determinant of susceptibility and agents with less frequency-dependent block preferable. The $S(-)$-enantiomers, ropivacaine or levobupivacaine, are the drugs of choice in the younger patients. Case reports have shown that recovery is rapid after ropivacaine-induced cardiotoxicity [59,60]. The clinical manifestation of cardiac toxicity usually occurs at the same time or even before the appearance of convulsions. Impaired ventricular conduction is seen with QRS widening, bradycardia, torsade de pointes followed by either ventricular fibrillation or asystole. Decrease in contractility is not the major problem after a rapid rise in serum concentration. Treatment includes standard resuscitation measures (oxygenation and external chest compression) and adrenaline in small incremental boluses (2–4 μg/kg). If ventricular fibrillation occurs, defibrillation (4 J/kg) must be performed. In the case of bupivacaine, resuscitation may need to be prolonged. Recent reports have suggested that the use of lipid infusions may be beneficial [61].

Prevention of toxicity includes slow, fractional injection and frequent aspiration tests. The use of a test dose with a solution containing adrenaline is recommended by some authors. It is important to remember, however, that false negatives occur in about one-third of the cases and that adding adrenaline may be harmful. In the case of indwelling catheter administration for postoperative pain relief, continuous administration is preferred to repeat bolus injections, which may lead to a peak-and-trough phenomenon. Moreover, continuous administration is safer than bolus injection if the catheter migrates. In older children, the practice of PCRA (patient-controlled regional anaesthesia) is an excellent solution as the boluses are small enough to be safe.

ADJUNCTS TO LOCAL ANAESTHETICS

A number of adjuncts are used to prolong the analgesic duration of various paediatric nerve blocks. In a recent survey approximately 60 per cent of paediatric anaesthetists regularly used an adjunct when performing caudal blockade, with ketamine, clonidine and opioids being the most frequently used [62].

Other agents (e.g. midazolam, neostigmine and magnesium) have been used but none appears to confer any clinical advantages. The use of these drugs or any other new alternatives should at this time be used only in a clinical trial and should be adopted into practice only if they prove to be associated with an improved risk–benefit ratio compared with current options [63].

Neuroaxial nerve blocks

PHARMACOKINETICS OF NEUROAXIALLY ADMINISTERED ADJUNCTS

Available data for opioids and clonidine are given in Table 14.6. Unfortunately, no data are currently available for ketamine.

Caudal and epidural administration (Table 14.7 and Fig. 14.3)

OPIOIDS

The caudal administration of 33–50 μg/kg of preservative-free morphine is optimum as higher doses do not enhance the duration or quality of analgesia but increase the incidence of side-effects [70]. For certain indications (e.g. cardiac surgery, liver transplantation) the use of caudal morphine without concomitant administration of local anaesthetics has been advocated [71]. The most frequently used dose of fentanyl is 1 μg/kg [72–74]. Although a number of other opioids have also been used they do not appear to have advantages compared with morphine and fentanyl. Some, such as buprenorphine, are associated with an unacceptably high incidence of postoperative nausea and vomiting (PONV; 80 per cent) [75].

In continuous epidural infusions, fentanyl is the most favoured option but the use of sufentanil has also been described [76–78]. Addition of fentanyl to achieve a final concentration of 1–2 μg/mL to the local anaesthetic solution is frequently recommended (corresponding to an infusion rate of approximately 5–10 μg/kg over 24 hours) [79–80]. The practice of adding fentanyl to continuous epidural infusions is widespread but a randomised multicentre study failed to show any beneficial effect of adjunct

Table 14.6   Pharmacokinetic information of neuroaxially administered adjunct drugs

	Dose	Measured parameters	Reference
Morphine			
Caudal	50 μg/kg	C_{max}: 21 ± 5 ng/mL	64
		T_{max}: 10 minutes	
		C_{3h}: 4.1 + 2.6 ng/mL	
Epidural	50 μg/kg	C_{max}: 27 ± 9 ng/mL	65
		T_{max}: 10 ± 0.3 minutes	
		$T_{1/2}$: 74 ± 42 minutes	
		V_d: 2.9 ± 0.9 L/kg	
		Clearance: 28 ± 3 mL/min/kg	
		AUC: 1371 ± 148 ng/min/mL	
Intrathecal	20 μg/kg	CSF concn 6 hours: 2860 ± 540 ng/mL	66
		12 h: 640 ± 220 ng/mL	
		18 h: 220 ± 150 ng/mL	
Fentanyl			
Caudal	20 μg/kg	C_{max}: 0.21 ng/mL	67
		T_{max}: 30 minutes	
Epidural	Bolus: 1.5 μg/kg		68
	Infusion: 5 μg/kg per 24 hours	C_{max}: 0.12–0.25 ng/mL after bolus	
		T_{max}: 30 minutes (range: 20–60)	
		C_{24h}, range: 0.10–0.25 ng/mL	
		C_{48h}, range: 0.14–0.26 ng/mL	
Sufentanil			
Epidural	Bolus: 0.6 μg/kg	C_{max}: 0.03–0.07 ng/mL after bolus	68
	Infusion: 2 μg/kg per 24 hours	T_{max}: 20 minutes (range: 20–30)	
		C_{24h}, range: 0.04–0.05 ng/mL	
		C_{48h}, range: 0.02–0.06 ng/mL	
Clonidine			
Epidural	2 μg/kg	C_{max} median: 0.62 ng/mL	69
		(95% CI): 0.53–0.71 ng/mL	
		T_{max} median: 108 minutes (95% CI): 61–152 minutes	
		$T_{1/2}$ median: 396 minutes (95% CI): 221–540 minutes	
		AUC median: 423 ng/min/mL (95% CI): 334–535 ng/min/mL	
		95% absorption median: 1.6 hours (95% CI): 0.9–4.7 hours	
		Bioavailablity: 102% (95% CI): 87–146%	

AUC, area under the concentration–time curve; 95% CI, 95 per cent confidence interval; C_{max} is the maximum observed concentration after single-shot injection; CSF, cerebrospinal fluid; $T_{1/2}$ is the terminal half-life; T_{max} is the time to C_{max}; C_{3h}, C_{24h} and C_{48h} are the concentrations observed 3 hours, 24 hours and 48 hours, respectively, after the beginning of administration; V_d, volume of distribution.

fentanyl when it was used together with low concentrations of levobupivacaine (0.0625–0.125 per cent) for abdominal surgery [80]. In contrast, epidural morphine, being more water soluble, attains higher CSF concentrations than lipophilic opioids and has been shown to be effective in small doses (1–4 μg/kg/h) [81].

The use of opioids as adjuncts to caudal and epidural blocks has recently been questioned, because of the risk of respiratory depression but even more so because of the high incidence of other side-effects that accompany the use of neuraxial opioids (e.g. pruritus, PONV, urinary retention and paralytic ileus) [82]. It is, however, possible to minimise side-effects by titration of the infusion to analgesic need and the use of urinary catheters inserted at the time of operation [83].

CLONIDINE

This α_2-adrenoceptor agonist has repeatedly been shown to approximately double the analgesic duration of caudal blocks [84,85] and has also been shown to enhance the efficacy of dilute long-acting LAs (e.g. 0.1 per cent ropivacaine) [86]. Systemic absorption of caudally injected clonidine can result in secondary effects, such as reduced need for volatile agents and/or opioids and improved haemodynamic stability [87], but may also cause slightly increased levels of postoperative sedation of limited duration [69].

For single injection in caudal blocks 1–2 μg/kg is most frequently used [69,84,86]. In an epidural dose–response study co-infusion of >0.1 μg/kg/h of clonidine with ropivacaine 0.1 per cent was found both to improve

Table 14.7 Dose recommendations for some frequently used adjunct drugs

Drug	Dose
Morphine	
Caudal/epidural bolus	33–50 μg/kg
Fentanyl	
Caudal/epidural bolus	1.0–1.5 μg/kg
Epidural infusion	5 μg/kg/24 h
Sufentanil	
Epidural bolus	0.6 μg/kg
Epidural infusion	2 μg/kg/24 h
Clonidine	
Caudal/epidural bolus	1–2 μg/kg
Epidural infusion	≥0.1 μg/kg/24 h
Ketamine	
Caudal bolus, racemic ketamine	0.25–0.5 mg/kg
Caudal bolus, S(+)-ketamine	0.5–1.0 mg/kg

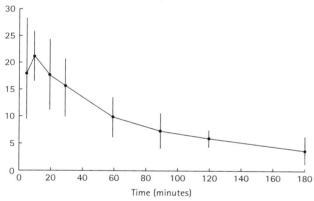

Figure 14.3 Plasma concentrations of morphine following caudal administration (from Wolf *et al.* [64]).

analgesia and to increase postoperative haemodynamic stability [88,89].

An epidural bolus injection results in either a fast or a slow absorption pattern. This difference may result from the volume and characteristics of the abundant epidural fat that is present in children. Regardless of absorption pattern, complete bioavailability of an epidurally injected dose of clonidine can be expected [69].

KETAMINE

For prolongation of postoperative analgesia following single-injection caudal blockade, ketamine appears to be the best adjunct currently available [90]. Both preservative-free racemic and S(+)-ketamine preparations can be used. Even using doses within the normal dose range may result in psychotropic side-effects in the early postoperative period but such reactions are usually only of a minor to

moderate degree [91,92]. The use of S(+)-ketamine may be preferable since it is claimed to be associated with a reduced risk for psychotropic side-effects. S(+)-Ketamine is available only as a preservative-free preparation.

Caudal administration of ketamine alone also results in effective postoperative analgesia. Preservative-free racemic ketamine 0.5 mg/kg and S(+)-ketamine 1.0 mg/kg have been reported to produce similar postoperative pain relief to bupivacaine 0.25 per cent with adrenaline [93,94]. Furthermore, the combined use of S(+)-ketamine (0.5–1.0 mg/kg) and clonidine (1–2 μg/kg) without LA is capable of giving approximately 24 hours of adequate postoperative analgesia following inguinal hernia repair [95,96].

Only non-neuroaxial pharmacokinetic data are currently available for ketamine in children [97]; however, 0.5–1.0 mg/kg of S(+)-ketamine and 0.25–0.5 mg/kg of preservative-free racemic ketamine are suggested doses [91, 92, 97].

Intrathecal administration

Intrathecal administration of adjuncts is much less common than caudal or epidural use in paediatric patients. However, some indications for this treatment option have been reported.

MORPHINE

Early publications on the administration of intrathecal morphine in children reported a significant incidence of respiratory depression and other side-effects. In recent years doses have been reduced and the risk of side-effects has subsequently been diminished [98]. At present, the main indications for the use of intrathecal morphine are improved pain relief after major back operations (e.g. scoliosis and rhizotomy surgery) [98,99], paediatric cardiac surgery [100,101] and frontal encephalocele repair [102]. For these indications morphine is most often given without concomitant LAs although co-administration of LAs may be used for cardiac surgery [103]. Dose–response data for paediatric back surgery have identified 5–10 μg/kg as the optimal dose for safe and effective postoperative analgesia [98,99].

CLONIDINE

This drug is rarely administered by the intrathecal route in children but its use has been reported to enhance the effect of spinal anaesthesia in ex-premature babies as well as in school-aged children [104,105]. In the dose-ranging study in ex-prematures a dose of 1 μg/kg was found to double the duration of the block without any significant side-effects [105].

Peripheral nerve blocks

In adults various drugs have been used as adjuncts for peripheral nerve blocks. Although a number of publications claim a positive effect of such co-administration conflicting data exist and no consensus has so far been reached concerning this issue [106, 107].

Publications regarding adjunct drug use for peripheral nerve blocks in children are scarce. The adjunct use of clonidine has been described for ilio-inguinal/ilio-hypogastric nerve block but data are inconclusive [104,106]. Promising data have been published with regard to adjunctive use of clonidine for local infiltration in the tonsillar fossae in children undergoing tonsillectomy. In this study co-administration of ropivacaine and clonidine 1 µg/kg was associated with significantly lower pain scores, both at rest and on swallowing, for up to 5 days postoperatively compared with saline placebo or ropivacaine alone [107].

REFERENCES

Key references

Bösenberg AT, Thomas J, Cronje L *et al*. Pharmacokinetics and efficacy of ropivacaine for continuous epidural infusion in neonates and infants. *Paediatr Anaesth* 2005; **15**(9): 739–49.

Hager H, Marhofer P, Sitzwohl C *et al*. Caudal clonidine prolongs analgesia from caudal *S*(+)-ketamine in children. *Anesth Analg* 2002; **94**(5): 1169–72.

Lerman J, Nolan J, Eyres R *et al*. Efficacy, safety, and pharmacokinetics of levobupivacaine with and without fentanyl after continuous epidural infusion in children: a multicenter trial. *Anesthesiology* 2003; **99**(5): 1166–74.

Mazoit JX, Dalens BJ. Pharmacokinetics of local anaesthetics in infants and children. *Clin Pharmacokinet* 2004; **43**: 17–32.

Mazoit JX, Decaux A, Bouaziz H, Edouard A. Comparative ventricular electrophysiologic effect of racemic bupivacaine, levobupivacaine, and ropivacaine on the isolated rabbit heart. *Anesthesiology* 2000; **93**: 784–92.

References

1. Denson DD, Mazoit JX. Physiology and pharmacology of local anesthetics. In: Sinatra RS. *Acute pain mechanisms and management*. St Louis, MO: Mosby, 1992: 124–39.
2. Cartwright PD, Fyhr P. The manufacture and storage of local anesthetics. *Reg Anesth* 1988; **13**: 1–12.
3. Mazoit JX, Dalens BJ. Pharmacokinetics of local anaesthetics in infants and children. *Clin Pharmacokinet* 2004; **43**: 17–32.
4. Tucker GT, Boyes RN, Bridenbaugh PO, Moore DC. Binding of anilide-type local anesthetics in human plasma. I. Relationships between binding, physicochemical properties, and anesthetic activity. *Anesthesiology* 1970; **33**: 287–303.
5. Denson DD, Coyle DE, Thompson GA, Myers JA. Alpha1-acid glycoprotein and albumin in human serum bupivacaine binding. *Clin Pharmacol Ther* 1984; **35**: 409–15.
6. Mazoit JX, Denson DD, Samii K. Pharmacokinetics of bupivacaine following caudal anesthesia in infants. *Anesthesiology* 1988; **68**: 387–91.
7. Booker PD, Taylor C, Saba G. Perioperative changes in alpha1-acid glycoprotein concentrations in infants undergoing major surgery. *Br J Anaesth* 1996; **76**: 365–8.
8. Meunier JF, Goujard E, Dubousset AM *et al*. Pharmacokinetics of bupivacaine after continuous epidural infusion in infants with and without biliary atresia. *Anesthesiology* 2001; **95**: 87–95.
9. Sitbon P, Laffon M, Lesage V *et al*. Lidocaine plasma concentrations in pediatric patients after providing airway topical anesthesia from a calibrated device. *Anesth Analg* 1996; **82**: 1003–6.
10. Taddio A, Ohlsson A, Einarson TR *et al*. Systematic review of lidocaine-prilocaine cream (EMLA) in the treatment of acute pain in neonates. *Pediatrics* 1998; **101**: E1.
11. Russell SC, Doyle E. A risk–benefit assessment of topical percutaneous local anaesthetics in children. *Drug Safety* 1997; **16**: 279–87.
12. Wachi A, Kudo S, Sato K. Characteristics of cerebrospinal fluid circulation in infants as detected with MR velocity imaging. *Child Nerv Syst* 1995; **11**: 227–30.
13. Higuchi H, Adachi Y, Kazama T. 2004; Factors affecting the spread and duration of epidural anesthesia with ropivacaine. *Anesthesiology* 101: 451–60.
14. Burm AGL. Clinical pharmacokinetics of epidural and spinal anesthesia. *Clin Pharmacokinet* 1989; **16**: 283–311.
15. Lönnqvist PA, Westrin P, Larsson BA *et al*. Ropivacaine pharmacokinetics after caudal block in 1–8-year-old children. *Br J Anaesth* 2000; **85**: 506–11.
16. Chalkiadis GA, Eyres RL, Cranswick N *et al*. Pharmacokinetics of levobupivacaine 0.25% following caudal administration in children under 2 years of age. *Br J Anaesth* 2004; **92**: 218–22.
17. van Obbergh LJ, Roelants FA, Veyckemans F, Verbeeck RK. In children, the addition of epinephrine modifies the pharmacokinetics of ropivacaine injected caudally. *Can J Anaesth* 2003; **50**: 593–8.
18. Flandin-Bléty C, Barrier G. Accidents following extradural analgesia in children. The results of a retrospective study. *Paediatric Anaesth* 1995; **5**: 41–46.
19. Gantenbein M, Attolini L, Bruguerolle B *et al*. Oxidative metabolism of bupivacaine into pipecolylxylidine in humans is mainly catalyzed by CYP3 A. *Drug Metab Dispos* 2000; **28**: 383–5.
20. Arlander E, Ekstrom G, Alm C *et al*. Metabolism of ropivacaine in humans is mediated by CYP1A2 and to a minor extent by CYP3A4. An interaction study with fluvoxamine and ketoconazole as *in vivo* inhibitors. *Clin Pharmacol Ther* 1998; **64**: 484–91.
21. Hines RN, McCarver DG. The ontogeny of human drug-metabolizing enzymes: phase I oxidative enzymes. *J Pharm Exp Ther* 2002; **300**: 355–60.
22. Hansen TG, Ilett KF, Reid C *et al*. Caudal ropivacaine in infants: population pharmacokinetics and plasma concentrations. *Anesthesiology* 2001; **94**: 579–584.
23. Rapp HJ, Molnar V, Austin S *et al*. September; Ropivacaine in neonates and infants: a population pharmacokinetic

evaluation following single caudal block. *Paediatr Anaesth* 2004; **14**: 724–32.

24. Bösenberg AT, Thomas J, Cronje L *et al.* Pharmacokinetics and efficacy of ropivacaine for continuous epidural infusion in neonates and infants. *Paediatr Anaesth* 2005; **15**: 739–49.

25. McCann ME, Sethna NF, Mazoit JX *et al.* The pharmacokinetics of epidural ropivacaine in infants and young children. *Anesth Analg* 2001; **93**: 893–7.

26. Luz G, Wieser C, Innerhofer P *et al.* Free and total bupivacaine plasma concentrations after continuous epidural anaesthesia in infants and children. *Paediatr Anaesth* 1998; **8**: 473–8.

27. Wulf H, Peters C, Behnke H. The pharmacokinetics of caudal ropivacaine 0.2% in children. A study of infants aged less than 1 year and toddlers aged 1–5 years undergoing inguinal hernia repair. *Anaesthesia* 2000; **55**: 757–60.

28. Catterall WA. Molecular mechanisms of gating and drug block of sodium channels. *Novartis Found Symp* 2002; **241**: 206–18.

29. Longobardo M, Delpon E, Caballero R *et al.* Structural determinants of potency and stereoselective block of hKv1.5 channels induced by local anesthetics. *Mol Pharmacol* 1998; **54**: 162–9.

30. Gonzalez T, Arias C, Caballero R *et al.* Effects of levobupivacaine, ropivacaine and bupivacaine on HERG channels: stereoselective bupivacaine block. *Br J Pharmacol* 2002; **137**: 1269–79.

31. Hirota K, Browne T, Appadu BL, Lambert DG. Do local anaesthetics interact with dihydropyridine binding sites on neuronal 1-type Ca^{2+} channels? *Br J Anaesth* 1997; **78**: 185–8.

32. Komai H, Lokuta AJ. Interaction of bupivacaine and tetracaine with the sarcoplasmic reticulum Ca^{2+} release channel of skeletal and cardiac muscles. *Anesthesiology* 1999; **90**: 835–43.

33. Vabnick I, Novakovic SD, Levinson SR *et al.* The clustering of axonal sodium channels during development of the peripheral nervous system. *J Neurosci* 1996; **16**: 4914–22.

34. Rasband MN, Trimmer JS. Developmental clustering of ion channels at and near the node of Ranvier. *Dev Biol* 2001; **236**: 5–16.

35. Raymond SA, Thalhammer JG, Strichartz GR. Axonal excitability. endogenous and exogenous modulation. In: Dimitrijevic R, ed. *Altered sensation and pain. Recent achievement in restorative neurology, Vol. 3*. Basel: Karger, 1990.

36. Benzon HT, Strichartz GR, Gissen AJ *et al.* Developmental neurophysiology of mammalian peripheral nerves and age-related differential sensitivity to local anaesthetics. *Br J Anaesth* 1988; **61**: 754–60.

37. Kohane DS, Sankar WN, Shubina M *et al.* Sciatic nerve blockade in infant, adolescent, and adult rats: a comparison of ropivacaine with bupivacaine. *Anesthesiology* 1998; **89**: 1199–208.

38. Booth D, Evans DJ. Anticonvulsants for neonates with seizures. *Cochrane Database Syst Rev* 2004; (4): CD004218.

39. de La Coussaye J, Brugada J, Allessie MA. Electrophysiologic and arrhythmogenic effects of bupivacaine. A study with high-resolution ventricular epicardial mapping in rabbit hearts. *Anesthesiology* 1992; **77**: 32–41.

40. Mazoit JX, Decaux A, Bouaziz H, Edouard A. Comparative ventricular electrophysiologic effect of racemic bupivacaine, levobupivacaine, and ropivacaine on the isolated rabbit heart. *Anesthesiology* 2000; **93**: 784–92.

41. Simon L, Kariya N, Edouard A *et al.* Effect of bupivacaine on the isolated rabbit heart: developmental aspect on ventricular conduction and contractility. *Anesthesiology* 2004; **101**: 937–44.

42. Iida H, Watanabe Y, Dohi S, Ishiyama T. Direct effects of ropivacaine and bupivacaine on spinal pial vessels in canine. Assessment with closed spinal window technique. *Anesthesiology* 1997; **87**: 75–81.

43. Burke D, Joypaul V, Thomson MF. Circumcision supplemented by dorsal penile nerve block with 0.75% ropivacaine: a complication. *Reg Anesth Pain Med* 2000; **25**: 424–7.

44. Vladimirov M, Nau C, Mok WM, Strichartz G. Potency of bupivacaine stereoisomers tested *in vitro* and *in vivo*. biochemical, electrophysiological, and neurobehavioral studies. *Anesthesiology* 2000; **93**: 744–55.

45. Groban L, Deal DD, Vernon JC *et al.* Does local anesthetic stereoselectivity or structure predict myocardial depression in anesthetized canines? *Reg Anesth Pain Med* 2002; **27**: 460–8.

46. Odoom JA, Sturk A, Dokter PWC *et al.* The effects of bupivacaine and pipecoloxylidide on platelet function in vitro. *Acta Anaesthesiol Scand* 1989; **33**: 385–8.

47. Hollmann MW, Gross A, Jelacin N, Durieux ME. Local anesthetic effects on priming and activation of human neutrophils. *Anesthesiology* 2001; **95**: 113–22.

48. Beloeil H, Asehnoune K, Moine P *et al.* Bupivacaine's action on the carrageenan-induced inflammatory response in mice: cytokine production by leukocytes after *ex-vivo* stimulation. *Anesth Analg* 2005; **100**: 1081–6.

49. Leduc C, Gentili ME, Estèbe JP *et al.* Inhibition of peroxidation by local anesthetic in an inflammatory rat model with carrageenan. *Anesth Analg* 2002; **95**: 992–6.

50. Rowbotham MC, Reisner-Keller LA, Fields HL. Both intravenous lidocaine and morphine reduce the pain of postherpetic neuralgia. *Neurology* 1991; **41**: 1024–8.

51. Linchitz RM, Raheb JC. Subcutaneous infusion of lidocaine provides effective pain relief for CRPS patients. *Clin J Pain* 1999; **15**: 67–72.

52. Dadure C, Motais F, Ricard C *et al.* Continuous peripheral nerve blocks at home for treatment of recurrent complex regional pain syndrome I in children. *Anesthesiology* 2005; **102**: 387–91.

53. Freedman JM, De-Kun I, Drasner K *et al.* Transient neurologic symptoms after spinal anesthesia. *Anesthesiology* 1998; **89**: 633–41.

54. Newman RJ, Radda GK. The myotoxicity of bupivacaine, a ^{31}P NMR investigation. *Br J Pharmacol* 1983; **79**: 395–9.

55. Zink W, Missler G, Sinner B *et al.* Differential effects of bupivacaine and ropivacaine enantiomers on intracellular Ca^{2+} regulation in murine skeletal muscle fibers. *Anesthesiology* 2005; **102**: 793–8.

56. Sztark F, Nouette-Gaulain K, Malgat M *et al*. Absence of stereospecific effects of bupivacaine isomers on heart mitochondrial bioenergetics. *Anesthesiology* 2000; **93**: 456–62.

57. Murat I, Esteve C, Montay G *et al*. Pharmacokinetics and cardiovascular effects of bupivacaine during epidural anesthesia in children with Duchenne muscular dystrophy. *Anesthesiology* 1987; **67**: 249–52.

58. Brown DL, Ransom DM, Hall JA *et al*. Regional anesthesia and local anesthetic-induced systemic toxicity. seizure frequency and accompanying cardiovascular changes. *Anesth Analg* 1995; **81**: 321–8.

59. Klein SM, Pierce T, Rubin Y *et al*. Successful resuscitation after ropivacaine-induced ventricular fibrillation. *Anesth Analg* 2003; **97**: 901–3.

60. Huet O, Eyrolle LJ, Mazoit JX, Ozier YM. Cardiac arrest after injection of ropivacaine for posterior lumbar plexus blockade. *Anesthesiology* 2003; **99**: 1451–3.

61. Weinberg G. Lipid rescue resuscitation from local anaesthetic cardiac toxicity. *Toxicol Rev* 2006; **25**: 139–45.

62. Sanders JC. Paediatric regional anaesthesia, a survey of practice in the United Kingdom. *Br J Anaesth* 2002; **89**: 707–10.

63. Lonnqvist PA. Adjuncts to caudal block in children – Quo vadis? *Br J Anaesth* 2005; **95**: 431–3.

64. Wolf AR, Hughes D, Hobbs AJ, Prys-Roberts C. Combined morphine–bupivacaine caudals for reconstructive penile surgery in children: systemic absorption of morphine and postoperative analgesia. *Anaesth Intens Care* 1991; **19**: 17–21.

65. Attia J, Ecoffey C, Sandouk P *et al*. Epidural morphine in children: pharmacokinetics and CO_2 sensitivity. *Anesthesiology* 1986; **65**: 590–4.

66. Nicholas DG, Yaster M, Lynn AM *et al*. Disposition and respiratory effects of intrathecal morphine in children. *Anesthesiology* 1993; **79**: 73–8.

67. Manach A, Estebe JP, le Naoures A Bentue-Ferre D *et al*. Determination of fentanyl in the plasma during caudal anesthesia in children. *Cah d'anésthesiol* 1987; **35**: 409–11.

68. Lejus C, Schwoerer D, Furic I *et al*. Fentanyl versus sufentanil: plasma concentrations during continuous epidural postoperative infusion in children. *Br J Anaesth* 2000; **85**: 615–17.

69. Ivani G, Bergendahl HT, Lampugnani E *et al*. Plasma levels of clonidine following epidural bolus injection in children. *Acta Anaesthesiol Scand* 1998; **42**: 306–11.

70. Krane EJ, Tyler DC, Jacobson LE. The dose-response of caudal morphine in children. *Anesthesiology* 1989; **71**: 48–52.

71. Rosen KR, Rosen DA. Caudal epidural morphine for control of pain following open heart surgery in children. *Anesthesiology* 1989; **70**: 418–21.

72. Campbell FA, Yentis SM, Fear DW, Bissonnette B. Analgesic efficacy and safety of a caudal bupivacaine–fentanyl mixture in children. *Can J Anaesth* 1992; **39**: 661–4.

73. Constant I, Gall O, Gouyet L *et al*. Addition of clonidine or fentanyl to local anaesthetics prolongs the duration of

surgical analgesia after single shot caudal block in children. *Br J Anaesth* 1998; **80**: 294–8.

74. Baris S, Karakaya D, Kelsaka E *et al*. Comparison of fentanyl–bupivacaine or midazolam–bupivacaine mixtures with plain bupivacaine for caudal anaesthesia in children. *Paediatr Anaesth* 2003; **13**: 126–31.

75. Khan FA, Memon GA, Kamal RS. Effect of route of buprenorphine on recovery and postoperative analgesic requirement in paediatric patients. *Paediatr Anaesth* 2002; **12**: 786–90.

76. Benlabed M, Ecoffey C, Levron JC *et al*. Analgesia and ventilatory response to CO_2 following epidural sufentanil in children. *Anesthesiology* 1987; **67**: 948–51.

77. Kokki H, Ruuskanen A, Karvinen M. Comparison of epidural pain treatment with sufentanil–ropivacaine infusion with and without epinephrine in children. *Acta Anaesthesiol Scand* 2002; **46**: 647–53.

78. Kart T, Walther-Larsen S, Svejborg TF *et al*. Comparison of continuous epidural infusion of fentanyl and bupivacaine with intermittent epidural administration of morphine for postoperative pain management in children. *Acta Anaesthesiol Scand* 1997; **41**: 461–5.

79. Lejus C, Surbled M, Schwoerer D *et al*. Postoperative epidural analgesia with bupivacaine and fentanyl: hourly pain assessment in 348 paediatric cases. *Paediatr Anaesth* 2001; **11**: 327–32.

80. Lerman J, Nolan J, Eyres R *et al*. Efficacy, safety, and pharmacokinetics of levobupivacaine with and without fentanyl after continuous epidural infusion in children: a multicenter trial. *Anesthesiology* 2003; **99**: 1166–74.

81. Berde CB. Epidural analgesia in children. *Can J Anaesth* 1994; **41**: 555–60.

82. Lönnqvist PA, Ivani G, Moriarty T. Use of caudal-epidural opioids in children: still state of the art or the beginning of the end? *Paediatr Anaesth* 2002; **12**: 747–9.

83. Lloyd-Thomas AR, Howard RF. A pain service for children. *Paediatr Anaesth* 1994; **4**: 3–15.

84. Lee JJ, Rubin AP. Comparison of a bupivacaine–clonidine mixture with plain bupivacaine for caudal analgesia in children. *Br J Anaesth* 1994; **72**: 258–62.

85. Jamali S, Monin S, Begon C *et al*. Clonidine in pediatric caudal anesthesia. *Anesth Analg* 1994; **78**: 663–6.

86. Ivani G, De Negri P, Conio A *et al*. Ropivacaine–clonidine combination for caudal blockade in children. *Acta Anaesthesiol Scandi* 2000; **44**: 446–9.

87. Nishina K, Mikawa K, Shiga M, Obara H. Clonidine in paediatric anaesthesia. *Paediatr Anaesth* 1999; **9**: 187–202.

88. De Negri P, Ivani G, Visconti C *et al*. The dose–response relationship for clonidine added to a postoperative continuous epidural infusion of ropivacaine in children. *Anesth Analg* 2001; **93**: 71–76.

89. Bergendahl HTG, Lonnqvist PA, De Negri P *et al*. Increased postoperative arterial blood pressure stability with continuous epidural infusion of clonidine in children. *Anesth Analg* 2002; **95**: 1121–2.

90. Cook B, Grubb DJ, Aldridge LA, Doyle E. Comparison of the effects of adrenaline, clonidine and ketamine on the

duration of caudal analgesia produced by bupivacaine in children. *Br J Anaesth* 1995; **75**: 698–701.

91. Semple D, Findlow D, Aldridge LM, Doyle E. The optimal dose of ketamine for caudal epidural blockade in children. *Anaesthesia* 1996; **51**: 1170–2.

92. Panjabi N, Prakash S, Gupta P, Gogia AR. Efficacy of three doses of ketamine with bupivacaine for caudal analgesia in pediatric inguinal herniotomy. *Reg Anesth Pain Med* 2004; **29**: 28–31.

93. Naguib M, Sharif AM, Seraj M *et al.* Ketamine for caudal analgesia in children: comparison with caudal bupivacaine. *Br J Anaesth* 1991; **67**: 559–64.

94. Marhofer P, Krenn CG, Plochl W *et al.* S(+)-ketamine for caudal block in paediatric anaesthesia. *Br J Anaesth* 2000; **84**: 341–5.

95. Hager H, Marhofer P, Sitzwohl C *et al.* Caudal clonidine prolongs analgesia from caudal S(+)-ketamine in children. *Anesth Analg* 2002; **94**: 1169–72.

96. Passariello M, Almenrader N, Canneti A *et al.* Caudal analgesia in children: S(+)-ketamine vs. S(+)-ketamine plus clonidine. *Paediatr Anaesth* 2004; **14**: 851–5.

97. Malinovsky JM, Servin F, Cozian A *et al.* Ketamine and norketamine plasma concentrations after i.v., nasal and rectal administration in children. *Br J Anaesth* 1996; **77**: 203–7.

98. Gall O, Aubineau JV, Berniere J *et al.* Analgesic effect of low-dose intrathecal morphine after spinal fusion in children. *Anesthesiology* 2001; **94**: 447–52.

99. Harris MM, Kahana MD, Park TS. Intrathecal morphine for postoperative analgesia in children after selective dorsal root rhizotomy. *Neurosurgery* 1991; **28**: 519–22.

100. Jones SE, Beasley JM, Macfarlane DW *et al.* Intrathecal morphine for postoperative pain relief in children. *Br J Anaesth* 1984; **56**: 137–40.

101. Suominen PK, Ragg PG, McKinley DF *et al.* Intrathecal morphine provides effective and safe analgesia in children after cardiac surgery. *Acta Anaesthesiol Scand* 2004; **48**: 875–2.

102. Tobias JD, Mateo C, Ferrer MJ *et al.* Intrathecal morphine for postoperative analgesia following repair of frontal encephaloceles in children: comparison with intermittent, on-demand dosing of nalbuphine. *J Clin. Anesth* 1997; **9**: 280–4.

103. Hammer GB, Ramamoorthy C, Cao H *et al.* Postoperative analgesia after spinal blockade in infants and children undergoing cardiac surgery. *Anesth Analg* 2005; **100**: 1283–8.

104. Kaabachi O, Ben Rajeb A, Mebazaa M *et al.* Spinal anesthesia in children: comparative study of hyperbaric bupivacaine with or without clonidine. *Ann Fr Anesth Reanim* 2002; **21**: 617–21.

105. Rochette A, Raux O, Troncin R *et al.* Clonidine prolongs spinal anesthesia in newborns: a prospective dose-ranging study. *Anesth Analg* 2004; **98**: 56–9.

106. Ivani G, Conio A, De Negri P *et al.* Spinal vs peripheral effects of adjunct clonidine: comparison of the analgesic effect of a ropivacaine–clonidine mixture when administered as a caudal or ilioinguinal-iliohypogastric nerve blockade for inguinal surgery in children. *Paediatr Anaesth* 2002; **12**: 680–4.

107. Giannoni C, White S, Enneking FK, Morey T. Ropivacaine with or without clonidine improves pediatric tonsillectomy pain. *Arch Otolaryngol Head Neck Surg* 2001; **127**: 1265–70.

Muscle relaxants

GEORGE H MEAKIN

KEY LEARNING POINTS

- Paediatric patients differ from adults in their response to muscle relaxants because of developmental changes in neuromuscular transmission and body composition.
- The neuromuscular junction of the human infant is sensitive to the effects of non-depolarising muscle relaxants because of a lack of acetylcholine in developing motor nerves. However, this is largely compensated for by the distribution of the drugs into a larger volume of extracellular fluid, so that the same per kilogram doses can be used in patients of all ages.
- The postjunctional membrane of the neuromuscular junction has a fully mature appearance in the human infant and

responds normally to the depolarising muscle relaxant suxamethonium. Infants and children therefore require significantly greater per kilogram doses of suxamethonium compared with adults because of the distribution of the drug into a larger volume of extracellular fluid.
- Muscle relaxants are among the safest drugs given by paediatric anaesthetists, although anaphylactoid and anaphylactic reactions may occur. Specific drugs and doses can be chosen to suit the clinical circumstances.

INTRODUCTION

Muscle relaxants (neuromuscular blocking drugs) produce relaxation of skeletal muscles by interrupting transmission of impulses at the neuromuscular junction. On the basis of their modes of action at the neuromuscular junction they can be classified as depolarising or non-depolarising. Depolarising muscle relaxants mimic the actions of acetylcholine (ACh) at postjunctional receptors. Non-depolarising relaxants bind to postjunctional receptors without activating them; thus they are competitive inhibitors of ACh. Muscle relaxants are often given in doses many times greater than the dose required to produce 95 per cent depression of twitch (ED_{95}) in order to achieve satisfactory tracheal intubating conditions in less than 2 minutes. The administration of these large doses is possible only because muscle relaxants, in contrast to the agents commonly used to induce and

maintain anaesthesia, are relatively free of cardiovascular effects

One of the earliest reports of the use of muscle relaxants in paediatric anaesthesia summarised their advantages as follows [1]:

1. They provide a means of effecting and maintaining control of respiration throughout the operation.
2. The patient is completely relaxed and the work of the surgeon facilitated.
3. The quantity of toxic anaesthetic agents is greatly reduced.

To this list we may add:

4. They facilitate excellent control of the airway by means of a tracheal tube.

5. The ability to use full doses of analgesic drugs.
6. Complete reversibility.

In view of all these advantages, it is hardly surprising that a balanced technique of anaesthesia, consisting of a hypnotic, opioid and relaxant, continues to be popular for neonates, small infants and other high-risk patients.

However, neonates differ significantly from adults in the way that they respond to muscle relaxants; specifically, they appear to be resistant to the depolarising drug suxamethonium and sensitive to the non-depolarising drug tubocurarine. If paediatric anaesthetists are to use muscle relaxants effectively they must understand the basis of such differences and their clinical implications. Accordingly, the first section of this chapter describes the major factors responsible for the altered responses of paediatric patients to muscle relaxants. Later sections review the clinical pharmacology of selected muscle relaxants and their antagonists as it pertains to neonates, infants and children.

FACTORS AFFECTING PAEDIATRIC RESPONSES TO NEUROMUSCULAR BLOCKING DRUGS

Development of the neuromuscular system

In humans, as in other animals, the development of skeletal muscles proceeds in a proximo-distal and rostro-caudal sequence. Thus, the muscles of the trunk appear before those of the limbs, while those of the hand and foot are the last to appear. Muscles of the upper limb develop at about 6 weeks of gestational age, slightly earlier than those of the lower limb [2].

Muscle fibre types

During development, muscle fibres differentiate into one of two main types [3]. Type I fibres are rich in oxidative enzymes and correspond to the slowly contracting 'red' muscles of animals. Type II fibres are rich in glycolytic enzymes and correspond to the rapidly contracting 'white' muscles of animals. Because of their high oxidative capacity, type I fibres are relatively resistant to fatigue; conversely, type II fibres are fatigue susceptible. In human peripheral muscles, type II fibres are the first to develop at around 20 weeks' gestation. From 26 weeks to 30 weeks there is a progressive increase in the proportion of type I fibres, so that by 30 weeks there are approximately equal numbers of type I and type II fibres, as in the adult. However, the diaphragm at full term contains only 25 per cent of type I fibres, and the adult proportion of 50 per cent is not attained until the age of 8 months (Fig. 15.1) [4]. The relative lack of type I fibres in the infant diaphragm makes it susceptible to fatigue. This, together with a reduced respiratory reserve and an increased oxygen requirement, makes it mandatory to ensure that the effect of any muscle relaxant given to patients in this age group is fully reversed at the end of anaesthesia.

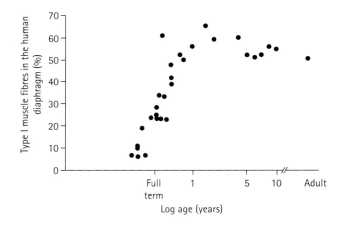

Figure 15.1 Variation in type I (slow-twitch, high-oxidative) muscle fibres with age in the human diaphragm [4]. Redrawn with permission from the American Physiological Society.

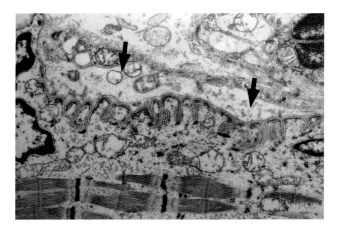

Figure 15.2 Motor end-plate at 31 weeks' gestation. Two nerve terminals are shown (arrows). The motor endplate has deep folds typical of the mature neuromuscular junction. Mitochondria and muscle fibre striations are clearly seen [5].

Neuromuscular junction

The development of the human neuromuscular junction has been studied using immunohistological staining methods that distinguish acetylcholine receptors (AChRs) [5]. At about 8 weeks' gestational age, AChRs occupy almost the entire surface of the myotubes, or primitive muscle fibres. Following the onset of innervation at 9 weeks, the AChR reactive areas contract to form primitive motor end-plates on one side of the muscle fibres. From 9 weeks to 16 weeks, the number of nerve terminals opposite one motor end-plate is greater than three, consistent with polyneuronal innervation; by 25 weeks, this number has decreased to 1.5–2, reflecting the transition from poly- to mononeuronal innervation. From 25 weeks to 31 weeks the motor end-plates attain mature appearance, although they continue to grow in size until the end of the first year of life (Fig. 15.2).

Acetylcholine receptor

The nicotinic AChR in mammalian muscles exists in foetal and adult forms [6,7] The foetal form is similar to the receptor isolated from the electric eel and is composed of five subunits: α, β, γ and δ [8]. In the adult form the γ subunit is replaced by a subunit designated ε. When two molecules of ACh combine with the α subunits the central pore opens allowing mainly sodium ions to enter the cell. The foetal receptor has a mean open time of about 6 ms when combined with acetylcholine, while the adult type has an open time of about 1.5 ms. The longer open time of the foetal receptor allows more sodium ions to enter the cell, resulting in a larger depolarising potential. Effectively, the foetal receptor is sensitive to the agonist ACh and resistant to antagonists such as tubocurarine. The reason for the expression of two types of ACh receptor is unknown, but it has been suggested that the presence of a receptor that is sensitive to ACh may compensate for reduced stores of the transmitter in immature nerve endings, thereby facilitating foetal movements which are essential for normal neuromuscular development [9].

The number and disposition of AChRs on developing muscle fibres are regulated by neural 'trophic' factors and muscle activity. The neurotrophic factors appear to be more important in establishing and maintaining early synaptic clusters, while muscle activity plays a critical role in the developmental loss of the predominantly foetal type extrajunctional receptors [10]. Before innervation the foetal receptor predominates and during synapse formation the two receptor classes coexist. At later stages of synapse formation the foetal receptors are fully replaced by those of the adult type [6]. Foetal AChRs are not normally detected on human muscle fibres after 31 weeks of gestational age [5]. However, they may reappear at extrajunctional sites in pathological states associated with prolonged inactivity (e.g. burns, denervation injury or prolonged muscle paralysis) giving rise to an exaggerated response to suxamethonium and a reduced response to non-depolarising muscle relaxants [11,12].

Maturation of neuromuscular transmission

In 1963, it was demonstrated that in neonates, in contrast to adults, the response of the hypothenar muscles to 50 Hz tetanic stimulation of the ulnar nerve was poorly sustained and was frequently followed by a period of post-tetanic exhaustion lasting from 5 min to 15 min [13]. Subsequently, it was shown that fade (i.e. decrement in the height of tetanus) occurred at the lower stimulation rate of 20 Hz in premature infants [14], while a rate of 50–100 Hz produced fade in infants up to 3 months of age [15]. These observations indicate that maturation of neuromuscular transmission is incomplete at birth.

Experiments in young rats suggest that the main deficiency in neuromuscular transmission in newborns is a reduction in the availability of ACh in developing motor

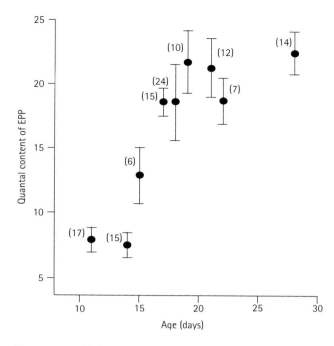

Figure 15.3 Variation in quantal content of the end-plate potential with age in phrenic nerve–hemidiaphragm preparations from young rats [16]. Redrawn by permission of Oxford University Press.

nerves. Thus, the quantal content of the evoked endplate potential in phrenic nerve–diaphragm preparations from 11-day-old rats was found to be only one-third of that in preparations from 21-day-old rats (Fig. 15.3) [16]. Furthermore, the threefold reduction in ACh release in preparations from 11-day-old rats corresponded with an identical increase in the sensitivity of the preparation to tubocurarine [17]. A similar reduction in the release of ACh from motor nerves could explain the threefold increase in sensitivity of the neuromuscular junction of the human neonate to tubocurarine and other non-depolarising muscle relaxants. A prejunctional locus for the weakness in neuromuscular transmission in human neonates is consistent with the mature appearance of the motor end-plate and the absence foetal ACh receptors from 31 weeks' gestational age (see above). It is also consistent with the apparently normal response of the motor end-plate to suxamethonium the newborn period.

Variation in cardiac output

Figure 15.4 shows the variation in cardiac output with age [18]. At birth, cardiac output is around 200 mL/kg/min. Thereafter it declines gradually during childhood to around 100 mL/kg/min by adolescence. The higher cardiac output in paediatric patients translates into faster circulation times, which in turn means that relaxants and other drugs will be distributed to and from their site of action more rapidly.

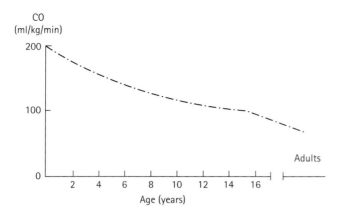

Figure 15.4   Variation in cardiac output with age [18]. Redrawn with permission from Blackwell Publishing.

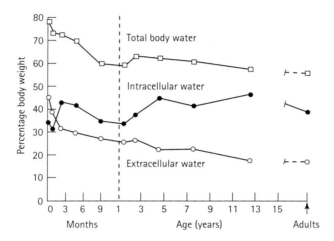

Figure 15.5   Changes in body water compartments with age [19].

Changes in extracelluar fluid volume

Figure 15.5 shows the changes in body water compartments with age [19]. At birth total body water constitutes 80 per cent of the body weight, but this declines dramatically in the first year to about 60 per cent. Most of this reduction is accounted for by a decrease in extracellular fluid, which declines from 45 per cent at birth to 26 per cent of body weight by the age of 1 year. There is then a further gradual reduction in extracellular fluid volume during childhood, down to about 19 per cent of body weight in the adult. As muscle relaxants are highly ionised drugs that penetrate cell membranes poorly, the increase in extracellular fluid in infants and children corresponds to an increase in the volume of distribution of these drugs.

DEPOLARISING MUSCLE RELAXANTS

Suxamethonium

Suxamethonium is the only depolarising muscle relaxant in clinical use. Its molecular structure resembles two

Table 15.1   The ED_{90} (effective dose in 90 per cent of patients) of suxamethonium in mg/kg is greater in neonates, infants and children than in adults. However, the ED_{90} does not change with age when expressed in mg/m^2

	mg/kg	mg/m^2
Neonates	0.517	8.24
Infants	0.608	12.04
Children	0.352	8.45
Adults	0.290	11.94

Paediatric data from Meakin *et al.* [24]; adult data from Smith *et al.* [25].

molecules of ACh joined back to back by an ester linkage. A unique combination of rapid onset and ultrashort duration of action makes it especially useful for rapid sequence and emergency intubations. Elimination depends on hydrolysis by butyrylcholinesterase (also known as plasma cholinesterase or pseudocholinesterase).

There have been no conventional studies of the pharmacokinetics of suxamethonium owing to the lack of a suitable assay; however, first-order elimination kinetics can be assumed from the linear relationship between log dose and duration of effect, and elimination rate constants can be calculated from the slope of the line [20,21]. The elimination rate constants calculated for infants, children and adults are 0.41, 0.38 and 0.17/minute respectively [22], which correspond to elimination half-times of 1.7, 1.8 and 4.3 minutes.

Using a device to measure airway pressure, it was found that neonates required at least twice the dose of suxamethonium to produce respiratory effects comparable to those obtained in adults [1]. This was later confirmed in a study using depression of thumb twitch, which showed that suxamethonium 1 mg/kg in infants was equipotent with 0.5 mg/kg in children [23]. However, a dose–response study undertaken in 1989 showed that the effective doses for 90 per cent depression of twitch response (ED_{90}) in neonates, infants and children were all greater than those previously obtained in adults under similar anaesthetic conditions (Table 15.1) [24,25]. In view of the higher effective doses and a marked variability in response to small doses of suxamethonium, the authors recommended intubating doses of 3 mg/kg for neonates and infants and 2 mg/kg for children. Following these doses, the onset of 95 per cent block occurs in 30–40 seconds and the duration of complete neuromuscular block is similar or somewhat less than that produced by suxamethonium 1 mg/kg in adults (6–8 minutes) [26].

The increased dose requirement of suxamethonium in younger patients is thought to result from its rapid distribution into an enlarged volume of extracellular fluid rather than an altered response to the action of the drug at postjunctional ACh receptors [23]. The fact that expressing the dose of suxamethonium in mg/m^2 abolishes the differences in dose requirements between the age groups supports this suggestion, because extracellular fluid volume and surface area bear a close relationship throughout life (Table 15.1) [19].

Suxamethonium is also effective when given intramuscularly. This unique property among clinically available relaxants probably relates to the thin shape and small size of the suxamethonium molecule, which has only one-quarter and one-half of the molecular weight of the benzylquinolinium and aminosteroidal relaxants respectively [27]. These physical characteristics are believed to facilitate diffusion from the muscle into the blood and from the blood to the effect compartment at the neuromuscular junction. Intramuscular suxamethonium can be particularly valuable if laryngospasm occurs in a child undergoing inhalation induction of anaesthesia prior to establishing intravenous access. In such circumstances, suxamethonium 4 mg/kg injected into the deltoid muscle relieves laryngospasm within 60 seconds and the block resolves in about 20 minutes [28]. Infants aged less than 6 months require 5 mg/kg of suxamethonium to achieve the same degree of neuromuscular block as children given 4 mg/kg, but recovery is faster in infants [29]. Intramuscular suxamethonium is also indicated for tracheal intubation when a suitable vein is inaccessible. Using the above doses, satisfactory intubating conditions will be achieved after 3–4 minutes.

Since suxamethonium is hydrolysed by butyrylcholinesterase, a deficiency in this enzyme may result in prolonged block. Butyrylcholinesterase deficiency is usually an inherited condition due to the presence of one or more abnormal genes. In the mild form, which affects 1/25 of the population, the patient is heterozygous for one of three abnormal genes (atypical, silent or fluoride resistant) and suxamethonium-induced block is prolonged for only a few minutes, which is usually undetected. In the more severe forms, which affect about 1/2500 of the population, both genes are abnormal and the suxamethonium-induced block may last for 2–4 hours, requiring ventilation and sedation to be continued until spontaneous resolution of the block occurs. Although neonates and infants aged less than 6 months have only half the level of butyrylcholinesterase activity of adults this does not prolong the effect of suxamethonium [30].

SIDE-EFFECTS

The unique mode of action of suxamethonium (sustained depolarisation) and its activity at muscarinic acetylcholine receptors are responsible for the large number of side-effects.

Mild, transient increases in heart rate are frequently observed after the administration of suxamethonium. The tachycardia is more pronounced during anaesthesia with sevoflurane than with halothane [31]. Of greater concern is the occasion bradycardia caused by the action of suxamethonium on the sinoatrial node. This is especially common in infants, in whom it is reliably attenuated by prior administration of atropine 20 μg/kg or glycopyrrolate 10 μg/kg [32].

Muscle fasciculations, which are frequently seen after administration of suxamethonium in adults, are generally milder in children and absent in infants. This may be due to the progressively larger extracellular fluid volume and smaller muscle mass in younger patients. Also, postoperative muscle pain, which may correlate with the severity of fasciculations in adults [33], is less frequent in children, and there is little increase in intragastric pressure. However, an increase in intraocular pressure, which is independent of fasciculations, occurs 1 minute after the administration of suxamethonium and lasts 6 minutes in both children and adults [34]. The increase in intraocular pressure appears to be due mainly to the cycloplegic action of suxamethonium, which deepens the anterior chamber and increases resistance to outflow of aqueous humour. In view of the risk of extrusion of global contents that may result from a sudden rise of intraocular pressure, it is inadvisable to use suxamethonium in children with open eye injury. Rocuronium 0.6 mg/kg may be a good alternative for rapid sequence induction in these patients [35,36].

The administration of suxamethonium to healthy children increases the plasma potassium concentration by about 0.2 nmol/L [37]. This small increase in potassium concentration, caused by the depolarising action of the relaxant at motor end-plates, is usually well tolerated and does not produce cardiovascular effects. In contrast, severe hyperkalaemia leading to arrhythmia or cardiac arrest may follow the administration of suxamethonium to patients with burns, paraplegia, trauma or disuse atrophy [38]. In these conditions, prolonged immobility leads to the appearance of large numbers of extrajunctional (foetal-type) acetylcholine receptors on the surface of skeletal muscle fibres, so that the whole muscle becomes capable of releasing potassium during suxamethonium-induced depolarisation [11,12]. These events appear to be a reversal of the normal developmental sequence in which muscle activity is the major factor responsible for the loss extrajunctional receptors (p. 229) [10]. Patients with cerebral palsy or meningomyelocele respond normally to suxamethonium and do not demonstrate hyperkalaemia [39,40].

Myoglobinaemia [41] and increases in serum creatine kinase [42] indicate that muscle damage may occur following suxamethonium. Neither the incidence nor the severity of fasciculations correlate with the occurrence of myoglobinaemia, but may be correlated with the increase in serum creatine kinase [43]. In boys with Duchenne or Becker muscular dystrophy or other types of myopathy, suxamethonium may produce rhabdomyolysis and hyperkalaemia with cardiac arrest [44]. Children with various myotonic syndromes may develop sustained muscle contraction causing rigidity of the jaw and respiratory muscles, which probably represents an extreme response to the normal pharmacological actions of suxamethonium (see below).

Masseter muscle spasm (MMS), defined as a severe and prolonged (more than 2 minutes) episode of resistance to mouth opening following suxamethonium administration, is a frequent early indication of malignant hyperpyrexia [45]. Historically, 50 per cent of patients who have been diagnosed with MMS and referred for *in vitro* contracture testing have proven to be malignant hyperpyrexia susceptible.

However, MMS may be difficult to distinguish from the increase in masseter muscle tone that occurs as a normal pharmacological response to suxamethonium in nearly all children and the majority of adults [46,47]. This myotonic effect of suxamethonium is consistent with the fact that it is primarily an agonist at the neuromuscular junction with actions mimicking those of ACh. In children, the increase in masseter muscle tension peaks at 15–70 seconds and lasts up to 2 minutes despite abolition of the twitch response [48]. It also occurs in peripheral muscles, but the onset is less rapid than in the masseter group [48,49]. The use of a large dose of suxamethonium (2 mg/kg) and delaying the intubation attempt until 60 seconds after injection of suxamethonium (20–30 seconds after the cessation of fasciculations) may reduce the incidence of clinically detectable jaw tension at laryngoscopy in children [26,50]. Increased jaw tension with suxamethonium is also less frequently detected when anaesthesia is induced with thiopental rather than halothane [51].

The difficulty of diagnosing MMS with certainty has led to two very different approaches to its immediate management. Some anaesthetists favour discontinuing elective anaesthesia and surgery whenever there is MMS following suxamethonium administration [52,53]. Others favour continuing the procedure with non-triggering agents while monitoring end-expired carbon dioxide, venous and/or arterial blood gases, blood pressure, heart rate, temperature and muscle tone [54]. If early signs of malignant hyperpyrexia appear the case is cancelled and treatment begun with dantrolene. In any case of MMS the duration of the jaw stiffness should be recorded and the patient should remain in hospital postoperatively for determination of serum myoglobin and 12- and 24-hour creatine kinase levels. When full recovery has occurred the patient should be referred for determination of their malignant hyperpyrexia status by muscle biopsy (see Chapter 29) [45,52].

CLINICAL USE OF SUXAMETHONIUM

The use of suxamethonium during routine anaesthesia in children is declining, primarily because of its poor side-effect profile [55,56]. Of particular concern have been the instances of life-threatening malignant hyperpyrexia and reports of rare, but often fatal, hyperkalaemic cardiac arrests in young boys with undiagnosed muscular dystrophy [57]. As a result of these reports, in 1994, the US Food and Drug Administration (FDA) and the manufacturers of suxamethonium agreed with clinicians to amend the package insert for suxamethonium to read:

'Since there may be no signs or symptoms to alert the practitioner to which patients are at risk, it is recommended that the use of suxamethonium in children should be reserved for emergency intubation and instances where immediate securing of the airway is necessary, e.g. laryngospasm, difficult airway, full stomach, or for intramuscular use when a suitable vein is inaccessible.'

Interestingly, the incidence of reporting of sudden deaths in children with unrecognised muscular dystrophies differed between countries and paediatric institutions. For example, one large paediatric hospital in Canada had no record of such deaths; similarly, none had been reported to the National Malignant Hyperpyrexia Referral Centre (MHRC) in the UK [58]. These differences may reflect the greater use of intravenous. induction methods in children in Canada and the UK compared with the USA, where all published cases of cardiac arrest had occurred following suxamethonium given after induction with halothane. Notwithstanding the lack of reporting of deaths in the UK, a subsequent survey showed that 7 out of 15 cardiac arrests following suxamethonium in children between 1965 and 1993 were, or were likely to be, caused by myopathies [58].

NON–DEPOLARISING MUSCLE RELAXANTS

Non-depolarising muscle relaxants owe their pharmacological activity to highly ionised quaternary ammonium groups which bind to the α subunits of the ACh receptor preventing depolarisation by ACh. Because two molecules of ACh are required to interact simultaneously with the α subunits to initiate depolarisation, the presence of even one molecule of a non-depolarising relaxant is sufficient to block activation of the receptor.

In mature mammals there is a large margin of safety in neuromuscular transmission. In peripheral muscles, 70–80 per cent of ACh receptors must be blocked before any decrease in the response to motor nerve stimulation is observed [59]. The diaphragm has an even greater margin of safety and continues to function with 90 per cent of its ACh receptors occupied [60]. However, neuromuscular transmission begins to fail in the diaphragms of young animals when only 40 per cent of receptors are blocked [16].

In 1955, it was observed that the respiratory effects of tubocurarine were greater in neonates than in adults [1]. However, subsequent studies produced conflicting results about the sensitivity of paediatric patients to non-depolarising relaxants. Depending upon the anaesthetic conditions, the end-point chosen to define effect and the dosing criteria, authors judged that neonates and infants were sensitive [61–63], were not sensitive [64–66] or were resistant [67] to the effects of these drugs. A confounding factor in many of the studies was the uncontrolled use of volatile anaesthetics, which are known to interfere with neuromuscular transmission [68].

The question was largely resolved in 1982 by a combined study of the pharmacokinetics and pharmacodynamics of tubocurarine in neonates, infants, children and adults [69]. The pharmacokinetic parameters are shown in Table 15.2. From this it can be seen that, while the plasma clearance of tubocurarine did not vary with age, the steady-state volume of distribution was greater in neonates and infants, reflecting a relative increase in the volume of extracellular fluid. Consequently, the half-time of elimination

Table 15.2 Variation in the pharmacokinetics of tubocurarine with age

	Cl (mL/kg/min)	V_{dss} (L/kg)	$T_{\frac{1}{2}\beta}$ (min)
Neonates	3.7	0.74	174
Infants	3.3	0.52	130
Children	4.0	0.41	90
Adults	3.0	0.30	89

Data from Fisher *et al.* [69].
Cl, clearance; V_{dss}, steady-state volume of distribution; $T_{\frac{1}{2}\beta}$, half-time of elimination.

Table 15.3 Steady-state concentration of tubocurarine for 50 per cent depression of electromyograph (EMG) twitch (C_{pss50}), steady-state volume of distribution (V_{dss}) and dose for 50 per cent depression of twitch (D_{50}) calculated from the other two parameters [69]

	C_{pss50} (μg/mL)	×	V_{dss} (L/kg)	=	D_{50} (μg/kg)
Neonates	0.18		0.74		155
Infants	0.27		0.52		158
Children	0.42		0.41		163
Adults	0.53		0.30		152

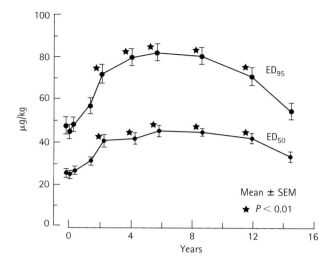

Figure 15.6 Variation in the effective doses of vecuronium for 50 per cent and 95 per cent depression of electromyograph (EMG) twitch with age in paediatric patients. The values are significantly greater in children aged 2–13 years compared with younger and older patients [72].

of tubocurarine was also longer in neonates (according to the relationship $T_{\frac{1}{2}\beta} = 0.693V_d/Cl$), which correlates with a reported increase in the duration of action of tubocurarine in this age group [66].

In order to determine whether neonates were sensitive to tubocurarine, the steady-state concentration of tubocurarine corresponding to 50 per cent depression of electromyograph (EMG) twitch (C_{pss50}) was determined. The results suggested that the neuromuscular junction of the neonate was approximately three times as sensitive and that of the infant twice as sensitive to the effects of tubocurarine compared with adults. However, when the dose corresponding to 50 per cent depression of EMG twitch (D_{50}) was calculated for each patient by multiplying the C_{pss50} by the steady-state volume of distribution (V_{dss}) there were no significant differences between the groups (Table 15.3). It was concluded that, while neonates were sensitive to tubocurarine in terms of requiring a lower plasma concentration to produce a given effect, this was countered by an increased volume of distribution, such that dose requirement did not vary significantly with age. Evidence from young rats suggests that the increased sensitivity of the neuromuscular junction of the human neonate and infant to non-depolarising muscle relaxants is the result of reduced release of ACh from immature motor nerves (Fig. 15.3).

While subsequent studies seem to confirm that the infant's sensitivity to non-depolarising muscle relaxants is

balanced by their greater volume of extracellular fluid (ECF), it is clear that this relationship does not remain constant throughout childhood [70–72]. Thus, when effective dose is plotted against age, the graph is found to be biphasic with dose requirements increasing during infancy to a peak in childhood, and thereafter decreasing to adulthood (Fig. 15.6). The increasing dose requirement during infancy and early childhood probably reflects maturation of neuromuscular transmission, while the decreasing dose requirement from later childhood to adulthood appears to mirror the decline in weight-normalised ECF volume. However, the variation in the effective dose of non-depolarising relaxants during childhood is small (0.2–0.6 × ED_{95}) in comparison with the dose required for tracheal intubation (2–3 × ED_{95}), so that the same dose can be used in patients of all ages.

The available non-depolarising muscle relaxants can be classified according to their chemical structure into benzylquinolinium or aminosteroidal compounds. These compounds have strikingly different side-effect profiles. Benzylquinolium drugs are associated with histamine release and hypotension, while aminosteroidal compounds are associated with tachycardia and hypertension. Non-depolarising muscle relaxants can be further classified according to their clinical duration of action (i.e. time taken to 25 per cent recovery of control twitch height) into long-, intermediate- and short-acting drugs (Table 15.4) [73].

Following their introduction in the early 1980s the intermediate-duration drugs atracurium and vecuronium rapidly became the most frequently used muscle relaxants in the UK and the USA [74]. Atracurium remains especially popular with paediatric anaesthetists because of its reliable offset of action in patients of all ages. Vecuronium has largely been superseded by rocuronium, a drug with a

Table 15.4 Definitions of adjectives describing non-depolarising neuromuscular blocking agents. Onset = time to maximum block. Durarion = time to 25% recovery of control switch height [73]

Adjectives	Time (minutes)	
	Minimum	Maximum
Onset		
Ultrarapid	Not needed	<1
Rapid	1	2
Intermediate	2	4
Slow	4	Not needed
Duration		
Ultrashort	Not needed	8
Short	8	20
Intermediate	20	50
Long-acting	>50	Not needed

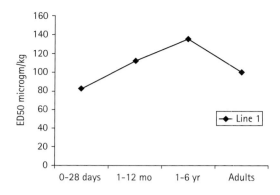

Figure 15.7 Variation of ED_{50} (effective dose – produces desired effect in 50 per cent of population) of atracurium with age. Data from Meakin *et al.* [70] and Basta *et al.* [81].

similar duration of action to vecuronium but a more rapid onset. Long-acting drugs tend to be reserved for extensive surgical procedures, especially those in which controlled ventilation is planned postoperatively.

Benzylquinolinium compounds

ATRACURIUM

Atracurium is a bisquaternary benzylquinolinium diester with an intermediate duration of clinical action. The molecule is eliminated mainly by Hofmann elimination, a process dependent on pH and temperature [75]. Ester hydrolysis is involved in a second degradation step, but its contribution to total elimination may be negligible [76]. The only pharmacologically active metabolite is laudanosine. High doses of laudanosine produce central nervous excitation and seizures in animals, but such effects are unlikely with the doses used in clinical practice [77].

The clinical pharmacokinetics of atracurium have been studied in infants and children [78]. In contrast to tubocurarine (see Table 15.2), the plasma clearance of atracurium was found to be greater in infants (9.1 mL/kg/min) compared with children (5.1 mL/kg/min). This feature presumably relates to the fact that atracurium degradation by Hofmann elimination proceeds more rapidly in the larger volume of ECF found in younger patients. As with other relaxants, the volume of distribution of atracurium was increased in infants (0.18 L/kg), compared with children (0.14 L/kg), but the net result of these changes was a reduction in elimination half-time from 19.1 minutes (children) to 13.6 minutes (infants).

The effects of age and volatile anaesthetic agents on the potency of atracurium have been investigated by several authors [70,71,79,80]. The ED_{95} values of atracurium in infants, children and adolescents were in the ranges 156–170 μg/kg, 170–350 μg/kg and 157–180 μg/kg respectively. Anaesthesia with halothane or isoflurane reduced the ED_{95}

of atracurium in children by about 30 per cent from that required during thiopental–N_2O–opioid anaesthesia. When measured during thiopental–N_2O–opioid anaesthesia, the ED_{50} of atracurium was 82 μg/kg in neonates, 112 μg/kg in infants and 135 μg/kg in children compared with 100 μg/kg in adults [70,81] (Fig 15.7). Following a standard intubating dose of atracurium 0.5 mg/kg, onset of maximum block occurred in 1.1 minutes in neonates, 1.2 minutes in infants and 1.7 minutes in children compared with 3.7 minutes in adults. Recovery to 25 per cent of the control twitch height occurred in 28.7 minutes in neonates, 35.9 minutes in infants and 33.7 minutes in children compared with 43.6 minutes in adults. Prompt recovery in the neonates and infants is a major advantage of atracurium when used in paediatric anaesthesia.

Rapid degradation by non-enzymatic means makes atracurium a suitable drug for administration by continuous infusion [79,82,83]. In studies in children, the average infusion rate required to maintain 90–99 per cent neuromuscular block was 9 μg/kg/min with thiopental–N_2O–opioid anaesthesia, 7–8 μg/kg/min with halothane anaesthesia and 6 μg/kg/min with isoflurane anaesthesia. No signs of accumulation were apparent during or after cessation of the infusion. The infusion requirement of atracurium in neonates is about 25 per cent less than that in older infants and children [83]. Prolonged use of atracurium in paediatric intensive care patients results in increased infusion requirements. This increase probably reflects upregulation of ACh receptors as a result of prolonged immobility [11]. In a study in 12 ventilated children, atracurium infusion rates increased from an average of 8 μg/kg/min to 27 μg/kg/min over 72 h [84] Absence of drug accumulation was indicated by prompt recovery from neuromuscular block upon discontinuing the infusion.

The adverse effects associated with atracurium relate mainly to histamine release [85]. This commonly results in a macular rash or erythema along the course of the vein of injection, which may subsequently spread peripherally. Occasionally, the rash may be accompanied by more serious histamine-mediated effects such as hypotension, tachycardia or bronchospasm. The cardiovascular changes are dose related and usually occur at doses more than twice the ED_{95}.

CISATRACURIUM

Cisatracurium is the $1R$-cis, $1'R$-cis isomer of atracurium, and one of 10 steroisomers that make up the commercially available atracurium mixture. Like atracurium, it is an intermediate duration relaxant that undergoes spontaneous degradation in the body by Hofmann elimination producing clinically insignificant amounts of laudanosine [86]. Cisatracurium and atracurium share a similar pharmacokinetic profile, suggesting that equipotent doses of these agents should have a similar duration of action [87,88].

The potency of cisatracurium is about three times that of atracurium [89]. When measured in children during thiopental–N_2O–opioid anaesthesia, the ED_{95} of cisatracurium is 0.045 mg/kg, which is similar to that found in adults [90]. Increased potency is associated with greater specificity of drug action and fewer side effects [91]; accordingly, cisatracurium has less propensity for histamine release and provides greater cardiovascular stability than atracurium. Doses of cisatracurium of $3 \times ED_{95}$ in children and up to $8 \times ED_{95}$ in adults produce no signs of histamine release or significant changes in heart rate or blood pressure [92,93]. Nevertheless, rare cases of severe anaphylaxis have occurred after cisatracurium, as with other non-depolarising muscle relaxants [94,95]. The main disadvantage of increased potency is a slower onset of action [96]. In adults undergoing N_2O–opioid anaesthesia, the onset of maximum neuromuscular block following doses of $2 \times ED_{95}$ of atracurium and cisatracurium are 3.7 minutes and 5.2 minutes respectively [81,89,97]. Accordingly, a dose of about $3 \times ED_{95}$ of cisatracurium (0.15 mg/kg) is required to produce intubating conditions at 2 minutes comparable to those obtained with atracurium $2 \times ED_{95}$ in both adults and children [98,99].

The time course of action of cisatracurium has been studied in paediatric patients during N_2O–opioid anaesthesia [92]. Following a dose of 0.15 µg/kg, onset of maximum block occurred more rapidly in infants than in children (2.0 minutes versus 3.0 minutes), while recovery to 25 per cent of control twitch height occurred more rapidly in children than in infants (36 minutes versus 43 minutes) The 25 per cent recovery time in children was comparable to that reported for atracurium 0.5 mg/kg under similar anaesthetic conditions [70,80]. However, the clinical duration in infants appeared to be 5–10 minutes longer after cisatracurium 0.15 mg/kg than after atracurium 0.5 mg/kg, which could have clinical importance in infants undergoing short surgical procedures. Onset and recovery times following cisatracurium 0.15 mg/kg appear to be somewhat shorter in infants and children than in adults [92].

For longer cases, cisatracurium can be used by continuous infusion. The mean infusion rate to maintain 90–99 per cent block in infants and children undergoing thiopental–N_2O–opioid anaesthesia is about 2.0 µg/kg/min [90].

This is consistent with data showing that infants and children require similar rates of atracurium infusion to maintain a constant level of neuromuscular block [83].

MIVACURIUM

Mivacurium is a short-acting non-depolarising muscle relaxant with a bisquaternary benzylquinolinium diester structure resembling that of atracurium. It is a mixture of three steroisomers and its two active isomers (*trans–trans* and *cis–trans* diesters) are rapidly hydrolysed in the plasma by butyrylcholinesterase into pharmacologically inactive compounds. The *in vitro* rate of hydrolysis of mivacurium in human plasma is 70–90 per cent of that of suxamethonium with an estimated half-time of 2.6 minutes [100,101]. Plasma clearance of mivacurium decreases with age, which is consistent with the faster recovery times and greater infusion requirements reported in infants and children compared with adults [102].

The potency of mivacurium has been determined in infants and children during both N_2O–halothane and N_2O–opioid anaesthesia [103–105]. The ED_{95} values for children varied between 89 µg/kg and 110 µg/kg while those for infants tended to be less, varying between 65 µg/kg and 94 µg/kg [106,107]. After a dose of approximately $2 \times ED_{95}$ of mivacurium in infants and children, onset of maximum block occurs in 1–2 minutes and recovery to 25 per cent of control twitch height occurs in 9–10 minutes [104,106]. These onset and recovery times are less than those reported in adults (time to maximum block and 25 per cent recovery in adults, 2.5 minutes and 14 minutes respectively) [108].

Mivacurium 0.2 mg/kg provides satisfactory intubating conditions in 98 per cent of children 90 seconds after administration during thiopental–N_2O anaesthesia [105]. In contrast, satisfactory intubating conditions were found in only 65 per cent and 80 per cent of adult patients 120 seconds and 150 seconds after mivacurium 0.2 mg/kg [109]. In order to obtain satisfactory intubation conditions in 94 per cent of adult patients at 150 seconds a dose of mivacurium 0.25 mg/kg is required [108]. The shorter time to satisfactory intubating conditions in children, despite the smaller dose, probably reflects the more rapid onset of action of neuromuscular blockade in these patients.

In view of the short duration of action of mivacurium, administration by continuous infusion may be the most practical way of maintaining neuromuscular block. When measured during N_2O–opioid anaesthesia, mivacurium infusion rates for infants and children are somewhat greater than twice those for adults (13.7 and 15.8 versus 6.0 µg/kg/min) [108,110,111] bcause of increased plasma clearance in younger patients [102]. Infusion requirements may be reduced by 20–60 per cent when using volatile anaesthetic agents [112,113]. Absence of cumulative effects is shown by the observation that infusion requirements do not change over time and that recovery following cessation of a controlled infusion is prompt and predictable.

Since mivacurium is hydrolysed by butyrylcholinesterase, a deficiency in this enzyme may result in prolonged block [106,114]. In patients heterozygous for an abnormal butyrylcholinesterase gene, mivacurium-induced block is prolonged by about 50 per cent, but this is unlikely to be a clinical problem. In patients in whom both genes are abnormal mivacurium-induced block may last from 2 hours to 4 hours, requiring treatment by sedation or continuing anaesthesia, and controlled ventilation. Once recovery has commenced, as shown by a response to peripheral nerve stimulation, it may be hastened by administering an anti-cholinesterase drug.

In 18 infants and young children, mivacurium 0.2 mg/kg produced a small (7 per cent) decrease in mean diastolic blood pressure and a small (13 per cent) increase in heart rate [115]. Slight cutaneous flushing was also observed in one child. These data suggest that mivacurium, like atracurium, has significant histamine-releasing properties, which may be evident at therapeutic doses.

Aminosteroidal compounds

PANCURONIUM

Pancuronium is a potent, long-acting, bisquaternary aminosteroidal muscle relaxant lacking the histamine releasing and hypotensive properties of tubocurarine [116,117]. The bisquaternary structure favours postganglionic muscarinic block and the production of vagolytic effects. As pancuronium is mainly eliminated via the kidney its duration of action may be prolonged in patients with renal failure.

When measured during N_2O–halothane anaesthesia, the ED_{95} of pancuronium in infants is about 46 μg/kg in infants, 58 μg/kg in children and 45 μg/kg in adults [118,119]. These values are about 60 per cent less than those obtained in infants, children and adolescents undergoing thiopental–N_2O–opioid anaesthesia [120], although all three studies cited show the same biphasic pattern of age-dependent variation in dose. In children anaesthetised with halothane, a dose of 0.12 mg/kg ($2 \times ED_{95}$) produced 95 per cent depression of controlled twitch height in about 2 minutes with recovery to 25 per cent control twitch height taking over 1 hour [121]. Increases in heart rate of 30–40 per cent and systolic blood pressure of 10–15 per cent were also found after this dose of pancuronium. The vagolytic effect of pancuronium may be an advantage in infants, in whom bradycardia is highly undesirable, or in patients undergoing anaesthesia with high-dose opioids, which tend to decrease heart rate and blood pressure. The latter group may include cardiac and other high-risk cases, in whom the use of pancuronium to facilitate postoperative ventilation can reduce oxygen consumption by up to 13 per cent [122].

VECURONIUM

Vecuronium is a monquaternary aminosteroid relaxant produced by N-demethylation in the 2-piperidino substitution of pancuronium [123]. This single alteration to the molecular structure of pancuronium results in a molecule with greater selectivity of pharmacological profile, a shorter duration of action and a less cumulative effect. Unlike pancuronium, which is heavily dependent on the kidney as its principal route of elimination, vecuronium is largely eliminated unchanged by the liver.

The pharmacokinetics of vecuronium have been studied in infants, children and adults [124]. As with tubocurarine (see Table 15.2), the plasma clearance of vecuronium did not vary with age, but the volume of distribution was increased in infants (0.36 L/kg) compared with children (0.20 L/kg) and adults (0.27 L/kg). As a result, the mean residence time (a parameter similar to half-time of elimination) was also increased in infants compared with the other two groups (66 minutes versus 34 minutes and 52 minutes, respectively).

Age-related variation in the dose of vecuronium has been demonstrated in paediatric patients undergoing thiopental–N_2O–opioid anaesthesia (see Fig. 15.6) [72]. As with other non-depolarising relaxants, a biphasic distribution of the effective doses was seen with the ED_{95} in infants (49 μg/kg) being similar to that in adolescents (55 μg/kg) while the dose in children was greater (maximum 82 μg/kg at 5–7 years). A standard intubating dose of 0.1 mg/kg of vecuronium (about $2 \times ED_{95}$) produced over 90 per cent neuromuscular blockade for almost an hour in neonates and infants compared with only 18 minutes in children [125]. Vecuronium is therefore a long-acting muscle relaxant in neonates and infants because of its increased residence time and potency in these age groups (see Table 15.4).

Intubating conditions after vecuronium 0.1 mg/kg have been studied in children induced with thiopental or halothane [126]. No significant differences were found between the groups. Intubation conditions were rated satisfactory (good to excellent) in 93 per cent of children at 90 seconds. In three studies of healthy infants and children, intubating doses of vecuronium 0.07–0.1 mg/kg produced no significant changes in heart rate or blood pressure or signs of histamine release [126–128]. Cardiovascular stability has been demonstrated in adults given three to four times the recommended intubation dose [123].

Minimal cardiovascular effects and histamine release have made vecuronium a popular choice for ventilating critically ill children. In a study in which the rate of infusion was adjusted to maintain only one twitch of the train-of-four (TOF), neonates and infants required 45 per cent less vecuronium (mean infusion rate 55 μg/kg/h) than older children (mean infusion rate 99.7 μg/kg/h) and had faster recovery to TOF ratio 0.7 (mean of 45 minutes versus 65 minutes) with no evidence of prolonged weakness after cessation of the infusion [129]. In contrast, muscle weakness lasting up to 7 days has been reported following prolonged vecuronium infusion in adult intensive care patients. [130,131] Common features in these patients were the administration of high doses of vecuronium, the occurrence of renal failure and high plasma concentrations of 3-hydroxy-vecuronium, the main metabolite of vecuronium and a potent (50–80 per cent of vecuronium) neuromuscular blocking drug. Prolonged weakness following long-term use of neuromuscular blocking agents occurs more commonly following aminosteroid drugs than with benzylquinolinium compounds. Continuous monitoring of neuromuscular block in critically ill patients reduces the likelihood of prolonged muscle weakness due to overdosage of neuromuscular blocking agents or the accumulation of active metabolites.

ROCURONIUM

Rocuronium (rapid-onset -*curonium*) is a monoquaternary relaxant structurally related to vecuronium. The drug is characterised by a rapid onset and intermediate duration of action. Rapid onset is the result of reduced potency, which necessitates an increase in dose, and hence the injection of larger numbers of drug molecules [96,132]. Rocuronium undergoes minimal metabolism and is eliminated mainly unchanged in bile and urine. Accordingly, its duration of action can be markedly prolonged in patients with hepatorenal disease.

The pharmacokinetics and pharmacodynamics of rocuronium have been compared in infants and children recovering from elective surgery in a paediatric intensive care unit (PICU) [133]. The plasma clearance was found to be less in infants (4.2 mL/kg/min) compared with children (6.7 mL/kg/min), while the volume of distribution was greater in infants (0.231 L/kg) compared with children (0.165 L/kg). As a result the mean residence time was longer in infants (56 minutes) than in children (26 minutes). The observation that infants required a lower concentration of rocuronium in the effect compartment to produce 50 per cent neuromuscular block compared with children (1.2 mg/L versus 1.7 mg/L) was consistent with earlier observations on tubocurarine and vecuronium [69,124].

Potency studies in children during N_2O–halothane or N_2O–opioid anaesthesia suggest that the ED_{95} of rocuronium is approximately 300–400 µg/kg, which is around six to seven times the ED_{95} of vecuronium [35,134–136]. When compared during N_2O–opioid anaesthesia, the ED_{95} of rocuronium was found to be significantly less in infants [255 µg/kg] than in children (402 µg/kg) or adults (350 µg/kg) [136].

The onset and duration of action of a standard intubation dose of rocuronium 0.6 mg/kg (about $2 \times ED_{95}$) have been determined in infants and children [134,137]. While there was no difference in the time to maximum block between the groups [64 seconds versus 78 seconds), recovery to 25 per cent of control twitch height took much longer in the infants than in the children (41.9 minutes versus 26.7 minutes). These results confirm that rocuronium, like vecuronium, has a longer duration of action in infants because of its increased potency and longer mean residence time. However, unlike vecuronium, rocuronium retains the characteristics of intermediate duration relaxant in infants, as defined in Table 15.4.

Intubating conditions with rocuronium 0.6 mg/kg have been assessed in children following induction of anaesthesia

with halothane, thiopental and propofol [134,138,139]. In all three studies, rocuronium 0.6 mg/kg produced satisfactory intubating conditions in 100 per cent of patients at 60 seconds. In a further study, the authors used probit analysis to determine the effective time to satisfactory intubating conditions in 90 per cent of children following rocuronium 0.6 mg/kg. This time, the 'ET_{90}', was found to be 61 seconds (upper 95 per cent confidence interval 70 seconds). Rocuronium would appear to be an acceptable alternative to suxamethonium for rapid sequence induction after a careful assessment of the airway to exclude possible difficulty with intubation [140].

Doses of $1–2 \times ED_{95}$ of rocuronium in children have been shown to produce an 11–18 per cent increase in heart rate with no change in systolic or diastolic blood pressure [135]. This small, transient increase in heart rate is clinically unimportant. Reports from France and Norway have suggested a frequent incidence of anaphylaxis with rocuronium [141,142]. However, authors in Australia and the UK have suggested that the incidence of these reactions simply reflects an increase in the clinical use of rocuronium or a difference in reporting patterns between countries [143,144]. This view seems to be supported by a recent study which found that the incidence of reported anaphylactic reactions with rocuronium in the USA in 1999–2002 did not differ from that with vecuronium and was significantly less than the frequency of reports from other countries [145].

RAPACURONIUM

Rapacuronium, a further analogue of vecuronium, became available in the USA in 1999. Its characteristics of rapid onset and short duration of action are thought to be the result of low potency which is also known to be associated with reduced specificity and an increase in side effects [91]. Ten months after its release, postmarketing surveillance revealed an increased incidence of bronchospasm and increased airway pressure which seemed to be especially severe in paediatric patients [146–149]. As a result the drug was voluntarily withdrawn from sale by the manufacturers in March 2001.

ANTAGONISM OF NON–DEPOLARISING MUSCLE RELAXANTS

Any significant residual non-depolarising neuromuscular block at the conclusion of anaesthesia should be antagonised using a reversal agent. This is especially important in infants because of their increased oxygen requirements and reduced respiratory reserve. Pharmacological reversal may not be necessary when using an intermediate-or short-acting relaxant; however, if it is omitted neuromuscular transmission should be assessed to ensure adequate spontaneous recovery has taken place (e.g. by assessment of muscle tone, ability to open eyes, lift head, move limbs).

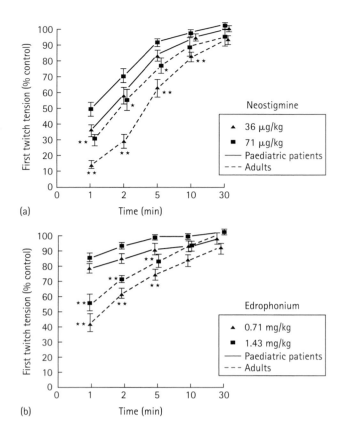

Figure 15.8 Recovery of the first twitch tension as a percentage of control in paediatric patients and adults after one of two doses of neostigmine (a) or edrophonium (b). Significant differences between paediatric and adult patients after the same dose of antagonist: *$P < 0.05$; **$P < 0.01$ [149].

The commonly used reversal agents, neostigmine and edrophonium, are antagonists of acetylcholinesterase that bind to the enzyme by electrostatic forces between the positively charged nitrogen in the molecules and the negatively charged anionic site of the enzyme. In addition, neostigmine transfers a carbamyl group to the esteratic site of the enzyme. Edrophonium has a more rapid onset of action compared with neostigmine, but larger doses are required to ensure sustained effect.

The rates of recovery from a 90 per cent pancuronium-induced neuromuscular block after one of two doses of neostigmine (36 μg/kg and 71 μg/kg) or edrophonium (0.71 mg/kg and 1.43 mg/kg) have been compared in paediatric patients and adults (Fig 15.8) [150]. Recovery after edrophonium was significantly faster than that after neostigmine for the first 2 minutes following injection, but doubling the doses of the antagonists had no significant effect on recovery. Recovery after either antagonist was significantly faster in paediatric patients than in adults [151]. These results suggest that in the presence of 10 per cent recovery of twitch height, about 35 μg/kg of neostigmine or 0.7 mg/kg of edrophonium should provide maximal antagonism in all age groups. For convenience, the somewhat larger doses of 50 μg/kg of neostigmine or 1 mg/kg of edrophonium are

usually given. Atropine 20 μg/kg or glycopyrrolate 10 μg/kg should be administered before, or with, the anticholinesterase to prevent muscarinic effects.

Sugammadex

Sugammadex (Org 25969) is a modified γ-cyclodextrin that specifically antagonises rocuronium-induced neuromuscular block. It does this by forming tight 1:1 complexes with rocuronium in the plasma, thereby inducing a rapid transfer of free rocuronium from the effect compartment. This chelation, or encapsulation, mechanism is so rapid and complete that Sugammadex 8 mg/kg can antagonise profound rocuronium-induced block in adults within 2 minutes [152]. As it does not directly involve the cholinergic system, reversal is not accompanied by the cardiovascular side effects usually seen with anticholinesterase drugs, and pretreatment with muscarinic inhibitors is unnecessary. At the time of writing Sugammadex is undergoing phase 3 clinical trials in adults and children.

REFERENCES

Key references

Goudsouzian NG, Standaert FG. The infant and the myoneural junction. *Anesth Analg* 1986; **65**: 1208–17.

Hesselmans LFGM, Jennekens FGI, Van Den Oord CJM *et al*. Development of innervation of skeletal muscle fibers in man: relation to acetylcholine receptors. *Anat Rec* 1993; **236**: 553–62.

Meakin GH, McKiernan EP, Morris P, Baker RD. Dose–response curves for suxamethonium in neonates, infants and children. *Br J Anaesth* 1989; **62**: 655–8.

Meakin GH, Shaw EA, Baker RD, Morris P. Comparison of atracurium-induced neuromuscular blockade in neonates, infants and children. *Br J Anaesth* 1988; **60**: 171–5.

Wareham AC, Morton RH, Meakin GH. Low quantal content of the endplate potential reduces safety factor for neuromuscular transmission in the diaphragm of the newborn rat. *Br J Anaesth* 1994; **72**: 205–9.

References

1. Stead AL. The response of the newborn infant to muscle relaxants. *Br J Anaesth* 1955; **27**: 124–30.

2. Mastaglia FL. The growth and development of the skeletal muscles. In: Davis JA, Dobbing J, eds. *Scientific foundations of paediatrics*. London: William Heinmann Medical Books, 1974: 350.

3. Dubowitz V. Enzyme histochemistry of skeletal muscle. *J Neurol Neurosurg Psychiatry* 1965; **28**: 516–24.

4. Keens TG, Bryan AC, Levinson H, Ianuzzo CD. Developmental patterns of muscle fibre types in human ventilatory muscles. *J Appl Physiol* 1978; **44**: 909–13.

5. Hesselmans LFGM, Jennekens FGI, Van Den Oord CJM et al. Development of innervation of skeletal muscle fibers in man: relation to acetylcholine receptors. Anat Rec 1993; 236: 553–62.

6. Mishina M, Takai T, Imoto K et al. Molecular distinction between foetal and adult forms of muscle acetylcholine receptor. Nature 1986; 321: 406–11.

7. Jamarillo F, Scheutze SM. Kinetic difference between embryonic- and adult-type acetylcholine receptors in rat myotubes. J Physiol 1988; 396: 267–96.

8. Goudsouzian NG, Standaert FG. The infant and the myoneural junction. Anesth Analg 1986; 65: 1208–17.

9. Jamarillo F, Vicini S, Schuetze SM. Embryonic acetylcholine receptors guarantee spontaneous contractions in rat developing muscles. Nature 1988; 335: 66–8.

10. Schuetze SM, Role LW. Developmental regulation of nicotinic acetylcholine receptors. Annu Rev Neurosci 1987; 10: 403–57.

11. Fambrough DM. Control of acetycholine receptors in skeletal muscle. Physiol Rev 1979; 59: 165–227.

12. Martyn JAJ. The neuromuscular junction – basic receptor pharmacology. In: Fukushima K, Ochiai R, eds. Muscle relaxants: physiologic and pharmacologic aspects. London: Springer, 1995: 37–47.

13. Churchill-Davidson HC, Wise RP. Neuromuscular transmission in the newborn infant. Anesthesiology 1963; 24: 271–8.

14. Koenigsberger MR, Patten B, Lovelace RE. Studies of neuromuscular function in the newborn: a comparison of myoneural function in the full term and premature infant. Neuropaediatrie 1973; 4: 350–61.

15. Crumrine RS, Yodlowski EH. Assessment of neuromuscular function in infants. Anesthesiology 1981; 54: 29–32.

16. Wareham AC, Morton RH, Meakin GH. Low quantal content of the endplate potential reduces safety factor for neuromuscular transmission in the diaphragm of the newborn rat. Br J Anaesth 1994; 72: 205–9.

17. Meakin GH, Morton RH, Wareham AC. Age-dependent variation in response to tubocurarine in the isolated rat diaphragm. Br J Anaesth 1992; 68: 161–3.

18. Rudolph AM. Congenital diseases of the heart. Chicago: Year Book Medical Publishers, 1974.

19. Friis-Hansen B. Body water compartments in children: changes during growth related changes in body composition. Pediatrics 1961; 28: 169–81.

20. Levy G. Kinetics of pharmacologic activity of succinylcholine in man. J Pharm Sci 1967; 56: 1687–8.

21. Levy G. Pharmacokinetics of succinylcholine in newborns. Anesthesiology 1970; 32: 551–2.

22. Cook DR, Wingard LB, Taylor FH. Pharmacokinetics of succinylcholine in infants, children and adults. Clin Pharmacol Ther 1976; 20: 493–8.

23. Cook DR, Fischer CG. Neuromuscular blocking effects of succinylcholine in infants and children. Anesthesiology 1975; 42: 662–5.

24. Meakin GH, McKiernan EP, Morris P, Baker RD. Dose–response curves for suxamethonium in neonates, infants and children. Br J Anaesth 1989; 62: 655–8.

25. Smith CE, Donati F, Bevan DR. Dose–response curves for succinylcholine: single versus cumulative techniques. Anesthesiology 1988; 69: 338–42.

26. Meakin G, Walker RWM, Dearlove OR. Myotonic and neuromuscular blocking effects of increased doses of suxamethonium in infants and children. Br J Anaesth 1990; 65: 816–8.

27. Bevan DR, Donati F. Muscle relaxants of the future. Semin Anaesth 1992; 11: 123–30.

28. Liu LMP, DeCook TH, Goudsouzian NG et al. Dose response to intramuscular succinylcholine in children. Anesthesiology 1981; 55: 599–602.

29. Liu LMP, Goudsouzian NG. Neuromuscular effect of intramuscular succinylcholine in infants. Anesthesiology 1982; 57: A413.

30. Zsigmond EK, Downes JR. Plasma cholinesterase activity in newborns and infants. Can Anaesth Soc J 1971; 18: 278–85.

31. Reiger A, Hass I, Striebel HW et al. Marked increases in heart rate associated with sevoflurane but not halothane following suxamethonium administration in children. Eur J Anaesthesiol 1996; 13: 616–21.

32. Lerman J, Chinyanga HM. The heart rate response to succinylcholine in children: a comparison of atropine and glycopyrrolate. Can Anaesth Soc J 1983; 30: 377–81.

33. Waters DJ, Mapleson WW. Suxamethonium pains: hypothesis and observations. Anaesthesia 1971; 26: 127–41.

34. Craythorne NWB, Rottenstein HS, Dripps RD. The effect of succinylcholine on intraocular pressure in adults, infants and children during general anesthesia. Anesthesiology 1960; 21: 59–63.

35. Hopkinson JM, Meakin G, McCluskey A, Baker RD. Dose–response relationship and effective time to satisfactory intubation conditions after rocuronium in children. Anaesthesia 1997; 52: 428–32.

36. Stoddart PA, Mather SJ. Onset of neuromuscular blockade and intubating conditions one minute after the administration of rocuronium in children. Paediatr Anaesth 1998; 8: 37–40.

37. Keneally JP, Bush GH. Changes in serum potassium after suxamethonium in children. Anaesth Intensive Care 1974; 2: 147–150.

38. Gronert GA, Theye RA. Pathophysiology of hyperkalemia induced by succinylcholine. Anesthesiology 1975; 43: 88–99.

39. Dierdorf SF, McNiece WL, Rao CC et al. Effect of succinylcholine on plasma potassium in children with cerebral palsy. Anesthesiology 1985; 62: 88–90.

40. Dierdorf SF, McNiece WL, Rao CC et al. Failure of succinylcholine to alter plasma potassium in children with myelomeningocele. Anesthesiology 1986; 64: 272–3.

41. Ryan JF, Kagen LJ, Hyman AL. Myoglobinaemia after a single dose of succinylcholine. N Engl J Med 1971; 285: 824–7.

42. Cozanitis DA, Erkola O, Klemola UM, Makela V. Precurarisation in infants and children less than three years of age. Can J Anaesth 1987; 34(1): 17–20.

43. Karhunen U. Serum creatine kinase levels after succinlycholine in children with 'muscle, eye and brain disease'. Can J Anaesth 1988; 35: 90–2.

44. Larach MG, Rosenberg MD, Gronert GA, Allan CA. Hyperkaemic cardiac arrests during anesthesia in infants and children with occult myopathies. *Clin Pediatr* 1997; **36**: 9–16.

45. Hopkins PM. Masseter muscle spasm. In: Pollard BJ, ed. *Handbook of clinical anaesthesia*. Edinburgh: Churchill Livingstone, 2004: 767–8.

46. van der Spek AFL, Fang WB, Ashton-Miller JA *et al*. The effects of succinylcholine on mouth opening. *Anesthesiology* 1987; **67**: 459–65.

47. Leary NP, Ellis FR. Masseteric muscle spasm as a normal response to suxamethonium. *Br J Anaesth* 1990; **64**: 488–92.

48. Plumley MH, Bevan JC, Saddler JM *et al*. Dose-related effects of succinylcholine on the adductor pollicis and masseter muscles in children. *Can J Anaesth* 1990; **37**(1): 15–20.

49. van der Spek AF, Fang WB, Ashton-Miller JA *et al*. Increased masticatory muscle stiffness during limb muscle flaccidity associated with succinylcholine administration. *Anesthesiology* 1988; **69**(1): 11–6.

50. Hannallah RS, Kaplan RF. Jaw relaxation after a halothane/succinylcholine sequence in children. *Anesthesiology* 1994; **81**(1): 99–103.

51. Lazzell VA, Carr AS, Lerman J *et al*. The incidence of masseter muscle rigidity after succinylcholine in infants and children. *Can J Anaesth* 1994; **41**(6): 475–9.

52. Rosenberg H, Shutack JG. Variants of malignant hyperthermia. Special problems for the paediatric anaesthesiologist. *Paediatr Anaesth* 1996; **6**: 87–93.

53. Rosenberg H. Trismus is not trivial. *Anesthesiology* 1987; **67**(4): 453–5.

54. Berry FA, Lynch C 3rd. Succinylcholine and trismus. *Anesthesiology* 1989; **70**(1): 161–3.

55. Delphin E, Jackson D, Rothstein P. Use of succinylcholine during elective pediatric anesthesia should be reevaluated. *Anesth Analg* 1987; **66**: 1190–2.

56. Hatcher IS, Stack CG. Postal survey of the anaesthetic techniques used for paediatric tonsillectomy surgery. *Paediatr Anaesth* 1999; **9**: 311–5.

57. Rosenberg H, Gronert GA. Intractable cardiac arrest in children given succinylcholine. *Anesthesiology* 1992; **77**: 1054.

58. Hopkins PM. Use of suxamethonium in children. *Br J Anaesth* 1995; **75**: 675–7.

59. Paton WDM, Waud DR. The margin of safety of neuromuscular transmission. *J Physiol* 1967; **191**: 59–90.

60. Waud BE, Waud DR. The margin of safety of neuromuscular transmission in the muscle of the diaphragm. *Anesthesiology* 1972; **37**: 417–22.

61. Lim HS, Davenport HT, Robson JG. The response of infants and children to muscle relaxants. *Anesthesiology* 1964; **25**: 161–8.

62. Bush GH, Stead AL. The use of d-tubocurarine in neonatal anaesthesia. *Br J Anaesth* 1962; **34**: 721–8.

63. Walts LF, Dillon JB. The response of newborns to succinylcholine and *d*-tubocurarine. *Anesthesiology* 1969; **28**: 372–6.

64. Churchill-Davidson HC, Wise RP. The response of the newborn infant to muscle relaxants. *Can Anaesth Soc J* 1964; **11**: 1–6.

65. Matteo RS, Lieberman IG, Salanitre E *et al*. Distribution, elimination and action of *d*-tubocurarine in neonates, infants, children and adults. *Anesth Analg* 1984; **63**: 799–804.

66. Long G, Bachman L. Neuromuscular blockade by *d*-tubocurarine in children. *Anesthesiology* 1967; **28**: 723–9.

67. Goudsouzian NG, Donlon JV, Savarese JJ, Ryan JF. Re-evaluation of dosage and duration of action of *d*-tubocurarine in the pediatric age group. *Anesthesiology* 1975; **43**: 416–25.

68. Miller RD, Way WL, Dolan WM *et al*. The dependence of pancuronium and *d*-tubocurarine-induced neuromuscular blockades on alveolar concentrations of halothane and Forane. *Anesthesiology* 1972; **37**: 573–81.

69. Fisher DM, O'Keefe C, Stanski DR *et al*. Pharmacokinetics and pharmacodynamics of *d*-tubocurarine in infants, children and adults. *Anesthesiology* 1982; **57**: 203–8.

70. Meakin GH, Shaw EA, Baker RD, Morris P. Comparison of atracurium-induced neuromuscular blockade in neonates, infants and children. *Br J Anaesth* 1988; **60**: 171–5.

71. Brandom BW, Woefel SK, Cook DR *et al*. Clinical pharmacology of atracurim in infants. *Anesth Analg* 1984; **63**: 309–12.

72. Meretoja OA, Wirtavuori K, Neuvonen PJ. Age-dependence of the dose–response curve of vecuronium in pediatric patients during balanced anesthesia. *Anesth Analg* 1988; **67**: 21–6.

73. Bedford RF. From the FDA. *Anesthesiology* 1995; **82**: 33A.

74. Meakin GH. Recent advances in myorelaxant therapy. *Paediatr Anaesth* 2002; **11**: 523–31.

75. Stenlake JB, Waigh RD, Urwin J *et al*. Atracurium: conception and inception. *Br J Anaesth* 1983; **55**: 3S–10S.

76. Weindlmayr-Goettel M, Gilly H, Kress HG. Does ester hydrolysis change the *in vitro* degradation rate of cisatracurium or atracurium? *Br J Anaesth* 2002; **88**: 555–62.

77. Chapple DJ, Miller AA, Ward JB, Wheatley PL. Cardiovascular and neurological effects of laudanosine. *Br J Anaesth* 1987; **59**: 218–25.

78. Brandom BW, Stiller RL, Cook DR *et al*. Pharmacokinetics of atracurium in anesthetized infants and children. *Br J Anaesth* 1986; **58**: 1210–3.

79. Brandom BW, Cook DR, Woelfel SK *et al*. Atracurium infusion requirements in children during halothane, isoflurane, and narcotic anesthesia. *Anesth Analg* 1985; **64**: 471–6.

80. Goudsouzian NG, Liu LMP, Gionfriddo M, Rudd GD. Neuromuscular effects of atracurium in infants and children. *Anesthesiology* 1985; **62**: 75–9.

81. Basta SJ, Ali HH, Savarese JJ *et al*. Clinical pharmacology of atracurium besylate (BW 33A): a new non-depolarizing muscle relaxant. *Anesth Analg* 1982; **61**: 723–9.

82. Goudsouzian NG, Martyn J, Rudd GD *et al*. Continuous infusion of atracurium in children. *Anesthesiology* 1986; **64**: 171–4.

83. Kalli I, Meretoja OA. Infusion of atracurium in neonates, infants and children. A study of dose requirements. *Br J Anaesth* 1988; **60**: 651–4.

84. Kushimo OT, Darowski MJ, Morris P, Meakin G. Dose requirements of atracurium in paediatric intensive care patients. *Br J Anaesth* 1991; **67**: 781–3.

85. Bevan DR, Bevan JC, Donati F. *Muscle relaxants in clinical anaesthesia*. Chicago: Year Book Medical Publishers, 1988.

86. Lien CA, Schmith VD, Belmont MR *et al*. Pharmacokinetics of cisatracurium in patients receiving nitrous oxide/opioid/barbiturate anesthesia. *Anesthesiology* 1996; **84**: 300–8.

87. Lien CA, Schmith VD, Belmont MR *et al*. Pharmacokinetics/ dynamics of 51W89 in healthy patients during opioid anesthesia. *Anesthesiology* 1994; **81**: A1082.

88. Ward S, Neill EAM, Weatherley BC, Corall IM. Pharmacokinetics of atracurium besylate in healthy patients (after a single i.v. bolus dose). *Br J Anaesth* 1983; **55**: 113–18.

89. Belmont MR, Lien CA, Quessy S *et al*. The clinical neuromuscular pharmacology of 51W89 in patients receiving nitrous oxide/opioid/barbiturate anesthesia. *Anesthesiology* 1995; **82**: 1139–45.

90. de Ruiter J, Crawford MW. Dose–response relationship and infusion requirement of cisatracurium besylate in infants and children during nitrous oxide-narcotic anesthesia. *J Clin Anesth* 2001; **94**: 790–2.

91. Wierda JMKH, Proost JH. Structure-onset relationship of steroidal neuromuscular blocking agents. In: Fukushima K, Ochiai R, eds. *Muscle relaxants: physiologic and pharmacologic aspects*. Tokyo: Springer, 1995; 163–6.

92. Taivainen T, Meakin GH, Meretoja OA *et al*. The safety and efficacy of cisatracurium 0.15 mg/kg during nitrous oxide–opioid anaesthesia in infants and children. *Anaesthesia* 2000; **55**: 1047–51.

93. Lien CA, Belmont RA, Abalos A *et al*. The cardiovascular effects and histamine-releasing properties of 51W89 in patients receiving nitrous oxide/opioid/barbiturate anesthesia. *Anesthesiology* 1995; **82**: 1131–8.

94. Legros CB, Orliaguet GA, Mayer M-N *et al*. Severe anaphylactic reaction to cisatracurium in a child. *Anesth Analg* 2001; **92**: 648–9.

95. Briassoulis G, Hatzis T, Mammi P, Alikatora A. Persistent anaphylactic reaction after induction with thiopentone and cisatracurium. *Paediatr Anaesth* 2000; **10**: 429–34.

96. Bowman WC, Rodger IW, Houston J *et al*. Structure: action relationships among some desacetoxy analogues of pancuronium and vecuronium in the anesthetized cat. *Anesthesiology* 1988; **69**: 57–62.

97. Foldes FF, Nagashima H, Boros M *et al*. Muscular relaxation with atracurium, vecuronium and Duador under balanced anaesthesia. *Br J Anaesth* 1983; **55**: 97s–103s.

98. Littlejohn IH, Abhay K, El Sayed A *et al*. Intubating conditions following 1R-*cis*, 1'R-*cis* atracurium (51W89): a comparison with atracurium. *Anaesthesia* 1995; **50**: 499–502.

99. Meakin G, Meretoja OA, Perein's RR. Tracheal intubating conditions and pharmacodynamics following cisatracurium in infants and children undergoing halothane and thiopental–fentanyl anaesthesia. *Paediatr Anaesth* 2007; **17**: 113–20.

100. Cook DR, Stiller RL, Weakly JN *et al*. *In vitro* metabolism of mivacurium chloride (BW B1090U) and succinylcholine. *Anesth Analg* 1989; **68**: 452–6.

101. Saverese JJ, Ali HH, Basta SJ *et al*. The clinical neuromuscular pharmacology of mivacurium chloride (BW B1090U). *Anesthesiology* 1988; **68**: 723–32.

102. Markakis DA, Lau M, Brown R *et al*. The pharmacokinetics and steady state pharmacodynamics of mivacurium in children. *Anesthesiology* 1998; **88**(4): 978–83.

103. Sarner JB, Brandom BW, Woelfel SK *et al*. Clinical pharmacology of mivacurium chloride (BW B1090U) in children during nitrous oxide-halothane and nitrous oxide-narcotic anesthesia. *Anesth Analg* 1989; **68**: 116–21.

104. Goudsouzian NG, Alifimoff JK, Eberly C *et al*. Neuromuscular and cardiovascular effects of mivacurium in children. *Anesthesiology* 1989; **70**: 237–42.

105. McCluskey A, Meakin G. Dose–response and minimum time to satisfactory intubation conditions after mivacurium in children. *Anaesthesia* 1996; **51**: 438–41.

106. Goudsouzian NG, Denman W, Schwartz A *et al*. Pharmacodynamic and hemodynamic effects of mivacurium in infants anesthetized with halothane and nitrous oxide. *Anesthesiology* 1993; **79**: 919–25.

107. Woelfel SK, Brandom BW, McGowan FX, Cook DR. Clinical pharmacology of mivacurium in pediatric patients less than 2 years old during nitrous oxide-halothane anesthesia. *Anesth Analg* 1993; **77**: 713–20.

108. Shanks CA, Fragen RJ, Pemberton D *et al*. Mivacurium-induced neuromuscular blockade following single bolus doses and with continuous infusion during either balanced or enflurane anesthesia. *Anesthesiology* 1989; **71**: 362–6.

109. Maddenini VR, Mirakhur RK, McCoy EP *et al*. Neuromuscular effects and intubating conditions following mivacurium: a comparison with suxamethonium. *Anaesthesia* 1993; **48**: 940–5.

110. Meretoja OA, Taivainen T, Wirtavuori K. Pharmacodynamics of mivacurium in infants. *Br J Anaesth* 1994; **73**: 490–3.

111. Meretoja OA, Olkkola KT. Pharmacodynamics of mivacurium in children using a computer-controlled infusion. *Br J Anaesth* 1993; **71**: 232–7.

112. Alifimoff JK, Goudsouzian NG. Continuous infusion of mivacurium in children. *Br J Anaesth* 1989; **63**: 520–4.

113. Woloszczuk-Gebicka B. Mivacurium infusion requirement and spontaneous recovery of neuromuscular transmission in children anaesthetized with nitrous oxide and fentanyl, halothane, isoflurane or sevoflurane. *Paediatr Anaesth* 2002; **12**: 511–8.

114. Maddenini VR, Mirakhur RK. Prolonged neuromuscular block following mivacurium. *Anesthesiology* 1993; **78**: 1181–4.

115. Woelfel SK, Brandom BW, McGowan FX, Cook DR. Clinical pharmacology of mivacurium in pediatric patients less than two years old during nitrous oxide-halothane anesthesia. *Anesth Analg* 1993; **77**: 713–20.

116. Baird WLM, Reid AM. The neuromuscular blocking properties of a new steroid compound, pancuronium bromide: a pilot study in a man. *Br J Anaesth* 1967; **39**: 775–80.

117. Nightingale DA, Bush GH. A clinical comparison between tubocurarine and pancuronium in children. *Br J Anaesth* 1973; **45**: 63–70.

118. Laycock JRD, Bevan DR, Donati F. The potency of pancuronium at the adductor pollicis and diaphragm in infants and children. *Anesthesiology* 1988; **68**: 908–11.

119. Blinn A, Woelfel SK, Cook DR *et al*. Pancuronium dose-response revisited. *Paediatr Anaesth* 1992; **2**: 153–5.

120. Meretoja OA, Luosto T. Dose-response characteristics of pancuronium in neonates, infants and children. *Anesth Intensive Care* 1990; **18**: 455–9.

121. Montgomery CJ, Steward DJ. A comparative evaluation of intubating doses of d-tubocurarine, pancuronium and vecuronium in children. *Can J Anaesth* 1988; **35**: 36–40.

122. Palmisano BW, Fisher DM, Willis M, Gregory GA, Ebert PA. The effect of paralysis on oxygen consumption in normoxic children after cardiac surgery. *Anesthesiology* 1984; **61**: 518–22.

123. Baird WLM, Savage DS. Vecuronium – the first years. *Clin Anesthesiology* 1985; **3**: 347–60.

124. Fisher DM, Castagnoli BA, Miller RD. Vecuronium kinetics and dynamics in anesthetized infants and children. *Clin Pharmacol Ther* 1985; **37**: 402–6.

125. Meretoja OA. Is vecuronium a long-acting neuromuscular blocking agent in neonates and infants? *Br J Anaesth* 1989; **62**: 184–7.

126. Ferres CJ, Crean PM, Mirakhur RK. An evaluation of Org NC 45 (vecuronium) in paediatric anaesthesia. *Anaesthesia* 1983; **38**: 943–7.

127. Goudsouzian NG, Martyn JJA, Liu LMP, Gionfriddo M. Safety and efficacy of vecuronium in adolescents and children. *Anesth Analg* 1983; **62**: 1083–8.

128. Fisher DM, Miller RD. Neuromuscular effects of vecuronium (ORG NC45) in infants and children during N_2O, halothane anesthesia. *Anesthesiology* 1983; **58**: 519–23.

129. Hodges UM. Vecuronium infusion requirements in paediatric patients in intensive care units: the use of acceleromyography. *Br J Anaesth* 1996; **76**: 23–8.

130. Kupfer Y, Namba T, Kaldawi E, Tessler S. Prolonged weakness after long-term infusion of vecuronium bromide. *Ann Intern Med* 1992; **117**: 484–6.

131. Segredo V, Caldwell JE, Matthay MA *et al*. Persistent paralysis in critically ill patients after long-term administration of vecuronium. *N Engl J Med* 1992; **327**: 524–8.

132. Wierda JMKH, Beaufort AM, Kleef UW *et al*. Preliminary investigations of the clinical pharmacology of three short-acting non-depolarizing neuromuscular blocking agents, Org 9453, Org 9489 and Org 9487. *Can J Anaesth* 1994; **41**: 213–20.

133. Wierda JM, Meretoja OA, Taivainen T, Proosk JH. Pharmacokinetics and pharmacokinetic–dynamic modelling of rocuronium in infants and children. *Br J Anesth* 1997; **78**: 690–5.

134. Woelfel SK, Brandon BW, Cook DR, Sarner JB. Effects of bolus administration of ORG-9426 in children during

nitrous oxide-halothane anesthesia. *Anesthesiology* 1992; **76**: 939–42.

135. Bikhazi G, Marin F, Halliday NJ, Deepika K, Foldes FF. The pharmacodynamics of rocuronium in pediatric patients anesthetized with halothane. *J Anesth* 1994; **8**: 256–60.

136. Meretoja OA, Taivainen T, Erkola O, Rautoma P, Juvakoski M. Dose–response and time-course of effect of rocuronium bromide in paediatric patients. *Eur J Anaesthesiol* 1995; **12**(11): 19–22.

137. Woelfel SK, Brandom BW, McGowan FX, Gronert BJ, Cook DR. Neuromuscular effects of 600 mg/kg of rocuronium in infants during nitrous oxide-halothane anaesthesia. *Paediatr Anaesth* 1994; **4**: 173–7.

138. Fuchs-Buder T, Tassonyi E. Intubating conditions and time course of rocuronium-induced neuromuscular block in children. *Br J Anaesth* 1996; **77**: 335–8.

139. Naguib M, Samarkandi AH, Ammar A, Turkistani A. Comparison of suxamethonium and different combinations of rocuronium and mivacurium for rapid tracheal intubation in children. *Br J Anaesth* 1997; **79**: 450–5.

140. McCourt KC, Samela L, Mirakhur RK *et al*. Comparison of rocuronium and suxamethonium for use during rapid sequence induction of anaesthesia. *Anaesthesia* 1998; **53**: 867–71.

141. Laxenaire MC, Mertes PM. Anaphylaxis during anaesthesia. Results of a two-year survey in France. *Br J Anaesth* 2001; **87**: 549–58.

142. Baillard C, Korinek AM, Galanton V *et al*. Anaphylaxis to rocuronium. *Br J Anaesth* 2002; **88**: 600–2.

143. Rose M, Fisher M. Rocuronium: high risk for anaphylaxis? *Br J Anaesth* 2001; **86**: 678–82.

144. Watkins J. Incidence of UK reactions involving rocuronium may simply reflect market use. *Br J Anaesth* 2002; **87**: 522.

145. Bhananker SM, O'Donnell JT, Salemi JR, Bishop MJ. The risk of anaphylactic reactions to rocuronium in the United States is comparable to that of vecuronium: an analysis of Food and Drug Administration reporting of adverse events. *Anesth Analg* 2005; **101**: 819–22.

146. Goudsouzian NG. Rapacuronium and bronchospasm. *Anesthesiology* 2001; **94**: 727–8.

147. Kron SS. Severe bronchospasm and desaturation in a child associated with rapacuronium. *Anesthesiology* 2001; **94**: 923–4.

148. Naguib M. How serious is the bronchospasm induced by rapacuronium? *Anesthesiology* 2001; **94**: 924–5.

149. Meakin GH, Pronske EH, Lerman J *et al*. Bronchospasm after rapacuronium in infants and children. *Anesthesiology* 2001; **94**: 926–7.

150. Meakin G, Sweet PT, Bevan JC, Bevan DR. Neostigmine and edrophonium as antagonists of pancuronium in infants and children. *Anesthesiology* 1983; **59**: 316–21.

151. Ferguson A, Egerszegi P, Bevan DR. Neostigmine, pyridostigmine and edrophonium as antagonists of pancuronium. *Anesthesiology* 1980; **53**: 390–4.

152. Gijsenbergh F, Ramael S, Houwing N, van Iersel T. First human exposure of Org 25969, a novel agent to reverse the action of rocuronium bromide. *Anesthesiology* 2005; **103**: 695–703.

Adjuncts to anaesthesia

HILARY GLAISYER

KEY LEARNING POINTS

- Currently, antimuscarinics are not used routinely and are reserved for a small minority of patients who need reduction of their secretions or protection against bradycardia.
- Up to 50 per cent of school-age children have postoperative nausea and vomiting (PONV) – this can cause unanticipated readmission following day-case surgery.
- PONV prophylaxis in a high-risk group may be justified because it reduces costs and improves patient satisfaction – but not for children at low risk.

- Evidence suggests that the most effective prophylaxis against or treatment of PONV may be:
  - the avoidance of all contributory factors, and
  - a serotonin antagonist combined with dexamethasone.
- Clonidine has analgesic and sedative properties that may calm and sedate children in recovery.

INTRODUCTION

Despite the introduction of new drugs, anaesthesia and surgery are still associated with nausea, vomiting and autonomic side-effects. The choice of drugs available to counter these problems has expanded greatly and some drugs have become useful adjuncts because they have multifaceted beneficial effects. This chapter will focus, in the main, on drugs that have specific antimuscarinic and antiemetic properties. Hypertension and tachycardia are also common during surgery and, although they are usually controlled by increasing the doses of analgesia or hypnosis components of anaesthesia, drugs with specific cardiovascular effects are useful and indicated occasionally. Clonidine has several useful properties and the value of this unusual drug as an adjunct will be discussed here. Anaesthetics, sedatives and analgesics that, in addition to their primary role, also act as adjuncts are covered in other chapters.

ANTIMUSCARINICS

In the past, the use of antimuscarinic drugs has been widespread in adult and paediatric anaesthesia. Initially, they were introduced to reduce troublesome airway secretions caused by ether and chloroform and then subsequently to prevent bradycardia. Modern anaesthetic drugs are much less irritant to the airway, do not stimulate excessive secretions and cause less cardiovascular depression. Thus currently, in paediatric anaesthesia, antimuscarinics are not used routinely and are reserved for the small minority of patients who need reduction of their secretions or protection against bradycardia; both atropine and glycopyrrolate are standard agents.

Atropine

Atropine can be administered via the oral, intramuscular (IM), intravenous (IV), subcutaneous or rectal routes.

The oral or IM routes are most commonly used for pre-medication. Following an IM dose of 20 μg/kg, the peak plasma concentration and clinical effects (increased heart rate and rise in core temperature) occur at 25 minutes [1]. After an oral dose, peak plasma levels are achieved after 90 minutes and an equipotent dose is more than 30–40 μg/kg [1,2]. The plasma half-life is 2–3 hours. Fifty per cent of the dose is protein bound.

Atropine causes a tachycardia and prevents bradycardia by blocking the vagus nerve. It also directly stimulates the medulla, higher centres and the respiratory centre. Irritability, confusion and coma are possible with overdose. Sweat, bronchial and salivary glands are paralysed and bronchial smooth muscle is relaxed, increasing slightly the anatomical and physiological dead space. It can dilate cutaneous blood vessels and cause a flushed appearance. Lower oesophageal sphincter tone is reduced which may allow regurgitation of gastric contents.

Glycopyrrolate

Glycopyrrolate is a synthetic quaternary ammonium compound and does not cross the blood–brain barrier. Central effects are minimal. The increase in heart rate is less marked than atropine, but the antisialogogue effect is greater [3]. The onset of action is similar to atropine, but the drying effect after an IV injection is much more prolonged. This makes IV glycopyrrolate useful when IM injection is inappropriate. The most commonly used dose is 10 μg/kg which, if given by the IM route, produces clinical effects by 30 minutes.

Roles in clinical practice

Previously, antimuscarinics were used to premedicate all children. This is no longer considered necessary and these drugs now have a much more defined and restricted role. Effective premedication doses are 20 μg/kg IM or 30 μg/kg orally of atropine and 10 μg/kg IM or IV of glycopyrrolate. Intramuscular injections should be avoided unless other routes are impractical or unreliable.

INDICATIONS

Many anaesthetists use antimuscarinic premedication in very small premature or ex-premature babies to prevent bradycardia and reduce secretions; the IM route may be appropriate because intravenous access is often difficult in these patients. Both the management of a difficult airway (including fibre-optic intubation) and airway surgery may be easier if the airway is dry because secretions can obstruct the view or cause laryngospasm. Also, the action of topical liocaine may be more effective when applied to a dry glottis [4]. In the sitting and prone positions for neurosurgery, salivation is potentially dangerous because the

tape securing the tracheal tube may be loosened by saliva and, in these circumstances, an antisialogogue can prevent this hazard. Other possible indications include particular operations or procedures associated with an appreciable risk of bradycardia; squint surgery and posterior fossa neurosurgery are good examples.

Halothane anaesthesia causes a fall in cardiac output by reducing both the heart rate and myocardial contraction. Premedication with antimuscarinics helps to preserve the heart rate and hence reduce the fall in cardiac output. This is especially important in small infants [5]. Atropine is no longer used to prevent bradycardia associated with a single dose of suxamethonium because an increasing body of evidence has demonstrated that the fall in heart rate is minimal, short-lived and clinically insignificant [6].

CONTRAINDICATIONS

Antimuscarinics can cause a rise in core temperature and cutaneous flushing. It has been suggested that these drugs should be avoided in febrile patients, although the rise in core temperature is usually less than 1°C only at 1 hour [2]. The drying effect increases the viscosity of airway secretions, which can lead to mucus retention and plugging; this should be avoided in suppurative respiratory conditions such as cystic fibrosis. The tachycardia induced by antimuscarinics may be undesirable in some cardiac conditions such as valvular and supravalvular aortic stenosis.

ANTIEMETICS

Postoperative nausea and vomiting (PONV) is a leading cause of morbidity in children [7]. Up to 50 per cent of school-age children have PONV and it is a major cause of unanticipated overnight admission following day-case surgery [8]. Its prevention is thus important not only for patient comfort but also for economic and social reasons. Many factors influence PONV and only some are under the control of the anaesthetist. Only perioperative antiemetic therapy will be considered here.

Vomiting is a complex response controlled by the emetic centre which has an input from several areas within the central nervous system. These input areas are rich in dopamine (D_2), muscarine, serotonin ($5HT_3$), histamine and opioid receptors. Such a wide variety of receptors explains the range of drug groups that influence PONV. It also explains the limited efficacy of a drug with a single mechanism of action. Except for serotonin receptor antagonists, other antiemetic drugs in clinical use affect more than one receptor group.

Measuring PONV has methodological problems in nonverbal children because scaling tools may not be sensitive or reliable enough; for example, nausea without vomiting can be extremely unpleasant and difficult to detect. The measured primary outcome variable in many paediatric studies is the presence of postoperative vomiting (POV) within the first 24 hours [9].

When comparing the efficacy of drugs, some investigators have used the term 'number needed to treat' (NNT) which is the number of patients who need to receive treatment in order to benefit one patient [10]. It is equivalent to the inverse of the absolute risk reduction (absolute risk reduction = risk in control group − risk in treated group) and is independent of baseline risk (baseline risk = risk in control group). Nevertheless, the NNT does not indicate the baseline risk; it indicates only the absolute reduction. Confusion can arise with the term relative risk (relative risk = risk in treated group/risk in control group) which is highly dependent upon baseline risk. Another important statistic is the 'odds ratio' (OR) which can also be confusing, but is mathematically useful in logistic regression and is commonly used in meta-analysis [9]. 'Odds' is a ratio of probabilities and OR is a ratio of probability ratios. For example, if in a sample population 80 children out of 100 vomit, the odds equals the ratio of probabilities of vomiters versus non-vomiters (e.g. odds = 80/100 divided by 20/100, i.e. 80/20, or 4 and this means that children in the sample are four times more likely to vomit than not). The OR tends to produce counterintuitive results: for example, if a drug changes the vomiting incidence to 20 in 100 similar children (odds = 20/80 or 0.25) the OR is 0.25/4 (or approximately 0.06). Note that there is an apparent exaggeration of drug effect because, whereas the incidence of vomiting has been reduced by only a factor of four, the OR is 0.06 which means that the drug has reduced the odds of vomiting by a factor of 17.

Readers should note that in the following discussions, unless otherwise stated, both the NNT and the OR refer to the efficacy of prophylaxis or prevention and not to the treatment of children who are vomiting.

Antimuscarinics

The vestibular apparatus and the solitary nucleus are rich in muscarinic receptors. Antagonism of these is effective in preventing the emetic effects of vestibular stimulation. Atropine crosses the blood–brain barrier and is therefore more effective than glycopyrrolate [11]. Scopolamine (hyoscine), administered by transdermal patch, reduces the incidence of PONV in children receiving morphine analgesia [12]. The side-effects of scopolamine, which can be significant, include dry mouth, sedation, confusion and visual disturbance [12].

Antihistamines

These are weak but inexpensive antiemetic agents. They are not associated with extrapyramidal side-effects but do cause sedation and hence may be inappropriate for children having day-case surgery. Cyclizine, a piperazine derivative, has been widely used to treat motion sickness and is probably the most commonly used perioperative antiemetic in the UK. Some studies show it to be effective [13] while in

others it fares no better than placebo [14,15]. Pain on injection and local irritation make it an unpleasant drug to administer to children postoperatively [15]. It also causes a tachycardia, probably owing to vagal inhibition. Other oral antihistamines such as cinnarizine, meclazone and promethazine are available for the treatment of motion sickness and may be relevant in children travelling to and from hospital. Alimemazine (formerly known as trimeprazine) was a standard sedative premedicant with antiemetic properties.

Phenothiazines

Phenothiazines act by blocking central dopamine and histamine receptors and all cause a degree of sedation. Prochlorperazine and perphenazine have been used for PONV in the past but are little used now. Chlorpromazine is reserved for nausea and vomiting of terminal illness. Promethazine and chlorpromazine are combined with pethidine to form 'Pethidine compound injection' which is a potent IM sedative.

Droperidol

Droperidol, a butyrophenone and an antagonist of central dopaminergic receptors have been shown to be effective in the prophylaxis of PONV; the estimated NNT is 4–5 [16]. It is no longer available following a Food and Drug Administration (FDA) 'black box warning' of cardiac rhythm changes secondary to prolonged QT syndrome.

Metoclopramide

Metoclopramide, a benzamide, has antiemetic and pro kinetic gastric effects, and both may contribute to a reduction in PONV. Antiemetic effects are mediated through antagonism of central dopaminergic (D_2) receptors. In a review of five prospective randomised controlled studies in children, 0.25 mg/kg was shown to be beneficial; the NNT was 6 [16,17]. No patients suffered movement disorders. Metoclopramide has been shown to be inferior to ondansetron in PONV prophylaxis [16].

Serotonin receptor antagonists

These drugs have been successfully used in children for the treatment of nausea and vomiting induced by chemotherapy. Serious side-effects are extremely rare, the most common being headache and constipation. Although haemodynamic disturbance, including bradycardia and hypotension, has been reported in adults following rapid injection this has not been published in children [16,18]; there are, however, UK 'Yellow card' (adverse drug reactions) reports of bradycardia in children. In a meta-analysis of ondansetron by Tramer and colleagues, who reviewed 53 trials, the best single dose for PONV was 100 µg/kg [19]. Sadhasivam and colleagues have since performed a dose–response study of ondansetron for strabismus surgery and noted the optimal dose to be 75 µg/kg [20]. This dose significantly reduced the incidence and severity of emesis and improved patient satisfaction compared with placebo. The NNT for successful prophylaxis was 2.

Ondansetron is more effective as an antiemetic than as an antinausea agent [21,22]. In controlled, randomised, double-blinded studies it has been shown to reduce the incidence of POV in children undergoing a wide variety of surgery, including tonsillectomy [23,24], strabismus surgery, inguinal hernia repair or orchidipexy [25], otoplasty [26], genitourinary [15] and orthopaedic procedures [27]. It is consistently better than placebo, metoclopramide, droperidol and cyclizine [15,16].

Newer 5HT$_3$ antagonists include granisetron, dolasetron and tropisetron. All these have longer plasma half-lives than ondansetron but appear to have similar duration of action. Data in children are limited and it is unclear if they have any clinical advantage.

The timing of antiemetic administration may influence any prophylactic effect. It has been suggested that early blockade of the chemoreceptor trigger zone, before surgery, may better prevent PONV rather than at the end of surgery [28]. However, there is counter-evidence to show that antiemetics can be effective when given at the conclusion of surgery [29]. Indeed, a recent study found that ondansetron was more effective when administered at the end of a procedure rather than at the beginning [30].

Dexamethasone

The mechanism of action of dexamethasone as an antiemetic is not clearly understood but a combination of prostaglandin antagonism [31], release of endorphins [32] and tryptophan depletion [33] has been suggested. Despite this lack of understanding, the antiemetic effects of dexamethasone have been extensively demonstrated and are widely accepted.

Dexamethasone is inexpensive, has a prolonged biological half-life [34] and lacks side-effects when used as a single injection. In a systematic review by Henzi and colleagues, dexamethasone was found to be effective against early and late PONV in children, with an NNT of 3.8 and no clinically relevant toxicity [35]. The combination of dexamethasone and ondansetron further decreases the risk of PONV [35] and this combination is likely to be the most effective prophylactic currently available antiemetic intervention.

Recently, dexamethasone has been used to aid recovery following tonsillectomy. This deserves emphasis because tonsillectomy is one of the commonest paediatric surgical procedures and, despite changes in anaesthetic technique, it is associated with POV, poor oral intake and pain. In 2003, using meta-analysis of randomised studies, the Cochrane Collaboration Group established that a single intraoperative dose of dexamethasone (dose range 0.15–1 mg/kg) significantly reduced morbidity associated with tonsillectomy [17,36,37]. The observed effects included reduction in PONV and an earlier return to eating. Any reduction in pain could not be shown because of unreported data and inconsistent outcome measures. There were no reports of adverse reactions. The optimum dose is unknown and awaits dose-finding studies. In 2006, another review of the literature has estimated efficacy of all methods of antiemetic prophylaxis in children after tonsillectomy and it concluded that the OR with and without dexamethasone was 0.23 [9].

Given the frequency with which tonsillectomy is performed, and the low cost and relative safety, the evidence supports the routine use of a single dose of dexamethasone for paediatric tonsillectomy. Dexamethasone also has a prophylactic effect on PONV in children after strabismus surgery [38–40].

Clonidine

In addition to its other properties clonidine can be used specifically for its antiemetic effect. In a study of children having strabismus surgery, oral clonidine premedication (4 µg/kg) reduced PONV from 34 per cent (placebo) to 11 per cent [41]. Oral clonidine has nearly 100 per cent bioavailability [42].

Antiemetics and the management of PONV

AVOIDABLE ASSOCIATED FACTORS

The association of opioids with PONV is well known and important. In many circumstances their use can be avoided or minimised by using a multimodal approach with para cetamol, non-steroidal anti-inflammatory drugs (NSAIDs) and local anaesthesia. The risk of PONV may also be reduced by avoiding any inhalational agent (especially nitrous oxide) and by using propofol total intravenous anaesthesia (TIVA). Although such an approach may not be practical and may be no better than using antiemetics, it should, nevertheless, be considered in individuals if PONV has been difficult to manage previously. Dehydration provokes PONV and IV hydration should also be considered.

NON-PHARMACOLOGICAL TECHNIQUES

The P6 acupoint is located between the flexor tendons on the wrist and its stimulation, either by needles or by transcutaneous electrical stimulation, can relieve nausea in some individuals. The mechanism of action is unknown. A meta-analysis of 19 studies has shown that P6 stimulation is better than placebo in preventing early PONV only in adults [43]. No benefit has been seen in children [9,43].

PROPHYLAXIS

There is no clear consensus on the relative benefit of management strategies for the prevention of PONV. Routine administration of antiemetic drugs to all children does not seem justifiable as most do not suffer from PONV [44]. Older drugs can produce significant side-effects, and the serotonin antagonists are prohibitively expensive for widespread use in many institutions. While some believe that the benefit of routine prophylaxis has not been proven even in high-risk cases [45], most clinicians broadly agree that prophylaxis is better than waiting for symptoms to become established.

An evidence-based analysis by Olutoye and Watcha suggested that prophylaxis in the high-risk population is justified because it reduces costs and improves patient satisfaction – but not for children at low risk [8]. Children at highest risk are those of school age, with a past history of PONV and those having specific procedures (e.g. squint surgery or tonsillectomy) [7]. Watcha and Smith found that prophylactic ondansetron was cost-effective when the frequency of PONV exceeded 33 per cent; prophylactic droperidol, which is no longer available, was cost-effective even if the frequency was only 10 per cent [46]. Despite their proven effectiveness many institutions do not use antiserotonin drugs for prophylaxis and reserve them for treatment only [47].

Given, in general, the limited efficacy of antiemetics and the large number of drugs with different modes of action, it seems reasonable to assume that a combination of antiemetics may be more effective than any single drug. If combining the drugs reduces their doses, side-effects can be minimised. Antiemetic drug combinations have been shown to be effective in chemotherapy patients and adults after surgery. A multimodal approach, based on avoiding all factors known to increase PONV and coupled with a combination of antiemetics, has been extremely effective in reducing early PONV from 76 per cent (of women having laparoscopy) to 2 percent [48]. This rigorous approach needs to be studied in high-risk children.

In children the combination of dexamethasone and a serotonin antagonist [38,49,50], and metoclopramide and ondansetron [51], have a superior antiemetic effect to a serotonin antagonist alone. Also, in the past, the combination of oral droperidol and metoclopramide was superior to either drug alone [52].

There seems little doubt that a child at high risk of, or with established PONV would benefit from (a) the avoidance of all agents that could contribute to sickness, and (b) a serotonin antagonist combined with dexamethasone as either prophylaxis or treatment. The clear advantage of prophylaxis for patients at lower risk has not been established. However, new and expensive drugs may be used increasingly if they have minimal side-effects and financial restraints are not overbearing.

There is no consensus in the literature on the role of the older less effective drugs, of which none has been found to be reliably superior to any other, and the main consideration may be the seriousness of side-effects.

CONTROL OF TACHYCARDIA AND HYPERTENSION

Analgesic and hypnotic drugs should be sufficiently effective to prevent or control the sympathetic activation caused by surgery. Remifentanil [7,53] and propofol, for example, are highly effective and suitably short-acting to manage almost any situation. Nevertheless, excessive doses of these drugs may not be necessary or appropriate and therefore drugs with specific cardiovascular depression effects can be useful. Controlled hypotension is required only rarely and will not be discussed in detail here; for reference, Tobias has reviewed modern techniques [54].

Clonidine

This drug, an α_2 partial agonist, can be administered by mouth or intravenously and causes sedation, analgesia and vasodilatation [42,55–58]. Intravenous clonidine (up to 1.25 µg/kg) has been used safely to cause a moderate decrease in blood pressure [55] but probably should be titrated carefully to avoid hypotension. High doses have caused bradycardia and hypertension in adults but these are rare side-effects in children. Dexmedetomidine is a more specific α_2 agonist and, like clonidine, is a useful cardiovascular calming and sedative adjunct. In addition, either of these drugs may calm and sedate children who appear to have delirium in recovery [59].

β Blockers

Propranolol is an effective drug that is occasionally useful to modify unexplained tachycardia and has been a standard treatment for cyanotic spells in infants with tetralogy of Fallot. It may cause hypoglycaemia especially after prolonged fasting [60]. Esmolol, a very short-acting and potent blocker, needs to be infused carefully and has been used in the postoperative control of hypertension after cardiac surgery in infants [61] and in the management of thyrotoxic crisis [62].

REFERENCES

Key references

Bolton CM, Myles PS, Nolan T, Sterne JA. Prophylaxis of postoperative vomiting in children undergoing tonsillectomy: a systematic review and meta-analysis. *Br J Anaesth* 2006; **97**(5): 593–604.

Domino KB, Anderson EA, Polissar NL, Posner KL. Comparative efficacy and safety of ondansetron, droperidol, and metoclopramide for preventing postoperative nausea and vomiting: a meta-analysis. *Anesth Analg* 1999; **88**(6): 1370–9.

Isik B, Arslan M, Tunga AD, Kurtipek O. Dexmedetomidine decreases emergence agitation in pediatric patients after sevoflurane anesthesia without surgery. [Erratum appears in *Paediatr Anaesth* 2006; **16**(7): 811]. *Paediatr Anaesth* 2006; **16**(7): 748–53.

McAuliffe G, Bissonnette B, Cavallé-Garrido, Boutin C. Heart rate and cardiac output after atropine in anaesthetised infants and children. *Can J Anaesth* 1997; **44**: 154–9.

Tramer MR, Moore RA, Reynolds DJ, McQuay HJ. A quantitative systematic review of ondansetron in treatment of established postoperative nausea and vomiting. *BMJ* 1997; **314**(7087): 1088–92.

References

1. Gervais HW, El Gindi M, Radermacher PR *et al.* Plasma concentration following oral and intramuscular atropine in children and their clinical effects. *Paediatr Anaesth* 1997; **7**: 13–8.

2. Saarnivaara L, Kautto UM, IISalo E, Pihlajamaki K. Comparison of pharmacokinetic and pharmacodynamic parameters following oral or intramuscular atropine in children. Atropine overdose in two small children. *Acta Anaesthesiol Scand* 1985; **29**(5): 529–36.

3. Warran P, Radford P, Manford ML. Glycopyrrolate in children. *Br J Anaesth* 1981; **53**(12): 1273–6.

4. Whittet HB, Hayward AW, Battersby E. Plasma lignocaine levels during paediatric endoscopy of the upper respiratory tract. Relationship with mucosal moistness. *Anaesthesia* 1988; **43**(6): 439–42.

5. McAuliffe G, Bissonnette B, Cavallé-Garrido, Boutin C. Heart rate and cardiac output after atropine in anaesthetised infants and children. *Can J Anaesth* 1997; **44**: 154–9.

6. McAuliffe GL, Bissonnette B, Boutin C. Should the routine use of atropine before succinylcholine in children be reconsidered? *Can J Anaesth* 1995; **42**(8): 724–9.

7. Rose JB, Watcha MF. Postoperative nausea and vomiting in paediatric patients. *Br J Anaesth* 1999; **83**(1): 104–17.

8. Olutoye O, Watcha MF. Management of postoperative vomiting in pediatric patients. *Int Anesthesiol Clin* 2003; **41**(4): 99–117.

9. Bolton CM, Myles PS, Nolan T, Sterne JA. Prophylaxis of postoperative vomiting in children undergoing tonsillectomy: a systematic review and meta-analysis. *Br J Anaesth* 2006; **97**(5): 593–604.

10. Cook RJ, Sackett DL. The number needed to treat: a clinically useful measure of treatment effect. *BMJ* 1995; **310**(6977): 452–4.

11. Salmenpera M, Kuoppamaki R, Salmenpera A. Do anticholinergic agents affect the occurrence of postanaesthetic nausea? *Acta Anaesthesiol Scand* 1992; **36**(5): 445–8.

12. Doyle E, Byers G, McNicol LR, Morton NS. Prevention of postoperative nausea and vomiting with transdermal hyoscine in children using patient-controlled analgesia. *Br J Anaesth* 1994; **72**: 72–6.

13. Cholwill JM, Wright W, Hobbs GJ, Curran J. Comparison of ondansetron and cyclizine for prevention of nausea and vomiting after day-case gynaecological laparoscopy. *Br J Anaesth* 1999 Oct; **83**(4): 611–4.

14. Watts SA. A randomized double-blinded comparison of metoclopramide, ondansetron and cyclizine in day-case laparoscopy. *Anaesth Intensive Care* 1996; **24**(5): 546–51.

15. O'Brien CM, Titley G, Whitehurst P. A comparison of cyclizine, ondansetron and placebo as prophylaxis against postoperative nausea and vomiting in children. *Anaesthesia* 2003; **58**(7): 707–11.

16. Domino KB, Anderson EA, Polissar NL, Posner KL. Comparative efficacy and safety of ondansetron, droperidol, and metoclopramide for preventing postoperative nausea and vomiting: a meta-analysis. *Anesth Analg* 1999; **88**(6): 1370–9.

17. Henzi I, Walder B, Tramer MR. Metoclopramide in the prevention of postoperative nausea and vomiting: a quantitative systematic review of randomized, placebo-controlled studies. *Br J Anaesth* 1999; **83**(5): 761–71.

18. Rose JB, McCloskey JJ. Rapid intravenous administration of ondansetron or metoclopramide is not associated with cardiovascular compromise in children. *Paediatr Anaesth* 1995; **5**: 121–4.

19. Tramer MR, Reynolds DJ, Moore RA, McQuay HJ. Efficacy, dose–response, and safety of ondansetron in prevention of postoperative nausea and vomiting: a quantitative systematic review of randomized placebo-controlled trials. *Anesthesiology* 1997; **87**(6): 1277–89.

20. Sadhasivam S, Shende D, Madan R. Prophylactic ondansetron in prevention of postoperative nausea and vomiting following pediatric strabismus surgery: a dose–response study. *Anesthesiology* 2000; **92**(4): 1035–42.

21. Tramer MR, Moore RA, Reynolds DJ, McQuay HJ. A quantitative systematic review of ondansetron in treatment of established postoperative nausea and vomiting. *BMJ* 1997; **314**(7087): 1088–92.

22. Tramer MR. A rational approach to the control of postoperative nausea and vomiting: evidence from systematic reviews. Part II. Recommendations for prevention and treatment, and research agenda. *Acta Anaesthesiol Scand* 2001; **45**(1): 14–19.

23. Litman RS, Wu CL, Catanzaro FA. Ondansetron decreases emesis after tonsillectomy in children. *Anesth Analg* 1994; **78**: 478–81.

24. Morton NS, Camu F, Dorman T *et al.* Ondansetron reduces nausea and vomiting after paediatric adenotonsillectomy. *Paediatr Anaesth* 1997; **7**: 37–45.

25. Calamandrei M, Andreuccetti T, Crescioli M *et al.* Effects of ondansetron and metoclopramide on postoperative nausea and vomiting after epidural anesthesia in children. *Cah Anesthesiol* 1994; **42**(1): 19–23.

26. Paxton D, Taylor RH, Gallagher TM, Crean PM. Postoperative emesis following otoplasty in children. *Anaesthesia* 1995; **50**: 1083–5.

27. Goodarzi M. A double blind comparison of droperidol and ondansetron for prevention of emesis in children undergoing orthopaedic surgery. *Paediatr Anaesth* 1998; **8**(4): 325–9.

28. Watcha MF, White PF. Postoperative nausea and vomiting. Its etiology, treatment, and prevention. *Anesthesiology* 1992; **77**(1): 162–84.

29. Alon E, Himmelseher S. Ondansetron in the treatment of postoperative vomiting: a randomized, double-blind comparison with droperidol and metoclopramide. *Anesth Analg* 1992; **75**(4): 561–5.

30. Tang J, Wang B, White PF *et al.* The effect of timing of ondansetron administration on its efficacy, cost-effectiveness, and cost-benefit as a prophylactic antiemetic in the ambulatory setting. *Anesth Analg* 1998; **86**(2): 274–82.

31. Kris MG, Gralla RJ, Tyson LB *et al.* Controlling delayed vomiting: double-blind, randomized trial comparing placebo, dexamethasone alone, and metoclopramide plus dexamethasone in patients receiving cisplatin. *J Clin Oncol* 1989; **7**(1): 108–14.

32. Rich WM, Abdulhayoglu G, DiSaia PJ. Methylprednisolone as an antiemetic during cancer chemotherapy – a pilot study. *Gynecol Oncol* 1980; **9**(2): 193–8.

33. Young SN. Mechanism of decline in rat brain 5-hydroxytryptamine after induction of liver tryptophan pyrrolase by hydrocortisone: roles of tryptophan catabolism and kynurenine synthesis. *Br J Pharmacol* 1981; **74**(3): 695–700.

34. Haynes R. Adenocorticotrophic hormone: adrenocortical steroids and their synthetic analogs – inhibitors of the synthesis and actions of adenocortical hormones. In: Gilman A, Gilman LS, Rall TW, Murad F, eds. *The pharmacological basis of therapeutics.* 8th edn. New York: Pergamon Press, 1990: 1447–8.

35. Henzi I, Walder B, Tramer MR. Dexamethasone for the prevention of postoperative nausea and vomiting: a quantitative systematic review. *Anesth Analg* 2000; **90**(1): 186–94.

36. Rose JB, Martin TM, Corddry D *et al.* Ondansetron reduces the incidence and severity of poststrabismus repair vomiting in children. *Anesth Analg* 1994; **79**: 486–9.

37. Steward DL, Welge JA, Myer CM. Steroids for improving recovery following tonsillectomy in children. *Cochrane Database Syst Rev* 2003; (1): CD003997.

38. Splinter WM, Rhine EJ. Low-dose ondansetron with dexamethasone more effectively decreases vomiting after strabismus surgery in children than does high-dose ondansetron. *Anesthesiology* 1998; **88**: 72–5.

39. Pappas AL, Sukhani R, Hotaling AJ *et al.* The effect of preoperative dexamethasone on the immediate and delayed postoperative morbidity in children undergoing adenotonsillectomy. *Anesth Analg* 1998; **87**(1): 57–61.

40. Aouad MT, Siddik SS, Rizk LB *et al.* The effect of dexamethasone on postoperative vomiting after tonsillectomy. *Anesth Analg* 2001; **92**(3): 636–40.

41. Mikawa K, Nishina K, Maekawa N *et al.* Oral clonidine premedication reduces vomiting in children after strabismus surgery. *Can J Anaesth* 1995; **42**(11): 977–81.

42. Nishina K, Mikawa K, Shiga M, Obara H. Clonidine in paediatric anaesthesia. *Paediatr Anaesth* 1999; **9**(3): 187–202.

43. Lee A, Done ML. The use of nonpharmacologic techniques to prevent postoperative nausea and vomiting: a meta-analysis. *Anesth Analg* 1999; **88**(6): 1362–9.

44. White PF, Watcha MF. Postoperative nausea and vomiting: prophylaxis versus treatment. *Anesth Analg* 1999; **89**(6): 1337–9.

45. Tramèr M, Moore A, McQuay H. Prevention of vomiting after paediatric strabismus surgery: a systematic review using the numbers-needed-to-treat method. *Br J Anaesth* 1996; **75**: 556–61.

46. Watcha MF, Smith I. Cost-effectiveness analysis of antiemetic therapy for ambulatory surgery. *J Clin Anesth* 1994; **6**(5): 370–7.

47. Paech MJ, Pavy TJ, Kristensen JH, Wojnar-Horton RE. Postoperative nausea and vomiting: development of a management protocol. *Anaesth Intensive Care* 1998; **26**(2): 152–5.

48. Scuderi PE, James RL, Harris L, Mims GR III. Multimodal antiemetic management prevents early postoperative vomiting after outpatient laparoscopy. *Anesth Analg* 2000; **91**(6): 1408–14.

49. Lopez-Olaondo L, Carrascosa F, Pueyo FJ *et al.* Combination of ondansetron and dexamethasone in the prophylaxis of postoperative nausea and vomiting. *Br J Anaesth* 1996; **76**(6): 835–40.

50. Fujii Y, Saitoh Y, Tanaka H, Toyooka H. Prophylactic therapy with combined granisetron and dexamethasone for the prevention of post-operative vomiting in children. *Eur J Anaesthesiol* 1999; **16**(6): 376–9.

51. Kathirvel S, Shende D, Madan R. Comparison of anti-emetic effects of ondansetron, metoclopromide or a combination of both in children undergoing surgery for strabismus. *Eur J Anaesthesiol* 1999; **16**(11): 761–5.

52. Kymer PJ, Brown RE Jr, Lawhorn CD *et al.* The effects of oral droperidol versus oral metoclopramide versus both oral droperidol and metoclopramide on postoperative vomiting when used as a premedicant for strabismus surgery. *J Clin Anesth* 1995; **7**(1): 35–9.

53. Degoute CS, Ray MJ, Gueugniaud PY, Dubreuil C. Remifentanil induces consistent and sustained controlled hypotension in children during middle ear surgery. *Can J Anaesth* 2003; **50**(3): 270–6.

54. Tobias JD. Controlled hypotension in children: a critical review of available agents. *Paediatr Drugs* 2002; **4**(7): 439–53.

55. Lonnqvist PA, Bergendahl H. Pharmacokinetics and haemodynamic response after an intravenous bolus injection of clonidine in children. *Paediatr Anaesth* 1993; **3**: 359–64.

56. Ambrose C, Sale S, Howells R *et al.* Intravenous clonidine infusion in critically ill children: dose-dependent sedative

effects and cardiovascular stability. *Br J Anaesth* 2000; **84**(6): 794–6.

57. Inomata S, Kihara S, Miyabe M *et al.* The hypnotic and analgesic effects of oral clonidine during sevoflurane anesthesia in children: a dose–response study. *Anesth Analg* 2002; **94**(6): 1479–83.

58. Arenas-Lopez S, Riphagen S, Tibby SM *et al.* Use of oral clonidine for sedation in ventilated paediatric intensive care patients. *Int Care Med* 2004; **30**(8): 1625–9.

59. Isik B, Arslan M, Tunga AD, Kurtipek O. Dexmedetomidine decreases emergence agitation in pediatric patients after sevoflurane anesthesia without surgery. [Erratum appears in *Paediatr Anaesth* 2006; **16**(7): 811]. *Paediatr Anaesth* 2006; **16**(7): 748–53.

60. Bush GH, Steward DJ. Severe hypoglycaemia associated with preoperative fasting and intraoperative propranolol. A case report and discussion. *Paediatr Anaesth* 1996; **6**: 415–7.

61. Wiest DB, Garner SS, Uber WE, Sade RM. Esmolol for the management of pediatric hypertension after cardiac operations. *J Thorac Cardiovasc Surg* 1998; **115**(4): 890–7.

62. Knighton JD, Crosse MM. Anaesthetic management of childhood thyrotoxicosis and the use of esmolol. *Anaesthesia* 1997; **52**: 62–76.

PART **II**

BASIC TECHNIQUES

Preoperative assessment

LIAM BRENNAN

KEY LEARNING POINTS

- Careful preoperative evaluation is essential for safe, efficient, paediatric anaesthetic practice.
- Using preadmission nurse-led and clinician-led assessment clinics may streamline the evaluation process.
- Good preoperative paediatric assessment requires a thorough knowledge of the common diseases of childhood that affect anaesthetic care.

- Excellent clinical, diagnostic and communication skills applicable to children are the cornerstones of the assessment process.

INTRODUCTION

Thorough preoperative evaluation is a fundamental concept in anaesthetic practice: ensuring full patient evaluation, thereby delivering perioperative care safely and efficiently, with minimal distress for children and their families. This is particularly important for paediatric patients as the margins for error during anaesthesia compared with adults are much less because of the smaller physiological reserve of younger patients, especially infants. Efficiency is one of the watchwords of modern health care; poor preoperative assessment results in delayed operating schedules and short-notice cancellations with wastage of scarce resources. Assessment in advance of the day of surgery may provide the opportunity to optimise a child's condition, thereby minimising preventable cancellations, decreasing distress and inconvenience for children and parents [1].

How does the assessment process for children differ from the adult model? First, children must be assessed in conjunction with their parents or principal adult carer. The younger child cannot give a history; even for the articulate older child, a discussion with the parents is important for clarification.

Moreover, it allows both generations to ask questions about anaesthesia as part of informed consent. Second, the paediatric anaesthetist has to consider a different spectrum of medical problems. In adult practice, anaesthetists are mainly concerned with assessing the consequences of chronic illness, predominantly involving the cardiorespiratory systems. Although chronic disorders do occur, they have a much lower incidence in children. The predominant disease processes in childhood are the consequences of congenital defects or acute problems, particularly infectious diseases. There are increasing numbers of children with problems such as morbid obesity, which previously was confined to adulthood and is now providing new challenges for the paediatric anaesthetist [2].

When, where and by whom should the preoperative assessment be performed? In a perfect world, the anaesthetist responsible for the case, well in advance of the proposed procedure, would assess every child; however, time constraints and the logistics of contemporary health care make this ideal an impossible goal. For straightforward minor and intermediate day-case procedures performed on healthy children, nurse-led assessment using carefully constructed questionnaires works well [3]. A safety net for equivocal cases requires input from experienced medical staff and, of course, all children need to be seen and examined by the anaesthetist on the day of surgery. Children with complex medical problems or those having major operative procedures require detailed assessment, best performed in a preassessment clinic. If this is not possible, the child must be admitted to hospital to allow adequate time for assessment and investigation.

CLINICAL EVALUATION

The preoperative evaluation of children is based upon a careful history, including current medication, an appropriate physical examination and review of relevant clinical investigations. In addition, a history of allergic problems should be sought.

The history

In the otherwise healthy surgical paediatric patient the review of medical history is likely to be short; nevertheless, the interview is still important to ensure that no important details of the past medical history are missed and to develop a rapport with the child and parents or carers.

Access to previous medical notes and anaesthetic records is essential to ensure safe care; previous anaesthetic problems can be identified and any complex medical problems that may affect anaesthesia can be anticipated. A discussion about the child's previous anaesthetic experiences is important. The anaesthetist should enquire about the method of anaesthetic induction used, its acceptability to the child, any behavioural problems in the perioperative period and any postoperative complications such as nausea and vomiting that are influenced by anaesthesia. A history of familial anaesthetic-related conditions should be sought, including malignant hyperthermia, pseudocholinesterase deficiency, metabolic disorders with anaesthetic significance such as hepatic porphyrias and any suggestion of an inherited muscular dystrophic disorder. A full drug and allergy history should also be obtained. Requirements for preoperative fasting should be explained (see Chapter 18) at preoperative assessment and adherence to the policy must be confirmed on the day of admission.

For infants an antenatal and neonatal history (prematurity and gestational age) should be sought. The ex-preterm infant requires careful preoperative assessment by experienced personnel. A full discussion of the problems of prematurity associated with anaesthesia is found in Chapter 8.

Social, cultural and religious issues may also need to be discussed. For example, for day-case patients the distance the family live from the hospital may preclude ambulatory management. Parents who are Jehovah's witnesses may have issues with their child receiving blood products in the perioperative period. If transfusion is likely to be needed,

this highly sensitive issue should be discussed well in advance of elective surgery with the surgeon, parents, child (if appropriate) and a representative of the local Hospital Liaison Committee for Jehovah's Witnesses. The well-being of the child is paramount; if the parents refuse to give permission it may be necessary to apply to the High Court to obtain a 'Specific Issue Order' under Section 8 of The Children's Act 1989 to allow the use of a blood transfusion. In emergencies, where the child is likely to succumb without immediate blood transfusion, there may not be enough time to seek legal guidance. In these circumstances, the clinician, having obtained a second opinion from a colleague and documented the details in the medical notes, should proceed with the transfusion, following the general guidelines outlined in Chapter 24. The courts are highly likely to uphold the decision of the doctor in such a scenario [4].

For adolescents it may be necessary, tactfully, to obtain a history of smoking, alcohol usage and even recreational drug abuse. The possibility of pregnancy in teenage girls may need to be considered. Difficult issues such as these should be discussed with sensitivity, respecting the confidential nature of the information imparted by the young person and divulging it to others only with their consent [5].

Given the child's medical condition and the complexity of the proposed surgery, if admission to intensive care is likely, this should be discussed with the parents and child. The scarcity of paediatric critical care resources outside of specialist centres usually precludes the child with complex medical and surgical needs being managed in district hospitals, even if the surgical and anaesthetic teams are competent to deliver the intraoperative care.

DRUG HISTORY

The anaesthetist should enquire about current and past medications. Some drugs may have significant implications for perioperative care, for example, non-steroidal anti-inflammatory drugs (NSAIDs) or aspirin affects platelet function; others may demand modification of the anaesthetic technique – for example, avoiding high-inspired oxygen, which may lead to pulmonary fibrosis in patients receiving bleomycin.

There is an increasing tendency for children to be given herbal or homeopathic preparations. In a recent survey in the USA, 7.5 per cent of children presenting for surgery in a Californian city were receiving alternative medicines [6]. Use of alternative remedies should be discussed in the preoperative assessment as they are potential causes of unexpected adverse events occurring in the perioperative period. For example, *Echinacea,* commonly used in the prevention and treatment of upper respiratory tract infections, may cause severe allergic reactions and it it should be used with caution in the asthmatic patient [7]. In addition, garlic, ginkgo and ginseng may be associated with excessive bleeding, ephedra with cardiovascular instability and ginseng may also cause hypoglycaemia [8].

IMMUNISATION

Controversy surrounds the management of the recently immunised child presenting for general anaesthesia. Systemic effects from recent immunisation (Hib [*Haemophilus influenza* type b], MMR [measles–mumps–rubella] and quadruple vaccine) such as fever, coryza and malaise may mimic the symptoms of upper respiratory infection, which, depending on their severity, may constitute a relative contraindication to anaesthesia [9]. Side-effects of immunisation such as fever, vomiting and pain may be confused with postoperative complications, as may rarer but more severe reactions, for example, convulsions and encephalopathy, both of which may be delayed by up to 2 weeks with some vaccines. Although there is no evidence that recent immunisation is a direct contraindication to anaesthesia, some authors have recommended that elective procedures should be postponed for variable periods from 2 days to 2 weeks, depending on the vaccine used. Government agencies do not appear to have uniform advice on this subject: the New Zealand Health Ministry concur with the postponement advice but the Australian authorities do not agree and the USA and the UK have no official policy on this issue [10].

ALLERGIES

A careful history of known allergies to drugs and other substances that may be encountered during hospital admission should be sought. An increasing incidence of perioperative anaphylactic reactions to natural latex has been reported [11,12] since the first reported case in 1989 [13]. Allergy to latex may be the most common cause of intraoperative anaphylaxis in children, whereas in adults muscle relaxants are the commonest precipitant. In a large French survey, latex allergy accounted for 19 per cent of perioperative allergic reactions [14]. The anaesthetist should be wary in high-risk groups and ask for specific symptoms of clinical latex allergy such as lip swelling or tingling, bronchospasm or eye swelling with rubber balloons or other latex-containing toys. One should also enquire about sensitivity to certain foodstuffs notably kiwi fruit, bananas, avocado and chestnuts as they have cross-reactivity with latex proteins. The care of those with latex allergy is addressed in Chapter 29; if these recommendations are followed there is no reason why day care cannot be offered to these patients, although a longer period of postoperative observation is advised.

Physical examination

All children should be examined before anaesthesia, with the main emphasis being on the airway (including the dentition), cardiovascular, respiratory and, where indicated, the neurological systems. In addition, the anaesthetist may wish to assess potential locations for venous access and inspect sites for performing regional anaesthetic nerve blocks. In addition to yielding diagnostic information – albeit rarely in healthy children – the physical examination also serves two other important purposes: first, it is often reassuring to anxious parents that the anaesthetist has made a thorough assessment of their child's condition before surgery and, second, the act of examination helps to familiarise the younger child especially with handling by the anaesthetist prior to arrival in the operating suite.

It is important to respect the modesty particularly of older children during physical examination and ensure appropriate privacy during dressing and undressing. Younger children often get distressed when required to disrobe and they should be undressed only to the extent required to allow an adequate examination. This is particularly important for infants who lose body heat rapidly when uncovered.

Investigations

Routine preoperative investigations such as urinalysis, haemoglobin estimation and serum electrolytes are unnecessary for the healthy child presenting for minor or intermediate surgery. They have no justification on clinical, economic or humanitarian grounds [15]. The current practice is to target investigations at specific patient groups who have pre-existing medical problems that may influence anaesthetic management.

Although mild degrees of anaemia are more prevalent in the infant age group there is little evidence that this increases perioperative morbidity or alters management particularly for day-case procedures [16,17]. An exception to this view is the neonate or ex-premature infant in whom a haematocrit of less than 30 per cent may be associated with a higher incidence of postoperative apnoea [18]. Preoperative haemoglobin measurement for these patients is therefore regarded as essential by some clinicians.

There is still some debate outside the UK about the advisability of performing routine coagulation profiles before certain procedures in children such as adenotonsillectomy and neuroaxial blockade. The evidence supporting this practice is tenuous with numerous studies confirming that in the absence of a positive history of bleeding problems screening tests are unnecessary [19,20]. However, in situations where even minimal postoperative bleeding could be critical (e.g. some neurosurgical procedures) or when it may be difficult to obtain a history of bleeding tendency because of language difficulties, or in young infants, coagulation screening may be justified.

Children from racially susceptible groupings are usually tested for sickle cell disease and other common haemoglobinopathies. Sickle cell disease is most prevalent in West and Central Africa but also occurs in north-east Saudi Arabia and east central India. It has also been described in southern Mediterranean populations. The incidence of sickle cell disease among African–Americans is under 1 per cent. If the sodium metabisulphite screening test (Sickledex) is positive a haemoglobin electrophoresis should be performed to determine the precise genotype and so allow accurate assessment of perioperative risk. It is important to note that the Sickledex test is not accurate in neonates because of the high percentage of foetal haemoglobin in this age group [21]. Haemoglobin electrophoresis is not a rapid investigation and to prevent unnecessary cancellation of elective procedures it should be done well in advance of admission. A positive screening test in the context of emergency surgery requires careful consideration in close collaboration with a senior haematologist to ensure safe perioperative management (see Chapter 7).

Accurate preoperative weighing of children is vital as many anaesthetic interventions and all drug dosages are calculated on a weight basis. Drug dose errors occur more frequently in children and many of these problems arise because of inaccurate estimates of body weight. Visual estimation of body weight is notoriously inaccurate, particularly in the infant population [22]. Formula-based estimates using the age of the patient are becoming dangerously irrelevant as the epidemic of childhood obesity grows [23]. When weighing the child is impossible or impracticable, particularly in emergencies, measuring the height/length of the child, using a Broslow tape, allows reasonably accurate weight estimation [24].

SELECTED CONDITIONS

The following is a discussion of some common problems that the anaesthetist needs to assesss at the preoperative interview. Preoperative preparation and medication are discussed in the Chapter 18.

The child with a heart murmur

One of the commonest dilemmas in paediatric anaesthesia is the finding of a previously undiagnosed cardiac murmur. Heart murmurs are common in the preschool child and there are reports of 8–80 per cent of children having auscultatory abnormalities [25]: although most of these murmurs have no clinical significance, a small minority may represent a cardiac abnormality that poses significant haemodynamic risk during anaesthesia or predisposes to bacterial endocarditis.

How does one distinguish an innocent from a pathological heart murmur? A full medical history should be obtained from the parents, seeking symptoms outlined in Table 17.1. If the child is completely asymptomatic then it is unlikely that the murmur will complicate anaesthesia although prophylactic antibiotics may still be required. For neonates and young infants the clinical features of serious congenital heart disease may be subtle. A history of recurrent chest infections, cyanosis, tachypnoea, sweating and difficulties with feeding, leading to failure to thrive, are suggestive of a significant abnormality in the baby with a heart

Table 17.1 Worrying symptoms and signs associated with a cardiac murmur

Symptoms	Signs
Failure to thrive	Tachycardia
Dyspnoea	Tachypnoea
Poor exercise tolerance	Cyanosis
Recurrent respiratory infections	Finger clubbing
Cyanotic episodes	Hepatomegaly
Syncope	Precordial thrills
Chest pain	Decreased or absent femoral pulses

Table 17.2 Some features of innocent and pathological cardiac murmurs

	Innocent	Pathological
Timing	Systolic (venous hum continuous)	Systolic or diastolic
Precordial thrill	Never	Sometimes
Quality of murmur	Blowing/musical/vibratory	Variable
Variation with posture	Often	Rarely
Cardiac symptoms and signs	Rarely	Commonly

murmur (Table 17.1). Outside of infancy, the clinical features of a serious heart lesion may be more obvious, including decreased exercise tolerance compared with peers, repeated chest infections, failure to thrive, cyanosis and finger clubbing (Table 17.1).

The auscultatory features of innocent and pathological murmurs are summarised in Table 17.2. At the outset, it is important to emphasise that it is difficult, if not impossible, on clinical grounds alone to unequivocally differentiate between an innocent murmur and a murmur caused by a significant cardiac abnormality. However, innocent murmurs tend to be soft or blowing in quality, systolic in timing and vary with posture. A venous hum is heard in both systole *and* diastole at the base of the heart with the child in the sitting position but disappears on lying flat. Pathological murmurs are often loud, pansystolic or pandiastolic in timing and are nearly always associated with symptoms and signs of cardiac disease as outlined above. The presence of a palpable thrill always indicates a significant lesion. The exception is severe aortic stenosis or hypertrophic obstructive cardiomyopathy (HOCM) which may be asymptomatic but still pose a considerable perioperative risk. Fortunately, the electrocardiogram (ECG) is abnormal in both these conditions (demonstrating left axis deviation and left ventricular hypertrophy) and hence is included in the widely quoted algorithm for assessing heart murmurs in children (Fig. 17.1).

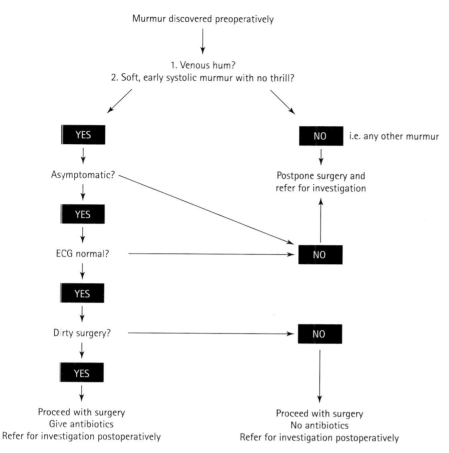

Figure 17.1 Algorithm for preoperative management of cardiac murmurs in children older than 1 year. From McEwan *et al.* [26], with permission.

One should be wary of dismissing murmurs as innocent in children with syndromes that are recognised as being associated with congenital heart disease, e.g. Down syndrome, CHARGE association, VATER association, Turner syndrome and DiGeorge syndrome (see Chapter 28). Always obtain a cardiological opinion if there is any doubt about the character of a murmur. Echocardiography is easy to perform and can rapidly clarify the situation. Newly discovered murmurs in infancy require special consideration. Any child under 1 year old with a murmur should always be referred for cardiological assessment as at this young age a potentially significant lesion may not yet have declared itself [26].

Prophylactic antibiotics must be prescribed for all children with suspected or proven cardiac defects or after previous corrective cardiac surgery. The antibiotic regimen used should follow national protocols; in the UK the regimen published in the *British National Formulary for Children* is most commonly followed (http://www.bnf.org/bnf/) [27]. If in doubt, antibiotics should be administered as the risks of bacterial endocarditis developing after high-risk surgery (e.g. dental, oral and upper respiratory tract procedures, all lower gastrointestinal tract and some upper gastrointestinal tract procedures and all genitourinary procedures) are significant without prophylaxis and the consequences of established endocarditis are associated with a high mortality.

Asthma

The prevalence of childhood asthma has risen sharply in recent decades although this upward trend may have slowed or already peaked [28]. Nearly every elective paediatric operating list seems to include a child with a history of asthma and this is supported by the observation that up to 30 per cent of young teenagers report asthmatic symptoms in the previous year [29]. The fundamental causes of asthma are unknown but genetic predisposition, atopy, prenatal and early life environment (including passive smoking) all appear to contribute to the condition [30].

Asthma is not a single clinical entity but has a broad spectrum of precipitants and a severity ranging from an infrequent mild wheeze to life-threatening respiratory failure that requires ventilation. Adverse events during anaesthesia for children with asthma are fortunately rare but it is essential for the anaesthetist to recognise those with more severe disease. This allows these higher-risk patients to be fully assessed and their condition optimised before anaesthesia and, if necessary, to arrange for their surgery to take place in an inpatient rather than in a day-case environment.

Although there is a strong association between atopy (i.e. immunoglobulin E [IgE]-mediated hypersensitivity) and asthma, it is recognised that many children who wheeze do not have atopic asthma. A large respiratory study from the USA distinguished between the classic atopic asthmatics and so-called transient wheezers and non-atopic wheezers [31]. Transient wheezers are usually children in the first few years of life who wheeze in response to viral infections. These infection-induced episodes usually resolve before starting school. Non-atopic wheezers are children who continue to wheeze beyond early childhood, often in response to respiratory infections, but their symptoms are less likely to persist than in the atopic asthmatic. In addition, other conditions may present with wheeze such as tracheomalacia and bronchomalacia, which are unresponsive to bronchodilator medication. Is this categorisation of airway disease useful in clinical practice? There is no routine test that distinguishes these different forms of airway disease. However, the preschool child who presents with intermittent asthmatic symptoms that are only associated with respiratory infections and have been improving since infancy is likely to indicate the transient wheeze syndrome. Such children can be safely managed in a day-case environment provided that they are not in the midst of an acute exacerbation.

Assessment of the severity and control of the child's asthma are important at the preoperative visit. These two issues are closely linked, as mild asthma that is poorly controlled may appear severe in terms of frequent and persistent symptoms. Conversely, a severely asthmatic child may have excellent symptom control but require inhaled or even oral steroids to maintain this level of stability [30]. Severity is assessed by the amount of medication required to achieve symptom control; this ranges from the mildly asthmatic child requiring occasional inhaled short-acting β_2-agonist medication to the severely disabled child needing high-dose inhaled or oral steroid therapy plus a long-acting β_2 agonist and a leukotriene receptor antagonist.

Symptom control is assessed by taking a careful history and examining the respiratory system. A previous history of severe or life-threatening asthma, particularly if requiring intensive care with or without mechanical ventilation, is indicative of a very vulnerable group of children. These patients may require preoptimisation with increased steroid therapy under the supervision of a respiratory paediatrician before proceeding even with minor procedures under anaesthesia. Examination of the asthmatic child should focus on signs of respiratory distress including tachypnoea, use of accessory respiratory muscles, and the presence of wheeze or localised signs on chest auscultation.

At the preoperative visit, the child should be well and the asthma controlled on the patient's current medication. If this is not the case, elective surgery should be postponed and the child's condition optimised. Emergency surgery in the midst of an asthma exacerbation is hazardous. In the time available before surgery, the anaesthetist should work closely with paediatric colleagues to improve the child's respiratory status. Everyone, including the parents and child if appropriate, should be warned that postoperative high-dependency/intensive care might be required. Anaesthesia, particularly that requiring tracheal intubation, may exacerbate symptoms in the unstable asthmatic resulting in cough, worsening bronchospasm, increased risk of pneumothorax during intraoperative ventilation and the potential for postoperative respiratory failure.

Investigations are not of great benefit in the preoperative assessment of the younger asthmatic. The preschool child cannot cooperate consistently with lung function testing to produce meaningful results and chest radiographs are rarely useful unless there are focal signs on auscultation or a pneumothorax is suspected. However, peak flow and forced expiratory volume in 1 second (FEV_1) measurements may be useful for the older child while remembering that it is important to refer to nomograms that relate the normal ranges of these parameters to age and size of patient. Measuring inflammatory markers in blood, urine or expired air may help in the diagnosis or monitoring of asthma; although promising, at the time of writing these tests largely remain a research tool.

Consideration should be given at the preoperative visit to the advisability of using NSAIDs in the asthmatic child for perioperative pain relief, as there is concern that these drugs may worsen asthmatic symptoms. However, NSAID sensitivity appears much less common in children than in adults and several studies attest to the safe use of NSAIDs in asthmatic children [32]. A recent systematic review of the published literature on this subject in children and adults recommends avoiding all NSAIDs in asthmatic patients with a history of adverse reaction to any NSAID, particularly those with the triad of NSAID sensitivity, asthma and nasal polyps [33]. The same review also recommends that NSAIDs should be used with caution in asthmatic patients who have not previously received this class of medication and suggest that the first dose should be taken under medical supervision.

Diabetes mellitus

Diabetes mellitus is the commonest endocrine disorder of children with an incidence of 1:500 and a peak incidence of first diagnosis at 7 years [25]. Although 90 per cent of childhood diabetics are type 1 (insulin-dependent disease) there is an increasing incidence of the type 2 form (non-insulin-dependent disease) particularly in affluent societies. In the USA 30 per cent of adolescents aged 12–19 years with diabetes have type 2 disease, an increase in incidence that has paralleled the increase in childhood obesity in that country [34,35]. The incidence of type 1 disease is also increasing with a two- to threefold rise in some populations over the past decade. The reasons for the increase in this class of the disease are unclear but it is a concern that many of these new cases are occurring in the under-5-year-old-age group [36].

In addition to the well-described type 1 and type 2 patterns of disease, maturity-onset diabetes of youth (MODY) is an inherited form of type 2 diabetes. It is transmitted as an autosomal dominant and presents in late childhood or adolescence with a relatively mild, slowly progressive course that eventually become insulin requiring. Glucose intolerance may also be a feature of some chromosomal and other genetic conditions (e.g. Down and Prader–Willi syndromes). It may also feature as part of the clinical picture of intrinsic pancreatic disorders such as cystic fibrosis or occur as a complication of steroid drug therapy.

Childhood diabetes is being managed with increasingly complex insulin regimens as diabetologists strive to mimic the natural pancreatic endocrine function. This approach has gained popularity as it has been realised that maintaining tight glycaemic control helps minimise end-organ damage in later life, which is the hallmark of this disease. This means that, at the preoperative visit, the anaesthetist may be confronted with a complex prescription of up to three different insulins with short, intermediate and ultra-long durations of action administered by multiple daily injections or by continuous subcutaneous infusion.

Although diabetic management has become more complex in recent times, the overall aims of safe perioperative management have remained unchanged – namely, to avoid hypoglycaemia and excessive hyperglycaemia. The dangers of unrecognised hypoglycaemia in the unconscious patient are widely appreciated but even short periods of excessive hyperglycaemia can be detrimental. High blood glucose is associated with impaired immune function, systemic infection and poor wound healing.

The perioperative management of diabetes should be tailored to the type, extent and urgency of the surgery taking into account the current glycaemic control. Diabetic control can be assessed by questioning the child and parent about the incidence of large glucose swings, perusing personal records of blood glucose measurements and reviewing glycated haemoglobin (HbA1c) measurements. The HbA1c measurements provide information about diabetic control in the preceding 6–8 weeks. The ideal range for HbA1c varies with age: for children younger than 5 years 7–9 per cent is acceptable whereas, for the teenager, 6–8 per cent is optimal [37]. Poorly controlled diabetics, especially if experiencing frequent episodes of ketoacidosis, should be admitted to hospital early for stabilisation before surgery by the paediatric diabetic team. Teenage diabetics can be a particularly difficult group to deal with for anaesthetic management. Pubertal hormonal changes, rapid growth and problems with compliance with insulin therapy combine to make glucose control notoriously erratic in these young patients.

Minor surgery in well-controlled diabetic children may safely proceed on a day-stay basis. The usual dose of ultra-long-acting insulin is administered the day before surgery. On the morning of surgery, breakfast should be withheld and short and intermediate insulin omitted. It is important that excessive starvation be avoided by careful liaison between the hospital and the parents preoperatively. The child should be admitted to hospital and scheduled first on the morning operating list. Blood glucose should be checked on arrival and occasionally serum creatinine and electrolytes if there is concern about hydration or renal function. Fortunately, end-organ damage secondary to diabetes is rare in the paediatric age group and so apart from assessing glycaemic control other preoperative investigations are not usually required before elective surgery. In theatre, blood glucose should be monitored frequently but usually no additional insulin or parenteral glucose is required during short operative procedures. Postoperatively, blood glucose monitoring is maintained and the child should be encouraged to eat breakfast with a suitable covering dose of short-acting insulin. Provided that the child has eaten an adequate amount without vomiting and the blood glucose is in the normal to high normal range then same-day discharge can be considered. However, day-case management is unsuitable for the newly diagnosed diabetic, younger children (<5 years old) and for procedures with a high incidence of post-operative vomiting (e.g. adenotonsillectomy).

For more major surgery, when restarting oral feeding is likely to be delayed, earlier preoperative admission will be required so that an intravenous glucose and insulin regimen can be commenced before surgery. This regimen should be commenced and managed in close collaboration with the paediatric diabetic team following an agreed local protocol. Children receive between 0.01 and 0.1 units/kg/h of short-acting insulin combined with a 5 per cent glucose, 0.45 per cent saline infusion, potassium replacement and regular blood glucose measurements to maintain blood glucose at 7–10 mmol/L [38]. An example of a protocol for the perioperative management of diabetes in children is shown in Table 17.3.

Emergency surgery in diabetics is associated with large fluctuations in blood glucose. An insulin/glucose regimen should be started early for these children with careful surveillance for developing ketoacidosis. It should be remembered that abdominal symptoms could be the presenting symptoms of diabetic ketoacidosis (DKA) either in a

Table 17.3 Recommendations for the management of type 1 diabetes mellitus*

Blood glucose (mmol/l)	Insulin rate (IU/kg/h)	Advice
<4.0	0	Contact doctor, stop insulin, treat hypoglycaemia
4.1–7.0	0.01	
7.1–9.0	0.03	
9.1–12.9	0.05	
13.0–28.0	0.1	Check ketones
>28.0	0.1	Check intravenous lines and connections, call doctor

*Standard volumes (determined by weight) of maintenance fluids, glucose 5 per cent and saline 0.45 per cent 500 mL containing 10 mmol KCl, are given to accompany the insulin infusion.

known diabetic or as first presentation of the disease. The anaesthetist may need to remind their surgical colleagues that abdominal symptoms may be due to the metabolic imbalance rather than a pathology needing surgical intervention. Anaesthesia in the presence of DKA is hazardous. The child should be appropriately fluid resuscitated before surgery, with blood glucose lowered to 17 mmol/L or less and abnormal serum electrolytes vigorously corrected [38]. Clearly, the decision to proceed to operation in this situation should be made only by a senior surgeon and the anaesthetist should liaise closely with the paediatric medical team in the preoperative resuscitation phase. High-dependency or full intensive care will be required in the perioperative period for these patients.

Upper respiratory tract infection

The assessment of the child with upper respiratory tract infection (URTI) and the decision whether to proceed is one of the most controversial issues in paediatric anaesthesia. URTI occurs with a frequency of up to eight episodes per year in the normal child or even more in the under-fives attending nursery school [39]. Although many of these clinical episodes are of viral aetiology, some children may have identical symptoms resulting from non-infective seasonal rhinitis or adenoidal hypertrophy. Distinguishing between these different groups of children with a 'runny nose' can be difficult and requires careful history taking and good clinical acumen if unnecessary cancellation is to be avoided.

The traditional approach to the child with a URTI presenting for elective surgery was to defer the procedure until the child was asymptomatic. This advice was largely based on data from a large study that suggested an increase in perioperative airway complications (e.g. coughing, laryngospasm, desaturation episodes, atelectasis) in the presence of true infection particularly if the trachea was intubated [40]. A subsequent study concluded that that it was prudent to cancel surgery for up to 6 weeks to avoid these complications and this approach became standard practice for most of the next decade [41].

Should we subscribe to a blanket cancellation policy for children with URTI? Although many of the older studies reported increased adverse perioperative events in children with URTI, none had identified the risk factors that predicted these events and few considered the long-term postoperative outcomes associated with these problems [42]. Contemporary studies have addressed these important questions so that the advisability of whether to proceed with anaesthesia can be assessed for the *individual* child.

The risk–benefit issues of this problem are considered in a study of more than 15 000 children listed for day-case procedures [43]. The authors estimated that, if all children with mild URTI were postponed, then 2000 cases would have been cancelled to prevent 15 episodes of laryngospasm. In reality only 0.5 per cent of children in this cohort had their surgery deferred. A longitudinal study of more than 1000 children with URTI in the preceding 4 weeks identified the risk factors for adverse respiratory events. These included the use of a tracheal tube, history of prematurity, history of asthma, airway surgery, paternal smoking and copious airway secretions. Perhaps the most important finding from this study was that despite perioperative adverse events there were *no* significant problems for these children following discharge home [44]. The lack of residual respiratory morbidity is supported by other studies and the absence of cases in the medical malpractice literature implicating URTI in serious adverse events [45,46]. However, although morbidity following discharge is infrequent, there are sporadic reports of death in children with URTI after surgery [47] and there is an unknown incidence of myocarditis associated with the viraemic phase of some coryzal illnesses, which may rarely have fatal consequences [48].

Other important facets of this discussion are considered in a recent study that looked at adverse respiratory events in children who did not have evidence of URTI [49]. This study found a 21 per cent incidence of adverse respiratory events in children aged 1–14 and these occurred more frequently during ENT procedures involving younger children, particularly when anaesthetised by anaesthetic trainees rather than specialist paediatric anaesthetists. The study concludes that the procedure, age of the child and quality of perioperative care are important factors implicated in perioperative respiratory morbidity and it is likely that these factors will be at least as important in children with a recent URTI.

How should we approach the preoperative assessment of a child with a recent URTI? If we agree that an indiscriminate cancellation policy is inappropriate, the anaesthetist will need to assess each child with URTI carefully and weigh up the risks and benefits for the individual case. This requires a detailed history and appropriate clinical examination conducted by an experienced anaesthetist. An algorithm for the assessment and anaesthetic management of children with URTI from a recent comprehensive review article is shown in Fig. 17.2.

Essentially, the anaesthetist should question the parents about the child's respiratory symptoms. This helps the clinician distinguish between infectious and non-infectious aetiologies, assess severity of symptoms, and decide whether the child is in the midst of the illness or in the convalescent phase. In a large study from the USA, confirmation of a URTI by a parent was found to be a better predictor of perioperative laryngospasm than relying on symptom criteria alone [43]. Symptoms and signs of severe infection should alert the anaesthetist that all but the most urgent operations should be deferred (Table 17.4). When a child is essentially well with minimal respiratory symptoms and awaiting minor surgery or is overtly sick, the decision to proceed or cancel the procedure is relatively easy. The difficulty arises when, as is more often the case, the child's clinical status lies somewhere between these two extremes. In this situation, the anaesthetist may be wise to take a more conservative approach for children with a history of asthma or prematurity particularly if from the

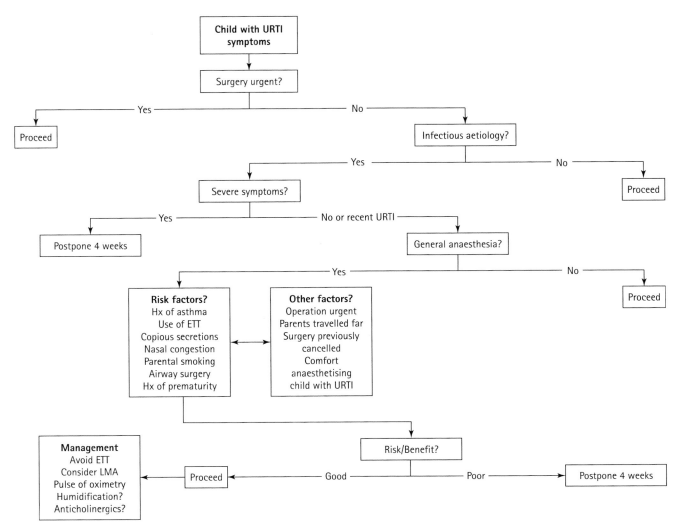

Figure 17.2   Algorithm for the assessment of the child with an upper respiratory tract infection. URTI, upper respiratory tract infection; Hx, history; ETT, tracheal tube; LMA, laryngeal mask airway. From Tait and Malviya [42], with permission.

Table 17.4   Symptoms and signs of severe upper respiratory tract infection

Unwell, lethargic child
Pyrexia >37.5°C
Purulent nasal secretions
Productive cough
Abnormal auscultatory signs

infant age group and if they require airway surgery or need tracheal intubation. All of these factors are associated with an increased incidence of perioperative complications. Social factors may also need to be considered as part of the decision-making process; the disruption to child-care arrangements, the distance the child has travelled for surgery and whether the child has been previously cancelled due to illness may all need to be taken into account. For the child who experiences multiple URTIs each year it may be difficult to target a symptom-free window for elective

surgery. The decision to proceed in the face of social pressures should be made only by the most experienced clinicians who are confident that they are not compromising patient safety in this situation.

Are investigations useful in deciding whether to proceed or cancel a procedure? Laboratory and radiological investigations can confirm the presence of a respiratory tract infection but a normal white blood cell count or normal chest radiograph does not exclude significant respiratory infection. In reality, investigations are of little practical value in busy clinical practice. The decision to proceed or not to proceed with surgery in the presence of respiratory symptoms still largely remains a matter of clinical judgement.

If it is decided to defer the operation, how long should the cancellation period be? There is still no consensus on the optimal time to wait before rescheduling surgery but most authorities agree that any child with severe symptoms should have surgery postponed for at least 4 weeks. This is on the basis that the risk of respiratory complications remains increased for this period of time after URTI [44].

Shorter periods of cancellation of 1–2 weeks quoted for milder symptomatology are less convincing as it is likely that many of these children, certainly those having minor procedures, could be safely anaesthetised without excess morbidity.

REFERENCES

Key references

Black AE. Medical assessment of the paediatric patient. *Br J Anaesth* 1999; **83**(1): 3–15.

Chadwick V, Wilkinson KA. Diabetes mellitus and the paediatric anaesthetist. *Paediatr Anaesth* 2004; **14**(9): 716–23.

Doherty GM, Chisakuta A, Crean P, Shields MD. Anesthesia and the child with asthma. *Paediatr Anaesth* 2005; **15**(6): 446–54.

McEwan AI, Birch M, Bingham R. The preoperative management of the child with a heart murmur. *Paediatr Anaesth* 1995; **5**(3): 151–6.

Tait AR, Malviya S, Voepel-Lewis T *et al.* Risk factors for perioperative adverse events in children with upper respiratory tract infections. *Anesthesiology* 2001; **95**: 299–306.

References

1. Brennan LJ. Modern day-case anaesthesia for children. *Br J Anaesth* 1999; **83**(1): 91–103.

2. Smith HL, Brennan LJ, Meldrum DJ. Childhood obesity: a challenge for the anaesthetist? *Paediatr Anaesth* 2002; **12**(9): 750–61.

3. Rushforth H, Bliss A, Burge D, Glasper EA. A pilot randomised controlled trial of medical versus nurse clerking for minor surgery. *Arch Dis Child* 2000; **83**(3): 223–6.

4. Association of Anaesthetists of GB and Ireland. *Management of anaesthesia for Jehovah's Witnesses*, 2nd edn. London: AAGBI, 2005.

5. Loughrey J. Medical information, confidentiality and a child's right to privacy. *Legal Stud* 2003; **23**: 510–35.

6. Everett LL, Birmingham PK, Williams GD *et al.* Herbal and homeopathic medication use in pediatric surgical patients. *Paediatr Anaesth* 2005; **15**(6): 455–60.

7. Huntley AL, Thompson Coon J, Ernst E. Safety of herbal medicinal products derived from *Echinacea* species: a systematic review. *Drug Saf* 2005; **28**: 387–400.

8. Ang-Lee MK, Moss J, Yuan CS. Herbal medicines and perioperative care. *JAMA* 2001; **286**(2): 208–16.

9. van der Walt JH, Roberton DM. Anaesthesia and the recently vaccinated child. *Paediatr Anaesth* 1996; **6**(2): 135–41.

10. van der Walt JH, Jacob R, Zoanetti DC. Infectious diseases of childhood and their anesthetic implications. *Paediatr Anaesth* 2004; **14**(10): 810–19.

11. Kelly KJ, Pearson MI, Kurup VP *et al.* A cluster of anaphylactic reactions in children with spina bifida during general anaesthesia: epidemiologic features, risk factors and latex hypersensitivity. *J Allerg Clin Immunol* 1994; **94**: 53–61.

12. Murat I. Latex allergy: where are we? *Paediatr Anaesth* 2000; **10**(6): 577–9.

13. Gerber AC, Jorg W, Zbinden S *et al.* Severe intraoperative anaphylaxis to surgical gloves: latex allergy, an unfamiliar condition. *Anesthesiology* 1989; **71**: 800–2.

14. Laxenaire MC. Epidemiology of anaesthetic anaphylactoid reactions. Fourth multicentre inquiry (July 1994-December 1996). *Ann Fr Anesth Reanim* 1998; **18**: 796–810.

15. Hannallah RS. Preoperative investigations. *Paediatr Anaesth* 1995; **5**(5): 325–9.

16. Meneghini L, Zandra N, Zannette G *et al.* The usefulness of routine preoperative laboratory tests for one day surgery in healthy children. *Paediatr Anaesth* 1998; **8**(1): 11–15.

17. Ansermino JM, Than M, Swallow PD. Pre-operative tests in children undergoing plastic surgery. *Ann RCS Eng* 1999; **81**(3): 175–8.

18. Cote CJ, Zaslevsky A, Downes JJ *et al.* Postoperative apnoea in former preterm infants after inguinal herniorraphy. *Anesthesiology* 1995; **82**: 809–22.

19. Roux CL, Lejus C, Surleb M *et al.* Is haemostasis biological screening always useful before performing a neuroaxial blockade in children? *Paediatr Anaesth* 2002; **12**(2): 118–23.

20. Eberl W, Wendt I, Schroeder HG. Preoperative coagulation screening prior to adenoidectomy and tonsillectomy. *Klinische Pädiatrie* 2005; **217**(1): 20–4.

21. Marchant WA, Walker I. Anaesthetic management of the child with sickle cell disease. *Paediatr Anaesth* **13**(6): 2003; 473–89.

22. Kesugi T, Okada N, Sakai K *et al.* Accuracy of visual estimation of body height and weight in supine paediatric patients. *Paediatr Anaesth* 2002; **12**(6): 489.

23. Dearlove CB, Dearlove O. Visual estimation of children's weights. *Anaesthesia* 1999; **54**(12): 128–129.

24. Black K, Barnett P, Wolfe R, Young S. Are methods to estimate weight in children accurate? *Emerg Med* 2002; **14**: 160–5.

25. Black AE. Medical assessment of the paediatric patient. *Br J Anaesth* 1999; **83**(1): 3–15.

26. McEwan AI, Birch M, Bingham R. The preoperative management of the child with a heart murmur. *Paediatr Anaesth* 1995; **5**(3): 151–6.

27. Paediatric Formulary Committee. *British national formulary for children*. London: BMJ Publishing/RCPCH, 2006.

28. Toelle BG, Ng K, Belousova E *et al.* Prevalence of asthma and allergy in schoolchildren in Belmont, Australia. *BMJ* 2004; **328**: 386–7.

29. Anderson HR, Ruggles R, Strachan DP *et al.* Trends in prevalence of symptoms of asthma, hay fever and eczema in 12–14-year-olds in the British Isles, 1995–2002: questionnaire survey. *BMJ* 2004; **328**: 1052–3.

30. Doherty GM, Chisakuta A, Crean P, Shields MD. Anesthesia and the child with asthma. *Paediatr Anaesth* 2005; **15**(6): 446–54.

31. Taussig LM, Wright AL, Holberg CJ *et al.* Tucson children's respiratory study: 1980 to present. *J Allerg Clin Immunol* 2003; **111**: 661–75.

32. Short JA, Barr CA, Palmer CD *et al.* Use of diclofenac in children with asthma. *Anaesthesia* 2000; **55**: 334–7.

33. Jenkins C, Costello J, Hodge L Systematic review of prevalence of aspirin induced asthma and its implications for clinical practice. *BMJ* 2004; **328**: 434–40.

34. Glaser NS. Non-insulin dependent diabetes in childhood and adolescence. *Pediatr Clin North Am* 1997; **44**: 307–25.

35. Fagot-Campagna A, Saaddine JB, Flegal KM, Beckles GL. Diabetes, impaired fasting glucose, and elevated HbA1c in US adolescents: the 3rd National Health and Nutrition Examination Survey. *Diabetes Care* 2001; **24**: 834–7.

36. Gardener SG, Bingley PJ, Sawtell PA *et al*. Rising incidence of insulin-dependent diabetes in children under 5 years in the Oxford region: time trend analysis. *BMJ* 1997; **315**: 713–17.

37. Rhodes ET, Ferrari LR, Wolfsdorf JI. Perioperative management of pediatric surgical patients with diabetes mellitus. *Anesth Analg* 2005; **101**: 986–99.

38. Chadwick V, Wilkinson KA. Diabetes mellitus and the paediatric anaesthetist. *Paediatr Anaesth* 2004; **14**(9): 716–23.

39. Gwaltney J. The common cold. In: Mandell G, Bennett J, Dolin R, eds. *Principles and practice of infectious diseases*. New York: Churchill Livingstone, 1995: 561–6.

40. Cohen MM, Cameron CB. Should you cancel the operation when a child has an upper respiratory tract infection? *Anesth Analg* 1991; **72**: 282–8.

41. van der Walt JH. Anaesthesia in children with viral respiratory tract infections. *Paediatr Anaesth* 1995; **5**(4): 257–62.

42. Tait AR, Malviya S. Anesthesia for the child with an upper respiratory infection: still a dilemma? *Anesth Analg* 2005; **100**: 59–65.

43 Schreiner MS, O'Hara I, Marakakis DA, Politis GD. Do children who experience laryngospasm have an increased risk of upper respiratory tract Infection? *Anesthesiology* 1996; **85**: 475–80.

44. Tait AR, Malviya S, Voepel-Lewis T *et al*. Risk factors for perioperative adverse events in children with upper respiratory tract infections. *Anesthesiology* 2001; **95**: 299–306.

45. Morray J, Geiduschek J, Caplan R *et al*. A comparison of pediatric and adult anesthesia closed malpractice claims. *Anesthesiology* 1993; **78**: 461–7.

46. Parnis SJ, Barker DS, van der Walt JH. Clinical predictors of anaesthetic complications in children with respiratory tract infections. *Paediatr Anaesth* 2001; **11**(1): 29–40.

47. Konarzewski WH, Ravindran N, Findlow D, Timmis PK. Anaesthetic death of a child with a cold. *Anaesthesia* 1992; **47**: 624.

48. Bloch EC. Anaesthetic death of a child with a cold. *Anaesthesia* 1993; **48**(2): 171.

49. Mamie C, Habre W, Delhumeau C *et al*. Incidence and risk factors of perioperative respiratory adverse events in children undergoing elective surgery. *Paediatr Anaesth* 2004; **14**(3): 218–24.

18

Preoperative preparation and medication

KAR-BINH ONG

KEY LEARNING POINTS

- Many children are not anxious at induction but standard anxiolysis with oral midazolam should be considered in many situations.
- Preoperative preparation with skilled nurses and play therapists reduces anxiety.

- Preoperative fasting should be minimised to reduce unnecessary hunger and thirst.
- Children with asthma or epilepsy should receive their standard medications before anaesthesia.

INTRODUCTION

Preoperative preparation aims to reduce anxiety, minimise discomfort or distress and, most importantly, to ensure that the child's physical status is optimised to maximise safety. This chapter covers the common preoperative medications, fasting and the management of common medical conditions.

PREOPERATIVE MEDICATIONS

Anxiolytic premedication

The methods of reducing anxiety in frightened children are discussed in Chapter 25. A review is presented below of the common anxiolytic drugs that may be useful for routine use in children who are considered to be neither particularly frightened nor uncooperative.

In many hospitals, anxiolytic drugs are not used routinely because, although they may be generally helpful, children are not usually sufficiently anxious to justify the tasks of drug prescription, drug administration, and the observation and supervision of sedated children before anaesthesia

is induced. However, anxiolytic drugs are potentially important in any preparation process and two common scenarios should be considered. An anxiolytic or sedative drug can be administered on the ward but this will need to be given at an appropriate time before induction, which may cause delay. Transport of a sedated child to the operating theatre on a trolley by a porter also has the potential to cause delay. Alternatively, children can receive a drug in an area next to the operating theatre. This area could be the anaesthetic induction room but these rooms are not available in many countries. A separate receiving area may be available, staffed by nurses who can assess children and parents and use behavioural techniques and premedicants appropriately. In some countries parents are not allowed to be present at induction so that short-acting drugs such as midazolam [1,2], ketamine [3] or fentanyl [4,5] have been used routinely to reduce the distress of separation.

BENZODIAZEPINES

Increasingly, midazolam has become the drug of choice for reducing anxiety in children weighing less than 20 kg during the preoperative period [6]. Its popularity is related to the low frequency of serious side effects and its short onset.

Midazolam is usually given orally although sublingual, buccal and intranasal routes have also been used. An oral dose of 0.5 mg/kg is usually effective and higher doses have been associated with an increased frequency of side-effects [7]. The ideal interval between the administration of oral midazolam and induction of anaesthesia is 20–30 minutes, although significant anxiolytic effects have been reported within 15 minutes [8]. It has a bitter taste that can be masked with various sweetening agents. For example, midazolam can be mixed with paracetamol elixir. Paradoxical excitement [9–11] can be troublesome and may be related to the time after administration; the incidence and timing are unknown.

Other short-acting benzodiazepines such as temazepam may be useful in older children. Oral temazepam can be given (0.5–1 mg/kg) 1 hour before induction, either as a tablet or as an elixir. Studies have shown that it causes variable calming and it may not be as effective as alimemazine [12,13] but it has few side-effects and has little effect on recovery time [14].

OTHER SEDATIVE DRUGS

Other premedicants are discussed in detail in Chapter 25. Chloral hydrate and triclofos (25–50 mg/kg) are predictable but they are impractical in children larger than 12 kg because the volume of drug required is unpalatable. Clonidine can be given orally before induction and has the advantage of reducing agitation both before [15] and after sevoflurane [16]. However, an oral dose (4 μg/kg) takes approximately 60–90 minutes to take full effect, it may not be as effective as midazolam in calming before induction and it prolongs recovery [17]. It does have analgesic [17], antiemetic [18,19] and calming properties [20] but these can be achieved with intravenous administration during anaesthesia, which may be more reliable and convenient. Melatonin is another potentially useful standard oral sedative that has the advantage of having few, if any, side-effects [21,22]. It reduces anxiety and may be associated with fewer postoperative behavioural problems than midazolam [22]. An oral dose of 0.2 mg/kg has also been shown to reduce the dose of propofol required to induce anaesthesia when given 50 minutes before the onset of anaesthesia [23].

NON-PHARMACOLOGICAL METHODS OF REDUCING ANXIETY

The presence of parents at induction, play therapy, hypnotherapy and music therapy may all be considered as helpful standard techniques. Even though some anxious parents may not be able to calm their children, parental presence has become widely accepted. Parents themselves must be included in the standard preparation for anaesthesia. They need information and reassurance and these are crucial tasks in the assessment interview. Further preparation such as visits to the operating theatre before the day of surgery, written information, videos and interactive websites can all be offered at preoperative assessment clinics.

These methods are covered in detail in Chapter 25. In general, non-pharmacological methods of anxiolysis are valuable but time-consuming.

Other preoperative medications

TOPICAL LOCAL ANAESTHETICS

Whenever intravenous induction is planned, topical local anaesthetics such as EMLA (Eutectic Mixture of Local Anaesthetics) or Ametop are extremely useful in reducing the pain of intravenous cannulation. EMLA contains 2.5 per cent lidocaine and 2.5 per cent prilocaine in an oily base that promotes skin penetration and it should be applied at least 1 hour beforehand. Longer applications may be more effective [24] and the sensory block can last for 120–140 minutes after it is removed. Side-effects include blanching of the skin and vasoconstriction, which may make intravenous cannulation more difficult. Ametop is a gel formulation of 4 per cent amethocaine and should be applied onto the skin 30–45 minutes before venepuncture. It has superior analgesic effects to EMLA [25,26] and it may cause less vasoconstriction.

SIMPLE ANALGESICS

Paracetamol and non-steroidal anti-inflammatory drugs (NSAIDs) can be given preoperatively as a simple method of achieving postoperative analgesia for minor surgical procedures. Paracetamol is well absorbed orally and the recommended loading dose is 20 mg/kg. Ibuprofen and diclofenac can also be given orally before induction at doses of 5 mg/kg and 1 mg/kg respectively. These drugs should be given at least 30 minutes before induction, but, as with all oral drugs, perioperative nausea and vomiting may affect bioavailability and therefore alternative routes of administration (intravenous, rectal) may be more reliable and should be considered.

ANTIMUSCARINICS

Atropine and glycopyrrolate are now used less frequently as premedications and are no longer prescribed routinely. They may still have a role as antisialagogues whenever secretions need to be reduced, such as before airway surgery. These drugs are covered in detail in Chapter 16.

H_2-RECEPTOR ANTAGONISTS

H_2-receptor antagonists such as ranitidine reduce the volume and acidity of gastric contents and may help reduce the risk of pneumonitis if there is pulmonary aspiration. In paediatric anaesthetic practice, these drugs are used infrequently because acid aspiration pneumonitis is so rare. In a study of children prepared for elective surgery ranitidine reduced gastric acidity but not volume [27]. Ranitidine may be beneficial in reducing the effects of anaphylaxis in cases where there is a risk of latex allergy.

PREOPERATIVE FASTING

In children, the incidence of pulmonary aspiration of gastric contents ranges from 1 to 9 cases in 10 000 anaesthetics [28–30]. Although pulmonary aspiration is rare, a period of preoperative fasting has traditionally been required before elective surgery in order to maximise gastric emptying and, consequently, to reduce the risks of aspiration. However, prolonged preoperative fasting causes thirst, hunger and irritability [31,32]. In neonates and small infants, fasting risks hypoglycaemia. Long periods (greater than 8 hours) of fasting in infants can result in dehydration causing haemodynamic instability during anaesthesia [33]. Given the disadvantages of prolonged fasting, care should be taken to minimise fasting times, and children may be comforted by being allowed clear fluids 2 hours before induction. A reasonable guideline is presented in Table 18.1.

Normal gastric emptying

The risk of aspiration pneumonitis has been assumed to be related to the volume and acidity of gastric contents. Preoperative fasting has therefore been considered important and guidelines have been developed based on studies of how quickly the stomach can empty after the ingestion of various solids and liquids.

CLEAR FLUIDS

Gastric emptying of liquids has a first-order exponential relationship with time. In children, this process is largely complete 2–3 hours after ingestion. Several studies have shown that children given clear fluids 2–3 hours before surgery have gastric contents of similar volume and pH compared with those who have been fasted for much longer periods [34–36]. A recent Cochrane review [32] concluded that giving healthy children clear fluids up to 2

hours before surgery does not increase gastric volume or acidity. Moreover, the review did not find a relationship between the volume of fluid intake and residual gastric volume. Healthy infants less than 1 year of age also do not appear to have increased gastric volumes or acidity when fed clear fluids up to 2 hours before surgery [37]. Clear fluids have been defined either as a fluid through which it is possible to read newsprint or as a non-particulate fluid without fat. Examples of clear fluids include water, glucose water, apple juice, orange squash, tea without milk and black coffee.

BREAST MILK

In animals pulmonary aspiration of human breast milk can cause significant lung injury [38]. Human breast milk usually empties from the infant stomach in a biphasic manner, with an initial rapid phase followed by a steady, slower phase [39]. The length of time required for complete emptying from the stomach of healthy infants is not precisely known but there is evidence that significant quantities of breast milk can be found 2 hours after ingestion [37]. A 3- to 4-hour fast for breast milk should be adequate based on data from a study of residual gastric volumes and a study using real-time ultrasonography [40,41]. Nevertheless, the rate of emptying varies between infants and is influenced by the fat and protein content of milk, which may vary according to time of day.

Current recommendations from the Association of Anaesthetists of Great Britain and Ireland (AAGBI) [42] and the American Society of Anesthesiologists (ASA) [43] state that children should be fasted for at least 4 hours in the case of breast milk. National surveys of current practice in the UK and the USA [44,45] have shown that, although the majority of centres adhere to these recommendations, some have shortened fasting times for breast milk to 3 hours [46].

FORMULA MILK

Formula milk is derived usually from cows' milk although soya-based products are available. As with breast milk, the gastric emptying of infant formula can show a biphasic pattern, with a slower constant phase that obeys zero-order

Table 18.1 Minimum safe fasting times for children having elective surgery

	Clear fluids	Breast milk	Formula milk	Solids
Children over 1 year	2 hours	–	6 hours	6 hours
Infants aged 6–12 months	2 hours	4 hours (3 hours may be adequate)	6 hours	6 hours
Infants under 6 months	2 hours	4 hours (3 hours may be adequate)	6 hours (4 hours may be adequate)	6 hours

kinetics [39]. However, in some infants, there is a mono-phasic pattern of emptying, with the formula milk leaving the stomach at a constant rate [39]. Most types of formula milk take longer to empty from the stomach of infants than breast milk. Rates of gastric emptying vary according to the content of the milk so that casein-predominant milk (with its higher protein content) empties at a slower rate than whey-predominant milk [47].

Cow's milk reacts with gastric juices and separates into solid and liquid phases and this is the reason why fasting times have been the same as for solid food. Current recommendations in both the UK and the USA agree that fasting should be at least 6 hours after both cows' and formula milk. However, there is evidence that gastric volumes are similar at 4 hours after formula milk, compared with those 2 hours after clear fluids, in healthy infants [48], and this has prompted some centres to shorten fasting times for infant formula to 4 hours in infants under 6 months of age [46,48]. There has been a reported case of pulmonary aspiration in an infant who had formula milk 4 hours before surgery but other factors were important in this case in addition to the fasting time [49]. Nevertheless shortening fasting times in infants may increase the risk of pulmonary aspiration. For older children, there is no evidence to support shortening of fasting times for formula or cows' milk to 4 hours, and the current 6-hour fasting time should be adhered to.

SOLID FOOD

There are few studies of gastric emptying of solid food in children. Adult data suggest that solid food leaves the stomach at a constant rate that is influenced by the proportion of carbohydrate, fat and protein. Current national guidelines [42,43] recommend that children should not eat any solid food for 6 hours before anaesthesia. Children given biscuits 2–4 hours before surgery have been found to have identifiable food residue within their stomachs, unlike children who were fasted for longer periods [50]. There is no evidence to support any shortening of recommended fasting times.

Delayed gastric emptying

There is evidence that children who sustain a traumatic injury have significant volumes of gastric aspirate even when they have been fasted for over 8 hours [51]. Data suggest that gastric residual volume is more dependent on the interval from food intake to time of injury than from food intake to induction of anaesthesia. Therefore, any child who requires urgent surgery after a major injury should be managed as if they have a full stomach, unless there has been a long period between food intake and time of injury.

Anxiety and pain may also affect the rate of gastric emptying but this has not been extensively studied in children. Attempts to correlate gastric volumes with preoperative anxiety scores in children have produced some surprising results. In one study, children with high anxiety scores were found to have significantly lower gastric volumes than children with low anxiety scores [52]. Anxiolytic or sedative drugs do not appreciably delay gastric emptying. For example, oral premedication with midazolam does not affect the volume or pH of gastric contents [53].

COMMON MEDICAL CONDITIONS

Asthma

The preoperative assessment of asthma is discussed in Chapter 17. The aim of preparation should be to minimise the risk of perioperative bronchospasm. A retrospective study has suggested that intraoperative bronchospasm in asthmatic children is unlikely provided that they have been adequately prepared [54,55]. Elective surgery should be delayed if there is bronchospasm or if there has been a recent episode of bronchospasm or respiratory tract infection. Children with asthma should be given their usual medications before anaesthesia. The additional administration of a nebulised β_2 agonist 1–2 hours before surgery may be beneficial. Oral corticosteroids such as prednisolone have been advocated [54] for children with moderate or severe asthma undergoing surgery and these should be started 5 days beforehand at a dose of 1 mg/kg/day.

Epilepsy

Epilepsy affects up to 5 per cent of children. Preparation aims to minimise the risk of seizures during the perioperative period. Any children with well-controlled epilepsy, who are having non-neurosurgical operations, need to receive their usual anticonvulsant medications. Perioperative control of convulsions is not usually troublesome in these patients but if they are unable to take oral medications after surgery advice about alternative anticonvulsants should be sought. In children who are undergoing anaesthesia for the investigation or surgical treatment of epilepsy, control of seizures may be extremely difficult and neurologists should be involved in the optimisation of the anticonvulsant drug regimen. Checking blood levels of anticonvulsants may be necessary. In some children convulsions may remain uncontrolled or intractable during the perioperative period. Anticonvulsants may reduce the conscious level and, consequently, the dose of anaesthetic should be modified to avoid prolonged recovery. The choice of anaesthesia drugs is discussed in Chapter 38.

Children with epilepsy often have associated behavioural problems and developmental delay. Sedative premedication drugs and other forms of anxiolysis may therefore be useful.

A ketogenic diet is used in some children to modify refractory seizures. This is a high-fat, low-carbohydrate diet which aims to increase plasma levels of ketones. It can be effective in some children, although its mechanism of action remains unclear. The ketogenic diet has several implications for anaesthesia. First, children on this diet may have abnormal blood chemistry such as hypoalbuminaemia, hypocalcaemia or metabolic acidosis [55]. There is a potential risk of peri-operative hypoglycaemia, although the risk is probably not clinically significant [56] it is reasonable to check a blood glucose level during anaesthesia. Medications containing sugar or sugar substitutes are relatively contraindicated with the ketogenic diet because the carbohydrate load in these drugs may make the diet less effective. This includes paracetamol elixir and some blood products contain dextrose.

Diabetes

The perioperative management of diabetes is covered in detail in Chapter 17.

Long-term steroids

Large doses of steroids over long periods may cause adrenal insufficiency by suppression and atrophy of the hypothalamic–pituitary–adrenal axis. The glucocorticoid stress response to surgery (and critical illness) can be suppressed and may manifest as cardiovascular collapse during the recovery period as a result of an addisonian crisis. For this reason perioperative steroid supplementation generally is recommended in patients who are having or recently have had steroid therapy. Children who have stopped taking steroids within 2 months of surgery should still be given supplementary steroids as the activity of the hypothalamic–pituitary–adrenal axis may take some time to return to normal.

Nevertheless, perioperative steroid cover is based on data from adult patients and there is very little evidence that steroid supplementation is necessary. It is likely that the majority of children having minor surgery do not need any increase in their usual steroid treatment – but this has yet to be evaluated. Children having major surgery or stressful treatments should have steroid supplementation. Guidelines for steroid supplementation used at my institution are presented in Table 18.2. The doses quoted were derived from studies investigating plasma cortisol concentrations after intravenous hydrocortisone in children with critical illness [57] and the doses are probably excessively high. Lower doses have been proposed in adults [58].

Table 18.2   Steroid cover for surgery

1. Children on steroids should receive:
   - Hydrocortisone (IV) 1 mg/kg at induction
   - Hydrocortisone (IM or IV) 6-hourly for 1–4 days after surgery depending on the type of surgery
2. Children who have stopped steroids within 2 months of surgery should receive:
   - Hydrocortisone (IV) 1 mg/kg at induction
   - Hydrocortisone (IM or IV) 6-hourly for 1–2 days after surgery
3. Children who have stopped steroids for more than 2 months do not need any steroid cover

PREVENTION OF PERIOPERATIVE VENOUS THROMBOEMBOLISM

There are few published guidelines for the prevention of perioperative deep vein thrombosis and pulmonary embolus in children. This reflects the low incidence of these complications in children compared with adults. Nevertheless, when these complications do occur in children they result in significant morbidity and mortality [59].

Incidence

Data from a Canadian register of thromboembolic disease suggest that the incidence of deep vein thrombosis or pulmonary embolus in children is 5.3 cases per 10 000 hospital admissions or 0.07 cases per 10 000 children in the general population [60]. Estimates of the incidence of deep vein thrombosis in children from the USA range from 1.2 cases to 5 cases per 10 000 hospital admissions [61,62]. There are few studies of the incidence of venous thromboembolic complications relating specifically to paediatric surgical patients. Although the incidence of these complications is low (about one-tenth of that seen in the adult population), it appears to be rising. This may be due to increased awareness of the problem but may also be because of other contributing factors including the more frequent use of central venous catheters in children. In addition, children with complex congenital conditions, some of which are associated with thromboembolism, may be surviving longer.

Venous thromboembolism may be less likely in children compared with adults because of a reduced capacity to produce thrombin, higher levels of the thrombin inhibitor α_2-macroglobulin and enhanced antithrombotic mechanisms in vessel walls.

Risk factors

Deep vein thromboses and pulmonary emboli occur more frequently in infants and in teenagers [60,63] but the reasons for this have not been well studied. Teenage girls are at greater risk than teenage boys [63]. When children of all ages are considered, however, there is no difference between the genders [60]. Factors associated with venous thromboembolic complications in children [60,64,65] are summarised in Table 18.3.

Inherited thrombophilias such as factor V Leiden deficiency, antithrombin III deficiency, protein S deficiency and protein C deficiency are associated with an increased risk of thromboembolic complications in adult patients. The evidence that these are important in children is less clear. In one prospective cohort study [66], the risk of thrombosis in children with a single thrombophilic defect was estimated to be low. Most children in this study were heterozygous for the defects; homozygotes are likely to be at much greater risk. Other investigators have demonstrated that factor V

Table 18.3 Risk factors for venous thromboembolism in children

Congenital	Acquired
Factor V Leiden mutation	Indwelling central venous catheter
Prothrombin gene mutation	Trauma
Antithrombin III deficiency	Immobilisation
Protein S deficiency	Surgery
Protein C deficiency	Previous history of thromboembolism
	Infection
	Cancer, leukaemia
	Chemotherapy
	Bone marrow transplantation
	Total parenteral nutrition
	Systemic lupus erythematosus
	Obesity
	Nephrotic syndrome
	Oral contraceptive pill (teenagers)

mutation, antithrombin deficiency and protein C deficiency are independent risk factors for childhood venous thrombosis [67].

The presence of an indwelling central venous catheter is probably the single most important risk factor for the development of deep vein thrombosis and pulmonary embolus in children [60]. Central venous catheters damage vessel walls and affect blood flow. In addition, the solutions infused are often thrombogenic. The location of a central venous catheter can influence the risk. Catheters placed in the subclavian vein appear to be associated with a greater risk of thrombosis than those placed in the jugular vein [68]. In addition, the technique used for insertion of the central line may also be important. Subclavian lines inserted using a percutaneous technique may be associated with a higher risk of thrombosis than lines placed using a venous cut-down technique [68].

Prophylaxis

All children should be encouraged to mobilise during the postoperative period. Dehydration should be avoided and central venous catheters should be removed as soon as they are no longer required. The majority of children undergoing surgery do not need any other measures to prevent deep vein thrombosis and pulmonary embolus. In the older child who is at risk, physical devices such as elastic compression stockings and pneumatic compression boots (e.g. Flotron) may be beneficial but they are often not available in appropriate sizes for children. Children with a known risk of thromboembolism should receive heparin. Increasingly, unfractionated heparin has been replaced by low-molecular-weight heparin; this can be given as a subcutaneous injection and

has more predictable pharmacokinetics than unfractionated heparin. The anticoagulant effect of low-molecular-weight heparin is mediated largely by its anti-factor-Xa activity. Dose-finding studies have therefore tended to measure levels of anti-factor-Xa activity in relation to the dose of heparin. Preparations of low-molecular-weight heparin include enoxaparin and reviparin. The suggested dose of enoxaparin for prophylaxis against thromboembolism is 0.5 mg/kg every 12 hours for children over 5 kg [69,70]. Larger doses (0.75 mg/kg every 12 hours) may be required in infants under 5 kg in order to achieve the same anticoagulant effects. Reviparin should be administered at a dose of 30 U/kg every 12 hours for children over 3 months of age and at a dose of 50 U/kg every 12 hours for infants under 3 months. Monitoring by anti-factor-Xa activity assays is recommended [70]. Bleeding complications may be seen but these tend to be relatively minor with recommended prophylaxis doses.

REFERENCES

Key references

Andrew M, David M, Adams M et al. Venous thromboembolic complications (VTE) in children: first analyses of the Canadian registry of VTE. *Blood* 1994; **83**(5): 1251–7.

Brady M, Kinn S, O'Rourke K et al. Preoperative fasting for preventing perioperative complications in children. *Cochrane Database Syst Rev* 2005; **2**: CD005285.

Kain ZN, Hofstadter MB, Mayes LC et al. Midazolam: effects on amnesia and anxiety in children. *Anesthesiology* 2000; **93**(3): 676–84.

Litman RS, Wu CL, Quinlivan JK. Gastric volume and pH in infants fed clear liquids and breast milk prior to surgery. *Anesth Analg* 1994; **79**: 482–5.

Zachary CY, Evans R. Perioperative management for childhood asthma. *Ann Allergy Asthma Immunol* 1996; **77**: 468–72.

References

1. Karl HW, Rosenberger JL, Larach MG, Ruffle JM. Transmucosal administration of midazolam for premedication of pediatric patients: comparison of the nasal and sublingual routes. *Anesthesiology* 1993; **78**: 885–91.

2. Kogan A, Katz J, Efrat R, Eidelman LA. Premedication with midazolam in young children: a comparison of four routes of administration. *Paediatr Anaesth* 2002; **12**(8): 685–9.

3. Weber F, Wulf H, el Saeidi G. Premedication with nasal S-ketamine and midazolam provides good conditions for induction of anesthesia in preschool children. *Can J Anaesth* 2003; **50**(5): 470–5.

4. Howell TK, Smith S, Rushman SC et al. A comparison of oral transmucosal fentanyl and oral midazolam for premedication in children. *Anaesthesia* 2002; **57**(8): 798–805.

5. Tamura M, Nakamura K, Kitamura R et al. Oral premedication with fentanyl may be a safe and effective alternative to oral midazolam. Eur J Anaesthesiol 2003; **20**(6): 482–6.

6. Kain ZN, Mayes LC, Bell C et al. Premedication in the United States: a status report. Anesth Analg 1997; **84**: 427–32.

7. Coté CJ, Cohen IT, Suresh S et al. A comparison of three doses of a commercially prepared oral midazolam syrup in children. Anesth Analg 2002; **94**(1): 37–43.

8. Kain ZN, Hofstadter MB, Mayes LC et al. Midazolam: effects on amnesia and anxiety in children. Anesthesiology 2000; **93**(3): 676–84.

9. Sanders JC. Flumazenil reverses a paradoxical reaction to intravenous midazolam in a child with uneventful prior exposure to midazolam. Paediatr Anaesth 2003; **13**(4): 369–70.

10. Golparvar M, Saghaei M, Sajedi P, Razavi SS. Paradoxical reaction following intravenous midazolam premedication in pediatric patients – a randomized placebo controlled trial of ketamine for rapid tranquilization. Paediatr Anaesth 2004; **14**(11): 924–30.

11. Mancuso CE, Tanzi MG, Gabay M. Paradoxical reactions to benzodiazepines: literature review and treatment options. Pharmacotherapy 2004; **24**(9): 1177–85.

12. Padfield NL, Twohig MM, Fraser AC et al. Temazepam and trimeprazine compared with placebo as premedication in children. An investigation extended into the first 2 weeks at home. Br J Anaesth 1986; **58**(5): 487–93.

13. Thomas DL, Vaughan RS, Vickers MD et al. Comparison of temazepam elixir and trimeprazine syrup as oral premedication in children undergoing tonsillectomy and associated procedures. Br J Anaesth 1987; **59**(4): 424–30.

14. Obey PA, Ogg TW, Gilks WR et al. Temazepam and recovery in day surgery. Anaesthesia 1988; **43**(1): 49–51.

15. Constant I, Leport Y, Richard P et al. Agitation and changes of Bispectral Index and electroencephalographic-derived variables during sevoflurane induction in children: clonidine premedication reduces agitation compared with midazolam. Br J Anaesth 2004; **92**(4): 504–11.

16. Tesoro S, Mezzetti D, Marchesini L, Peduto VA. Clonidine treatment for agitation in children after sevoflurane anesthesia. Anesth Analg 2005; **101**(6): 1619–22.

17. Fazi L, Jantzen EC, Rose JB et al. A comparison of oral clonidine and oral midazolam as preanesthetic medications in the pediatric tonsillectomy patient. Anesth Analg 2001; **92**(1): 56–61.

18. Handa F, Fujii Y. The efficacy of oral clonidine premedication in the prevention of postoperative vomiting in children following strabismus surgery. Paediatr Anaesth 2001; **11**(1): 71–4.

19. Mikawa K, Nishina K, Maekawa N et al. Oral clonidine premedication reduces vomiting in children after strabismus surgery. Can J Anaesth 1995; **42**(11): 977–81.

20. Malviya S, Voepel-Lewis T, Ramamurthi RJ et al. Clonidine for the prevention of emergence agitation in young children: efficacy and recovery profile. Paediatr Anaesth 2006; **16**(5): 554–9.

21. Naguib M, Samarkandi AH. Premedication with melatonin: a double-blind, placebo-controlled comparison with midazolam. Br J Anaesth 1999; **82**(6): 875–80.

22. Samarkandi A, Naguib M, Riad W et al. Melatonin vs. midazolam premedication in children: a double-blind, placebo-controlled study. Eur J Anaesthesiol 2005; **22**: 189–96.

23. Naguib M, Samarkandi AH, Moniem MA et al. The effects of melatonin premedication on propofol and thiopental induction dose–response curves: a prospective, randomized, double-blind study. Anesth Analg 2006; **103**(6): 1448–52.

24. Morgan-Hughes NJ, Kirton CB. EMLA – is one hour long enough? Anaesthesia 2001; **56**(5): 495–6.

25. Browne J, Awad I, Plant R et al. Topical amethocaine (Ametop™) is superior to EMLA for intravenous cannulation. Can J Anaesth 1999; **46**(11): 1014–18.

26. Arrowsmith J, Campbell C. A comparison of local anaesthetics for venepuncture. Arch Dis Child 2000; **82**: 309–10.

27. Maekawa N, Nishina K, Mikawa K et al. Comparison of pirenzepine, ranitidine, and pirenzepine-ranitidine combination for reducing preoperative gastric fluid acidity and volume in children. Br J Anaesth 1998; **80**: 53–7.

28. Warner MA, Warner MD, Warner DO et al. Perioperative pulmonary aspiration in infants and children. Anesthesiology 1999; **90**(1): 66–71.

29. Olsson GL, Hallen B, Hambraeus-Jonzon K et al. Aspiration during anaesthesia: a computer-aided study of 185,358 anaesthetics. Acta Anaesthesiol Scand 1986; **30**: 84–92.

30. Tiret L, Nivoche Y, Hatton F et al. Complications related to anaesthesia in infants and children: a prospective survey of 40,420 anaesthetics. Br J Anaesth 1988; **61**: 263–9.

31. Schreiner MS, Triebwasser A, Keon TP. Ingestion of liquids compared to preoperative fasting in pediatric outpatients. Anesthesiology 1990; **72**(4): 593–7.

32. Brady M, Kinn S, O'Rourke K et al. Preoperative fasting for preventing perioperative complications in children. Cochrane Database Syst Rev 2005; **2**: CD005285.

33. Friesen RH, Wurl JL, Friesen RM et al. Duration of preoperative fast correlates with arterial blood pressure response to halothane in infants. Anesth Analg 2002; **95**: 1572–6.

34. Splinter WM, Stewart JA, Muir JG. The effect of preoperative apple juice on gastric contents, thirst, and hunger in children. Can J Anaesth 1989; **36**(1): 55–8.

35. Splinter WM, Schaefer JD, Zunder IH. Clear fluids three hours before surgery do not affect the gastric fluid contents of children. Can J Anaesth 1990; **37**(5): 498–501.

36. Crawford M, Lerman J, Christensen S, Farrow-Gillespie A. Effects of duration of fasting on gastric fluid pH and volume in healthy children. Anesth Analg 1990; **71**: 400–3.

37. Litman RS, Wu CL, Quinlivan JK. Gastric volume and pH in infants fed clear liquids and breast milk prior to surgery. Anesth Analg 1994; **79**: 482–5.

38. O'Hare B, Chin C, Lerman J, Endo J. Acute lung injury after instillation of human breast milk into rabbits' lungs: effects of pH and gastric juice. Anesthesiology 1999; **90**(4): 1112–18.

39. Cavell B. Gastric emptying in infants fed human milk or infant formula. Acta Paediatr Scand 1981; **70**: 639–41.

40. van der Walt JH, Foate JA, Murrell D et al. A study of preoperative fasting in infants aged less than 3 months. Anaesth Intensive Care 1990; **18**(4): 527–31.

41. Sethi AK, Chatterji C, Bhargava SK *et al.* Safe pre-operative fasting times after milk or clear fluid in children: a preliminary study using real-time ultrasound. *Anaesthesia* 1999; **54**(1): 51–9.

42. The Association of Anaesthetists of Great Britain and Ireland. *Pre-operative assessment: the role of the anaesthetist.* London: AAGBI, 2001.

43. American Society of Anesthesiologists Task Force on Preoperative Fasting. Practice guidelines for preoperative fasting and the use of pharmacologic agents to reduce the risk of pulmonary aspiration: application to healthy patients undergoing elective procedures: a report by the American Society of Anesthesiologists Task Force on Preoperative Fasting. *Anesthesiology* 1999; **90**(3): 896–905.

44. Ferrari LR, Rooney FM, Rockoff MA. Preoperative fasting practices in pediatrics. *Anesthesiology* 1999; **90**(4): 978–80.

45. Emerson BM, Wrigley SR, Newton M. Pre-operative fasting for paediatric anaesthesia. *Anaesthesia* 1998; **53**: 326–30.

46. Cook-Sather SD, Litman RS. Modern fasting guidelines in children. *Best Pract Res Clin Anaesthesiol* 2006; **20**(3): 471–81.

47. Billeaud C, Guillet J, Sandler B. Gastric emptying in infants with or without gastro-oesophageal reflux according to the type of milk. *Eur J Clin Nutr* 1990; **44**: 577–83.

48. Cook-Sather SD, Harris KA, Chiavacci R *et al.* A liberalized fasting guideline for formula-fed infants does not increase average gastric fluid volume before elective surgery. *Anesth Analg* 2003; **96**: 965–9.

49. Kawabata T, Tokumine J, Nakamura S, Sugahara K. Unanticipated vomiting and pulmonary aspiration at anaesthesia induction in a formula-fed 4-month old infant. *Anesthesiology* 2004; **100**: 1330–1.

50. Meakin G, Dingwall AE, Addison GM *et al.* Effects of fasting and oral premedication on the pH and volume of gastric aspirate in children. *Br J Anaesth* 1987; **59**(6): 678–82.

51. Bricker SRW, McLuckie A, Nightingale DA. Gastric aspirates after trauma in children. *Anaesthesia* 1989; **44**: 721–4.

52. Kawana S, Uzuki M, Nakae Y, Namiki A. Preoperative anxiety and volume and acidity of gastric fluid in children. *Paediatr Anaesth* 2000; **10**: 17–21.

53. Riva J, Lejbusiewicz G, Papa M *et al.* Oral premedication with midazolam in paediatric anaesthesia. Effects on sedation and gastric contents. *Paediatr Anaesth* 1997; **7**(3): 191–6.

54. Zachary CY, Evans R. Perioperative management for childhood asthma. *Ann Allergy Asthma Immunol* 1996; **77**: 468–72.

55. McNeely JK. Perioperative management of a paediatric patient on the ketogenic diet. *Paediatr Anaesth* 2000; **10**: 103–6.

56. Valencia I, Pfeifer H, Thiele EA. General anesthesia and the ketogenic diet: clinical experience in nine patients. *Epilepsia* 2002; **43**(5): 525–9.

57. Charmandari E, Lichtarowicz-Krynska EJ, Hindmarsh PC *et al.* Congenital adrenal hyperplasia: management during critical illness. *Arch Dis Child* 2001; **85**: 26–8.

58. Nicholson G, Burrin JM, Hall GM. Per-operative steroid supplementation. *Anaesthesia* 1998; **53**: 1091–104.

59. Monagle P, Adams M, Mahoney M *et al.* Outcome of pediatric thromboembolic disease: a report from the Canadian Childhood Thrombophilia Registry. *Pediatr Res* 2000; **47**(6): 763–6.

60. Andrew M, David M, Adams M *et al.* Venous thromboembolic complications (VTE) in children: first analyses of the Canadian registry of VTE. *Blood* 1994; **83**(5): 1251–7.

61. Buck JR, Connors RH, Coon WW *et al.* Pulmonary embolism in children. *J Pediatr Surg* 1981; **16**: 385–91.

62. Rohrer MJ, Cutler BS, MacDougall E *et al.* A prospective study of the incidence of deep venous thrombosis in hospitalized children. *J Vasc Surg* 1996; **24**(1): 46–50.

63. Stein PD, Kayali F, Olson RE. Incidence of venous thromboembolism in infants and children: data from the national hospital discharge survey. *J Pediatr* 2004; **145**(4): 563–5.

64. David M, Andrew M. Venous thromboembolic complications in children. *J Pediatr* 1993; **123**(3): 337–46.

65. Parasuraman S, Goldhaber SZ. Venous thromboembolism in children. *Circulation* 2006; **113**: 12–16.

66. Tormene D, Simioni P, Prandoni P *et al.* The incidence of venous thromboembolism in thrombophilic children: a prospective cohort study. *Blood* 2002; **100**(7): 2403–5.

67. Nowak-Göttl U, Junker R, Hartmeier M *et al.* Increased lipoprotein (a) is an important risk factor for venous thromboembolism in childhood. *Circulation* 1999; **100**: 743–8.

68. Male C, Chait P, Andrew M *et al.* Central venous line-related thrombosis in children: association with central venous line location and insertion technique. *Blood* 2003; **101**: 4273–8.

69. Dix D, Marzinotto V, Leaker M *et al.* The use of low molecular weight heparin in pediatric patients: review of a single institution experience. *J Pediatr* 2000; **136**: 439–45.

70. Sutor AH, Chan AKC, Massicote P. Low-molecular-weight heparin in pediatric patients. *Semin Thromb Hemost* 2004; **30**(suppl 1): 31–9.

19

Equipment and basic anaesthesia techniques

JANE LOCKIE, DAVID DEBEER

KEY LEARNING POINTS

Airway equipment

- Specialist equipment is required for paediatric anaesthesia.
- Differences in anatomy and physiology mean that scaled-down versions of adult equipment are not always suitable.
- Recent data have challenged the mandatory use of uncuffed tracheal tubes for children.

Basic techniques

- Preparation is the key to avoiding complications.
- Parents are the best carers for their children and should be involved as much as possible.
- Airway complications are common in children under 6 years of age and particularly so in infants.
- A modified rapid sequence inductions technique is suitable for use in children.

INTRODUCTION

The aim of this chapter is to review the equipment required for paediatric anaesthesia and describe some approaches to standard anaesthetic techniques. Planning of anaesthesia technique, communication with patients, parents, operators and the anaesthesia team are emphasised. The importance of airway management skills in paediatric practice is discussed.

Anaesthesia should not be embarked upon without due consideration for the equipment needed, the environment and the anaesthesia team available. For recommendations relating to the care of children and young people in the hospital setting see Chapter 48.

AIRWAY EQUIPMENT

Masks

FACEMASKS

Facemasks are used for inhalational induction of anaesthesia, preoxygenation and during spontaneous or controlled ventilation. The most widely used facemasks are made of clear plastic with inflatable cushioned rims (Fig. 19.1); they have advantages over reusable black rubber masks in that they are latex free, have a soft inflatable rim that can be adjusted to provide a good seal on the face, and allow observation of a patient's colour and expiratory condensate and detection of secretions or regurgitated matter. They do have a larger dead space compared with the Rendell–Baker Soucek mask, though this is not clinically significant as there is a minimal relationship between the size of the facemask and the functional dead space [1]. Cushion masks may be scented to aid acceptance for inhalational induction. A specially designed facemask is available for fibre-optic intubation. These have an off-centre connector to the breathing system to allow the passage of a fibre-optic scope through the mask centrally (see Chapter 21, Fig 21.4).

NASAL MASKS

Although nasal masks, such as the Goldman nasal mask, may be used in children undergoing dental anaesthesia, they have largely been superseded by the laryngeal mask airway, which has been shown to provide a superior airway and better quality anaesthesia [2].

Airways

OROPHARYNGEAL AIRWAYS

Guedel oropharyngeal airways are useful adjuncts for maintaining upper airway patency but should not be regarded as a substitute for poor airway technique. They are available in a range of sizes from 000 to 4 for use in neonates to large children. An appropriately sized oropharyngeal airway must be used as an incorrect size may compound upper airway obstruction. This can be assessed by placing the airway against the side of the child's face; the correct size is that which extends from the angle of the mandible to the level of the incisors at the corner of the mouth. Airway insertion needs an adequate depth of anaesthesia as coughing and laryngospasm may be provoked. It should be inserted with care in infants and young children to avoid traumatising pharyngeal structures.

NASOPHARYNGEAL AIRWAYS

Nasopharyngeal airways are not routinely used in paediatric practice; however, they may be a useful in patients with loose teeth or poor mouth opening and in those in whom an oral airway does not relieve airway obstruction. Becuase they are better tolerated by the semi-awake child than an oropharyngeal airway, they are useful in children with obstructive sleep apnoea. While a range of flanged soft rubber airways are available, a nasopharyngeal airway can be constructed by shortening a standard tracheal tube of the appropriate size. This should be 1 mm less than the appropriately sized tracheal tube (see below). It is important that a nasopharyngeal airway is the correct length. This can be assessed by measuring the distance from the nasal tip to the external auditory meatus. The nasopharyngeal airway should be well lubricated prior to insertion so as to avoid trauma to the nasal mucosa or adenoids and

once inserted it should be safely secured to prevent accidental displacement into the nasopharynx. The size and length (centimetres) should be recorded to facilitate accurate suctioning.

LARYNGEAL MASK AIRWAY

The laryngeal mask airway (LMA) is well established in paediatric practice, not only for routine, but also for difficult, airway management. Of the sizes (1–6) available, 1–3 are most suited to paediatric practice. These are scaled-down versions of the adult prototype and, despite there being significant anatomical differences between infants and small children and adults, cadaveric studies have shown that the pharyngeal shape, which is most relevant for laryngeal mask use, is similar [3]. Size selection is according to weight (Table 19.1).

The 'classic' LMA is made of silicone and is latex free. It is capable of withstanding autoclaving and can be reused up to 40 times (as recommended by the manufacturer). Each mask should have a record card to register each sterilisation cycle. Whatever the technique of insertion used, a small amount of water-soluble lubricant should be placed on the posterior aspect of the mask. Once inserted, it is important to fix the LMA securely in place, as accidental dislodgement may occur, particularly in younger children where there is a significant portion of the tube protruding from the mouth. The safety and efficacy of LMAs in children have been shown in a number of large studies [4,5]. Over-inflation of the cuff should be avoided; if an unacceptable leak persists after inflation with the recommended volume of air, try repositioning or use a larger LMA. When positioned correctly, the epiglottis and oesophagus should be outside the mask, though this is not always the case. Fibre-optic bronchoscopies performed through 'clinically well-positioned size 1 LMAs' have shown a clear laryngeal opening in only 27 per cent of patients, with the epiglottis being either impinged in the bars of the LMA or folded down by the LMA in 57 per cent and 38 per cent of patients, respectively [6]. In infants there should be a low threshold for changing to a tracheal tube, as correct LMA

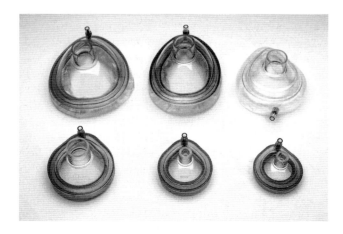

Figure 19.1 Clear facemasks with inflatable rims.

Table 19.1 Appropriate sizes of paediatric laryngeal mask airways (LMAs)*

Size of classic LMA	Weight of patient (kg)	Maximum cuff inflation volume (mL)
1	<5	4
1.5	5–10	7
2	10–20	10
2.5	20–30	14
3	30–50	20

*Intavent Orthofix Ltd, Maidenhead, UK, 2006.

placement is less likely and delayed airway obstruction secondary to movement is more likely.

A number of modifications have been made to the LMA classic.

The magnetic resonance imaging compatible laryngeal mask airway

An magnetic resonance imaging (MRI) compatible mask is available. The pilot balloon (yellow) does not have a metal spring in the self-sealing valve, so that image artefact is reduced to a minimum.

The reinforced laryngeal mask airway (LMA Flexible)

A reinforced laryngeal mask airway has been designed for use in head, neck and oral surgery and is available in sizes 2, 2½, 3, 4 and 5 (Fig. 19.2). The mask is attached to a flexible, non-kinking metallic tube that is longer and has a smaller internal diameter than the standard version. The resulting increase in flow resistance makes them less suitable for use with spontaneous ventilation over prolonged periods.

The intubating laryngeal mask airway

An intubating laryngeal mask airway (ILMA) has been developed to enable blind tracheal intubation. At present, It is only made in size 3 and above, which limits its use in children.

The Pro-Seal laryngeal mask airway

The LMA Pro-Seal is a new laryngeal mask airway that has a second posterior cuff and an oesophageal drainage tube. This allows a higher seal pressure than the LMA classic for the same intra-cuff pressure and permits drainage of gastric secretions. It is available in sizes 1½ upwards. Although the sizes below 3 do not have a posterior cuff, they have been shown to be effective airway devices in children, isolating the glottis from the oesophagus when correctly positioned. The performance of the size 2 Pro-Seal LMA has been shown to be similar to that of the size 3 (which does have a posterior cuff) in terms of insertion success, efficacy of seal, tidal volume, fibre-optic position and gastric tube placement [7]. A greater depth of anaesthesia is required for insertion of the LMA Pro-Seal compared with the LMA classic.

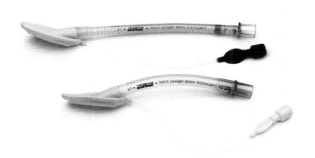

Figure 19.2   Size 2½ reinforced (above) and classic (below) laryngeal mask airways.

The single-use laryngeal mask airway

In response to concerns regarding possible transmission of new-variant Creutzfeldt–Jakob disease (vCJD) to patients via reusable devices, the single-use LMA has been developed; it is made from latex-free, clear, polyvinyl chloride (PVC). For patent reasons most single-use LMAs do not have epiglottic bars and therefore there is a theoretical risk of obstruction of the tube by the epiglottis.

Tracheal tubes

Despite the widespread use of the laryngeal mask airway, the gold standard for airway management in children remains the tracheal tube, especially when using controlled ventilation, where controversy over the safety of the LMA continues.

SIZE OF TRACHEAL TUBE

The narrowest part of the child's upper airway is the cricoid cartilage and not the vocal cords. This forms a complete ring around the airway so that any oedema of the airway from trauma at intubation may lead to narrowing of the lumen, with a resulting increase in airflow resistance. In order to prevent damage to the tracheal mucosa and possible subglottic stenosis, it is important that the correct size of tracheal tube is used, especially in neonates and infants. A number of formulae have been devised to predict the appropriate size; however, the most reliable method is to ensure that the tube passes through the glottis and cricoid ring without resistance, and that there is a small audible leak at an inflating pressure of $20\,cmH_2O$. This assumes that the mucosal capillary pressure is 20–25 mmHg. If there is no leak or there is an inappropriately large leak, the tracheal tube should be changed.

Above the age of 1 year, a commonly used formula is as follows:

$$\text{Internal diameter (mm)} = \frac{\text{Age (years)}}{4} + 4.5.$$

As this is only a guide, tubes 0.5 mm above and below the predicted size should always be available. Below the age of 2 years, formulaic prediction of tracheal tube size is less reliable and both age and weight should be taken into account. A normal full-term neonate ($\geqslant 3\,kg$) will usually take a 3.5, while the appropriate size for a smaller neonate is a 3.0 (2–3 kg) or 2.5 ($<2\,kg$). From the age of 3 months to 6 months, a size 4.0 will usually be required and a size 4.5 for a 1-year-old child. Predicting tracheal tube size by matching the external diameter of the tube to the child's index finger has been shown to be unreliable [8].

Uncuffed tracheal tubes are traditionally used in children under about 8 years of age, although the necessity for this has recently been challenged (see below). As the cricoid cartilage is circular in this age group, a correctly sized uncuffed tube will prevent aspiration and allow assisted ventilation without excessive air leak. In the older child, as in the adult, the narrowest part of the upper airway is the glottis, which is hexagonal in cross-section. A standard tracheal tube, round in cross-section and small enough to fit through the narrowest part of the glottis, will have a large leak around it, thus necessitating use of a tube with an inflatable cuff.

LENGTH OF TRACHEAL TUBE

Owing to the relatively short length of the trachea in paediatric patients, use of the correct length of tracheal tube is essential if endobronchial intubation or inadvertent extubation are to be avoided. Ideally, the tip of an uncuffed tracheal tube should lie in the mid-trachea and a number of mathematical formulae have been devised in order to help in determining the correct length. Depth of insertion is usually referred to by the centimetre marking at the teeth of corner of the mouth. A useful formula is as follows:

$$\text{Length} = \frac{\text{Age (years)}}{2} + 12 \text{ cm (oral tubes)}.$$

$$\text{Length} = \frac{\text{Age (years)}}{2} + 15 \text{ cm (nasal tubes)}.$$

For a normal ful-term neonate (3.0–3.5 kg), the tracheal tube should be advanced to 10 cm, while the appropriate length for a smaller neonate (2–3 kg) is 8–9 cm or 7 cm (<2 kg). From the age of 3 months to a year of age, a length of 11–13 cm will be adequate. Other methods include: insertion of the tracheal tube to a predetermined depth in centimetres equating to three times the internal diameter of the tube in millimetres [9]; deliberate endobronchial intubation followed by withdrawal of the tube 2 cm above the carina [10]; or alignment of the distal tracheal tube marker (usually one or two solid black lines) at the level of the vocal cords [11]. In a prospective study comparing these three methods in 60 infants and children undergoing fluoroscopic procedures, the mainstem method was shown to have the highest rate of appropriate tracheal tube placement [12], although it should be borne in mind that auscultation may fail to detect endobronchial intubation in up to 11.8 per cent of patients [13]. In patients for whom prolonged intubation is required, such as those in an intensive care unit (ICU), a chest X-ray is mandatory.

USE OF CUFFED TUBES IN SMALL CHILDREN

Recently, there has been renewed interest in the use of cuffed tracheal tubes in small infants and children. Concerns associated with the use of uncuffed tubes include: multiple intubations with incorrect sizes, difficult ventilation in patients with poor lung compliance, inaccurate capnography, difficulties with low flow techniques, environmental pollution and the risk of aspiration [14]. The use of a larger tracheal tube in an attempt to limit the air leak and facilitate effective ventilation, may risk laryngotracheal injury. In a French postal survey on the use of cuffed and uncuffed tracheal tubes in infants and children, 25 per cent of respondents routinely used cuffed tracheal tubes for more than 80 per cent of their patients, while 37 per cent used them in less than 20 per cent of cases [15]. A number of publications have suggested that the use of cuffed tubes in small children is safe. In a study of 210 children under the age of 5 years, including 27 neonates, there were no reported problems following intubation with cuffed tubes for a mean period of 13 days [16]. In a prospective, randomised study of 488 children under the age of 8 years undergoing routine general anaesthesia, no differences in postoperative complications were found between those receiving cuffed and those receiving uncuffed tubes [17]. Of interest is the fact that there was a significantly increased incidence of multiple intubation attempts in children receiving uncuffed tubes (23 per cent versus 1.2 per cent). However, it is important to remember that cuffed tubes can cause damage in children. High cuff pressure may result in mucosal damage and stenosis so the use of high-volume, low-pressure cuffs is recommended. Cuff pressure may also change, particularly during nitrous oxide anaesthesia [18]. A revised formula for calculating the appropriate size of a cuffed tracheal tube is:

$$\text{Internal diameter (mm)} = \frac{\text{Age (years)}}{4} + 3.$$

TUBE FIXATION

Cutting tracheal tubes to length requires reinsertion of the connector, which may result in damage to the tube. It is therefore common practice at the authors' institutions to use uncut tubes. It is important that the tube is secured to the patient in such a way that significant movement is not permitted, and that due care is taken to ensure that the length of tube protruding from the mouth does not kink. The authors' preference is to site a Guedel airway alongside the tracheal tube to stabilise it and prevent significant lateral movement. The tracheal tube is then secured by means of two 'trouser-shaped' lengths of strong adhesive tape: one end of each adheres to the tube and the other end to either the mandible or the maxilla. The attached breathing system should then be secured in a tube holder.

TYPES OF TRACHEAL TUBES

The majority of tracheal tubes are made of implant-tested PVC and are available in a range of sizes (internal diameter 2–10 mm). There are now a wide variety of tracheal tubes available for use in children.

Polar (RAE) tracheal tube

The polar or RAE tube, designed by Ring, Adair and Elwyn, has a preformed shape to enable secure fixation to the chin or forehead with the connector well away from the face. They are useful for head and neck surgery, as they do not interfere with operator access. Oral tubes are available in a north-or south-facing pattern. The nasal tube is north facing only and is particularly useful as it allows complete access to the mouth. The main disadvantage is the fixed length of the intraoral or intranasal section, as occasionally the appropriately sized tube is too long, increasing the risk of bronchial intubation. If this happens, the tube should be withdrawn slightly and a dental roll placed underneath at the chin before being secured with strong adhesive tape. The RAE tube has one or two Murphy's eyes (cuffed or uncuffed, respectively) to ensure adequate ventilation should the tube be advanced too far into the trachea or the head is flexed. Polar tubes can be temporarily straightened should a gum elastic bougie or suction catheter need to be used.

Armoured tracheal tube

The armoured tracheal tube is used in neurosurgery, patients in the prone position or for surgical procedures in which there is a lot of head and neck movement. The walls of this tube contain a metal spiral to prevent kinking or occlusion, though it is still vulnerable to kinking at the junction of the tube and connector. As the external diameter is greater than for standard tubes, a tube half a size smaller than calculated should be used. Furthermore, owing to their increased flexibility, a malleable introducer or metal stylet may need to be used to aid intubation.

Cole tracheal tube

Although the Cole tracheal tube is very seldom used in anaesthesia, it is still used in some neonatal units. The tube has a relatively wide intraoral section, which narrows distally so that the appropriate diameter passes through the vocal cords (Fig. 19.3). As the shoulder of the tube rests on the vocal cords, endobronchial intubation is prevented, but damage to the cords can occur should it slip downwards. It can be of value in infants with subglottic stenosis (see Chapter 33).

Laser-resistant tracheal tube

Standard tracheal tubes are not suitable for use in laser airway procedures as they are readily ignited. Metal laser tracheal tubes, designed to withstand the effect of both carbon dioxide and KTP laser beams, are available for single or multiple use down to size 3.0 internal diameter. The cuffed tubes should have their PVC cuffs filled with saline as an air filled cuff may ignite.

TRACHEAL TUBE CONNECTORS AND CATHETER MOUNTS

Although there are a variety of connectors available, male to female 15 mm ISO connectors are now usually used in

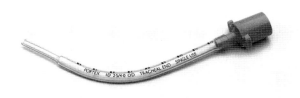

Figure 19.3 'Cole' pattern tracheal tube.

theatre to connect the tracheal tube to the breathing circuit. The male connector attaches to the tracheal tube via a tapered cone, which has a slightly larger diameter than the tube to ensure a snug fit. Before use, the connector should be advanced into the tube slightly to ensure a firm connection. The tracheal tube is connected to the breathing system via a plastic angle piece or catheter mount, which has a female connector with an internal diameter of 15 mm and an outer diameter of 22 mm. The catheter mount provides a flexible link between the breathing system tubing and the facemask, laryngeal mask airway or tracheal tube and minimises the transmission of accidental movements of the breathing system to the tracheal tube. However, this must be balanced against the increase in dead space that the catheter mount contributes. Non-ISO connectors such as the metal Magill connector, often used with nasal tubes in the past, are no longer used at the authors' institutions. Catheter mounts are seldom used in paediatric practice owing to the increase in dead space that they create.

SUCTION CATHETERS

A range of suction catheters should always be available as the narrow lumens of paediatric tracheal tubes may become obstructed. The appropriate size of suction catheter is determined by the following formula [19]:

$$\text{Suction catheter} = 2 \times \text{internal diameter}$$
$$\text{(French size)} \qquad \text{(mm) of tracheal tube}$$

Laryngoscopes and blades

A wide variety of laryngoscope blades are available that differ in both longitudinal shape and cross-section. While choice of a particular blade is largely a matter of personal preference, it is also important to take into consideration the anatomy of the paediatric airway.

STRAIGHT LARYNGOSCOPE BLADES

The large, floppy epiglottis and more cephalad position of the larynx mean that neonates and infants younger than 6 months are easier to intubate using a straight-bladed laryngoscope. The laryngoscope blade is advanced into the mouth as far as possible, lifting the epiglottis directly in the process, and then withdrawn slowly to reveal the laryngeal inlet. This technique may be associated with bradycardia since the straight blade is in contact with the posterior surface of the epiglottis, which is innervated by the vagus nerve. There are a number of straight laryngoscope blades available and personal preference often dictates which blade is used (Fig. 19.4). The Robertshaw and Seward blades are popular since their open cross-sectional profile enables easy intraoral manipulation of a nasal tube. In contrast, the C-shaped cross-section of the Miller laryngoscope blade restricts such manipulation. However, the

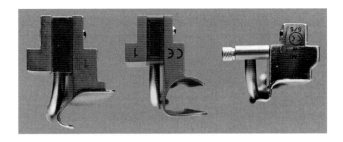

Figure 19.4 A cross-section of straight laryngoscope blades: Robertshaw, Miller, Seward from left to right.

extended curve at the tip of the blade facilitates easy anterior lifting of the epiglottis and this blade remains a popular choice among paediatric anaesthetists. The Magill blade is set at an angle of 10° to the handle and has an open rear profile, while the Anderson–Magill modification has an adjustable hook that facilitates easier manipulation of the handle and allows manipulation of the larynx with the fifth digit of the left hand. The Wisconsin blade has an open U-shaped rear profile, which enhances visualisation of the larynx. The Oxford blade has a slightly curved distal end, a rounded C-shaped cross-section and a flat flange, which makes it very useful in infants with cleft palate.

CURVED LARYNGOSCOPE BLADE (MACINTOSH BLADE)

In infants older than 6 months and children, a curved Macintosh laryngoscope blade should be used. The blade is advanced along the tongue into the vallecula and the laryngoscope then lifted upwards, thereby elevating the epiglottis and exposing the vocal cords. The Macintosh blade is available in five sizes (neonate No. 0, infant No. 1, child No. 2, adult No. 3 and large adult No. 4) and has a bulbous tip to assist in lifting the larynx. A left-sided Macintosh blade is also available for use in children with right-sided facial deformities, such as hemifacial microsomia. Other modifications to the Macintosh laryngoscope include the polio blade which fits to the handle at an obtuse angle (120°) and a shorter 'stubby' handled version, both of which improve access when intubating children with restricted neck mobility or in whom there is limited access to the chest.

SPECIALISED LARYNGOSCOPES

MacCoy laryngoscope

The McCoy laryngoscope was developed in the early 1990s as an aid to difficult intubation in adults. It is based on the standard Macintosh blade but has a hinged tip that is elevated by depressing a lever attached to the handle (see Chapter 21, Fig 21.5). This may be used to elevate a large epiglottis that is obstructing the view of the laryngeal inlet. A paediatric version based on the Seward straight blade is now available for use in infants and children (sizes 1 and 2), though it has not yet been widely studied.

Bullard laryngoscope

The Bullard laryngoscope is a rigid fibre-optic laryngoscope that allows visualisation of the laryngeal inlet without the need for alignment of the oral, pharyngeal, and laryngeal axes. It is particularly useful in patients with limited neck movement or mouth opening, such as those with unstable cervical spine fractures, temporomandibular joint (TMJ) immobility and micrognathia (Pierre Robin syndrome) as it requires minimal head and neck manipulation and only 6 mm of mouth opening [20]. The Bullard laryngoscope is available in both an adult version (patient height >1.5 m) and paediatric size (patient height <1.5 m) (see Chapter 21, Fig 21.7). Recently a laryngoscope for use in infants has been released. A stylet should be used to guide the tracheal tube during orotracheal intubation. This can be the dedicated unmalleable wire stylet attached directly to the laryngoscope or an independent malleable stylet, which is passed through a dedicated channel.

Aids to intubation

GUM ELASTIC BOUGIES

Gum elastic bougies are useful in patients in whom it is difficult to attain a good view of the laryngeal inlet. The bougie is passed through the vocal cords or alternatively posterior to the epiglottis and into the trachea and then a tracheal tube is 'railroaded' over it.

STYLETS/INTRODUCERS

Stylets are composed of malleable metal and can be inserted into a standard tracheal tube to direct the tip through the vocal cords or alternatively can be used to reinforce a flexible tube. It is important that the tip of the stylet does not protrude beyond the end of the tracheal tube as this may result in trauma during intubation.

MAGILL FORCEPS

The Magill forceps have offset handles and are specifically designed for ease of use within the mouth and oropharynx and are available in both small and large sizes. They are particularly useful in directing the tracheal tube through the vocal cords during nasal intubation. Care should be taken not to damage the tracheal tube cuff during this manoeuvre. The Magill forceps may also be used to insert a throat pack and to remove foreign bodies in the oropharynx.

ANAESTHESIA MACHINE

Most paediatric patients can be anaesthetised using the standard adult continuous flow anaesthesia machine. These should be equipped with an antihypoxia device so as to ensure that a minimum of 25 per cent oxygen is delivered at all times. In addition it is important to be able to deliver air in situations in which nitrous oxide or a high-inspired oxygen concentration is undesirable. The anaesthetic machine should be equipped with full monitoring and be checked thoroughly prior to use according to local guidelines.

Breathing systems

The 'ideal' paediatric anaesthetic breathing system should have minimal resistance to gas flow with no valves or very low resistance valves, minimal dead space and minimal gas turbulence [21]. The quest for such a system has resulted in the development of a number of different anaesthetic delivery systems, which have traditionally been classified as being open, semi-open, closed or semi-closed. This classification is not only confusing, but more importantly does not afford a clear understanding of the functional differences between the various breathing systems. A more clinically useful classification divides anaesthetic breathing systems into two broad categories: those that contain a means by which carbon dioxide is absorbed (absorber systems) and those that do not (non-absorber systems). These categories can be subdivided further according to the direction of gas flow within the system into either unidirectional or bidirectional flow systems [22].

NON-ABSORBER BIDIRECTIONAL BREATHING SYSTEMS

Of the non-absorber breathing systems, bidirectional flow systems are the most commonly used in anaesthesia. These breathing systems do not have a CO_2 absorption device and therefore, if rebreathing is to be avoided, the fresh gas flow must be sufficient to flush the expired CO_2 out of the system. Numerous breathing systems are available, each differing in the arrangement of their component parts, particularly with respect to the position of the reservoir bag and adjustable pressure-limiting valve (APL). Mapleson's classification categorises these breathing systems from A to F in order of increasing requirement of fresh gas flow to prevent rebreathing during spontaneous ventilation [23]. These can be subdivided into afferent, efferent and junctional reservoir systems depending on which limb of the breathing system allows for the predominant movement of gas flow.

EFFERENT RESERVOIR BREATHING SYSTEMS

Jackson Rees modification of Ayre's T-piece (Mapleson F)

The most commonly used breathing system in paediatric anaesthesia, especially neonatal and infant anaesthesia, is the Mapleson F system or Jackson Rees modification of the Ayre's T-piece [24] (Fig. 19.5). It may be used in patients up to a weight of 20–25 kg. It differs from the original T-piece by having an open-ended reservoir bag attached to the end

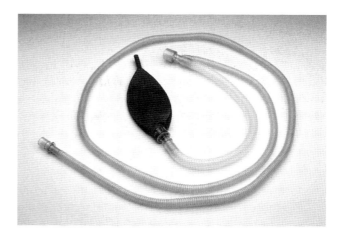

Figure 19.5   Disposable T-piece circuit.

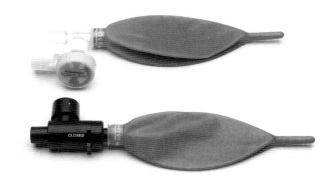

Figure 19.6   Two patterns of T-piece scavenging system.

of an extended expiratory limb. The reservoir bag allows easy observation of spontaneous breathing and the means to deliver controlled ventilation. It may also be partly occluded to apply continuous positive airway pressure (CPAP) or removed and the T-piece connected to a mechanical ventilator. Although the Jackson Rees T-piece approximates closely to the 'ideal' paediatric breathing system in being lightweight and having a low-volume, low-resistance expiratory limb with no valves, there are some drawbacks. One is the difficulty in scavenging anaesthetic gases from the open reservoir bag during spontaneous ventilation, though this can be effected using a specially made valve (Fig. 19.6). This is a lightweight, low-resistance device with an adjustable thumb control to allow spontaneous or controlled ventilation and is used with a closed-tail reservoir bag and either an active or a passive gas-scavenging system. As the T-piece has no pressure relief valve itself, there is a risk of high pressure developing within the system when the valve is fully closed. However, at gas flows of less than 6 L/min, a pinhole in the inner valve limits the build up of pressure to below 30 cmH_2O. Another drawback of the Jackson Rees T-piece and the Mapleson D and E systems is their relative inefficiency during spontaneous ventilation, requiring high fresh gas flows in order to avoid rebreathing. A number of factors determine the composition of gases in the expiratory limb, and therefore the gas mixture of the next inspiration. These include CO_2 production (which is related to both the size and metabolic status of the patient), respiratory rate and pattern, tidal volume, expiratory reservoir volume and fresh gas flow. If the expiratory pause is too short or indeed absent, as is the case with small infants during rapid spontaneous breathing, there is insufficient time for the fresh gas to flush out alveolar gas from the expiratory limb before the next breath unless the fresh gas flow is increased. Similarly, if the tidal volume increases, the increased volume of alveolar gas reaching the expiratory limb will result in rebreathing unless there is a sufficient expiratory pause or else an increase in the fresh gas flow. The volume of the expiratory limb must also exceed the patient's tidal volume. If the fresh gas flow is too low, rebreathing will increase with respiratory rate, though the $PaCO_2$ initially remains stable despite an increase in the minute ventilation [25]. There are a number of formulae that can be used to determine the minimum fresh gas flow required to avoid rebreathing during spontaneous and controlled ventilation (Table 19.2); however, the safest and most accurate is to continuously monitoring the end-tidal CO_2. It should be borne in mind that in small infants, particularly those less than 8 kg, end-tidal CO_2 measurements may be underestimated when they are ventilated with a T-piece owing to dilution of expired gases by fresh gas [26]. As is evident from Table 19.2, the Jackson Rees T-piece is more efficient for controlled ventilation.

BAIN BREATHING SYSTEM (MAPLESON D)

The Bain breathing system is a coaxial form of the Mapleson D system. Fresh gas flows through an inner tube to the patient end of the breathing system while exhaled gases are conveyed to the reservoir bag and expiratory valve at the machine end of the breathing system via an outer corrugated tube, where they are easily scavenged. The reservoir bag may be removed and the system connected to a ventilator such as the Penlon Nuffield anaesthesia ventilator. The inner tube should be inspected carefully before use to ensure that it is not disconnected at the proximal end of the breathing system or excessive rebreathing will result. As the fresh gas is delivered to the patient end of the breathing circuit, the length of coaxial tubing can be varied without affecting the physical properties of the system. Bain breathing systems with longer coaxial tubing are available for use in head and neck surgery as well as in the MRI suite where the anaesthetic machine needs to remain outside the magnetic field. The Bain breathing system is relatively inefficient during spontaneous ventilation and high fresh gas flows of at least two to three times the minute ventilation are required in order to avoid significant rebreathing. It is not suitable for spontaneous ventilation in children weighing less than 20 kg owing to the resistance of the expiratory valve. The system is much more efficient during controlled ventilation where normocapnia may be achieved with a fresh gas flow of only 70 mL/kg/min however, it should not be used for controlled ventilation in infants because of the high compliance of the expiratory limb compared with the relatively small tidal volumes.

Afferent reservoir breathing systems

MAPLESON A BREATHING SYSTEM (MAGILL AND LACK SYSTEMS)

The Mapleson A or Magill breathing system, while no longer in common use in the UK, deserves brief mention as the enclosed version of the system still has its proponents. The system consists of a reservoir bag at the machine end of the breathing system, a length of corrugated tubing and an APL at the patient end of the breathing system. It is particularly efficient during spontaneous ventilation, requiring a fresh gas flow of only 0.7–1.0 times the patient's minute ventilation to avoid rebreathing. However, it is inefficient when used for controlled ventilation and high fresh gas flows of at least twice the patient's minute ventilation are required in order to avoid rebreathing. The close proximity of the position of the APL to the patient's face is cumbersome and makes scavenging difficult. The Lack modification of the Magill system has the valve positioned at the machine end of the breathing system, making scavenging easy, and is available in coaxial and parallel format. The Magill breathing system is not suitable for children less than 20 kg because of the large apparatus dead space and resistance of the APL.

Table 19.2 Fresh gas flows required with the Jackson Rees T-piece to avoid rebreathing during spontaneous and controlled ventilation

Type of ventilation	Weight (kg)	FGF (mL)	Minimum FGF (L)	Minute ventilation (mL/kg/min)	Reference
Spontaneous	10–30	1000 + 100 mL/kg	–	–	27
Spontaneous		15 × respiratory rate (/min) × weight (kg)	–	–	28
Controlled	10–30	1000 + 100 mL/kg	3.0	1.5 × FGF	27
Controlled	3–20	1000 + 200 mL/kg	–	200	29

FGF, fresh gas flow.

Enclosed afferent reservoir breathing system

The enclosed afferent reservoir (EAR) breathing system is the most efficient non-absorber breathing system. It is essentially a Mapleson A system enclosed within a plastic container and consists of a set of bellows on the afferent limb of the breathing system and a one-way valve on the expiratory limb, which is linked to the container. During spontaneous ventilation, the EAR behaves like a Magill system. Controlled ventilation is achieved by increasing the pressure within the container and compressing the bellows, while at the same time closing the expiratory valve to avoid venting fresh gas as occurs with the standard Magill system. Meakin and colleagues have shown that, in children over 10 kg, the EAR is highly efficient in both spontaneous and controlled ventilation, owing to conservation of dead space gas. A fresh gas flow equal to normal alveolar ventilation ($0.6 \times \sqrt{\text{weight [kg]}}$ in L/min) was shown to be adequate for either mode of ventilation [30]. This is a third less than the fresh gas flow required when using a T-piece.

Hybrid systems

HUMPHREY ADE BREATHING SYSTEM

The Humphrey ADE system is a hybrid system incorporating the Mapleson A, D and E systems. It consists of parallel breathing hoses connected to the fresh gas flow outlet of the anaesthesia machine via a manifold, a reservoir bag and an APL. A lever on the manifold can be used to convert the system from the Mapleson A (Lack modification) to the D/E (Bain type) system, so that it can be used for spontaneous ventilation with the Mapleson A system (lever up) and for controlled ventilation with the D/E mode (lever down) using a ventilator such as the Penlon Nuffield anaesthetic ventilator. Although a paediatric version of this system has been evaluated in children [31], it has not established itself in paediatric anaesthetic practice.

Absorber unidirectional breathing systems

CIRCLE ABSORPTION BREATHING SYSTEM

Low-flow anaesthesia using carbon dioxide absorption is now widely used in paediatric anaesthetic practice and is the subject of a number of comprehensive reviews [32,33]. The advantages include conservation of heat and moisture, decreased anaesthetic gas consumption and reduced operating theatre pollution compared with non-absorber breathing systems. It also facilitates the use of standardised equipment, as the adult circle system, fitted with flexible lightweight 15-mm diameter tubing and a smaller reservoir bag, is suitable for paediatric patients of all ages. Initial concerns about the safety of low-flow anaesthesia, namely accidental hypoxia, underdosage or overdosage of volatile

agents and hypercapnia as a result of soda lime exhaustion, have largely been eliminated following the mandatory use of oxygen saturation and volatile agent monitors. Compound A, a degradation product of sevoflurane resulting from its reaction with carbon dioxide absorbents, may accumulate in the circle. While this compound is nephrotoxic in rats, the same effect has not been demonstrated in clinical practice [32]. However, as the concentration of compound A in absorber breathing systems increases with decreased fresh gas flow, the Food and Drug Administration (FDA) of the USA has recommended that a minimum fresh gas flow of 2 L/min be used with sevoflurane [34]. Other concerns regarding the use of absorber breathing systems, particularly in small children, relate to the potential for increased resistance to breathing and leaks in the breathing system. However, the work of breathing imposed by the paediatric circle system in spontaneously breathing children aged 2–6 years was found to be no different to that of the Bain or Jackson Rees system [35]. As with other breathing systems, ventilation should ideally be controlled when the circle system is used in small infants and neonates. Leaks in the breathing system may be associated with the use of uncuffed tracheal tubes in children. Although the airway sealing afforded by both uncuffed tracheal tubes and laryngeal mask airways has been shown to be adequate for low-flow anaesthesia in children [36], significantly lower flow rates were achieved with a laryngeal mask airway or cuffed tracheal tube compared with an uncuffed tracheal tube in children undergoing pressure-controlled ventilation [37].

Humidifiers

Heat and moisture exchangers (HMEs) are now routinely used in paediatric anaesthesia. They not only protect the patient from inhaling infective or hazardous particles and prevent cross-contamination when the breathing system is used for more than one patient, but also warm and humidify the inspired anaesthetic and respiratory gases. This is important to prevent adverse changes in the upper airways and possible pulmonary complications resulting from thick secretions. Neonates and infants have an even greater need for the benefits of an HME filter than do older children and adults. They may be more susceptible to nosocomial pneumonias and other infections, and they also lose heat more rapidly from the inhalation of dry gases as their minute ventilation to body surface area is twice that of adults [38]. The use of filters in this group of patients has been the subject of a recent review [39].

The filtration efficiency of paediatric breathing system filters has recently been brought into question following an evaluation of neonatal, paediatric and adult breathing system filters that suggested that paediatric filters may allow greater penetrance than the equivalent adult models at preset flow rates [40]. However, the Association of Paediatric Anaesthetists of Great Britain and Ireland (APAGBI) has pointed out that the flow rate used in these tests

(15 L/min) is proportionately much greater than that used to test adult filters (30 L/min) and has therefore suggested that the tests be repeated using lower, more representative flow rates. This testing demonstrated that penetrance levels are much closer to those for adult filters [41] under these conditions, although the optimum performance remains unknown.

With regard to humidification, it has been shown that, in infants ventilated with a circle system, passive airway humidification with an HME filter resulted in an initial relative humidity of 45 per cent, a level close to the minimum threshold of 50 per cent that is reported to preserve ciliary function. In this study, the relative humidity increased to approximately 80 per cent after 1 hour of anaesthesia, a level similar to the 90 per cent achieved in patients receiving active airway humidification and warming [42].

Although paediatric breathing system filters have been designed to have as small a dead space and low a resistance as possible, problems may arise particularly when they are used for neonates and small infants. Paediatric filters offer greater resistance to gas flow than adult ones, as measured by the pressure drop across the filter at a set flow rate [40]. The increased resistance will also add positive end-expiratory pressure to the breathing system and may go on to cause obstruction if they become occluded with secretions. Tracheal tubes, catheter mounts, angle pieces and other components of the breathing circuit may also add resistance; the calculated resistance of a paediatric HME filter, however, is markedly lower than that of a paediatric tracheal tube [43]. As neonates and infants are usually intubated and ventilated during general anaesthesia, the ventilator compensates for the increased airway resistance.

Anaesthesia ventilators

Intermittent positive pressure ventilation is commonly used in paediatric anaesthesia and can be delivered either manually or by mechanical means.

MANUAL VENTILATION

The ability to hand ventilate neonates and infants by means of a T-piece circuit is an essential skill in paediatric anaesthesia. In experienced hands, important information may be gained with regard to changes in lung compliance as well as to mechanical problems such as disconnection or occlusion. It is particularly useful during surgical procedures such as neonatal tracheoesophageal fistula repair, where sudden changes in pulmonary compliance can be compensated for and surgical access to the fistula can be optimised, with intermittent lung inflation. Controlled manual ventilation should not be used as the only form of respiratory monitoring as even experienced paediatric anaesthetists may not be able reliably to detect changes in pulmonary compliance in neonates when using the feel of the reservoir bag alone [44].

MECHANICAL VENTILATION

The majority of children can be ventilated using standard adult anaesthetic ventilators provided that they are equipped with paediatric breathing system tubing and appropriate adjustments to the ventilatory parameters are made prior to the initiation of controlled ventilation. Ideally, a paediatric anaesthesia ventilator should have the following characteristics:

- ability to deliver volume-and pressure-controlled ventilation
- easy to change from controlled to manual ventilation
- compatible with circle breathing system
- ability to deliver small tidal volumes
- ability to deliver rapid respiratory rates
- ability to deliver variable positive end-expiratory pressure (PEEP)
- ability to deliver variable inspiratory flow rates and I:E ratio
- ability to deliver an oxygen: air mixture
- accurate pressure and volume monitoring and alarms including oxygen concentration and disconnect alarms.

Although there are numerous classifications for mechanical ventilators, in the simplest terms they can act as either pressure or flow generators. Flow generators deliver a predetermined inspiratory tidal volume irrespective of the inspiratory pressure, while pressure generators deliver a predetermined inspiratory pressure and are therefore able to compensate for leaks in the breathing system. In paediatric anaesthesia, pressure-controlled ventilation is usually the preferred mode of ventilation as there is often a leak around the tracheal tube and the risk of barotrauma is reduced. For ease of description it is convenient to classify the ventilators commonly used in paediatric anaesthesia according to the principles upon which they work: 'mechanical thumbs', 'intermittent blowers' and 'bag squeezers'.

Mechanical thumbs

The intermittent occlusion of the expiratory limb of a T-piece forms the basis of T-piece occluder or 'mechanical thumb' ventilators such as the Sechrist, Babylog and Bear Cub. The ventilator is connected to the expiratory limb of the T-piece with fresh gas flow being delivered into the breathing system in the usual manner. As the fresh gas flow must equal the inspiratory rate, this mode of ventilation is very wasteful of fresh gas in large patients and its use should therefore be restricted to children weighing less than 20 kg [45].

Intermittent blowers: Penlon Nuffield 200 ventilator

Despite the increased use of more sophisticated microprocessor-controlled anaesthesia ventilators, 'intermittent blowers' such as the Penlon Nuffield 200 are still used in paediatric practice. This is due in part to its ease of use and compatibility with the T-piece, Bain and circle breathing systems. The Penlon Nuffield 200 ventilator is driven by compressed gas, either oxygen or air, which is independent of the fresh gas flow. The control module, which directs the flow of driving gas into the patient valve, consists of an airway pressure gauge, independent inspiratory and expiratory time dials, inspiratory flow control dial and an on–off switch. The patient valve has a spring-loaded piston with a ventilator connection, a port for tubing to connect to the breathing system reservoir bag mount and an exhaust port. With the unmodified patient valve connected, the Penlon Nuffield 200 functions as a flow generator. The tidal volume is determined by the inspiratory flow rate (0.25 and 1.0 L/second) and the inspiratory time, while the respiratory rate can be varied from 10 to 85 breaths per minute by altering the inspiratory:expiratory times. As it is not possible to reduce the inspiratory flow rates to a level low enough to generate appropriately small tidal volumes for infants and young children, the Penlon Nuffield 200 ventilator in its unmodified form should not be used to ventilate children weighing less than 25 kg. In patients above this weight, the Penlon Nuffield 200 ventilator is usually used in conjunction with a Bain or circle breathing system.

When the standard valve is replaced by a Newton valve, the Penlon Nuffield 200 ventilator is converted from a flow generator to a pressure generator and is suitable for use in neonates and infants. The Newton valve consists of a ventilator connection, patient connection and fixed orifice gas outlet. It therefore acts simply as a fixed leak allowing some of the inspiratory flow to go to the patient while venting the remainder through the fixed orifice. The modified ventilator is used in conjunction with the T-piece breathing system, the ventilator being connected to the expiratory limb of the T-piece in place of the reservoir bag. It is important that the inspiratory flow dial is on the lowest setting (0.25 L/s) before connecting the ventilator to the T-piece so as to avoid the possibility of inadvertent barotrauma. Once connected, the inspiratory flow can then be increased until adequate chest movement, and thus tidal volume, is obtained. As the flow rate selected is no longer the flow rate delivered to the patient, as is the case with a standard valve, the tidal volume can no longer be calculated from the flow and inspiratory time settings. The modified Penlon Nuffield 200 ventilator is capable of delivering tidal volumes of between 10 and 300 mL at frequencies of 10–85 breaths per minute. The inspiratory pressure is shown on the airway pressure gauge and should ideally be less than 20 cmH$_2$O. A PEEP valve may be added to the gas outlet, with the level of PEEP being indicated on the pressure gauge.

The Penlon Nuffield 200 ventilator with Newton valve does have a number of disadvantages, however. As the ventilator functions as a pressure generator, the peak inspiratory pressure may not change when lung compliance decreases or there is occlusion of the breathing system. Furthermore, the ventilator sound remains unchanged with disconnection or occlusion of the breathing system. Low levels of PEEP are generated which may become significant when high inspiratory flows are used in larger children. As the driving gas may dilute the anaesthetic gases, it is important that the tubing connecting the ventilator to the breathing system is at least 90 cm long [46]. Having a driving gas that is separate from the fresh gas flow may also lead to a situation where satisfactory chest movement is achieved with no fresh gas flowing. As the modified Penlon Nuffield 200 ventilator has no inbuilt alarms, continuous monitoring of ventilation by means of chest movement, capnography and pulse oximetry is mandatory.

Bag squeezers

'Bag squeezers' or bellows-type ventilators are commonly used in conjunction with a circle breathing system and may be either pneumatic or mechanical. Pneumatic 'bag squeezers', such as the Servo 900 series and Ohmeda 7900 ventilators, use a separate gas supply to provide the driving pressure needed to compress the reservoir bag ('bag-in-a-bottle') or bellows of the breathing system, while mechanical 'bag squeezers' use a motor or piston to drive the bellows. When using some 'bag squeezer' ventilators, it is important to appreciate the effect alterations in fresh gas flow may have on the delivered tidal volume during volume-controlled ventilation. Fresh gas entering the breathing system during the inspiratory phase of respiration is added to the tidal volume delivered by the ventilator bellows and therefore makes a contribution to the total minute ventilation. As a result, the delivered minute ventilation may be altered without changing the ventilator settings. This effect has been shown to be greater in small children, some patients experiencing a 40 per cent difference in delivered minute ventilation when the fresh gas flow was changed from 1.5 L/minute to 6.0 L/minute, without any change in the ventilator settings [47]. This effect does not occur during pressure-controlled ventilation as the excess fresh gas flow is vented through the pop-off valve.

Electronically controlled ventilators

Microprocessor-based, electronically controlled 'bag squeezers' are now commonly used in paediatric anaesthesia. In addition to volume and pressure control ventilation, many of the newer anaesthesia ventilators are also capable of more sophisticated modes of ventilation such as synchronised intermittent mandatory ventilation (SIMV) with pressure support and pressure support with apnoea backup. Furthermore, as most have an integrated compensatory mechanism, consistent delivery of set tidal volumes is ensured. This is achieved by automatically adjusting for changes in fresh gas flows and small leaks in the breathing system, changing lung compliance or compression losses in the ventilator, absorber and bellows. This eliminates the effect a change of fresh gas flow has on minute ventilation as described above.

Vascular access

PERIPHERAL INTRAVENOUS CANNULAE

Non-tapered Teflon or polyurethane over-the-needle cannulae are available in a range of designs and gauges. Some

Table 19.3 Peripheral venous cannulae

Gauge of cannula (G)	Maximum flow (mL/h)
24	13
22	31
20	54
18	80
16	180
14	270

have a spring mechanism that retracts the needle into a plastic barrel once the vein is cannulated in order to prevent needle-stick injury. A 22G cannula is sufficient for most infants and children for fluid and drug administration, although a 24G cannula may be more appropriate in premature neonates and in those with difficult venous access. Larger cannulae should be inserted into children in whom significant blood loss is anticipated in order to facilitate the rapid transfusion of fluid (Table 19.3). In all but minor surgical cases, it is wise to secure two venous access sites, particularly if one is suboptimal. One of these may then be used postoperatively as a dedicated peripheral line for patient-controlled analgesia (PCA) or nurse-controlled analgesia (NCA) drug administration. The techniques and preferred sites for venous access are described later in this chapter.

INTRAOSSEOUS NEEDLE

The intraosseous route provides rapid, safe and effective vascular access during paediatric resuscitation or, during anaesthesia, when peripheral access is not available. Purpose-made intraosseous needles are available in sizes 18G (0–6 months), 16G and 14G. The common feature is a trocar to prevent plugging of the lumen with bone. Standard bone marrow aspiration needles can also be used. It is usual to position the needle manually, applying pressure with an oscillating motion but bone injection guns are available that 'fire' the needle directly into the bone. There is very little experience of these in children.

PERIOPERATIVE TEMPERATURE CONTROL

The maintenance of normothermia is an important consideration in paediatric anaesthesia. Hypothermia increases oxygen consumption by non-shivering thermogenesis in neonates and infants and shivering in children, it increases sympathetic stimulation, impairs immune function, delays wound healing, impairs coagulation, reduces platelet function, increases acidosis, blood loss and transfusion requirements, and decreases drug metabolism [48]. Although mild hypothermia (core temperature 34–36°C) has not been shown to impair respiratory function or post-anaesthetic recovery in healthy infants and children undergoing minor

surgery [49], the situation may be different in patients who are unwell or in those undergoing major surgery.

Measurement of core body temperature

Core body temperature should be monitored continuously during anaesthesia in children. This is important not only to prevent intraoperative hypothermia but also to avoid hyperthermia in those patients who are being actively heated. While core body temperature may be measured at a number of sites, nasopharyngeal temperature is the most commonly used. This approximates to brain temperature but may underestimate core temperature in the presence of a significant leak around the tracheal tube. Rectal temperature probes may also be used, but these tend to be inaccurate in the presence of faeces. Oesophageal and bladder temperature measurement are other options but are less commonly used intraoperatively. In addition to core body temperature monitoring, the measurement of skin temperature may be useful in providing information about peripheral perfusion during major surgery by means of the core–peripheral temperature difference. In recovery, intermittent temperature measurement is commonly performed using cutaneous chemical colorimetric or infrared tympanic membrane thermometers.

Maintaining core body temperature

Radiation loss from the skin is the main source of heat loss during surgery and may be reduced significantly by increasing the ambient temperature. The extent to which this is required depends on the age of the patient as the thermo-neutral environment (ambient temperature at which there is no increased oxygen consumption in order to maintain body temperature) is considerably higher in neonates and infants compared with older children (26°C and 21°C, respectively). Instead of increasing the ambient temperature in the operating room to the point where the working environment may become unbearable, the room temperature is often maintained at about 21°C and efforts concentrated instead on warming the patient's microenvironment. Another important consideration is the avoidance of unnecessary patient exposure. In particular, the relatively large head of infants represents a large surface area for heat loss and should therefore be covered if at all possible. Any form of covering can reduce radiant and convective heat losses; the material used appears to be less important than the total area of skin covered [50]. A number of active warming devices may also be used.

OVERHEAD RADIANT WARMERS

Overhead radiant heaters with servomechanism temperature control may be used during induction of anaesthesia and surgical preparation as well as for warming up small infants postoperatively. In order to avoid thermal injury it is important that the heater is at an appropriate distance from the patient, the control sensor is always applied to the warmed skin and that a maximum temperature of 37°C is used.

WARMING MATTRESS

Warming mattresses may use either warm air or warm water to reduce conductive heat loss. The latter have been shown to be effective in maintaining normothermia in patients with a body surface area of 0.5 m² or less than 10 kg body weight [51]. However, they are less effective in older children as the decreasing ratio of body surface area to body weight in older children makes the transfer of heat inefficient at safe temperatures. For the same reason, they are ineffective for rewarming a patient. When using a warming mattress, the temperature should not exceed 39°C and direct contact between the patient and mattress avoided by ensuring that a sheet is interposed between the two.

FORCED-AIR WARMING SYSTEM

The most effective and widely accepted active patient warming device is the forced-air convective warming system. This system relies on filtered warm air being blown into a specialised disposable perforated cover, which remains in direct contact with exposed skin. These covers are available in a variety of shapes and sizes and are supplied with two plastic drapes, which may be used to reduce evaporative heat losses. The forced-air warming system has been shown to be more effective than circulating-water mattresses in preventing hypothermia in young children undergoing major surgery [52]. These devices are also effective when only a portion of the body surface area can be covered [53]. So effective is the forced-air warming system that continuous monitoring of temperature is required in order to avoid hyperthermia. These devices should not be used without a cover as blowing hot air directly onto the patient under the surgical drapes may result in injury.

AIRWAY HEATING AND HUMIDIFICATION

The importance of providing warmed humidified anaesthetic gases to paediatric patients through the use of an HME filter has been discussed previously. However, it is worth emphasising that, as 75 per cent of respiratory heat loss results from the high latent heat of vaporisation of water, humidification of inspired gases is more important than warming them [54].

FLUID WARMERS

Heat loss due to the administration of cold intravenous fluids or blood transfusions may be prevented by using an intravenous warming device. Conventional fluid warmers are not very efficient in children because at slow infusion rates the warmed fluid cools down to room temperature as heat is lost along the length of intravenous tubing between the warmer and the patient. This problem has been largely overcome by new inline countercurrent heat exchange fluid warming systems such as the Level 1 Hotline (Smiths Medical International Ltd), in which warm water circulates around the delivery line thereby eliminating patient line cool down. The Hotline has been shown to be particularly effective in warming fluids at low flow rates but is able to deliver normothermic fluids at rates ranging from 50 to 6000 mL/hour for saline to 50–6000 mL/hour for blood [55]. The coaxial fluid warming system has also been shown to be more effective in warming the small volumes of albumin and blood that are needed during neonatal surgery, than either immersion in a water bath at 37°C or placing prefilled syringes between a circulating water mattress and a forced-air warming blanket [56]. As there is a danger of air embolism due to microbubble formation resulting from the decreased solubility of gases in warmed fluid, a gas eliminator may be added to the patient end of the Hotline fluid warmer. In view of the fact that the disposable tubing is expensive, this system is only cost-effective if relatively large volumes of fluid are being administered at low flow rates to small children.

BASIC TECHNIQUES

Equipment preparation and planning

The preparation of drugs and equipment (see above) requires knowledge of the child's age and weight. All children should be weighed; where this is not possible the formula weight (kg) = (age + 4) × 2 can be used for patients aged 1–7 years, although this underestimates the weight of most children in the developed world. Drug distribution, however, is dependent on lean body mass and the formula can be useful to estimate this in obese children. It is useful to have a rough mental estimate of the child's likely weight, as mistakes can occur, for example weight may be recorded in the wrong units. In emergency situations where weighing may not be available a tape measure can be used to estimate the patient's height, from which a weight can be calculated.

Before commencing anaesthesia, the anaesthetist should prepare drugs and equipment for the patient and check both emergency equipment and drugs. Doses of emergency drugs should be calculated in advance, as it is easy to make errors in acute situations. Alternatively, for single cases, emergency drugs (suxamethonium and atropine) may be pre-prepared on an individual weight basis. Ephedrine is not a standard emergency drug in paediatric anaesthesia.

The nature of the proposed procedure should be discussed with the operator as it is impossible to provide good quality anaesthesia and operating conditions without a thorough understanding of the forthcoming intervention.

The anaesthesia plan should be discussed with the anaesthetic assistant. An appropriately sized tracheal tube and suitable laryngoscope should always be available no matter which method of airway management is proposed. A final check of fasting, consent and patient identification should be made just prior to induction.

Induction of anaesthesia

Two methods of induction are predominantly used in children: intravenous or inhalational. Intramuscular ketamine or rectal thiopental induction may also be used but these techniques are usually reserved for special situations and will not be discussed further.

COMPARISON BETWEEN INHALATIONAL AND INTRAVENOUS TECHNIQUES

Both types of induction are satisfactory and will depend on patient preference; however, institutional preferences and the anaesthetist's training and experience will also influence the choice. Where possible patients should be offered a choice of technique, informed by demonstrations from a play specialist. Some patients state a clear preference for one or the other, but they should not be asked to make an immediate decision. A calm discussion between the child and parent while waiting to be called to theatre allows the patient to engage, make a decision and present their choice to the anaesthetist on arrival in theatre. Positive engagement 'it's my choice' makes induction easier as the child feels control over their destiny at this difficult time. Sometimes a 'needle-phobic' patient is actually afraid of everything but will focus on the needle initially. They can become agitated before induction even though they appeared to be willing to cooperate during discussion on the ward. Although there may be a higher incidence of anxiety during cannulation for intravenous induction, the difference is not measurable by the time of recovery [57]. Furthermore, postoperative behavioural disturbance may not be related to apparent anxiety at induction and one study has shown more negative recollections of entire hospital treatment in those who had inhalational compared with intravenous induction, even when the induction appeared smooth [58].

The incidence of hypoxia is less in inhalational induction (not surprisingly as O_2 is being administered) but there is no initial intravenous (IV) access for drug administration. Vascular access requires two anaesthetists or a highly skilled assistant so that one can manage the airway while the other gains intravenous access. Alternatively, definitive airway management takes place without vascular access; should laryngospasm occur in this circumstance intramuscular or intraosseous drugs would have to be given – not an ideal situation. For anxious patients it can be useful to obtain venous access on the ward as this separates the cannulation from the induction of anaesthesia.

In any location, successful intravenous access cannot always be achieved on the first or even subsequent attempts and inhalational induction may then be necessary. It is important not to make too many attempts before deciding to change techniques

In some circumstances the clinical picture will influence the choice of induction (e.g. inhalational for a difficult airway or intravenous for rapid sequence induction). It is important that paediatric anaesthetists should become skilled in both techniques and choose the one that suits the individual patient and situation.

INHALATIONAL INDUCTION

Sevoflurane

The agent used most commonly in the developed world for inhalational induction is sevoflurane. An overpressure technique is commonly used; sevoflurane 8 per cent is administered to the child via the anaesthesia circuit and facemask. It is non-irritant to the airway and is said to be sweet smelling [59]. Alternatively, it can be incrementally increased by 1 per cent every few breaths. Unless there is a contraindication, N_2O in O_2 is used as the carrier gas as this will speed induction. Apnoea may occur following sevoflurane induction but it has been shown that even with apnoea or total airway obstruction the patient may lighten because of redistribution of sevoflurane [60]. This feature combined with lack of airway irritation and cardiovascular stability make sevoflurane a suitable choice for induction of anaesthesia in those with a suspected difficult or partially obstructed airway.

A single vital capacity breath technique may also be used from about the age of 5 years. The child must exhale completely to their residual capacity then take a full breath from a circuit primed with 8 per cent sevoflurane in N_2O and O_2. They must then hold their breath. This technique has been described as providing the fastest time of induction with sevoflurane in patients pre-medicated with midazolam [61].

Halothane

Halothane use has diminished in the developed world. However, worldwide its long safety record and economic advantage mean that it is still commonly used. Some promote its use for the management of difficult airways in small babies where it can provide excellent conditions for airway examination (see Chapter 33). The pharmacology of volatile agents is discussed in detail in Chapter 10.

INTRAVENOUS INDUCTION

For a detailed description of IV induction agents see Chapter 11.

Propofol is the most commonly used drug for intravenous induction in children who require much higher doses than adults; 3–5 mg/kg is needed to permit safe insertion of an LMA. In addition, its rapid redistribution in children means that it needs to be given more rapidly than in adults. Induction is rapid and smooth although there can be involuntary movements. The main disadvantage is

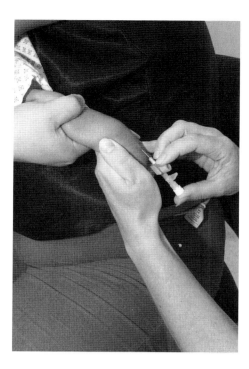

Figure 19.7   Cannulation of a hand vein with child on parent's lap.

pain on injection, which is reduced but not abolished in the lipid formulations. Many methods are described for reducing pain on injection but the addition of lidocaine to the syringe or pretreatment with lidocaine are the most widely adopted.

Thiopental is also suitable for intravenous induction, although its use has declined. The principal advantages are smooth induction and absence of pain on injection, which is particularly relevant when injecting through established small cannulae. Recovery is slightly delayed when compared with propofol but this is less noticeable in young children and procedures lasting over an hour [62].

Positioning for induction

Healthy children of a suitable weight to be lifted once unconscious (less than about 20 kg) can be induced on their parent's lap. Children and parents feel secure during this method of induction but the parents need to be prepared for both the rapidity of the onset of anaesthesia and the speed required to move the child onto the trolley. This position is particularly useful for gaining intravenous access (Fig. 19.7) and anaesthesia can be induced following cannulation in the same position. Most children will readily accept a pulse oximeter before anaesthesia (indeed, many are intrigued by it). Ideally, the electrocardiogram (ECG) and blood pressure (BP) cuff should also be applied but, if the child is anxious, it can be simpler to add them as soon as they are asleep.

Inhalational induction can also be performed with the patient on the parent's lap. A clear facemask can be used as described above or alternatively the anaesthetist can administer the gases using their cupped hand as a shaped

facemask. If, as is usual in this technique, the circuit is a T-piece and a filter is used, it is important to occlude the tail of the bag to prevent the gases being diverted down the expiratory limb. This technique results in more environmental pollution but can be useful for more frightened patients.

Older cooperative children may prefer to breathe 70 per cent nitrous oxide through a close-fitting mask for a few minutes, prior to the introduction of a volatile agent, as it is odourless and provides good sedation.

Throughout induction, the parent should be encouraged to talk to and reassure their child. In some institutions the play specialists will accompany patients to theatre and they can be very useful for helping with distraction techniques. Communication on the ward beforehand about the play specialist's contribution will avoid conflicts and avoid misleading information being given to patients.

Immediately following induction and placing the child horizontal, the parent should be encouraged to leave the anaesthetic environment. They should be given reassurance by dedicated staff (who should remain with them for a short while) as many find the process very distressing. Try to avoid phrases such as 'say goodbye' – particularly if the surgery is major. A better choice is 'you can leave now and we'll look after him or her for you'. Parents are reassured by being given an approximate time for the whole procedure (induction to recovery in the post-anaesthesia care unit [PACU], an overestimate is wise as anxiety occurs when it takes longer than originally thought.

Airway management

Good airway management is central to the safe conduct of paediatric anaesthesia. Critical incidents in paediatric anaesthesia continue to be caused by difficulties with airway management despite the low incidence of unanticipated airway difficulty. Adverse respiratory events have been shown to be related more to experience of staff, type of surgery (e.g. ear, nose and throat procedures) and airway management and commonly occur in ASA 1 and 2 patients. Critical incidents due to airway difficulties are usually said to be more common in infants but one study showed increased risk up to 6 years of age [63].

AIRWAY OPENING MANOEUVRES AND SKILLS

Positioning

Children less than 3 years of age will be maintained in the neutral position more easily without a pillow. In infants or neonates a small head-ring may help keep the head in the neutral position. A shoulder roll may be required in addition to a head ring in neonates with protuberant occiputs.

When applying a facemask to the paediatric patient great care must be taken not to compress the soft tissues under the chin, at the floor of the mouth. Pressure here will push the tongue upwards onto the palate and exacerbate airway obstruction. Very little force is required to maintain a child's airway; more important is distending pressure provided with a well-fitting mask. Care with this manoeuvre will provide a patent airway in most children under anaesthesia.

A jaw thrust is a most effective manoeuvre to open the structures at the back of the pharynx but it requires two people to manage the airway: one to hold the jaw and the mask and the other to ventilate (if required) and operate the anaesthetic machine. Lateral positioning of the child may also help [64].

Use of airway adjuncts

The infant tongue commonly 'sticks' to the roof of the mouth and an oropharyngeal airway will clear this and reproduce the airway opening manoeuvres described above. They should be inserted with care in smaller children to avoid damage to the oropharynx or tonsils; they are not tolerated at light planes of anaesthesia. Nasopharyngeal airways are not routinely used in paediatric practice but can be usefully left *in situ* during emergence in children with obstructive sleep apnoea.

Facemask anaesthesia

Modern cushion masks can be used very satisfactorily for short cases. There is a tendency to use laryngeal masks for all cases to free up the anaesthetist's hands. It should be remembered that this practice may increase airway complications [63].

Laryngeal mask airways

Laryngeal mask airways have revolutionised both adult and paediatric anaesthesia since their introduction to clinical practice in the late 1980s and provide good airway management for a wide variety of clinical situations. There is an increased incidence of complications with the use of sizes 1 and 1.5 but this age group has a higher risk of airway difficulties with any technique. For all but the shortest cases a tracheal tube is likely to provide a more secure airway in children less than 10 kg.

Adequate depth of anaesthesia should be confirmed before insertion by checking that the jaw is relaxed and the pupils small and central. Induction of anaesthesia with a bolus dose of propofol 4 mg/kg allows rapid insertion.

The manufacturer's instruction for insertion of the classic LMA is to have the cuff fully deflated and introduce the mask without rotation until resistance is felt. It has been suggested that it is easier to have the cuff partly inflated, insert the mask on its side and rotate once through the gap between the tonsils [65]. Concomitant use of a jaw thrust can also help with either insertion technique. Using lidocaine rather than water-soluble gel to lubricate the LMA does not reduce the incidence of sore throat. Sore throat will be increased with overinflation of the LMA cuff, which may also cause damage to the pharyngeal structures.

Laryngeal masks can be used for airway management in the vast majority of straightforward paediatric cases including the use of the reinforced version for some shared airway cases (e.g. dental procedures) where they provide better airway protection from soiling than a plain tracheal tube and throat pack [66]. In addition they can be invaluable for difficult airway management (see Chapter 21). Laryngeal mask airways are generally used with a spontaneously breathing patient but positive pressure ventilation through a well-fitting LMA in a relaxed patient should not increase gastric distension. Laryngeal masks can dislodge during the procedure, however, and the risks and benefits of ventilating through an LMA rather than a tracheal tube are still debated.

Vigilance is required in any case where an LMA is used as airway obstruction can occur during the procedure because of either laryngospasm or dislodgement. They should probably be avoided if access to the airway will be difficult.

Tracheal intubation

To allow laryngoscopy and intubation there must be sufficient depth of anaesthesia and relaxation of the vocal cords. This can be achieved in a number of ways.

Deep volatile anaesthesia is used where there is a reason to maintain spontaneous respiration (e.g. in a case of anticipated difficult intubation). Sevoflurane is the most commonly chosen agent and intubation can be achieved when the pupils are small and central.

General anaesthesia plus a non-depolarising muscle relaxant particularly for cases where muscle relaxation is also required for the procedure (e.g. intra-abdominal surgery).

A combination of propofol with short-acting opiate (e.g. alfentanil or remifentanil) may be chosen where muscle relaxation is not required but a tracheal tube would be beneficial (e.g. some intraoral surgery); this avoids the use of suxamethonium and its side-effects.

Technique

Infants less than 3–6 months have a longer epiglottis and are easier to intubate with a straight blade. In this technique, the blade of the laryngoscope is positioned posterior to the epiglottis, which is lifted forward to expose the larynx. The combination of greater resting parasympathetic tone in young children and direct vagal stimulation of the underside of the epiglottis makes bradycardia more likely and many anaesthetists administer atropine to avoid this. From 6 months of age a standard technique using Macintosh blades is very satisfactory. Following intubation the tracheal tube must be carefully checked and secured.

Laryngospasm

Laryngospasm is caused by glottic closure due to a reflex constriction of laryngeal muscles. The incidence is much higher in paediatric anaesthesia than in adults. All airway complications including laryngospasm are more common in children with upper respiratory tract infections and in those passively exposed to cigarette smoke. High-risk periods during anaesthesia are during induction and emergence, particularly where the airway is stimulated at an insufficient depth of anaesthesia. Younger children are at greater risk.

Their oxygen consumption is also greater so hypoxia ensues more quickly.

Recognition

With partial airway obstruction there will be a characteristic stridulous noise accompanied by increased respiratory effort, nasal flaring, intercostal or subcostal recession, and decreased tidal volumes as monitored by the movement in the reservoir bag of the anaesthesia circuit. Complete obstruction is silent and there will be no movement of the reservoir bag. Hypoxia rapidly ensues.

Prevention

Laryngospasm incidence is decreased with good anaesthetic technique and is related to the experience of the anaesthetist. Ensuring adequate depth of anaesthesia before instrumentation of the airway or other stimulation of the patient is key.

Treatment

- Act quickly.
- Apply PEEP via the anaesthesia circuit to distend the soft tissues of the upper airway.
- Position the airway but minimise soft tissue pressure, which is stimulating and counterproductive.
- Alert your assistant that you may need a tracheal tube and intubation drugs.
- Increase the depth of anaesthesia, ideally with propofol (1 mg/kg), which will also act as a direct laryngeal muscle relaxant
- If the above measures fail give suxamethonium preceded by atropine before profound hypoxia ensues

MANAGEMENT OF EXTUBATION AND LARYNGEAL MASK REMOVAL (Table 19.4)

Apart from special situations (e.g. ophthalmic surgery) paediatric patients should be extubated awake when their protective reflexes have returned.

With modern anaesthesia patients are very rarely deeply anaesthetised using a volatile agent and therefore safe 'deep' extubation, which requires a minimum alveolar concentration (MAC) value of at least 1.5, is unusual. Laryngeal mask airways are well tolerated until the patient is awake and swallowing, and some studies have shown this results in fewer airway complications than removal while the patient is still anaesthetised [67], although this may depend on the anaesthetic agent used [68]. During emergence from anaesthesia emergency equipment and drugs should remain to hand and a suitable assistant should remain present. In emergency cases where the child may have a full stomach this is the most likely time for vomiting to occur.

RAPID SEQUENCE INDUCTION IN CHILDREN

There is lack of clarity with regard to both the requirement for and the method of rapid sequence induction. Recent studies have shown that there is a variety of opinion as to how emergency cases that are at risk of having a 'full stomach' should be managed [69,70]. Experienced paediatric specialists seem to be less likely to propose a classic rapid sequence induction.

It is well known that experimental data suggest that aspiration of a volume of more than 0.4 mL/kg of gastric contents with a pH of less than 2.5 can result in pneumonitis. Any child requiring emergency anaesthesia for illness or injury should be regarded as being at risk of potential aspiration with volumes in excess of this value. Furthermore, there does not appear to be a reliable safe time interval from last oral intake either before the injury or illness or before anaesthesia [71].

The 'gold standard' way of avoiding aspiration in these circumstances is the classic rapid sequence induction (RSI) with cricoid pressure. There are several problems with this in paediatric practice, and these are outlined below

Pre-oxygenation

The purpose of pre-oxygenation is to de-nitrogenate the functional residual capacity (FRC) to give the greatest possible reserve of O_2 should difficulty with intubation occur. The O_2 consumption is greater in children and may be three times higher in infants or small children but the FRC is of proportionally similar size. Making an uncooperative child cry by applying a facemask may increase O_2 consumption even further.

Intravenous induction

Intravenous induction may prolong recovery, particularly in neonates. In addition, hypoxia is a potent stimulator for vomiting and intravenous induction in children is more associated with hypoxia. Thus, many paediatric anaesthetists adopted the practice of inhalational induction with cricoid pressure.

Suxamethonium

The advantages are rapid muscle relaxation and a quick recovery, but in both children and adults there are many adverse effects (see Chapter 15).

Cricoid pressure

The cricoid ring is well formed at birth but is higher at the level of C4. Cricoid pressure may be incorrectly applied if the cartilage is not identified before induction of anaesthesia and forces used are unknown and may not be correct [72].

Avoiding ventilation while waiting for the relaxant to work

This is recommended to avoid inflating the stomach but the time required for the suxamethonium to work, followed by intubation before commencing ventilation, may easily exceed the capacity of the O_2 stores in the FRC to maintain saturation in arterial blood (SaO_2), particularly in the neonate or small child. It has been shown that cricoid pressure prevents gastric insufflation during positive pressure ventilation with a facemask [73]. To avoid hypoxia therefore, it is common and reasonable to inflate the lungs of the neonate or small infant gently even in the context of a rapid sequence induction.

If the argument above is accepted, the reasons for continuing to use suxamethonium become less compelling and competitive neuromuscular blockade becomes an acceptable alternative.

Cuffed or uncuffed tube

A well-fitting uncuffed tube is said to offer protection from airway soiling as there will be small positive pressure and a flow of gases around the tube out through the larynx. This mechanism is presumably lost if a spontaneously breathing technique is chosen after intubation. There is renewed interest in cuffed tubes in children (see page 276) and in the emergency patient they offer the advantage that the correct fit should be achieved at the initial intubation. They should certainly be considered if there is poor chest compliance, although the smaller lumen may inhibit clearance of copious secretions.

Management of extubation

This is the time of highest risk so awake extubation is recommended (Table 19.4).

Table 19.4 Recommendations for modified rapid sequence induction

- Aspirate the nasogastric tube (if present) and leave on free drainage
- Pre-oxygenate if the child will tolerate the mask easily
- Identify the cricoid ring before anaesthesia and ask your assistant to apply cricoid pressure as consciousness is lost
- Perform a rapid sequence induction
- Give suxamethonium (2 mg/kg in infants and neonates)
- Gently ventilate with cricoid pressure on (ensure a clear airway by meticulous attention to airway-opening manoeuvres). You will buy more time, avoid hypoxia and identify a patient who is difficult to ventilate (and therefore you need help) a little earlier
- Consider a cuffed tube if appropriate size and type available
- Extubate awake

Vascular access

The use of topical anaesthetic cream prior to cannulation is now standard paediatric practice. Two creams are currently available: EMLA and Ametop. EMLA is a eutectic mixture of 2.5 per cent lidocaine and prilocaine in a 1:1 ratio formulated in an oil-in-water emulsion. It requires 1 hour to be effective. After 30–60 minutes skin blanching is seen, due to vasoconstriction, which can make cannulation more difficult [74]. Ametop is a gel preparation of 4 per cent tetracaine (amethocaine) which should be removed after 45 minutes, although it is still helpful even with a shorter

application. The effect of both creams remains after removal but that of Ametop lasts longer (up to 4–6 hours). A recent Cochrane review of several studies concludes that Ametop is superior to EMLA for all time periods of application [75]. Erythema is common with Ametop but this may be due to the vasodilator properties; however, frank blistering with cutaneous bullae can occur in some children. The latter is not seen with EMLA. The prilocaine in EMLA may convert haemoglobin to methaemoglobin so caution is advised in infants less than 3 months old who may not have full activity of the methaemoglobin reductase enzyme. In practice, this is not a problem if the skin is intact. Ametop is not recommended for babies under 1 month. Tetracaine is metabolised by non-specific esterases both in the skin and systemically.

It is clearly important to identify the correct position for application of the cream and children are often happy for you to draw on their hand or arm to indicate this.

There have been case reports of children either licking the cream or rubbing it into their eyes. A bandage placed over the occlusive dressing in young or uncooperative children should prevent these problems. Even where an inhalational induction is planned it is worth considering applying topical anaesthetic cream as this facilitates venous access at lighter planes of anaesthesia.

Vascular access is mandatory for all cases for drug and fluid administration. Good quality cannulae are readily available in a variety of sizes (see page 283).

TIPS FOR SUCCESS AT GAINING VASCULAR ACCESS

- Practice!
- Consider all possible sites in advance. Look carefully before selecting a vein to cannulate. Ideally, select a possible site on the ward for topical cream application. Remember, there may be more visible veins in the feet than the hands. Volar wrist veins can be very useful in the neonate or infant. The long saphenous vein may not be visible but is very reliable in position and may be felt just anterior to the medial malleolus at the ankle (Fig. 19.8).
- An experienced assistant makes a big difference; they should be instructed to stretch the skin over the site to be cannulated and not to squeeze the limb too hard to avoid occluding the arterial supply.
- In the older child with difficult veins Entonox can be helpful to reduce their anxiety while cannulation is attempted.
- Good positioning of the patient (e.g. in the parent's lap) can help to minimise limb movement, allowing the assistant to concentrate on the squeeze of the limb. All cannulas and syringes should be kept out of the child's view until cannulation is achieved. Many children find the actual squeezing of the limb unpleasant so they should be told what is happening.
- Don't rely solely on the adhesive dressing during induction as the child may move the limb suddenly.

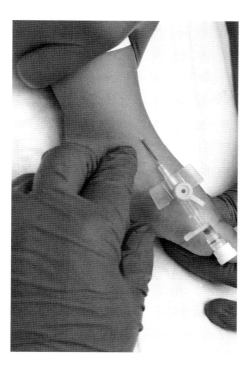

Figure 19.8 The long saphenous vein. The finger of the left hand is on the medial malleolus.

Hold the child's hand or foot gently with your thumb on the cannula and, if the child's limb moves, move with them.

- Consider an inhalational induction in a child with difficult veins but remember the length of anaesthesia without vascular access may be prolonged by this approach. You may need two anaesthetists.

Techniques for difficult vascular access are described in Chapter 22. In the urgent situation intraosseous access should be obtained.

MAINTENANCE OF ANAESTHESIA

Anaesthesia is most commonly maintained using a volatile agent supplemented with either a local block or an opiate. Total intravenous anaesthesia is becoming more popular, however, as paediatric pharmacokinetic algorithms are now available (see Chapter 11). Although older children can breathe spontaneously through a LMA or facemask for many procedures, infants and small children are better managed with positive pressure ventilation for all but the briefest anaesthetics for reasons that are fully reviewed in Chapter 2.

Monitoring is discussed in Chapter 20.

Attention to temperature control is essential in children and temperature should be monitored in all but the shortest procedures. Children are thermolabile and, although hypothermia is usually emphasised, hyperthermia also occurs and should be actively managed.

Fluid management is discussed in Chapter 4.

RECOVERY

Recovery of a child from anaesthesia should take place in a suitable, child-friendly, environment near to the operating theatres or procedure rooms. Recovery staff must be aware of and be able to manage the common complications of general anaesthesia described below. Parents may help to calm their own distressed children and they should be encouraged to attend as early as possible.

Recovery staff should be competent in airway control, oxygen therapy and the recognition of signs that may presage deterioration [76,77]. A full range of monitoring appropriate for the surgery performed should be available. For simple cases in healthy children a pulse oximeter is often sufficient but non-invasive blood pressure and ECG monitors should be used in addition if cardiovascular instability is possible. Discharge from recovery should be according to local protocol as it will depend on local organisation and resources. An example of discharge criteria is included in Table 19.5.

A strategy for pain relief must be implemented using a multimodal approach (see Chapter 27). Additional 'rescue' analgesia must be available. Fortunately, nausea and vomiting are not common in the first 30 minutes of recovery but 5–10 per cent of children may vomit and antiemetics must be available, together with drug prescriptions and a strategy for later. If intravenous drugs are planned the IV access must therefore be protected with soft and secure bandaging. Body temperature should be checked and suitable passive or active methods of temperature control used. Feeding often comforts infants and young children and this should be done as soon as possible. Intravenous fluids must be used if there is an appreciable delay.

Airway complications are common in recovery. Laryngospasm has been discussed above. Stridor can occur after tracheal extubation and is probably caused by inflammation in the airway at the level of the cricoid ring. It may be more common if there has been a recent upper respiratory tract infection and in Down syndrome children [78]. In the author's experience this problem is rare but the incidence, in the literature, varies between 0.1 per cent [79] and 1 per cent [80,81]. The management is supportive and to treat the airway oedema with nebulised adrenaline and intravenous dexamethasone (see Chapter 33). Other causes of stridor should be considered such as foreign body or retained throat pack. Pulmonary aspiration during induction, maintenance and recovery is fortunately unlikely in children – its incidence is probably less than 1:1000. Moreover significant morbidity is rare and its management should be supportive; in most cases the child can cough out any material aspirated. Treatment is not necessary unless there is a pyrexia or physical signs of pulmonary aspiration. Management is otherwise supportive and no different from adult practice. Occasionally, bronchoscopy is necessary to remove inhaled solid matter.

Obstructive sleep apnoea can be troublesome and is a common problem before and after tonsillectomy. Few children need intensive care but the recovery and ward staff

Table 19.5   Criteria for discharge after anaesthesia from the recovery ward*

Consider discharging the patient once the following targets have been met or on specific agreement with the anaesthetist/ward nurse:	
Vital signs	Patient has spontaneous, regular respirations and a self-supporting clear airway
	The SpO$_2$ is within normal patient limits, oxygen has been prescribed if necessary
	Heart rate and blood pressure are stable and within preoperative limits
	Central and peripheral temperatures are within normal limits
Conscious state	Patient is awake or easily rousable
	Patient is comfortable or any pain adequately controlled
	Nausea/vomiting is absent or adequately controlled
Surgical details	Wound is dry or with minimal exudate
	Catheters and drains are patent and drainage is within anticipated limits
	Intravenous hydration has been prescribed if required
	If appropriate, the patient is free from neurovascular compromise
	Documentation is complete

SpO$_2$, pulse oximetry.
*Edited extracts from the Clinical Procedure Guideline of Great Ormond Street Hospital: *Recovery: Care Of The Child*, 2006.

will need a clear strategy on who can be managed on the general ward (see Chapter 33). Ex-preterm infants and neonates are at greater risk of apnoea related to their maturity and, in general, they should stay in hospital for monitoring for at least 12 hours after anaesthesia (see Chapter 8).

REFERENCES

Key references

Aguilera IM, Patel D, Meakin GH, Masterson J. Perioperative anxiety and postoperative behavioural disturbances in children undergoing intravenous or inhalation induction of anaesthesia. *Paediatr Anaesth* 2003; **13**: 501–7.

Bordet F, Allaouchiche B, Lansiaux S *et al*. Risk factors for complications during general anaesthesia in paediatric patients. *Paediatr Anaesth* 2002; **12**: 762–9.

Bricker SR, McLuckie A, Nightingale DA. Gastric aspirates after trauma in children. *Anaesthesia*. 1989; **44**: 721–4.

Jackson Rees G. Anaesthesia in the newborn. *Br J Anaesth* 1950; **2**: 1419–22.

James I. Cuffed tubes in children. *Paediatr Anaesth* 2001; **11**: 259–63.

Lopez-Gil M, Brimacombe J, Alvarez M. Safety and efficacy of the laryngeal mask airway. A prospective survey of 1400 children. *Anaesthesia* 1996; **51**: 969–72.

Shenoy GH, Meakin GH, Masterson JJ. Comparison of the work of breathing imposed by three anaesthetic breathing systems in children. *Paediatr Anaesth* 2002; **12**: 826–27.

References

1. Miller D, Adams AP, Light D. Dead space and paediatric anaesthetic equipment: a physical lung model study. *Anaesthesia* 2004; **59**: 600–6.

2. Bailie R, Barnett MB, Fraser JF. The Brain laryngeal mask – a comparative study with the nasal mask in paediatric dental outpatients. *Anaesthesia* 1991; **46**: 358–60.

3. Brain AIJ. The development of the Laryngeal mask – a brief history of the invention, early clinical work from which the laryngeal mask evolved. *Eur J Anaesthesiol* 1991; **4**: 5–17.

4. Mason DG, Bingham RM. The laryngeal mask airway in children. *Anaesthesia* 1990; **45**: 760–3.

5. Lopez-Gil M, Brimacombe J, Alvarez M. Safety and efficacy of the laryngeal mask airway. A prospective survey of 1400 children. *Anaesthesia* 1996; **51**: 969–72.

6. Dubreuil M, Lasson M, Plaud B *et al*. Complications and fibreoptic assessment of size 1 laryngeal mask airway. *Anesth Analg* 1993; **76**: 527.

7. Lopez-Gil M, Brimacombe J. The Proseal™ laryngeal mask airway in children. *Paediatr Anaesth* 2005; **15**: 229–34.

8. van den Berg AA, Mphanza T. Choice of tracheal tube size for children: finger size or age related formula? *Anaesthesia* 1997; **52**: 695–703.

9. Hatch DJ. Paediatric anaesthetic equipment. *Br J Anaesth* 1985; **57**: 672–84.

10. Bloch EC, Ossey K, Ginsberg B. Tracheal intubation in children: a new method for assuring correct depth of tube placement. *Anesth Analg* 1988; **67**: 590–2.

11. Goel S, Lim SL. The intubating depth marker: the confusion of the black line. *Paediatr Anaesth* 2003; **13**: 579–83.

12. Mariano ER, Ramamoorthy C, Chu LF *et al*. A comparison of three methods for estimating appropriate tracheal tube depth in children. *Paediatr Anaesth* 2005; **15**: 846–51.

13. Verghese ST, Hannallah RS, Slack MC *et al*. Auscultation of bilateral breath sounds does not rule out endobronchial intubation in children. *Anesth Analg* 2004; **99**: 56–8.

14. James I. Cuffed tubes in children. *Paediatr Anaesth* 2001; **11**: 259–63.

15. Orliaguet GA, Renaud E, Lejay M *et al*. Postal survey of cuffed or uncuffed tubes for paediatric tracheal intubation. *Paediatr Anaesth* 2001; **11**: 277–81.

16. Newth CJL, Rachman B, Patel N *et al*. Cuffed versus uncuffed endotracheal tubes in pediatric intensive care. *Am J Respir Crit Care Med* 2000; **161**: A78.

17. Khine HH, Corddry DH, Kettrick RG *et al*. Comparison of cuffed and uncuffed endotracheal tubes in young children. *Anesthesiology* 1997; **86**: 627–31.

18. Felten ML, Schmautz E, Delaporte-Cerceau S *et al*. Endotracheal tube cuff pressure is unpredictable in children. *Anesth Analg* 2003; **97**: 1612–6.

19. Advanced Life Support Group. *Advanced paediatric life support – the practical approach*. London: BMJ 1997.

20. Watts ADJ, Gelb AW, Bach DB, Pelz DM. Comparison of the Bullard and Macintosh laryngoscopes for endotracheal intubation of patients with a potential cervical spine injury. *Anesthesiology* 1997; **87**:1335–42.

21. Ward C, ed. *Ward's anaesthetic equipment*. London: WB Saunders, 1998.

22. Miller DM. Anaesthetic breathing systems. *Br J Anaesth* 1988; **60**: 555–64.

23. Mapleson WW. The elimination of rebreathing in various semiclosed anaesthetic systems. *Br J Anaesth* 1954; **26**: 323–32.

24. Jackson Rees G. Anaesthesia in the newborn. *Br J Anaesth* 1950; **2**: 1419–22.

25. Vekckemans F. Equipment, monitoring, and environmental conditions, In: Bissonnette B, Dalens B, eds. *Paediatric anaesthesia*. New York: McGraw-Hill, 2002.

26. Badgewell JM, Heavner JE, May WS *et al*. End-tidal PCO_2 monitoring in infants and children ventilated with either a partial rebreathing of a non-rebreathing circuit. *Anesthesiology* 1987; **66**: 405–10.

27. Froese AB, Rose DK. A detailed analysis of T-piece systems. In: Steward DJ, ed. *Aspects of paediatric anaesthesia*. Amsterdam: Excerpta Medica, 1982; 101–36.

28. Lindahl SGE, Hulse MJ, Hatch DJ. Ventilation and gas exchange during anaesthesia and surgery in spontaneously breathing infants and children. *Br J Anaesth* 1984; **56**; 121–9.

29. Hatch DJ, Yates AP, Lindahl SGE. Flow requirements and rebreathing during mechanically controlled ventilation in a T-piece (Mapleson E) system. *Br J Anaesth* 1987; **59**: 1533–40.

30. Meakin G, Jennings AD, Beatty PCW *et al*. Fresh gas flow requirements of an enclosed afferent reservoir breathing system in anaesthetized spontaneously breathing children. *Br J Anaesth* 1992; **68**: 333–7.

31. Orlikowski CEP, Ewart MC, Bingham RM. The Humphrey ADE system: evaluation in paediatric use. *Br J Anaesth* 1991; **66**: 253–7.

32. Baum JA, Aitkenhead AR. Low-flow anaesthesia. *Anaesthesia* 1995; **50**: 37–44.

33. Meakin GH. Low-flow anaesthesia in infants and children. *Br J Anaesth* 1999; **83**(1): 50–7.

34. Mazze RI, Jamison RL. Low-flow anaesthesia (1 L/min) sevoflurane: is it safe? *Anesthesiology* 1997; **86**: 1225–7.

35. Shenoy GH, Meakin GH, Masterson JJ. Comparison of the work of breathing imposed by three anaesthetic breathing systems in children. *Paediatr Anaesth* 2002; **12**: 826–27.

36. Frohlich D, Schwall B, Funk W, Hobbhan J. Laryngeal mask airway and uncuffed tubes are equally effective for low-flow or closed system anaesthesia in children. *Anesth Analg* 1997; **79**: 289–92.

37. Engelhardt T, Johnston G, Kumar MM. Comparison of cuffed, uncuffed tracheal tubes and laryngeal mask airways in low flow pressure controlled ventilation in children. *Paediatr Anaesth* 2006; **16**(2): 140–3.

38. Brock-Utne J. Editorial: humidification in paediatric anaesthesia. *Paediatr Anaesth* 2000; **10**: 117–19.

39. Whitelock DE, de Beer DAH. The use of filters with small infants. *Respir Care Clin North Am* 2006; **12**(2): 307–20.

40. Wilkes A. *Breathing system filters: an assessment of 104 breathing systems filters. MHRA Evaluation 04005*. London: MHRA, 2004.

41. Malan CA, Wilkes AR, Gildersleve C. An evaluation of the filtration performance of paediatric breathing system filters using sodium chloride particles at low flows. *Paediatr Anaesth* 2006; **16**: 1298–9.

42. Bissonnette B, Sessler DI. Passive or active inspired gas humidification increases steady-state temperatures in anesthetised infants. *Anesth Analg* 1989; **69**(6): 783–7.

43. Wilkinson K, Cranston D, Hatch D, Fletcher M. Assessment of a hygroscopic heat and moisture exchanger for paediatric use. *Anaesthesia* 1991; **46**: 296–9.

44. Spears RS, Yeh A, Fisher DM, Zwass MS. The 'educated hand'. Can an anesthesiologist assess changes in neonatal pulmonary compliance manually? *Anesthesiology* 1991; **75**(4): 693–6.

45. Veyckemans F. Equipment, monitoring, and environmental conditions. In: Bissonnette B, Dalens B, eds. *Paediatric anaesthesia: principles and practice*. New York: Mc Graw-Hill 2002.

46. Newton NI, Hillman KM, Varley JG. Automatic ventilation with the Ayre's T-piece. *Anaesthesia* 1981; **36**: 22–36.

47. Cote CJ. Pediatric breathing circuits and anesthesia machines. *Int Anesthesiol Clin* 1992; **30**: 51–61.

48. Sessler DI. Mild perioperative hypothermia. *N Engl J Med* 1997; **336**: 1730–7.

49. Bissonnette B, Sessler DI. Mild hypothermia does not impair postanesthetic recovery I. Infants and children. *Anesth Analg* 1993; **76**: 168–72.

50. Sessler DI, McGuire J, Sessler AM. Perioperative thermal insulation. *Anesthesiology* 1992; **74**: 875–9.

51. Goudsouzian NG, Morris RH, Ryan JF. The effects of a warming blanket on the maintenance of body temperature in anesthetized infants and children. *Anesthesiology* 1973; **39**: 351–3.

52. Kurz A, Kurz M, Poeschl G *et al*. Forced-air warming maintains intraoperative normothermia better than circulating-water mattresses. *Anesth Analg* 1993; **77**(1): 89–95.

53. Murat I, Berniere J, Constant I. Evaluation of the efficacy of a forced-air warmer (Bair Hugger) during spinal surgery in children. *J Clin Anesth* 1994; **6**(5): 425–9.

54. Booker PD. Equipment and monitoring in paediatric anaesthesia. *Br J Anaesth* 1999; **82**: 78–90.

55. Presson RG Jr, Bezruczko AP, Hillier SC, McNiece WL. Evaluation of a new fluid warmer effective at low to moderate flow rates. *Anesthesiology* 1993; **78**(5): 974–80.

56. Schultz J-A, Simms C, Bissonnette B. Methods for warming intravenous fluids in small volumes. *Can J Anaesth* 1998; **45**: 1110–5.

57. Aguilera IM, Patel D, Meakin GH, Masterson J. Perioperative anxiety and postoperative behavioural disturbances in children undergoing intravenous or inhalation induction of anaesthesia. *Paediatr Anaesth* 2003; **13**: 501–7.

58. Kotiniemi LH, Ryhanen PT. Behavioural changes and children's memories after intravenous, inhalation and rectal induction of anaesthesia. *Paediatr Anaesth* 1996; **6**: 201–7.

59. Sigston PE, Jenkins AMC, Jackson EA *et al*. Rapid inhalation induction in children: 8 per cent sevoflurane compared with 5 per cent halothane. *Br J Anaesth* 1997; **78**: 362–5.

60. Girgis Y, Frerk CM, Pigott D. Redistribution of halothane and sevoflurane under simulated conditions of acute airway obstruction. *Anaesthesia* 2001; **56**: 613–5.

61. Lejus C, Bazin V, Fernandez M *et al*. Inhalation induction using sevoflurane in children: the single-breath vital capacity technique compared to the tidal volume technique. *Anaesthesia* 2006; **61**: 535–40.

62. Runcie CJ, Mackenzie SJ, Arthur DS, Morton NS. Comparison of recovery from anaesthesia induced in children with either propofol or thiopentone. *Br J Anaesth* 1993; **70**: 192–5.

63. Bordet F, Allaouchiche B, Lansiaux S *et al*. Risk factors for complications during general anaesthesia in paediatric patients. *Paediatr Anaesth* 2002; **12**: 762–9.

64. Arai YC, Fukunaga K, Ueda W *et al*. The endoscopically measured effects of airway maneuvers and the lateral position on airway patency in anesthetized children with adenotonsillar hypertrophy. *Anesth Analg* 2005; **100**: 949–52.

65. Kundra P, Deepak R, Ravishankar M. Laryngeal mask insertion in children: a rational approach. *Paediatr Anaesth* 2003; **13**: 685–90.

66. Kaplan A, Crosby GJ, Bhattacharyya N. Airway protection and the laryngeal mask airway in sinus and nasal surgery. *Laryngoscope* 2004; **114**: 652–5.

67. Kitching AJ, Walpole AR, Blogg CE. Removal of the laryngeal mask airway in children: anaesthetized compared with awake. *Br J Anaesth* 1996; **76**: 874–6.

68. Pappas AL, Sukhani R, Lurie J *et al*. Severity of airway hyperreactivity associated with laryngeal mask airway removal: correlation with volatile anesthetic choice and depth of anesthesia. *J Clin Anesth* 2001; **13**: 498–503.

69. Marcus RJ, Thompson JP. Anaesthesia for manipulation of forearm fractures in children: a survey of current practice. *Paediatr Anaesth* 2000; **10**: 273–7.

70. Seidel J, Dorman T. Anesthetic management of preschool children with penetrating eye injuries: postal survey of pediatric anesthetists and review of the available evidence. *Paediatr Anaesth* 2006; **16**: 769–76.

71. Bricker SR, McLuckie A, Nightingale DA. Gastric aspirates after trauma in children. *Anaesthesia* 1989; **44**: 721–4.

72. Landsman I. Cricoid pressure: indications and complications. *Paediatr Anaesth* 2004; **14**: 43–7.

73. Laws EG, Campbell I. Inflation pressure, gastric insufflation and rapid sequence induction. *Br J Anaesth* 1987; **59**: 315–8.

74. Gajraj NM, Pennant JH, Watcha MF. Eutectic mixture of local anesthetics (EMLA) cream. *Anesth Analg* 1994; **78**: 574–83.

75. Lander JA, Weltman BJ, So SS. EMLA and amethocaine for reduction of children's pain associated with needle insertion. *Cochrane Database Syst Rev* 2006; **3**: CD004236.

76. Xue FS, Tong SY, Liao X *et al*. Observation of the correlation of postanaesthesia recovery scores with early postoperative hypoxaemia in children. *Paediatr Anaesth* 1999; **9**: 145–51.

77. Xue FS, Huang YG, Tong SY *et al*. A comparative study of early postoperative hypoxemia in infants, children, and adults undergoing elective plastic surgery. *Anesth Analg* 1996; **83**: 709.

78. Sherry K. Post-extubation stridor in Down's syndrome. *Br J Anaesth* 1983; **55**: 53–4.

79. Litman RS, Keon TP. Post-extubation stridor croup in children. *Anesthesiology* 1991; 75: **6**: 1122–3.

80. Koka BV, Jeon IS, Andre JM *et al*. Post-extubation croup in children. *Anesth Analg* 1977: **56**, 501–5.

81. Cohen MM, Cameron, Duncan PG. Pediatric anesthesia morbidity and mortality in the perioperative period. *Anesth Analg* 1990; **70**: 160–7.

Monitoring

MIKE BROADHEAD, MONTY MYTHEN

KEY LEARNING POINTS

- Non-invasive monitoring is essential in all cases—new pulse oximetry and capnography technology has improved accuracy.
- Single variable monitoring is less reliable than an integrated approach in which data from several monitors are combined against the background of the patient's disease process.
- The risks of invasive monitoring should be balanced against the potential gains.

- Echocardiography is a valuable monitor during cardiac surgery and other situations of major haemorrhage or haemodynamic instability.
- Respiratory compliance monitoring enables adjustment of optimal ventilation support.
- Processed EEG monitoring may be applicable in children but has not been validated in infants.

INTRODUCTION

Anaesthesia, sedation and intensive care enable clinicians to perform procedures that would otherwise be impossible. Better anaesthesia skills, understanding of pathophysiology, and modern surgical and medical intensive care have all, undoubtedly, contributed to a decline in morbidity and mortality, but a key element in safe practice involves the monitoring of vital functions.

As early as 1868 Dr Joseph Clover advised that the pulse be continuously palpated during anaesthesia to detect both irregularities and reduction in pulse volume [1] and, by 1896, continuous monitoring of both heart and breath sounds had been advocated [2]. While clinical assessment of the patient is still important today, technological advances have increased so that we are now reliant on monitoring. Many devices are readily available and so commonplace that minimum standards are practical and affordable. Indeed, minimum standards for monitoring are recommended in many countries by their respective anaesthetic societies, and are well known [3,4]. As technology has advanced so has the minimum standard of care. New monitoring techniques of today will become commonplace tomorrow if they make appreciable contributions to patient care.

This chapter discusses not only the essentials of paediatric monitoring but also important new technology that, one day, may become standard. For example, new monitors of neurological, cardiovascular and respiratory function used in intensive care units (ICUs) may soon be useful in anaesthesia. Most monitors have been developed in adults and adapted for children yet, because of size and physiological differences, some have had limited application and have needed specific development. Complications of invasive monitoring may be increased in children because of their size and fragility. It is a concern that new technology may be used widely before both validation and safety can be carefully considered and assessed. This should be avoided [5]. Our future clinical strategy should be to test validity against accepted standards in intensive care scenarios so that, in time, new technology may migrate into the practice of anaesthesia and sedation.

GENERAL CONSIDERATIONS

Anaesthesia, sedation and surgery can result in profound changes in the cardiovascular and respiratory systems. Basic clinical observations and measurement of blood pressure, heart rate, capillary return, peripheral temperature, respiratory rate and efficiency are all important yet minimum monitoring standards insist on continuous electrocardiography, regular and frequent measurement of blood pressure, oxygen saturation and end-tidal CO_2. The anaesthetist must be in constant attendance. The rationale for monitoring is simply based on historical case review and personal experience that persuade us to accept that monitoring improves safety and reduces morbidity and mortality. Direct evidence is difficult to find [6].

The expectation or likelihood of cardiorespiratory compromise will direct the level of monitoring. For example, rapid changes of blood pressure may need to be assessed by invasive rather than non-invasive monitoring. Additional monitoring of the central venous pressure (CVP), left atrial pressure (LAP), cardiac output (CO) and mixed central venous saturations may also be appropriate.

We assume that invasive monitoring reduces complications and improves survival, but the invasive monitors can themselves cause complications. In adults, for example, pulmonary artery catheters cause so many complications that overall outcome is not improved [7]. Drugs and therapies need to be introduced and adjusted carefully according to our monitoring. But there is considerable variation in the interpretation of the monitoring, even among well-trained specialists [8,9]. An integrated approach in which data from several monitors are combined against the background of the patient's disease process seems a reasonable approach [10]. However, no studies have tested the efficacy of integrated monitoring, though it is probably true that a single variable, in isolation, is prone to greater misinterpretation [11,12]. Furthermore, few monitoring techniques are fully validated with clear evidence of benefit. Faced with this uncertainty, the correct physiological values and response to a given signal may be debatable. Some may conclude that using more invasive monitoring during anaesthesia has no benefit but this negative outlook may also be detrimental; a pragmatic approach is to use it wisely and to accept that it can be misleading. If catheters have been inserted, it is reasonable to gain as much information from them as possible (i.e. cardiac output and mixed venous saturations) [13].

There is often no clear consensus on the appropriate level of monitoring because of the variation in disease state, experience and availability. Practice guidelines for specified situations in defined groups of patients may be helpful. This chapter gives an account of the current and potentially useful monitoring techniques applicable to paediatric anaesthesia.

CARDIOVASCULAR

Electrocardiogram

The electrocardiogram (ECG) is the most common tool used to examine heart rate, rhythm and myocardial health. In the full-term neonate, even though the right and left ventricular masses are equal, the right ventricle is approximately one-third thicker than the left. In the premature infant, however, there is less right ventricular dominance compared with a full-term neonate. By the age of 3–6 months the left ventricle has twice the mass of the right ventricle, and by school age the ratio is 2.5:1, which is similar to that of the adult. These changes are represented on the ECG. The QRS axis has right ventricular dominance in neonates and eventually becomes similar to that of an adult by school age. The size of the R wave may diagnose ventricular hypertrophy but in comparison with echocardiography it has poor predictive value (Fig. 20.1 and Table 20.1) [14,15]. The ST-segment changes are very uncommon but ischaemic heart disease can be detected in some children such as those who

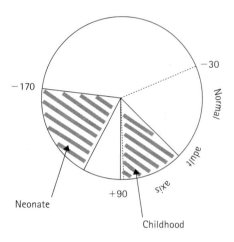

Figure 20.1 Normal range of QRS axis according to age. Normal range of axis in adult is +90° to −30°.

Table 20.1 Normal limits (median and 98th centile) of R-wave amplitude in leads V1 and V6

	V1 (mV)	V6 (mV)
0–1 month	–	–
1–3 months	0.9 (1.8)	1.2 (2.15)
3–6 months	1.0 (2.0)	1.3 (2.25)
6–12 months	0.9 (2.0)	1.25 (2.25)
1–3 years	0.85 (1.75)	1.3 (2.25)
3–5 years	0.8 (1.75)	1.5 (2.5)
5–8 years	0.7 (1.4)	1.65 (2.8)
8–12 years	0.5 (1.25)	1.6 (2.5)
12–16 years	0.4 (1.0)	1.5 (2.3)

have cardiomyopathy or myocarditis or who have had heart transplantation. Infants are particularly prone to bradycardia during anaesthesia and surgery and an ECG enables immediate assessment in order that treatment can be quick enough to prevent hypotension and permanent damage. Fortunately other serious arrhythmias are unlikely especially since sevoflurane has replaced the need for halothane [16].

HEART RATE VARIABILITY

Heart rate variability (HRV) measures the variation in the time between each successive normal heartbeat. Variability is caused by an active healthy autonomic nervous system. In illness the heart rate (and other variables such as blood pressure) becomes more regular and an early application of HRV was to detect foetal distress [17]. More recently, HRV has been investigated as a surrogate variable of conscious level [18–20] and sepsis.

The sequence of RR intervals not only can be analysed by simple statistics but also can be plotted to derive a waveform that can be further processed (e.g. by fast Fourier transformation) to achieve a power spectrum of constituent frequencies [17,21]. Two frequencies are prominent in normal RR sequences. The high-frequency (HF, 0.15–0.4 Hz) component is associated with vagal parasympathetic tone and is synchronous with pulmonary ventilation (i.e. respiratory sinus arrhythmia). The low-frequency (LF, 0.05–0.15 Hz) component may be sympathetic in part. To estimate power within frequency bands the ECG complex must have a clearly defined R wave and the measurement must be accurate to at least 5 milliseconds. Power estimation may not be feasible with less than 2 minutes of steady-state ECG because sufficient R waves are needed to generate a sequence of RR intervals to assess LF HRV [17,21].

Arterial blood pressure

NON-INVASIVE

The gold standard for assessment of blood pressure is the manual auscultation method. Automated oscillotonometry, with correct cuff size, is accurate in infants and children [22]. The cuff width should be almost as long as the circumference of the arm; if the cuff is too small it overestimates blood pressure. Large-sized cuffs result in less error.

Several devices continually monitor blood pressure non-invasively. The Colin tonometer (ScanMed Medical Instruments, Moreton-in-Marsh, UK) and the Finapres unit (Finapres Medical Systems, Amsterdam, the Netherlands) and, more recently, the Vasotrac (Medwave, Arden Hills, MN, USA) are all potentially useful but have some variation when compared with direct pressure measurement. The Colin tonometer uses a cuffed transducer over the skin of the radial artery. The cuff gradually inflates until the radial artery is partially occluded. Arterial pulsations are used to

calculate the blood pressure. The Finapres incorporates an optical plethysmograph within a small cuff inflated around a finger. The transmission of the infrared light through the finger is measured to generate feedback control of the cuff pressure, which counters the change in blood flow within the finger and keeps the infrared transmission constant. The change in cuff pressure therefore matches the arterial pressure waveform. Both these devices require calibration [23]. The Vasotrac monitor uses frequent gentle compression and decompression of the radial artery at the wrist over three or four heartbeats. The signal is processed by an algorithm which estimates systolic, diastolic and mean arterial blood pressures [24]. The display updates the arterial pressures every 12–15 heart beats. It has been successfully used in children following cardiac surgery.

INVASIVE

Systemic direct invasive pressure monitoring is common practice, particularly in intensive care. Unfortunately the catheters can cause thrombosis, embolism and infection, but these complications are usually outweighed by the ability to measure blood pressure when it is very low or high or changing rapidly. The catheters also allow repeated painless arterial blood gas analysis. The size of the cannula varies depending on the infant. The smallest cannulae are 26G, which are appropriate in radial arteries of very small premature infants, whereas 22G cannulae are suitable for the femoral or radial artery of a 3 kg neonate. Umbilical artery catheters can cause aortic thrombosis and sepsis but it is reasonable to leave them in place for up to 3 days provided that they are being used. Heparinised saline (1 mL/h) is necessary to maintain catheter patency. In very small infants this volume may contribute to the overall fluid balance [25].

Preload

Recently, it has become appreciated that the arterial systolic pressure wave changes during positive pressure ventilation [26] and that this can be used to measure the response to a fluid challenge. Cardiac output can be increased by a fluid volume challenge that increases ventricular filling (or end-diastolic volume) and thereby increases stroke volume. In theory, the volume could be guided by ventricular preload – which, in the normal heart, equates to atrial pressure – but preload is a poor predictor of response to a fluid challenge. Hearts with small left ventricular end-diastolic volumes may not increase their output in response to volume loading, whereas those with large end-diastolic volumes can. Tavernier and colleagues have found that systolic pressure variation was more useful in adults than either pulmonary artery occlusion pressure or echocardiography [27]. This has been termed 'preload responsiveness' and although it has not been validated in children it may be useful because arterial monitoring is commonplace whereas pulmonary catheters and echocardiography skills are not.

CENTRAL VENOUS PRESSURE

Central venous cannulation is useful when large changes in blood volume are anticipated. Measuring preload may help the anaesthetist to judge volume requirements better during resuscitation. Sampling of mixed venous blood is also potentially valuable [28]. Complications include inadvertent arterial cannulation, haemorrhage, perforation of the heart, tamponade, thrombosis and infection [29,30]. Ultrasound has become widely used as an aid to placing central lines [31] but it is likely that its value depends upon training, skill and experience. Leyvi and colleagues reported that ultrasound did not reduce traumatic complications but it did significantly improve the success rate, particularly in children over 1 year old [32]. In another study Verghese and colleagues found that that the success rate of internal jugular vein catheterisation in infants was 100 per cent when guided by ultrasound compared with 77 per cent in a control group in whom only palpation and surface landmarks were used – 25 per cent of the controls had accidental carotid artery punctures [33].

The correct positioning of the tip of the cannula is the subject of debate. Line tips within the confines of the pericardial sac may result in cardiac tamponade, whereas those outside may result in vessel perforation or thrombosis. On balance, current opinion suggests that the catheter tip may be safely sited in the upper atrium provided that it does not pass through the tricuspid valve or into the coronary sinus, and provided that its position is parallel to the atrial wall [34]. If inserted under image guidance it is usually not necessary to perform another chest radiograph [35]. Peripheral central line catheters cause less complications [36]. In neonates, the tip should not be within the right atrium because it is associated with tamponade [37]. Central catheters can cause permanent disability and death [25] and alternative methods of estimating intravascular volume status may be better, such as preload responsiveness (see above), intrathoracic blood volume and stroke volume index, and corrected flow time (see below).

LEFT ATRIAL PRESSURE

A catheter can be placed into the left atrium during cardiac surgery by the surgeon in order to assess postoperative left ventricular filling and function. Indirect estimation of LAP is also possible with a pulmonary artery catheter that can be floated and wedged (with or without a balloon) into a pulmonary capillary. Pulmonary capillary wedge pressure (PCWP) is assumed to equal LAP because pulmonary veins have no valves. The smallest size pulmonary artery catheter is 5 French gauge and this can be used in a 3 kg neonate.

Cardiac output

The thermodilution technique has been the gold standard but now new methods have become reliable [38]. However there is variation in the measurements which may be as much as 30 per cent and in comparison with thermodilution there may be a positive bias of 10 per cent [39].

PULMONARY ARTERY CATHETERS

Pulmonary artery (PA) catheters became established for adults in the 1970s and were useful for direct measurement of pulmonary artery pressure (PAP), PCWP and CO (by the indicator dilution techniques). Systemic and pulmonary vascular resistances (SVR and PVR, respectively), left and right ventricular stroke work, and stroke volume can be calculated. In critically ill children PA catheters have been used with some success to guide drug infusions and fluid therapy [40]. Measuring cardiac output in children is difficult not only because of size but also because of intracardiac shunting that causes recirculation of indicator. Results from a retrospective study in the 1996 suggests that their routine use in intensive care has an unacceptable complication rate [41]. Despite more recent prospective studies there is insufficient evidence to justify routine use [7] and this has led to the investigation of other less invasive techniques.

Extravascular lung water (EVLW) detected by radiological signs of pulmonary oedema can also be detected by indicator dilution techniques. Its importance has been demonstrated in adult ICU patients undergoing volume resuscitation for hypotension and in those receiving diuretic therapy for pulmonary oedema [42]. However, EVLW is not necessarily secondary to pulmonary oedema. Lung infiltrates unrelated to cardiac disease such as infection may significantly contribute to raised EVLW [43].

TRANSPULMONARY INDICATOR DILUTION

Transpulmonary indicator dilution (TPID) involves injection of an indicator into a central vein and its detection in the aorta or the femoral artery. It enables bedside measurement of CO and calculation of SVR in infants and children and the results match measurements derived by using the Fick principle [44,45]. Analysis of the aortic thermodilution curve enables calculation of global end-diastolic volume (GEDV) and intrathoracic blood volume (ITBV). Both these may be superior to CVP and PCWP as indicators for intravascular volume status and cardiac preload [46,47]. In children who have direct arterial pressure monitoring, TPID does not involve additional invasive catheters. It has been used successfully to assess stroke volume and cardiac output in neonates, and infants, in response to changes in preload [47].

PULSE CONTOUR ANALYSIS

This method uses a complex algorithm to estimate stroke volume, and therefore cardiac output, by analysis of the contour of the arterial line waveform. It is based on the principle that area under the pressure versus time curve correlates with the stroke volume. The PiCCO system

(Pulsion Medical Systems, Munich, Germany) incorporates TPID with pulse contour analysis. Transpulmonary indicator dilution is used for initial and periodic calibration and pulse contour analysis is then used for continuous measurements of the cardiac index (CI). The TPID correlates well with PA catheter thermodilution methods in adults [48,49] and also has been used successfully in children following cardiac surgery [50,51]. It may not be accurate enough when there are rapid changes in systemic vascular resistance and arrhythmias.

OESOPHAGEAL DOPPLER

Oesophageal Doppler (OesD) measures blood flow velocity in the descending aorta by means of a Doppler transducer incorporated in the tip of a flexible probe. Within the oesophagus, the probe needs to be rotated so that the transducer faces the aorta to obtain a characteristic aortic blood velocity signal. Its advantage is that the technique requires minimal training and is relatively non-invasive [52]. The probe is relatively large and delicate so that children need to be anaesthetised or deeply sedated for its insertion. Aortic blood flow (ABF) is calculated from the product of flow velocity (Vf) and aortic cross-sectional area (CSAa). The ABF in the descending aorta is only an estimate of CO because some blood flows to proximal aortic arch branches. The ABF is typically 70 per cent of CO and although this varies between patients and disease states it is relatively constant in the individual. The OesD estimation of CO is as reliable as thermodilution methods and there is no significant bias [38]. The technique may give more reproducible results than external suprasternal Doppler [53] and has become useful both in paediatric intensive care and during major surgery [54,55].

Cardiac output may also be derived from the minute distance (MD) which is the area under the velocity–time waveform (i.e. the curve integral). Blood flow during each pulse can be termed the stroke distance and represents the distance travelled by a column of blood during systole. The product of stroke distance and heart rate is the MD, and is the distance travelled by a column of blood in 1 minute. The product of aortic root diameter in systole (which can be estimated from a nomogram) and MD is an estimation of CO.

Another useful variable is the flow time. This is the time required from start of a waveform upstroke to the return to baseline. But since it is heart-rate dependent, the flow time is corrected (FTc) by dividing it by the square root of the cycle time. In hypovolaemia FTc is shortened, and lengthens as stroke volume increases. Thus, FTc can be used to assess preload but it is also altered by contractility and SVR so that caution is needed in its interpretation.

Although the adult literature suggests that OesD estimates of cardiac output match those derived from thermodilution, in children OesD is better as a monitor of trend rather than absolute values [39]. Greater accuracy may be possible with more accurate and real-time estimates of CSAa and Vf. Furthermore, children with abnormalities of

the left outflow tract such as coarctation, stenosis or dilatation, or those with patent ductus arteriosus, are probably not suitable for OesD estimates of CO.

THORACIC ELECTRICAL BIOIMPEDANCE SYSTEM

Thoracic electrical bioimpedance (TEB) measures the variation in impedance of a high-frequency, low-magnitude electrical current between electrodes placed either side of the chest. As blood flows in and out of the chest, a waveform of impedance is produced and cardiac output can be calculated using a validated algorithm. The CO estimations compare favourably with thermodilution and pulse contour waveform analysis [56,57] and the method has been used in children successfully [58,59].

ECHOCARDIOGRAPHY

In addition to anatomical diagnosis, echocardiography can be used to assess both global and regional ventricular function. Suitable echo signals can be achieved either from the surface (transthoracic) or from the oesophagus (trans-oesophageal). Two-dimensional echocardiography provides important information about cardiac function and structure, including ventricular cavity size, fractional shortening and regional wall motion abnormalities [60]. Any abnormalities, however, are only indirect markers of myocardial perfusion and they can persist for prolonged periods after cardiac function has returned. Transoesophageal echocardiography is now widely used [61] and is established in the perioperative management of paediatric cardiac patients [62–66]. Coloured signals can indicate both the direction and quantification of blood flow though shunts and valves. Oesophageal probes are now small enough to be used in neonates to assess cardiac surgical repair and cardiac function [67]. The disadvantages of echocardiography are that it takes skill and experience for accurate measurements and diagnoses. Too large probes can damage the oesophagus and compress the trachea.

Tissue perfusion

The difference between core and central temperature is a simple and useful monitor of the trend of skin blood flow and overall cardiac output. The efficiency of global perfusion can be inferred also from the following surrogate markers.

URINE OUTPUT

Urine production depends upon adequate blood pressure and therefore a fall in urine output could indicate a fall in CO or hypotension, or both. Urine output in excess of 1 mL/kg/h infers good renal blood flow and therefore monitoring it enables assessment of organ perfusion and helps keep track of fluid balance. The bladder should be catheterised in any patient with appreciable cardiovascular instability during anaesthesia [68].

BASE DEFICIT AND BLOOD LACTATE

Monitoring and defining metabolic acidosis are important parts of assessing adequacy of cardiac output. However, simple measurements of pH and base deficit (BD) cannot determine the cause of a metabolic acidosis. Metabolic acidosis, caused by tissue hypoxia, is usually marked by a rise in plasma lactate. The anion gap (AG) is the difference between the readily measured cations and anions in plasma and this difference is caused by unmeasured or *occult* anions such as lactate. Lactate measurement is now readily available but the residual difference may result from other anions found in sick patients such as ketones or poisons. Furthermore, the normal value for AG is largely due to the plasma albumin concentration and if this is low, which it often is in sick patients, the concentration of occult anions will appear lower than its true value. This has led to the albumin-corrected AG, which is simple to use at the bedside. In sick children undergoing intensive care, in whom hypoalbuminaemia is common, AG (corrected for low albumin) has a better correlation with tissue acidosis than BD [69,70].

A more complicated approach is to calculate the difference between the apparent strong ion difference (SIDa) and the anion component of the plasma buffers (bicarbonate, albumin, phosphate – called the effective SID) and the difference between these two is the *unmeasured* strong ion gap. Greater accuracy in determining the cause of acidosis may be possible using the method derived by Stewart (modified by Figge) who proposed combining arterial partial pressure of CO_2 ($PaCO_2$), SID and the total weak acid concentration. SID has been used in children following cardiac surgery in children [71].

$$AG = (Na^+ + K^+) - (HCO_3^- + Cl^-)$$

$$\text{Corrected AG} = AG + (0.25 \times (44 - [Alb]))$$

$$\text{Apparent SID} = (Na + K + Mg + Ca) - (Cl + lactate)$$

$$\text{Effective SID} = [HCO_3^-] + [Alb^-]^* + [Pi^-]^*$$

$$[Alb^-] = [Alb^-] \times ((0.123 \times pH) - 0.631)$$

$$[Pi^-]^* = [Pi^-] \times ((0.309 \times pH) - 0.469).$$

Use of lactate concentration alone may assess anaerobic metabolism but does not differentiate poor oxygen delivery from increased oxygen extraction by the tissues. Also, inborn errors of metabolism, changes in glucose metabolism and impairment of liver function have effects on lactate. Nevertheless, lactate is increasingly measured in shocked patients and has prognostic value in determining

outcome in critically ill paediatric surgical and non-surgical patients. An increase in lactate level of more than 3 mmol/L during cardiopulmonary bypass is associated with increased mortality [50,72–74].

MIXED VENOUS SATURATION

True mixed venous oxygen saturation ($S\bar{v}O_2$) is almost the same as the saturation of blood taken from any central line near or inside the right atrium [75]. Left-to-right intracardiac shunts may make interpretation of absolute values difficult, yet the trend still may be valuable. Venous oxygen saturation can be regarded as an index of both oxygen demand and supply. It depends upon oxygen uptake (VO_2), arterial oxygen saturation, cardiac output and haemoglobin, and all of these need to be considered if $S\bar{v}O_2$ is to be interpreted correctly. The evidence supporting the optimisation of $S\bar{v}O_2$ comes from data showing that the morbidity of critically ill patients can be reduced [76] and, recently, $S\bar{v}O_2$ has become an important index of tissue oxygenation in paediatric cardiac surgery [77,78]. However, $S\bar{v}O_2$ may be difficult to interpret in septic shock where there can be a paradoxical increase in $S\bar{v}O_2$ because tissue perfusion is so poor [28]. A normal $S\bar{v}O_2$, therefore, does not prove normal oxygen supply [12]. Fibre-optic catheters are now available for insertion into blood vessels to measure O_2 saturation continuously and this could be a useful tool in the early recognition of impaired tissue perfusion or sepsis.

RESPIRATORY

Auscultation

Monitoring respiration and heart rate with a stethoscope was recognised as being important as early as 1896 [2], and its use soon became commonplace. Auscultation is invaluable at detecting inadvertent bronchial intubation. In paediatric anaesthesia continuous precordial auscultation became standard practice because it was easy, cheap and reliable. Many anaesthetists still use auscultation either by an individually fitted ear-piece or by amplification of a microphone. Oesophageal stethoscopes are a further refinement and can be combined with a thermistor for monitoring core temperature. However, the practice of continuous auscultation has probably become obsolete with the arrival of reliable and affordable monitors of pulse oximetry and capnography. Confirmation of tracheal intubation is more reliable by capnography.

Pulse oximetry

Continuous measurement of peripheral haemoglobin oxygen saturation (SpO_2) is considered mandatory during anaesthesia, sedation and intensive care. During paediatric anaesthesia minor desaturations ($SpO_2 \leqslant 95$ per cent for more than 60 seconds) are common; one study found it occurred in one-third of paediatric patients [79]. Motion artefact is a significant problem and has recently been reduced with the development of new generation pulse oximeters using the Masimo SET algorithm (Masimo UK, Basingstoke). In the neonatal intensive care unit, these monitors were shown to record true desaturations and bradycardia better than conventional pulse oximeters [80].

There are some special considerations for pulse oximetry in neonates and small infants. The saturations measured on the right and left hands may be appreciably different because of venous blood shunting through a patent ductus arteriosus causing lower saturations in the left hand. Hyperoxia is a problem in premature neonates and leads to retinopathy of prematurity (ROP). Because of the sigmoid shape of the oxygen dissociation curve (and the characteristics of foetal haemoglobin) it is not possible to infer the partial pressure of arterial oxygen (PaO_2) accurately from the haemoglobin saturation. Nevertheless, pulse oximetry is relatively easy and is as good at preventing hyperoxia as arterial blood gas analysis or transcutaneous electrode monitoring. For infants less than 28 weeks (postconceptional age) the saturations can be kept between 70 and 90 per cent to minimise the risk of ROP – supplemental oxygen may be unnecessary. In older preterm infants supplemental oxygen may paradoxically prevent ROP [81]. The use of oxygen to achieve high saturations in term infants may also not be appropriate. Birth asphyxia neonates may do better if they have been resuscitated with air rather than 100 per cent oxygen – rushing to achieve high saturations in this group of patients may cause harm [82].

Transcutaneous monitoring of carbon dioxide tension

Arterial carbon dioxide tension ($PaCO_2$) can be estimated from the continuous measurement of transcutaneous carbon dioxide ($TcCO_2$) tension. Experience with $TcCO_2$ monitoring in paediatric intensive care and following cardiac surgery has also been published [83,84] and $TcCO_2$ has a good correlation with $PaCO_2$ [85]. Its use during anaesthesia, however, has problems: set-up and calibration requires over 10 minutes; skin perfusion has to be arterialised by warming (the sensor temperature has to be 43–44°C and must be moved every 3 or 4 hours to avoid thermal skin damage); skin perfusion needs to be good and constant. With these in mind it is clearly more suitable for the intensive care setting rather than in the operating theatre. It is unlikely that $TcCO_2$ will replace end-tidal monitoring of carbon dioxide ($P_{ET}CO_2$) but may be a useful adjunct in cases where $P_{ET}CO_2$ may not accurately represent $PaCO_2$. This is the case in neonatal transport, where conventional methods of detecting $P_{ET}CO_2$ have an unacceptable under-recording bias [86].

Capnography

Monitoring $P_{ET}CO_2$ is considered mandatory for anaesthesia especially in intubated patients. Some technical constraints make capnography less reliable in paediatrics. There are two types of capnograph: side-stream and in-line. In both, sufficient tidal gas may not be available for analysis to obtain a true end-tidal plateau when respiration is rapid or shallow, or whenever there is a large apparatus dead space or a leak around an uncuffed tracheal tube. With side-stream capnographs the $P_{ET}CO_2$ can also be diluted by a high aspiration flow rate [87]; standard flow rates of 150–200 mL/minute cause underestimation of $P_{ET}CO_2$ whenever the tidal volume is very small. New side-stream capnographs are much more accurate because the aspiration flow rate is reduced to 50 mL/minute into a 15-μL sensor [88] – called 'microstream' technology – and seem to reduce the $P_{ET}CO_2$–$PaCO_2$ gradients to a minimum in neonates with normal lungs. Even in very small infants (body weight <1000 g) $P_{ET}CO_2$ underestimates $PaCO_2$ only by less than 0.1 kPa [89,90]. However, $P_{ET}CO_2$ is still lower than $PaCO_2$ in the presence of pulmonary disease [91]. In intensive care the aspiration tubing commonly becomes blocked by condensation from active humidification. In-line capnography should be more accurate but the sample cell is heavy and bulky and therefore risks kinking small tracheal tubes.

Despite all these problems capnography is invaluable in the early detection of major complications including circuit disconnections and rebreathing, tracheal extubation, oesophageal intubation, hypoventilation and cardiac arrest [92].

End-tidal monitoring of carbon dioxide is also useful for monitoring respiratory function in sedated infants and children who do not have any artificial airway. Purpose-made nasal catheters are available that also combine the administration of oxygen. Microstream technology is important for accuracy. In these circumstances capnography can provide an early warning of airway obstruction, alveolar hypoventilation and bronchospasm, and therefore prevent hypoxaemia [93]. Capnography may improve the safety of sedation [94].

Ventilation

Airway pressure, both inspired and expired, must be monitored during positive pressure ventilation. These parameters inform the anaesthetist about changes in pulmonary function and guide therapy. Airway pressure monitoring can reliably detect disconnection. It may not detect airway obstruction, however, if the alarm limits are not set close enough to the unobstructed airway pressures. This is because the apparatus may have similar compliance to the lungs. Ventilation by hand can be more sensitive and allow detection of both obstruction of a tracheal tube and a change in lung compliance, although this also depends upon the compliance of the breathing system – a T-piece is less complaint and more sensitive than a Mapleson D system [95]. A disconnect alarm is essential during mechanical ventilation.

Monitoring respiratory mechanics

Anaesthesia changes respiratory dynamics and contributes to atelectasis in dependent parts of the lung during ventilation [96]. Appropriate positive pressure ventilation is necessary to prevent atelectasis but too much pressure ventilation can result in lung trauma. The concept of ventilator-induced lung injury is well established in the intensive care setting. Lung injury can result in a systemic inflammatory response leading to acute respiratory distress syndrome (ARDS) and death. Permissive hypoxia, permissive hypercapnia and low tidal volume ventilation (6 mL/kg) together contribute to a protective strategy of ventilation during intensive care [97]. To prevent or minimise lung trauma during ventilation, monitoring of lung mechanics is mandatory. The majority of ventilators in paediatric intensive care now allow accurate monitoring, not only of pressure and volume, but also flow – all of which can be displayed graphically.

Ventilators for anaesthesia are now beginning to incorporate spirometry systems to enable the anaesthetist to optimise compliance and gas exchange [98]. Pressure–volume and flow–volume loops illustrate the real-time relationships of pressure, volume and flow [99]. Changes in the respective loops displayed dynamically not only enable the clinician optimally to recruit alveoli, but also provide quick graphic warning of several adverse events.

PRESSURE–VOLUME LOOPS

Dynamic pressure–volume (P-V) loops reveal lower and upper inflection points (see Chapter 2). The lower inflection

point guides appropriate setting for positive end-expiratory pressure (PEEP), while the upper inflection point warns against over-distension of the lung respectively (Fig. 20.2). Changes in dynamic lung compliance such as abdominal distension, pnuemothorax, bronchospasm and endobronchial intubation result in changes in the P-V loops (Fig. 20.3).

FLOW–VOLUME LOOPS

Flow–volume (F-V) loops are particularly good at representing changes in resistance, and identifying air leaks from around the tracheal tube. The change in resistance may occur during inspiration (e.g. a blocked tracheal tube) or during expiration (e.g. bronchospasm) (Fig. 20.4).

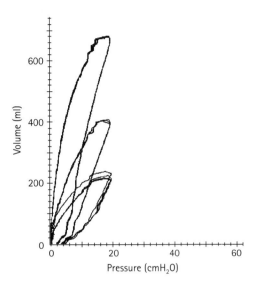

Figure 20.3 Pressure–volume loops from pressure-controlled ventilation. Changes in loop are caused by changes in compliance. From Lucangelo *et al.* [99].

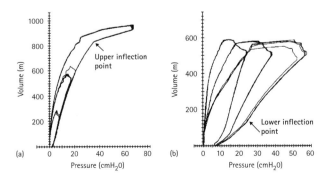

Figure 20.2 Pressure–volume loops from volume-controlled ventilation. (a) Pressure increase related to the volume increase, with identification of the upper inflection point. (b) Pressure increase related to the decrease in compliance. On the inspiratory limb, the lower inflection point (arrow) occurs at higher pressure as the compliance decreases. From Lucangelo *et al.* [99].

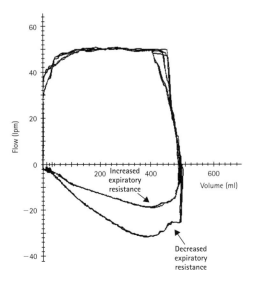

Figure 20.4 The effect of resistance on the expiratory limb only, with no effect on inspiratory flow. From Lucangelo *et al.* [99].

Flow–volume loops can reveal air leaks that would not be identified with P-V loops. The loop is characteristically incomplete because of loss in volume (Fig. 20.5).

Gas analysis

Continuous monitoring of inspired oxygen and anaesthetic gas or vapour concentrations is essential during anaesthesia. The accuracy of current infrared vapour analysis is limited to $\pm$ 0.1 per cent. Expired or end-tidal vapour analysis is extremely useful, provided that the inaccuracies of end-tidal gas sampling are appreciated. End-tidal vapour concentration may be the best indication that a patient is anaesthetised and remains anaesthetised after surgical stimulation.

CENTRAL NERVOUS SYSTEM

Acute brain injury is a common problem in intensive care and may occur following birth asphyxia, trauma or cardiac arrest. Management strategies try to reduce secondary neurological injury by achieving physiological stability. The adequacy of cerebral perfusion pressure (CPP) can be assessed by comparing intracranial pressure (ICP) with mean arterial pressure (MAP).

Intracranial pressure monitoring

The brain is enclosed in a non-expandable vault of bone. As the ICP rises, due perhaps to cerebral oedema or haemorrhage, blood flow is impeded so that brain ischaemia follows and eventually brain death becomes inevitable. Monitoring both ICP and MAP enables the clinician to manipulate the CPP to optimise cerebral perfusion. There are no randomised controlled trials in children but consensus practice and some published data suggest that intense cardiovascular monitoring combined with ICP monitoring may reduce the incidence of secondary injury after traumatic brain injury in children. Guidelines for the acute

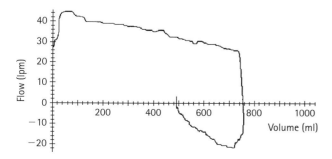

Figure 20.5 Air leak revealed by failed closure of flow–volume loop and failure to reach zero on the expiratory curve. From Lucangelo *et al.* [99].

medical management of trau-matic brain injury in children have been published [100].

Intracranial pressure monitoring can be achieved by inserting an intraventricular drain, or by probes placed in the parenchyma or in either the subarachnoid or extradural spaces. Intraventricular drains are prone to infection but enable drainage of cerebrospinal fluid (CSF). Intraparenchymal probes have the advantage that they have a low infection rate and can be easily inserted in an intensive care environment; they use either a small strain gauge pressure sensor (mounted at the tip of a thin catheter) or a fibre-optic catheter (the change in reflection of a light beam is pre-calibrated). They are accurate and show little change in baseline drift.

Intracranial pressure values of over 25 mmHg in adults are associated with poor outcome and so treatment should be vigorous to ensure adequate CPP. Types of ICP waves are observed. Type A waves are steep changes in ICP lasting 5–20 minutes. These are always pathological and are associated with severe brain injury. Other fluctuations in ICP may reflect changes in autoregulation, blood pressure, states of arousal, blood gases and temperature, and are not necessarily pathological. In children there are limited data to help guide the treatment of ICP but it has been suggested that ICP should be kept below 15 mmHg in infants, 18 mmHg in children up to 8 years and 20 mmHg in children over 8 years [101].

When CPP is used as a target, pressures ranging from 50 mmHg to 80 mmHg are thought to be safe. Higher as well as lower pressures may be detrimental and associated with a poor outcome. Other forms of monitoring such as transcranial Doppler, jugular venous bulb oximetry, microdialysis and brain tissue oximetry may guide perfusion but have not yet improved outcome [102].

Cerebral function by electroencephalogram monitoring

The electroencephalogram (EEG) is a complex waveform that can be interpreted to indicate changes in cortical function. This is most valuable during intensive care but has been used in paediatric cardiac surgery also.

First, the EEG is the only method of detecting epileptiform cortical discharges in a patient who is otherwise immobile. Second, major suppression of cortical electric activity occurs in coma caused by sedation and anaesthesia, cortical ischaemia, hypothermia and other less common metabolic pathology. Burst suppression precedes electrical silence and is characterised by periods of silence alternating with bursts of activity. The frequency components of an EEG signal can be broken down into constituent frequencies either by a system of filters at source or after digitisation by various methods including fast Fourier transformation analysis. The signal needs to be steady or continuous for such an approach to be useful – the presence of burst suppression, for example, either invalidates this approach or must be included in any mathematical algorithm. Electronic processing of an EEG with fast computers takes seconds and can be used to assess cortical activity continuously. Early processed EEG monitors (in the 1980s) used filters to exclude unwanted low and high frequencies and then measured the amplitude of the remaining signal. The cerebral function monitor (CFM) measures the minimum and maximum amplitude of a wide frequency band [103–105] and the cerebral functioning analysing monitor (CFAM) quantifies the amplitude of wide range of frequency bands (ranging from very low frequency of <1 Hz to the highest band of <20 Hz) [106]. It has been a standard tool in many paediatric intensive care units and is still used in specialist units caring for infants with encephalopathy related to birth asphyxia [107].

Near-infrared spectroscopy

Near-infrared spectroscopy (NIRS) is a continuous non-invasive method applying the principles of light transmission and absorption to determine tissue oxygen saturation [108]. It measures both oxygenated and deoxygenated haemoglobin (Hb). It also estimates the redox state of cytochrome aa_3 using an averaged value of arterial, venous and capillary blood (using the principle of the law of Lambert–Beer). Cytochrome aa_3 is crucial for oxidative phosphorylation and is responsible for approximately 90 per cent of cellular oxygen consumption. A decrease in cellular oxygen delivery results in a reduction of oxidative phosphorylation and decreased oxidation of cytochrome aa_3. Monitoring the redox state of cytochrome aa_3 therefore might be a key indicator of an impaired cellular oxidative metabolism. Although NIRS may be applied to almost any organ, it has mainly been used to study global and regional cerebral oxygenation [109,110].

Depth of anaesthesia

Two main outcomes are important in depth of anaesthesia monitoring. First, it is important to prevent patients being aware when they should be asleep. Awareness, however, is usually reported only by patients who can remember it and thus explicit recall is the second outcome and is frequently used as a measure of effectiveness. Awareness during surgery is possible if a patient is given inadequate anaesthesia and cannot move because of the effects of a muscle relaxant. If circulation to their arm is isolated before the muscle relaxant is given they can communicate by moving their arm [111,112]. This isolated forearm technique (IFT) has been achieved in children as young as age 5 years [113]. The incidence of awareness without recall is uncertain and fortunately, when it does occur, it is infrequently associated with pain. To complicate matters, recall of events during

inadequate anaesthesia is possible although rare even without muscle relaxants, and the memories can be very distressing [114]. Movement during anaesthesia has been used as an outcome in many studies but it is important to realise that movement alone is not a measure of conscious level. For example, spinal involuntary reflexes are not suppressed by the anaesthetised brain [115] – even complex movements can be coordinated without any proven activity within the cortex.

The incidence of explicit recall may be 1–2 per 1000 cases if depth of monitoring detection is limited to clinical signs of autonomic arousal and end-tidal anaesthetic agent analysis. Indeed, the incidence of awareness during anaesthesia may be even higher in children [116–118]. The potential devastating consequences of awareness have given rise to the development of cerebral monitors in an attempt to monitor depth of anaesthesia.

Early techniques were based on real-time signal processing of the EEG and were unreliable in adults. Techniques currently under development are still based on the EEG, but may be more reliable; they include auditory evoked potential (AEP), Bispectal Index (BIS) and spectral entropy. Each processes EEG and outputs a dimensionless index from 0 to 100 that aims to correlate with a behavioural score. Full validation of the techniques, particularly in children, is still to come. The EEG data of infants under anaesthesia are very limited [119] and clinical descriptors of consciousness have not been agreed. In adults, many studies have tested processed EEG in its ability to predict movement and for reasons already explained this may be unreasonable. Movement may be better predicted with AEP because it may correlate with the dose of anaesthesia rather than a cortical effect. The Narcotrend, which is another but less used processed EEG monitor, has recently been shown to have a very poor relationship to awareness detected using the IFT [120]; the performance of BIS and entropy have not yet been tested by the IFT.

AUDITORY EVOKED POTENTIALS

The AEP has been investigated since the 1980s, and is an EEG response to an auditory click caused by neural transmission through the brain stem, the midbrain and the cortex. Background EEG is removed by averaging the recordings after many clicks (typically 1024 clicks at 6 Hz) to produce a characteristic signal showing peaks and troughs (it may take 2–3 minutes to achieve). There are components from the brain stem, early cortical and late cortical transmission and they can be seen, respectively, in the first 20 milliseconds, 20–70 milliseconds and up to 500 milliseconds after the click. The early response is unchanged by clinical doses of anaesthesia, and the late response is easily suppressed by low doses. The early cortical or middle latency response (MLR), however, changes predictably with the depth of anaesthesia [121].

Quantitative analysis of MLR amplitude and latency depends on visual examination of the waveform and so is open to operator bias. The Alaris AEP monitor is an automated machine that can calculate an index within 2–6 seconds by analysing the AEP signals with a technique called autoregressive modelling [122]: the index ranges from 0 to 100, representing deep coma and alert state respectively. Electromyograph (EMG) interference may not be removed by signal averaging because contraction of the posterior auricular muscle can be triggered by noise and therefore the AEP is most reliable when muscle relaxants are used [123,124]. Few data are available in small children and although AEP measurement is possible in infants it is made less reliable by the presence of ECG interference [125].

Studies also indicate that the change in MLR varies with type of anaesthesia administered [126] and, in particular, opioids do not affect MLR directly but may do so by reducing surgical stimulation [127]. Benzodiazepines have little effect on MLR. There may be a complicated relationship between amplitude and latency for different anaesthetic agents and, if so, MLR monitoring will need careful interpretation.

BISPECTRAL INDEX

The BIS (Aspect Medical Systems, Newton, MA, USA) is an accepted measure of the hypnotic effect of anaesthetics and sedative drugs. It is a processed EEG that incorporates four main calculated variables into an algorithm (these are the power of selected frequency bands, the phase relationship between selected frequencies, burst suppression and EMG). A BIS score of less than 60 indicates sufficient cortical suppression to ensure unconsciousness (and lack of explicit recall) [128–130]. The algorithm is validated only in adults and may not be suitable for all anaesthesia drugs – ketamine is an exception, for example. Bispectral Index monitoring has gained in popularity for anaesthetised adults but it is still not in everyday use.

Studies in children suggest that BIS scores match behavioural scores as well as they do for adults. This is not so in infants in whom awakening occurs very quickly, even from low BIS scores. Various anaesthetic agents (volatile and intravenous) have different EEG signatures. Halothane anaesthesia administered to infants induces slow waves [131,132] whereas isoflurane may induce high-frequency activity [133]. Other reports suggest that propofol administered to children over 6 years generates the typical EEG changes seen in adults, as does sevoflurane in children over 4 months [134,135]. Indeed, various volatile anaesthetic agents at 1 MAC (minimal alveolar concentration) appear to generate slightly different BIS scores and, paradoxically, BIS can even increase with increasing MAC [136–142]. Note should be taken that MAC is probably a measure of spinal cord immobility rather than effect on the cortex. The effect of opioids is also complex. High doses reduce arousal (detected by BIS) because the nociceptive stimulus is reduced, whereas low doses of opiate themselves have minimal effect on BIS [143,144]. Such observations reduce the confidence of the monitor to judge depth of anaesthesia.

The technique cannot automatically be extrapolated to children because the central nervous system of children is constantly changing as the child develops. The awake EEG dominant frequency increases with age; it is 5 Hz at 6 months increasing to 10 Hz by adulthood. Children also have specific EEG patterns associated with the transition to and from natural sleep [119]. Under anaesthesia the BIS value for infants is different from that observed in children for a given state of arousal – although equating behavior of infants and children is problematic [145–147]. BIS values also rise for a given MAC as age decreases [148] but again this is difficult to interpret because MAC is related to spinal cord suppression. Other factors such as hypoglycaemia, cerebral ischaemia and hypothermia all decrease BIS. Abnormal EEG patterns after convulsions, in children with cerebral palsy and in severe brain injury, may also alter BIS [149].

Because BIS varies with age it is probably unwise to rely on it in children under the age of 2 years.

SPECTRAL ENTROPY

Entropy describes the irregularity, complexity and unpredictable characteristics of the EEG. It is independent of frequency and amplitude. It has a score of zero when the signal is completely regular and predictable and, when the patient is awake, the EEG is more disorganised, has more entropy and rises to a maximum of 100 [150]. Conversely, with increasing concentration of anaesthetic, entropy falls [151–153]. The concept of entropy is particularly attractive to monitoring depth of anaesthesia in children because the normal EEG varies with age. There are, however, limited studies in children. One small study showed a good correlation between entropy and BIS in children and toddlers, but poor correlation in infants [154]. The same group in a later study showed that both BIS and entropy scores vary with age, being lowest in infants less than 1 year for a given MAC of sevoflurane. Both BIS and entropy performed equally well but should be used with caution below 1 year of age [147].

NEUROMUSCULAR FUNCTION

Neuromuscular transmission alters as the child develops. The changing volume of drug distribution, the increased muscle mass and the maturation of the neuromuscular junction itself all serve to modify the size and duration of effect of neuromuscular blocking agents. Non-invasive monitors of neuromuscular block are available and enable the anaesthetist to test neuromuscular transmission via train of four (TOF), double burst, tetanic and post-tetanic stimulation. In the first few months of life tetanic and post-tetanic stimulation are less useful because even without relaxant drugs neonates, and in particular premature infants, are prone to tetanic fade and post-tetanic exhaustion.

Train-of-four stimulation at 2 Hz for 2 seconds repeated every 20 seconds can safely and reliably be used from birth, and is the preferred method for detecting neuromuscular blockade. In general, it is a good predictor of minute ventilation at the end of anaesthesia but it is influenced by factors other than relaxant drug concentration. It should be noted that the fourth twitch is usually lower in amplitude than the first in neonates [155]. Hypothermia reduces the height of all the twitches but not the ratio. Increases in twitch height can be seen with repeated TOF tests – probably owing to enhanced mechanical response independent of the neuromuscular junction. An in-depth review of neuromuscular transmission monitoring in children is recommended reading [156].

TEMPERATURE

During surgery and anaesthesia a number of factors conspire to impair normal thermoregulation and reduce the core temperature of patients. Anaesthesia (not ketamine) leads to impairment of hypothalamic function, vasoconstriction, shivering and reduced metabolic rate. Surgery causes large thermal losses. Much of the temperature fall occurs within the first hour of surgery [157]. Initially, there is a rapid fall in temperature resulting from loss of tonic vasoconstriction. Eventually, if hypothermia reaches a certain point, some vasoconstriction is triggered [158]. Children have a higher surface area to body weight ratio compared with adults, and so they lose heat more rapidly. Neonates and preterm babies are particularly susceptible to hypothermia [159].

There is a general consensus that maintaining normothermia may lead to fewer intraoperative and postoperative complications [160]. Certainly hypothermia in preterm babies and neonates at delivery is associated with increased morbidity and mortality [161]. Maintaining normothermia in this patient group may be especially important. Active warming is now commonplace in paediatric anaesthesia, using radiant heaters, warming blankets, convection heaters, humidification and warming of inspired gases, and warming of intravenous and irrigating fluids all serve to reduce the temperature fall during anaesthesia. Some forms of warming by convection are so effective that they may even result in hyperthermia [162]. Water-filled garments have been used in which water temperature can be automatically controlled to maintain a chosen core temperature. This approach may be useful in major surgery where thermal control is otherwise difficult [163].

Temperature monitoring is therefore essential in paediatrics to detect both hypothermia and inadvertent hyperthermia. Many sites are useful but each has its limitations. They include digital skin, forehead, axilla, bladder, rectum, oesophagus and nasopharynx. The temperature of the tympanic membrane could be regarded as the most representative measurement of brain temperature but the probe can cause perforation of the tympanic membrane. Measurements made in the nasopharynx, bladder and oesophagus are considered more precise than the axilla, forehead and rectum, and are much better than digital surface temperature [164]. Oesophageal temperature probes need to be inserted into the lower oesophagus to avoid being influenced by the temperature of inspired gases. Rectal temperature probes may cause perforation in neonates and should not be used in neutropenic patients.

GENERAL CONDUCT OF MONITORING AND RECORD-KEEPING DURING ANAESTHESIA

Monitoring is unproductive unless the anaesthetist is vigilant and reacts correctly. During almost all situations alarms should be set to assist vigilance. Occasionally, the setting of specific alarms is crucial; for example, capnography is the best method of warning of an air embolism during neurosurgery. Regular manual recording of physiological variables was previously the accepted standard for both anaesthesia and intensive care charts but automated electronic recording and printouts have now superseded this approach. During critical incidents it is not possible to record and react at the same time and so data from human memory are likely to be inaccurate. Moreover, the memory will often subconsciously record data that support a false diagnosis rather than record the true data that could be useful to obtain the correct diagnosis later. Electronic record-keeping is ideal but care should be taken to annotate some recordings that may be due to artefact, e.g. diathermy. Nevertheless, automatic record-keeping is a standard in many hospitals and it should be achieved widely in the foreseeable future.

REFERENCES

Key references

Cote CJ, Rolf N, Liu LM *et al.* A single-blind study of combined pulse oximetry and capnography in children. *Anesthesiology* 1991; **74**(6): 980–7.

De Waal EEC, Kalkman CJ. Haemodynamic changes during low-pressure carbon dioxide pneumoperitoneum in young children. *Paediatr Anaesth* 2003; **13**(1): 18–25.

Durward A, Tibby SM, Skellett S *et al.* The strong ion gap predicts mortality in children following cardiopulmonary bypass surgery. *Pediatr Crit Care Med* 2005; **6**(3): 281–5.

Lightdale JR, Goldmann DA, Feldman HA *et al.* Microstream capnography improves patient monitoring during moderate sedation: a randomized, controlled trial. *Pediatrics* 2006; **117**(6): e1170–8.

Verghese ST, McGill WA, Patel RI *et al.* Ultrasound-guided internal jugular venous cannulation in infants: a prospective comparison with the traditional palpation method. *Anesthesiology* 1999; **91**(1): 71–7.

References

1. Clover JT. Under administration of chloroform through the nostrils. *Lancet* 1868; i: 23.
2. Kirk R. On auscultation of the heart during chloroform narcosis. *BMJ* 1896; **2**: 1704–6.

3. Association of Anaesthetists of Great Britain and Ireland. *Recommendations for standards of monitoring during anaesthesia and recovery.* London: AAGBI, 2000.

4. American Society of Anaesthetists. *Standards for basic anesthetic monitoring.* San Francisco: ASA, 2005.

5. Thompson JP, Mahajan RP. Monitoring the monitors – beyond risk management. *Br J Anaesth* 2006; **97**(1): 1–3.

6. Young, D Griffiths J. Clinical trials of monitoring in anaesthesia, critical care and acute ward care: a review. *Br J Anaesth* 2006; **97**(1): 39–45.

7. Hall JB. Searching for evidence to support pulmonary artery catheter use in critically ill patients. *JAMA* 2005; **294**(13): 1693–4.

8. Iberti TJ, Daily EK, Leibowitz AB *et al.* Assessment of critical care nurses' knowledge of the pulmonary artery catheter. The Pulmonary Artery Catheter Study Group. *Crit Care Med* 1994; **22**(10): 1674–8.

9. Pulmonary Artery Catheter Consensus Conference: consensus statement. *New Horiz* 1997; **5**(3): 175–94.

10. Bellomo R, Uchino S. Cardiovascular monitoring tools: use and misuse. *Curr Opin Crit Care* 2003; **9**(3): 225–9.

11. Pinsky MR. Rationale for cardiovascular monitoring. *Curr Opin Crit Care* 2003; **9**(3): 222–4.

12. Bihari D, Gimson AE, Waterson M, Williams R. Tissue hypoxia during fulminant hepatic failure. *Crit Care Med* 1985; **13**(12): 1034–9.

13. Boldt J. Clinical review: hemodynamic monitoring in the intensive care unit. *Crit Care* 2002; **6**(1): 52–9.

14. Dickinson DF. The normal ECG in childhood and adolescence. *Heart* 2005; **91**(12): 1626–30.

15. Sharieff GQ, Rao SO. The pediatric ECG. *Emerg Med Clin North Am* 2006; **24**(1): 195–208, vii–viii.

16. Paris ST, Cafferkey M, Tarling M *et al.* Comparison of sevoflurane and halothane for outpatient dental anaesthesia in children. *Br J Anaesth* 1997; **79**(3): 280–4.

17. Berntson GG, Bigger JT Jr, Eckberg DL *et al.* Heart rate variability: origins, methods, and interpretative caveats. *Psychophysiology* 1997; **34**(6): 623–48.

18. Pomfrett CJ. Heart rate variability, BIS and 'depth of anaesthesia'. *Br J Anaesth* 1999; **82**(5): 659–62.

19. Sleigh JW, Donovan J. Comparison of bispectral index, 95 per cent spectral edge frequency and approximate entropy of the EEG, with changes in heart rate variability during induction of general anaesthesia. *Br J Anaesth* 1999; **82**(5): 666–71.

20. Pomfrett CJ, Sneyd JR, Barrie JR, Healy TE. Respiratory sinus arrhythmia: comparison with EEG indices during isoflurane anaesthesia at 0.65 and 1.2 MAC. *Br J Anaesth* 1994; **72**(4): 397–402.

21. Task Force of the European Society of Cardiology and the North American Society of Pacing and Electrophysiology. Heart rate variability: standards of measurement, physiological interpretation and clinical use. *Circulation* 1996; **93**(5): 1043–65.

22. Park MK, Menard SM. Accuracy of blood pressure measurement by the Dinamap monitor in infants and children. *Pediatrics* 1987; **79**(6): 907–14.

23. Birch AA, Morris SL. Do the Finapres and Colin radial artery tonometer measure the same blood pressure changes following deflation of thigh cuffs? *Physiol Meas* 2003; **24**(3): 653–60.

24. Cua CL, Thomas K, Zurakowski D, Laussen PC. A comparison of the Vasotrac with invasive arterial blood pressure monitoring in children after pediatric cardiac surgery. *Anesth Analg* 2005; **100**(5): 1289–94.

25. Hermansen MC, Hermansen MG. Intravascular catheter complications in the neonatal intensive care unit. *Clin Perinatol* 2005; **32**(1): 141–56, vii.

26. Gunn SR, Pinsky MR. Implications of arterial pressure variation in patients in the intensive care unit. *Curr Opin Crit Care* 2001; **7**(3): 212–7.

27. Tavernier B, Makhotine O, Lebuffe G *et al.* Systolic pressure variation as a guide to fluid therapy in patients with sepsis-induced hypotension. *Anesthesiology* 1998; **89**(6): 1313–21.

28. Ince C, Sinaasappel M. Microcirculatory oxygenation and shunting in sepsis and shock. *Crit Care Med* 1999; **27**(7): 1369–77.

29. Kees HP, Armand RG. Central venous catheter use. *Intensive Care Med* 2002; **V28**(1): 1–17.

30. Polderman K. Girbes A. Central venous catheter use. *Intensive Care Med* 2002; **V28**(1): 18–28.

31. Slama M, Novara A, Safavian A *et al.* Improvement of internal jugular vein cannulation using an ultrasound-guided technique. *Intensive Care Med* 1997; **23**(8): 916–9.

32. Leyvi G, Taylor DG, Reith E, Wasnick JD. Utility of ultrasound-guided central venous cannulation in pediatric surgical patients: a clinical series. *Paediatr Anaesth* 2005; **15**(11): 953–8.

33. Verghese ST, McGill WA, Patel RI *et al.* Ultrasound-guided internal jugular venous cannulation in infants: a prospective comparison with the traditional palpation method. *Anesthesiology* 1999; **91**(1): 71–7.

34. Fletcher SJ, Bodenham AR. Safe placement of central venous catheters: where should the tip of the catheter lie? *Br J Anaesth* 2000; **85**(2): 188–91.

35. Lucey B, Varghese JC, Haslam P, and Lee MJ. Routine chest radiographs after central line insertion: mandatory postprocedural evaluation or unnecessary waste of resources? *Cardiovasc Intervent Radiol* 1999; **22**(5): 381–4.

36. Racadio JM, Doellman DA, Johnson ND *et al.* Pediatric peripherally inserted central catheters: complication rates related to catheter tip location. *Pediatrics* 2001; **107**(2): e28.

37. Darling JC, Newell SJ, Mohamdee O *et al.* Central venous catheter tip in the right atrium: a risk factor for neonatal cardiac tamponade. *J Perinatol* 2001; **21**(7): 461–4.

38. Bein B, Worthmann F, Tonner PH *et al.* Comparison of esophageal Doppler, pulse contour analysis, and real-time pulmonary artery thermodilution for the continuous measurement of cardiac output. *J Cardiothorac Vasc Anesth* 2004; **18**(2): 185–9.

39. Chew M, Poelaert J. Accuracy and repeatability of pediatric cardiac output measurement using Doppler: 20-year review of the literature. *Intensive Care Med* 2003; **29**(11): 1889.

40. Carcillo JA, Davis AL, Zaritsky A. Role of early fluid resuscitation in pediatric septic shock. *JAMA* 1991; **266**(9): 1242–5.

41. Connors AF Jr, Speroff T, Dawson NV *et al*. The effectiveness of right heart catheterization in the initial care of critically ill patients. SUPPORT Investigators. *JAMA* 1996; **276**(11): 889–97.

42. Eisenberg PR, Hansbrough JR, Anderson D, Schuster DP. A prospective study of lung water measurements during patient management in an intensive care unit. *Am Rev Respir Dis* 1987; **136**(3): 662–8.

43. Isakow W, Schuster DP. Extravascular lung water measurements and hemodynamic monitoring in the critically ill: bedside alternatives to the pulmonary artery catheter. *Am J Physiol Lung Cell Mol Physiol* 2006; **291**(6): L1118–31.

44. Tibby SM, Hatherill M, Marsh MJ *et al*. Clinical validation of cardiac output measurements using femoral artery thermodilution with direct Fick in ventilated children and infants. *Intensive Care Med* 1997; **23**(9): 987–91.

45. Linton RA, Jonas MM, Tibby SM *et al*. Cardiac output measured by lithium dilution and transpulmonary thermodilution in patients in a paediatric intensive care unit. *Intensive Care Med* 2000; **26**(10): 1507–11.

46. Hofer CK, Furrer L, Matter-Ensner S *et al*. Volumetric preload measurement by thermodilution: a comparison with transoesophageal echocardiography. *Br J Anaesth* 2005; **94**(6): 748–55.

47. Schiffmann H, Erdlenbruch B, Singer D *et al*. Assessment of cardiac output, intravascular volume status, and extravascular lung water by transpulmonary indicator dilution in critically ill neonates and infants. *J Cardiothorac Vasc Anesth* 2002; **16**(5): 592.

48. Godje O, Thiel P, Lamm C *et al*. Less invasive, continuous hemodynamic monitoring during minimally invasive coronary surgery. *Ann Thorac Surg* 1999; **68**(4): 1532–6.

49. Godje O, Hoke K, Goetz AE *et al*. Reliability of a new algorithm for continuous cardiac output determination by pulse-contour analysis during hemodynamic instability. *Crit Care Med* 2002; **30**(1): 52–8.

50. Hamamoto M, Imanaka H, Kagisaki K *et al*. Is an increase in lactate concentration associated with cardiac dysfunction after the Fontan procedure? *Ann Thorac Cardiovasc Surg* 2005; **11**(5): 301–6.

51. Mahajan A, Shabanie A, Turner J *et al*. Pulse contour analysis for cardiac output monitoring in cardiac surgery for congenital heart disease. *Anesth Analg* 2003; **97**(5): 1283–8.

52. Murdoch IA, Marsh MJ, Tibby SM, McLuckie A. Continuous haemodynamic monitoring in children: use of transoesophageal Doppler. *Acta Paediatr Scand* 1995; **84**(7): 761–4.

53. Mohan UR, Britto J, Habibi P *et al*. Noninvasive measurement of cardiac output in critically ill children. *Pediatr Cardiol* 2002; **23**(1): 58–61.

54. Larousse E, Asehnoune K, Dartayet B *et al*. The hemodynamic effects of pediatric caudal anesthesia assessed by esophageal Doppler. *Anesth Analg* 2002; **94**(5): 1165–8.

55. Gueugniaud PY, Muchada R, Moussa M *et al*. Continuous oesophageal aortic blood flow echo-Doppler measurement during general anaesthesia in infants. *Can J Anaesth* 1997; **44**(7): 745–50.

56. Hirschl MM, Kittler H, Woisetschlager C *et al*. Simultaneous comparison of thoracic bioimpedance and arterial pulse waveform-derived cardiac output with thermodilution measurement. *Crit Care Med* 2000; **28**(6): 1798–802.

57. Spiess BD, Patel MA, Soltow LO, Wright IH. Comparison of bioimpedance versus thermodilution cardiac output during cardiac surgery: evaluation of a second-generation bioimpedance device. *J Cardiothorac Vasc Anesth* 2001; **15**(5): 567–73.

58. Braden DS, Leatherbury L, Treiber FA, Strong WB. Noninvasive assessment of cardiac output in children using impedance cardiography. *Am Heart J* 1990; **120**(5): 1166–72.

59. De Waal EEC, Kalkman CJ. Haemodynamic changes during low-pressure carbon dioxide pneumoperitoneum in young children. *Paediatr Anaesth* 2003; **13**(1): 18–25.

60. Cahalan MK, Litt L, Botvinick EH, Schiller NB. Advances in noninvasive cardiovascular imaging: implications for the anesthesiologist. *Anesthesiology* 1987; **66**(3): 356–72.

61. Kneeshaw JD. Transoesophageal echocardiography (TOE) in the operating room. *Br J Anaesth* 2006; **97**(1): 77–84.

62. Singh GK, Shiota T, Cobanoglu A *et al*. Diagnostic accuracy and role of intraoperative biplane transesophageal echocardiography in pediatric patients with left ventricle outflow tract lesions. *J Am Soc Echocardiogr* 1998; **11**(1): 47–56.

63. Shiota T, Omoto R, Cobanoglu A *et al*. Usefulness of transesophageal imaging of flow convergence region in the operating room for evaluating isolated patent ductus arteriosus. *Am J Cardiol* 1997; **80**(8): 1108–12.

64. Stevenson JG. Role of intraoperative transesophageal echocardiography during repair of congenital cardiac defects. *Acta Paediatr Scand Suppl* 1995; **410**: 23–33.

65. Xu J, Shiota T, Ge S *et al*. Intraoperative transesophageal echocardiography using high-resolution biplane 7.5 MHz probes with continuous-wave Doppler capability in infants and children with tetralogy of Fallot. *Am J Cardiol* 1996; **77**(7): 539–42.

66. Kavanaugh-McHugh A, Tobias JD, Doyle T *et al*. Transesophageal echocardiography in pediatric congenital heart disease. *Cardiol Rev* 2000; **8**(5): 288–306.

67. Denault AY, Couture S, McKenty *et al*. Perioperative use of transesophageal echocardiography by anesthesiologists: impact in noncardiac surgery and in the intensive care unit. *Can J Anaesth* 2002; **49**(3): 287–93.

68. Pinsky MR. Targets for resuscitation from shock. *Minerva Anesthesiol* 2003; **69**(4): 237–44.

69. Murry DM, Olhsson V, Fraser JI. Defining acidosis in postoperative cardiac patients using Stewart's method of strong ion difference. *Pediatr Crit Care Med* 2004; **5**(3): 240–5.

70. Hatherill M, Waggie Z, Purves L *et al*. Correction of the anion gap for albumin in order to detect occult tissue anions in shock. *Arch Dis Child* 2002; **87**(6): 526–9.

71. Durward A, Tibby SM, Skellett S *et al*. The strong ion gap predicts mortality in children following cardiopulmonary bypass surgery. *Pediatr Crit Care Med* 2005; **6**(3): 281–5.

72. Hatherill M, McIntyre AG, Wattie M, Murdoch IA. Early hyperlactataemia in critically ill children. *Intensive Care Med* 2000; **26**(3): 314–18.

73. Munoz R, Laussen PC, Palacio G *et al.* Changes in whole blood lactate levels during cardiopulmonary bypass for surgery for congenital cardiac disease: an early indicator of morbidity and mortality. *J Thorac Cardiovasc Surg* 2000; **119**(1): 155–62.

74. Hatherill M, Sajjanhar T, Tibby SM *et al.* Serum lactate as a predictor of mortality after paediatric cardiac surgery. *Arch Dis Child* 1997; **77**(3): 235–8.

75. Rivers EP, Ander DS, Powell D. Central venous oxygen saturation monitoring in the critically ill patient. *Curr Opin Crit Care* 2001; **7**(3): 204–11.

76. Marx G, Reinhart K. Venous oximetry. *Curr Opin Crit Care* 2006; **12**(3): 263–8.

77. Hoffman GM, Tweddell JS, Ghanayem NS *et al.* Alteration of the critical arteriovenous oxygen saturation relationship by sustained afterload reduction after the Norwood procedure. *J Thorac Cardiovasc Surg* 2004; **127**(3): 738–45.

78. Bradley SM, Atz AM. Postoperative management: the role of mixed venous oxygen saturation monitoring. *Semin Thorac Cardiovasc Surg Pediatr Card Surg Annu* 2005: 22–7.

79. Cote CJ, Rolf N, Liu LM *et al.* A single-blind study of combined pulse oximetry and capnography in children. *Anesthesiology* 1991; **74**(6): 980–7.

80. Hay WW Jr, Rodden DJ, Collins SM *et al.* Reliability of conventional and new pulse oximetry in neonatal patients. *J Perinatol* 2002; **22**(5): 360–6.

81. Sinha SK, Tin W. The controversies surrounding oxygen therapy in neonatal intensive care units. *Curr Opin Pediatr* 2003; **15**(2): 161–5.

82. Saugstad OD. Oxygen for newborns: how much is too much? *J Perinatol* 2005; **25**(suppl 2): S45–9; discussion S50.

83. Tobias JD, Wilson WR Jr, Meyer DJ. Transcutaneous monitoring of carbon dioxide tension after cardiothoracic surgery in infants and children. *Anesth Analg* 1999; **88**(3): 531–4.

84. Tobias JD, Meyer DJ. Noninvasive monitoring of carbon dioxide during respiratory failure in toddlers and infants: end-tidal versus transcutaneous carbon dioxide. *Anesth Analg* 1997; **85**(1): 55–8.

85. Nosovitch MA, Johnson JO, Tobias JD. Noninvasive intraoperative monitoring of carbon dioxide in children: endtidal versus transcutaneous techniques. *Paediatr Anaesth* 2002; **12**(1): 48–52.

86. Tingay DG, Stewart MJ, Morley CJ. Monitoring of end tidal carbon dioxide and transcutaneous carbon dioxide during neonatal transport. *Arch Dis Child Fetal Neonatal Ed* 2005; **90**(6): F523–6.

87. Kirpalani H, Kechagias S, Lerman J. Technical and clinical aspects of capnography in neonates. *J Med Eng Technol* 1991; **15**(4–5): 154–61.

88. Colman Y, Krauss B. Microstream capnograpy technology: a new approach to an old problem. *J Clin Monit Comput* 1999; **15**(6): 403–9.

89. Rozycki HJ, Sysyn GD, Marshall MK *et al.* Mainstream end-tidal carbon dioxide monitoring in the neonatal intensive care unit. *Pediatrics* 1998; **101**(4 Pt 1): 648–53.

90. Wu CH, Chou HC, Hsieh WS *et al.* Good estimation of arterial carbon dioxide by end-tidal carbon dioxide monitoring in the neonatal intensive care unit. *Pediatr Pulmonol* 2003; **35**(4): 292–5.

91. Hagerty JJ, Kleinman ME, Zurakowski D *et al.* Accuracy of a new low-flow sidestream capnography technology in newborns: a pilot study. *J Perinatol* 2002; **22**(3): 219–25.

92. Bhavani-Shankar K, Moseley H, Kumar AY, Delph Y. Capnometry and anaesthesia. *Can J Anaesth* 1992; **39**(6): 617–32.

93. Krauss B, Green SM. Procedural sedation and analgesia in children. *Lancet* 2006; **367**(9512): 766–80.

94. Lightdale JR, Goldmann DA, Feldman HA *et al.* Microstream capnography improves patient monitoring during moderate sedation: a randomized, controlled trial. *Pediatrics* 2006; **117**(6): e1170–8.

95. Tan SSW, Sury MRJ, Hatch DJ. The 'educated hand' in paediatric anaesthesia – does it exist? *Paediatr Anaesth* 1993; **3**: 291–5.

96. Magnusson L, Spahn DR. New concepts of atelectasis during general anaesthesia. *Br J Anaesth* 2003; **91**(1): 61–72.

97. Ricard JD, Dreyfuss D, Saumon G. Ventilator-induced lung injury. *Eur Respir J* 2003; **42**(suppl): 2s–9s.

98. Nunes S, Takala J. Evaluation of a new module in the continuous monitoring of respiratory mechanics. *Intensive Care Med* 2000; **26**(6): 670–8.

99. Lucangelo U, Bernabe F, Blanch L. Respiratory mechanics derived from signals in the ventilator circuit. *Respir Care* 2005; **50**(1): 55–65; discussion 65–7.

100. Adelson PD, Bratton SL, Carney NA *et al.* Guidelines for the acute medical management of severe traumatic brain injury in infants, children, and adolescents. *Pediatr Crit Care Med* 2003; **4**(3): S1–76.

101. Mazzola CA, Adelson PD. Critical care management of head trauma in children. *Crit Care Med* 2002; **30**(11 suppl): S393–401.

102. Steiner LA, Andrews PJ. Monitoring the injured brain: ICP and CBF. *Br J Anaesth* 2006; **97**(1): 26–38.

103. Dubois M, Savege TM, O'Carroll TM, Frank M. General anaesthesia and changes on the cerebral function monitor. *Anaesthesia* 1978; **33**(2): 157–64.

104. Schwartz MS, Colvin MP, Prior PF *et al.* The cerebral function monitor. Its value in predicting the neurological outcome in patients undergoing cardiopulmonary by-pass. *Anaesthesia* 1973; **28**(6): 611–8.

105. Maynard DE, Jenkinson JL. The cerebral function analysing monitor. Initial clinical experience, application and further development. *Anaesthesia* 1984; **39**(7): 678–90.

106. Frank M, Maynard DE, Tsanaclis LM *et al.* Changes in cerebral electrical activity measured by the Cerebral Function Analysing Monitor following bolus injections of thiopentone. *Br J Anaesth* 1984; **56**(10): 1075–81.

107. Gluckman PD, Wyatt JS, Azzopardi D *et al.* Selective head cooling with mild systemic hypothermia after neonatal encephalopathy: multicentre randomised trial. *Lancet* 2005; **365**(9460): 663–70.

108. Elwell CE. *A practical users guide to near infrared spectroscopy.* Hamakita-city: Hamamatsu Photonics KK, 1995.

109. Gottlieb EA, Fraser CD Jr, Andropoulos DB, Diaz LK. Bilateral monitoring of cerebral oxygen saturation results in

recognition of aortic cannula malposition during pediatric congenital heart surgery. *Paediatr Anaesth* 2006; **16**(7): 787–9.

110. Nollert G, Jonas RA, Reichart B. Optimizing cerebral oxygenation during cardiac surgery: a review of experimental and clinical investigations with near infrared spectro-photometry. *Thorac Cardiovasc Surg* 2000; **48**(4): 247–53.

111. Tunstall ME. Detecting wakefulness during general anaesthesia for caesarean section. *BMJ* 1977; **1**(6072): 1321.

112. Russell IF, Wang M. Isolated forearm technique. *Br J Anaesth* 1996; **76**(6): 884–6.

113. Byers GF, Muir JG. Detecting wakefulness in anaesthetised children. *Can J Anaesth* 1997; **44**(5 Pt 1): 486–8.

114. Domino KB, Posner KL, Caplan RA, Cheney FW. Awareness during anesthesia: a closed claims analysis. *Anesthesiology* 1999; **90**(4): 1053–61.

115. Antognini JF, Carstens E. *In vivo* characterization of clinical anaesthesia and its components. *Br J Anaesth* 2002; **89**(1): 156–66.

116. Iselin-Chaves I, Lopez U, Habre W. Intraoperative awareness in children: myth or reality? *Curr Opin Anesthesiol* 2006; **19**(3): 309–14.

117. Sebel PS, Bowdle TA, Ghoneim MM *et al.* The incidence of awareness during anesthesia: a multicenter United States study. *Anesth Analg* 2004; **99**(3): 833–9.

118. Davidson AJ, Huang GH, Czarnecki C *et al.* Awareness during anesthesia in children: a prospective cohort study. *Anesth Analg* 2005; **100**(3): 653–61.

119. Davidson AJ. Measuring anesthesia in children using the EEG. *Paediatr Anaesth* 2006; **16**(4): 374–87.

120. Russell IF. The Narcotrend 'depth of anaesthesia' monitor cannot reliably detect consciousness during general anaesthesia: an investigation using the isolated forearm technique. *Br J Anaesth* 2006; **96**(3): 346–52.

121. Thornton C. Evoked potentials in anaesthesia. *Eur J Anaesthesiol* 1991; **8**(2): 89–107.

122. Jensen EW, Lindholm P, Henneberg SW. Autoregressive modeling with exogenous input of middle-latency auditory-evoked potentials to measure rapid changes in depth of anesthesia. *Methods Inf Med* 1996; **35**(3): 256–60.

123. Thornton C, Sharpe RM. Evoked responses in anaesthesia. *Br J Anaesth* 1998; **81**(5): 771–81.

124. Wenningmann I, Paprotny S, Strassmann S *et al.* Correlation of the A-LineTM ARX index with acoustically evoked potential amplitude. *Br J Anaesth* 2006; **97**(5): 666–75.

125. Bell SL, Smith DC, Allen R, Lutman ME. Recording the middle latency response of the auditory evoked potential as a measure of depth of anaesthesia. A technical note. *Br J Anaesth* 2004; **92**(3): 442–5.

126. Dutton RC, Smith WD, Rampil IJ *et al.* Forty-hertz midlatency auditory evoked potential activity predicts wakeful response during desflurane and propofol anesthesia in volunteers. *Anesthesiology* 1999; **91**(5): 1209–20.

127. Tooley MA, Stapleton CL, Greenslade GL, Prys-Roberts C. Mid-latency auditory evoked response during propofol and alfentanil anaesthesia. *Br J Anaesth* 2004; **92**(1): 25–32.

128. Flaishon R, Windsor A, Sigl J, Sebel PS. Recovery of consciousness after thiopental or propofol. Bispectral index and isolated forearm technique. *Anesthesiology* 1997; **86**(3): 613–9.

129. Glass PS, Bloom M, Kearse L *et al.* Bispectral analysis measures sedation and memory effects of propofol, midazolam, isoflurane, and alfentanil in healthy volunteers. *Anesthesiology* 1997; **86**(4): 836–47.

130. Kearse LA Jr, Rosow C, Zaslavsky A *et al.* Bispectral analysis of the electroencephalogram predicts conscious processing of information during propofol sedation and hypnosis. *Anesthesiology* 1998; **88**(1): 25–34.

131. Kitahara Y, Kojima Y, Nozaki F. [Aperiodic analysis of EEG in children during halothane anesthesia.] *Masui* 1990; **39**(3): 396–402.

132. Sugiyama K, Joh S, Hirota Y *et al.* Relationship between changes in power spectra of electroencephalograms and arterial halothane concentration in infants. *Acta Anaesthesiol Scand* 1989; **33**(8): 670–5.

133. James PD, Volgyesi GA, Burrows FA. Alpha-pattern EEG during pediatric cardiac operations under isoflurane anesthesia. *Anesth Analg* 1986; **65**(5): 525–8.

134. Borgeat A, Dessibourg C, Popovic V *et al.* Propofol and spontaneous movements: an EEG study. *Anesthesiology* 1991; **74**(1): 24–7.

135. Rodriguez RA, Hall LE, Duggan S, Splinter WM. The bispectral index does not correlate with clinical signs of inhalational anesthesia during sevoflurane induction and arousal in children. *Can J Anaesth* 2004; **51**(5): 472–80.

136. Rampil IJ, Kim JS, Lenhardt R *et al.* Bispectral EEG index during nitrous oxide administration. *Anesthesiology* 1998; **89**(3): 671–7.

137. Hirota K, Kubota T, Ishihara H, Matsuki A. The effects of nitrous oxide and ketamine on the bispectral index and 95 per cent spectral edge frequency during propofol-fentanyl anaesthesia. *Eur J Anaesthesiol* 1999; **16**(11): 779–83.

138. Detsch O, Schneider G, Kochs E *et al.* Increasing isoflurane concentration may cause paradoxical increases in the EEG bispectral index in surgical patients. *Br J Anaesth* 2000; **84**(1): 33–7.

139. Puri GD. Paradoxical changes in bispectral index during nitrous oxide administration. *Br J Anaesth* 2001; **86**(1): 141–2.

140. Vereecke HE, Struys MM, Mortier EP. A comparison of bispectral index and ARX-derived auditory evoked potential index in measuring the clinical interaction between ketamine and propofol anaesthesia. *Anaesthesia* 2003; **58**(10): 957–61.

141. Edwards JJ, Soto RG, Thrush DM, Bedford RF. Bispectral index scale is higher for halothane than sevoflurane during intraoperative anesthesia. *Anesthesiology* 2003; **99**(6): 1453–5.

142. Davidson AJ, Czarnecki C. The Bispectral Index in children: comparing isoflurane and halothane. *Br J Anaesth* 2004; **92**(1): 14–7.

143. Iselin-Chaves IA, Flaishon R, Sebel PS *et al.* The effect of the interaction of propofol and alfentanil on recall, loss of

consciousness, and the Bispectral Index. *Anesth Analg* 1998; **87**(4): 949–55.

144. Guignard B, Menigaux C, Dupont X *et al.* The effect of remifentanil on the bispectral index change and hemodynamic responses after orotracheal intubation. *Anesth Analg* 2000; **90**(1): 161–7.

145. Bannister CF, Brosius KK, Sigl JC *et al.* The effect of bispectral index monitoring on anesthetic use and recovery in children anesthetized with sevoflurane in nitrous oxide. *Anesth Analg* 2001; **92**(4): 877–81.

146. Davidson AJ, McCann ME, Devavaram P *et al.* The differences in the bispectral index between infants and children during emergence from anesthesia after circumcision surgery. *Anesth Analg* 2001; **93**(2): 326–30.

147. Davidson AJ, Huang GH, Rebmann CS, Ellery C. Performance of entropy and Bispectral Index as measures of anaesthesia effect in children of different ages. *Br J Anaesth* 2005; **95**(5): 674–9.

148. Wodey E, Tirel O, Bansard JY *et al.* Impact of age on both BIS values and EEG bispectrum during anaesthesia with sevoflurane in children. *Br J Anaesth* 2005; **94**(6): 810–20.

149. Dahaba AA. Different conditions that could result in the Bispectral Index indicating an incorrect hypnotic state. *Anesth Analg* 2005; **101**(3): 765–773.

150. Viertio-Oja H, Maja V, Sarkela M *et al.* Description of the Entropy algorithm as applied in the Datex-Ohmeda S/5 Entropy Module. *Acta Anaesthesiol Scand* 2004; **48**(2): 154–61.

151. Vanluchene AL, Vereecke H, Thas O *et al.* Spectral entropy as an electroencephalographic measure of anesthetic drug effect: a comparison with bispectral index and processed midlatency auditory evoked response. *Anesthesiology* 2004; **101**(1): 34–42.

152. Ellerkmann RK, Liermann VM, Alves TM *et al.* Spectral entropy and bispectral index as measures of the electroencephalographic effects of sevoflurane. *Anesthesiology* 2004; **101**(6): 1275–82.

153. Schmidt GN, Bischoff P, Standl T, *et al.* Comparative evaluation of the Datex-Ohmeda S/5 Entropy Module and the Bispectral Index monitor during propofol-remifentanil anesthesia. *Anesthesiology* 2004; **101**(6): 1283–90.

154. Davidson AJ, Kim MJ, Sangolt GK. Entropy and bispectral index during anaesthesia in children. *Anaesth Intensive Care* 2004; **32**(4): 485–93.

155. Goudsouzian NG. Maturation of neuromuscular transmission in the infant. *Br J Anaesth* 1980; **52**(2): 205–14.

156. Saldien V, Vermeyen KM. Neuromuscular transmission monitoring in children. *Paediatr Anaesth* 2004; **14**(4): 289–92.

157. Imrie MM, Hall GM. Body temperature and anaesthesia. *Br J Anaesth* 1990; **64**(3): 346–54.

158. Sessler DI. Perioperative heat balance. *Anesthesiology* 2000; **92**(2): 578–96.

159. Bissonnette B. Temperature monitoring in pediatric anesthesia. *Int Anesthesiol Clin* 1992; **30**(3): 63–76.

160. Scott EM, Buckland R. A systematic review of intraoperative warming to prevent postoperative complications. *AORN J* 2006; **83**(5): 1090–104, 1107–13.

161. Watkinson M. Temperature control of premature infants in the delivery room. *Clin Perinatol* 2006; **33**(1): 43–53, vi.

162. Cassey JG, Armstrong PJ, Smith GE, Farrell PT. The safety and effectiveness of a modified convection heating system for children during anesthesia. *Paediatr Anaesth* 2006; **16**(6): 654–62.

163. Sury MR, Scuplak S. Water-filled garment warming of infants undergoing open abdominal or thoracic surgery. *Pediatr Surg Int* 2006; **22**(2): 182–5.

164. Cork RC, Vaughan RW, Humphrey LS. Precision and accuracy of intraoperative temperature monitoring. *Anesth Analg* 1983; **62**(2): 211–4.

SPECIAL TECHNIQUES

Management of the difficult airway

ANN E BLACK

KEY LEARNING POINTS

- Most children who have airways that are difficult to manage are identifiable preoperatively.
- Children who may be difficult to intubate are usually easily predicted. Unexpected difficult intubation is very rare.
- Spontaneous respiration should be maintained until the airway is either secured or fully assessed.
- Sedation should be avoided if the airway is compromised.
- There should always be a clear anaesthetic plan and a back-up plan.
- Management of a child with such issues will require meticulous planning and the help of an expert team.
- Ongoing training and regular practice of advanced techniques are essential.

Fibre-optic intubation

- Use a preoperative drying agent.
- Stabilise the child's head on a head ring.
- Use suction to clear the airway, particularly of oral secretions, before starting.
- Maintain jaw thrust or use soft traction on the tongue if using the nasal route.
- Position the camera screen in an ergonomic way so that you are looking ahead at the screen.
- Avoid causing trauma and bleeding as this makes obtaining a good view difficult.

INTRODUCTION

Difficult airway management in children may be defined as any condition in which holding a mask airway is awkward or in which bag-and-mask ventilation is hard to achieve with conventional equipment. Difficult intubation may be defined as tracheal intubation requiring more than three attempts, or abnormalities demanding advanced airway techniques. Fortunately, most children who present such difficulties can be identified preoperatively, because they have either a syndrome associated with airway abnormalities or a suggestive diagnosis (Table 21.1). In adults, the incidence of difficult direct laryngoscopy is 1.5–8.5 per cent, and failed intubations occur in 0.13–0.3 per cent [1]; equivalent figures for children are unknown but are believed to be considerably lower [2]. Difficult intubation in paediatric cardiac patients has been reported to be 1.25 per cent, with 50 per cent of these having syndromal abnormalities

[3]. The overall incidence of difficult intubation in children with cleft lip or palate is 4.7 per cent, most frequently in infants aged 1–6 months (7 per cent) [4].

Morbidity and mortality have been reported when difficulties arise in managing the paediatric airway. In closed claims reports (statistics derived from closed claims for damages associated with anaesthetic practice in the USA), there were nine cases of reported difficulties associated with difficult paediatric intubation and five associated with acid aspiration [5].

Even though guidelines are available for difficult airway management in adults, these are not directly transferable to the paediatric population and no specific difficult paediatric airway management algorithms have national recognition [6,7].

CAUSES OF DIFFICULT PAEDIATRIC INTUBATION

Children who are likely to be difficult to intubate fall into the following broad categories:

- facial syndromal features, e.g. micrognathia, microsomia, macroglossia, retrognathia (Pierre Robin, Treacher Collins or Goldenhar's syndrome)
- temporomandibular joint (TMJ) fusion (juvenile rheumatoid arthritis, TMJ fusion following septic arthritis of the joint), congenital abnormalities, arthrogryposis
- abnormal airway soft tissue
  - tumours, e.g. cystic hygroma, haemangioma, cervical teratoma
  - burns, contractures, caustic ingestion, epidermolysis bullosa
  - mucopolysaccharidosis (Hunter or Hurler syndrome)
- infection (epiglottitis, granuloma, papilloma)
- limited neck mobility, bony abnormality, Klippel–Feil syndrome, instability of the cervical spine, juvenile rheumatoid arthritis and trauma.

IDENTIFICATION OF THE CHILD WITH A DIFFICULT AIRWAY

Clinical history

The unexpected difficult airway in paediatric practice is unusual, and an anaesthetic review will reveal most of the clinical issues described above (for further detail, see preoperative assessment in Chapter 17). Previous anaesthetic records are a resource for future management; it is good practice always to record the Cormack and Lehane grade of laryngoscopy for each intubated patient. It is also helpful to note any specific beneficial techniques used during airway management.

Table 21.1 Principal conditions associated with difficult airway management*

Inherited	Pierre Robin syndrome
	Nagar syndrome
	Arthrogryposis
	Treacher Collins syndrome
	Goldenhar's syndrome
	Klippel–Feil syndrome
	Beckwith–Wiedemann syndrome
	Mucopolysaccharidoses
	Cystic hygroma, teratoma
	Dysmorphic facial features of unknown cause
	Epidermolysis bullosa
Acquired	Juvenile arthritis
	Septic arthritis of the temporo-mandibular joint with resultant micrognathia
	Caustic ingestion with airway burns
	Trauma
	Papillomatosis

*For further details and a more comprehensive list see Table 28.1 in Chapter 28.

If children have had major facial surgery, it is difficult to know whether their airway is likely to be easier or more difficult to manage at their next operation. The facial appearance may be greatly improved but the airway may remain difficult [8]. The presence of loose teeth or awkward gaps in dentition can be important, particularly when using advanced airway techniques.

Children with cleft lip and palate, particularly if bilateral, may be more difficult to intubate, as the laryngoscope or tracheal tube often slips into the cleft and may be difficult to direct (this is discussed in detail in Chapter 35). The cleft may be part of other syndromal combinations, e.g. Pierre Robin syndrome, where facial abnormalities increase the complexity of airway management.

The natural history of some syndromes is divergent: in Pierre Robin syndrome (Fig. 21.1), the mandible tends to grow with age and therefore direct laryngoscopy becomes easier, whereas the opposite is true in Treacher Collins syndrome, as facial growth remains limited and consequently laryngoscopy and tracheal intubation become increasingly difficult with age.

Among other features indicating airway compromise are poor feeding, apnoeas, cyanosis, airway obstruction, obstructive sleep apnoea (OSA), persisting oxygen requirement, stridor and pulmonary hypertension. Associated anomalies such as cardiac lesions, neck disorders and gastro-oesophageal reflux should be sought and may alter anaesthetic management. Clinical conditions giving rise to predictable problems include clotting abnormalities (mild local trauma may result in airway bleeding or preclude the use of a nasal tube), epidermolysis bullosa (fragile skin, scarring and contractures around the mouth and nose, poor dental tissues and laryngeal stenosis) and acute burns or severe facial skin infections that make airway access difficult and mask ventilation a challenge. Antenatal diagnosis of major cervical or facial swelling predicted to cause airway compromise has been reported and this early diagnosis allows planning of airway management at delivery [9].

The anaesthetic review should distinguish between patients in whom the airway itself will be difficult to manage (see Case study 21.1) and those in whom the airway is anticipated to be manageable but intubation difficult

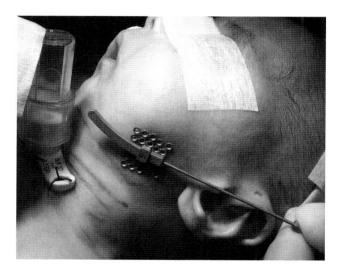

Figure 21.1   Pierre Robin syndrome: severe micrognathia gave rise to airway compromise which needed a tracheostomy; a mandibular distraction device has been fitted.

(see Case study 21.2). If there are signs of airway obstruction, try to define the likely level of the obstruction to assist airway management. For example, obstruction predominately at the nasopharyngeal level is readily resolved with insertion of a nasal prong, whereas oral airways or jaw lift helps when lower pharyngeal obstruction is present.

Management may also be difficult if the airway is to be shared with the surgeons, e.g. during bronchoscopy, or if the airway is compromised, e.g. following head and neck trauma or if there are infections such as epiglottitis. Incipient respiratory failure, caused by airway obstruction, is diagnosed mainly by serial clinical assessments, looking for increasing respiratory rate, subcostal or intercostal recession, tracheal tug, stridor and cyanosis (a late sign). Patients who need night-time nasal continuous positive airway pressure (CPAP) or who are already oxygen dependent are likely to have significant airway compromise. A history of OSA will indicate a likelihood of early airway obstruction following induction of anaesthesia. Obstructive sleep apnoea in adults is associated with an increased incidence of difficult intubation, although the reasons for this are unclear [10]. Adenotonsillar hypertrophy is the most common cause of OSA in children, but the incidence of OSA is increased with obesity, some craniofacial abnormalities, Down syndrome, many congenital syndromes and neuromuscular disease (for further details, see Chapter 28).

Clinical examination

Most clinical assessment tests used in adults to identify the difficult airway or potential difficult intubation have not

---

Case study 21.1 Difficult airway, difficult intubation

A 4-year-old boy presented with juvenile rheumatoid arthritis and adenotonsillar hypertrophy for major facial surgery. On review, he had temporomandibular joint fusion, no mouth opening and a rigid neck secondary to the arthritis. He slept upright at night, snored loudly and had brief apnoeic episodes during sleep. As expected on induction of anaesthesia, his airway was completely obstructed and it was not possible to use bag-and-mask ventilation successfully. Urgent insertion of a nasopharyngeal airway bypassed the nasopharyngeal obstructive component and provided a good airway so that anaesthesia could be continued. Fibre-optic intubation was achieved during spontaneous respiration and anaesthesia.

Case study 21.2 Easy airway, difficult intubation

A 3-year-old girl presented with fused temporomandibular joint secondary to septic arthritis as a neonate. Her mandible had grown poorly and she had marked micrognathia and minimal mouth opening. Following a gas induction, spontaneous respiration and subsequent bag-and-mask ventilation were easy; there was no relaxation of the soft tissues, and therefore elective nasal fibre-optic intubation was undertaken using a modified facemask. This was uneventful.

been validated for use in paediatric practice. Airway assessment includes the following:

- Visual review, particularly noting mandibular hypoplasia, retrognathia, microsomia, presence of facial or airway masses, or asymmetrical facies or ears. Measurement of thyromental distances has not been validated in paediatrics, and variations with age or size would make it difficult for this test to be useful in children.
- The ability of a child to slide the lower jaw anteriorly and bring the lower teeth in front of the upper teeth is a useful indicator of poor movement at the TMJ. Lack of movement here often heralds difficulty with laryngoscopy (Fig. 21.2).
- Mallampati assessment can be carried out in children who are able to cooperate, although, once again, it has not been validated for children. It may help to identify some potentially difficult cases.
- Limited mouth opening, whether due to congenital abnormalities, abnormal tissue, tumours, fibrosis, scarring as in epidermolysis bullosa or caustic burns, or inflammation as in juvenile rheumatoid arthritis, can make laryngoscopy difficult or impossible. Mouth opening of 1–2 cm may be sufficient for use of a small laryngeal mask airway (LMA), a light wand or the Bullard laryngoscope. Even very limited mouth opening may be useful, for instance, to allow a pair of Magill forceps in, thereby enabling traction on the tongue during fibre-optic intubation (FOI) and much improving the view via the nose.
- Nasal patency can be checked by asking the child to 'sniff' through each nostril separately while occluding the opposite nares, thus determining which is the most patent. This is likely to be the larger side, which would then be used for a nasal tube or for elective nasal FOI.
- Neck abnormalities and restriction of movement can contribute greatly to making direct laryngoscopy

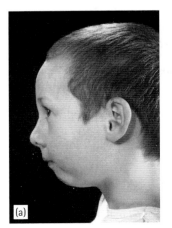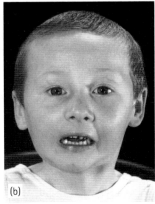

Figure 21.2 (a) A patient with micrognathia and temporomandibular joint fusion. (b) Maximum mouth opening.

difficult and are assessed in cooperative children as in adult practice.

Investigations

Children who have facial abnormalities have usually had a selection of imaging tests and investigations carried out. Imaging may have a useful role, particularly computed tomography (CT) and magnetic resonance imaging (MRI). Three-dimensional reconstruction of head, neck or chest X-rays may be useful. Nasendoscopy can be done in an awake patient and may provide useful information on the dynamic status of the airway. Sleep studies may identify the extent and mechanism of abnormal sleep patterns and the frequency and severity of the episodes of arterial desaturation during sleep. Occasionally a sleep study will be of help in identifying those children whose OSA is mainly caused by obstruction, as opposed to those who have apnoeas that are mainly central in origin. This will affect the anaesthetic plan for induction but also that for recovery management.

MANAGEMENT OF THE DIFFICULT AIRWAY

General principles

- Get the team organised and ensure that the equipment is available and checked.
- Maintain spontaneous respiration until the anaesthetist is confident that the airway is manageable.
- Avoid muscle relaxants if the airway is difficult to manage.
- Ask for help early on.

Preoperative preparation

SEDATIVE PREMEDICATION

This is relatively contraindicated in children with significant airway difficulties, especially in those with apnoeic episodes or obvious airway obstruction. There is some benefit from a carefully chosen dose of sedation, particularly if the child is very anxious or is having repeated anaesthetics. This has to be judged individually, but earlier anaesthetic records may be a useful guide. Midazolam (0.5 mg/kg, max. 15 mg) has been shown to be effective.

ANTIMUSCARINICS

The use of atropine or glycopyrronium (glycopyrolate) as premedication is now less common than it used to be, as the newer inhalational and intravenous (IV) anaesthetic agents are not as irritant to the airways, are less vagotonic and have less cardiac depressant effect, as described in Chapter 10. However, antimuscarinics are useful in patients undergoing airway investigations or requiring FOI. The antisialogue action decreases the incidence of complications such as coughing or laryngospasm at induction and emergence [10]. The drying effect reduces systemic absorption of lidocaine and enhances topical action, whilst there is also a clearer field for fibre-optic endoscopy. Atropine given orally 30–40 µg/kg (maximum dose 500 µg) is less predictable or effective as intramuscular (IM) administration 20 µg/kg (maximum dose 500 µg) but is psychologically better tolerated by children. Cholinoreceptor occupancy takes 90 minutes to peak after an oral dose compared with 25 minutes following IM administration [11].

Children with long-term tracheostomies are a special case. They have a secure airway and sedation may be considered. Many have profuse secretions and it can be difficult to access the airway perioperatively for suctioning. Secretions will build up, particularly during prolonged procedures, and ventilation would be compromised; therefore, an anticholinergic should be given preoperatively.

FASTING

Routine preoperative fasting times are used in children with potential difficult airways, but as acid aspiration syndrome is a risk in these patients, prophylaxis (e.g. ranitidine 1 mg/kg IV or 2 mg/kg orally) should be considered, especially in older children. Use of cricoid pressure may make direct laryngoscopy more difficult because of airway distortion [12]. Rapid-sequence induction (RSI) is used less in paediatric than in adult practice, probably because the incidence of complications related to aspiration is so low (see Chapter 19).

Consent

The anaesthetic plan is discussed with the parent and child, where possible, and questions are answered at this time. The options for airway management may be limited by surgical considerations (e.g. access required to the mouth, making nasal intubation more suitable) and this should be made clear. The risks and benefits of the surgery and anaesthetic need to be weighed up. Can a procedure be done without a general anaesthetic? If a tracheostomy may be needed, specialist ENT advice should be sought and the family will need time to consider the longer-term implications. It is helpful for such families to meet other children with tracheostomies so that they can understand the changes that it will make to their daily lives. Children who have difficult airways and severe obstructive symptoms are often considerably improved and able to thrive once a tracheostomy has been carried out.

Planning

If difficult airway management is anticipated, it is important to ensure that the anaesthetic team is able to deal with all the

potential strategies; developing and discussing a plan are essential, as is clear preparation. Is intubation always needed? Many surgical and imaging procedures can be successfully achieved without it and this approach may be safer than multiple difficult manipulations of the airway or attempts at intubation. If prolonged airway difficulties are experienced, it is wise to consider waking up the child and reassessing the situation and to re-plan surgery for a later date.

Documentation

All discussions with families should be documented on the anaesthetic chart and in the notes if undertaken in the preoperative assessment clinic. A child with a difficult airway should be easily identifiable when presenting for future anaesthetics; there must be clear notes of previous techniques used, whether successful or not. Parents should be informed so that they can pass the information on to subsequent anaesthetists. In addition, parents should be given a letter documenting the relevant issues and giving contact details for more information; wearing a MedicAlert bracelet should also be considered.

Monitoring

Even in a child who requests or is planned to have a gaseous induction, an IV cannula is sited, ideally before induction, or alternatively immediately afterwards. Routine monitoring is instituted early and used throughout anaesthesia. Patients with difficult airways may have a prolonged period in the anaesthetic room and should be fully monitored. Particular attention should be applied to the risk of awareness should intubation attempts be prolonged.

Following tracheal intubation, rapid confirmation of placement can be difficult. Clinical tests of chest movement or auscultation are potentially inconclusive and end-tidal capnography is essential. Positioning the tube above the carina and adequate fixation are important and will be related to the planned operation. In head and neck surgery, fixing to face or forehead may compromise surgical access and the tube can be secured by wiring it to the teeth (oral tubes) or stitching it to the nares (nasal tubes).

Awake/asleep intubation – the debate

Some older children are able to be managed awake, with sedation, for elective FOI. However, the majority are unable to cooperate with such a plan. Therefore, a technique of maintaining the airway and anaesthesia, while undertaking intubation, is required. Many anaesthetists do not favour awake techniques for intubation in children [13], although awake tracheostomy has been suggested for highly challenging cases, such as children with neck trauma and a full stomach.

Immediately post partum, many babies are intubated awake in the delivery suite. This practice has been extended to neonatal anaesthesia, particularly if airway management is likely to be difficult or if there is a tracheo-oesophageal fistula, where there may be a risk of difficulty with ventilation. Awake tracheal intubation in neonates is possible because their laryngeal reflexes are less sensitive. Spontaneous respiration can be maintained during laryngoscopy and the use of the oxyscope, a laryngoscope with a side channel for the administration of oxygen during intubation, resulted in a safe technique. This practice has been superseded by the availability of better anaesthetic agents and most intubations are now safely achieved with anaesthesia even in small babies.

Induction

Gaseous induction is recommended for children with difficult airways; a recent survey reported that over 90 per cent of anaesthetists chose this strategy [13]. If the airway is partially obstructed during induction, early use of CPAP allows deepening of the anaesthetic, while maintaining spontaneous respiration, after which an oral or nasal airway can be used.

SEVOFLURANE

Sevoflurane is the induction agent of choice and has been used extensively in children with difficult airways [14] (see Chapter 10).

HALOTHANE

This remains an occasional agent for the management of the difficult paediatric airway. Repeated halothane anaesthetics are a concern but the very small potential risk must be weighed against the useful characteristics of this agent. Halothane retains its use in difficult paediatric airway management because it is not irritant to the airway and, at deeper levels of anaesthesia, with spontaneous respiration maintained, airway reflexes are diminished such that intubating conditions are satisfactory without the need for muscle relaxants [15–17].

PROPOFOL

Propofol can also be used in many situations either as the sole induction agent or in combination with an inhalational agent. Some argue that gradual loss of the airway during inhalational induction is noticed more rapidly than during the acute apnoea associated with propofol. However, propofol is rapidly distributed and peak levels are transient, so that respiration returns rapidly, provided that modest doses (1–2 mg/kg) are used.

KETAMINE

Intramuscular or intravenous ketamine has also been reported to be useful as an induction agent, in that it allows laryngeal reflexes to be maintained during induction and intubation. Following ketamine induction, an inhalational agent can be gradually introduced [18].

RAPID–SEQUENCE INDUCTION

Rapid-sequence induction is used less frequently in children than in adults. It will be required in selected cases, particularly following trauma or prior to gastrointestinal surgery. Accidental aspiration of gastric contents into the airway is less common in children than in adults and is rarely associated with significant morbidity. In a large paediatric series, there was an incidence of 0.04 per cent, the majority of cases occurring in emergency patients, and only in one child was aspiration associated with difficult laryngoscopy [19]. Use of cricoid pressure may make the laryngeal view more difficult, as well as a tracheal intubation, so care must be taken not to exert excessive pressure, particularly in young children.

OPIATES

These should be used sparingly at induction, or not at all, as the effects may be unpredictable in young children. Unexpected apnoea associated with opiate use is unhelpful during induction in children with difficult airways.

Whatever the choice of induction agent, it is important to ensure that enough agent is given for adequate anaesthesia during the early stages when attempts at airway management may be prolonged.

Use of muscle relaxants

It is an important general principle that spontaneous ventilation should be maintained until the anaesthetist is confident of managing the airway. Then, if the airway is easy to manage, although tracheal intubation is anticipated to be difficult, it is reasonable to provide a short period of muscle relaxation in order to take over mask ventilation and provide the best conditions for direct laryngoscopy. In the easy airway, any of the non-depolarising relaxants can be used with care, but if concerns remain about the likelihood of achieving intubation then, unless contraindicated, suxamethonium will be the most useful drug.

Relaxants are less commonly used for tracheal intubation in routine paediatric practice and there are several alternatives for aiding tracheal tube advancement [20].These include deepening the anaesthetic with inhalational agent, a bolus of propofol 1 mg/kg, or a bolus of a short-acting opioid, alfentanil 15 μg/kg or remifentanil 1 μg/kg, in combination with propofol. In children with normal airways, it has been shown that there are no significant differences between the intubating conditions with these different agents [21].

During FOI, relaxants are often used, following identification of the carina, to facilitate railroading of the tracheal tube over the fibre-optic scope. The laryngeal reflexes remain brisk until the deeper planes of anaesthesia are achieved, and providing adequate relaxation at this step will greatly aid tube placement. In some children, particularly those with increased supraglottic soft tissue (e.g. those with mucopolysaccharidoses), there is an advantage to maintaining spontaneous respiration and pharyngeal tone, as the airway may be even more compromised by floppy soft tissue encroachment following the onset of neuromuscular block.

TECHNIQUES FOR AIRWAY MANAGEMENT

When choosing an airway management strategy it is important to differentiate the following:

- a child who has an airway that is easy to manage but who is difficult to intubate
- a child who has an airway that is difficult to manage and who may be difficult to intubate
- a child known to be easy to intubate, as direct laryngoscopy is documented to be straightforward, but the airway is easily lost on induction, usually because facemask fit is awkward.

The last type are not difficult to manage if they are preoxgenated and intubated early after induction.

Facemasks and airways

If the airway proves easy to maintain with bag-and-mask ventilation once the child has been anaesthetised, many avenues for management are available. If this is not the case and the child's airway proves difficult to manage then a rapid assessment must be made. Simple manoeuvres to improve the airway include:

- adjusting the head position, the tongue and the jaw
- trying different-sized oral airways
- trying different designs and positions of facemasks to achieve a better fit on a syndromal child's face
- using an LMA
- inserting a nasopharyngeal airway (often well tolerated early following induction – Fig. 21.3).

Usually one of these interventions provides an adequate airway and the anaesthetic can be deepened so that direct laryngoscopy can be tried before muscle relaxation is used. The adequacy of spontaneous respiration or assisted ventilation can be assessed and monitoring completed.

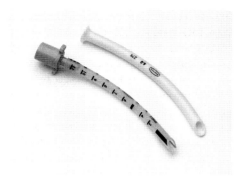

Figure 21.3   Nasal prongs and nasopharyngeal airway.

Laryngeal mask airway

The LMA provides a satisfactory airway in most children and has a specific role in children with a difficult airway [22]. Several different types are available, including classic, Proseal and disposable LMAs, which are available in various paediatric sizes. The LMA provides airway management suitable for many procedures. It is usually easily placed and provides an airway that can be monitored during either spontaneous respiration or ventilation. There may be a slight increase in the risk of mild gastric distension when positive pressure ventilation is used.

The LMA can be particularly useful in patients with mandibular hypoplasia and in those with soft tissue abnormalities, especially children with mucopolysaccharidoses, who can be very challenging to manage by other methods. Reported use in patients with facial or airway burns suggests an advantage, as additional potential trauma to the airway from tracheal intubation is avoided [23]. The LMA also has a role in resuscitation of children who cannot be intubated [24]. The LMA can be used in epidermolysis bullosa and, if carefully placed, may produce less trauma than intubation.

Positioning of the LMA is usually easy, provided that there is sufficient mouth opening. Different sizes may need to be tried and adequacy of ventilation checked. In a group of children with mucopolysaccharidoses, the LMA provided a good airway in 73 per cent and an adequate airway in 27 per cent, but visualisation of the larynx using a fibrescope via the LMA revealed a grade 1–2 view of the larynx in only 54 per cent [22]. By contrast, a grade I–II LMA fibrescope view has been reported in 94 per cent of children with normal airways [25].

Cuffed oropharyngeal airway

Cuffed oropharyngeal airways (COPAs) are available in various designs and sizes. These have been used in patients with difficult airways both to maintain the airway and as a conduit for fibre-optic scope (FOS)-guided tracheal intubation [26].

TECHNIQUES FOR THE MANAGEMENT OF DIFFICULT TRACHEAL INTUBATION

Introducers and exchange catheters

Probably the most useful adjunct to laryngoscopy is the airway bougie, which is mainly used as a tracheal tube guide when the larynx is anterior or the laryngeal view is suboptimal for any reason. It can also be used to exchange tracheal tubes and occasionally to facilitate blind intubation via an LMA. Many types of exchange catheters, e.g. Cook, are available, some of which are hollow and have an adaptor that allows insufflation of oxygen and monitoring of exhaled CO_2. They allow the intratracheal position to be confirmed, before the new tracheal tube is advanced over the catheter. More recently, fibre-optic intubating stylettes have become available, which can also be used with a monitor screen. The use of cardiac catheter wires, gastroscopy or ureteral dilator as guides for intubation has also been reported. A useful straightforward technique is the 'two-anaesthetist technique', whereby one anaesthetist uses a laryngoscope and manipulates the larynx to get the best view possible, while the other passes a bougie under direct vision into the larynx, which allows railroading of the tube.

Laryngoscopes

Many different patterns of laryngoscope blades are available for paediatric practice, as described in Chapter 19. Straight blades allowing lateral insertion to sweep aside supraglottic structures and give a good laryngeal view have their enthusiasts and this is the approach favoured by ENT surgeons. Different handles can be helpful. A short-handled laryngoscope can be very useful, particularly if there is tumour mass on the neck or chest, the child is in halo traction or has a thoracic plaster jacket, all of which compromise easy access with a conventional laryngoscope. Laryngoscopes such as the McCoy have paediatric-sized blades for all main age groups (Fig. 21.4).

If direct laryngoscopy provides an adequate laryngeal view but a tracheal tube will not pass, smaller tubes should be tried, but occasionally pathology such as subglottic stenosis or tracheal stenosis will prevent their passage. A Cole pattern tube may be useful in these circumstances, as the design provides a more rigid shouldered tube with a narrowed distal end, which is easy to pass. An alternative may be to avoid intubation altogether and use an LMA to manage the airway. Prolonged ventilation with an LMA in a child with a difficult airway has been reported and this strategy, or even returning to mask anaesthesia, will provide adequate airway control while deciding whether to wake the child up or proceed to tracheostomy.

LMA as an aid to tracheal intubation

The LMA has proved to be useful in the management of the difficult paediatric airway; in babies with severe

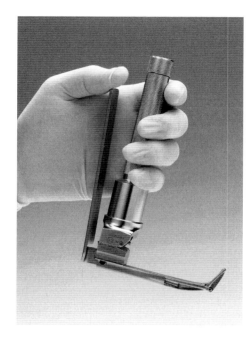

Figure 21.4 McCoy laryngoscope.

micrognathia it can be life-saving. It can be used both to maintain the airway during surgery and as a conduit for the placement of an orotracheal tube. Fibre-optic visualization via the LMA in children with known difficult airways has shown that in 54 per cent the LMA is positioned such that the tracheal inlet is visible [22], which is a lower percentage than in adults and therefore there is less likelihood of success (and more of damage) with blind passage of a tracheal tube into the larynx through an LMA. However, successful tracheal tube insertion through the LMA has been reported in children who were potentially difficult intubations [27]. If a tracheal tube is passed successfully into the trachea through the LMA, another tube, wedged into the proximal end of the patient's tracheal tube, should be used to advance the primary tube, after which the LMA can be removed.

Other techniques have been described, including using the LMA as an airway conduit in combination with a wire and an FOS (see below). The intubating LMA (ILMA) is available in sizes 3 and 4, which may be useful in older children, and patents are pending for paediatric versions of this device.

Blind nasal intubation

In younger children, the larynx is relatively anterior and the oesophagus more in line with a tube passed blindly through the nose (hence the ease of passing nasogastric tubes in children). This makes the technique of blind nasal intubation unreliable in this age group, although it is more successful in older adolescents. It may be possible to 'follow the breath sounds' and slowly advance the tube into the trachea and this can be aided by watching an end-tidal CO_2

trace monitored from a connector on the tracheal tube throughout intubation [28]. Blind nasal intubation can be a useful technique if resources are scarce and other alternatives are not readily available.

Fibre-optic intubation

Fibre-optic intubation remains the favoured technique for the management of difficult intubation when direct laryngoscopy has failed [13]. Equipment specially designed for paediatric intubation or bronchoscopy is widely available (Table 21.2), and good technique in FOI is considered a core skill for anaesthetists. Techniques learnt in adult practice can be transferred to paediatric practice with modification. Fibre-optic intubation is successful in children, and failure rates of 4.3 per cent and 0 per cent in children with mucopolysaccharidoses and other airway abnormalities have been reported [29,30]; however, it does require practice. Fibreoscopy may be easy but the main challenge lies in achieving intubation with the tracheal tube. Several studies in children with normal airways report that FOI is more difficult in the young. Failure of FOI was reported in 25 per cent of normal infants when using the 2.2 mm FOS [31], and in 18 per cent in a study of children aged 3 months to 8 years [32].

PREPARATION FOR FIBRE-OPTIC INTUBATION

A successful fibre-optic technique requires good planning. Use of a camera system enhances the image, allows team members to be involved and encourages teaching. Fibre-optic nasal intubation is often easier to achieve than oral intubation, as the normal anatomical alignment of nose to larynx helps, whereas, for oral intubation, more angling of the scope is required in order to access the anterior larynx. Usually, it is the surgical access needs that dictate the preferred approach.

Premedication with either atropine (20 μg/kg, maximum dose 500 μg) or glycopyrronium (4–8 μg/kg, maximum dose 200 μg) should be given to decrease secretions. Once asleep, a nasal mucosal vasoconstrictor such as 0.5 per cent ephedrine or 0.1 per cent xylometazoline is used to decrease bleeding.

Table 21.2 Features of paediatric fibre-optic scopes

Scope	Tracheal tube	Special features
2.2	2.5	No suction channel Whippy, easily damaged
2.5	3.0	Suction channel Improved optics More robust
3.8	4.5	Better optics Easier to manoeuvre Suction channel

MAINTAINING THE AIRWAY DURING FOI

Although awake FOI may be possible in some older children, most children will require anaesthesia for FOI and various techniques are available for maintaining the airway, thereby allowing spontaneous respiration, anaesthesia and oxygenation during FOI.

The anaesthetist maintaining and monitoring the airway during fibre-oscopy plays a crucial role and can improve the success rate by simple manoeuvres. They must ensure adequate ventilation and anaesthesia, maintain a jaw thrust whenever possible, and improve the posterior pharyngeal space by using an oral airway or holding the tongue forward. Depending on whether an oral or a nasal tracheal tube is required, the airway can be maintained in various ways. The easiest method is to place a nasopharyngeal airway in the contralateral nares and attach the breathing circuit to this, thus allowing access to either the other nares or the mouth. There are also specially designed facemasks (Fig. 21.5) for FOI or modified angle pieces for FOI which have a flexible port through which to pass the scope. The FOI airways are also available in various paediatric sizes for guiding oral FOI.

TECHNIQUES FOR FIBRE-OPTIC INTUBATION

Tube over the scope technique

Many different sizes of scopes are available; it is best to choose one that is not a snug fit (to avoid damaging the coating and bundles in the scope) but which is also large enough to be able to act as a guide on advancing the tube. The tracheal tube is mounted on the FOS, which is then passed through the nose or mouth. Once a clear view of the cords is achieved, it is essential to centre this view before trying to advance the tube. The FOS is then advanced until the carina is identified. While advancement of the FOS into the trachea is well tolerated, in order to advance the tracheal tube the laryngeal reflexes must be suppressed. How this is achieved depends crucially on whether the child's airway is sufficiently difficult to manage that the anaesthetic plan requires the maintenance of spontaneous respiration. If so, the main options are either to topicalise the larynx with lidocaine 1–2 per cent (but keeping the total dose within

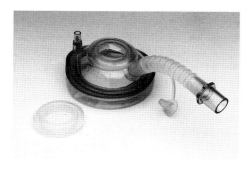

Figure 21.5 A VBM fibre-optic intubation facemask.

accepted levels of 3–4 mg/kg given via the scope) or to deepen the anaesthetic with either inhalational agents or small increments of propofol 0.5–2 mg/kg according to effect. If the airway is manageable then more options are available, including the use of a small bolus of opiate, e.g. remifentanil 1 μg/kg or alfentanil 15 μg/kg or, if appropriate, a muscle relaxant. Suxamethonium may have an occasional role here. If the airway is easy to maintain, although intubation is difficult, use of a longer-acting muscle relaxant may be satisfactory. The rapid onset of muscle relaxation with rocuronium 0.6 mg/kg can be useful in this setting.

Use of a wire technique via the suction port of the FOS

In this method it is not necessary to advance the scope into the trachea; instead it is positioned just above the vocal cords and a fine wire, such as a cardiac catheter wire, is manipulated through the suction channel and watched as it passes into the trachea. The scope can then be removed, while holding the wire in place, and a suitable tracheal tube is passed over the wire into the trachea. In larger children, an additional step is required; after wire placement, an exchange catheter such as a Cook catheter is passed over the wire to stiffen it and then an appropriate tracheal tube is fed over that. If this extra manoeuvre is not done, it is easy, with the larger tube, accidentally to push the tube and wire into the oesophagus. The guidewire technique has been reported to be very successful in children with difficult airways, particularly those with mucopolysaccharidoses. A series of 31 intubations in children who were known to be difficult was reported, all of which were successful [22].

Use of small-calibre scopes (e.g. 2.2 and 2.5 mm)

The 2.2 mm scope is designed for infant use; it is delicate and easily damaged. It is very flexible and allows use of a 2.5 mm internal diameter tracheal tube. Owing to the smaller number of fibre-optic bundles, the view obtained is less sharp than that from larger scopes, but adequate, even when used with a camera system. As this scope does not have a suction port, it is essential to clear the pharynx before starting [31]. These scopes can be used for diagnostic purposes and for intubation. The tracheal tube is placed over the scope and, once the scope has been advanced into the trachea and the carina identified, the tracheal tube is manipulated forwards off the FOS. When using the scope via the mouth, a guide such as an intubation airway is needed or the whippy scope will be difficult to keep aligned.

Scopes that are 2.5 mm or larger do have suction channels, which allow clearance of secretions and blood, installation of local anaesthetic, insufflation of oxygen and use of the guidewire technique described above.

Intubation via the LMA using the FOS

Numerous different techniques have been described [22,33,34]. Most commonly, an FOS is passed through the

LMA and a long wire is advanced under direct vision into the trachea via the suction channel, after which the LMA is removed and the tracheal tube advanced over the wire (Fig. 21.6). An airway exchange catheter may be needed.

Choice of tracheal tube for FOI

Choice of the most appropriate tracheal tube depends on the child and the surgical requirements. The FOS should be chosen such that it fits the tracheal tube rather than using a small scope in a large tube. This helps when feeding the tube off the scope, which is the most difficult part of the procedure [32]. Flexometallic tubes are very useful and, when they are advanced in a twisting motion, the slightly blunter bevel allows easier passage into the larynx. Cuffed tubes have a role even in small children, particularly if the TMJ is immobile and it is not possible to use a throat pack to allow adequate ventilation in the presence of a leak around the tracheal tube. The use of cuffed tracheal tubes in young children remains controversial but there are indications for this. Cuffed tubes are available in most sizes and types and increasingly have a role, particularly if a child requires postoperative ventilation where the cuff seal permits the monitoring of lung parameters [35]. There are many designs available and these are constantly improving [36].

BULLARD LARYNGOSCOPE

There are adult, mid-sized and paediatric versions of this rigid fibre-optic laryngoscope designed particularly for intubating the patient with a difficult airway. The scope allows an indirect view of the larynx, and then a tracheal tube can be advanced either over the specialist Bullard intubating stylet or using a bougie (Fig. 21.7). Successful use of the Bullard requires practice. It can be used in children with some limitation of mouth opening. It remains an expensive but interesting adjunct to the difficult airway equipment.

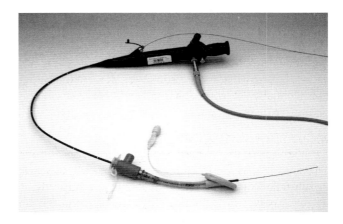

Figure 21.6 Paediatric 3.8 mm scope with wire through suction channel and laryngeal mask airway (LMA) in place, for fibre-optic intubation using LMA as a guide device.

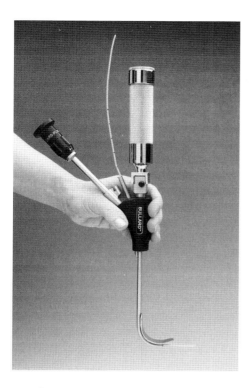

Figure 21.7   Paediatric Bullard laryngoscope with bougie.

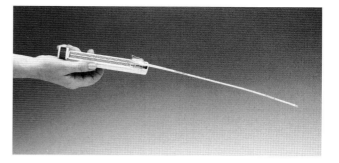

Figure 21.8   Light wand.

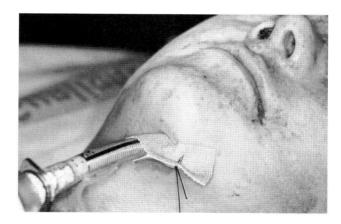

Figure 21.9   Submental intubation.

LIGHT WAND

This is used for oral intubation and is particularly indicated if there is some limitation of mouth opening or suspected instability of the cervical spine (Fig. 21.8). The tracheal tube is mounted on the wand and the illuminated tip is watched transcutaneously at the front of the neck as the wand is directed to the midline towards the larynx. An example of this equipment is the Trachlight.

LIGHTED TUBE STYLET

These are particularly useful outside the operating theatre situations when fibre-optic bronchoscopes are not available. Various external diameter stylets are available, from 2.5 mm up, and an appropriate size should be chosen to fit the tracheal tube snugly. More sophisticated equipment with fibre-optic lighted stylets and mini-screens is also available [37].

RIGID BRONCHOSCOPY

This technique is more commonly used by ENT surgeons, usually following general anaesthesia and topical anaesthesia of the larynx with lidocaine. It is possible to gain an adequate laryngeal view and feed a tracheal tube through to the trachea. This is particularly useful if there is a risk of complete airway obstruction, as in the case of large intra-thoracic masses causing tracheal compression.

SUBMENTAL INTUBATION

This technique allows good surgical access to the mouth, especially in patients in whom the nasal route is not applicable, and decreases the risk of accidental extubation. It is particularly useful for some maxillofacial procedures. The oral tracheal tube is passed initially as usual. Then, with the connector temporarily removed, a small surgical incision is made beneath the chin and through the submental tissues to the mouth. The tracheal tube is passed through this opening and reattached to the anaesthetic circuit (Fig. 21.9). Once surgery is completed, the tube is removed. The inframandibular incision heals well.

RETROGRADE INTUBATION

If access to the trachea has proved difficult via either the mouth or the nose, retrograde intubation may be a solution. While the child is anaesthetised and the airway maintained either with an LMA, nasal prong or facemask, a Tuohy needle is passed through the anterior cricothyroid membrane. An epidural catheter is passed cepalad and retrieved from the mouth [38,39]. This catheter may need to be supported using a Cook exchange catheter and then the tracheal tube is fed into the trachea via this airway device. A similar technique is to advance a catheter via a longstanding tracheostoma to the mouth and use this as a guide to advance an oral tube to the trachea [40].

THE DIFFICULT AIRWAY AFTER SURGERY

Extubation

At the end of surgery, once a regular pattern of respiration has returned, the next step is to achieve successful extubation; either 'deep' or 'light' extubation is satisfactory depending on the clinical scenario. Extubation between these markers is fraught with potential difficulties, particularly laryngospasm, coughing or airway irritation leading to apnoeas. In children with difficult airways, it is usually wise to ensure they are awake and responding appropriately before removing the tracheal tube.

Airway swelling related to surgery or due to airway manipulations is a hazard at extubation. Surgical alterations to the airway, such as closure of a cleft palate, may also make a child more at risk of postoperative airway obstruction. Supplemental oxygen, a nasopharyngeal airway, pulse oximeter and apnoea monitors may be required. Some babies or children will need care in either a high-dependency or paediatric intensive care unit (PICU). If severe postoperative airway swelling is anticipated, the tracheal tube is left *in situ* and the child cared for in a PICU. Dexamethasone (0.25 mg/kg, max. 8 mg) is given prior to extubation when a leak occurs around the tube. Postextubation complications are most common in the smallest infants when the decrease in area of the airway becomes clinically significant with only a small amount of oedema.

Stridor

Following difficulties with intubation, local laryngeal swelling may result in stridor, particularly in infants. Management includes 100 per cent oxygen by facemask with CPAP, steroid (e.g. dexamethasone 0.25 mg/kg, maximum 8 mg) and nebulised adrenaline (5 mg in 10 mL 0.09% or normal saline – employ ECG monitoring during use). The incidence varies and risk factors are listed in Table 21.3.

Monitoring postoperatively

Postoperative monitoring is required if there is a history of apnoeas or desaturations. The main groups frequently affected by this are the premature or ex-premature baby and children at risk of airway obstruction. These patients are monitored with respiratory rate, pulse oximetry and apnoea monitors. Some children will also require overnight monitoring in a high-dependency area. It is wise to keep an LMA at the bedside if this would be useful should the airway

Table 21.3 Factors potentially affecting the incidence of postextubation stridor

Previous airway pathology
Local trauma, repeated attempts at intubation
Use of large tubes, lack of leak around a tracheal tube
Use of cuffed tubes
Local trauma to the cricoid
Presence, or recent history, of upper respiratory tract infection symptoms preoperatively
Episodes of hypoperfusion, sepsis
Long-term intubation

become compromised. Early identification of respiratory difficulty is important and, if seen, requires a return to theatre, where airway equipment is available.

FAILED INTUBATION

There will be a small subgroup of children whose airways are so difficult to manage that an elective tracheostomy is required. This can be a life-saving operation, and the possibility of a tracheostomy should be discussed clearly in advance. If a child with a known difficult airway is likely to have more airway compromise following major craniofacial or maxillofacial surgery, they may be better managed with an elective tracheostomy to cover the surgical period, particularly if repeated airway, or head or neck, surgery is planned over an extended period.

In children with difficult airways, the surgeon may also struggle to perform a tracheostomy under pressing conditions; an experienced otolaryngologist is needed in these circumstances. Awake tracheostomy is suggested for selected situations [41]; however, the majority can be safely done asleep. The airway is maintained as well as is possible with either a tracheal tube, if feasible, or an LMA, nasopharyngeal airway or, in some circumstances, a facemask. Tracheostomy is used less frequently than in the past. This is because we have more techniques that can be used to manage the airway and there is known to be increased morbidity and mortality for children with tracheostomy. Some planned surgery in children with compromised airways will need to be scheduled around an elective tracheostomy prior to their major surgery.

In the emergency situation, cricothyroidotomy may be life saving, particularly if the patient has both an airway that is likely to be difficult to maintain and a trachea that is difficult to intubate. Cricothyroidotomy is part of the management options in the Advanced Paediatric and Trauma Life Support training, although it is a technique that is difficult in the emergency situation and increasingly difficult in smaller patients and is mainly recommended for children above 12 years. In babies it is harder to identify the landmarks, the tissues are softer and the small size of the cricothyroid membrane makes access difficult [42]. Whilst cricoidotomy is a technique that can be practised on a teaching model, it is used very infrequently and evidence of successful use is mainly anecdotal. Specially designed kits for achieving this are available. Some centres use elective cricothyroidotomy for airway management during anaesthesia in children with severe airway difficulties, such as those with burns contractures or trauma of the face and neck.

Various emergency methods for ensuring adequate oxygenation have been described. Insertion of one or more transtracheal IV cannulae to be used for oxygenation has been reported (Fig. 21.10). The use of the Sanders injector in paediatric practice is controversial. There are inherent risks, particularly of barotrauma (pneumothorax or pneumomediastinum and surgical emphysema). Gaining some oxygenation may be easier than ensuring adequate expiration and the arterial CO_2 may rise, but this is relatively well tolerated in children for short periods.

COMPLICATIONS ASSOCIATED WITH DIFFICULT AIRWAY MANAGEMENT

Even in expert hands, the management of the difficult paediatric airway can be challenging and may require considerable resources of time, equipment and skilled personnel. There is a specific risk of awareness and care must be taken to avoid this by delivering an adequate anaesthetic during attempts at intubation. Failure to do so is a recognised feature of claims for awareness. Each technique may have potential morbidity associated with it and potential complications (these are summarised in Table 21.4).

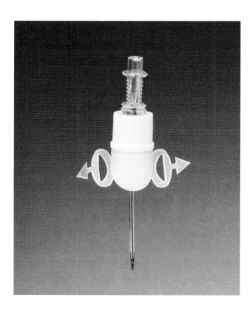

Figure 21.10 Transtracheal needle set.

Table 21.4 Potential complications associated with difficulties in managing the paediatric airway

Early complications
Laryngospasm, hypoxia, cough, wheeze
Trauma, airway oedema and stridor
Haemorrhage
Perforation: pneumothorax, pneumomediastinum, pharyngeal perforation
Accidental aspiration syndrome
Awareness
Dental damage or loss
Local mouth or nasal trauma, related to route of attempted intubation
Vocal cord damage, local paralysis
Damage to equipment, especially fibre-optic scopes
Failure of technique, which may result in the need to waken the patient or 'emergency' tracheostomy/cricothyroidotomy
Hypoxia, death

Late complications
Airway scarring
Subglottic stenosis
Psychological trauma

EQUIPMENT

All departments managing children should have a difficult paediatric airway trolley. Routine anaesthetic equipment as found in the anaesthetic room does not need to be included and this will avoid over-complexity of the trolley contents. The difficult intubation trolley contents will vary but may include those listed in Table 21.5.

TRAINING AND MAINTAINING AIRWAY SKILLS

As an anaesthetist, it is essential to have a clear plan at the start of the anaesthetic, so that the whole team understands their role in helping with managing the case. It is important to have a trained and experienced team. Meticulous notes must be kept and any special tips for future airway management documented.

Learning skills can be difficult [43]. In-theatre training backed up by e-learning, practical courses and skills workshops are all valuable. Paediatric manikins are available to practise airway and particularly intubation skills. Use of the paediatric medical simulator to practise airway skills and scenarios is expanding and is particularly useful when training is required for events that are rare, as outlined in Chapter 49. Airway training equipment is also available, from intubation training models to fibre-optic skills trainers such as the Oxford Box. The anaesthetist and team will

Table 21.5 The difficult intubation trolley. The contents will vary but may include the items listed. All equipment is kept in varying sizes appropriate to the clinical work of the area

Bougies
Intubating facemasks
Intubating oral airways
Intubating angle connectors
Nasal prong airways
Specialist laryngoscopes: McCoy, Miller, oxyscope, Bullard, polio blade, etc.
Airway exchange catheters, wires for exchange use. Epidural set for retrograde technique
ILMA3, -4
Trachlight
Fibre-optic scopes (FOS; may be held in a separate cupboard for storage but available for use with the difficult airway trolley; portable FOS particularly useful)
Camera and attachments
Light source
Spare batteries, demist solution for FOS
Transtracheal catheter sets
Equipment for cricothyroidotomy
High-flow ventilation system – Manujet

require ongoing practice and regular updates. It is important that the different airway techniques are integrated into regular anaesthetic practice where possible. Maintaining skills and learning new techniques are both crucial to providing an excellent service for this challenging group of children.

REFERENCES

Key references

Frei FJ, Ummenhofer W. Difficult intubation in paediatrics. *Paediatr Anaesth* 1996; **6**(4): 251–63.
Henderson JJ, Popat MT, Latto IP, Pearce AC. Difficult Airway Society guidelines for management of the unanticipated difficult intubation. *Anaesthesia* 2004; **59**(7): 675–94.
James I. Cuffed tubes in children. *Paediatr Anaesth* 2001; **11**(3): 259–63.

References

1. Crosby ET, Cooper RM, Douglas MJ *et al.* The unanticipated difficult airway with recommendations for management. *Can J Anaesth* 1998; **45**(8): 757–76.
2. Frei FJ, Ummenhofer W. Difficult intubation in paediatrics. *Paediatr Anaesth* 1996; **6**(4): 251–63.
3. Akpek EA, Mutlu H, Kayhan Z. Difficult intubation in pediatric cardiac anesthesia. *J Cardiothorac Vasc Anesth* 2004; **18**(5): 610–12.
4. Xue FS, Zhang GH, Li P *et al.* The clinical observation of difficult laryngoscopy and difficult intubation in infants with cleft lip and palate. *Paediatr Anaesth* 2006; **16**(3): 283–9.
5. Caplan RA, Posner KL, Ward RJ, Cheney FW. Adverse respiratory events in anesthesia: a closed claims analysis. *Anesthesiology* 1990; **72**(5): 828–33.
6. Practice guidelines for management of the difficult airway: an updated report by the American Society of Anesthesiologists Task Force on Management of the Difficult Airway. *Anesthesiology* 2003; **98**(5): 1269–77.
7. Henderson JJ, Popat MT, Latto IP, Pearce AC. Difficult Airway Society guidelines for management of the unanticipated difficult intubation. *Anaesthesia* 2004; **59**(7): 675–94.
8. Roche J, Frawley G, Heggie A. Difficult tracheal intubation induced by maxillary distraction devices in craniosynostosis syndromes. *Paediatr Anaesth* 2002; **12**(3): 227–34.
9. Hullett BJ, Shine NP, Chambers NA. Airway management of three cases of congenital cervical teratoma. *Paediatr Anaesth* 2006; **16**(7): 794–8.
10. Siyam MA, Benhamou D. Difficult endotracheal intubation in patients with sleep apnea syndrome. *Anesth Analg* 2002; **95**(4): 1098–102.
11. Gervais HW, el Gindi M, Radermacher PR *et al.* Plasma concentration following oral and intramuscular atropine in children and their clinical effects. *Paediatr Anaesth* 1997; **7**(1): 13–18.
12. Engelhardt T, Strachan L, Johnston G. Aspiration and regurgitation prophylaxis in paediatric anaesthesia. *Paediatr Anaesth* 2001; **11**(2): 147–50.
13. Brooks P, Ree R, Rosen D, Ansermino M. Canadian pediatric anesthesiologists prefer inhalational anesthesia to manage difficult airways. *Can J Anaesth* 2005; **52**(3): 285–90.
14. Holm-Knudsen R, Eriksen K, Rasmussen LS. Using a nasopharyngeal airway during fibre-optic intubation in small children with a difficult airway. *Paediatr Anaesth* 2005; **15**(10): 839–45.
15. Bagshaw ON, Stack CG. A comparison of halothane and isoflurane for gaseous induction of anaesthesia in infants. *Paediatr Anaesth* 1999; **9**(1): 25–9.
16. Black A, Sury MR, Hemington L *et al.* A comparison of the induction characteristics of sevoflurane and halothane in children. *Anaesthesia* 1996; **51**(6): 539–42.
17. Sury MR, Black A, Hemington L *et al.* A comparison of the recovery characteristics of sevoflurane and halothane in children. *Anaesthesia* 1996; **51**(6): 543–6.
18. Przybylo HJ, Stevenson GW, Vicari FA *et al.* Retrograde fibreoptic intubation in a child with Nager's syndrome. *Can J Anaesth* 1996; **43**(7): 697–9.
19. Warner MA, Warner ME, Warner DO *et al.* Perioperative pulmonary aspiration in infants and children. *Anesthesiology* 1999; **90**(1): 66–71.
20. Simon L, Boucebci KJ, Orliaguet G *et al.* A survey of practice of tracheal intubation without muscle relaxant in paediatric patients. *Paediatr Anaesth* 2002; **12**(1): 36–42.
21. Robinson DN, O'Brien K, Kumar R, Morton NS. Tracheal intubation without neuromuscular blockade in children: a comparison of propofol combined either with alfentanil or remifentanil. *Paediatr Anaesth* 1998; **8**(6): 467–71.

22. Walker RW. The laryngeal mask airway in the difficult paediatric airway: an assessment of positioning and use in fibreoptic intubation. *Paediatr Anaesth* 2000; **10**(1): 53–8.

23. McCall JE, Fischer CG, Schomaker E, Young JM. Laryngeal mask airway use in children with acute burns: intraoperative airway management. *Paediatr Anaesth* 1999; **9**(6): 515–20.

24. Sarti A. New pediatric resuscitation guidelines: new evidence or new ideas? *Paediatr Anaesth* 2006; **16**(6): 607–10.

25. Rowbottom SJ, Simpson DL, Grubb D. The laryngeal mask airway in children. A fibreoptic assessment of positioning. *Anaesthesia* 1991; **46**(6): 489–91.

26. Szmuk P, Ezri T, Narwani A, Alfery DD. Use of CobraPLA as a conduit for fibre-optic intubation in a child with neck instability. *Paediatr Anaesth* 2006; **16**(2): 217–18.

27. Inada T, Fujise K, Tachibana K, Shingu K. Orotracheal intubation through the laryngeal mask airway in paediatric patients with Treacher Collins syndrome. *Paediatr Anaesth* 1995; **5**: 129–32.

28. Ng A, Vas L, Goel S. Difficult paediatric intubation when fibreoptic laryngoscopy fails. *Paediatr Anaesth* 2002; **12**(9): 801–5.

29. Blanco G, Melman E, Cuairan V *et al.* Fibreoptic nasal intubation in children with anticipated and unanticipated difficult intubation. *Paediatr Anaesth* 2001; **11**(1): 49–53.

30. Walker RMW, Allen DL, Rothera MR. A fibreoptic intubation technique for children with mucopolysaccharidoses using the laryngeal mask airway. *Paediatr Anaesth* 1997; **7**: 421–6.

31. Wrigley SR, Black AE, Sidhu VS. A fibreoptic laryngoscope for paediatric anaesthesia. A study to evaluate the use of the 2.2 mm Olympus (LF-P) intubating fibrescope. *Anaesthesia* 1995; **50**(8): 709–12.

32. Hakala P, Randell T, Meretoja OA, Rintala R. Orotracheal fibreoptic intubation in children under general anaesthesia. *Paediatr Anaesth* 1997; **7**: 371–4.

33. Hasan MA, Black AE. A new technique for fibreoptic intubation in children. *Anaesthesia* 1994; **49**: 1031–3.

34. Weiss M, Gerber AC, Schmitz A. Continuous ventilation technique for laryngeal mask airway (LMA) removal after fibre-optic intubation in children. *Paediatr Anaesth* 2004; **14**(11): 936–40.

35. James I. Cuffed tubes in children. *Paediatr Anaesth* 2001; **11**(3): 259–63.

36. Weiss M, Balmer C, Dullenkopf A *et al.* Intubation depth markings allow an improved positioning of endotracheal tubes in children. *Can J Anaesth* 2005; **52**(7): 721–6.

37. Pfitzner L, Cooper MG, Ho D. The Shikani Seeing Stylet for difficult intubation in children: initial experience. *Anaesth Intensive Care* 2002; **30**(4): 462–6.

38. Przybylo HJ, Stevenson GW, Vicari FA *et al.* Retrograde fibreoptic intubation in a child with Nager's syndrome. *Can J Anaesth* 1996; **43**: 679–99.

39. Nicholson SC, Black AE, Kraras CM. Management of a difficult airway in a patient with Hurler–Scheie syndrome during cardiac surgery. *Anesth Analg* 1992; **75**: 830–2.

40. Arima H, Sobue K, Tanaka S *et al.* Difficult airway in a child with spinal muscular atrophy type I. *Paediatr Anaesth* 2003; **13**(4): 342–4.

41. Mohiuddin S, Martin TW, Mayhew JF. Difficult airway management of a child impaled through the neck. [letter; comment.] *Paediatr Anaesth* 2002; **12**(4): 378–9.

42. Navsa N, Tossel G, Boon JM. Dimensions of the neonatal cricothyroid membrane – how feasible is a surgical cricothyroidotomy? *Paediatr Anaesth* 2005; **15**(5): 402–6.

43. Erb T, Marsch SC, Hampl KF, Frei FJ. Teaching the use of fibre-optic intubation for children older than two years of age. *Anesth Analg* 1997; **85**(5): 1037–41.

Difficult venous access

STEVE SCUPLAK, DEREK J ROEBUCK

KEY LEARNING POINTS

- Careful fixation of peripheral cannulae will prolong their effective duration.
- Intraosseous access has a high success rate and a low incidence of complications.
- Central venous catheters inserted via the internal jugular vein have the highest success rate and the lowest incidence of complications.
- Central venous catheter insertion should be visualised using real-time ultrasound whenever possible.
- Landmark insertion techniques should be taught, supported by anatomical demonstration using real-time ultrasound.

INTRODUCTION

Venous access is a crucial part of modern paediatric anaesthesia and intensive care. Despite the apparent simplicity of venous access procedures, they can be extremely difficult in unfavourable circumstances. Various strategies are available to help, including imaging guidance, especially real-time ultrasound, for central venous access. These techniques make simple cases safer [1], and allow percutaneous central access in circumstances (e.g. venous occlusion at, or central to, all the usual access points) where it would otherwise be impossible.

CANNULATION OF PERIPHERAL VEINS

The desired end-point for adequate intravascular access in the vast majority of anaesthetic interventions is the cannulation of a peripheral vein, and anxiety is always heightened until this is achieved. In adult anaesthesia, this anxiety is removed in most cases by performing cannulation prior to induction of anaesthesia; however, in paediatric anaesthesia, a different strategy is required. In all patients receiving gaseous induction of anaesthesia, a clear plan of action should be formulated prior to commencement in case intravascular access is needed urgently, most usually to administer muscle relaxants and enable rapid control of the airway. This process should work in a similar way to a failed intubation drill, but the question posed will be: What will I do in this patient, in this situation, to gain rapid intravascular access?

All patients should be assessed immediately prior to induction and a preferred site for rapid cannulation identified. If cannulation proves unsuccessful then a definitive decision has to be taken about whether to persist with peripheral vein cannulation or change tactics. The safest and quickest alternative to intravenous (IV) access is the intraosseous route. The other major routes available are intramuscular (IM) injection, and after intubation certain drugs can be given endotracheally. Fluid can be administered with great care via peripheral arterial access, but some drugs may cause ischaemia via this route. The superior sagittal sinus has even been used for emergency blood transfusion in an infant with an open anterior fontanelle [2].

Peripheral cannulae

Peripheral venous access alone may not be adequate if the calibre of the cannula is insufficient to provide the desired infusion rates, or if continuous monitoring or sampling is required. Peripheral cannulation may be inappropriate if access is required for an extended period of time or if the fluid to be infused requires central venous administration (e.g. parenteral nutrition and vasoactive drugs).

The flow of liquids through tubes is governed by Poiseuille's law, so that the length of a cannula, the viscosity of the fluid and the pressure drop across it are directly related. By far the most important factor is the internal radius of the tube (r), as flow is proportional to r^4. Cannulae are graded according to their external diameter, so the thickness of the catheter wall needs to be considered. For most paediatric cases, a 22-gauge cannula is adequate, and for neonates and small infants 24 gauge will suffice. The 24-gauge devices available vary greatly in wall thickness and therefore in their internal radii. Thin-walled cannulae are easier to insert and provide higher flow rates, but they lack inherent strength and are more liable to damage on passage through the skin and to destructive kinking. Flow rates for various cannulae are given in Table 19.3 in Chapter 19.

The suitability of sites for cannulation depends on their ease of visual or tactile identification, anatomical consistency and freedom from major complications. The dorsum of the hand is the most common site, but the dominant thumb-sucking side should be avoided in order to reduce postoperative distress. Cannulation near a joint should be avoided as the mobility increases instability when secure fixation is difficult. Several other sites are worth special mention. The palmar aspect of the wrist has many visible small veins due to the paucity of overlying fat. The long saphenous vein at the ankle is of substantial size and constant position in all ages and can be palpated or accessed blindly anterior to the medial malleolus. The external jugular vein is often clearly visible but successful puncture is sometimes difficult as the vessel is thick walled and mobile with an awkward angle of approach. Scalp veins are easily located but fixation is difficult and may provoke major parental anxiety. In the antecubital fossa, inadvertent intra-arterial placement must be avoided.

Techniques to facilitate peripheral cannulation include proximal venous occlusion by the use of a tourniquet or assistant, hanging the limb over the side of the anaesthetic trolley and asking patients to clench their fist. Heating the limb (usually with a warm towel) causes venous distension and has been shown to reduce the number of attempts required for cannulation in adults [3]. Transillumination using a cold-light fibre-optic technique can improve visualisation and facilitate venous access [4], especially on the

dorsum of the hand; however, burns have been reported and the equipment is bulky and awkward to use. Transepidermal glyceryl trinitrate (GTN) has been employed successfully to enhance cannulation in adults and this has been confirmed in children [5]. GTN ointment, mixed with the standard eutectic mixture of local anaesthetic cream, significantly enhanced venous dilatation and ease of cannulation. Topical GTN has been shown to have adverse effects in neonates and should not be used in this age group [6].

Superficial veins can be visualised with real-time ultrasound. This can be used to identify suitable sites for blind percutaneous access, or for real-time guidance of needle placement. Surgical cutdown is waning in popularity in the face of readily available alternatives and should be attempted only as an adjunct to continuing attempts with other methods. Any major vein may be used but the preferred access site is the long saphenous vein. In one study [7], the mean time taken to complete the procedure by the surgeon depended on the patient's age: 11 minutes for neonates, 8 minutes at 1 month to 5 years, and 6 minutes at 6–16 years. The range of times to completion, however, was wide, with some procedures taking up to 90 minutes.

Umbilical vein cannulation

Umbilical vein catheters (UVCs) are is easy to insert in the first days of life. The normal umbilical cord has two arteries and one vein. The vein can be identified by its larger size and thin wall, and is usually found at the 12 o'clock position. Catheterisation may be short term, for resuscitation until peripheral access is secured. In this case the catheter need be placed only 3–5 cm beyond the mucocutaneous junction so that inadvertent placement in the portal circulation is avoided.

Longer-term access requires more accurate line placement with radiological assessment, the ideal tip position being in the inferior vena cava above the diaphragm or just inside the right atrium. Umbilical vein catheters are normally inserted blindly to a predetermined length, and are frequently (20–37 per cent) misplaced in the portal circulation, most commonly in the liver but occasionally in the spleen. Complications of intraportal UVC tip position include hepatic necrosis and portal hypertension. Tsui et al. [8] have developed an interesting technique to prevent malposition of UVCs, using the catheter itself as an electrocardiographic electrode and monitoring the changing morphology of the P-wave. An alternative is to use ultrasound to confirm the position of the catheter tip. Multiple-lumen catheters are available, and reduce the need for peripheral cannulation, but the most commonly used UVC is a 5Fr single-lumen line.

Infection is a common complication of UVCs and a duration limit of 14 days is commonly applied. A recent study compared longer-term use (up to 28 days) with elective replacement after 7–10 days with a percutaneous central line [9]. Infection and complication rates were similar in both groups, so longer-term use may be justified. Other complications, such as thrombus formation and perforation of the surrounding tissue, are common to all centrally placed lines.

Neonatal long lines

Neonatal long lines (NLLs) are fine (2–3Fr) silicone elastomer (Silastic) catheters, which can be inserted into a peripheral vein and threaded to a central position. They offer an attractive means of venous access compared with repeated insertion of peripheral cannulae, and decrease the rate of catheter-related sepsis [10]. In general, they are inserted from the upper limbs, although saphenous and scalp vein approaches are also possible [11].

The tip of the NLL should be left outside the pericardial reflection in order to decrease the risk of cardiac tamponade [12]. For lines inserted from a supracardiac approach, this means that the tip must be more than 1 cm above the cavoatrial junction in premature neonates, and 2 cm in term infants [12]. The position of the tip should be confirmed by a chest radiograph, best achieved by opacification of the NLL with a very small amount of non-ionic contrast, e.g. iohexol with iodine content 300 mg/mL (Omnipaque 300). Neonatal long lines have a tendency to occlude. There is no evidence that continuous infusion of heparin through NLLs is advantageous [13].

Other peripherally inserted central venous catheters

In older children, larger diameter (3–6Fr) peripherally inserted central venous catheters PICCs can be used. These have one or two lumina, and may have a valve (to prevent reflux of blood) at the tip of the catheter or at its hub (Fig. 22.1).

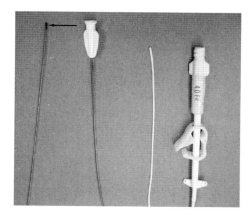

Figure 22.1 Peripherally inserted central venous catheters (PICCs). The Groshong-type catheter (left) has a valve to prevent reflux of blood at its distal end (arrow). The open-ended catheter (right) must be flushed with dilute heparin to prevent clotting in the catheter, but has the advantage that it can be inserted over a guidewire if necessary.

Peripherally inserted central venous catheters are usually inserted through veins in the upper limbs, but lower limb or scalp veins may also be used. The catheter is introduced through a large cannula or a peel-away sheath. The tip of the PICC should be left in a central position, defined as the superior vena cava, the upper right atrium or the inferior vena cava at or above the level of the diaphragm [14]. In the best hands, without fluoroscopic guidance, a central tip position is achieved in 86 per cent of insertions [15]. Non-central tip position is associated with a markedly increased risk of complications [14], and the use of fluoroscopy at the time of insertion is therefore recommended when this is possible. Procedural complications of PICC insertion are rare and usually not serious.

In general, PICCs are appropriate for treatment durations of weeks to months, and the longer-term use of PICCs as an alternative to tunnelled central venous catheters (CVCs) is associated with a predictable increase in mechanical complications and infection [16]. Peripherally inserted central verous catheters are particularly useful to avoid the pain and distress of repeated cannulation and to preserve peripheral veins in long-term patients.

CENTRAL VENOUS ACCESS

Indications for central venous access

The indications for short-term central venous access in anaesthesia and intensive care include inability to secure adequate peripheral access, monitoring of central venous pressure, frequent blood sampling (in the absence of intra-arterial access) and administration of sclerosant or vasoactive drugs. The usual indications for long-term central venous access are:

- parenteral nutrition
- haemodialysis
- chemotherapy
- antibiotic treatment
- enzyme replacement
- the infusion of blood products.

Choice of access site

The sites of first choice for most CVCs are the internal jugular veins (IJVs). These are easier to access than the subclavian veins, especially if ultrasound is used, and the risk of pneumothorax or haemothorax is much lower. In addition, thrombosis and permanent occlusion are probably more likely and more clinically significant following subclavian vein puncture. This may be especially important in children with chronic renal failure, because preservation of veins for future haemodialysis catheters is crucial, and also because subclavian stenosis is an important cause of failure of upper limb dialysis fistulas.

External jugular veins may be punctured with or without ultrasound guidance [17], although, when imaging is not used, there is sometimes difficulty advancing a catheter or guidewire into the subclavian vein from this approach.

The subclavian veins can be punctured from either a supraclavicular or infraclavicular approach, with or without ultrasound guidance. Their use may be indicated when the IJVs are occluded, or needed for other purposes, or in children with a tracheostomy, where the lateral puncture site may reduce the rate of infection compared with the use of IJVs.

The common femoral veins are relatively easy to puncture, and immediate complications are rare. This has led to their widespread use for insertion of short CVCs in neonates and infants. Although this is convenient, especially in emergencies, short femoral CVCs commonly cause iliofemoral venous occlusion in small children and infants [18]. The severity of immediate symptoms (swelling and colour change of the affected limb) depends on the development of collateral venous drainage. Iliac venous occlusion occasionally causes significant long-term problems of venous insufficiency or difficult venous access (e.g. in children who require right heart catheterisation). Stenzel et al. [19] compared femoral with non-femoral central venous catheter insertion in a prospective trial involving 395 critically ill children. Systemic infections attributable to the catheters were recognised for 2.5 per cent of femoral catheters and 2.1 per cent of non-femoral catheters, suggesting that this is not a major issue. In addition, all complications at the time of insertion were in the non-femoral group. Heparin-bonded catheters may significantly reduce femoral catheter-related thrombosis and infection [20].

Central venous access devices

SHORT CVCs (INCLUDING TEMPORARY HAEMODIALYSIS CATHETERS)

These catheters are inserted directly over a guidewire. Non-tunnelled short CVCs are simple to insert and reliable, and are consequently widely used in anaesthesia and intensive care. When it is anticipated that a CVC will be required for more than about 7–10 days, however, a tunnelled device or PICC may be more appropriate.

HICKMAN AND SIMILAR CATHETERS

These catheters have one, two or three lumina, and range in size from 0.9 mm (2.7Fr) to 4.0 mm (12Fr). A Dacron tissue in-growth cuff lies on the part of the catheter in the subcutaneous tunnel, in order to decrease the risks of accidental removal and ascending infection.

HAEMODIALYSIS CATHETERS

Most long-term haemodialysis catheters are similar to Hickman catheters, but have two lumina with offset openings, to prevent recirculation of blood during dialysis.

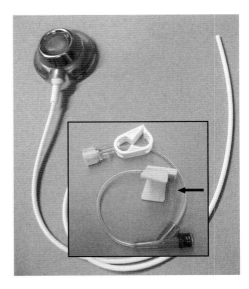

Figure 22.2 A venous port device. The inset shows the access system, with a non-coring (Huber) needle (arrow).

VENOUS PORT DEVICES

These devices have no external catheter; the venous catheter is instead connected to a subcutaneous reservoir, the superficial surface of which is covered by a thick silicone membrane. This can be accessed percutaneously with a non-coring (Huber) needle (Fig. 22.2). Port devices are less likely than tunnelled CVCs to become infected, cannot be accidentally removed, and facilitate activities such as showering and swimming. They are preferable for most children who require access only intermittently (e.g. weekly or less often), including those with haematological diseases and cystic fibrosis. They are less appropriate in children who cannot tolerate regular needle access, or who require continuous or frequent access, e.g. those who need parenteral nutrition or very intensive chemotherapy.

CATHETER DIAMETER

The appropriate diameter of the catheter to be used will depend on the child's size and the indications for insertion. Haemodialysis catheters need to be relatively large to allow sufficiently high flow rates. For other indications, small catheters (<5Fr) may be appropriate in infants, as the risk of complications is higher when large catheters are used [21].

CARE OF CVCs

Bloodstream infections associated with intravascular catheters are the most commonly reported nosocomial infection in paediatric intensive care [22]. There is evidence that specific measures (universal barrier precautions at the time of catheter insertion, chlorhexidine skin disinfection, catheters impregnated with an antibiotic, handwashing campaigns and physical barriers between patient beds) can significantly reduce nosocomial infection rates [23]. Introduction of these steps was associated with a 63 per cent decline in the rate of catheter-associated bloodstream infection.

LANDMARK TECHNIQUES FOR CENTRAL VENOUS ACCESS

Internal jugular veins

The IJV is a large, relatively superficial vein that provides a reliable site for central venous access. It runs in the carotid sheath from the jugular foramen at the base of the skull to a point between the clavicular and sternal heads of the sterno-cleidomastoid muscle. For most of its course, it lies deep to the medial edge of sternocleidomastoid. The relationship of the IJV to the carotid is variable, but higher in the neck at the level of the cricoid cartilage the IJV tends to be more lateral, becoming more anterior to the carotid artery as it descends into the root of the neck [24]. The technique to gain access blindly into the IJV must therefore be adapted according to the level of the puncture. The IJV may be visible or palpable low in the neck, aiding a more direct approach. Distension of the vessel will aid successful placement. This can be achieved by tilting the table head-down, by infusing fluids or simply by gentle compression of the liver.

In higher approaches to the IJV, the carotid pulsation is the important landmark for needle insertion. The path of the needle should be superficial to the carotid, passing laterally deeper into the neck below sternocleidomastoid in the direction of the ipsilateral nipple. This approach aims to pierce the IJV with safety whether it is anterior or lateral to carotid, because the needle is heading away from the carotid impulse. Cannulation can be achieved with a standard cannula-over-needle or needle-guidewire (Seldinger) technique. It is important to appreciate that the IJV is highly compressible, and needle pressure alone often results in the collapse of the vessel, so that the anterior and posterior walls are simultaneously punctured. If this occurs, blood can be aspirated only on withdrawal of the needle, when the two walls are pulled apart and the lumen reappears.

Subclavian veins

The high incidence of complications renders the subclavian veins less popular for blind cannulation. Complication rates from 3 per cent to as high as 34 per cent have been recorded, varying with age, side of puncture and indication [25,26].

The technique used to gain needle access differs slightly between children and adults. Positioning the head in the neutral position, without a shoulder roll, increases the cross-sectional diameter of the vessel [27] and, along with head-down tilt, should optimise conditions. The needle entry site is 1 cm below the midpoint of the clavicle. The needle should be stepped down the clavicle, passing under it as superficially as possible, then directed towards the suprasternal notch [28]. If this is unsuccessful, the vein may be found

on withdrawal. Finck et al. [29] used the landmark technique and achieved only an 80 per cent success rate in small infants (<6 months). These findings were confirmed by Yao et al. [30], who were only successful in 83 per cent of patients less than 5 kg, and 96 per cent of those weighing between 5 and 10 kg. Citak et al. [31] reported 100 per cent success in mostly older children, but with a significant rate of inadvertent arterial puncture and pneumothorax.

Common femoral veins

Femoral access avoids most of the intrathoracic complications of CVC insertion, and is relatively safe in inexperienced hands, with the major immediate complication being inadvertent arterial puncture [28]. The landmark for insertion is the femoral artery, with the vein lying medially. The vein should be punctured just below the inguinal ligament. The femoral vessels in small infants are relatively small, until they grow with weight bearing. Femoral venous catheterisation, therefore, is often complicated by obstruction with lower limb swelling and discoloration in neonates [32]. Previous catheterisation of a femoral vessel often results in subsequent attempts proving difficult, so the other side or another site should be used [33]. Even in critically ill preterm babies, blind femoral access appears to be a valuable technique. Chen [34] studied 49 critically ill preterm infants weighing less than 1000 g: catheterisation was successful in 80 per cent, with approximately 50 per cent of these completed within 10 minutes.

IMAGE–GUIDED CENTRAL VENOUS ACCESS

Real-time ultrasound guidance allows quick and safe central venous access in almost all children. We believe that, compared with landmark techniques, ultrasound reduces the rate of complications (specifically inadvertent arterial puncture, haematoma and pneumothorax) and increases the chance of success at the first attempted point of access. There is some evidence to support this [1]. In children who have had previous CVCs and possible venous occlusion, ultrasound allows the operator to select a patent vein for puncture. There is now a clear shift in anaesthetic practice towards the use of real-time ultrasound.

Equipment

ULTRASOUND EQUIPMENT

A high-frequency ($\geq$7 MHz) linear-array transducer ('probe') is used for puncture of the internal jugular and common femoral veins in most children. In small children and infants, small footplate ('hockey stick') transducers are ideal (Fig. 22.3). These transducers are also appropriate for puncture of brachial veins for PICC insertion. A probe cover is used to maintain sterility during the procedure.

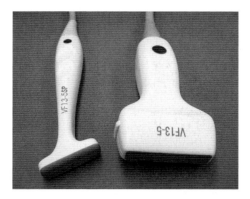

Figure 22.3 High-frequency ultrasound transducers. The small footplate ('hockey stick') transducer (left) is ideal for central venous access in infants or peripheral puncture in small children. The standard linear-array transducer (right) is used for central venous puncture in older children.

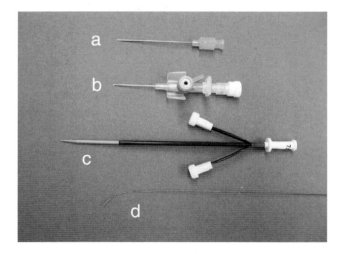

Figure 22.4 Equipment for insertion of a tunnelled central venous catheter in an infant. The vein is punctured with a 21-gauge needle (a) or a 22-gauge cannula (b). A peel-away sheath (c) is then inserted over a 0.46 mm (0.018 inch) guidewire, in this case a Cope nitinol mandril wire (Cook, Bjaeverskov, Denmark) (d).

FLUOROSCOPY

Fluoroscopy is particularly useful for difficult cases, where guidewire manipulations or venographic guidance may be needed. Even in simple cases it reduces the risk of catheter tip malposition, and removes the need for a post-procedure chest radiograph [35]. We routinely use fluoroscopy for insertion of tunnelled CVCs.

EQUIPMENT FOR CVC INSERTION

In small children, it is probably best to puncture central veins with small needles. We always use a 21-gauge one-part needle or 22-gauge cannula (Fig. 22.4) in children less than 10 kg. Both of these accept a 0.46 mm (0.018 inch) guidewire. The best guidewires, e.g. the Cope nitinol

mandril wire (Cook, Bjaeverskov, Denmark), have a stiff shaft and a short, floppy, gently curved tip (Fig. 22.4). The wire must be advanced until its stiff part is in the vein in order to allow insertion of a catheter or peel-away sheath. The floppy tip can be steered to some extent under fluoroscopic guidance. A thicker, 0.89 or 0.97 mm (0.035 or 0.038 inch), guidewire is required for certain peel-away sheaths, such as those for tunnelled haemodialysis catheters.

In small children, or when small veins are accessed in older children, the 0.46 mm guidewire can be exchanged for a 0.89 mm wire using a coaxial dilator system (Micropuncture Introducer Set, Cook). Puncture of larger veins with a bigger (19- or 18-gauge) needle permits immediate use of a thicker guidewire, making insertion of the peel-away sheath much more straightforward. Peel-away sheaths (Fig. 22.4) are almost always used when a tunnelled catheter is inserted. They are available in a wide range of sizes, from 3.5Fr to over 20Fr. In theory, the stated size of a sheath is equal to the diameter of a catheter that can be introduced through it. This should be checked in advance when using unfamiliar combinations of sheath and catheter.

Basic ultrasound techniques

CHOICE OF ULTRASOUND PLANE FOR IMAGING AND PUNCTURE

The geometric arrangement of needle, probe and vein will depend on the location of the vein and the size of the patient. There are at least three main methods:

Technique 1: the needle is advanced along the line of the vein, puncturing its superficial surface, with the probe held perpendicular to the needle and vein (Fig. 22.5a,b). This technique is most useful for the common femoral veins, infraclavicular puncture of the medial part of the subclavian vein and for insertion of PICCs into the arm veins.

Technique 2: the probe is held in the same plane as the needle, with each almost perpendicular to the long axis of the vein, which is then punctured from an anterolateral approach (Fig. 22.6). This technique can be used for tunnelled IJV catheters, when it produces a gracefully curved subcutaneous tunnel. In infants this may be important to prevent kinking of the catheter.

Technique 3: the probe, needle and vein all lie in the same plane (Fig. 22.5c,d). This technique has the significant disadvantage of producing a misleading partial-volume averaging artefact. This causes the needle to appear to be in the vein when it is in fact lying alongside it. It may, however, be appropriate for large veins such as the left brachiocephalic (see below).

INSERTION TECHNIQUES

The skin is prepared and draped according to standard surgical practice. Buffered lidocaine (or levobupivacaine 2.5 mg/mL

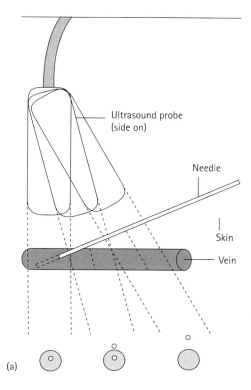

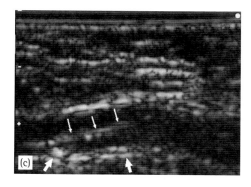

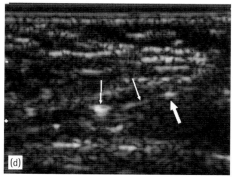

Figure 22.5 (Continued)   (c) Ultrasound image in the long axis of the vein. Following apparently successful puncture, the guidewire (thick arrows) has been advanced along a subintimal plane, raising an intimal flap (thin arrows). (d) After withdrawing the guidewire, the needle tip (thick arrow) has been repositioned in the lumen, and the wire readvanced (thin arrows). The usual cause of failure to advance a guidewire in a patent vein is that the needle is too far in.

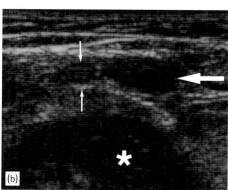

Figure 22.5   Basic technique for venous puncture (technique 1 in text). The needle is advanced along the line of the vein, puncturing its superficial surface, with the probe held perpendicular to both the needle and the vein. (a) Drawing showing the transducer, vein and needle (top) and schematics of the ultrasound images obtained as the transducer is tilted (bottom). (Modified from Barnacle [46]). (b) The right common femoral artery (small arrows) and vein (large arrow), seen in transverse section anterior to the non-ossified femoral head (asterisk) in an infant.

if general anaesthesia is used) is injected at the puncture site and the subcutaneous tunnel if one is required. A stab incision is made in a skin crease at the entry point of the puncture needle with a number 11 scalpel blade. This may be widened slightly with artery forceps if a large catheter is used. We usually tunnel the catheter before the puncture, where appropriate, but alternatively the puncture can be performed

first. The catheter is pulled out through the stab incision and wrapped in antiseptic-soaked gauze. The puncture needle, with a small syringe attached, is inserted through the stab incision, taking care not to damage the catheter, and the vein is punctured with a sharp stabbing motion. This ensures that its tip enters the lumen cleanly. If the opposite wall of the vein is punctured, the needle can be withdrawn into the lumen with ultrasound guidance. The operator can confirm that the tip of the needle is intraluminal by demonstrating free movement on ultrasound, without a 'tent' of intima over its tip (Fig. 22.5c,d), and by free aspiration of venous blood. The angle of entry of the needle may then be altered slightly so that it is pointing centrally. The guidewire is advanced into the vein, using ultrasound and/or fluoroscopic guidance if necessary.

Tips for access at the usual sites

ARM VEINS

The easiest upper limb veins to puncture with ultrasound guidance are those that accompany the brachial and axillary arteries (the venae comitantes of the brachial artery and the axillary vein). It is almost always best to do this with the probe perpendicular to the vein (technique 1 above). In smaller children, venous spasm may hinder the progress of a PICC, usually near the shoulder. Injection of vasodilators is rarely successful, but the spasm may resolve spontaneously after 10 minutes or so. It is often difficult to negotiate the junction of the cephalic and subclavian veins, and a curved-tip hydrophilic guidewire (e.g. Radiofocus, Terumo Europe, Leuven, Belgium) may be helpful in this situation.

INTERNAL JUGULAR VEINS (FIGS 22.6 AND 22.7)

In small children (when using fluoroscopic guidance) it may be useful to advance the guidewire through the right atrium (RA) and down the inferior vena cava if this is easy to do. Use of the Cope nitinol mandril wire may facilitate this technique, which makes insertion of the peel-away sheath or catheter easier and safer. Following removal of the needle, the peel-away sheath or catheter is advanced over the guidewire under fluoroscopic control. It is mandatory to fix the guidewire relative to the patient at this stage. If it is allowed to advance with the peel-away sheath or catheter, these may then cause serious damage to the superior vena cava or heart.

When a tunnelled catheter is inserted, the guidewire and the dilator of the peel-away sheath are then removed. Mechanical ventilation with positive end-expiratory pressure effectively prevents air entering the peel-away sheath at this stage, but great care should be taken to avoid air

embolism (e.g. by pinching the sheath or using a valved sheath) if the patient is breathing spontaneously. The catheter is advanced through the sheath, which is then split and removed. The position of the catheter tip is confirmed with fluoroscopy, and adjusted if necessary. Tip position will depend on the type of catheter and local preferences. The tips of short-term CVCs are usually left in the lower superior vena cava. On fluoroscopy this is at about the level of the carina. The tips of tunnelled CVCs are usually left in the upper RA, at about the T7 level. It is more accurate to use fluoroscopy than to cut the catheter at the level of the nipple.

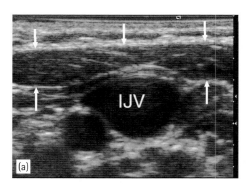

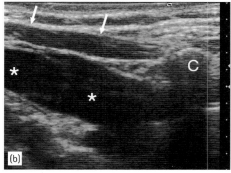

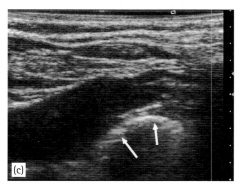

Figure 22.7 Left internal jugular (IJV) and left brachiocephalic veins. Transverse (a) and sagittal (b) images low in the neck show the left IJV lying anterolateral to the left common carotid artery and deep to the left sternocleidomastoid muscle (arrows). The valve which is commonly seen low in the IJV lies between the asterisks. The clavicle (C) is also shown. Transverse section at a more caudal level (c) shows the left brachiocephalic (innominate) vein, which may be punctured directly, as long as care is taken to avoid the apex of the left lung (arrows). Note: standard radiological view. Anaesthetists will normally have a cephalocaudal view, when the IJV will be to the left of the image and the CCA to the right.

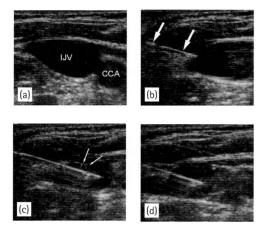

Figure 22.6 Basic technique for venous puncture (technique 2 in the text). (a) Transverse ultrasound image of the neck showing the right internal jugular vein (IJV) and common carotid artery (CCA). (b) The vein (large arrows) is punctured from an anterolateral approach, taking care to keep the needle aligned with the ultrasound probe. (c) Very commonly, the needle will raise an intimal 'tent' (small arrows). It is usually possible to aspirate blood, but if the guidewire is introduced at this point it will take a subintimal path (see Fig. 22.5). (d) If the needle is twisted and/or advanced abruptly a short distance, its tip will break through the intima and lie freely in the lumen. The guidewire can now be advanced. Note: standard radiological view. Anaesthetists will normally have a cephalocaudal view, when the IJV will be to the right of the image and the CCA to the left.

SUBCLAVIAN VEINS

A combination of the first and third configurations of the ultrasound transducer and needle can be used for infraclavicular puncture of the subclavian vein. In infants, this implies a more lateral skin entry site than that described for the landmark technique. Fluoroscopy is helpful to confirm that the guidewire is advancing centrally and not into the ipsilateral IJV or contralateral brachiocephalic vein.

COMMON FEMORAL VEINS

The first configuration is used for femoral vein puncture. The transducer can be rotated into the long axis of the vein to confirm that the guidewire is advancing, if necessary.

Unconventional central venous access

Long-term central venous access tends to become a problem in certain children, particularly those who need haemodialysis or parenteral nutrition. Various approaches to this problem are available. The simplest is often to puncture one of the brachiocephalic veins (Fig. 22.7c), which are often patent even when the ipsilateral internal jugular and subclavian veins are occluded [36].

Long-standing occlusions are always associated with the development of collateral veins. These small veins can often be used for central venous access following ultrasound-guided puncture. In the neck, these include the jugular arch and anterior jugular veins, which become prominent when there is obstruction of the IJVs. The use of these veins is facilitated by fluoroscopy and 'road-mapping' venography. Alternatively, the obturator veins can be punctured in the adductor compartment of the thigh, and used to bypass occlusions of the femoral and external iliac veins.

If access at these sites is unsuccessful, we recommend attempting recanalisation (discussed below) before proceeding to IVC access. Ultrasound-guided transhepatic access to the IVC is mainly used for cardiac interventions but is occasionally appropriate for insertion of CVCs, particularly in older children [37,38]. In young children (less than about 2 years old) there is a tendency for transhepatic catheters to migrate into the peritoneal cavity, although intraperitoneal bleeding seems to be rare. Despite its obvious disadvantages, transhepatic access is usually technically straightforward. The translumbar approach to the IVC requires more skill, as well as fluoroscopic guidance, and is rarely necessary [37,39].

Recanalisation of occluded veins

When ultrasound and fluoroscopy are available, it is often possible to recanalise occluded large veins [40]. The technique involves puncture of a convenient vein peripheral to the occlusion, and insertion of a dilator or catheter. Venography is performed through the dilator, and also through a catheter on the other side of the obstructed segment if necessary. This can be used as a road map to guide the incremental alternating advance of the catheter and a guidewire through the occluded segment ('blunt recanalisation'). Relatively stiff guidewires, such as the Radiofocus, are required for chronic occlusions, but floppy-tipped wires, such as the Cope nitinol wire (see Fig. 22.4), work well in fresh thrombus. Pulmonary thromboembolism is a theoretical risk, but has not been reported. The dilator tip may become extravascular during unsuccessful recanalisation, but this does not appear to cause significant haemorrhage. Sharp recanalisation with an intravascular needle can be attempted if blunt recanalisation of a short occlusion is unsuccessful, but may require biplane fluoroscopy. Balloon dilatation of the occluded segment is sometimes adequate to maintain patency. Stents should be inserted only if necessary.

INTRAOSSEOUS ACCESS

In emergency and trauma care, intraosseous needle access is rapidly gaining favour as the preferred alternative route to intravascular access, when peripheral IV access is difficult. The technique is part of standard resuscitation protocols, such as those in the *Advanced Paediatric Life Support* textbook [28]. Even though the procedure is rarely performed, it can easily be taught with a satisfactory success rate and few complications [41]. Intraosseous lines have even been used in resuscitation and stabilisation of preterm and full-term neonates and have been found to be effective with no long-term side-effects [41]. Less experienced personnel found intraosseous access easier and significantly quicker than umbilical venous catheterisation [42].

Two types of needle are available to puncture the outer cortical bone: a specialised intraosseous needle or a standard bone marrow needle (Fig. 22.8). An automated gun device is also available in both paediatric and adult versions. The site of insertion is dictated by the risks of complications. Anatomical studies in neonates have shown that the optimal site for insertion in the tibia is 10 mm distal to the tibial tuberosity [43]. More proximal sites increase the risk of damage to the growth plate, and distally the cortical bone thickens and insertion is more difficult. Radiological follow-up studies indicate that there is no long-term effect on tibial growth.

The potential complications of intraosseous insertion are rare but predictable. As well as potential damage to the growth plate, infection may be introduced and fractures may occur. Compartment syndrome can occur due to damage to the bone or extravasation of fluids. Fat or bone marrow emboli are a risk, but animal studies suggest that infusions are safe.

Studies have compared intraosseous, central venous and peripheral venous infusions of emergency drugs in animals. Epinephrine, sodium bicarbonate (1 mmol/kg), calcium chloride, 50 per cent dextrose, hydroxyethyl starch and lidocaine, when given by the intraosseous route, had equivalent magnitudes of peak effects and drug levels to the other routes [44].

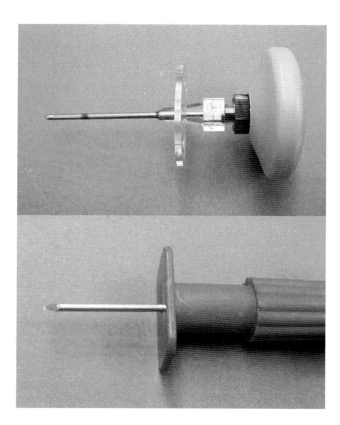

Figure 22.8   Intraosseous needles. Top: specialised intraosseous needle (Cook, Bjaeverskov, Denmark); bottom: standard bone marrow needle (Sternum Temno, Allegiance Healthcare, Troy, MI, USA).

One animal study compared IV, intraosseous and IM suxamethonium [45]. Six sheep were anaesthetised and acted as their own control. The average times to 100 per cent loss of forefoot twitch were 93.3 ± 34 seconds for IV, 100.8 ± 24.2 seconds for intraosseous and 291 ± 109 seconds for IM injection. The quicker response to intraosseous than to IM injection was significant and should translate to reduced morbidity in clinical practice. For this reason, intraosseous needles should be readily available wherever anaesthesia is practised and should be a part of resuscitation equipment.

Finally, intraosseous needles can be aspirated and the sampled blood analysed. The values obtained for haemoglobin, sodium, chloride, glucose, bilirubin, pH and bicarbonate are highly predictive of a venous sample. Potassium is moderately predictive, but PCO_2, PO_2 and platelet and leukocyte counts are significantly different.

REFERENCES

Key references

Bhutta A, Gilliam C, Honeycutt M *et al*. Reduction of bloodstream infections associated with catheters in paediatric intensive care unit: stepwise approach. *BMJ* 2007; **334**: 362–5.

Butler-O'Hara M, Buzzard CJ, Reubens L *et al*. A randomized trial comparing long-term and short-term use of umbilical venous

catheters in premature infants with birth weights of less than 1251 g. *Pediatrics* 2006; **118**(1): e25–35.

Janik JE, Conlon SJ, Janik JS. Percutaneous central access in patients younger than 5 years: size does matter. *J Pediatr Surg* 2004; **39**(8): 1252–6.

References

1. Hind D, Calvert N, McWilliams R *et al*. Ultrasonic locating devices for central venous cannulation: meta-analysis. *BMJ* 2003; **327**(7411): 361.

2. Graupman P. Using the superior sagittal sinus for emergency venous access in an infant. Case report. *J Neurosurg* 2006; **104**(3 suppl): 195–6.

3. Lenhardt R, Seybold T, Kimberger O *et al*. Local warming and insertion of peripheral venous cannulas: single blinded prospective randomised controlled trial and single blinded randomised crossover trial. *BMJ* 2002; **325**(7361): 409–10.

4. Bellotti GA, Bedford RF, Arnold WP. Fiberoptic transillumination for intravenous cannulation under general anesthesia. *Anesth Analg* 1981; **60**(5): 348–51.

5. Teillol-Foo WL, Kassab JY. Topical glyceryl trinitrate and eutectic mixture of local anaesthetics in children. A randomised controlled trial on choice of site and ease of venous cannulation. *Anaesthesia* 1991; **46**(10): 881–4.

6. Maynard EC, Oh W. Topical nitroglycerin ointment as an aid to insertion of peripheral venous catheters in neonates. *J Pediatr* 1989; **114**(3): 474–6.

7. Iserson KV, Criss EA. Pediatric venous cutdowns: utility in emergency situations. *Pediatr Emerg Care* 1986; **2**(4): 231–4.

8. Tsui BC, Richards GJ, Van Aerde J. Umbilical vein catheterization under electrocardiogram guidance. *Paediatr Anaesth* 2005; **15**(4): 297–300.

9. Butler-O'Hara M, Buzzard CJ, Reubens L *et al*. A randomized trial comparing long-term and short-term use of umbilical venous catheters in premature infants with birth weights of less than 1251 g. *Pediatrics* 2006; **118**(1): e25–35.

10. Liossis G, Bardin C, Papageorgiou A. Comparison of risks from percutaneous central venous catheters and peripheral lines in infants of extremely low birth weight: a cohort controlled study of infants <1000 g. *J Matern Fetal Neonatal Med* 2003; **13**(3): 171–4.

11. Racadio JM, Johnson ND, Doellman DA. Peripherally inserted central venous catheters: success of scalp-vein access in infants and newborns. *Radiology* 1999; **210**(3): 858–60.

12. Nowlen TT, Rosenthal GL, Johnson GL *et al*. Pericardial effusion and tamponade in infants with central catheters. *Pediatrics* 2002; **110**(1 Pt 1): 137–42.

13. Shah P, Shah V. Continuous heparin infusion to prevent thrombosis and catheter occlusion in neonates with peripherally placed percutaneous central venous catheters. *Cochrane Database Syst Rev* 2005; (3): CD002772.

14. Racadio JM, Doellman DA, Johnson ND *et al*. Pediatric peripherally inserted central catheters: complication rates related to catheter tip location. *Pediatrics* 2001; **107**(2): E28.

15. Fricke BL, Racadio JM, Duckworth T et al. Placement of peripherally inserted central catheters without fluoroscopy in children: initial catheter tip position. Radiology 2005; 234(3): 887–92.

16. Matsuzaki A, Suminoe A, Koga Y et al. Long-term use of peripherally inserted central venous catheters for cancer chemotherapy in children. Support Care Cancer 2006; 14(2): 153–60.

17. Soong WJ, Jeng MJ, Hwang B. The evaluation of percutaneous central venous catheters – a convenient technique in pediatric patients. Intensive Care Med 1995; 21(9): 759–65.

18. Talbott GA, Winters WD, Bratton SL, O'Rourke PP. A prospective study of femoral catheter-related thrombosis in children. Arch Pediatr Adolesc Med 1995; 149(3): 288–91.

19. Stenzel JP, Green TP, Fuhrman BP et al. Percutaneous femoral venous catheterizations: a prospective study of complications. J Pediatr 1989; 114(3): 411–5.

20. Krafte-Jacobs B, Sivit CJ, Mejia R, Pollack MM. Catheter-related thrombosis in critically ill children: comparison of catheters with and without heparin bonding. J Pediatr 1995; 126(1): 50–4.

21. Janik JE, Conlon SJ, Janik JS. Percutaneous central access in patients younger than 5 years: size does matter. J Pediatr Surg 2004; 39(8): 1252–6.

22. Richards MJ, Edwards JR, Culver DH, Gaynes RP. Nosocomial infections in pediatirc intensive care units in the United States. National nosocomial infections surveillance system. Pediatrics 1999; 103: e39.

23. Bhutta A, Gilliam C, Honeycutt M et al. Reduction of bloodstream infections associated with catheters in paediatric intensive care unit: stepwise approach. BMJ 2007; 334: 362–5.

24. Mallinson C, Bennett J, Hodgson P, Petros AJ. Position of the internal jugular vein in children. A study of the anatomy using ultrasonography. Paediatr Anaesth 1999; 9(2): 111–4.

25. Casado-Flores J, Valdivielso-Serna A, Perez-Jurado L et al. Subclavian vein catheterization in critically ill children: analysis of 322 cannulations. Intensive Care Med 1991; 17(6): 350–4.

26. Casado-Flores J, Barja J, Martino R et al. Complications of central venous catheterization in critically ill children. Pediatr Crit Care Med 2001; 2(1): 57–62.

27. Lukish J, Valladares E, Rodriguez C et al. Classical positioning decreases subclavian vein cross-sectional area in children. J Trauma 2002; 53(2): 272–5.

28. Mackway-Jones KME, Molyneux E, Phillips B, Wieteska S. Practical procedures – circulation. In: ALS Group, eds. Advanced paediatric life support 4. London: BMJ Books, 2005: 235–40.

29. Finck C, Smith S, Jackson R, Wagner C. Percutaneous subclavian central venous catheterization in children younger than one year of age. Am Surg 2002; 68(4): 401–4.

30. Yao ML, Chiu PC, Hsieh KS et al. Subclavian central venous catheterization in infants with body weight less than 10 kg. Acta Paediatr Taiwan 2004; 45(6): 324–7.

31. Citak A, Karabocuoglu M, Ucsel R, Uzel N. Central venous catheters in pediatric patients – subclavian venous approach as the first choice. Pediatr Int 2002; 44(1): 83–6.

32. Wardle SP, Kelsall AW, Yoxall CW, Subhedar NV. Percutaneous femoral arterial and venous catheterisation during neonatal intensive care. Arch Dis Child Fetal Neonatal Ed 2001; 85(2): F119–22.

33. Celermajer DS, Robinson JT, Taylor JF. Vascular access in previously catheterised children and adolescents: a prospective study of 131 consecutive cases. Br Heart J 1993; 70(6): 554–7.

34. Chen KB. Clinical experience of percutaneous femoral venous catheterization in critically ill preterm infants less than 1,000 g. Anesthesiology 2001; 95(3): 637–9.

35. Janik JE, Cothren CC, Janik JS et al. Is a routine chest x-ray necessary for children after fluoroscopically assisted central venous access? J Pediatr Surg 2003; 38(8): 1199–202.

36. Roebuck DJ, Ade-Ajayi N, McLaren CA, Kleidon T. Ultrasound-guided brachiocephalic (innominate) vein puncture for central venous access in children [abstract]. Pediatr Radiol 2004; 34: S129–S130.

37. Azizkhan RG, Taylor LA, Jaques PF et al. Percutaneous translumbar and transhepatic inferior vena caval catheters for prolonged vascular access in children. J Pediatr Surg 1992; 27(2): 165–9.

38. Bergey EA, Kaye RD, Reyes J, Towbin RB. Transhepatic insertion of vascular dialysis catheters in children: a safe, life-prolonging procedure. Pediatr Radiol 1999; 29(1): 42–5.

39. Robertson LJ, Jaques PF, Mauro MA et al. Percutaneous inferior vena cava placement of tunneled silastic catheters for prolonged vascular access in infants. J Pediatr Surg 1990; 25(6): 596–8.

40. Roebuck DJ, Kleidon T, McLaren CA, Barnacle AM. Central venous access by recanalisation of occluded central veins [abstract]. Pediatr Radiol 2005; 35: S76.

41. Ellemunter H, Simma B, Trawoger R, Maurer H. Intraosseous lines in preterm and full term neonates. Arch Dis Child Fetal Neonatal Ed 1999; 80(1): F74–5.

42. Abe KK, Blum GT, Yamamoto LG. Intraosseous is faster and easier than umbilical venous catheterization in newborn emergency vascular access models. Am J Emerg Med 2000; 18(2): 126–9.

43. Boon JM, Gorry DL, Meiring JH. Finding an ideal site for intraosseous infusion of the tibia: an anatomical study. Clin Anat 2003; 16(1): 15–8.

44. Orlowski JP, Porembka DT, Gallagher JM et al. Comparison study of intraosseous, central intravenous, and peripheral intravenous infusions of emergency drugs. Am J Dis Child 1990; 144(1): 112–7.

45. Moore GP, Pace SA, Busby W. Comparison of intraosseous, intramuscular, and intravenous administration of succinylcholine. Pediatr Emerg Care 1989; 5(4): 209–10.

46. Barnacle AM, Kleidon TM, Roebuck DJ. The use of ultrasound in central venous access in children. Ultrasound 2005; 13: 93–9.

Resuscitation

ROBERT BINGHAM

KEY LEARNING POINTS

- Most cardiac arrests in children are secondary to cardiovascular or respiratory failure.
- The primary cause is usually detectable and treatable.
- The earlier the treatment is initiated, the better the outcome.
- Interruption to chest compressions should be minimised during cardiopulmonary resuscitation.

- Ventricular fibrillation may occur in up to 27 per cent of in-hospital paediatric arrests.
- Automated external defibrillators are safe to use in children over 1 year of age.
- Resuscitation duration of greater than 30 minutes is associated with extremely poor outcome.

INTRODUCTION

Anaesthetists can be involved in the resuscitation of children for a number of reasons: a child they are anaesthetising could have a cardiac arrest, they might be a member of a hospital's cardiac arrest team, or they could be involved in the delivery of care in an intensive care unit. Fortunately, it is rare to have to resuscitate a child – one study puts the incidence of cardiac arrest under anaesthesia at 1.4/10 000 [1] – so an individual can undergo an entire career without encountering it. This presents the problem of training in the skills and knowledge required for successful resuscitation and the retention of those skills. Fortunately, most countries now have courses designed for this purpose – Pediatric Advanced Life Support (PALS), European Paediatric Life Support (EPLS) and Advanced Paediatric Life Support (APLS) are good examples. All paediatric anaesthetists should undertake such training and update their knowledge at regular intervals.

The purpose of this chapter is not to teach resuscitation, however, as this is much better done by the courses. It is intended to provide an explanation of the process of producing resuscitation guidelines and to outline the evidence base that underpins them.

RESUSCITATION GUIDELINES

Background

Resuscitation guidelines are formulated by a process of international consensus. There is no clinical justification for having different ones for different areas, and as health professionals are increasingly moving between countries it is clearly advantageous to keep guidelines uniform. Evidence on resuscitation interventions is, of course, accumulating all the time, but, like other areas of medicine, advances are generally made in small steps rather than giant leaps. It would also be impossible to modify the guidelines every time another piece of evidence emerged so, by general agreement, there is a 5-yearly review of the literature and a revision of the guidelines where necessary. Occasionally evidence emerges that merits an interim report, an example being the statement on the use of automated defibrillators in children published in 2003 [2]. The evidence review takes place under the auspices of a body called the International Liaison Committee on Resuscitation (ILCOR), which itself comprises representatives from all the world's resuscitation councils. The process is expensive and is largely funded by the American Heart Association (AHA).

In advance of the 5-yearly reviews, ILCOR determines the topics to be examined and assigns two experts to conduct independent literature searches and evidence-based evaluations. For the 2005 round there were 276 individual topics examined. Following this, there is a consensus conference involving the expert reviewers, which results in the production of a *Consensus on Science and Treatment Recommendation* (CoSTR) document from which resuscitation councils develop the guidelines themselves [3].

Traditionally, different resuscitation sequences are employed for children versus adults, as the aetiology of the cardiac arrest is different and adult resuscitation is focused around the treatment of primary cardiac arrest in ventricular fibrillation (VF). In children, VF is uncommon, accounting for only about 7–10 per cent of cardiac arrest overall, and the most common arrest rhythms are asystole or pulseless electrical activity (PEA), usually preceded by progressive bradycardia [4]. This is, in turn, the result of respiratory or circulatory failure, and thus cardiac arrest is usually a secondary event in children. The best way of treating this is to identify the primary process in its early stages and institute measures to prevent further progression; this is the focus of the paediatric resuscitation courses mentioned earlier. Both respiratory and circulatory failure have early compensated phases as the body's homeostatic mechanisms attempt to maintain a normal oxygen delivery to vital organs. As the disease progresses, these mechanisms are exhausted and a decompensated phase occurs, which is rapidly followed by cardiorespiratory failure and arrest. Early warning scoring systems, which use physiological parameter observations to warn staff of deterioration, show promise in alerting carers before decompensation has occurred.

Significant improvement in outcome can be achieved if clinical decline is detected early. Outcomes are very poor once the heart has stopped (>5 per cent good-quality survival at 1 year) but earlier intervention, even in the bradycardic pre-arrest phase, will increase survival to about 70 per cent and over [5,6].

Other factors that favourably affect outcome are witnessed arrest, respiratory failure aetiology, the presenting rhythm (primary VF has better outcomes than asystole), and a duration of resuscitation of >20 minutes [6–8].

Basic Life Support (Fig. 23.1)

Basic Life Support (BLS) was initially defined as the performance of cardiopulmonary resuscitation (CPR) without specialist equipment or drugs. The definition was then extended to include some airway adjuncts, such as face shields and pocket masks. Recently, with the wide availability of automated external defibrillators (AEDs), designed to be used by lay people, it has been accepted that the use of these should also be part of BLS.

Despite differences in aetiology between adult and paediatric cardiac arrest, a major focus of recent guideline reviews has been an attempt to simplify the advice in order to promote better assimilation and retention of knowledge. Areas of difference create potential confusion and should be avoided unless absolutely necessary. It is well known that many children who require resuscitation outside hospital receive no intervention until a health professional arrives, as people fear causing harm. Since bystander CPR is known to improve survival, it is important to encourage onlookers to initiate resuscitation, and so guideline simplicity is vital [9]. To this end, an area of particular focus has been the ratio of

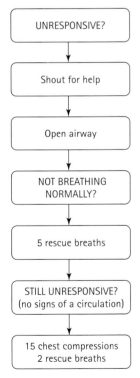

Figure 23.1 Paediatric Basic Life Support algorithm, published with kind permission from the Resuscitation Council (UK). CPR, cardiopulmonary resuscitation.

chest compressions to ventilation. It has traditionally been assumed that children require more ventilation during resuscitation than adults as they have a proportionally greater oxygen requirement and a high incidence of respiratory causes for the arrest. Past guidelines advocated five compressions for each breath for children under 8 years old and 15 compressions to 2 breaths for those over 8 years. An increasing body of evidence from experimental and adult investigation, however, has highlighted that rescuers tend to overventilate during resuscitation, with potentially detrimental consequences. A paediatric manikin study also showed that, with the 5:1 ratio, the time spent in transition between compression and ventilation was significant. Consequently, minute ventilation was similar to that achieved with a 15:2 ratio – where less time is wasted – but the number of chest compressions was significantly less [10].

Further evidence demonstrated potentially deleterious effects of excessive ventilation resulting from the resultant increases in right atrial pressure (RAP) [11]. Coronary perfusion is marginal during CPR. It is dependent on coronary perfusion pressure, which is the difference between aortic root pressure and RAP. Rises in RAP due to excessive ventilation therefore reduce coronary blood flow. Determining the correct pulmonary ventilation during CPR is complex. Pulmonary blood flow is low in this circumstance and pulmonary ventilation should be similarly low to match it. There is little chance of effectively removing CO_2, so the focus should be on ensuring that alveoli are open and filled with oxygen. If ventilation is reduced and more chest compressions are performed the blood flow will increase but the oxygen content of the blood will fall. Theoretically it should be possible to calculate the optimum balance between blood flow and oxygen content. This was done by Babbs and Kern [12] and they concluded that, in adults, there should be 15 chest compressions for each inflation (or 30 for two inflations) [12]. In a separate study, using the same calculations, Babbs and Nadkarni [13] calculated that children require proportionately more inflation breaths and that the requirement increases with diminishing age. It would be far too complex to have a scale of compression/ventilation ratios according to age, yet it is necessary to provide a ratio in the guideline, so an average of 15 compressions to 2 inflations was selected as the optimum for children and this is the recommendation for teams of health professionals responding to paediatric emergencies.

The importance of any particular ratio on survival is not known, but experimental data suggest that it is not particularly great. One study demonstrated that performing either chest compression with no ventilation or ventilation with no compression resulted in survival rates that were not significantly different from those generated by 'optimum' CPR. The important point was that any resuscitation intervention significantly improved survival [14].

People learning adult CPR are thus now told that they can use the same techniques in children, in order to encourage them to initiate resuscitation. The only concern with this approach is that, in Europe, the adult guidelines now start with chest compressions, and rescuers are told to leave the victim to 'phone for help if they are alone' (in order to expedite the arrival of a defibrillator). These two actions are not optimal for child victims, particularly if they are in the bradycardic pre-arrest state. Three minor modifications to the adult technique are therefore suggested to make it significantly more appropriate for use in children:

- Perform initial rescue breaths before starting chest compression.
- If alone, perform CPR for 1 minute before leaving to 'phone for help'.
- When performing chest compression, compress the chest by approximately one-third of its anteroposterior diameter.

Other simplifications to previous guidelines include the use of the same chest compression landmarks for all age groups (one finger's breadth above the xiphisternum) [15] and standardisation of the age range for the use of paediatric techniques (if the rescuer thinks the victim is a child, they should use the paediatric guideline). Small differences remain between resuscitation for infants and that for older children, however, mainly due to the particularities of infant anatomy. When two rescuers are present, chest compression is more effective in infants if it is performed by encircling the chest with the hands and compressing the lower sternum with both thumbs. During manoeuvres to treat choking, abdominal thrusts should be avoided in infants as the liver and spleen are not protected by the ribcage.

The algorithm for the management of choking has also been considerably simplified (Fig. 23.2). Foreign body airway obstruction (FBAO) is common, particularly in pre-school children. Although there are no data on the optimum management of choking, the success of manoeuvres intended to provide a sudden, large increase in intrathoracic pressure has been documented in numerous case reports. There is no evidence to support a particular order for these attempts, so the most important feature of the algorithm has to be simplicity, to facilitate learning and retention. Current advice is to start

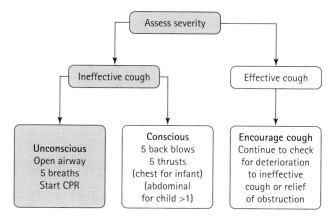

Figure 23.2 Paediatric foreign body airway obstruction treatment, published with kind permission from the Resuscitation Council (UK). CPR, cardiopulmonary resuscitation.

with back blows in conscious victims of all ages – indeed, this is the natural response of most lay people to this situation. If these are not successful, proceed to abdominal thrusts (Heimlich manoeuvre). In infants, in whom these may be dangerous, chest thrusts are advised in place of abdominal thrusts. In unconscious victims, CPR (which is, of course, a series of chest thrusts interspersed with attempts to ventilate) should be performed in all age groups.

AUTOMATED EXTERNAL DEFIBRILLATORS

As mentioned earlier, an interim statement was issued about the use of AEDs in children as evidence accumulated that they were effective, even in younger children [2]. Previous guidelines had suggested that AEDs could be used in children over 8 years of age. Younger children were not included, as AEDs are designed for adult use and deliver a shock with full adult energy levels. In addition, the arrhythmia analysis programmes were developed for adult arrhythmias and there was concern that they may advise an inappropriate shock. From the late 1990s onwards, investigations into the latter point began to generate evidence that many AED arrhythmia analysis programmes were suitable for children and, in particular, the specificity was found to be 100 per cent, i.e. the machine would not advise a shock unless the victim had a shockable rhythm [16]. This finding was combined with case reports of children, who were known to be in VF, not being defibrillated – and thus dying – as ambulance treatment protocols prohibited the use of AEDs in under-8s.

The remaining concern about the toxicity of high energy levels in small children had been studied in animals and shown to be unfounded [17]. For children over 1 year of age, the AED will reliably analyse the ECG and advise a shock only if it is required. Even if a full adult shock is delivered in this circumstance, it is extremely unlikely to cause damage. Indeed, for a child in VF, the most dangerous energy level is 0 J/kg! There remains a small concern about arrhythmia analysis in children under 1 year due to their rapid normal heart rates. An adult energy level shock delivered inappropriately in this circumstance may certainly cause harm, so there is no current recommendation for (or against) the use of AEDs in infants. Fortunately, VF is very rare in this age group. Some manufacturers claim that their machines are suitable for use in infants and these may therefore be used, provided that the manufacturer's instructions are followed. Attenuation systems have been developed to modify adult AEDs for use in children under 8 years of age. These are usually in the form of paediatric defibrillation pads or a switch on the machine, which reduces its output, typically to 50 J. These systems have recently been studied and found to be effective; they should be used in children under 8 years, if available [18]. However, defibrillation should not be delayed while one is obtained.

Advanced Life Support

Advanced Life Support (ALS) involves the use of drugs and equipment for the definitive management of cardiopulmonary

arrest. As in BLS there is a paucity of good-quality evidence to underpin the recommendations in children. Most of the guidelines are based on extrapolation from adult, animal or theoretical work.

For the reasons outlined earlier for BLS, the paediatric ALS algorithm (Fig. 23.3) is now simpler and is similar to the adult algorithm – the main difference is the extra emphasis on oxygenation at the beginning, as hypoxia is a common precipitant of paediatric arrest.

AIRWAY

It has been assumed that the tracheal tube is the 'gold standard' for airway management for paediatric emergencies; however, this does not stand up to careful scrutiny. A large prospective controlled study of outcome in children, randomised to receive tracheal intubation or bag-and-mask ventilation in out-of-hospital cardiac arrest, found that there were no significant outcome differences between the groups [19]. In addition, a small number of children in the tracheal tube group had undetected oesophageal intubation, all of whom died. Bag-and-mask ventilation is perfectly satisfactory during the initial phases of CPR and prolonged attempts to intubate the trachea are likely to result in harm.

There is increasing interest in the use of cuffed tracheal tubes in all areas of paediatric practice (see Chapter 19). In resuscitation, the potential advantages are that there is no necessity to change tubes because of a size disparity and that a cuffed tube facilitates positive pressure ventilation in children with poor lung compliance. The use of CO_2 detection to confirm tracheal tube placement is recommended, although during cardiac arrest, expired CO_2 may not be detected, even from a correctly placed tracheal tube, if the pulmonary blood flow is too low [20]. Capnography should always be available for transfer of intubated children.

There are numerous case report of use of the laryngeal mask airway (LMA) for the resuscitation of children with supraglottic airway abnormalities (e.g. Pierre Robin syndrome). The LMA clearly has a role in this situation for those experienced in its use. It is less clear whether this device offers advantages for airway management during paediatric resuscitation in general. Data from adult studies show that inexperienced providers can safely use the LMA for airway control [21]. There are no similar studies in children, but evidence from the use of LMAs in paediatric anaesthesia suggests that there is greater difficulty with insertion and complication rates are high until experience in the technique is obtained. Furthermore, malpositioning and downfolding of the epiglottis are more common in children and the incidence increases with decreasing age. The LMA is not therefore currently recommended for general use in the resuscitation of children.

There are numerous other supraglottic airway devices (combitube, laryngeal tube, cuffed oropharyngeal airway) that have been promoted for use during anaesthesia, but

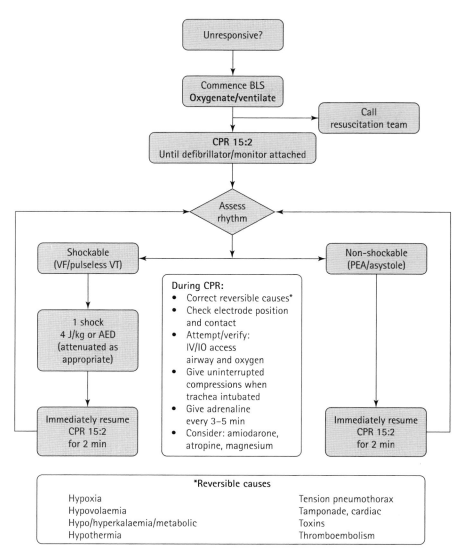

Figure 23.3 Paediatric Advanced Life Support algorithm, published with kind permission from the Resuscitation Council (UK). AED, automated external defibrillator; BLS Basic Life Support; CPR, cardiopulmonary resuscitation; IO, intraosseous; IV, intravenous; PEA, pulseless electrical activity.

there are currently no studies of their use in paediatric resuscitation.

BREATHING

As discussed above, there is a great tendency to over-ventilation during CPR. When a tracheal tube is in place, chest compressions can continue uninterrupted and a ventilation rate of approximately 12/minute is adequate for all ages. The most important objective is to open the alveoli with a high concentration of oxygen. In this circumstance, it is important to ensure that the chest is inflating properly. If there is any doubt, it may be preferable to revert to a 15:2 sequence.

The most commonly used ventilation device is a self-inflating bag system. These have the great advantage that they will function in the absence of a gas supply. Most paediatric anaesthetists, however, will be comfortable to use a T-piece circuit assuming that there is a piped or cylinder oxygen supply. Although there is an emerging debate about

the dangers of high oxygen concentrations, particularly during resuscitation at birth, 100 per cent oxygen is still the ventilation gas of choice.

CIRCULATION

Gaining circulatory access can be the most demanding aspect of resuscitating a child. There is often intense peripheral vasoconstriction and veins can be impossible to cannulate. Fortunately, intraosseous (IO) access is simple and effective and this should be the route of choice unless an obvious peripheral vein is available [22]. Intraosseous cannulation is an old technique, which resurfaced in the 1990s. The usual site is the anteromedial surface of the tibia, although other sites (e.g. femoral or tibial condyles) have also been described. All currently used resuscitation drugs and fluids can be infused via this route and blood samples obtained can be used for blood gas analysis, haematological and biochemical assay, and cross-matching. Intraosseous cannulae should not be sited in a fractured bone or in children with osteogenesis imperfecta. With careful use, complications (bone fracture, compartment syndrome, infection) are rare.

Lipid-soluble resuscitation drugs (adrenaline, naloxone, atropine and lidocaine) can be delivered via the lungs. It is usually recommended that the drugs are administered down a catheter through a tracheal tube and are either mixed with or followed by a bolus of 0.9% or normal saline. A much larger dose is required than for IV administration (e.g. adrenaline 100 μg/kg). In practice, this is a very unreliable route, resulting in unpredictable drug levels. It is preferable to obtain IO access.

FLUIDS

Fluid administration is discussed in detail in Chapter 4. For initial resuscitation, the most important features of a resuscitation fluid are that they are isotonic with plasma and that they are easy to store and thus readily available. Isotonic saline solutions are ideal. Most children requiring resuscitation will benefit from a fluid bolus of 20 mL/kg, but a brief history of the antecedent events should be obtained to eliminate those who have pre-existing circulatory overload. Some clinicians are happy to continue resuscitation with crystalloid solutions but others may prefer to move to colloid solutions after the initial phase.

RESUSCITATION DRUGS

Adenosine

An endogenous purine nucleotide, adenosine is useful in the management of supraventricular tachycardia, as it transiently blocks conduction through the atrioventricular (AV) node and either terminates the arrhythmia or slows the ventricular rate and thus helps diagnose the underlying problem [23]. Because of its extremely short half-life (about 10 seconds), it should be administered as close to the heart as possible and followed immediately by a flush of saline. A number of side-effects have been described: unpleasant sensations including chest tightness, severe bronchospasm and worsening of the arrhythmia in Wolf–Parkinson–White (WPW) syndrome. Adenosine should be used with great care in denervated hearts (e.g. after heart transplantation) as the effect may be exaggerated.

Adrenaline

This is the main resuscitation drug used in children; it is used on both the shockable and non-shockable sides of the ALS algorithm (see Fig. 23.3), since it induces potent vasoconstriction and therefore increases coronary and cerebral perfusion pressures. In VF, it improves contractility and increases the amplitude and frequency of the fibrillation, thus increasing the likelihood of successful defibrillation. There has been much debate about the optimum dose of adrenaline during CPR in children. One publication found enhanced survival in a study group using 100 μg/kg compared with that in a retrospective control group using 10 μg/kg [24]. This finding prompted the inclusion of a recommendation to use the higher dose if conventional doses had failed in earlier guidelines. Subsequent research, however, has failed to corroborate the initial finding and a large, prospective, randomised controlled trial demonstrated no survival improvement with high-dose adrenaline, together with a possible reduction in survival in a subgroup with hypoxic/ischaemic arrest [25]. The resuscitation dose of adrenaline is thus 10 μg/kg; larger doses should be avoided except in rare circumstances, such as adrenoceptor blocker overdose or where downregulation of adrenoceptors is likely, such as following prolonged infusions of catecholamines.

Amiodarone

The antiarrhythmic action of amiodarone is mediated through several mechanisms; it slows AV conduction, prolongs the QT interval and the refractory period, and is a competitive inhibitor at adrenergic receptors. In adults, amiodarone has been shown to be superior to lidocaine in facilitating defibrillation. Amiodarone has also been used successfully in children for the treatment of arrhythmias, particularly junctional ectopic tachycardia following cardiac surgery [26]. It is now recommended as the preferred antiarrhythmic in the treatment of resistant VF in children, and is given just before the fourth shock is delivered. Although it should be given as a bolus during CPR, amiodarone is usually administered as a slow infusion in the management of perfusing arrhythmias, as it causes hypotension. This side-effect is reduced in a recently developed aqueous formulation [27].

Atropine

The use of atropine during paediatric resuscitation is common but it is likely to be of use in circumstances only where high vagal tone is implicated, as in severe bradycardia following intubation or traction on the extraocular muscles. Atropine can be used in the treatment of bradycardia due to hypoxia/ischaemia, but its administration should not delay the optimum treatment, which is oxygenation followed by adrenaline. The minimum dose should be 100 μg, as paradoxical bradycardia mediated though a central mechanism has been described [28].

Calcium

Although calcium increases myocardial contractility and has been used following cardiopulmonary bypass in children to enhance cardiac output, there is no demonstrated benefit in either electromechanical dissociation or asystole [29,30]. Calcium is indicated for resuscitation in the presence of ionised hypocalcaemia – a relatively common occurrence in children, particularly those in intensive care units or on dialysis.

Magnesium

This cation is indicated in the management of documented or strongly suspected hypomagnesaemia and in the treatment of refractory polymorphic ventricular tachycardia (torsade de pointes) [31].

Sodium bicarbonate

Acidosis is a common accompaniment to cardiac arrest and it is universal in secondary cardiac arrest, which is the usual form in children. Nevertheless, since the buffering capacity of bicarbonate depends on the generation and elimination of CO_2, it is of limited use during CPR as the pulmonary blood flow is too low to clear the evolved CO_2 effectively, which may then cross cell membranes and, paradoxically, generate an intracellular acidosis. In addition, the high sodium content (1000 mmol/L) may generate osmotic shifts and result in unacceptably high plasma sodium levels. Since adrenaline is partially inactivated by acidosis, however, a dose of bicarbonate can be considered, once ventilation and compressions are established, if initial adrenaline doses have failed to restore spontaneous circulation. Bicarbonate is also indicated for the treatment of hyperkalaemia and in tricyclic antidepressant overdose.

Vasopressin

It has been suggested that the intense vasoconstriction mediated by the actions of vasopressin at the V_1 receptor may be beneficial during resuscitation, as it will increase coronary perfusion pressure without the potentially undesirable β-adrenergic actions of adrenaline [32,33]. This is particularly the case when myocardial ischaemia is likely, as in coronary artery disease. Since the evidence for this supposition is lacking even in adults, vasopressin cannot currently be recommended for use in paediatric resuscitation.

DEFIBRILLATION IN CHILDREN

Although VF is uncommon in children overall, it may occur in up to 37 per cent of in-hospital arrests [7], particularly in hospitals with a cardiology or cardiac surgery programme. AEDs have been mentioned earlier and, although they are increasingly used, it is recommended that manual defibrillators be used for the resuscitation of children in hospitals. There are a large variety of manual defibrillators available, but all new machines now deliver a biphasic energy waveform, as this has been shown to be effective at lower energy levels and cause less myocardial dysfunction than the older monophasic waveform in adult and experimental studies. Although this is assumed to be the same for children, data are limited, so the optimum defibrillation dose is unknown. The recommended energy level of 4 J/kg is based on a single observational study and is probably an overestimate of the energy required, so in the USA and Australasia an initial dose of 2 J/kg is suggested [34]. There is evidence that even much greater defibrillation shocks (10–15 J/kg) do not cause harm, however, so in Europe, for simplicity and to maximise first shock success, a single energy level of 4 J/kg is advised for all shocks [35].

Traditionally, defibrillation has been performed with the use of hand-held paddles. Adult paddles (8–12 cm diameter) are suitable for most children as long as they can be adequately separated on the chest wall [36]. In very small children and infants, it is possible to deliver the shock 'front to back' if adequate paddle separation cannot be achieved. It is preferable, though, to use conventionally positioned infant paddles (4.5 cm diameter) in this situation [37]. The paddles need to be in good contact with the skin and this is facilitated by firm pressure. A conducting interface is essential; electrode gel is messy and risks spreading across the chest with consequent arcing of the current, particularly in small children. It is preferable to use purpose-made conducting pads as defibrillation is considerably simplified (particularly during surgery) by the use of adhesive pads, which remain in place for the course of the resuscitation. These reduce the risk of accidental shock, arcing and sparking, and minimise the time external chest compression (ECC) is interrupted (see below). It is even possible to continue ECC while the defibrillator is charging.

THE ALS SEQUENCE

Background

The ALS sequence was revised considerably between the 2000 and 2005 literature reviews; much of this was in response to the realisation that during most resuscitation attempts there were long pauses during which ECC was interrupted. There are two main consequences of this, both of which are detrimental to a successful outcome:

- Coronary perfusion pressure falls – coronary perfusion depends on a pressure gradient between the aortic root and the right atrium (coronary sinus). Since ECC develops small stroke volumes, it takes a number of compressions to generate a reasonable aortic root pressure. When ECC is stopped, this falls to baseline immediately and the process must start again [38]. This is a further reason why compression ratios with a larger number of consecutive compressions are preferable to those with frequent interruptions (e.g. 15:2 rather than 5:1).
- The right heart dilates – when compressions stops, the pressures in the circulation equalise and the blood flows from the elastic walled left ventricle and arteries to the venous capacitance vessels and eventually the right heart, which becomes very dilated. This results in a raised RAP (further diminishing coronary perfusion pressure) and a distended right ventricle, which in turn deviates the ventricular septum and compresses the left ventricular cavity. In this circumstance, even if the left ventricle contracts, it will generate little or no stroke volume, there will be no coronary perfusion and the recovery will not be sustained unless blood in the right heart is conducted via the pulmonary circulation to the left heart.

It is clear, therefore, that any interruption in ECC is detrimental to successful resuscitation and should be avoided, and the 2005 ALS algorithm reflects this. Chest compression is continuous, the only interruption being for ventilation and a brief check of the ECG every 2 minutes and for defibrillation if the rhythm is shockable. Following delivery of a shock,

ECC is resumed immediately (with no ECG check). ECC should be restarted, even if the rhythm is seen to change, as, for the reasons described above, the heart will not be able to support the circulation immediately. The only other reason to interrupt chest compression is if the child starts to breathe normally or move spontaneously. Continuous chest compression is tiring if performed for long periods and the quality declines, so it is important to change rescuer frequently (such as at each of the 2-minute ECG checks).

Rhythm check

The purpose of the ECG check every 2 minutes is to ascertain if the rhythm is shockable. In most paediatric cardiac arrests, it will not be. If the rhythm is shockable, a single shock is delivered. Although previous guidelines have recommended three stacked shocks, adult data strongly suggest that modern defibrillators will successfully defibrillate the heart on the first occasion if the circumstances are favourable [39]. If a single shock is not successful, it is likely that more chest compressions or medication is required to create the conditions in which the heart can be defibrillated. If the heart has not restarted after the second shock, a dose of adrenaline should be administered and this should be repeated every 3–5 minutes (just before each second rhythm check). If a further shock is unsuccessful, a dose of amiodarone should be given; thus the management of VF in children is the same as for adults, except for the energy levels.

Although the treatment is the same, the aetiology is likely to be different. Adult VF is usually due to myocardial ischaemia secondary to coronary artery disease – this is extremely unusual in children, in whom electrolyte disturbances, drug toxicity and hypothermia are more likely causes. A search should therefore be made for reversible causes, which are usefully remembered by the mnemonic 4Hs and 4Ts:

- Hypoxia
- Hypovolaemia
- Hyper-/hypokalaemia – or other electrolyte disturbances
- Hypothermia
- Tension pneumothorax
- Tamponade (cardiac)
- Toxic (or therapeutic) substances
- Thromboembolism (pulmonary or coronary).

The reversible causes should also be sought in the non-shockable side of the algorithm as, together with the administration of adrenaline, this is the mainstay of treatment.

Management of Arrhythmias

Arrhythmias are uncommon in children, but they are more likely during surgery and anaesthesia. Most arrhythmias can be managed successfully using the simple approach outlined in Fig. 23.4.

The most important initial management of any arrhythmia is to ensure oxygenation and ventilation and to consider and treat reversible causes (see above). Under anaesthesia, likely causes are electrolyte disturbances, drug toxicity and mechanical stimulation of the heart (e.g. by central line guidewire). A quick assessment should be made of the adequacy of the cardiac output. Is it absent? Is there compensated or decompensated circulatory failure? If the cardiac output is absent, the management follows the ALS algorithm. In the compensated state (normal blood pressure and organ perfusion), advice can be sought if necessary and, although the situation can deteriorate, there is no necessity to treat immediately. Simple manipulation of vagal tone can be safely used in the compensated state. Atropine can be administered for bradyarrhythmias and vagal manoeuvres such as Valsava's or facial application of iced water for tachyarrhythmias [40].

In the decompensated state (evidence of poor organ perfusion), treatment has to be initiated rapidly.

BRADYARRHYTHMIAS

For bradyarrhythmias, it is essential to confirm adequate oxygenation. If the heart rate is less than 60/minute, ECC should be commenced. Following this, the treatment options are atropine or adrenaline. If the likely cause is hypoxia/ischaemia then adrenaline is the first choice. An initial dose of 2–5 µg/kg can be administered before proceeding to the full resuscitation dose (10 µg/kg) if necessary. Atropine should be used if high vagal tone is likely but *in extremis* the administration of adrenaline should not be delayed. Pacing is only of use in the extremely unusual circumstance of AV block or sinus node dysfunction.

TACHYARRHYTHMIAS

The management of decompensated tachyarrhythmia is more complex. Although tachyarrhymias are generally divided into broad and narrow complex, in practice this is not as useful in children as it is for adults because paediatric tachycardias, even broad complex ones, are more likely to be supraventricular in origin – ventricular tachycardia is rare [41]. One important distinction in narrow complex tachycardia, however, is between sinus and supraventricular tachycardia (SVT). As children's heart rates are already high, an increase can lead to rates close to those of SVT. Table 23.1 lists the features distinguishing sinus tachycardia from SVT. The ECG features can be difficult to interpret and information gleaned from the history, e.g. speed of onset, may be more useful.

The management of decompensated shock with SVT is by removing any precipitating cause (e.g. direct atrial stimulation) and synchronised cardioversion, initially at 0.5–1 J/kg, increasing to 2 J/kg. An alternative, particularly in conscious children, is adenosine (100 µg/kg, maximum 6 mg, increasing to 200 µg/kg, maximum 12 mg). Adenosine must be used with care, if at all, in asthmatics, heart transplant recipients and those with WPW syndrome.

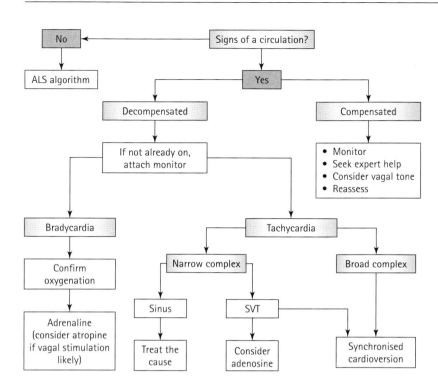

Figure 23.4 Algorithm detailing the approach to arrhythmias in children, published with kind permission from the Resuscitation Council (UK) . ALS, Advanced Life Support; SVT, supraventricular tachycardia.

VENTRICULAR TACHYCARDIA

As mentioned above, ventricular tachycardia (VT) is rare in children, but may occur in association with anaesthesia (particularly local anaesthetic toxicity) and with electrolyte disturbances. Decompensated shock is usual in VT and the treatment is again removal of the precipitating cause and synchronised cardioversion. Adenosine will not convert the rhythm but may be used to differentiate between VT and SVT, as the ventricular rate will reduce with the consequent AV block in SVT. One form of polymorphic VT – torsade de pointes (so called because the ECG resembles a twisted comb) – responds to the administration of magnesium ions [31].

LOCAL ANAESTHETIC TOXICITY

Overdose with local anaesthetics, particularly bupivacaine, can cause severe arrhythmias, including cardiac arrest in any rhythm. Resuscitation can be extremely difficult, as bupivacaine binds tightly to the myocardium. Resuscitation may be prolonged and should be continued, as myocardial and neurological outcome should be favourable if good-quality CPR is initiated promptly. Extracorporeal membrane oxygenation (ECMO) should be considered if it is available. Animal work has suggested that lipid infusion can hasten unbinding of the drug from the myocardium and there is a human case report of successful resuscitation from ropivacaine toxicity after a bolus of 2 mL/kg of 20 per cent Intralipid, followed by infusion of approximately 0.2 mL/kg/h (the experimental study used twice this dose) [42].

Table 23.1 Distinguishing features of sinus tachycardia and supraventricular tachycardia (SVT)

	Sinus tachycardia	SVT
History	Associated illness	No associated illness
Onset	Gradual	Sudden
Heart rate (HR)	<200	>220
P waves	Present	May not be seen
HR variability	Present	Absent

POST-RESUSCITATION CARE

The immediate aim of care after successful return of spontaneous circulation is to minimise organ damage, particularly of the brain. Achieving this requires the prompt restoration of normal physiology – this may necessitate fluid and inotropic support and, except after the briefest of arrests, will involve positive pressure ventilation. It also seems logical to measure and correct any electrolyte disturbances. Elevated blood glucose levels are associated with poor neurological outcome in adults following cardiac arrest and stroke [43]. Tight glucose control, using insulin if necessary, is thus advocated for adults. There are no comparable data for children and fear of their propensity for hypoglycaemia, which will also worsen outcome [44], has inhibited any strong recommendation for insulin treatment. Glucose levels should initially be managed through control of administration.

Seizures will result in large increases in cerebral oxygen consumption and measures for their detection and control should be in place.

Hyperthermia will similarly increase oxygen consumption in all organs and should be treated aggressively. A large multicentre trial (Hypothermia after Cardiac Arrest Study Group) demonstrated that adults who remain comatose following VF arrest benefit from mild hypothermia (32–34°C) for 12–24 hours [45]. In addition, there are data to support the safety, and some suggestion of benefit, of induced hypothermia and selective head cooling following resuscitation at birth [46,47]. Although there is no direct evidence in favour of hypothermia in the paediatric age group, avoidance of active warming during and immediately following resuscitation (unless temperature <32°C) is a reasonable option.

STOPPING RESUSCITATION

The decision to terminate a resuscitation attempt is a difficult one and there are no absolute rules, as individual case reports have documented survival in exceptional circumstances. Good-quality survival is unlikely after 30 minutes of resuscitation, however, unless there are favourable circumstances such as:

- the arrest was witnessed and resuscitation started promptly
- good-quality CPR has continued throughout
- the rhythm is shockable
- there is hypothermia (e.g. cold water drowning)
- there is drug (e.g. local anaesthetic) toxicity
- ECMO is available and the primary condition is reversible.

The decision will depend on the individual circumstances and can be made only by the team leader in conjunction with any available staff members involved in the child's care.

PARENTAL PRESENCE

Parents generally want to be present during a resuscitation attempt on their child [48]. There is evidence that, if they are present, they are more clearly able to understand the efforts being made. Also, if the outcome is unsuccessful, they are with their child at the moment of death, which helps the grieving process [49]. It is important to have a member of staff detailed to look after the family, whose role is to support them, prepare them for what they will see and explain the reasons for the procedures being performed. This can be done while tracheal intubation and vascular access are being performed and the parents can be then be brought in when the resuscitation is well established. Staff members involved in the resuscitation may feel threatened, but the parents' presence may also promote professionalism and help staff to see the child in the context of the family [50].

'DO NOT ATTEMPT RESUSCITATION' (DNAR) ORDERS

It is inappropriate to initiate resuscitation when death is inevitable (as in end-stage malignancy), it has no chance of succeeding or the quality of life following a successful attempt will be unacceptable. In order to avoid this, children in these categories should have a DNAR order so that staff know not to call the clinical emergency team. The order should be established following discussion with the parents or guardian and, if possible, with the children themselves. Everyone should be aware that a DNAR order does not exclude other active management, either therapeutic or palliative.

Do not attempt resuscitation orders should be clear to all the staff involved in the care of the child and should be reviewed regularly and following changes in the child's condition.

REFERENCES

Key references

Gausche M, Lewis RJ, Stratton SJ et al. Effect of out-of-hospital pediatric endotracheal intubation on survival and neurological outcome: a controlled clinical trial. J Am Med Assoc 2000; 283(6): 783–90.

Kern KB, Hilwig RW, Berg RA et al. Importance of continuous chest compressions during cardiopulmonary resuscitation: improved outcome during a simulated single lay-rescuer scenario. Circulation 2002; 105(5): 645–9.

Morray JP, Geidushek JM, Ramamoorthy C et al. Anesthesia related cardiac arrest in children: Initial findings of the pediatric perioperative cardiac arrest (POCA) registry. Anesthesiology 2000; 93(1): 6–14.

The International Liaison Committee on Resuscitation (ILCOR). Consensus on science with treatment recommendations for pediatric and neonatal patients: pediatric basic and advanced life support. Pediatrics 2006; 117(5): 955–77.

Young KD, Seidel JS. Pediatric cardiopulmonary resuscitation: a collective review. Ann Emerg Med 1999 1999; 33(2): 195–205.

References

1. Morray JP, Geidushek JM, Ramamoorthy C et al. Anesthesia related cardiac arrest in children: Initial findings of the pediatric perioperative cardiac arrest (POCA) registry. Anesthesiology 2000; 93(1): 6–14.

2. Samson R, Berg R, Bingham R et al. Use of automated external defibrillators for children: an update. An advisory statement from the Pediatric Advanced Life Support Task Force, International Liaison Committee on Resuscitation. Resuscitation 2003; 57(3): 237–43.

3. The International Liaison Committee on Resuscitation (ILCOR). Consensus on science with treatment recommendations for

pediatric and neonatal patients: pediatric basic and advanced life support. *Pediatrics* 2006; **117**(5): 955–77.

4. Young KD, Gausche-Hill M, McClung CD *et al*. A prospective, population-based study of the epidemiology and outcome of out-of-hospital pediatric cardiopulmonary arrest. *Pediatrics* 2004; **114**(1): 157–64.

5. Young KD, Seidel JS. Pediatric cardiopulmonary resuscitation: a collective review. *Ann Emerg Med* 1999 1999; **33**(2): 195–205.

6. Lopez-Herce J, Garcia C, Dominguez P *et al*. Characteristics and outcome of cardiorespiratory arrest in children. *Resuscitation* 2004; **63**(3): 311–20.

7. Samson RA, Nadkarni VM, Meaney PA *et al*. Outcomes of in-hospital ventricular fibrillation in children. *N Engl J Med* 2006; **354**(22): 2328–39.

8. Donoghue AJ, Nadkarni V, Berg RA *et al*. Out-of-hospital pediatric cardiac arrest: an epidemiologic review and assessment of current knowledge. *Ann Emerg Med* 2005; **46**(6): 512–22.

9. Kuisma M, Suominen P, Korpela R. Paediatric out-of-hospital cardiac arrests: epidemiology and outcome. *Resuscitation* 1995; **30**(2): 141–50.

10. Dorph E, Wik L, Steen PA. Effectiveness of ventilation-compression ratios 1:5 and 2:15 in simulated single rescuer paediatric resuscitation. *Resuscitation* 2002; **54**(3): 259–64.

11. Aufderheide TP, Lurie KG. Death by hyperventilation: a common and life-threatening problem during cardiopulmonary resuscitation. *Crit Care Med* 2004; **32**: S345–51.

12. Babbs CF, Kern KB. Optimum compression to ventilation ratios in CPR under realistic, practical conditions: a physiological and mathematical analysis. *Resuscitation* 2002; **54**(2): 147–57.

13. Babbs CF, Nadkarni V. Optimizing chest compression to rescue ventilation ratios during one-rescuer CPR by professionals and lay persons: children are not just little adults. *Resuscitation* 2004; **61**(2): 173–81.

14. Berg RA, Hilwig RW, Kern KB *et al*. Simulated mouth-to-mouth ventilation and chest compressions (bystander cardiopulmonary resuscitation) improves outcome in a swine model of prehospital pediatric asphyxial cardiac arrest. *Crit Care Med* 1999; **27**(9): 1893–9.

15. Clements F, McGowan J. Finger position for chest compressions in cardiac arrest in infants. *Resuscitation* 2000; **44**(1): 43–6.

16. Cecchin F, Jorgenson DB, Berul CI *et al*. Is arrhythmia detection by automatic external defibrillator accurate for children? Sensitivity and specificity of an automatic external defibrillator algorithm in 696 pediatric arrhythmias. *Circulation* 2001; **103**(20): 2483–8.

17. Babbs CF, Tacker WA, Van Vleet JF *et al*. Therapeutic indices for transchest defibrillator shocks: effective, damaging, and lethal electrical doses. *Am Heart J* 1980; **99**(6): 734–8.

18. Atkins D, Jorgenson D. Attenuated pediatric electrode pads for automated external defibrillator use in children. *Resuscitation* 2005; **66**(1): 31–7.

19. Gausche M, Lewis RJ, Stratton SJ *et al*. Effect of out-of-hospital pediatric endotracheal intubation on survival and neurological outcome: a controlled clinical trial. *J Am Med Assoc* 2000; **283**(6): 783–90.

20. Bhende MS, Thompson AE. Evaluation of an end-tidal CO_2 detector during pediatric cardiopulmonary resuscitation. *Pediatrics* 1995; **95**(3): 395–9.

21. Stone B. The use of the laryngeal mask airway by nurses during cardiopulmonary resuscitation. Results of a multicentre trial. *Anaesthesia* 1994; **49**(1): 3–7.

22. Orlowski JP, Porembka DT, Gallagher JM *et al*. Comparison study of intraosseous, central intravenous, and peripheral intravenous infusions of emergency drugs. *Am J Dis Child* 1990; **144**(1): 112–7.

23. Losek JD, Endom E, Dietrich A *et al*. Adenosine and pediatric supraventricular tachycardia in the emergency department: multicenter study and review. *Ann Emerg Med* 1999; **33**(2): 185–91.

24. Goetting MG, Paradis NA. High-dose epinephrine improves outcome from pediatric cardiac arrest. *Ann Emerg Med* 1991; **20**(1): 22–6.

25. Perondi M, Reis A, Paiva E *et al*. A comparison of high-dose and standard-dose epinephrine in children with cardiac arrest. *N Engl J Med* 2004; **350**(17): 1722–30.

26. Michael JG, Wilson WR, Jr, Tobias JD. Amiodarone in the treatment of junctional ectopic tachycardia after cardiac surgery in children: report of two cases and review of the literature. *Am J Ther* 1999; **6**(4): 223–7.

27. Somberg JC, Timar S, Bailin SJ *et al*. Lack of a hypotensive effect with rapid administration of a new aqueous formulation of intravenous amiodarone. *Am J Cardiol* 2004; **93**(5): 576–81.

28. Dauchot P, Gravenstein JS. Effects of atropine on the electrocardiogram in different age groups. *Clin Pharmacol Ther* 1971; **12**(2): 274–80.

29. Stueven HA, Thompson B, Aprahamian C *et al*. The effectiveness of calcium chloride in refractory electromechanical dissociation. *Ann Emerg Med* 1985; **14**(7): 626–9.

30. Stueven HA, Thompson B, Aprahamian C *et al*. Lack of effectiveness of calcium chloride in refractory asystole. *Ann Emerg Med* 1985; **14**(7): 630–2.

31. Tzivoni D, Banai S, Schuger C *et al*. Treatment of torsade de pointes with magnesium sulfate. *Circulation* 1988; **77**(2): 392–7.

32. Voelckel WG, Lurie KG, McKnite S *et al*. Comparison of epinephrine and in a pediatric porcine model of asphyxial cardiac arrest. *Crit Care Med* 2000; **28**(12): 3777–83.

33. Mann K, Berg RA, Nadkarni V. Beneficial effects of vasopressin in prolonged pediatric cardiac arrest: a case series. *Resuscitation* 2002; **52**(2): 149–56.

34. Gutgesell HP, Tacker WA, Geddes LA *et al*. Energy dose for ventricular defibrillation of children. *Pediatrics* 1976; **58**(6): 898–901.

35. Gurnett CA, Atkins DL. Successful use of a biphasic waveform automated external defibrillator in a high-risk child. *Am J Cardiol* 2000; **86**(9): 1051–3.

36. Atkins DL, Kerber RE. Pediatric defibrillation: current flow is improved by using 'adult' electrode paddles. *Pediatrics* 1994; **94**(1): 90–3.

37. Atkins DL, Sirna S, Kieso R *et al.* Pediatric defibrillation: importance of paddle size in determining transthoracic impedance. *Pediatrics* 1988; **82**(6): 914–8.

38. Kern KB, Hilwig RW, Berg RA *et al.* Importance of continuous chest compressions during cardiopulmonary resuscitation: improved outcome during a simulated single lay-rescuer scenario. *Circulation* 2002; **105**(5): 645–9.

39. Poole JE, White RD, Kanz KG *et al.* Low-energy impedance-compensating biphasic waveforms terminate ventricular fibrillation at high rates in victims of out-of-hospital cardiac arrest. LIFE Investigators. *J Cardiovasc Electrophysiol* 1997; **8**(12): 1373–85.

40. Sreeram N, Wren C. Supraventricular tachycardia in infants: response to initial treatment. *Arch Dis Child* 1990; **65**(1): 127–9.

41. Benson D, Jr., Smith W, Dunnigan A *et al.* Mechanisms of regular wide QRS tachycardia in infants and children. *Am J Cardiol* 1982; **49**: 1778–88.

42. Litz RJ, Popp M, Stehr SN *et al.* Successful resuscitation of a patient with ropivacaine-induced asystole after axillary plexus block using lipid infusion. *Anaesthesia* 2006; **61**(8): 800–1.

43. Kent TA, Soukup VM, Fabian RH. Heterogeneity affecting outcome from acute stroke therapy: making reperfusion worse. *Stroke* 2001; **32**(10): 2318–27.

44. Salhab WA, Wyckoff MH, Laptook AR *et al.* Initial hypoglycemia and neonatal brain injury in term infants with severe fetal acidemia. *Pediatrics* 2004; **114**(2): 361–6.

45. Hypothermia after Cardiac Arrest Study Group. Mild therapeutic hypothermia to improve the neurologic outcome after cardiac arrest. *N Engl J Med* 2002; **346**(8): 549–56.

46. Gluckman PD, Wyatt JS, Azzopardi D *et al.* Selective head cooling with mild systemic hypothermia after neonatal encephalopathy: multicentre randomised trial. *Lancet* 2005; **365**(9460): 663–70.

47. Compagnoni G, Pogliani L, Lista G *et al.* Hypothermia reduces neurological damage in asphyxiated newborn infants. *Biol Neonate* 2002; **82**(4): 222–7.

48. Boie ET, Moore GP, Brummett C *et al.* Do parents want to be present during invasive procedures performed on their children in the emergency department? A survey of 400 parents. *Ann Emerg Med* 1999; **34**(1): 70–4.

49. Robinson SM, Mackenzie-Ross S, Campbell Hewson GL *et al.* Psychological effect of witnessed resuscitation on bereaved relatives . *Lancet* 1998; **352**(9128): 614–7.

50. Jarvis AS. Parental presence during resuscitation: attitudes of staff on a paediatric intensive care unit. *Intensive Crit Care Nurs* 1998; **14**(1): 3–7.

24

Blood transfusion and conservation

ELIZABETH JACKSON

KEY LEARNING POINTS

- Transfusion transmitted infection, especially viral infection, is now extremely rare.
- Variant Creutzfeldt–Jakob disease is transmissible through blood transfusion and is an emerging problem mainly in the UK. Measures have been taken to reduce the risk, especially in children.
- Human error is an important cause of transfusion-related morbidity and mortality. Errors in patient identification and failure to recognise special transfusion requirements (e.g. irradiated products) are the commonest problems.
- All transfusions of allogenic products must be fully justified and this is particularly important in children because of their long life expectancy.

- Reduction in the use of allogeneic blood in surgical patients can be achieved through: (a) treatment of preoperative iron deficiency; (b) acceptance of low transfusion thresholds; (c) autologous transfusion techniques; and (d) pharmacological agents.
- There is a lack of good-quality evidence to guide practice for most patient groups, particularly in relation to autologous transfusion techniques. The use of and choice of these techniques are largely based on availability, surgical preference and costs.

INTRODUCTION

Blood transfusion and approaches to minimise unnecessary exposure to donor blood are an important part of the perioperative management of many children undergoing complex surgery. Safety is of particular importance in children, given that they usually have a high probability of recovery [1].

RISKS AND COMPLICATIONS OF BLOOD TRANSFUSION

An understanding of the risks of blood transfusion is necessary for the recognition and management of problems

related to transfusion and to enable the provision of information to patients and parents in relation to consent. The main risks of transfusion are summarised in Table 24.1.

Transmission of infection

BACTERIAL CONTAMINATION

Bacterial contamination of blood products can occur if donor skin flora are introduced at the time of collection or the donor has bacteraemia. It may also occur during processing of the blood product. Platelets are more likely to transmit bacterial infection than other blood components, as they are stored at higher temperatures. Improvements in the collection procedure for donations [2] have reduced the risk of bacterial contamination. Products should be inspected for visual discoloration and the integrity of packaging checked before use. The possibility of bacterial contamination should be considered if the patient develops fever, tachycardia and hypotension shortly after commencing a transfusion. The transfusion should be discontinued and supportive treatment instituted. Broad-spectrum antibiotics should be given until blood culture confirms the organism involved [2].

VIRAL INFECTIONS

Human immunodeficiency virus (HIV), hepatitis B virus (HBV) and hepatitis C virus (HCV) can all be transmitted through blood transfusion. The combination of excluding donors with behaviour that may put them at high risk of infection and increasingly sophisticated screening tests that reduce the marker-negative window phase of infection has greatly reduced the risk of transmission of these infections in developed countries. Current estimates of the residual risk of infected blood units entering the blood supply in the UK are given in Table 24.2 [3]. In the UK, blood is also routinely

Table 24.1   Risks of blood transfusion

Transmission of infection
Bacterial
Viral
Prion

Immunological
Acute haemolytic transfusion reactions
Delayed haemolytic transfusion reactions
TA-GvHD
TRALI
Non-specific febrile reactions
Anaphylactic reactions
Development of HLA antibodies; platelet refractoriness
PTP
Immunomodulation

HLA, human leukocyte antigen; PTP, post-transfusion purpura; TA-GvHD, transfusion-associated graft-versus-host disease; TRALI, transfusion-associated acute lung injury.

tested for human T-lymphotropic virus type 1 (HTLV-1). Several other viruses have been transmitted by transfusion, including hepatitis A and West Nile virus. The latter is a sufficient problem in some countries, including the USA, to warrant screening. Imported plasma products used for children in the UK are subjected to viral inactivation processes that virtually eliminate the risk of viral infection.

The transmission of cytomegalovirus (CMV) infection is a potential problem in immunocompromised patients, including preterm babies. Leukodepletion greatly reduces the likelihood of transmission. In the UK the current national guidelines are that infants (age 1 year) should have CMV-negative products and there are local policies in place that cover other patient groups, e.g. transplant recipients [4].

PRIONS: VARIANT CREUTZFELDT–JAKOB DISEASE

Variant Creutzfeldt–Jakob disease (vCJD) is a fatal degenerative neurological disease first encountered in England in 1996 and is caused by the trans-species transmission of the prion responsible for bovine spongiform encephalopathy (BSE). Evidence that vCJD can be transmitted by transfusion has accumulated first from animal studies and now from case reports in humans [5]. There is currently no test available to detect vCJD in donated blood and the risks have not been quantified.

In the UK, a number of steps have been taken to reduce the risks of transfusion-related transmission of vCJD. In 1999 universal leukodepletion was introduced and, more recently, a policy has been adopted of not accepting blood donors who have themselves received blood products. Extra measures have been taken to reduce the risks in children, because those born after January 1996 will not have been exposed to BSE in the food chain. Only virally inactivated fresh frozen plasma (FFP) imported from the USA, where BSE has never been a problem, should be issued for use in children. Exposure to plasma is also limited by using red cells stored in optimal additive solution rather than whole blood. Countries where BSE has never been a problem protect patients by excluding donors who have lived in affected European countries. Animal research suggests that selective absorption of prions from donated blood might be an approach to reducing the risk of transmission of vCJD in the future [6].

Table 24.2   Estimates of the frequency of HIV, HBV and HCV infectious donations issued per million donations and 1 per x million donations after testing in the UK, 2003–04 [3] where x is the number in the column

	HIV		HBV		HCV	
	Per million	1 in x million	Per million	1 in x million	Per million	1 in x million
All donors	0.19	5.22	2.02	0.50	0.03	29.03
New donors	0.44	2.26	6.11	0.16	0.15	6.79
Repeat donors	0.16	6.16	1.54	0.65	0.02	46.99

HBV, hepatitis B virus; HCV, hepatitis C virus; HIV, human immunodeficiency virus.

Immunologically mediated risks of transfusion

ACUTE AND DELAYED HAEMOLYTIC TRANSFUSION REACTIONS

The most severe acute haemolytic reactions usually occur as a result of immunological destruction of donated red cells because of ABO incompatibility. ABO incompatibility is always due to avoidable errors. Failure adequately to identify the patient either at the point of transfusion or at the time of blood sampling accounts for most cases; laboratory-based errors account for the remainder [7,8].

In the anaesthetised child, severe acute haemolysis due to ABO incompatibility presents with cardiovascular collapse with or without fever and may be accompanied by abnormal bleeding as a consequence of disseminated intravascular coagulation (DIC). Haemoglobinaemia and haemoglobinuria occur. If the diagnosis is suspected, the transfusion should be discontinued and supportive treatment instituted. A forced diuresis with alkalinisaton of the urine will help prevent renal failure. The donor unit and a blood sample from the recipient should be sent to the blood bank to confirm or refute the diagnosis and allow the issuing of compatible blood. If transfusion is required prior to confirmation of the patient's blood group, consideration should be given to using group O rhesus-negative blood.

Transfusion may result in antibodies being produced to the many other red cell antigens other than the ABO antigens. These alloantibodies may be a problem during subsequent transfusions as they may result in delayed haemolysis 1–14 days after transfusion. The antibodies are not always identified on standard antibody screens, as the levels may be too low for detection prior to the transfusion, which itself stimulates a rise in levels. They seldom cause severe clinical problems.

Alloantibody generation is less common in young children and virtually never seen in infants under 4 months. However, neonates may have maternal alloantibodies that have passed across the placenta and been acquired in the mother as a consequence of either transfusion or pregnancy. For this reason, when a neonate requires transfusion, maternal blood should ideally be screened for atypical red cell antibodies [4]. Accidental administration of rhesus-positive blood to a rhesus-negative girl may result in rhesus antibodies that are a potential major problem during pregnancy when she is older. If this error is recognised at the time, treatment with anti-D, with or without exchange transfusion, is indicated.

Neonates with necrotising enterocolitis occasionally become systemically infected with neuraminidase-producing organisms that can damage red cell proteins exposing the T-cryptoantigen. This T-activation is easily diagnosed by laboratory testing. Adult but not neonatal plasma usually contains anti-T IgM antibody that is potentially haemolytic

[9]. Red cells in optimal additives contain minimal plasma and can be transfused as needed. Plasma containing products including platelets should be avoided if possible because of the risks of haemolysis. Where available, low-titre anti-T plasma products may be preferred, and in the event of clinically significant haemolysis exchange transfusion may be required [4].

TRANSFUSION–ASSOCIATED GRAFT–VERSUS–HOST DISEASE

Transfusion-associated graft-versus-host disease (TA-GvHD) results from engraftment of donor T lymphocytes in the recipient whose immune system is unable to reject them. Transfusion-associated GvHD occurs in either immuno-compromised patients or immunocompetent individuals where there is a close tissue type match between recipient and donor, such as in the case of directed donations from relatives.

Patients at risk of TA-GvHD must have all red cell, platelet and granulocyte products irradiated to prevent this usually fatal complication of transfusion. Leukodepletion is not sufficient. The possibility that irradiated products may be required should be considered in all patients with congenital or acquired immunocompromise, including those undergoing treatment for malignancy and bone marrow transplantation. Requirements should be checked with the relevant teams caring for the patient. Table 24.3 summarises the main indications for irradiated products. Note that children with HIV and those with solid tumours do not need irradiated products [4].

One condition in which patients at risk of TA-GvHD may require transfusion before the diagnosis of congenital immunodeficiency can be confirmed or refuted is DiGeorge anomaly. In this disorder there is a combination of thymic hypoplasia, parathyroid hypoplasia and cardiac defects, particularly interrupted aortic arch and conotruncal abnormalities. There needs to be awareness of this association

Table 24.3 Indications for irradiated blood products

Product specific
All granulocytes
All HLA-matched products
Donations from first- and second-degree relatives

Recipient specific
Congenital immunodeficiency
Infants under 1 year of age who received an IUT
Hodgkin's disease (indefinitely from diagnosis)
Patients treated with purine analogues
Bone marrow transplant recipients including conditioning period*
Bone marrow donors – 7 days preharvest until harvest complete

---

HLA, human leukocyte antigen; IUT, intrauterine transfusion.
*Duration of requirement post-transplantation depends on many variables and should be checked with the relevant clinical team.

and, if there is any doubt, irradiated products should be used until the diagnosis can be excluded [4].

TRANSFUSION-RELATED ACUTE LUNG INJURY

Transfusion-related acute lung injury (TRALI) can result from the transfusion of any blood product that contains plasma. The onset is within 6 hours of the transfusion [10]. Although the pathogenesis is not fully understood, TRALI is believed to occur when donor antibodies (to antigens on white cells, especially human leukocyte antigens [HLA]) activate recipient neutrophils sequestered in the pulmonary vasculature. The activation of neutrophils culminates in capillary endothelial damage and the increased permeability characteristic of acute respiratory distress syndrome. HLA incompatibility of the donor and recipient has been documented in most of the reported cases of TRALI in children [11]. Children with TRALI usually recover within 72–96 hours with supportive treatment, although fatalities have been reported [1,11].

The blood product most frequently implicated in TRALI is fresh frozen plasma (FFP), usually from multiparous female donors who have developed antibodies to paternal antigens in pregnancy [11]. In the UK, the incidence of TRALI is decreasing, which is consistent with the policy introduced in 2004 of using male donors, where possible, for the preparation of FFP and the plasma contribution to platelet pools [7,8].

OTHER IMMUNE-RELATED RISKS AND COMPLICATIONS

Mild febrile reactions are common during blood transfusion, particularly in multiply transfused patients. They are attributed to the interaction of antibodies in the recipient with donor white cell antigens and to the accumulation of cytokines, lipids or complement in the donor product. Febrile reactions are less common with leukodepleted products. Similarly, minor urticarial reactions are common. Major anaphylactic reactions are rare but are seen particularly in patients who have antibodies to IgA as a consequence of congenital IgA deficiency [12].

Blood transfusion can result in the development of anti-HLA antibodies that lead to rapid destruction of transfused platelets and platelet refractoriness. This complication is less common with the leukodepleted blood. Rarely, transfusion of red cells or platelets results in the formation of alloantibodies to human platelet antigens and post-transfusion purpura due to severe thrombocytopenia that develops 5–9 days post-transfusion.

Allogeneic blood transfusion has a non-specific immunosuppressive action and it is possible that this may influence postoperative infection rates and recurrence rates for malignancy [13]. There is no conclusive evidence of these effects in children and the advent of leukodepletion probably makes this less relevant as most of the effects are believed to be leukocyte mediated.

REDUCING THE RISKS OF BLOOD TRANSFUSION

Data from haemovigilance programmes show that blood transfusion safety has improved in recent years, particularly in relation to the transmission of infection. The current focus is on reducing the risk of human error as many of the adverse events now reported are potentially avoidable. Table 24.4 summarises the report of the UK haemovigilance scheme for 2005 [7]. The most frequently reported serious transfusion problem was the administration of an incorrect blood component, of which there were 485 reports. Common problems of particular relevance to paediatric practice were failure to recognise the need for irradiated products and 'wrong blood events' where patients received blood of the incorrect group or intended for another patient. Failure to check the patient's identity at the time of sampling or transfusion and inadequate use of patient name bands were highlighted as particular areas of concern. Meticulous attention to good transfusion practices, especially in emergency situations, is an important part of reducing the risk of transfusion [2,7].

INTRAOPERATIVE BLOOD TRANSFUSION

Allogeneic blood from volunteer donors is a limited resource that can never be entirely free of risk. It is therefore important that all transfusions are fully justified and reasonable steps are taken to minimise exposure to donated products. The acceptance of transfusion triggers significantly below normal haemoglobin values is now established practice and represents the simplest method of reducing the use of blood during surgery and in the postoperative period. Most of the research to support this approach has been done in adults [14] and clear evidence-based transfusion thresholds for children undergoing surgery are not available. However, it is generally accepted that neonates and infants under 4 months of age need special consideration and that

Table 24.4 Summary of the serious hazards of transfusion (SHOT) annual report 2005 [7]

Reported complication	Number (n = 609)	Deaths (n = 5)
IBCT – 'wrong blood'	485	2
Acute transfusion reaction	68	1
Delayed transfusion reaction	28	
TRALI	23	2
Transfusion transmitted infection		
Viral (HBV)	1	
Bacterial	2	
Post-transfusion purpura	2	

HBV, hepatitis B virus; IBCT, incorrect blood component transfused; TRALI, transfusion-related acute lung injury.

thresholds based on adult practice are appropriate after 4 months of age [4,15].

Guidelines for transfusion published by the Association of Anaesthetists of Great Britain and Ireland [16] suggest that:

- transfusion is not normally indicated if the haemoglobin concentration is above 10 g/dL
- a haemoglobin concentration of 7 g/dL or less is a strong indication for transfusion
- transfusion is essential when the haemoglobin level decreases to 5 g/dL
- a haemoglobin concentration of 8 g/dL is safe even for patients with significant cardiorespiratory disease
- symptomatic patients should be transfused.

Similar guidelines have been issued by the Canadian Medical Association [17] and the American Society of Anesthesiologists [18], although the latter were not intended to apply to children.

Ultimately the decision to transfuse during surgery does not rest on the haemoglobin level alone, but is based on coexisting pathology, the likelihood of continued intraoperative and postoperative bleeding and on physiological parameters. Cyanotic congenital heart disease is seldom seen in adults and requires special consideration, as a haemoglobin level greater than 10 g/dL will usually be appropriate.

It has been suggested that in the developing world, where the risks of transfusion may be very high, a transfusion threshold of 5 g/dL may be appropriate provided that there is cardiovascular stability with a stable acid–base status [19]. Studies in healthy adult volunteers subjected to acute normovolaemic haemodilution show that this level of acute anaemia is well tolerated and it is reasonable to assume similar results would be obtained in healthy children [20].

Appropriate transfusion thresholds for the first 4 months of life are higher than for older children due to physiological differences between this age group and adults. Neonates and infants have higher oxygen consumption per kilogram and a higher cardiac output to blood volume ratio than adults. The neonatal myocardium operates at a near maximal level of performance, with increases in cardiac output being predominantly rate rather than stroke volume dependent. Normal haemoglobin values are significantly higher at birth and decrease gradually over the first few months of life to reach their lowest values at around 2–3 months of age. In addition, at birth foetal haemoglobin is the main haemoglobin and has a higher affinity for oxygen than adult haemoglobin. This results in decreased extraction of oxygen by the tissues. Foetal haemoglobin levels fall rapidly during the first few months of life with only trace amounts present by 6 months of age. In preterm infants, low haemoglobin levels are a risk factor for postoperative apnoea [21].

Suggested transfusion thresholds [4] for infants under 4 months of age are summarised in Table 24.5. These were not published with specific reference to surgical patients and were intended to form the basis of local protocols for neonatal units rather than as rigidly applied transfusion

Table 24.5 Transfusion thresholds for infants under 4 months of age [4]

Anaemia in first 24 hours	Haemoglobin 12 g/dL (Hct ≈0.36)
Neonates receiving intensive care	Haemoglobin 12 g/dL
Chronic oxygen dependency	Haemoglobin 11 g/dL
Late anaemia, stable patient	Haemoglobin 7 g/dL
Acute blood loss	10% blood volume

Table 24.6 Estimated blood volume (EBV) in children

Age	EBV (mL/kg)
Premature	90–100
Term neonate	80–90
Over 3 months	70
Very overweight	65

triggers. Acute surgical blood loss in excess of 10 per cent of the blood volume in a well neonate is not likely to require a red cell transfusion, provided that the haemoglobin concentration remains above 12 g/dL and the circulating volume is maintained.

To apply transfusion thresholds, it is useful to estimate the maximum allowable blood loss (MABL) [22]. This is calculated as follows:

$$MABL = EBV(Hct_0 - Hct_L)/Hct_0$$

where EBV is the estimated blood volume, Hct_0 is the starting haematocrit and Hct_L is the lowest acceptable haematocrit. (A haemoglobin level of 7 g/dL equates to a haematocrit of about 0.21.) The EBV is calculated from the body weight and depends on age (Table 24.6).

Blood losses should be measured where possible. Haemoglobin or haematocrit measurements using near-patient testing devices are helpful in determining the need for transfusion. Losses below the maximum allowable can be replaced with crystalloid or colloid. In the UK, red cells for intraoperative use are provided in optimal additive solution and have a haematocrit of about 0.55–0.60 [2]. In the absence of ongoing losses, about 4 mL/kg will be required to raise the haemoglobin level by 1 g/dL. In the presence of ongoing losses, in excess of the MABL, about 0.5–0.6 mL of red cells in optimal additive solution per millilitre of additional blood lost will be required to maintain a haematocrit around 0.30. In small children, transfusion to a normal haemoglobin level can often be achieved with transfusion from a single unit. In larger children, the need for further blood should be carefully considered after each unit to avoid unnecessary exposure to an additional donor for a small volume transfusion.

MASSIVE BLOOD TRANSFUSION

Massive blood loss is arbitrarily defined as the loss of one blood volume within a 24-hour period. An alternative definition, which may be more helpful in the surgical setting, is the loss of 50 per cent of the blood volume within 3 h. Guidelines on the management of massive blood loss, based on an appraisal of the literature and expert consensus, have recently been published by the British Committee for Standards in Haematology [23].

The main considerations during massive blood transfusions are:

- the maintenance of blood volume and haemoglobin concentration to ensure adequate tissue perfusion and oxygenation
- the use of blood components to correct coagulation defects
- the management of metabolic disturbances.

Good communication with the blood transfusion laboratory is important as blood components may take time to organise, particularly if there are special requirements.

Volume replacement should be guided by physiological variables, e.g. heart rate, blood pressure, central venous pressure, urine output, core and peripheral temperature difference, and acid–base status. Measured blood losses are of limited value in most circumstances. The selection of appropriate blood components should be guided by laboratory and near-patient testing data with haemoglobin or haematocrit levels, platelet counts and coagulation indices measured frequently. This is particularly important in small patients who require aliquots of blood products based on their weight rather than the use of whole packs of blood products. Table 24.7 summarises the goals of blood component therapy and gives the recommended quantities of blood components to be transfused in children based on published guidelines [4,23]. Blood products should be warmed to prevent hypothermia, which has deleterious effects on both oxygen delivery, due to displacement of the oxyhaemoglobin dissociation curve and coagulation [23].

Management of coagulation defects

Coagulation defects during massive transfusion are mainly the result of dilution of platelets and clotting factors. Studies in children suggest that the platelet count can be expected to fall to about 60 per cent of its starting value after the loss of one blood volume. Further falls to 40 per cent of the starting value will occur after the loss of two blood volumes, and to 30 per cent of the starting platelet count when three blood volumes have been lost. There is, however, considerable inter-patient variability [24]. It follows that patients who start with high platelet counts are less likely to need platelet transfusions than those who start at the lower end of the normal range; hence a baseline platelet count is useful for procedures where major blood loss is expected. In general, a platelet count of 50×10^9/L is adequate if no further bleeding is anticipated and platelet function is normal [25]. Guidelines suggest a platelet

Table 24.7 Blood component therapy for massive blood loss

Goal	Procedure
Maintain haemoglobin >8 g/dL	Red cell transfusion
	Group O rhesus-negative, group-specific or cross-matched blood depending on urgency
	Consider cell salvage
	Warm all fluids
Maintain platelet count	Anticipate platelet count $<50 \times 10^9$/L after two blood volumes
$>75 \times 10^9$/L*	Platelet transfusion
$>100 \times 10^9$/L for CNS or multiple trauma	Dose: weight <15 kg, 10–20 mL/kg; weight >15 kg, single apheresis unit/pool
Maintain PT, APTT	Anticipate PT and APPT >1.5 × control after 1–1.5 blood volumes
<1.5 × mean control	FFP transfusion
	Dose: 10–20 mL/kg
	Keep ionised Ca^{2+} >1.13 mmol/l
Maintain fibrinogen	If not corrected by FFP give cryoprecipitate
>1.0 g/L	Dose: weight <15 kg, 5 mL/kg; weight 15–30 kg, 5 units; weight >30 kg, 10 units

APTT, activated partial thromboplastin time; CNS, central nervous system; FFP, fresh frozen plasma; PT, prothrombin time.
*Allows a margin of safety to ensure platelets $>50 \times 10^9$/L.

transfusion trigger of 75×10^9/L to provide a margin of safety and a level of 100×10^9/L in patients with multiple trauma or central nervous system injuries [23]. Where platelet dysfunction is likely, such as after cardiopulmonary bypass or in chronic renal failure, empirical platelet transfusion may be required if microvascular bleeding is present.

Clinically important dilution of clotting factors should be anticipated with the loss of 1.5 blood volumes [23]. The level of fibrinogen falls to a critical level of 1.0 g/L first, followed by the fall of other labile clotting factors to critical levels after the loss of about two blood volumes. Coagulation should be monitored with serial measures of prothrombin time (PT), activated partial thromboplastin time (APTT) and plasma fibrinogen level. Activated prothrombin time and APPT greater than 1.5 times the normal for age and a fibrinogen level less than 1 g/L are correlated with an increased risk of bleeding [26] and generally require treatment. First-line treatment is with FFP, which, if given in sufficient quantities, will correct fibrinogen and most coagulation factor deficiencies. If the fibrinogen level remains below 1.0 g/L then cryoprecipitate, which provides fibrinogen in a more concentrated form, should be considered. However, this exposes the patient to multiple donors.

A further consideration in the UK is that FFP issued for use in children is imported to reduce the risk of vCJD but cryoprecipitate is not. Cryoprecipitate is no longer available in some parts of Europe, where virally inactivated fibrinogen concentrate is used instead.

Ideally, the use of platelets, FFP and cryoprecipitate should be guided by laboratory measurements. During rapid blood loss, it may be necessary to order blood products before the results of coagulation tests are available. It is reasonable to give FFP after one blood volume is lost if there is continued bleeding and the rapid turnaround of coagulation tests is not guaranteed. Suggested starting volumes are given in Table 24.7. Near-patient testing with the thromboelastograph (TEG) provides information about clot formation and lysis as well as a rapid means of assessing the effectiveness of interventions. The TEG has mainly been studied in cardiac surgical patients and its usefulness in the management of massive transfusion has not been established in adults or children.

Recombinant factor VIIa (rVIIa) is licensed for use in haemophiliacs with inhibitors to treat active bleeding or as prophylaxis for surgery. Recombinant factor VIIa promotes haemostasis at several locations within the clotting cascade. There are many reports of its off-licence use in the setting of massive blood transfusion, including case reports in children [22]. A systematic review has concluded that the use of rVIIa in patients with severe bleeding is promising and relatively safe (incidence of thrombotic complications, 1–2 per cent) [27]. The clinical use of rVIIa is likely to be limited as it is expensive with a short half-life such that multiple doses are required. Until good evidence from controlled trials is available, it is reasonable to consider the use of rVIIa in massive haemorrhage that cannot be surgically controlled, provided that there is no heparin or warfarin effect and there has been adequate replacement of clotting factors [2,23].

Metabolic complications

The metabolic consequences of transfusion are mainly an issue with large volume transfusions at rates that exceed 3 mL/kg/min for red cells and 1.5–2 mL/kg/min for FFP. The commonest problem is a reduced ionised calcium due to citrate toxicity [28] and this is most likely to be seen when large volumes of FFP are given, particularly in the presence of liver function abnormalities where citrate metabolism is slowed. Hypocalcaemia results in haemodynamic instability due to myocardial dysfunction and vasodilatation. The neonatal heart is particularly vulnerable. During massive transfusion, ionised calcium levels should be monitored using near-patient testing and hypocalcaemia should be treated with intravenous calcium. Calcium chloride rather than gluconate has been recommended on the basis that it is not dependent on liver metabolism [23]. Data in children suggest that, provided that equipotent doses of calcium chloride and gluconate are used, they are equally effective [29]. Appropriate treatment is 5–10 mg/kg calcium chloride or 15–30 mg/kg

calcium gluconate by slow intravenous injection, preferably via a central venous line. Calcium must not be allowed to mix with citrated blood products.

Hyperkalaemia may occur during massive transfusion due to the high extracellular potassium concentration in stored red cell products. Neonates and infants may experience cardiac arrest during large-volume transfusions, particularly if hypovolaemia is present [30,31]. The problem is more likely with irradiated and older blood. Treatment with calcium, bicarbonate and glucose with insulin may be required.

Hypomagnesaemia may occur with massive blood transfusions and, like hypocalcaemia, is a manifestation of citrate toxicity. Ventricular arrhythmias should suggest the diagnosis. Treatment is with intravenous magnesium sulphate (25–50 mg/kg, maximum dose 2 g).

Stored blood contains raised dissolved levels of carbon dioxide and elevated levels of lactic acid that can cause a transient combined respiratory and metabolic acidosis. Despite this, the development of metabolic acidosis during massive transfusion is more likely to be due to inadequate perfusion or underlying pathology such as sepsis.

AUTOLOGOUS BLOOD TRANSFUSION

Autologous transfusions are those where the blood to be transfused is obtained from the recipient either before or during the procedure. There are three approaches to autologous transfusion:

- preoperative autologous donation
- acute normovolaemic haemodilution
- autologous cell salvage.

Interest in autologous transfusion was at its greatest in the 1980s and 1990s, as a result of concern over transfusion-related HIV and HCV infections. These risks have been greatly reduced and, as a consequence, blood has become an increasingly expensive and limited resource. This, coupled with the emergence of vCJD, has led to renewed interest in autologous transfusion techniques. The literature regarding the effectiveness of the interventions is generally viewed as being of indifferent quality, largely due to inadequate randomisation and lack of blinding of outcome assessments [32,33]. All of the techniques have been described in children.

Preoperative autologous donation

Preoperative autologous donation (PAD) is the process whereby patients scheduled for major surgery donate their own blood for the procedure. If taken in sufficient time before the procedure, regeneration of red cells should occur. Multiple donations are made depending on the predicted transfusion requirements. Blood is processed and stored in the same manner as allogeneic donations.

The evidence base for PAD is small and mainly based on work in adults. A systematic review of PAD found that, although the probability of receiving allogeneic blood was reduced, the overall probability of receiving a transfusion (allogeneic or autologous) was increased [33,34]. This was mainly a consequence of lower preoperative haemoglobin levels in the PAD patients, as well as the tendency to transfuse autologous blood at higher haemoglobin levels. As patients receiving PAD blood are still exposed to the risks of bacterial contamination and errors resulting in the transfusion of the incorrect unit, it is recommended that the transfusion threshold for predonated blood should be the same as for allogeneic blood [17,35]. Preoperative autologous donation should be offered only when it is possible to guarantee the operative dates, as multiple donations are often required to achieve the desired volumes and the storage time is limited to 35 days as with allogeneic blood. Accurate prediction of losses is required to avoid too much or too little blood being collected [36].

The use of PAD has been reported in children as young as 3 months of age weighing less than 7 kg [37], although most of the paediatric studies have been in older children undergoing elective scoliosis surgery. The large and relatively predictable blood losses in this type of surgery, which is mainly undertaken in healthy older children, make it particularly suited to autologous blood techniques. As iron deficiency is common in children, supplemental iron with or without erythropoietin (EPO) has been used in most studies. Recent research suggests that the addition of EPO can improve the effectiveness of PAD in reducing allogeneic blood requirements in adolescents undergoing scoliosis surgery [38–40]. Unfortunately, EPO is expensive.

Most studies in children conclude that the donation procedure is well tolerated, although reactions including syncope have been reported [41]. Some programmes describe the replacement of the lost volume with saline, but this exposes the child to the risk of errors related to incorrect fluid administration. Practical problems with difficult venous access and a lack of cooperation or parental anxiety are recognised issues [41]. The use of deep sedation or general anaesthesia to facilitate donation in infants and toddlers has been reported [42] but is not an accepted practice and has been criticised on the grounds of risk and cost. Studies in adolescents undergoing scoliosis surgery have found high compliance rates, equal or superior to rates in adults [43].

The British Committee for Standards in Haematology (BCSH) has recently published a literature review and guidelines on PAD, including its use in children [35]. Scoliosis surgery is the only surgical procedure in children in which they recommend that PAD be considered. They do not recommend PAD for children under 10 years of age. The guidelines provide full details of the procedures required for the collection and testing of blood in order to comply with the UK Blood Safety Regulations 2005 and relevant European Commission Blood Directives [44]. There is greater enthusiasm for PAD in certain other countries, again mainly for children undergoing major orthopaedic surgery [45].

Directed donation (i.e. blood from a parent or close relative), though not autologous, is sometimes requested by families who may believe that it confers benefit over blood from volunteer donors. In countries that have good criteria for the selection of volunteer donors and use sophisticated tests to screen for viral infections, there is no evidence to support this view and it is possible that directed donation is less safe [46]. There are particular immunological issues with directed donations from close relatives. Blood from first- and second-degree relatives must be irradiated to avoid the risk of TA-GvHD due to close HLA matching. Maternal blood may have antibodies to paternally derived white cell HLA antigens and this may increase the risk of TRALI [11]. Neonates may have maternally derived antibodies to paternal red cell antigens that can result in delayed haemolytic reactions if they are transfused with paternal blood. Directed donation is strongly discouraged in the UK and the Blood Transfusion Service provides information to support discussions with families [2]. Compliance with UK legislation [44] means that, in practice, directed donations need to be collected by the National Blood Transfusion Service, and relatives who do not satisfy the criteria for volunteer donors are not accepted.

Acute normovolaemic haemodilution

Acute normovolaemic haemodilution (ANH) is a technique in which blood is removed from the patient shortly before the anticipated surgical loss and the circulating volume is maintained with crystalloid or colloid. The surgery then takes place while the patient is anaemic, thus minimising red cell losses. The collected blood, which is whole and contains clotting factors and platelets, is returned either when a transfusion trigger is reached or at the end of the procedure. The blood is transfused in reverse order of harvesting, i.e. the units with the highest haematocrit are returned last.

Acute normovolaemic haemodilution has been practised for over 30 years and it has been suggested, at least in adults, that it is an inexpensive and effective means of reducing exposure to allogeneic blood [18]. However, there remain questions as to the safety and efficacy of the procedure. There is a shortage of high-quality evidence from randomised controlled trials [47]. Interpretation is complicated by the fact that ANH has frequently been combined with other blood conservation strategies, including other autologous transfusion techniques. In addition, changes in transfusion practice, in particular the acceptance of lower transfusion triggers, combined with changes in surgical techniques, complicate the interpretation of much of the earlier work. A meta-analysis of ANH in adults demonstrated efficacy in terms of a reduction in the volume of blood transfused and in the likelihood of exposure to allogeneic blood [48]. However, the authors concluded, given the substantial and unexplained differences between studies, that the evidence to support the technique was inconclusive. A more recent meta-analysis concluded that the available evidence did not support a reduction in the risk of allogeneic blood transfusion in the perioperative period, while it showed a modest benefit in terms of the amount of blood transfused when compared with no blood conservation. The authors concluded that the literature supported only modest benefit, that the safety was unproven and that widespread adoption could not be encouraged [49].

Acute normovolaemic haemodilution offers practical advantages over PAD. It reduces collection costs and inconvenience to the patient, whilst the technique can be used in urgent as well as elective surgery. The blood is kept with the patient, and crossmatching and testing for viral agents are not required. There is minimal risk of significant bacterial contamination as the blood is not stored for prolonged periods. The risk of accidental administration of the wrong blood is virtually eliminated as ANH blood remains with the patient and is never stored in a blood bank, as this would pose an unacceptable risk to other patients.

Research suggests that the adaptation to acute anaemia during ANH depends on lowered blood viscosity and a reduced systemic vascular resistance, with increased cardiac output resulting in increased capillary blood flow and oxygen extraction [20,50]. The limits of safe haemodilution in children are discussed in a review by Woloszczuk-Gebicka, who concluded that, although children are quite resilient to haemodilution, haemoglobin levels below 6 g/dL cannot be recommended [51]. There are particular reservations about the technique in neonates and very young infants, as they have high baseline cardiac outputs and limited ability to increase their stroke volume, which is the usual adaptive mechanism in older children [52]. In addition, the high oxygen affinity of foetal haemoglobin limits oxygen extraction by the tissues in the neonate and young infant. Mathematical modelling and clinical studies show that ANH will be effective only if both blood loss and the difference between the baseline haematocrit and acceptable post-dilution haematocrit are large [48,53]. The lower haemoglobin levels of young children will therefore limit the effectiveness of ANH.

Most of the reports of ANH in children are in older children undergoing scoliosis surgery. There are a number of retrospective case–control studies demonstrating a reduction in the use of donated blood [54–56]. Acute normovolaemic haemodilution was combined with autologous donation and/or cell salvage in some studies and there have been significant changes in surgical and anaesthetic techniques since these studies were published. Concerns about spinal cord perfusion and the risk of cord damage have led to caution about extreme haemodilution in scoliosis surgery [22]. A small series of younger children down to 1 month of age having liver or tumour surgery has also been reported [57,58]. A prospective randomised trial of ANH in children having craniofacial surgery failed to demonstrate a reduction in the use of allogeneic blood [59].

If ANH is undertaken in small children, considerable attention to detail is required, as the practical problems are greater than in adults. Blood usually needs to be taken from an arterial or central venous line rather than a peripheral line. The amount of blood to be withdrawn to reach the target haematocrit needs to be carefully calculated. A target haematocrit of 0.30 has been suggested [51], although lower values have been used [59]. In small children it is necessary to adjust the amount of anticoagulant in the blood collection bag and to measure the amount of blood removed carefully, to ensure the correct blood to anticoagulant ratio.

Intraoperative cell salvage

Cell salvage involves the collection and retransfusion of autologous red cells lost during the intraoperative period. Blood losses are suctioned from the surgical field, anticoagulated and collected in a reservoir prior to processing. During processing, waste is separated from the red cells, which are then washed and suspended in saline ready to be returned to the patient. There are no clotting factors and no platelets in the returned blood. Like ANH, cell salvage requires minimal preoperative planning and does not inconvenience the patient. This technique has the further advantage that it can be rapidly set up in the event of unexpected massive haemorrhage. Effectiveness depends on the ability of the surgical team to collect blood and this is likely to depend on both the operation and the commitment of the surgeon to the technique. Cell salvage should not be used when the operating field is contaminated with bacteria, e.g. where there is bowel perforation or in operations where bowel may be opened. Malignancy used to be considered an absolute contraindication to cell salvage, although this is no longer the case in adult practice [60]. It is not known whether cell salvage is safe in children having tumour surgery and it cannot be recommended at present.

The evidence to support the use of cell salvage is limited, with all the larger studies being in adults. A Cochrane Review on the role of cell salvage in minimising perioperative allogeneic blood transfusion concluded that it appeared justified in orthopaedic surgery and probably in cardiac surgery [32]. Small non-randomised studies in children have reported cell salvage as being effective in avoiding transfusion in cerebral palsy patients undergoing major hip surgery [61] and in reducing, but not avoiding, the use of allogeneic blood in infants undergoing craniosynostosis surgery [62,63]. Research in children undergoing scoliosis surgery suggests that cell salvage may confer no additional benefit when combined with PAD or ANH [56,64].

The main problem with cell salvage in small children is that the absolute amount of blood collected is often insufficient to allow immediate processing with many of the available cell salvage devices because they have large collecting bowls. The studies in younger children have used devices with small collecting bowls (125–135 mL) or continuous autotransfusion systems (CATS) that require the collection of only 30 mL of shed blood to begin processing [65]. Small patients are at a disadvantage in terms of the cost-effectiveness of cell salvage, as this is related to the number of allogeneic units of blood saved.

OTHER APPROACHES TO REDUCING THE USE OF ALLOGENEIC BLOOD

Detection and treatment of preoperative iron deficiency

The lower the initial haemoglobin level, the greater the likelihood of transfusion during surgery. It therefore makes sense to diagnose and treat iron deficiency anaemia and optimise iron stores prior to elective surgery in which blood loss is anticipated. Iron deficiency anaemia is common in children, especially young children [66] and adolescent girls. Oral iron is the treatment of choice.

Preoperative erythropoietin

Human recombinant EPO has been used in the preoperative period to increase red cell mass as either a single modality or in combination with autologous transfusion to reduce exposure to allogeneic blood. In a non-randomised study of infants undergoing craniofacial surgery, 11 out of 30 patients in the EPO group avoided blood transfusion, but all the infants in the control group were transfused. The mean preoperative haematocrit in the EPO group was 0.43 compared with 0.34 in the control group [67]. As discussed above, EPO may be used to improve the effectiveness of PAD in scoliosis patients and its use in combination with ANH has also been described. A historical case–control study of preoperative EPO in combination with PAD in children aged 2–14 years undergoing cardiac surgery also showed a reduced need for allogeneic blood products [41]. There are reports of EPO being used in children who are Jehovah's Witnesses undergoing a variety of surgical procedures.

Erythropoietin is expensive and not currently licensed for routine preoperative use in children in the UK. Nor is it recommended for routine use in PAD [35]. A wide range of doses have been used, usually for about 3 weeks preoperatively. If EPO is used, consideration should be given to combining it with oral iron, as poor iron stores may limit its effectiveness.

Pharmacological approaches

A variety of pharmacological interventions have been used in an attempt to reduce blood loss and decrease or prevent the need for blood products in patients undergoing major surgery. A summary of the studies in children undergoing cardiac and non-cardiac surgery has been published by Guay et al. [68]. Aprotinin and tranexamic acid have a role in paediatric cardiac surgery (see Chapter 40). There is less evidence to support the use of aprotinin in other paediatric surgical patients. Conflicting results have been obtained in two small studies of scoliosis patients [69,70]and research in children undergoing liver transplantation demonstrated no benefit [71].

Two placebo-controlled studies of tranexamic acid in scoliosis surgery have failed to demonstrate a benefit in reducing allogeneic blood use. Neilipovitz et al. [72] used a dose of 10 mg/kg followed by an infusion of 1 mg/kg/h in combination with cell salvage and preoperative donation. There was no difference in intraoperative blood loss between the groups but there was a modest reduction in perioperative blood requirements in the tranexamic acid group. This did not translate to a reduction in the number of patients receiving allogeneic blood, possibly due to the low power of the study. In the second study, Sethna et al. [73] used high-dose tranexamic acid (100 mg/kg followed by 10 mg/kg/hour) in combination with cell salvage and modest hypotension. For patients with idiopathic scoliosis, there was no significant difference in blood loss or transfusion requirements between the treatment and placebo groups. For patients with secondary scoliosis there was a reduction in blood loss and blood transfusion requirements with tranexamic acid. The study groups were small and the placebo group contained more patients with Duchenne muscular dystrophy, which is known to be associated with particularly large blood losses. The authors acknowledged that a larger randomised controlled trial would be necessary to reach conclusive results about the benefits of tranexamic acid in scoliosis surgery. Desmopressin has also been studied; however, there are no data to support its use in the absence of platelet abnormalities.

The excellent results with rVIIa in haemophiliacs has led to interest in its use to improve haemostasis in high-risk surgical patients and a few studies have been undertaken in adults [74]. Even if the safety of this approach is confirmed, at the present time this drug is sufficiently expensive to preclude routine use as a means of avoiding exposure to a modest number of donated blood products.

Anaesthetic and surgical techniques

Deliberate hypotension has been used to reduce blood loss, mainly in scoliosis and major maxillofacial surgery. The popularity of deliberate hypotension has declined and techniques involving profound hypotension are no longer widely practised due to safety considerations. The role of blood pressure control in scoliosis surgery is discussed in Chapter 37. Surgeons can limit blood usage through meticulous attention to haemostasis and through the use of topical sealants where appropriate (e.g. topical fibrin glue).

REDUCING ALLOGENEIC BLOOD USE IN PRACTICE

The approaches to minimising transfusions with donated blood products have been described and are summarised in Table 24.8. In practice it is common to combine techniques in a multimodal approach. The simplest methods applicable to most elective patients are the treatment of preoperative iron deficiency anaemia and the acceptance of haemoglobin values below normal in the postoperative

Table 24.8 Approaches to reducing allogeneic blood use in surgical patients

Preoperative
Diagonosis and treatment of anaemia (oral iron)
Erythropoietin
Predeposit autologous donation

Intraoperative
Transfusion triggers and local policies
Surgical technique
Anaesthetic technique
Autologous blood
   Acute normovolaemic haemodilution
   Intraoperative cell salvage
Pharmacological approaches
   Aprotinin
   Tranexamic acid
   Recombinant factor VIIa

Postoperative
Reduce blood tests
Oral iron

period . The acceptable lowest haemoglobin level should be individualised; however, a level of 7 g/dL is adequate in most children aged over 4 months. Low transfusion thresholds are also applicable to most emergency patients.

There is limited evidence on which to base recommendations for the use of autologous transfusion techniques and pharmacological agents to reduce blood loss. The best studied groups of paediatric patients are those undergoing cardiac or scoliosis surgery. The management of cardiopulmonary bypass, including autologous transfusion, and the use of aprotinin and tranexamic acid in cardiac surgical patients are discussed in Chapter 40. There is evidence to support the use of autologous transfusion techniques for children undergoing scoliosis surgery. However, in practice the use of PAD, ANH and cell salvage even in this group of patients appears to be largely based on local availability, surgical preference and costs. There is no conclusive evidence to support the use of pharmacological agents in patients undergoing scoliosis surgery.

Case reports in Jehovah's Witnesses and a number of small studies have demonstrated that with a multimodal approach it is possible to eliminate the use of allogeneic blood even in small patients undergoing surgery with large blood losses. Combinations of preoperative iron and EPO, low transfusion thresholds and the use of PAD or ANH with cell salvage are described. Because small children are exposed to fewer donors per blood volume lost than adults, blood-conserving techniques in terms of both donor exposure and cost will be less beneficial. Given the current quality of allogeneic blood, it is not clear that some of the more extreme regimens described in small patients undergoing major surgery are justified. Erythropoietin is not licensed for routine preoperative use in children in the UK. There

are practical difficulties associated with PAD and ANH in small children and, if they are used, meticulous attention to detail is essential.

In the UK the only group of paediatric patients in whom it is recommended that PAD should be considered at present is children over 10 years of age having scoliosis surgery. There is limited evidence to support the use of cell salvage in small children, mainly from a study of patients undergoing craniofacial surgery. Newer cell salvage devices that permit processing of as little as 30 mL blood may result in cell salvage being more widely used in smaller children in the future.

REFERENCES

Key references

Barcelona SL, Thompson AA, Coté CJ. Intraoperative pediatric blood transfusion therapy: a review of common issues. Part I: hematologic and physiologic differences from adults; metabolic and infectious risks. *Paediatr Anaesth* 2005; **15**(9): 716–26.

British Committee for Standards in Haematology. Guidelines for policies on alternatives to allogeneic blood transfusion. 2007. Online: available via www.bcshguidelines.com.

Department of Health. *Handbook of transfusion medicine*, 4th edn. London: The Stationery Office, 2007.

Gibson BE, Todd A, Roberts I *et al.* Transfusion guidelines for neonates and older children. *Br J Haematol* 2004; **124**(4): 433–53.

Woloszczuk-Gebicka B. How to limit allogeneic blood transfusion in children. *Paediatr Anaesth* 2005; **15**(11): 913–24.

References

1. Gibson B, Stainsby D, Todd A *et al.* Serious hazards of transfusion in children – analysis of 7 years' data from SHOT. 2004. Online: available at www.shot-uk.org.
2. Department of Health. *Handbook of transfusion medicine*, 4th edn. London: The Stationery Office, 2007.
3. Joint UKBTS/NIBSC Professional Advisory Committee. Position Statement. Estimated frequency (or risk) of HIV, HCV or HBV infectious donations entering the UK blood supply. 2005. Online: available via www.transfusionguidelines.org.uk
4. Gibson BE, Todd A, Roberts I *et al.* Transfusion guidelines for neonates and older children. *Br J Haematol* 2004; **124**(4): 433–53.
5. Wroe SJ, Pal S, Siddique D, Hyare H *et al.* Clinical presentation and pre-mortem diagnosis of variant Creutzfeldt–Jakob disease associated with blood transfusion: a case report. *Lancet* 2006; **368**(9552): 2061–7.
6. Gregori L, Gurgel PV, Lathrop JT *et al.* Reduction in infectivity of endogenous transmissible spongiform encephalopathies present in blood by adsorption to selective affinity resins. *Lancet* 2006; **368**(9554): 2226–30.

7. The Serious Hazards of Transfusion Steering Group. Serious hazards of transfusion annual report 2005. 2006. Online: available at www.shot-uk.org

8. The Serious Hazards of Transfusion Steering Group. Serious hazards of transfusion annual report 2004. 2005. Online: available at www.shot-uk.org

9. Ramasethu J, Luban N. T activation. *Br J Haematol* 2001; **112**(2): 259–63.

10. Kleinman S, Caulfield T, Chan P *et al.* Toward an understanding of transfusion-related acute lung injury: statement of a consensus panel. *Transfusion* 2004; **44**(12): 1774–89.

11. Church GD, Price C, Sanchez R, Looney MR. Transfusion-related acute lung injury in the paediatric patient: two case reports and a review of the literature. *Transfus Med* 2006; **16**(5): 343–8.

12. Sandler SG, Mallory D, Malamut D, Eckrich R. IgA anaphylactic transfusion reactions. *Transfus Med Rev* 1995; **9**(1): 1–8.

13. Landers DF, Hill GE, Wong KC, Fox IJ. Blood transfusion-induced immunomodulation. *Anesth Analg* 1996; **82**(1): 187–204.

14. Hill SR, Carless PA, Henry DA *et al.* Transfusion thresholds and other strategies for guiding allogeneic red blood cell transfusion (Review). *Cochrane Database of Syst Rev* 2000; (1): CD002042.

15. Hume HA, Limoges P. Perioperative blood transfusion therapy in pediatric patients. *Am J Ther* 2002; **9**(5): 396–405.

16. Association of Anaesthetists of Great Britain and Ireland. *Blood transfusion and the anaesthetist – red cell transfusion.* London: AAGBI, 2001.

17. Expert Working Group. Guidelines for red blood cell and plasma transfusion for adults and children. *Can Med Assoc J* 1997; **156**(11 suppl): 1–24.

18. American Society of Anesthesiologists Task Force on Blood Component Therapy. Practice Guidelines for blood component therapy. *Anesthesiology* 1996; **84**(3): 732–47.

19. Barcelona SL, Thompson AA, Coté CJ. Intraoperative pediatric blood transfusion therapy: a review of common issues. Part I: hematologic and physiologic differences from adults; metabolic and infectious risks. *Paediatr Anaesth* 2005; **15**(9): 716–26.

20. Weiskopf RB, Viele MK, Feiner J *et al.* Human cardiovascular and metabolic response to acute, severe isovolemic anemia. *J Am Med Assoc* 1998; **279**(3): 217–21.

21. Coté CJ, Zaslavsky A, Downes JJ *et al.* Postoperative apnea in former preterm infants after inguinal herniorrhaphy. A combined analysis. *Anesthesiology* 1995; **82**(4): 809–22.

22. Barcelona SL, Thompson AA, Coté CJ. Intraoperative pediatric blood transfusion therapy: a review of common issues. Part II: transfusion therapy, special considerations, and reduction of allogenic blood transfusions. *Paediatr Anaesth* 2005; **15**(10): 814–30.

23. Stainsby D, MacLennan S, Thomas D *et al.* British Committee for Standards in Haematology: guidelines on the management of massive blood loss. *Br J Haematol* 2006; **135**(5): 634–41.

24. Coté CJ, Liu LM, Szyfelbein SK *et al.* Changes in serial platelet counts following massive blood transfusion in pediatric patients. *Anesthesiology* 1985; **62**(2): 197–201.

25. Contreras M. Consensus conference on platelet transfusion. Final statement. *Blood Rev* 1998; **12**(4): 239–40.

26. Ciavarella D, Reed RL, Counts RB *et al.* Clotting factor levels and the risk of diffuse microvascular bleeding in the massively transfused patient. *Br J Haematol* 1987; **67**(3): 365–8.

27. Levi M, Peters M, Buller HR. Efficacy and safety of recombinant factor VIIa for treatment of severe bleeding: a systematic review. *Crit Care Med* 2005; **33**(4): 883–90.

28. Dzik WH, Kirkley SA. Citrate toxicity during massive blood transfusion. *Transfus Med Rev* 1988; **2**(2): 76–94.

29. Coté CJ, Drop LJ, Daniels AL, Hoaglin DC. Calcium chloride versus calcium gluconate: comparison of ionization and cardiovascular effects in children and dogs. *Anesthesiology* 1987; **66**(4): 465–70.

30. Buntain SG, Pabari M. Massive transfusion and hyperkalaemic cardiac arrest in craniofacial surgery in a child. *Anaesth Intens Care* 1999; **27**(5): 530–3.

31. Brown KA, Bissonnette B, McIntyre B. Hyperkalaemia during rapid blood transfusion and hypovolaemic cardiac arrest in children. *Can J Anaesth* 1990; **37**(7): 747–54.

32. Carless PA, Henry DA, Moxey AJ *et al.* Cell salvage for minimising perioperative allogeneic blood transfusion. *Cochrane Database Sys Rev* 2006; (4): CD001888.

33. Department of Health. Better blood transfusion: appropriate use of blood. *Health Service Circular 2002/009.* 2002. London: Department of Health.

34. Henry DA, Carless PA, Moxey AJ *et al.* Pre-operative autologous donation for minimising allogeneic blood transfusion (review). *Cochrane Database Sys Rev* 2001; (4): CD003602.

35. British Committee for Standards in Haematology. Guidelines for policies on alternatives to allogeneic blood transfusion. 2007. Online: available via www.bcshguidelines.com.

36. Bess RS, Lenke LG, Bridwell KH *et al.* Wasting of preoperatively donated autologous blood in the surgical treatment of adolescent idiopathic scoliosis. *Spine* 2006; **31**(20): 2375–80.

37. Thompson HW, Luban NL. Autologous blood transfusion in the pediatric patient. *J Pediatr Surg* 1995; **30**(10): 1406–11.

38. Franchini M, Gandini G, Regis D *et al.* Recombinant human erythropoietin facilitates autologous blood collections in children undergoing corrective spinal surgery. *Transfusion* 2004; **44**(7): 1122–4.

39. Garcia-Erce JA, Munoz M, Bisbe E *et al.* Predeposit autologous donation in spinal surgery: a multicentre study. *Eur Spine J* 2004; **13**(suppl 1): S34–39.

40. Garcia-Erce JA, Solano VM, Saez M, Muoz M. Recombinant human erythropoietin facilitates autologous blood donation in children undergoing corrective spinal surgery. *Transfusion* 2005; **45**(5): 820–1.

41. Sonzogni V, Crupi G, Poma R *et al.* Erythropoietin therapy and preoperative autologous blood donation in children undergoing open heart surgery. *Br J Anaesth* 2001; **87**(3): 429–34.

42. Velardi F, Di Chirico A, Di Rocco C *et al.* 'No allogeneic blood transfusion' protocol for the surgical correction of craniosynostoses. II. Clinical application. *Child Nerv Sys* 1998 Dec; **14**(12): 732–9.

43. Murray DJ, Forbes RB, Titone MB, Weinstein SL. Transfusion management in pediatric and adolescent scoliosis surgery. Efficacy of autologous blood. *Spine* 1997; **22**(23): 2735–40.

44. Office of Public Sector Information. *The blood safety and quality regulations.* London: HMSO, 2005.

45. Letts M, Perng R, Luke B *et al.* An analysis of a preoperative pediatric autologous blood donation program. *Can J Surg* 2000; **43**(2): 125–9.

46. Wales PW, Lau W, Kim PC. Directed blood donation in pediatric general surgery: is it worth it? *J Pediatr Surg* 2001; **36**(5): 722–5.

47. Shander A, Perelman S. The long and winding road of acute normovolemic hemodilution. *Transfusion* 2006; **46**(7): 1075–9.

48. Bryson GL, Laupacis A, Wells GA. Does acute normovolemic hemodilution reduce perioperative allogeneic transfusion? A meta-analysis. The International Study of Perioperative Transfusion. *Anesth Analg* 1998; **86**(1): 9–15.

49. Segal JB, Blasco-Colmenares E, Norris EJ, Guallar E. Preoperative acute normovolemic hemodilution: a meta-analysis. *Transfusion* 2004; **44**(5): 632–44.

50. van IM, van der Waart FJ, Erdmann W, Trouwborst A. Systemic haemodynamics and oxygenation during haemodilution in children. *Lancet* 1995; **346**(8983): 1127–9.

51. Woloszczuk-Gebicka B. How to limit allogeneic blood transfusion in children. *Paediatr Anaesth* 2005; **15**(11): 913–24.

52. Weldon BC. Blood conservation in pediatric anesthesia. *Anesthesiol Clin North Am* 2005; **23**(2): 347–61.

53. Weiskopf RB. Efficacy of acute normovolemic hemodilution assessed as a function of fraction of blood volume lost. *Anesthesiology* 2001; **94**(3): 439–46.

54. Du TG, Relton JE, Gillespie R. Acute haemodilutional autotransfusion in the surgical management of scoliosis. *J Bone Joint Surg [Br]* 1978; **60**(2): 178–80.

55. Olsfanger D, Jedeikin R, Metser U *et al.* Acute normovolaemic haemodilution and idiopathic scoliosis surgery: effects on homologous blood requirements. *Anaesth Intens Care* 1993; **21**(4): 429–31.

56. Copley LA, Richards BS, Safavi FZ, Newton PO. Hemodilution as a method to reduce transfusion requirements in adolescent spine fusion surgery. *Spine* 223; **24**(3): 219–22.

57. Schaller RT, Jr, Schaller J, Furman EB. The advantages of hemodilution anesthesia for major liver resection in children. *J Pediatr Surg* 1984; **19**(6): 705–10.

58. Adzick NS, deLorimier AA, Harrison MR *et al.* Major childhood tumor resection using normovolemic hemodilution anesthesia and hetastarch. *J Pediatr Surg* 1985; **20**(4): 372–5.

59. Hans P, Collin V, Bonhomme V *et al.* Evaluation of acute normovolemic hemodilution for surgical repair of craniosynostosis. *J Neurosurg Anesthesiol* 2000; **12**(1): 33–6.

60. Thomas MJ. Infected and malignant fields are an absolute contraindication to intraoperative cell salvage: fact or fiction? *Transfus Med* 1999; **9**(3): 269–78.

61. Nicolai P, Leggetter PP, Glithero PR, Bhimarasetty CR. Autologous transfusion in acetabuloplasty in children. *J Bone Joint Surg [Br]* 2004; **86**(1): 110–2.

62. Fearon JA. Reducing allogenic blood transfusions during pediatric cranial vault surgical procedures: a prospective analysis of blood recycling. *Plast Reconstr Surg* 2004; **113**(4): 1126–30.

63. Jimenez DF, Barone CM. Intraoperative autologous blood transfusion in the surgical correction of craniosynostosis. *Neurosurgery* 1995; **37**(6): 1075–9.

64. Siller TA, Dickson JH, Erwin WD. Efficacy and cost considerations of intraoperative autologous transfusion in spinal fusion for idiopathic scoliosis with predeposited blood. *Spine* 1996; **21**(7): 848–52.

65. Deva AK, Hopper RA, Landecker A *et al.* The use of intraoperative autotransfusion during cranial vault remodeling for craniosynostosis. *Plast Reconstr Surg* 2002; **109**(1): 58–63.

66. Sherriff A, Emond A, Bell JC, Golding J, ALSPAC Study Team. Should infants be screened for anaemia? A prospective study investigating the relation between haemoglobin at 8, 12, and 18 months and development at 18 months. *Arch Dis Child* 2001; **84**(6): 480–5.

67. Helfaer MA, Carson BS, James CS *et al.* Increased hematocrit and decreased transfusion requirements in children given erythropoietin before undergoing craniofacial surgery. *J Neurosurg* 1998; **88**(4): 704–8.

68. Guay J, de Moerloose P, Lasne D. Minimizing perioperative blood loss and transfusions in children. *Can J Anaesth* 2006; **53**(6 suppl): 67.

69. Cole JW, Murray DJ, Snider RJ *et al.* Aprotinin reduces blood loss during spinal surgery in children. *Spine* 2003; **28**(21): 2482–5.

70. Khoshhal K, Mukhtar I, Clark P *et al.* Efficacy of aprotinin in reducing blood loss in spinal fusion for idiopathic scoliosis. *J Pediatr Orthoped* 2003; **23**(5): 661–4.

71. Rentoul TM, Harrison VL, Shun A. The effect of aprotinin on transfusion requirements in pediatric orthotopic liver transplantation. *Pediatr Transpl* 2003; **7**(2): 142–8.

72. Neilipovitz DT, Murto K, Hall L *et al.* A randomized trial of tranexamic acid to reduce blood transfusion for scoliosis surgery. *Anesth Analg* 2001; **93**(1): 82–7.

73. Sethna NF, Zurakowski D, Brustowicz RM *et al.* Tranexamic acid reduces intraoperative blood loss in pediatric patients undergoing scoliosis surgery. *Anesthesiology* 2005; **102**(4): 727–32.

74. Friederich PW, Henny CP, Messelink EJ *et al.* Effect of recombinant activated factor VII on perioperative blood loss in patients undergoing retropubic prostatectomy: a double-blind placebo-controlled randomised trial. *Lancet* 2003; **361**(9353): 201–5.

25

Management of the uncooperative frightened child

PHILIP M D CUNNINGTON

KEY LEARNING POINTS

- Preoperative anxiety is common, yet a minority of children are difficult to manage at induction.
- The anaesthesia team must know how to manage an uncooperative frightened child.
- The emphasis of management should be prevention.

- Uncooperative children need a perioperative plan and care by a multidisciplinary team.
- Postoperative negative behaviour is common and is related to distress – it is usually mild and transient, but can be prolonged.

INTRODUCTION

Few children are uncooperative unless they are frightened, distressed or psychologically disturbed. In paediatric anaesthesia, two troublesome behavioural scenarios are common and are associated with each other. First, managing an uncooperative frightened child at induction has always been distressing and tests the social and practical skills of the anaesthesia team. Second, more recently, delayed troublesome postoperative behaviour has been recognised as a problem that is related to distress during induction. It can persist for weeks or longer and sometimes, fortunately rarely, there are more prolonged or permanent psychological effects. Within the last 15 years, much work has helped to assess these problems, to identify children at special risk and to investigate potentially beneficial interventions. The management of uncooperative children should focus on prevention. This chapter explains the extent of behavioural problems related to anaesthesia, how to prevent them and how to manage uncooperative behaviour at induction of anaesthesia.

BEHAVIOURAL EFFECTS OF ANAESTHESIA AND SURGERY

The concept of anaesthesia and surgery causing distress and harmful psychological side-effects is not new, yet despite significant advances in the safety and quality of anaesthesia there has not, until recently, been comparable attention paid to reducing distress [1]. Unfamiliar surroundings, strange smells and noises, and separation from their parents may provoke a range of emotions in children that are expressed differently depending upon age, coping skills and previous experience. In the 1950s it was appreciated that distress was most common in children under 3 years old [2,3]. Since then hospital practice has changed enormously. Now, most operations are day-care procedures in child-friendly environments and with minimal parent–child separation. However, studies in the 1990s found that children were still distressed by their hospital experience: 65–88 per cent of children had delayed negative behavioural effects the day after surgery [4]. In one study of 551 children, 47 per cent were distressed on the day of minor day surgery and 9 per cent still had behavioural changes 4 weeks later [5]. Another study found that the incidence of negative or maladaptive postoperative behavioural changes (including general anxiety, night-time crying, enuresis, separation anxiety and temper tantrums) occurred in up to 53 per cent of children 2 weeks following surgery, reducing to 20 per cent 6 months later [6]. The strongest associated factor was preoperative anxiety [6], which may also be associated with postoperative delirium [7,8].

Sleep can also be disturbed. In a study of 192 children having outpatient surgery, 47 per cent had sleep disturbances, although this could have been due to pain [9]. By far the commonest behavioural problem seems to be separation anxiety, but only a very few develop serious long-term psychological problems or post-traumatic stress disorder (PTSD) (10). Nevertheless, negative memories of past anaesthetic experiences can persist into adult life [11].

Human behaviour is complex. Expression of perioperative anxiety can be verbal or behavioural, subtle or extreme. Yet some negative behaviours may sometimes be beneficial because they may serve to limit a child's helplessness and retain a sense of control [4] – they help the child to adapt to the new situations. If so, blocking behavioural change with sedation may interfere with an adaptive response. Furthermore, not all behavioural changes are negative [10]. Positive changes, observed after tonsillectomy, can include improved sleep, increased activity, decreased fear and decreased temper tantrums. These may be because of reduced pain and symptoms from upper airway obstruction.

Physiological effects of anxiety

In adults, associations have been found among preoperative anxiety, postoperative pain, analgesic requirements and prolonged hospital stay. The stress response to surgery may cause a negative nitrogen balance, delayed wound healing and immunosuppression. Children may be more vulnerable because of limited energy reserves and high energy requirements, and therefore reducing extreme anxiety may be helpful [12]. There is evidence to suggest that preoperative anxiety may increase anaesthetic requirements in adults but this has not been investigated in children. Inhalational inductions are more difficult in crying children, not only because the child avoids breathing the vapour but also because crying can cause nasal obstruction and hyperventilation which can exacerbate any airway obstruction. Increasing the inspired concentration of vapour may be necessary, but care must be taken to reduce it as soon as possible when the child is asleep so as to avoid unexpected cardiovascular depression.

Age-related behaviour and anxiety

By understanding how children develop and respond to stress, we may be better able to communicate with them and develop age-appropriate interventions. Behaviour development is described in detail in Chapter 1 but a brief overview follows here. Anxiety-related behaviours in the perioperative period are age dependent. Crying is common in toddlers, but older children may be mute and look frightened (tachypnoea, tachycardia and pallor) and in extreme cases may become combative.

LESS THAN 6 MONTHS

Young infants accept parental surrogates readily so that separation anxiety does not appear until around 5 or 6 months of age. They are usually calmed by holding, rocking and a gentle voice.

6 MONTHS TO 3 YEARS

During this period, children start to become attached to their caregivers and are less willing to be separated from them. They are too young to understand explanations but are comforted by soothing interventions and distraction from their parents. This is the age where premedication may start to become helpful.

3–6 YEARS

At this age, children begin to accept separation and understand simple brief explanations and reassurance about their body integrity. Giving an explanation may be more important than the content. Explanations should be 'concrete', i.e. where, when and how, and should contain sens-ory information such as noise, taste, smell and feel. Play therapy is useful at this age.

7–12 YEARS

These children need peer acceptance and enjoy being rewarded for their achievements. They are also aware of parental control over their health. The most successful interventions enhance feelings of control and include distraction (only if accepted by the child), positive self-talk and rewards. Play, story books, photographs and videos can all be useful. More sophisticated and intensive coping strategies, such as relaxation, guided imagery and desensitisation, help to combat anticipatory anxiety.

ADOLESCENCE

This stage is complex. An adolescent can behave like a child trapped in an adult body. Increased personal identity, the need for privacy, greater body awareness and independence must all be respected, as must the fear of losing control or loss of face. They may have adult coping mechanisms but can also be afraid of awareness, pain, not waking up and death. Interventions need to increase their self-control so that they learn coping skills and participate in decisions.

Table 25.1   Summary of the main observational scales and questionnaires used to measure perioperative anxiety, distress and behavioural problems

Scale	Purpose	Details	Characteristics and limitations
Modified Yale Preoperative Anxiety Scale (M-YPAS) [17]	Assesses distress in the preoperative holding area	Observations of: – activity – vocalisation – emotional expression – arousal – parental dependence	For children >2 years of age Takes a minute to complete Applicable to rapidly changing states
Induction compliance checklist [18]	Assesses cooperation at induction	Observations of 10 behaviour items	1–9 years of age
State–Trait Anxiety Inventory (STAI) [19]	Standard assessment of anxiety	Self-report questionnaire of 20 items. Includes subscales for: – trait (baseline) – state (situational) anxiety	Takes 5–10 minutes; not useful in young children or in rapidly changing situations
EASI scale child temperament [20]		Observations on: – emotionality – activity – sociability – impulsivity	
Monitor Blunter Style Scale (MBSS) [21]	Assesses coping style of children in stressful scenarios	Observations on: – information-seeking or avoiding (high and low monitors) – distractors or non-distractors (high and low blunters)	
Post-Hospital Behavioural Questionnaire (PHBQ) [22]	Assesses child's behaviour at home after surgery	Questionnaire for parents to assess: – general anxiety – separation anxiety – sleep disorders – eating problems – aggression – apathy	Observations on their children may be biased

ABNORMAL BEHAVIOUR

Many children presenting for anaesthesia and surgery have abnormal behaviour associated with neurodisability, behavioural disorders, autism and mental health problems, and they present a huge challenge.

PREVENTION OF ANXIETY AND RELATED BEHAVIOURAL PROBLEMS

Assessment

Prediction of children's behaviour is notoriously difficult [13]. The preoperative visit may help to determine the factors associated with anxiety but there is a wide variation in character and situations [14–16]. Various observational scales have been used to assess anxiety, temperament and

coping styles, and these are summarised in Table 25.1. Self-report questionnaires are obviously not appropriate for small children and some other scales are not flexible or quick enough to detect changes in the perioperative period. Early assessment of children may be able to direct anxious children (and parents) to behavioural therapy or anxiolytic premedication (or both) – certainly many children do not need these interventions, which can be time-consuming. The following are important risk factors of uncooperative behaviour and delayed effects of perioperative distress.

CHILDREN THEMSELVES

Children aged between 1 and 5 years are at greatest risk of developing perioperative anxiety. Separation anxiety peaks at 1 year and those over 5 years are better equipped to deal with unpredictable situations [4]. Poor social adaptive capability (shy and inhibited temperament) is an independent predictor of perioperative anxiety [23]. Previous bad experiences with medical services, such as vaccinations, predict perioperative anxiety. Parental prediction of cooperation may also be valuable.

PARENTS

Parents can both reduce and increase stress in their children by their own behaviour [24]. Maternal anxiety has been associated with increased postoperative behavioural problems [25]. Parental anxiety is highest when the mother is more anxious than the father, if the child is an infant, if there are repeated admissions and if the child is anxious [26,27]. Parents who use avoidance coping mechanisms or who have relationship problems tend to be more anxious. Delayed behavioural problems may be more common in children who do not have siblings and if their parents decline day-case surgery [28,29].

THE PROCEDURE

The type of surgery is also important. Genitourinary surgery is associated with the highest incidence of postoperative behavioural problems, whilst minor ear, nose and throat surgery is associated with the lowest incidence [6]. However, a meta-analysis found that surgical type did not affect the incidence of postoperative behavioural problems [30]. Interestingly, an overnight hospital stay does not increase the overall incidence of postoperative behavioural disturbances compared with day surgery [31]. A painful intravenous (IV) induction may cause more distress than an inhalational method at the time, but there is no significant increase in postoperative behavioural problems [32]. Although sevoflurane induction may be tolerated better than halothane, there may be no difference in the incidence of emergence delirium, postoperative behaviour or sleep disturbances [33].

Non-pharmacological interventions

PREOPERATIVE PREPARATION PROGRAMMES

Preoperative preparation programmes (PPPs) are well known to reduce anxiety. A meta-analysis of 27 publications showed that children who had undergone preoperative behavioural interventions had less negative behavioural outcomes [34]. However, PPPs are costly and may be necessary only in selected children. They may not be beneficial in children under 3 years old and may cause distress in previously hospitalised children or in those who are unusually anxious (high EASI [Emotionality, Activity, Sociability and Impulsivity Scale of child temperament] scores) [35]. Frightened children may benefit from a more intensive and individual programme of desensitisation, learning coping skills and reassurance through practice. Children over 6 years have been found to gain greatest benefit if they visit more than 5

days before surgery; surprisingly, the effect of visiting 1 day beforehand can be worse than not visiting at all, probably because children need time to process the information, adapt and develop coping skills [35]. Parents also benefit and even a simple video presentation can help [36].

Three types of programme interventions have been compared: a tour of the operating room, a videotape and practising coping skills. At anaesthesia 2 weeks later, practising coping skills achieved a reduction in anxiety in children and parents at the time of separation, but children's behaviour at induction was similar in all three groups. They also found that children who asked more questions seemed to benefit from extra information and that, in contrast, children who were quiet did not want information but could be helped by distraction.

The type of information needs to be considered. Sensory (visual, olfactory and tactile) elements sometimes are more important than facts [37,38].

THE PREOPERATIVE VISIT

The preoperative visit is fundamental to planning an anaesthetic. The process should be a tridirectional exchange of information among the anaesthetist, the child and the parents. It is well known that preoperative visits can reduce anxiety and that an interview should take place in a non-threatening, child-friendly environment where there are books to help give information and toys to provide distraction. In 1994, McGraw [1] suggested that both the content and non-verbal aspects of communication with children are valuable and he suggested the following rules:

- Do not be condescending.
- Do not convey the notion that their feelings are 'childish'.
- Do not laugh unless you are quite sure they intend it to be humorous.
- Squatting or kneeling may present a less imposing image.
- Discuss their care in terms that they can understand.

Informed consent requires discussion of risk but how much information is necessary or appropriate is often difficult to judge. Both excess and inadequate discussion of risks can cause anxiety in adults. In a study of children scheduled for surgery more than 95 per cent of their parents preferred detailed information and they were not made more anxious [39]. Nevertheless there is a balance between informing all patients about all risks and being able to consider appropriate and individual needs. Pre-assessment clinics are ideal places to exchange information by discussion or by other means; however, there are practical limitations because the timing of the meeting is important.

PARENTAL PRESENCE AT INDUCTION

Parental presence at induction (PPAI) has the potential to reduce separation anxiety but it has been controversial [40].

Although early studies found that parents helped to reduce their children's anxiety, a more recent study found no appreciable difference [25]. However, the conditions of induction were different in these studies and some of the observational tools used were not tested for validity and reliability. In a study using the M-YPAS scale, parental presence had little effect except in children over 4 years whose parents were not anxious [29].

In the UK it is routine to allow PPAI [41,42], perhaps because anaesthesia is usually induced in dedicated rooms, unlike in the USA where operating theatres are used instead. In the USA, most anaesthetists believe that parental presence is beneficial but few parents are allowed in the operating theatre [43]. In France, parental presence at induction is unusual. Opinions obviously vary due to cultural factors not only between nations but also between hospitals and professions.

Midazolam premedication may be more effective than PPAI in calming children and in achieving their compliance – and also in reducing anxiety in their parents [18]. In a further study, the combination of PPAI and midazolam had no advantage over midazolam without PPAI except that parents were calmer if they were present [24]. Parental presence at emergence may have no appreciable effect on either the incidence or severity of emergence distress in their children [44].

Some parents are distressed by witnessing their child going limp at induction and then having to accept separation. Nevertheless, despite their anxiety they feel duty bound to be present and believe that they can help [45]. Interestingly only a minority of parents who bring their children back for subsequent anaesthesia choose midazolam sedation for them [46]. Other potential disadvantages of PPAI include unpredictable or dangerous parental behaviour, the need for them to be accompanied by a staff member, and distraction or additional stress for the anaesthetist. There is also either the need for a separate induction room or the potential loss of sterility in theatre.

PLAY THERAPY

Play services help children not only by giving pleasure but also by enabling them to explore, interact and learn. Children can be prepared for specific procedures by using models, books and other visual aids [13,47]. These not only calm children but allow the transfer of information, and the development of coping strategies and trusting relationships with staff. At least one study showed that children who had play preparation before induction remained calmer and were more cooperative [48]. Preparation with play is especially useful for children having repeated distressing procedures. The timing is also important and preparation is more effective if it is started before the day of admission [47].

HYPNOSIS

Hypnosis can be defined as a pleasant natural calm state of altered consciousness or trance. The trance is induced by focusing the patient's attention on something and then, by a process of suggestion, they become calm and sleepy; it can be achieved only with good communication and cooperation. There are a few important differences in hypnotherapy techniques between children and adults. The most important is ensuring that the language and images are appropriate to the developmental level of the child. Many therapists find that children are more ready than adults to accept the process of suggestion and dissociation. Children under 4 years tend not to be suitable but they may be calmed by storytelling and suggestion by metaphors from fairytales. Above about 7 years of age, children usually have sufficient attention span to be able to listen to a story to enable a more formal induction of a hypnotic state. They may comply with arm levitation or eye fixation. In adolescents, inducing hypnosis is similar to that in adults, but they are anxious about loss of control and this can cause them to 'break out' of their trance.

Many anaesthetists use distraction or fantasy stories similar to hypnosis to calm children. 'Imagine you are an astronaut breathing special air' is a good example of a script. There have been several reports of hypnosis being used to improve trust and coping in children [49,50] and also to reduce postoperative analgesia requirements [51].

A recent study evaluated hypnosis [52] in which children (age 2–12 years) were randomised to receive either hypnosis (with placebo) or midazolam. There were fewer anxious children in the hypnosis group during induction (39 vs 68 per cent) and hypnosis reduced the frequency of postoperative behaviour disorders by approximately half on day 1 (30 vs 62 per cent) and day seven (26 vs 59 per cent). The hypnotic technique by the anaesthetist took 30 minutes. It is possible that hypnosis was not the true cause of better behaviour but rather simple pleasant attention and rapport.

ACUPUNCTURE

Children are unlikely to accept acupuncture but applying it to parents can help. In a randomised study, mothers who had acupuncture were calmer at induction of anaesthesia for their child than those who had sham acupuncture, and their children were significantly more compliant [53].

MUSIC

Bright lights, loud noises and unfamiliar people can increase a child's anxiety. In a randomised study, children submitted to dimmed lights, soft music (Bach) and one anaesthetist, rather than the standard operating theatre environment, were significantly calmer [54]. In a further study, children were randomised to placebo, oral midazolam or interactive music therapy [55]. Music was no better than oral placebo at reducing anxiety, and midazolam was the most effective. However, one of the music therapists had a greater calming effect than her colleagues, which suggests that many factors are important in behaviour modification.

Personal stereos can be useful both on the journey to theatre and during induction (author's personal observations).

PSYCHOLOGISTS

For many children, anxiety associated with anaesthesia or a procedure is transient and has no long-term sequelae. However, some children, especially those requiring multiple painful procedures, suffer considerable anticipatory anxiety and distress, and are at risk of developing long-term behavioural problems. These children and their parents may need help from a psychologist. The psychologist can explore their understanding of the problem and their worries. Special techniques include:

- relaxation – this includes progressive muscle relaxation and the use of directed fantasy stories; the child chooses the pace of the therapy
- distraction – this may be by parents, staff and the use of dolls, music or stories
- desensitisation – this involves graded exposure to the feared procedure/object and again the child remains in control; the aim is to achieve a lower state of physiological arousal with the feared procedure/object and a progressive diminution of the fear
- modelling – information is provided to develop coping strategies.

Pharmacological interventions

It is generally assumed that sedative premedication reduces perioperative anxiety, in particular that it facilitates separation from parents, and that it reduces negative behavioural outcomes. However, sedation has two potentially separate effects: reducing conscious level and modifying behaviour. Midazolam, triclofos and opioids have been shown to calm children without necessarily altering conscious level [56,57]. The commonest used is midazolam [43]. The following is a brief overview of the alternative drugs used for calming or sedating children.

MIDAZOLAM

Midazolam, a short-acting benzodiazepine, produces reliable dose-dependent anxiolysis 10–15 minutes after an oral dose. It has an elimination half-life of 1.5–2 hours and produces minimal cardiovascular and respiratory effects. It can be administered via other routes. Intranasal midazolam produces a rapid response but is unpleasant because it causes a burning sensation, whereas the sublingual route is more acceptable and is equally effective in about 20 minutes [58]. It can be sprayed into the nose via an atomiser attachment to a syringe (much less uncomfortable than drops) and requires less cooperation than oral administration [59]. Rectal and intramuscular midazolam are rarely necessary. The optimum dose of oral midazolam has been found to be 0.5 mg/kg, with higher doses producing blurred vision, ataxia, disinhibition and dysphoria [60]. The timing of premedication is important and, because of practical difficulties, this may lead its omission. It causes maximal effects at 30–45 minutes yet can cause significant anterograde amnesia as early as 10 minutes after administration and anxiolysis by 15 minutes [61] and this should encourage its use in many situations. The disadvantage of its bitter taste may be overcome by the use of a suitable sweetening agent. The delay in recovery and discharge times are of minor clinical significance and have not been reproduced by every study. Midazolam may not always be beneficial – one study found that it was associated with more delayed negative behaviours [62].

OTHER BENZODIAZEPINES

The following oral drugs are potentially useful:

- Temazepam (0.5–1 mg/kg, maximum dose 20 mg) is short acting and used for older children; it is administered 1 hour before surgery.
- Diazepam (0.2–0.3 mg/kg, max. dose 20 mg) is long acting, has an elimination half-life of 20–40 hours and causes an effect by 1 hour.
- Lorazepam (50 µg/kg, max. 4 mg), also long-acting, has an even slower onset and needs to be administered 2 hours preoperatively; it is inappropriate for day-case surgery.

ALIMEMAZINE

This phenothiazine (formerly known as trimeprazine) has sedative, antimuscarinic and antiemetic effects (2 mg/kg). Its use has waned following reports of cardiovascular and respiratory depression (3–4 mg/kg). It is not as effective as midazolam [63].

KETAMINE

An oral dose of ketamine (8 mg/kg) can produce sedation after about 10 minutes [64] and it can be combined with midazolam which may reduce the emetic side-effect [65]. Intramuscular ketamine may be necessary in uncooperative children, but, because of pain and the risk of injury to both patient and staff, it is a method of last resort.

CHORAL HYDRATE AND TRICLOFOS

Chloral hydrate (50–100 mg/kg) is as effective as midazolam but because of its bitter taste is poorly tolerated by some children. It is rapidly metabolised in the body to its main active metabolite, trichloroethanol. However, triclofos, the phosphoric ester of trichloroethanol, shares the same active metabolite and is a more palatable syrup. It is particularly useful in children less than 15 kg.

OPIOIDS

Morphine, papaveretum and pethidine were considered reliable calming premedicant drugs in the past but now the desire to avoid painful intramuscular injections and post-operative nausea and vomiting (PONV) has virtually eliminated their use. These were once standard sedative premedicants. There has been recent interest in fentanyl because an oral dose of 15–20 μg/kg produces sedation after 20 minutes and has a peak effect at 30–45 minutes. In a randomised, placebo-controlled trial, oral transmucosal fentanyl was as effective as midazolam in aiding compliance with anaesthesia, was preferred by more children and had better emergence characteristics [66]. However, it caused more vomiting, pruritus and oxygen desaturation.

CLONIDINE

Clonidine, an α_2-adrenoceptor agonist, is well absorbed orally and has an elimination half-life of 12.5 hours. A dose of 4 μg/kg is as effective as midazolam in producing anxiolysis and sedation and may be better at reducing post-operative pain, PONV, shivering, agitation and confusion [67]. Adverse haemodynamic effects may occur infrequently.

BARBITURATES

Oral barbiturate premedication is no longer in widespread use in the UK. It tends to cause sleep rather than calm behaviour and has an incidence of paradoxical reactions [68,69].

MANAGEMENT OF THE UNCOOPERATIVE CHILD AT INDUCTION OF ANAESTHESIA

Consent

The laws of consent vary between countries and the following is a summary of the current law in the UK. In 1969, the Family Law Reform Act gave children the right to consent to medical treatment once they reached the age of 16 years. It also gave doctors the right to treat those less than 16 years of age if they were sufficiently mature, and had enough understanding to make their own choices. Following the well-publicised 'Gillick' court case in 1985 and the Children Act in 1989, the concept of emerging competence has been accepted. However, for uncooperative children, the issue is less clear in terms of refusal to consent. In England, parents can consent for their children even if they have refused and are deemed competent up to the age of 18 years. However, in Scotland, young people older than 16 years are given the same right to consent or refuse consent as adults and this also applies to a competent child even if they are less than 16 years old.

Nevertheless, refusal by a competent child to consent for an elective procedure should be respected. Parents and clinical staff must then try to persuade the child to change his or her mind. If a non-competent child refuses consent for an elective procedure then a discussion should take place with the parents and carers. If there is agreement to proceed, this should be documented, including the reasons for it. When a competent child refuses consent in an emergency situation, there should be discussion to make sure that the patient understands the benefits of treatment and implications of refusal. If they still refuse then, in England, the child can be overruled if the treatment is in his or her 'best interests'. If there is time, the decision should be taken after consultation with hospital legal advisors, who may recommend referral to a Family Court judge for a rapid opinion. In the UK, refusals by competent children have always been overruled by the courts. In these circumstances, treatment under anaesthesia should be limited only to that which is necessary.

In Scotland, a competent child cannot be overruled, but the concept of 'competency' would be questioned if the child was refusing treatment that was obviously in his or her best interests.

Restraint

The use of restraint is highly controversial and raises some interesting moral and ethical dilemmas. Restraint may be defined as the positive application of force, with the intention of overpowering the child, applied without the child's consent – guidance has been published by the Royal College of Nursing [70]. The difference between restraint and holding a child still depends upon the degree of force required and the intention, implying that the child has given his or her permission. Obviously restraint could be regarded as physical assault and consent should be obtained from the parents. A parent may feel that temporary restraint can be justified if the treatment is clearly of benefit. If restraint is necessary, it should be performed expertly, quickly and using appropriate practical techniques. Local policy and guidelines are helpful. Parental consent is essential and must be recorded.

General approach to the uncooperative child

The emphasis should be aimed at achieving the child's assent by careful preparation to prevent or avoid the problem rather than face it unprepared at induction. Not all children need the full application of all methods aimed to reduce anxiety and distress – fortunately only a few children require a psychologist yet most children benefit from play therapy (Fig. 25.1). Difficult children require a coordinated, committed approach across a multidisciplinary team. The most important aspect of prevention is education. Anaesthetists need to take the lead in educating colleagues about the potential psychological damage of anaesthesia and surgery.

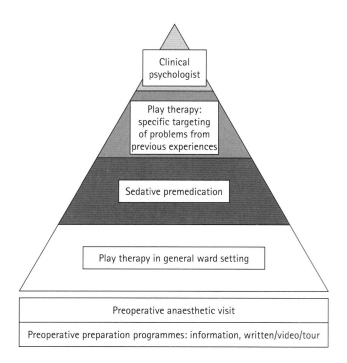

Figure 25.1   Pyramid of increasing therapeutic intervention.

Parents may need to understand that their own behaviour, preparation, coping style and anxiety can affect their child's psychological well-being. They could be sent information with their admission letter or at preadmission clinic, and encouraged to attend a PPP. Ward staff are in an ideal position to identify at-risk children. By making them aware of the risk factors, they are well placed to help to manage a difficult child and to involve play therapists at an early stage. They will be caring for the children postoperatively and should be able to detect altered behaviour. Surgeons can start the education process by giving written information in their clinics that helps to increase the parent's and child's knowledge.

What to do with the uncooperative child at induction?

Despite good preparation, it is inevitable that some children become unexpectedly uncooperative. Algorithms or strategies may be useful in this situation because they help clinical staff who may also be stressed. Figures 25.2

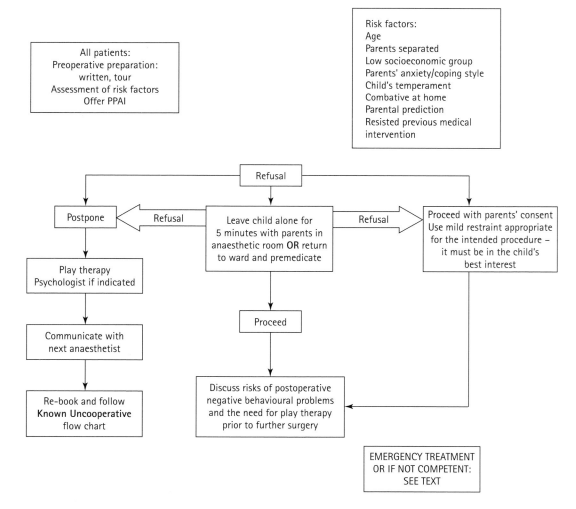

Figure 25.2   Management of a child who is presumed to be cooperative.

and 25.3 outline strategies for 'presumed cooperative' as distinct from 'presumed uncooperative' children; they are meant only to guide, and the reader should appreciate that there may be many exceptions.

PRESUMED COOPERATIVE

Only a minority of children should be uncooperative for their first anaesthetic but, if they are, it is important to try to make their experience as pleasant as possible. Even second-timers can have unexpected changes in behaviour. The emphasis of persuasion should be by positive reinforcement and reward rather than any punitive threat. The anaesthetist can try to salvage the situation with the help of the parents and ward staff by using use coercion or distraction. One person should talk to the child rather than several people all talking at the same time. Hopefully this can re-establish rapport by asking what they like, dislike, have as hobbies or do at school. Appropriately decorated anaesthetic rooms supplied with suitable books and toys help to calm the situation. Gentle persistent persuasion is the best approach and a trusted nurse or play therapist may be most persuasive. If not, then an attempt at premedication may be successful either in the anaesthetic room or on the ward.

For non-urgent, elective surgery it is reasonable to postpone surgery, especially if the child could benefit from play therapists or psychologists and there is a realistic chance that further preparation will improve the conditions. This is particularly justified if repeated anaesthetics are planned because getting it right on the first occasion may prevent or minimise subsequent problems. Older children may need to be allowed time alone with their parents to clarify the situation. If anaesthesia proceeds, parents will need to be warned of postoperative behavioural problems and that it may be useful to see the play therapist afterwards. The child's behaviour should be recorded to prevent the same problem in the future.

PRESUMED UNCOOPERATIVE

Uncooperative children are, without doubt, challenging. They may have communication problems or learning difficulties, such as children with autism [71], cerebral palsy (see Chapter 36) or Down Syndrome. These children and their

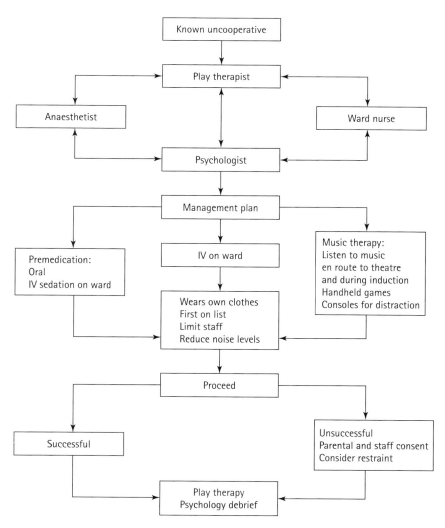

Figure 25.3   Management of a child who is presumed to be uncooperative. IV, intravenous.

parents need time with play therapists or psychologists and a plan should be agreed with the anaesthetist. Occasionally the anaesthetic technique needs to adjust to the specific needs of a child, e.g. IV sedation could be administered on the ward [71]. In children who are clearly not competent, when all methods have failed, and with parental and staff consent, restraint may need to be justified. All details should be recorded. If the child's non-competence is not accepted by anyone involved, it is wise to delay anaesthesia until agreement is achieved. Discussion with legal advisors may be necessary. The size of the child is a practical constraint because it may not be possible to restrain someone over 30 kg without risking physical damage to the child and staff [72]. Parents may request that their child be restrained and it is important to realise that they may not be making the best choice. For example, even though there may have been behavioural problems in the past, restraint is not appropriate once the child starts to show competence. The urgency of the operation is obviously an important consideration and must direct everyone to act in the child's best interests.

AFTER-CARE

If there have been problems, especially if restraint is necessary, the child and parents should be debriefed and further support offered. Often a postoperative visit a few hours later can re-establish rapport and it is important to reward the child for showing any good behaviour. All details of the induction should be recorded and a plan suggested for any future anaesthetic. Follow-up by telephone or at a clinic visit should check for major or persistent behavioural problems.

Clinical scenarios

Two common examples are presented that help to summarise the principles of a sympathetic approach to the uncooperative frightened child. Unfortunately, some children continue to be frightened and methods of calming seem to be ineffective. Nevertheless, it is important to continue to make all reasonable attempts to help children and their parents.

SCENARIO 1

A 6-year-old boy was listed for circumcision. The parents had not told him of his operation 'for fear of upsetting him'. He was clinging to his mother who was anxious – her father had died after an operation. The anaesthetist explained the possibility of behavioural problems if the child was distressed at induction. He recommended that the child was told about the operation. Later, the child became upset and refused to take midazolam or allow local anaesthetic cream to be applied.

The case was postponed so that the family could meet the play therapist on a subsequent day. They were shown a video which interested their child, but he still felt anxious.

With models and toys, the play therapist could show him what would happen. He was told about the medicine, which would make him 'a little bit sleepy' – he said he would take it. He was re-admitted, premedicated with midazolam and subsequently underwent an uneventful IV induction. Postoperatively he was happy and smiling and a telephone interview revealed no other sequelae, other than some disturbed nights for the first week.

SCENARIO 2

A 10-year-old girl was listed for adjustment of her external fixator following trauma to her right leg. She had also suffered a head injury which had left her with mild learning disability. She had become increasingly distressed with each inhalational induction despite premedication. On the previous induction, she would not take her premedication and refused to leave the ward. She had been distressed and violent. A psychologist assessed and discussed her fears. She hated the anaesthetic mask and did not recognise the anaesthetic staff because they were dressed in scrubs. She had severe anticipatory anxiety with blood tests. She also disliked the bitter taste of midazolam and refused to take it.

With persuasion, she underwent a programme of desensitisation which was successful in allowing local anaesthetic cream to be applied. However, she remained highly anxious and still refused to leave the ward. The anaesthetist visited the ward, wearing theatre scrubs and, by using coping techniques designed by the psychologist, an IV cannula was inserted the night before surgery. The next morning the anaesthetist sedated her with IV midazolam on the ward. Transfer to the anaesthetic room was achieved and anaesthesia proceeded uneventfully. Postoperatively she appeared more happy and self-confident. She underwent reinforcing sessions to minimise anticipatory anxiety about leaving the ward. The same anaesthesia plan worked well for subsequent operations.

REFERENCES

Key references

Armstrong TS, Aitken HL. The developing role of play preparation in paediatric anaesthesia. *Paediatr Anaesth* 2000; **10**(1):1–4.

Cote CJ, Cohen IT, Suresh S *et al*. A comparison of three doses of a commercially prepared oral midazolam syrup in children. *Anesth Analg* 2000; **94**(1): 37–43.

Kain ZN, Caldwell-Andrews AA, Wang SM *et al*. Parental intervention choices for children undergoing repeated surgeries. *Anesth Analg* 2003; **96**(4): 970–5.

Kain ZN, Caldwell-Andrews AA, Weinberg ME *et al*. Sevoflurane versus halothane: postoperative maladaptive behavioral changes: a randomized, controlled trial. *Anesthesiology* 2005; **102**(4): 720–6.

McCluskey A, Meakin GH. Oral administration of midazolam as a premedicant for paediatric day-case anaesthesia. *Anaesthesia* 1994; **49**:782–5.

References

1. McGraw T. Preparing children for the operating room: psychological issues. *Can J Anaesth* 1994; **41**: 1094–103.

2. Jackson K. Psychologic preparation as a method of reducing the emotional trauma of anesthesia in children. *Anesthesiology* 1951; **12**(3): 293–300.

3. Eckenhoff JE. Relationship of anaesthesia to postoperative personality changes in children (historical abstract). *Paediatr Anaesth* 1994; **4**: 248.

4. Kain ZN, Mayes LC, O'Connor TZ, Cicchetti DV. Preoperative anxiety in children. Predictors and outcomes. *Arch Pediatr Adolesc Med* 1996; **150**(12): 1238–45.

5. Kotiniemi LH, Ryhänen PT, Valanne J *et al*. Postoperative symptoms at home following day-case surgery in children: a multicentre survey of 551 children. *Anaesthesia* 1997; **52**: 963–9.

6. Kain ZN, Wang SM, Mayes LC *et al*. Distress during the induction of anesthesia and postoperative behavioral outcomes. *Anesth Analg* 1999; **88**(5): 1042–7.

7. Aono J, Mamiya K, Manabe M. Preoperative anxiety is associated with a high incidence of problematic behavior on emergence after halothane anesthesia in boys. *Acta Anaesth* Scand 1999; **43**(5): 542–4.

8. Kain ZN, Caldwell-Andrews AA, Maranets I *et al*. Preoperative anxiety and emergence delirium and postoperative maladaptive behaviors. *Anesth Analg* 2004; **99**(6): 1648–54.

9. Kain ZN, Mayes LC, Caldwell-Andrews AA *et al*. Sleeping characteristics of children undergoing outpatient elective surgery. *Anesthesiology* 2002; **97**(5): 1093–101.

10. Kotiniemi LH, Ryhänen PT, Moilanen IK. Behavioural changes in children following day-case surgery: a 4-week follow-up of 551 children. *Anaesthesia* 1997; **52**: 970–6.

11. Vessey JA, Bogetz MS, Caserza CL *et al*. Parental upset associated with participation in induction of anaesthesia in children. *Can J Anaesth* 1994; **41**: 276–80.

12. McCann ME, Kain ZN. The management of preoperative anxiety in children: an update. *Anesth Analg* 2001; **93**(1): 98–105.

13. Thomas J. Brute force or gentle persuasion? *Paediatr Anaesth* 2005; **15**(5): 355–7.

14. Holm-Knudsen RJ, Carlin JB, McKenzie IM. Distress at induction of anaesthesia in children. A survey of incidence, associated factors and recovery characteristics. *Paediatr Anaesth* 1998; **8**(5): 383–92.

15. Caldas JC, Pais-Ribeiro JL, Carneiro SR. General anaesthesia, surgery and hospitalization in children and their effects upon cognitive, academic, emotional and sociobehavioral development – a review. *Paediatr Anaesth* 2004; **14**(11): 910–15.

16. Watson AT, Visram A. Children's preoperative anxiety and postoperative behaviour. *Paediatr Anaesth* 2003; **13**(3): 188–204.

17. Kain ZN, Mayes LC, Cicchetti DV *et al*. The Yale Preoperative Anxiety Scale: how does it compare with a 'gold standard'? *Anesth Analg* 1997; **85**(4): 783–8.

18. Kain ZN, Caramico LA, Mayes LC *et al*. Preoperative preparation programs in children: a comparative examination. *Anesth Analg* 1998; **87**(6): 1249–55.

19. Spielberger CD. *STAIC: preliminary manual for the State-Trait Anxiety Inventory for Children ('How I feel questionnaire')*. Palo Alto, CA: Consulting Psychologists Press, 1973.

20. Buss AH, Plomin R. *Temperament: early developing personality traits*. Hillsdale, NJ: Lawrence Erlbaum Associates, 1984.

21. Miller SM. Monitoring and blunting: validation of a questionnaire to assess styles of information seeking under threat. *J Pers Soc Psychol* 1987; **52**(2): 345–53.

22. Vernon DT, Schulman JL, Foley JM. Changes in children's behavior after hospitalization. Some dimensions of response and their correlates. *Am J Dis Child* 1966; **111**(6): 581–93.

23. Kain ZN. Postoperative maladaptive behavioral changes in children: incidence, risks factors and interventions. *Acta Anaesthesiol Belg* 2000; **51**(4): 217–26.

24. Kain ZN, Mayes LC, Wang SM *et al*. Parental presence and a sedative premedicant for children undergoing surgery: a hierarchical study. *Anesthesiology* 2000; **92**(4): 939–46.

25. Bevan JC, Johnston C, Haig MJ *et al*. Preoperative parental anxiety predicts behavioural and emotional responses to induction of anaesthesia in children. *Can J Anaesth* 1990; **37**: 177–82.

26. Shirley PJ, Thompson N, Kenward M, Johnston G. Parental anxiety before elective surgery in children. A British perspective. *Anaesthesia* 1998; **53**(10): 956–9.

27. Litman RS, Berger AA, Chhibber A. An evaluation of preoperative anxiety in a population of parents of infants and children undergoing ambulatory surgery. *Paediatr Anaesth* 1996; **6**: 443–7.

28. Kain ZN, Ferris CA, Mayes LC, Rimar S. Parental presence during induction of anaesthesia: practice differences between the United States and Great Britain. *Paediatr Anaesth* 1996; **6**: 187–93.

29. Kain ZN, Mayes LC, Caramico LA *et al*. Parental presence during induction of anesthesia: a randomized controlled trial. *Anesthesiology* 1996; **84**: 1060–7.

30. Thompson RH, Vernon DT. Research on children's behavior after hospitalization: a review and synthesis. *J Dev Behav Pediatr* 1993; **14**(1): 28–35.

31. Kotiniemi LH, Ryhänen PT, Moilanen IK. Behavioural changes following routine ENT operations in two-to-ten-year-old children. *Paediatr Anaesth* 1996; **6**: 45–9.

32. Aguilera IM, Patel D, Meakin GH, Masterson J. Perioperative anxiety and postoperative behavioural disturbances in children undergoing intravenous or inhalation induction of anaesthesia. *Paediatr Anaesth* 2003; **13**(6): 501–7.

33. Kain ZN, Caldwell-Andrews AA, Weinberg ME *et al.* Sevoflurane versus halothane: postoperative maladaptive behavioral changes: a randomized, controlled trial. *Anesthesiology* 2005; **102**(4): 720–6.

34. Vernon DT, Thompson RH. Research on the effect of experimental interventions on children's behavior after hospitalization: a review and synthesis. *J Dev Behav Pediatr* 1993; **14**(1): 36–44.

35. Kain ZN, Mayes LC, Caramico LA. Preoperative preparation in children: a cross-sectional study. *J Clin Anesth* 1996; **8**(6): 508–14.

36. Cassady JFJ, Wysocki TT, Miller KM *et al.* Use of a preanesthetic video for facilitation of parental education and anxiolysis before pediatric ambulatory surgery. *Anesth Analg* 1999; **88**(2): 246–50.

37. Webber GC. Patient education. A review of the issues. *Med Care* 1990; **28**(11): 1089–103.

38. Faust J, Melamed BG. Influence of arousal, previous experience, and age on surgery preparation of same day of surgery and in-hospital pediatric patients. *J Consult Clin Psychol* 1984; **52**(3): 359–65.

39. Kain ZN, Wang SM, Caramico LA *et al.* Parental desire for perioperative information and informed consent: a two-phase study. *Anesth Analg* 1997; **84**: 299–306.

40. Messeri A, Caprilli S, Busoni P. Anaesthesia induction in children: a psychological evaluation of the efficiency of parents' presence. *Paediatr Anaesth* 2004; **14**(7): 551–6.

41. Braude N, Ridley SA, Sumner E. Parents and Paediatr Anaesth: a prospective survey of parental attitudes to their presence at induction. *Ann R Coll Surg Eng* 1990; **72**: 41–4.

42. McCormick ASM, Spargo PM. Parents in the anaesthetic room: a questionnaire survey of departments of anaesthesia. *Paediatr Anaesth* 1996; **6**: 183–6.

43. Kain ZN, Caldwell-Andrews AA, Krivutza DM *et al.* Trends in the practice of parental presence during induction of anesthesia and the use of preoperative sedative premedication in the United States, 1995–2002: results of a follow-up national survey. *Anesth Analg* 2004; **98**(5): 1252–9.

44. Tripi PA, Palermo TM, Thomas S *et al.* Assessment of risk factors for emergence distress and postoperative behavioural changes in children following general anaesthesia. *Paediatr Anaesth* 2004; **14**(3): 235–40.

45. Ryder IG, Spargo PM. Parents in the anaesthetic room. A questionnaire survey of parents' reactions. *Anaesthesia* 1991; **46**: 977–9.

46. Kain ZN, Caldwell-Andrews AA, Wang SM *et al.* Parental intervention choices for children undergoing repeated surgeries. *Anesth Analg* 2003; **96**(4): 970–5.

47. Armstrong TS, Aitken HL. The developing role of play preparation in paediatric anaesthesia. *Paediatr Anaesth* 2000; **10**(1): 1–4.

48. Schwartz BH, Albino JE, Tedesco LA. Effects of psychological preparation on children hospitalized for dental operations. *J Pediatr* 1983; **102**(4): 634–8.

49. Hopayian K. A brief technique of hypnoanaesthesia for children in a casualty ward. *Anaesthesia* 1984; **39**(11): 1139–41.

50. Betcher AM. Hypno-induction techniques in pediatric anesthesia. *Anesthesiology* 1958; **19**(2): 279–81.

51. Bensen VB. One hundred cases of post-anesthetic suggestion in the recovery room. *Am J Clin Hypn* 1971; **14**(1): 9–15.

52. Calipel S, Lucas-Polomeni MM, Wodey E, Ecoffey C. Premedication in children: hypnosis versus midazolam. *Paediatr Anaesth* 2005; **15**(4): 275–81.

53. Wang SM, Maranets I, Weinberg ME *et al.* Parental auricular acupuncture as an adjunct for parental presence during induction of anesthesia. *Anesthesiology* 2004; **100**(6): 1399–404.

54. Kain ZN, Wang SM, Mayes LC *et al.* Sensory stimuli and anxiety in children undergoing surgery: a randomized, controlled trial. *Anesth Analg* 2001; **92**(4): 897–903.

55. Kain ZN, Caldwell-Andrews AA, Krivutza DM *et al.* Interactive music therapy as a treatment for preoperative anxiety in children: a randomized controlled trial. *Anesth Analg* 2004; **98**(5): 1260–6.

56. McCluskey A, Meakin GH. Oral administration of midazolam as a premedicant for paediatric day-case anaesthesia. *Anaesthesia* 1994; **49**: 782–5.

57. Morgan-Hughes JO, Bangham JA. Pre-induction behaviour of children. A review of placebo-controlled trials of sedatives. *Anaesthesia* 1990; **45**: 427–35.

58. Karl HW, Rosenberger JL, Larach MG, Ruffle JM. Transmucosal administration of midazolam for premedication of pediatric patients: comparison of the nasal and sublingual routes. *Anesthesiology* 1993; **78**: 885–91.

59. Davis PJ, Tome JA, McGowan FX *et al.* Preanesthetic medication with intranasal midazolam for brief pediatric surgical procedures. *Anesthesiology* 1995; **82**: 2–5.

60. Cote CJ, Cohen IT, Suresh S *et al.* A comparison of three doses of a commercially prepared oral midazolam syrup in children. *Anesth Analg* 2000; **94**(1): 37–43.

61. Kain ZN, Hofstadter MB, Mayes LC *et al.* Midazolam: effects on amnesia and anxiety in children. *Anesthesiology* 2000; **93**(3): 676–84.

62. McGraw T, Kendrick A. Oral midazolam premedication and postoperative behaviour in children. *Paediatr Anaesth* 1998; **8**: 117–121.

63. Patel D, Meakin G. Oral midazolam compared with diazepam-droperidol and trimeprazine as premedicants in children. *Paediatr Anaesth* 1997; **7**: 287–93.

64. Turhanoglu S, Kararmaz A, Ozyilmaz MA *et al.* Effects of different doses of oral ketamine for premedication of children. *Eur J Anaesthesiol* 2003; **20**(1): 56–60.

65. Darlong V, Shende D, Subramanyam MS *et al.* Oral ketamine or midazolam or low dose combination for premedication in children. *Anaesth Intensive Care* 2004; **32**(2): 246–9.

66. Howell TK, Smith S, Rushman SC *et al.* A comparison of oral transmucosal fentanyl and oral midazolam for premedication in children. *Anaesthesia* 2002; **57**(8): 798–805.

67. Bergendahl H, Lonnqvist PA, Eksborg S. Clonidine in paediatric anaesthesia: review of the literature and comparison with benzodiazepines for premedication (review). *Acta Anaesthesiol Scand* 2006; **50**(2): 135–43.

68. Simpson JH, West CD, Law PJ. Paediatric sedation for CT scanning: the safety and efficacy of quinalbarbitone in a district general hospital setting. *Br J Radiol* 2000; **73**(865): 7–9.

69. Malviya S, Voepel-Lewis T, Tait AR *et al*. Pentobarbital vs chloral hydrate for sedation of children undergoing MRI: efficacy and recovery characteristics. *Paediatr Anaesth* 2004; **14**(7): 589–95.

70. Royal College of Nursing. Restraining, holding still and containing children and young people. Guidance for nursing staff. London: Royal College of Nursing, 2003. Available online at: http://www2.rcn.org.uk/cyp/resources/a-z_of_resources/restraint.

71. van der Walt JH, Moran C. An audit of perioperative management of autistic children. *Paediatr Anaesth* 2001; **11**(4): 401–8.

72. Christiansen E, Chambers N. Induction of anesthesia in a combative child; management and issues. *Paediatr Anaesth* 2005; **15**(5): 421–5.

26

Regional anaesthesia

PETER MARHOFER, STEPHAN KETTNER, JUSTUS BENRATH, PER-ARNE LÖNNQVIST, DESIRÉ SCHABORT

KEY LEARNING POINTS

- Nerve blocks are central to the practice of paediatric anaesthesia.
- Optimally accurate puncture techniques are essential.
- Blocks should be placed 'as central as necessary as peripheral as possible'.
- The volume of local anaesthetic agent injected should be minimised.

- Ultrasound guidance is the most effective way to achieve these aims.
- Structured training and supervised practice are required to optimise nerve blockade skills.
- Specific guidelines for regional anaesthesia in children should be developed from paediatric data.

INTRODUCTION

One of the most desirable achievements in paediatric surgery is that children can sleep quietly without pain after the procedure. This would not be possible without combined techniques of general and regional anaesthesia. The advantages of regional anaesthesia include lower doses of systemic anaesthetics, no requirement for opioids, less need for postoperative ventilation after major thoracic or abdominal surgery, reduced time in the intensive care unit and inhibition of endocrinological stress responses.

There is a widespread misconception that optimally accurate puncture techniques are not necessary in children. It is believed that the local anaesthetic will easily spread to the site of action, given the small dimensions of the anatomical structures involved. This view is wrong; accurate puncture techniques should be developed in children precisely because their anatomical structures are highly vulnerable.

Other factors must be considered as well. The vertebral bone grows faster than the neuraxial structures during foetal growth. As a result, the terminal end of the spinal cord is located around the L3 level at birth, while the dural sac terminates at the S3–4 level. Ossification of the vertebral bodies is an ongoing process [1] that is not completed before 6 years of age [2]; there is, consequently, a risk of inadvertently administering local anaesthetic into bone during central blocks [3]. The spinal curves are not fully developed at birth. The cervical lordosis develops at 3–6 months and the lumbar lordosis at 8–9 months. Hence children of different ages require different needle orientations for spinal and epidural puncture. The relative volume of cerebrospinal fluid decreases from 4 mL/kg in newborns to 2 mL/kg in adults. The viscosity of epidural fat increases only gradually after birth. Local anaesthetics will therefore spread more extensively in children under 6 years. Finally, myelinisation of peripheral nerves and spinal tracts is not complete before age 12. As a result, younger children require smaller concentrations of local anaesthetic for effective analgesia [4].

Numerous techniques described in the literature for paediatric use have been performed more or less 'blind'.

The reported success rates are poor. Examples include ilioinguinal/iliohypogastric and rectus sheath blocks or axillary approaches to the brachial plexus. Ultrasonography enables us to improve most nerve block techniques to an unprecedented level of accuracy. Direct visualisation of peripheral nerve blocks is a very recent accomplishment but has nevertheless grown to a relatively mature stage of development. At the time of writing, some of the techniques are not fully peer reviewed. The reader is therefore specifically reminded that some elements of this chapter must reflect our subjective views, although data from all the techniques described here will be published in due course. The available evidence strongly indicates that all these techniques may be applied in clinical practice and, where ultrasound-guided techniques have been reported in peer-reviewed journals, the results have been superior to conventional techniques (e.g. ilioinguinal/iliohypogastric nerve blocks).

At our institution (Department of Anaesthesiology and Intensive Care, Medical University of Vienna, Austria), these techniques are already standard care and we now perform most regional anaesthesia under ultrasound guidance. Despite being convinced ourselves, we are also well aware that ultrasonography is not currently the standard guidance technique in paediatric regional anaesthesia. Therefore, the present chapter will also cover other techniques.

CENTRAL VERSUS PERIPHERAL BLOCKS

As central as necessary, as peripheral as possible

Most available studies on regional anaesthesia have described central neuraxial blocks in adults. These reports include spinal and continuous epidural approaches, typically performed at lumbar or thoracic levels. All these techniques are also suitable for children with appropriate modifications. Regional anaesthesia offers valuable and safe ways to achieve high-quality analgesia in children. Central blocks are, however, not minor procedures and this is even true of caudal analgesia. While the overall morbidity of central blocks is low, there are complications [5]. Their indications must be weighed together with the scope of the surgical procedure and any complications that might occur. Peripheral blocks are safer and anaesthetists should therefore take this alternative whenever possible. In other words, nerve blocks should always be placed as central as necessary and as peripheral as possible. This principle applies to adults, and there is no reason why it should not apply to children.

Complications of central blocks

The morbidity rate of central blocks is less than 1 per 1000 but varies greatly from technique to technique. The highest rates have been described for lumbar epidurals (4.6 per 1000) and intervertebral sacral epidurals (6.8 per 1000) [5]. Inadvertent dural puncture is the most common complication of central blocks, especially when epidural approaches at sacral intervertebral levels are selected. Intrathecal injection of the epidural dose results in total spinal anaesthesia. However, haemodynamic side-effects are less frequent than in adults and not usually life threatening for the child. Intravascular injection can lead to seizures or transient cardiac arrhythmias but this is uncommon.

Overdoses of local anaesthetics can give rise to delayed cardiac arrhythmias. Less toxic agents such as levobupivacaine or ropivacaine should be used whenever possible. Toxic effects of local anaesthetics are more pronounced in children (and especially small infants) than in adults (see Chapter 14). Regional anaesthesia at caudal levels carries a risk of puncturing the sacrum or rectum. However, these complications should be avoidable with care and attention to detail [5]. Caudal anaesthesia for penile surgery has been shown to reduce nausea and vomiting compared with parenteral analgesics but not compared with peripheral penile blocks [6]. Complications of spinal anaesthesia are often related to the distribution of local anaesthetic, which may spread unpredictably, thereby causing either inadequate or excessive nerve blockade.

Complications from epidurals may include urinary retention, leg weakness, haematoma and infection. The incidence of urinary retention seems to be higher when epidural opioids are used and the response to naloxone is normally poor. In our daily practice, urinary retention is a minor problem in patients with epidural catheters since they usually have urinary catheters for surgical indications. Unlike in adults, hypotension is rarely a complication of epidurals in children (especially under 8 years old). Moreover, the incidence of epidural haematomas, infections and direct trauma to the spinal cord is thankfully very low in children. No such events have been reported in large case series for epidural or spinal anaesthesia [5,7].

Implications of peripheral blocks

Peripheral nerve blocks have not been studied anywhere as extensively as have central blocks in children. A Medline search performed in November 2005 returned a total of 149 relevant hits for epidural and 25 for peripheral nerve blocks in paediatric anaesthesia. It is therefore apparent that most peripheral nerve blocks are rarely used in clinical practice.

Giaufré et al. [5] reported a total of 24 409 regional anaesthetics performed in children over a 1-year period, 15 013 of them being central blocks. Thus central blocks accounted for more than 60 per cent of all procedures; only 38 per cent were peripheral blocks. The complication rate was 0.9 per 1000 cases and none of these was attributable to peripheral bocks.

Nerve stimulators are currently the standard tool to locate nerves in adults. Different standards are applied in children, as many paediatric anaesthetists are reluctant to use nerve stimulators and they continue to use what are essentially 'blind' approaches, including anatomical landmarks or fascial click techniques as sole reference. These approaches are used for ilioinguinal/iliohypogastric nerve blocks and for other techniques that are today exclusively used with nerve stimulators in adults.

The success rates of peripheral nerve blocks have been disappointing in children. Success rates of 60–90 per cent have been described for landmark-based guidance techniques, nerve stimulation or nerve mapping [8]. Of course, whether a block is considered successful depends heavily on the investigator's judgement. Even though there is little consensus on the optimum method for evaluating it, information on pain and comfort is, however, indispensable because it gives us the feedback that we need to optimise our approaches.

ULTRASOUND FOR GUIDANCE

Avoiding risks and eliminating pain

Children benefit from ultrasound guidance, which achieves an excellent success of nerve blockade with remarkably low volumes of local anaesthetic [9]. Although intoxication with local anaesthetics is not known to be a significant problem in children, there is every reason to believe that these events are underreported and there are sound pharmacological reasons to assume greater risk of toxicity in young children (see Chapter 14). It therefore seems very reasonable to minimise the administered volumes.

The most obvious benefit in children is that anatomical structures can be effectively identified despite being more condensed than in adults. In addition, ultrasound guidance offers children advantages that have been demonstrated in adults. Most importantly, these procedures involve scarcely any pain and avoid muscle contractions, triggered by nerve stimulation (which can be very painful, especially in the presence of fractures). Furthermore, the spread of local anaesthetic can be monitored, intravascular or intraneural punctures are avoided, sensory and motor onset times are reduced, and effective nerve blockade lasts longer and can be achieved with smaller volumes of local anaesthetic.

We rely almost exclusively on portable ultrasound equipment, as mobility is very important (Fig. 26.1). In this way, ultrasound-guided techniques can be used wherever nerve blocks are needed in paediatric surgery. Contemporary units have a rugged design and are ready to use promptly after being switched on.

Most blocks can be performed with 5–10 MHz linear ultrasound transducers, but probes offering a frequency of 13 MHz have recently become available. Probes with a small surface are required to deal with the condensed anatomical structures in children and a very appropriate choice are hockey-stick probes with a surface length of 25 mm (Fig. 26.2). Higher frequencies improve visualisation of superficial nerve structures. Lower frequencies should be used for deeper (e.g. psoas) compartment blocks in larger children. For this specific indication, we use 2–5 MHz sector transducers.

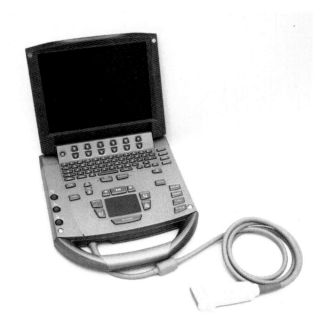

Figure 26.1   Transportable ultrasound system with a linear probe.

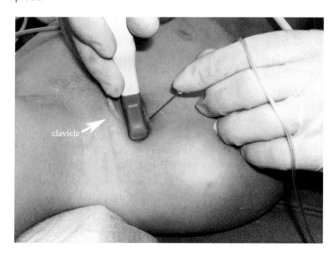

Figure 26.2   Cannula relative to the 'hockey-stick' probe in a cross-sectional technique for the infraclavicular approach to the brachial plexus.

There is a widespread misconception that only 'rich' institutions can afford ultrasound systems for regional anaesthesia. We challenge this view; portable units for less than half the price of regular anaesthesia systems are perfectly serviceable for all techniques described in this chapter.

There is a learning curve for ultrasound guidance techniques, however. Training should be sequential. Specialised workshops are offered in which the basic skills can be acquired in 2 days. The initial blocks on children should then be performed under competent supervision until the supervisor and instructor are happy that the appropriate experience level has been reached.

Cross-sectional technique

There are two major ultrasound techniques for nerve blockade: a cross-sectional technique and an in-line technique. The difference is in the needle position relative to the ultrasound transducer. For the cross-sectional technique, the needle orientation is transverse (Fig. 26.2). Visualisation in the ultrasound image is confined to the needle tip. The puncture angle must be selected such that the needle tip can be advanced precisely as deep as the target structure. Both the target structure and the position of the needle are reflected in the ultrasound image. Two criteria will identify the needle: the tissue it displaces and an acoustic shadow emerging dorsally at its tip.

The local anaesthetic must be injected very carefully to ensure that its spread is captured in the image. Note that the target nerves are blocked not by the needle but by the local anaesthetic. This may sound trivial, but anaesthetists tend to focus on the needle tip because all techniques developed in the past have relied on the position of the needle as the prime criterion for successful blockade. The injection must be immediately terminated if the local anaesthetic cannot be visualised because this signifies that the needle tip is outside the range of the ultrasound window.

The cross-sectional technique is used for most nerve blocks described in this chapter. It clearly offers a number of major advantages over in-line techniques despite the fact that the scope of visualisation is confined to the needle tip:

- Effective nerve blockade is most reliably achieved with a transverse needle orientation.
- It allows us to maintain well-established puncture angulations in developing our ultrasound-guided approaches to nerve blockade.
- Compared with in-line techniques, the needle has to be advanced significantly less far to reach the target structure. These punctures are therefore less traumatic and less painful, which also makes them the method of choice for blocks in awake children.

It is not crucial to the success of nerve blockade that the tip of the needle is located precisely in the ultrasound image. Certainly the position of the needle must be identified precisely to avoid complications, but this requirement can be met by visualising the tissue displaced by the needle and an acoustic shadow emerging dorsally at its tip rather than by visualising the needle directly.

In-line technique

The second option is to advance the needle longitudinally to the ultrasound probe. This will ideally allow the needle shaft to be visualised as well. However, orienting the probe relative to the needle is even more exacting with this approach because the needle has to be located strictly within the range of the emitted ultrasound signals to visualise its shaft.

Deviations as small as 1–2 mm will remove the needle from the image. There are only a few special applications for this technique in clinical practice.

System configuration

Experts in ultrasound-guided regional anaesthesia need to be adept at optimising images. Anaesthetists who need the following guidelines will have a much easier time performing the blocks discussed in this chapter.

IMAGE DEPTH

The quality of the ultrasound image is significantly reduced once the individual pixels become visible at larger magnifications. Therefore an appropriate balance must be found between overview and detail.

GAIN

The gain must be carefully optimised for the existing image depth. Some ultrasound systems offer independent gain settings for different sections of an image. This feature is known as time gain compensation. Other systems come with a less refined function of depth gain adjustment (surface/depth gain).

FOCUS

Vertical anatomical structures are significantly more condensed in children than in adults. Therefore the focus of the ultrasound image must be adjusted to capture the level of the target structures as distinctly as possible. High-end ultrasound systems offer an opportunity to select different focal zones. In other words, the zone of optimal resolution is progressively reduced as smaller focal zones are selected. A typical compromise would be to define two or three focal zones.

ISSUES AND RECOMMENDATIONS

PERIPHERAL VERSUS CENTRAL BLOCKADE

The fundamental decision to be made for regional anaesthesia is what region should be anaesthetised. The issue of central versus peripheral blocks is discussed in greater detail earlier in this chapter. To state our case once again: blocks should always be placed as peripheral as possible and as central as necessary.

CONTINUOUS VERSUS SINGLE-SHOT TECHNIQUE

Whether a single-shot or continuous technique should be used depends mainly on the postoperative setting. Good clinical practice is mandatory for catheter management, however, and robust local protocols involving a multidisciplinary paediatric pain team must be in place.

CONSENT

It is very important to offer accurate information and gain consent before performing local blocks. Exactly who should be informed is a function of age and social competence. As a general rule, however, the information needs to be conveyed to both the parent and, where appropriate, the child. The physician should seek to establish a good rapport with the child. It is not that difficult to create a trusting atmosphere in which the procedure will be simpler.

ACUTE VERSUS PLANNED SURGERY

There is a fundamental difference between acute and planned surgical procedures. Upper-limb fractures account for the majority of acute injuries in paediatric patients and are amenable to the use of local blocks, as are femoral fractures. Children with acute injuries who are in pain and accompanied by anxious parents call for rapid and effective action. Time must not be wasted in taking unnecessary preliminary steps such as premedication. The situation needs to be correctly assessed and any concomitant injuries must be identified.

PRESENCE VERSUS ABSENCE OF PARENTS

It is often helpful to encourage the parents' presence during nerve blockade performed under sedation. It is important that the entire anaesthetic procedure works smoothly in the parents' presence and it should therefore be performed by an anaesthetist experienced in the technique.

ANAESTHESIA VERSUS (NO) SEDATION

Eliminating the need for airway manipulation is a strong argument for regional anaesthesia in children. It is therefore necessary to overcome suboptimal techniques of regional nerve blockade. The spectrum of indications for purely regional techniques that avoid general anaesthesia has been growing over the past few years. Thus the safety of our children has been improved without affecting their comfort. This has been an important development.

Central blocks are usually performed under general anaesthesia. Signs of toxicity are therefore difficult to identify. Injecting adrenaline-loaded test doses into epidural vessels may not produce detectable cardiovascular changes in children, although T-wave elevation appears to be a better parameter than conventional haemodynamic criteria to detect intravascular injection [10]. Isoprenaline has been successfully used instead of adrenaline to improve the sensitivity of test doses [11]. We do not routinely use adrenaline-loaded test doses of local anaesthetic because they are not effective enough in detecting intravascular or subarachnoid injection.

Anaesthesia will also mask any warning signs of paraesthesia caused by nerve puncture. Ultrasonography can help to prevent both nerve puncture by visualising the needle tip and intrathecal injection by visualising the spread of infused substances [12,13].

Most peripheral nerve blocks can be performed without general anaesthesia. Absolute contraindications include some specific injury patterns and lengthy procedures such as replantation operations. Aside from these specific indications for general anaesthesia, a sedation regimen may or may not be applied for peripheral blocks. The child can remain alert if an atmosphere of trust has been created and if the anaesthetist is well prepared. Previous experience with the same child may be a factor. Sedation is the more typical scenario, however. Suitable medication can be used for this purpose (see Chapter 44), but note that in acute injury it is necessary to maintain airway control since acutely injured children are rarely hospitalised with an empty stomach [14]. Appropriate drugs and intubation equipment must be kept ready and within reach.

Monitoring can normally be confined to oxygen saturation and heart rate via pulse oximetry. The heart rate should be monitored by ECG if pulse oximetry is inadequate. Cuff monitors are not routinely used as they may be disturbing. The level of monitoring should be in line with the actual need. Children with haemodynamically relevant injuries will clearly require extended monitoring.

INDIRECT VERSUS DIRECT IDENTIFICATION OF NERVE STRUCTURES

Nerve stimulation and ultrasonography are currently the only two technologies that can be considered appropriate for most blocks. There are few remaining indications for techniques that rely solely on anatomical landmarks or loss of resistance. Penile nerve blocks are one example. Paraesthesia-based techniques are essentially obsolete.

The advantages of ultrasonography are discussed elsewhere in this chapter. Since ultrasound guidance has not yet been widely adopted at the time of writing, it cannot be regarded as the gold standard. The current minimum standard should be a modern nerve stimulator for peripheral nerve blocks and loss-of-resistance techniques for epidurals. Another popular method to identify peripheral nerves is transcutaneous nerve mapping. This technique does not, however, reveal how deeply the targeted nerve structures are located. Other techniques, such as electric stimulation to confirm the position of epidural catheters, are still experimental and do not currently have a role in everyday clinical practice.

The same technical and methodological standards of nerve stimulation should be applied as in adults. Current, state-of-the-art electric nerve stimulators have adjustable amperage, bandwidth and pulse duration. The bandwidth should be 0.1 ms if the child is alert, such that stimulation remains largely confined to A α motor fibres to avoid pain. In anaesthetised children, a bandwidth of up to 1 ms should be selected. The local anaesthetic is injected as soon as muscle feedback is elicited within an amperage range of

<0.3–$0.5\,mA$, indicating that the needle is presumably at a safe distance from the nerves.

PREPARATION OF MATERIALS

The materials for the block procedure must be duly prepared and checked. A suitable nerve stimulator must be present for conventional techniques of peripheral nerve blockade. Ultrasound-guided techniques involve the use of a probe and sterile ultrasound gel. A needle and an appropriate local anaesthetic must be prepared. Equipment for cleaning and surface anaesthesia of the area are also required. Air inclusions, no matter how tiny, can cause enormous artefacts in the ultrasound image. Therefore the needle system must be completely filled with local anaesthetic.

LOCAL ANAESTHETICS AND ADDITIVES (SEE ALSO CHAPTERS 14 AND 27)

A large number of studies on the use of pure enantiomers have been published over the past few years. Recent publications and pharmacological data indicate that ropivacaine and levobupivacaine are the best choice for most regional anaesthetic techniques; they are less toxic and offer longer block durations. They are also available in various concentrations to achieve differential blockade effects on sympathetic, sensory or motor responses (levobupivacaine, 0.125, 0.25 or 0.5 per cent; ropivacaine, 0.2, 0.475 or 0.75 per cent). Furthermore, they can be used to good effect for combined peripheral blocks under ultrasound guidance, thanks to their low toxicity and the fact that direct visualisation reduces injected volumes. Note that combination regimens in which two anaesthetics were used simultaneously have yielded low complication rates in most case series [5,7]. It is therefore wrong to believe that two anaesthetics might double the risk in children.

Other local anaesthetics have a narrow spectrum of indications, such as bupivacaine for penile nerve blocks. Additives intended to increase block duration and intensity have been extensively studied both in adults and in children. They have not been shown to influence the quality of peripheral nerve blocks but do have merits for central techniques, such as caudal or continuous epidural blocks (see Chapter 27).

NEEDLES AND CATHETERS

A major problem in the past was that appropriate paediatric equipment was not available for regional anaesthesia. Some manufacturers have since introduced appropriate needle material on realising that regional anaesthesia had become increasingly popular in children of all age groups. Today adequate equipment is available for most age groups.

We use 22–24G needles with a facet tip for peripheral blocks and 19–21G Tuohy needles with a 22–25G catheter for epidurals (Table 26.1). Some centres, however, find that these fine catheters are prone to displacement and prefer to

Table 26.1 Recommendations for epidurals

Age	Needle (G)	Catheter (G)
Preterm	21	25
0–6 months	21	25
6–24 months	20	24
24–84 months	19	23

use 18G needles with 21G catheters. Peripheral block techniques are invariably performed with facet needles and flexible injection tubes. This configuration is based on the immobile needle concept described by Winnie [15]. The facet design optimises the precision of needle guidance inside tissue. Less sharp cannulae such as Sprotte needles are disadvantageous in this situation.

Major efforts are also being made to develop special cannulae for ultrasound applications. Preliminary designs have already been introduced. These cannulae can be manufactured at lower cost as they feature no wiring and insulation for electric stimulation.

For caudal blocks, we also use a specially designed kit, including a 24G cannula 30 mm in length with an injection line, syringes and swabs. Continuous epidurals should be performed with Tuohy needles matched to age and body weight (Table 26.1).

STERILITY

We use the same sterile approach in children as in adults. For single-shot punctures under ultrasound guidance, a surface disinfectant is applied to the transducer in accordance with the manufacturer's recommendations. Then the puncture site is disinfected and covered with a sterile ultrasound gel. We favour the gels used on urinary catheters. All subsequent steps follow a no-touch strategy. Skilful manipulation is required to avoid all contact of the needle with the transducer or any other surfaces. For catheter techniques under ultrasonographic guidance, we employ a sterile drape, and the surface of the ultrasound probe is sealed with sterile wrapping (ultrasound gel is filled into a sterile cover, and then sterile gel is applied to the cover). We have never observed any infections with this sterile approach to regional anaesthesia.

CONTRAINDICATIONS

Regional anaesthesia is not normally recommended in patients with severe coagulopathies, neuromuscular conditions and psychiatric disorders. Note that these accepted contraindications do not necessarily apply in children. Techniques of regional anaesthesia may be particularly useful in children with neuromuscular conditions, in order to avoid general anaesthesia.

Absolute contraindications to epidural analgesia include severe malformations of the spinal cord or spine (e.g.

meningocele or complete spina bifida), coagulopathies and anticoagulative therapy. Relative contraindications include hydrocephalus, reduced intracranial compliance, elevated intracranial pressure, and severe convulsive or psychomotor disorders. At our institution, the presence of septic foci is no longer an absolute contraindication to epidural anaesthesia in children. This is another example illustrating that standards for regional anaesthesia in children will not necessarily coincide with those in adults [16].

Absence of consent is an absolute contraindication to performance of local blocks, but in our experience, most parents will agree with the suggested technique after being fully informed in an open conversation about its pros and cons.

NEURAXIAL BLOCKS

Central blocks account for over 50 per cent of all regional anaesthesia in children. These techniques offer an optimal level of perioperative analgesia but are invasive and carry risks. Their complications are discussed elsewhere in this chapter. A distinction should be made between single-shot blocks (such as caudals) and continuous epidurals. The former are easy to perform, the latter much more complex. Continuous techniques require optimal management and appropriate measures to avoid complications. A robust postoperative structure is needed to ensure that these requirements are met as the chain of neuraxial catheter management can only be as strong as its weakest link. It is therefore desirable that ward staff, surgeons and other personnel are trained, and take part, in catheter management.

Caudal anaesthesia

Caudal anaesthesia is the most frequently used technique of regional anaesthesia overall [5]. It is a single-injection technique performed through the sacral hiatus and the sacrococcygeal membrane into the caudal part of the epidural space. It is easy to learn; anaesthetists can achieve a success rate of 80 per cent after performing around 30 caudal blocks [17].

TECHNIQUE

The child is placed in a lateral position with the knees and hips flexed. The prone position may also be suitable but will complicate airway management. Landmarks to identify the sacrococcygeal membrane are the posterosuperior iliac spines and the sacral cornuae. These form an equilateral triangle with the apex of the sacral hiatus (Fig. 26.3).

The needle is advanced perpendicular to the skin through the sacrococcygeal membrane until the tissue palpably yields to the pressure as it penetrates the membrane, it is redirected by 20–30° in a rostral direction and carefully advanced into the sacral canal (not farther than 2–3 mm to avoid venous or dural puncture). The needle is left open for a few seconds to detect any reflux of blood or cerebrospinal

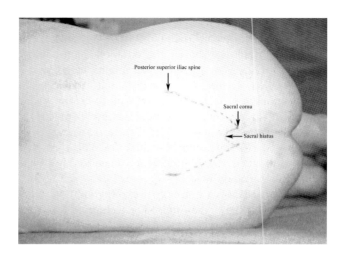

Figure 26.3 Landmarks for the caudal block with the child in a left lateral position.

fluid. If such reflux is noted, the needle is completely removed and the puncture started from scratch. The procedure should be abandoned if fluid is aspirated repeatedly. If the aspiration test is negative, the local anaesthetic is slowly injected into the epidural space.

Caudal anaesthesia is easier to learn than other techniques. Nevertheless venous punctures occur less frequently as the anaesthetist becomes more experienced. Caudal blocks can be performed with any needle gauges ranging from 25G in newborns to 22G in older children. Finer needles are less traumatic but may increase the risk of false-negative aspiration, venous puncture or dural tap. Short-bevelled needles can improve the sensing of membrane penetration, and they can also decrease the risk of venous puncture. Some authors prefer to use intravenous plastic cannulae, removing the stylet after membrane penetration and advancing only the blunt plastic cannula. We use the immobile needle technique as described by Winnie [15], with a flexible injection tube connected to a short-bevelled needle before puncture.

The failure rate of caudal anaesthesia is very low in infants but increases considerably in children older than 7 years [18]. Most failures occur when the sacral hiatus has not been correctly identified. Malpositioning of the needle in soft or hard tissue carries a risk of intraosseous injection and systemic toxicity. Failures in older children may also be due to fibrous septa that develop as the epidural space becomes enriched in connective fibres during childhood. These septa can give rise to unilateral or inadequate nerve blockade even if the local anaesthetic is correctly applied. The growth-related increases in size of the epidural space and in length of the spinal cord are considerable. Excessive amounts of local anaesthetics may therefore be needed to reach lumbar or thoracic levels through the caudal approach. Therefore we do not perform caudal anaesthesia in children with a body weight above 30 kg.

Catheters are rarely used at the caudal level, mainly because it is difficult to maintain sterility. Caudal anaesthesia is therefore essentially a single-shot technique. One concern is the relatively short duration of nerve blockade. The smaller the child, the shorter the duration; in newborns it is less than 2 hours [19]. In small infants, catheters are easier to insert via the caudal route than at lumbar levels. We therefore use caudal epidural catheters for major abdominal surgery in preterm neonates less than 1000 g. A 21G Tuohy needle with a 25G catheter is usually both suitable and convenient in this situation. The spread of local anaesthetic in the epidural space can be readily visualised by ultrasonography.

However, we do not normally use sonography for standard caudal blocks as the single-shot technique is neither difficult nor prone to failure. Injecting a test bolus under direct visualisation can be useful because this will reliably indicate whether the cannula has been correctly placed [20]. It is hardly ever useful, however, to visualise the sacral hiatus.

AWAKE CAUDAL ANAESTHESIA

Most caudal blocks are performed under general anaesthesia. Some indications can also be managed with the child awake or mildly sedated. These may include inguinal hernia repair, orthopaedic procedures on lower limbs, rectal biopsy, femoral vascular access (for central venous lines or diagnostic heart catheters) and magnetic resonance imaging (MRI).

A typical scenario would be hernia repair in premature newborns/infants who are at high risk for postoperative apnoea. According to a recent Cochrane Database report, however, there is not enough evidence to support the hypothesis that awake (caudal or spinal) regional anaesthesia decreases the incidence of postoperative apnoea in premature newborns/infants [21]. Another indication is insertion of femoral venous lines or diagnostic heart catheters. Surprisingly, awake caudal anaesthesia has been described for diagnostic brain MRI, where it can offer sedation while eliminating any need for airway management when access to the airway is limited [22].

To prepare for sedation and caudal anaesthesia, topical anaesthetic cream is applied to the venous and caudal puncture sites. Venous access is established, and the child is sedated with midazolam, $S(+)$-ketamine and/or propofol. Care must be taken to preserve spontaneous ventilation. We place children in a left lateral position (as described for caudal blocks under anaesthesia) and inject 1 mL/kg levobupivacaine 0.375 per cent. Onset time will be approximately 9 minutes; the duration of surgical anaesthesia (including motor blockade) varies from 90 minutes in babies to 180 minutes in children older than 6 months. As a rule, children under 6 months seem to sleep rather well without requiring additional sedation after caudal anaesthesia, whether as a side-effect of epidural application of local anaesthetics or because sensory afferents are blocked. Older children do not sleep and need additional sedation (e.g. propofol 6–8 mg/kg/h).

Epidural analgesia

Epidural analgesia in children was first described in 1954 but was not widely used until the late 1980s. Despite concerns about safety in anaesthetised patients, its popularity grew as Tuohy needles for paediatric use were introduced and more attention was focused on postoperative analgesia in children. Also, it was realised that dense afferent blocks might improve the outcome.

Today, the technique of epidural anaesthesia is considered safe. Children and infants (even preterm neonates) are increasingly managed in this way [7]. Epidurals minimise the use of opioids, which greatly facilitates postoperative management. The child can be extubated early, and there is less need for mechanical ventilation. There is some evidence that epidurals may improve the outcome of high-risk surgical procedures [23]. However, the current evidence is not strong enough to say the same of all major abdominal and thoracic procedures.

Epidurals can be performed at all cord levels, from thoracic downwards. Lumbar is the most popular level. We do not perform epidurals at the sacral level (the S2–3 intervertebral level), which carries a high risk of dural puncture [5,24]. For continuous postoperative epidural analgesia, catheter techniques are widely used. Bösenberg et al. [25] described a method of passing epidural catheters through the caudal route to thoracic levels. This method has not been not universally accepted, as it is time-consuming, and correct positioning of the catheter is often difficult to achieve.

Large case series have shown that epidurals at lumbar and thoracic levels are feasible in children [5,7]. Nevertheless, there is every reason to be cautious because the dura is closer to the spinal cord in children. Children under 6 months are particularly challenging. We wish to emphasise that epidural catheters in infants should be placed only by experienced paediatric anaesthetists who have undergone special training and developed appropriate manual skills. Well-trained personnel are needed for postoperative catheter management to protect the child against avoidable complications [5].

CONVENTIONAL TECHNIQUE

After induction of anaesthesia, the child is placed in a lateral position with knees, hips and spine flexed. To minimise the dose of local anaesthetic, the tip of the epidural catheter is placed close to the median dermatome at the surgical site. After identification of the appropriate spinous interspace and aseptic preparation, a small skin incision is made to facilitate insertion of a Tuohy needle. The needle is advanced through the skin and the stylet removed. Then a loss-of-resistance syringe filled with saline is attached and the needle is passed through the supraspinous and interspinous ligaments and ligamentum flavum.

Children usually have softer ligaments than adults and there is less scope for error. The main problem with the lateral body position is to remain in the median plane. Usually there is no need to select an oblique paramedian approach.

Rare exceptions are children with extreme scoliosis or vertebral malformation. Loss of resistance to saline is the most appropriate way to identify the epidural space. This will avoid complications such as venous air emboli, pneumoencephalos, neural compression or patchy analgesia. Saline will also eliminate the risk of temporary neurological deficits caused by subarachnoid injection of air. Any of these complications can be exacerbated by concurrent use of nitrous oxide.

The Tuohy needle is carefully advanced through the ligamentum flavum with constant pressure on the plunger of the syringe. At lumbar levels, the needle is introduced perpendicular to the skin. At thoracic levels, the needle has to be oriented at a rostal angle of 45–60° because spinous processes have a caudal slope. On sensing loss of resistance, 0.2–0.4 mL saline/kg body weight is injected to expand the epidural space. This will assist in placing the catheter, which may be difficult because the epidural space is very small in children. In infants under 6 months, it is only about 2 mm in diameter [26]. Dilution of the local anaesthetic is a disadvantage of saline injection to expand the space. It is appropriate to wait before retracting the needle, thus allowing the fluid to disperse and any reflux to settle. Not infrequently, saline will be leaking from the Tuohy needle, which creates a moment of uncertainty as to whether the dura may have been punctured. If it has not, the leakage will be brief and self-limiting.

At lumbar levels, body weight may relate to the depth of the epidural space (1 mm/kg body weight is a useful rule of thumb between the ages of 6 months and 10 years) [13,27]. Any needle positions significantly deeper than that should be regarded as an indication that the insertion angle is incorrect or that the needle has strayed from the midline.

At thoracic levels, the depth of the epidural space is less well investigated and is also complicated by the oblique insertion path. By the time of catheter placement, the depth of the epidural space should be known because it has been identified in the process of inserting the needle.

The catheter is advanced 1.5–3 cm into the epidural space. To avoid kinking at the skin, it is secured with a transparent occlusive dressing over a pre-cut gauze swab. Careful fixation is mandatory because catheters are prone to complications such as leakage, kinking or accidental removal. Leakage of local anaesthetic at the site of catheterisation is common when the epidural space is located less than 1 cm from the skin in small infants and it is not necessary to remove the catheter in this situation. Our policy is to maintain epidural analgesia for 72 hours after major surgical procedures in the chest or abdomen. The catheter must be checked by experienced personnel daily.

ULTRASOUND-GUIDED TECHNIQUE

Neuraxial imaging accelerates catheter placement and avoids bone contacts [12]. Visualising the epidural spread of local anaesthetic will reliably disclose the position of the needle and catheter. The child is placed in the same lateral position that is also used for the conventional technique. Both the puncture site and the ultrasound probe have to be aseptically prepared. A linear high-resolution probe (5–10 MHz) is used for ultrasound imaging. Hockey-stick probes are favourable in small children because they require less space.

The probe is applied in such a way that a paramedian and a longitudinal view are obtained. With this technique, the dura can be better visualised than the ligamentum flavum (Fig. 26.4). Therefore the anaesthetist should mainly rely on the dura as reference structure for the epidural puncture. Neuraxial structures are less well visible in ultrasound images of older children. The relative visibility of dura (at lumbar and thoracic levels) varies with age and body weight. It is excellent in newborns but decreases considerably in children older than 3 years (Table 26.2) [12]. We do not use ultrasonography for epidural puncture in patients older than 8 years.

Once the dura has been identified, the needle is inserted medial to the ultrasound probe. With this ultrasound technique, it is simple to assess the depth of the epidural space before puncture. The anaesthetist can therefore see at an early stage if the insertion angle is wrong or if the needle deviates from the midline. The needle can actually be visualised throughout the entire procedure in experienced hands. This helps to avoid complications such as dural tap.

As well as on ultrasound, this guidance technique for epidural punctures also relies on loss of resistance (which is in contrast to peripheral blocks). Thus objective visualisation of the target structure is combined with the tactile sensation of penetrating the ligamentum flavum. The imaging

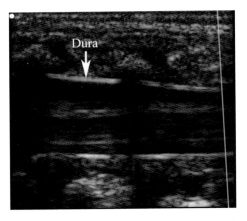

Figure 26.4 Ultrasonographic view of neuraxial structures with a 10 MHz linear probe in a 1-month-old baby. Below the dura is a hypoechoic area (subarachnoid space) and parallel horizontal lines (cauda equina) (left = cranial; depth of the figure = 15 mm).

Table 26.2 Neuraxial imaging by age groups

Age (months)	Weight (kg)	Visibility of dura (%)	
		Lumbar	Thoracic
0–3	4.1 ± 1.3	80 ± 14	70 ± 32
4–14	10.9 ± 2.5	58 ± 15	23 ± 13
15–35	14.0 ± 2.0	41 ± 13	29 ± 13
36–94	19.7 ± 2.8	30 ± 17	21 ± 13

technique will capture both the spread of the infused substance and the downward movement of the dura, which is the main criterion of correct needle positioning.

After passing the catheter (same technique as used without ultrasound guidance), its correct position is confirmed by visualising the spread of levobupivacaine injected through it. Finally it is fixed as described above.

Direct visualisation of the catheter is normally impeded by physical constraints, but the position of the catheter inside the epidural space can be verified perfectly well by monitoring the spread of local anaesthetic and subsequent downward movement of the dura.

Spinal anaesthesia

Techniques of spinal anaesthesia are not commonly used in children [5], although there are exceptions [28]. They offer good haemodynamic stability and a low incidence of headaches after dural puncture especially in small children. Furthermore, effective blockade can be achieved with minimal doses of local anaesthetics. The shorter duration of spinal blocks requires careful planning of postoperative analgesia. The technique itself is somewhat more demanding than caudal anaesthesia and involves a considerable failure rate even in the hands of experienced anaesthetists.

Spinal anaesthesia has been claimed to reduce the risk of postoperative apnoea that is associated with general anaesthesia in premature newborns/infants. Caudal blocks are a good alternative in this situation and are easier to perform. The same can be said of all indications for spinal anaesthesia. We abandoned spinals for routine use when ropivacaine and levobupivacaine became available, because the properties of these drugs rendered the higher doses needed for caudal blocks acceptable. More importantly, the consequences of inadvertently puncturing the spinal cord are severe.

TECHNIQUE

The child is placed in a lateral or sitting position. An experienced assistant is needed to look after the airway during the procedure. After aseptic preparation and infiltration of the skin with local anaesthetic, the dura is punctured between L4 and L5. Alternative levels are L3–4 or L5–S1. The needle is introduced perpendicular to the skin in what is basically a lumbar puncture technique. It is carefully advanced through the interspinous ligament and ligamentum flavum. Finally the dura mater is penetrated. Freely flowing cerebrospinal fluid indicates that the position of the needle is correct. After the local anaesthetic (levobupivacaine 0.5 per cent) has been slowly injected, the child is placed in the surgical position. Tilted and head-down positions must not be used.

These punctures should be performed with 24/25G spinal needles featuring a pencil-point design in children. In infants and young children, they should be 3.5 or 5 cm long. The standard 10 cm design may be indicated in older children and adolescents. Other needle types can be used

but should feature a stylet to prevent contamination of the subarachnoid space with soft-tissue cells. Hollow hypo dermic needles should be avoided for this reason.

Some authors have described a technique of continuous aspiration through a transparent extension line connected to the spinal needle. Our own preference is to remove the stylet after dural puncture and to check for freely flowing cerebrospinal fluid in the transparent plastic hub.

Recommendations

Recommendations for local anaesthetics and additives for central blocks are given in Addendum 26.1.

PARAVERTEBRAL BLOCKS

Access to the paravertebral space for nerve blockade is confined to the T1–12 levels. This approach can be used to establish nerve blockade for any type of surgery involving a unilateral thoracoabdominal incision. Examples include thoracotomy, breast surgery, subcostal abdominal incisions, renal surgery and appendectomy. It can also be successfully used for unilateral multiple rib fractures.

Two reports from the early 1990s described techniques in which this space was used for anaesthesia in children. Eng and Sabanathan [29] placed catheters in the paravertebral space of children for thoracic surgery. Lönnqvist used a modified Eason–Wyatt technique to cannulate the paravertebral space in children prior to surgical procedures [30]. Paravertebral blocks are currently at an early stage of investigation for postoperative pain relief following ductus ligation in premature children using a single-shot technique and for postoperative analgesia after congenital diaphragmatic hernia repair.

Regional anaesthesia through the paravertebral route offers a number of advantages over epidural anaesthesia performed at thoracic or lumbar levels. Sensory blockade remains confined to the surgical region and afferent blockade is more complete. Paravertebral blocks carry no risk of lower-limb weakness or paralysis; moreover, the absence of urinary retention eliminates the need for routine urinary catheterisation. In contrast to thoracic epidurals, there is no risk of accidental damage to the spinal cord. Sympathetic blockade is limited but does include the sympathetic chain, which is in contrast to epidural blocks, and there is no risk of blocking the cardio-accelerator fibres in a significant way. Consequently, paravertebral blocks provide good haemo dynamic stability. Coagulopathies are not an absolute contraindication to paravertebral blocks.

In a mixed population of 367 adults and children, the failure rate of paravertebral blocks was found to be 10 per cent [31]. Complications in that study included hypotension in 5 per cent of patients (all of whom were adults). Vascular puncture occurred in 4 per cent, inadvertent pleural puncture in 1 per cent and pneumothorax in 0.5 per cent of cases.

Paravertebral blocks were compared with lumbar epidurals for renal surgery in children [32]. This study showed that fewer patients required supplementary analgesics when managed by paravertebral block. Morphine consumption was also lower in that group. Good preliminary findings have recently also been reported from other European centres [33].

Anatomy

The paravertebral space is sealed off by the psoas muscle below the T12 level [34]. At the upper thoracic levels, paravertebral blocks can cause Horner's syndrome, so the space appears to communicate with fascial planes in the neck. Also, the various thoracic segments of the paravertebral space communicate with each other. Local anaesthetics will therefore spread to multiple segments upon injection [35]. The paravertebral space is limited by the vertebral body and disc medially, by the transverse process and costotransverse ligament dorsally, and by the parietal pleura anterolaterally (Fig. 26.5). Significant structures passing through the paravertebral space include the spinal nerve root and intercostal nerve, the sympathetic chain and the intercostal vessels. The pleura is very adhesive to the other structures, so there is some resistance to the introduction of a percutaneous catheter.

Technique

The puncture is conducted lateral to the spinous process with an appropriate Tuohy needle (20G in children under 3 years, 19G in children over 3 years) oriented perpendicular to the skin. The puncture level should be T5–6 for thoracotomy and T9–10 for renal surgery. The needle is advanced until contact with the transverse process is established and is then slowly moved above or below the process. A loss-of-resistance technique is used to pierce the costotransverse ligament and identify the paravertebral space. Then a catheter is inserted approximately 2 cm into the

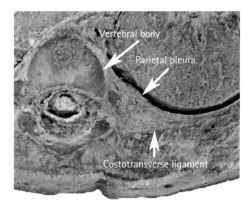

Figure 26.5 Transverse view of the paravertebral space at the T6 level. The paravertebral space shows a triangular form between the vertebral body, the parietal pleura and the costotransverse ligament.

space. Some manipulation of the Tuohy needle may be required before the catheter can be successfully inserted.

The lateral distance of the puncture site to the spinal process can be estimated by the formula $0.12 \times kg + 10.2 =$ distance in millimetres [36]. The distance from the skin surface to the paravertebral space can be estimated by the formula $0.53 \times kg + 21.2 =$ depth of paravertebral space in millimetres [37].

The local anaesthetic is injected after a negative aspiration test and a test dose. Bupivacaine 0.25 per cent at a dose level of 0.5 mL/kg has been shown to cover five or more segments [35]. After this bolus injection, continuous infusion is started with 0.25 mL/kg/hour of the same local anaesthetic solution and can be carried on for approximately 48 hours [38]. Blocks of this kind will typically cover the trunk unilaterally from the T4 to the T12 level [35].

SELECTIVE LIMB BLOCKS

Regional anaesthesia is a viable option for all types of arm surgery. Sometimes a brachial plexus catheter may be indicated for continuous analgesia and sympathetic blockade. Upper-limb blocks have never enjoyed widespread popularity in children, and, while there are no obvious reasons for this reluctance, lack of skills is certainly part of the explanation. It is difficult to collect experience with techniques not commonly used or extensively investigated; the technique may be underused because it is underreported.

The point of access to the brachial plexus depends mainly on the surgical procedure. Axillary blocks are suitable for any forearm interventions. Periclavicular blocks can be used to cover the upper arm; whether this should be infraclavicular or supraclavicular has to be decided case by case.

Peripheral nerve blocks for lower-limb procedures have not been popular in children, because caudal blocks offer an excellent alternative that does not normally involve significant complications. In addition, relatively few studies are available on peripheral blocks for lower-limb surgery and the scope of the studies that are available has been largely confined to investigating various types of local anaesthetics. Nevertheless, the general principle dictating that blocks should be performed as central as necessary and as peripheral as possible implies that selective lower-limb blocks should be part of the paediatric anaesthetist's repertoire.

Most of the available data on lower-limb blocks have been collected in adults. Both the puncture techniques and the volumes of local anaesthetic to be used in children have therefore usually been derived from adults. It is clear, however, that the close anatomical relationships in children call for the development of specific puncture techniques. It is also obvious that direct visualisation of the targeted nerves along with the surrounding anatomical structures offers clear advantages over other techniques that have been described. All techniques that rely on ultrasound guidance for lower-limb nerve blockade in children described on the following pages have yielded good results in clinical practice, even though they are not all well documented in the literature at the time of writing this chapter.

General neural anatomy

For detailed anatomy of the individual nerves, see Addendum 26.2.

BRACHIAL PLEXUS

This network is formed by the anterior roots of spinal nerves at C5–T1 and supplies sensory and motor information to the upper limbs. The roots leave the spinal canal behind the vertebral artery and pass through the transverse processes of the corresponding vertebral body. Beginning at this level, they form a superior (C5–6), intermediate (C7) and inferior (C8–T1) trunk. They then enter the posterior interscalene groove between the anterior and middle scalene muscles. Above the clavicle, each trunk divides into an anterior and posterior branch. (The subclavian artery enters the brachial plexus at the level of the first rib. Directly above the clavicle, the entire brachial plexus is lateral to the artery.)

The peripheral nerves emerge from the fascicles that are formed as these branches join in various ways at the level of the first rib. A lateral fascicle is formed by the anterior portions of the superior and middle trunks, a medial fascicle by the anterior portion of the inferior trunk and a posterior fascicle by the posterior portions of all three trunks. Note that the nomenclature for these fascicles (lateral, medial and posterior) applies to the axillary level only. Their respective positions are different directly below the clavicle (ventral, medial and inferior).

The brachial plexus is covered by connective tissue from its origin down to the axillary level. Septa formed by this connective tissue inside the plexus are apparently responsible for incomplete nerve blockade, particularly at the axillary level [39]. These septa are known to exist in adults but have never been investigated in children.

LUMBOSACRAL PLEXUS

This plexus extends through levels T12/L1–S3/4 and supplies sensory and motor information to the lower limbs. The lumbar plexus is formed by the ventral roots of spinal nerves T12/L1–4. It passes through the psoas muscle ventral to the transverse processes of the lumbar vertebrae. The iliohypogastric, ilioinguinal, genitofemoral and lateral femoral cutaneous nerves leave the plexus at a proximal level. The femoral nerve passes to the inguinal region between the greater psoas muscle and the quadratus lumborum and iliac muscles. Then it extends to the thigh lateral to the femoral artery. The sacral plexus is formed by fibres of the L4–5 and S1–4 cord segments. It crosses the greater sciatic foramen and divides at that level into a portion crossing the suprapiriformic part (gluteus superior nerve) and a larger portion crossing the infrapiriformic part (sciatic, posterior femoral cutaneous and gluteus inferior nerves). Only the sciatic and posterior femoral cutaneous nerves are relevant for regional anaesthesia.

Techniques and access routes

SUPRACLAVICULAR APPROACHES TO THE BRACHIAL PLEXUS

These approaches are indicated for upper-arm procedures, and they are well suited to continuous techniques. Paediatric applications have been reported [40]. Ultrasonography should be used as there is a considerable risk of puncturing the cervical pleura. Because of this hazard, the supraclaviciuar approach is used only when the plexus cannot be adequately visualised from an infraclavicular angle. Note, however, that this approach requires substantial experience.

INFRACLAVICULAR APPROACHES TO THE BRACHIAL PLEXUS

These techniques are indicated for surgical procedures above the elbow. They can also be used for forearm and hand procedures when the axillary approach is too painful. Caution should be exercised in the use of nerve stimulators for infraclavicular block techniques, despite some favourable reports [41,42]. Vertical approaches to infraclavicular plexus blockade carry a risk of piercing the cervical pleura if the needle penetrates halfway between the jugular incisure and the acromion [43]. These popular techniques are therefore not recommended.

Anatomy

The three fascicles enter the infraclavicular region at the clavipectoral trigonum lateral to the axillary artery and vein. The distance between the brachial plexus and the cervical pleura is very small in their median infraclavicular position (Fig. 26.6) and then increases in a lateral direction.

Conventional techniques

Fleischmann et al. [41] compared a lateral approach below the level of the coracoid process with an axillary approach under nerve stimulation. Nerve blockade was more effective with the infraclavicular technique. This applied to both sensory (musculocutaneous, axillary and medial brachial cutaneous nerves) and motor (musculocutaneous and axillary nerves) parameters. All infraclavicular blocks, but only 80 per cent of axillary blocks, were successful based on Vester-Andersen's criteria. The technique itself is relatively simple. A 40 mm facet needle is sagittally inserted to 0.5–1 cm below the coracoid process under peripheral muscle stimulation (Fig. 26.7). Slight repositioning in a cranial or caudal direction may be required.

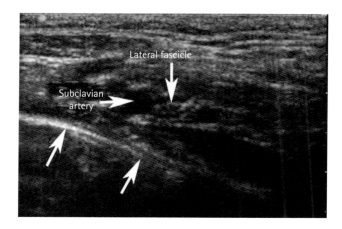

Figure 26.6 Lateral fascicle in the infraclavicular region; arrows indicate the cervical pleura (left side = medial, depth of the nerve structures = 11m).

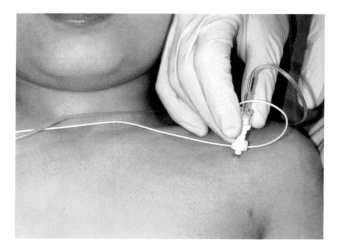

Figure 26.7 Nerve stimulator-guided lateral infraclavicular approach 0.5 cm caudal to the coracoid process.

Ultrasound-guided technique

Even though the results with nerve stimulation had been excellent, they could be improved further by using ultrasound guidance for lateral infraclavicular blockade in alert or mildly sedated children [44]. Mean onset times of sensory and motor blockade were reduced from 15 to 9 minutes. Mean block durations were extended by 1 hour. Perhaps more importantly, better visual analogue scores were obtained because muscle contractions as triggered by nerve stimulation were not present.

A 5–10 MHz linear ultrasound probe is advanced to the subclavian artery in the infraclavicular region. Note that the artery must be visualised as a round structure. The position of the brachial plexus is lateral to the artery. Its individual fascicles are difficult to spot. The lateral fascicle is usually identified first. Its location is the most ventro-medial relative to the posterior fascicle in this area. The brachial plexus will descend as the structures are laterally tracked to the medial border of the coracoid process. The pleura moves away in the process, and the nerve structures

become less visible as the high frequencies are cancelled by overlapping (major and minor pectoral) muscle structures.

The puncture site should coincide with the best attainable view of all anatomical structures. The needle is inserted along the short axis either below (see Fig. 26.2) or above the transducer. It is advanced to a point around the lateral or medial fascicle, where its tip is lateral to the subclavian artery. Puncturing below the transducer is easier since the clavicle is located above the transducer. The needle is advanced towards the pleura. Great care and tactile sensitivity are required to position the needle correctly. This technique is not strictly vertical. In very small children, the brachial plexus may be close to the pleura, even when the lateral infraclavicular approach is used.

The needle does not usually have to be repositioned because the spread of local anaesthetic will normally cover the artery. Therefore this approach is essentially a single-shot technique and differs in this respect from the axillary approach. Sometimes the local anaesthetic will not immediately spread as desired. After all, it has to pass through several muscle and fascia layers on its way to the plexus. Maldistribution usually occurs cranial to the plexus with the needle tip in a wrong layer. However, it will take only 0.2–0.3 mL of local anaesthetic to recognise the mistake. The needle is then advanced deeper. Placing the needle correctly is not always simple because the fasciae are very elastic in children. A good deal of experience will be required to implement the block quickly and safely nevertheless.

In our original study, we used a dose level of 0.5 mL/kg for this ultrasound-guided technique [44]. Recently we have reduced the dose to 0.3–0.4 mL/kg. Note that other block procedures can be optimised by reducing the volume to a minimum level at which the targeted nerve structures are fully covered with local anaesthetic. The infraclavicular technique, by contrast, requires a predefined volume of local anaesthetic because it is impossible to visualise all infraclavicular fascicles in a single ultrasound section. Therefore the overall distribution of local anaesthetic (including to the posterior and medial fascicles) cannot be visualised at a glance but requires careful repositioning of the ultrasound probe during injection.

AXILLARY APPROACHES TO THE BRACHIAL PLEXUS

Axillary approaches to the brachial plexus are indicated for surgical procedures below the cubital fossa. Treatment of forearm ischaemia is another indication [45]. Axillary approaches are easily the most common technique of brachial plexus blockade. Most anaesthetists are experienced with this method, and potential complications, such as intravascular puncture, can be easily managed. On the down-side, axillary nerve blocks are often incomplete and require painful arm positioning in the presence of fractures. An infraclavicular approach should be selected if this arm position is excessively painful.

Anatomy

The peripheral nerves are already present in the region where axillary blocks are performed. They surround the axillary artery. The musculocutaneous nerve, which originates from the lateral fascicle, is located between the short head of the biceps and the coracobrachial muscles. In smaller children, the musculocutaneous nerve may be close to the axillary artery and close to the median nerve along its further route.

Conventional technique

Interestingly, this technique has scarcely been reported in great detail, even though it is commonly used. Fisher *et al.* [46] advanced the needle tangentially to the neurovascular sheath very close to the chest area. They exclusively relied on a fascial click to ascertain the position of the needle. The mean volume of local anaesthetic was relatively large at 0.55 mL/kg. Supplemental simple analgesics had to be administered in 46 per cent of children. Jöhr [47] recommended a dose level of 0.75 mL/kg to be injected perivascularly in children under 8 years in what was also a blind approach. He mentioned additional indications of appropriate needle positioning, such as pulsation of the needle and a spindle-type distribution pattern of local anaesthetic. In larger children, he advocated the use of a nerve stimulator. Carre *et al.* [48] investigated the difference between single and multiple injections for axial plexus anaesthesia. With the aid of a nerve stimulator, they advanced the needle to either one or two nerves and injected 0.5 mL/kg of local anaesthetic. The success rate was better on multiple injections. The results are nevertheless disappointing because 34 and 26 per cent of sensory blocks were incomplete after single and multiple injections, respectively. Even worse, motor blockade was incomplete in 51 and 54 per cent of cases, respectively.

Ultrasound-guided technique

The local anaesthetic must be injected only after all relevant nerve structures (radial, median, ulnar and musculocutaneous nerves) have been clearly identified in the ultrasound image (Fig. 26.8). The first attempt is rarely successful. Usually the structures need to be tracked in a distal direction to be clearly identified. In doing so, the median nerve will always remain close to the artery. The ulnar nerve will always remain close to the surface on its way to the ulnar nerve sulcus. The radial nerve will quickly move deeper into the radial nerve sulcus.

Note that the ultrasound probe must be perpendicular to the body axis. The upper arm is optimally positioned for axillary blocks when it is in 90° abduction. As a result, caudal is on the right and cranial on the left of the image (Fig. 26.8). The needle orientation relative to the ultrasound probe is illustrated in Fig. 26.9. The puncture must be placed in the lower third near the distal end of the probe, such that all targeted nerves are easily accessible while the vessels remain protected. Unless the pressure exerted by the probe is very light, the venous vessels will be compressed and can no longer be visualised. Excessive pressure can also

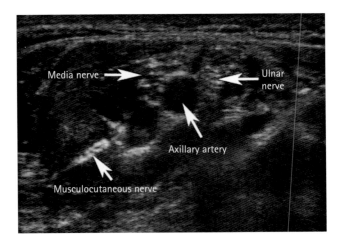

Figure 26.8 Ultrasonographic view of the axillary brachial plexus. The radial nerve is not visible in this transverse view (left side = cranial).

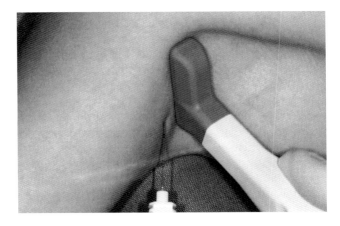

Figure 26.9 Needle orientation (transverse technique) for the ultrasonographic guided, axillary brachial plexus approach.

distort the positional relationships between nerves, as well as between nerves and vessels.

The radial nerve is routinely blocked first. It can always be found dorsal to the axillary artery. Then the needle is repositioned to block the ulnar and median nerves. These can be found superficial to the axillary artery. The musculocutaneous nerve has to be blocked separately in cases of early division from the lateral fascicle. It branches off the lateral fascicle and is commonly located between the short head of the biceps muscle and the coracobrachial muscle. In very small children, it may be close enough to the median nerve to be effectively blocked by the volume that has been injected for that nerve. Occasionally this effect is even seen in larger children.

The brachial cutaneous and medial antebrachial nerves can rarely be visualised directly in the ultrasound image because they are embedded in a fascial layer cranial to the rest of the brachial plexus. The medial antebrachial nerve branches off the medial fascicle. It is recommended that these nerves are blocked separately. Sometimes they can be visualised after puncturing the fascia and injecting 0.5 mL of local anaesthetic. However, the local anaesthetic can be expected to diffuse into this fascial space in very small children. The axillary nerve can be visualised medial to the humerus, close to the humeral circumflex artery. However, it is uncommon to block this nerve through axillary approaches to the brachial plexus. If its blockade is specifically required, a periclavicular approach should be used instead.

Our policy is to reduce the amount of local anaesthetic to the minimum level necessary for effective blockade; a volume of 0.2–0.3 mL/kg will normally suffice. The axillary route is basically suitable for catheter techniques although these catheters are difficult to stabilise especially in very small children. We therefore exclusively use the supraclavicular route for catheters.

Lower-limb blocks

FEMORAL NERVE (3-IN-1) BLOCK

This technique is used to block the femoral, obturator and lateral femoral cutaneous nerves simultaneously. Indications include all surgical procedures in sensory innervation areas of these three nerves. Combined with a sciatic nerve block, all surgical interventions in one lower limb can be covered.

Winnie et al. [49] first described a technique of inguinal perivascular three-in-one blockade in 1973. Whether this technique was really capable of blocking all three nerves was heavily debated for some time. Another controversial topic was the distribution of local anaesthetic. The original assumption had been that the local anaesthetic would spread from the inguinal puncture site proximally to the lumbar plexus along a muscle-fascia sheath. An MRI study demonstrated that this was clearly not the case [50]; the local anaesthetic was shown to spread in a lateral and medial direction only. Therefore smaller dose levels were required than had been previously assumed.

Our study group presented the first report on ultrasound guidance for 3-in-1 blocks in adults [51]. We also demonstrated that the quality of sensory blockade depends not so much on the volume of local anaesthetic as on the puncture technique [52]. What really matters is whether ultrasonography or nerve stimulation is used for guidance. As a consequence, the technique was also adopted for paediatric use because it is desirable to obtain effective nerve blockade with small amounts of local anaesthetic in children.

Anatomy

The femoral nerve passes below the inguinal ligament lateral to the femoral artery. Then it separates into several motor and sensory branches. The lateral femoral cutaneous nerve passes somewhat medial to the anterosuperior iliac spine in a distal direction. The obturator nerve crosses through the obturator foramen to the medial thigh.

Conventional technique

The 3-in-1 technique is relatively well documented for diagnostic muscle biopsies taken in children with suspected

malignant hyperthermia or neuromuscular disease [53–55]. Various authors have used single-shot or continuous techniques for perioperative analgesia in the treatment of femoral fractures [56–60]. Quite respectable success rates of up to 96 per cent have been achieved [57].

Initially, palpate the femoral artery. Note that the femoral nerve is located close to the artery. The puncture site should be slightly distal to the inguinal ligament. The needle is oriented cranially at an angle of 30°. Two fascial clicks will be noted as the needle penetrates the fascia lata and iliopectineal arch. The femoral nerve can be selectively blocked by 0.3 mL/kg local anaesthetic. A dose level of 0.5 mL/kg will additionally cover the lateral femoral cutaneous nerve and the anterior branch of the obturator nerve.

Ultrasound-guided technique

Ultrasonography offers a number of advantages over nerve stimulation for 3-in-1 blocks. The required volumes of local anaesthetic can be reduced and this implies that combined nerve blocks can be performed more safely. Femoral shaft fractures come to mind but, since the femoral shaft falls into the sensory distribution areas of the femoral and sciatic nerves, this latter nerve should be additionally blocked for fully effective analgesia. Direct visualisation is useful in itself because there is always a chance of nerve injury during puncture, and superficial nerves, such as the femoral, are especially at risk and so is the femoral artery, given its close proximity. Sonographic imaging creates an opportunity to direct the local anaesthetic laterally and medially for true 3-in-1 blockade. The femoral nerve can also be blocked selectively by reducing the amount of local anaesthetic.

A high-frequency ultrasound probe is advanced to a point immediately distal to the inguinal ligament where the femoral artery and nerve can be visualised (Fig. 26.10). The position of the nerve is lateral to the artery. The transducer is normally heavy enough to compress the femoral vein medial to the artery. The space between the artery and the nerve is occupied by the iliopectineal fascia, which is the deep folium of the inguinal ligament. The nerve is usually close to the skin, it separates into its distal branches nearby and should therefore be visualised close to the inguinal ligament. As in most peripheral blocks, the puncture is executed crosswise

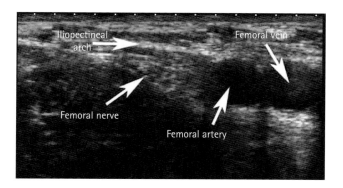

Figure 26.10 Ultrasonographic view of the femoral nerve and the femoral vessels in the inguinal area (left side = lateral).

to the transducer. The needle can be placed either lateral or medial to the femoral nerve. Since the nerve is so close to the artery, the needle must be carefully advanced if placed medially. The lateral alternative is safer. The volume of local anaesthetic injected depends on how many nerves are targeted. For selective blockade of the femoral nerve, it should just cover the surface. Complete 3-in-1 blocks require larger volumes and the local anaesthetic must visibly spread in a lateral and medial direction. Note that only the anterior ramus of the obturator nerve is blocked as a general rule; thus the 3-in-1 block is really a '2.5-in-1' block! The lateral femoral cutaneous nerve can be blocked only in larger children and with the help of a high-resolution transducer. The obturator nerve cannot normally be visualised because it is interposed between the adductor muscles, and both branches are very thin. Consequently, the anaesthetist has to rely on the lateral and medial distribution pattern of the local anaesthetic to target the obturator nerve.

Ultrasound-guided continuous technique (Fig. 26.11)

Continuous 3-in-1 blocks work very well, and have been described with conventional techniques of needle guidance [58,59]. The procedure for inserting the needle and injecting the local anaesthetic is identical to the single-shot approach, but subsequently the catheter is placed under sonographic monitoring below the iliopectineal fascia. The same approach can also be used to block the femoral nerve selectively. Most procedures are carried out without seeing the catheter directly, but a small test volume of local anaesthetic will reveal the spread direction and whether successful blockade can be expected if the position of the catheter is maintained. For selective blockade, 0.1–0.2 mL/kg of local anaesthetic in low concentration can be applied continuously right from the start. The recommended procedure for 3-in-1 blockade is to apply an initial bolus, but low concentrations of long-acting drugs, such as levobupivacaine 0.125 per cent or ropivacaine 0.2 per cent, twice daily will usually suffice. The bolus can be

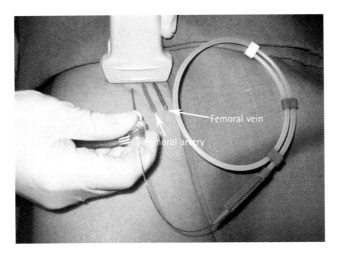

Figure 26.11 Ultrasonographic guided 3-in-1 catheter placement.

applied under direct visualisation to verify the position of the catheter.

NON-LIMB PERIPHERAL BLOCKS

A number of other peripheral blocks can be used in children. Abdominal wall blocks are useful to provide analgesia for a variety of common procedures including inguinal and umbilical hernia repair.

Current techniques for head blocks are poorly developed because they are purely based on anatomical landmarks and existing techniques have not been described in adequate detail. Efforts should be undertaken to improve this situation. A good anatomical knowledge is required to perform selective head blocks successfully and safely.

Intercostal and subcostal nerve blocks are widely used in adults. They are less popular in children, as there is an inherent risk of damaging the pleura. Sonographic guidance offers better safety. As a result, the spectrum of appropriate indications for these blocks may grow. Their full potential (e.g. for appendectomies) remains to be investigated.

Techniques and access routes

ILIOINGUINAL/ILIOHYPOGASTRIC NERVE BLOCK

This approach is indicated for surgical procedures in the inguinal region. Specific applications include herniotomy, hydrocele repair and appendectomy. It is common to block the ilioinguinal and iliohypogastric nerves jointly for procedures in regions supplied with sensory information by both nerves. The technique has been considered to offer the same effectiveness in the treatment of inguinal hernia and orchidopexy as caudal blocks [61]. The puncture for ilioinguinal/iliohypogastric is normally performed 10 mm medial to the anterosuperior iliac spine. The needle's location has traditionally been verified by a fascial click [62]. Failure rates of 20–30 per cent are the logical consequence [63]. This technique has also been reported to involve serious complications such as intestinal puncture and pelvic haematoma [64–66].

Anatomy

The anatomy of the lateral abdominal wall is rather complex. It has long been known that the positional relationships between nerves and muscles vary greatly in this region [67]. Reaching the vicinity of either nerve blind must be considered lucky rather than well done. It is definitely inappropriate to use this approach routinely. Schoor et al. [68] have clearly demonstrated this point in children. Most of the failed punctures in that study were located too far medially.

Both nerves pass through the lumbar fascia lateral to the quadratus lumborum muscle. Then they cross between the internal oblique and transversus abdominis muscles. The iliohypogastric nerve is located superior and medial to the ilioinguinal nerve. In the area of the anterosuperior iliac spine, it branches into two rami as its two terminal branches. The lateral cutaneous ramus passes through the internal oblique and external oblique muscles for sensory innervation of the anterior buttocks region. The medial cutaneous ramus crosses through the internal oblique muscle and the aponeurosis of the external oblique muscle. This ramus innervates the abdominal wall region above the symphysis. The ilioinguinal nerve supplies the skin region below the area supplied by the iliohypogastric nerve. It also supplies the anterior segments of the scrotum.

Ultrasound-guided technique

A safe and successful technique that should be adopted as standard in children was recently presented by Willschke et al. [9]. Ultrasonography should be performed with a high-frequency linear probe. The best location to visualise the ilioinguinal nerve is medial to the anterosuperior iliac spine. Our investigations have revealed a mean nerve-to-spine distance of 7 mm. The iliohypogastric nerve is located right next to the ilioinguinal nerve, the mean distance being only 3 mm. Note that, as often as not, only two muscle layers are present in the puncture area. These belong to the internal oblique and transversus abdominis muscles. The external oblique muscle is frequently only present as an aponeurosis in the puncture area. Also note that the nerves are located close to the peritoneum. The mean distance that we measured in our investigations was 3 mm (minimum 1 mm).

The needle is inserted transverse to the ultrasound probe between the internal oblique and transversus abdominis muscles (Fig. 26.12). A volume of 0.2 mL/kg will cover both nerves. This dose is considerably smaller than recommended in the literature, which makes the procedure much safer especially in infants against the background of very high serum levels reported for this technique [69]. It is seldom necessary to reposition the needle for the iliohypogastric nerve.

Combined anaesthesia consisting of inhalation anaesthesia with 1 MAC (minimum alveolar concentration) of anaesthetic gas and ultrasound-guided blockade of the ilioinguinal/iliohypogastric nerves yields a 96 per cent success rate. Complications such as intestinal puncture are avoided. The risk of accidental femoral blockade is eliminated thanks to the reduced dose level of local anaesthetic [70]. Willschke et al. [9] have clearly demonstrated that the distance between the anterosuperior iliac spine and the

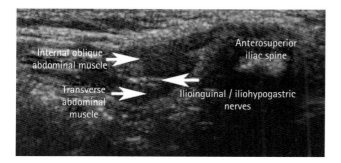

Figure 26.12   Ultrasonographic view of the ilioinguinal/iliohypogastric nerves.

ilioinguinal nerve, the depth of the ilioinguinal/iliohypogastric nerves, and the distance between the nerves and peritoneum do not correlate with parameters such as body weight or height.

RECTUS SHEATH BLOCK

This is a useful technique involving minimum doses of local anaesthetic for umbilical surgery. Indications include umbilical and paraumbilical hernia repair. Rectus sheath blocks are scarcely documented in the literature. Only small case series involving either two or four punctures are on record [71,72]. Injecting the local anaesthetic lateral to the umbilicus into the rectus abdominis muscle on both sides does not seem to be difficult. However, the nerve structures in this region are close to the peritoneal cavity. Therefore, we feel that an ultrasound-guided technique as outlined below should be used. Any blind techniques similar to those described for ilioinguinal/iliohypogastric nerve blockade would carry an excessive risk of intraperitoneal puncture.

Anatomy

The rectus abdominis muscle passes from the xiphisternum and costal cartilage down to the pubic crest. It is embedded in a fibrous sheath (linea semilunaris) formed by two aponeurotic layers of the transverse (external and internal oblique) abdominal muscles. The lateral border of the muscle-sheath complex descends from the tip of the ninth costal cartilage. The complex is anteriorly intersected by tendons at three levels: the xiphisternum, the umbilicus and midway between them. The rectus sheath is the posterior space between muscle and sheath. The ventral rami of the seventh to twelfth intercostal nerves pass anterior and downwards from the intercostal space. They pierce the posterolateral aspect of the rectus sheath and cross anteriorly through the muscle to supply the adjacent skin. The seventh and eighth intercostal nerves supply the motor innervation. Sensory information around the umbilicus is supplied by nerves at levels T9–11.

Ultrasound-guided technique

The umbilical and paraumbilical area is effectively blocked by two injections lateral to the umbilicus. The local anaesthetic should be administered at a dose of 0.1 mL/kg between the muscle and posterior sheath boundary under transverse visualisation of the paraumbilical region.

PENILE NERVE BLOC\K

This approach is the method of choice for circumcisions and other glans penis interventions [73,74]. Its effectiveness in these situations is on a par with caudal blocks [75]. Another useful indication is hypospadias surgery [76]. A 90 per cent success rate can be achieved after the first 40 penile blocks [77]. Potential complications include bleeding and inadvertent administration of adrenaline [78].

Anatomy

The penis is supplied by two terminal branches of sacral plexus nerves in its dorsal area and by sensory fibres from the genitofemoral and ilioinguinal nerves. Its dorsal nerves descend from below the pubic bone and cross the subpubic space dorsoventrally. They pass into the substance of the suspensory ligament and then enter the penis below the inner surface of Buck's fascia. The dorsal nerves can be blocked inside the subpubic pyramidal space proximal to the penis. This space is limited: cranially by the perineal membrane, iliac branches of the pubic bone and the symphysis pubis; laterally and caudally by the pelvic segment of the corpora cavernosa; and ventrally by both layers of the superficial abdominal fascia (the deep layer being Scarpa's fascia).

Technique

The penis is taped to both thighs. The puncture sites are located caudal to the symphysis at 11 and 1 o'clock. A 25 mm short-bevelled needle is used. The insertion route is somewhat sloped in a caudomedial direction. A fascial click will be felt as Scarpa's fascia is penetrated. At this point, the local anaesthetic is injected. Bupivacaine or levobupivacaine (0.25 per cent) 0.1 mL/kg without adrenaline should be used. Also, we place a subcutaneous weal at the dorsal raphe of the penis. Ropivacaine should not be used to avoid vasoconstriction [79].

INFRAORBITAL NERVE BLOCK

This nerve can be blocked for pain relief after lip repair, reconstructive procedures of the nose including the septum and endoscopic sinus surgery [80–82]. Injecting the local anaesthetic directly into intraorbital or intraocular areas must be carefully avoided.

Anatomy

The infraorbital nerve is the terminal branch of the second division of the trigeminal nerve. Emerging through the infraorbital foramen in front of the maxilla, it ramifies further into an inferior palpebral, an external nasal, an internal nasal and a superior labial branch. These four branches innervate the lower eyelid, the lateroinferior nose region, the nasal vestibule and the upper lip, including the vermilion and mucosa.

Technique

According to Bösenberg, the puncture site is approximately halfway between the angle of the mouth and the palpebral fissure [83]. An intraoral access route has also been described. The infraorbital foramen is palpated and the upper lip folded back. Then a 27G needle is inserted through the maxillary vestibule roughly parallel to the second molar. After advancing the needle tip to the level of the infraorbital foramen, the region is carefully aspirated. Then 0.5–1.0 mL of local anaesthetic is injected.

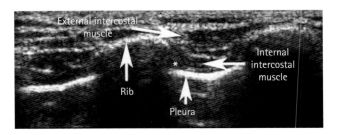

Figure 26.13 Transverse ultrasonographic view of the anatomy for the intercostal block (asterisk indicates the target for the local anaesthetic administration; left = cranial).

INTERCOSTAL AND SUBCOSTAL NERVE BLOCKS

These approaches are indicated for pain therapy after thoracotomy, rib fractures and abdominal wall surgery. Intercostal blocks should be performed only under direct visualisation in children because the risk of inadvertently puncturing the pleura is increased by the narrow anatomical relationships. The ultrasound-guided technique outlined below can reduce the resultant risk of pneumothorax.

Anatomy

The intercostal nerves are formed by the ventral rami of the spinal nerves. Their location in the dorsal chest region is at the sulcus of the ribs. Anterolaterally they are interposed between both intercostal muscle layers (internal and innermost intercostal muscles). Beginning at the posterior (nerves I–V) or anterior (nerves VI–XII) axillary line, the intercostal nerves separate into lateral cutaneous rami. They join the intercostal vessels in crossing the costal groove. A collateral nerve separates from the intercostal nerve and passes along the upper rib margin. The lateral cutaneous rami of nerves VII–XII innervate the anterior abdominal wall for motor and sensory supply.

Technique

The skin is punctured at the posterior axillary line with the child in a lateral position. A linear probe is used for sonographic visualisation. A transverse view of relevant anatomical structures is provided in Fig. 26.13. While the nerves themselves are usually too small to be visualised, they can still be blocked effectively by injecting a small volume (0.5–1 mL) of local anaesthetic between the intercostal muscles at the costal groove. A continuous technique has also been described [84]. However, more than two intercostal areas should preferably be blocked centrally with paravertebral or epidural techniques.

REFERENCES

Key references

Bösenberg AT, Bland BA, Schulte-Steinberg O *et al.* Thoracic epidural anesthesia via caudal route in infants. *Anesthesiology* 1988; **69**: 265–9.

Giaufré E, Dalens B, Gombert A. Epidemiology and morbidity of regional anesthesia in children: a one-year prospective survey of the French-Language Society of Pediatric Anesthesiologists. *Anesth Analg* 1996; **83**: 904–12.

Marhofer P, Sitzwohl C, Greher M, Kapral S. Ultrasound guidance for infraclavicular brachial plexus anaesthesia in children. *Anaesthesia* 2004; **59**: 642–6.

Puncuh F, Lampugnani E, Kokki H. Use of spinal anaesthesia in paediatric patients: a single centre experience with 1132 cases. *Paediatr Anaesth* 2004; **14**: 564–7.

Schuepfer G, Konrad C, Schmeck J *et al.* Generating a learning curve for pediatric caudal epidural blocks: an empirical evaluation of technical skills in novice and experienced anesthetists. *Reg Anesth Pain Med* 2000; **25**: 385–8.

References

1. Sze G, Baierl P, Bravo S. Evolution of the infant spinal column: evaluation with MR imaging. *Radiology* 1991; **181**: 819–27.
2. Verbout AJ. The development of the vertebral column. *Adv Anat Embryol Cell Biol* 1985; **90**: 1–122.
3. Zadra N, Giusti F. Caudal block in pediatrics. *Minerva Anestesiol* 2001; **67**: 126–31.
4. Dalens B. Acute pain in children and its treatment. *Ann Fr Anesth Reanim* 1991; **10**: 38–61
5. Giaufré E, Dalens B, Gombert A. Epidemiology and morbidity of regional anesthesia in children: a one-year prospective survey of the French-Language Society of Pediatric Anesthesiologists. *Anesth Analg* 1996; **83**: 904–12.
6. Allan CY, Jacqueline PA, Shubhda JH. Caudal epidural block versus other methods of postoperative pain relief for circumcision in boys. *Cochrane Database Syst Rev* 2003; CD003005.
7. Bösenberg AT. Epidural analgesia for major neonatal surgery. *Paediatr Anaesth* 1998; **8**: 479–83.
8. Bösenberg AT, Raw R, Boezaart AP. Surface mapping of peripheral nerves in children with a nerve stimulator. *Paediatr Anaesth* 2002; **12**: 398–403.
9. Willschke H, Marhofer P, Bösenberg AT. Ultrasonography for ilioinguinal/iliohypogastric nerve blocks in children. *Br J Anaesth* 2005; **95**: 226–30.
10. Kozek-Langenecker SA, Marhofer P, Jonas K *et al.* Cardiovascular criteria for epidural test dosing in sevoflurane- and halothane-anesthetized children. *Anesth Analg* 2000; **90**: 579–83.
11. Perillo M, Sethna NF, Berde CB. Intravenous isoproterenol as a marker for epidural test-dosing in children. *Anesth Analg* 1993; **76**: 178–81.
12. Marhofer P, Bösenberg A, Sitzwohl C *et al.* Pilot study of neuraxial imaging by ultrasound in infants and children. *Paediatr Anaesth* 2005; **15**: 671–6.
13. Willschke H, Marhofer P, Bösenberg AT. The impossibility of prediction of the depth of neonatal epidural space – proven with ultrasound. *Anesthesiology* 2005; **103**: A1379.
14. Bricker SR, McLuckie A, Nightingale DA. Gastric aspirates after trauma in children. *Anaesthesia* 1989; **44**: 721–4.
15. Winnie AP. An 'immobile needle' for nerve blocks. *Anesthesiology* 1969; **31**: 577–8.
16. Bösenberg AT, Ivani G. Regional anaesthesia – children are different. *Paediatr Anaesth* 1998; **8**: 447–50.
17. Schuepfer G, Konrad C, Schmeck J *et al.* Generating a learning curve for pediatric caudal epidural blocks: an empirical evaluation of technical skills in novice and experienced anesthetists. *Reg Anesth Pain Med* 2000; **25**: 385–8.
18. Dalens B, Hasnaoui A. Caudal anesthesia in pediatric surgery: success rate and adverse effects in 750 consecutive patients. *Anesth Analg* 1989; **68**: 83–9.
19. Jöhr M, Seiler SJ, Berger TM. Caudal anesthesia with ropivacaine in an awake 1.090-g baby. *Anesthesiology* 2000; **93**: 593.
20. Roberts SA, Guruswamy V, Galvez I. Caudal injectate can be reliably imaged using portable ultrasound – a preliminary study. *Paediatr Anaesth* 2005; **15**: 948–52.
21. Craven PD, Badawi N, Henderson-Smart DJ *et al.* Regional (spinal, epidural, caudal) versus general anaesthesia in preterm infants undergoing inguinal herniorrhaphy in early infancy. *Cochrane Database Syst Rev* 2003; CD003669.
22. Sites BD, Blike G, Cravero J *et al.* Single-dose caudal anaesthesia for two infants undergoing diagnostic brain magnetic resonance imaging: high risk and non-high risk. *Paediatr Anaesth* 2003; **13**: 171–4.
23. Meignier M, Souron R, Le Neel JC. Postoperative dorsal epidural analgesia in the child with respiratory disabilities. *Anesthesiology* 1983; **59**: 473–5.
24. Busoni P, Sarti A. Sacral intervertebral epidural block. *Anesthesiology* 1987; **67**: 993–5.
25. Bösenberg AT, Bland BA, Schulte-Steinberg O *et al.* Thoracic epidural anesthesia via caudal route in infants. *Anesthesiology* 1988; **69**: 265–9.
26. Willschke H, Marhofer P, Bösenberg AT. Ultrasound guided epidural anaesthesia in children – implementation of a new technique. *Anesthesiology* 2005; **103**: A1306.
27. Bösenberg AT, Gouws E. Skin-epidural distance in children. *Anaesthesia* 1995; **50**: 895–7.
28. Puncuh F, Lampugnani E, Kokki H. Use of spinal anaesthesia in paediatric patients: a single centre experience with 1132 cases. *Paediatr Anaesth* 2004; **14**: 564–7.
29. Eng J, Sabanathan S. Continuous paravertebral block for postthoracotomy analgesia in children. *J Pediatr Surg* 1992; **27**: 556–7.
30. Lönnqvist PA. Continuous paravertebral block in children. Initial experience. *Anaesthesia* 1992; **47**: 607–9.
31. Lönnqvist PA, MacKenzie J, Soni AK, Conacher ID. Paravertebral blockade. Failure rate and complications. *Anaesthesia* 1995; **50**: 813–5.
32. Lönnqvist PA, Olsson GL. Paravertebral vs epidural block in children. Effects on postoperative morphine requirement after renal surgery. *Acta Anaesthesiol Scand* 1994; **38**: 346–9.
33. Richardson J, Lönnqvist PA. Thoracic paravertebral block. *Br J Anaesth* 1998; **81**: 230–8.
34. Lönnqvist PA, Hildingsson U. The caudal boundary of the thoracic paravertebral space. A study in human cadavers. *Anaesthesia* 1992; **47**: 1051–2.

35. Lönnqvist PA, Hesser U. Radiological and clinical distribution of thoracic paravertebral blockade in infants and children. *Paediatr Anaesth* 1993; **3**: 83–7.

36. Lönnqvist PA, Hesser U. Location of the paravertebral space in children and adolescents in relation to surface anatomy assessed by computed tomography. *Paediatr Anaesth* 1992; **2**: 285–9.

37. Lönnqvist PA, Hesser U. Depth from the skin to the thoracic paravertebral space in infants and children. *Paediatr Anaesth* 1994; **4**: 99–100.

38. Lönnqvist PA. Plasma concentrations of lignocaine after thoracic paravertebral blockade in infants and children. *Anaesthesia* 1993; **48**: 958–60.

39. Thompson GE, Rorie DK. Functional anatomy of the brachial plexus sheaths. *Anesthesiology* 1983; **59**: 117–22.

40. Pande R, Pande M, Bhadani U *et al.* Supraclavicular brachial plexus block as a sole anaesthetic technique in children: an analysis of 200 cases. *Anaesthesia* 2000; **55**: 798–802.

41. Fleischmann E, Marhofer P, Greher M. Brachial plexus anaesthesia in children: lateral infraclavicular vs axillary approach. *Paediatr Anaesth* 2003; **13**: 103–8.

42. De Jose Maria B, Tielens LK. Vertical infraclavicular brachial plexus block in children: a preliminary study. *Paediatr Anaesth* 2004; **14**: 931–5.

43. Greher M, Retzl G, Niel P. Ultrasonographic assessment of topographic anatomy in volunteers suggests a modification of the infraclavicular vertical brachial plexus block. *Br J Anaesth* 2002; **88**: 632–6.

44. Marhofer P, Sitzwohl C, Greher M, Kapral S. Ultrasound guidance for infraclavicular brachial plexus anaesthesia in children. *Anaesthesia* 2004; **59**: 642–6.

45. Breschan C, Kraschl R, Jost R *et al.* Axillary brachial plexus block for treatment of severe forearm ischemia after arterial cannulation in an extremely low birth-weight infant. *Paediatr Anaesth* 2004; **14**: 681–4.

46. Fisher WJ, Bingham RM, Hall R. Axillary brachial plexus block for perioperative analgesia in 250 children. *Paediatr Anaesth* 1999; **9**: 435–8.

47. Jöhr M. *Axilläre Plexusanästhesie, Kinderanästhesie.* München: Jena, Urban & Fischer, 2001: 200–3.

48. Carre P, Joly A, Cluzel Field B. Axillary block in children: single or multiple injection? *Paediatr Anaesth* 2000; **10**: 35–9.

49. Winnie A, Ramamurthy S, Durrani Z. The inguinal perivascular technique of lumbar plexus anesthesia. 'The 3-in-1 block.' *Anesth Analg* 1973; **52**: 989–93.

50. Marhofer P, Nasel C, Sitzwohl C, Kapral S. Magnetic resonance imaging of the distribution of local anesthetic during the three-in-one block. *Anesth Analg* 2000; **90**: 119–24.

51. Marhofer P, Schrögendorfer K, Koinig H. Ultrasonographic guidance improves sensory block and onset time of three-in-one blocks. *Anesth Analg* 1997; **85**: 854–7.

52. Marhofer P, Schrogendorfer K, Wallner T. Ultrasonographic guidance reduces the amount of local anesthetic for 3-in-1 blocks. *Reg Anesth Pain Med* 1998; **23**: 584–8.

53. Gielen M, Viering W. Lumbar plexus block for muscle biopsy in malignant hyperthermia patients. Amide local anaesthetics may be used safely. *Acta Anaesthesiol Scand* 1986; **30**: 581–583.

54. Rosen K, Broadman LM. Anaesthesia for diagnostic muscle biopsy in an infant with Pompe's disease. *Can Anaesth Soc J* 1986; **33**: 790–4.

55. Maccani RM, Wedel DJ, Melton A, Gronert GA. Femoral and lateral femoral cutaneous nerve block for muscle biopsies in children. *Paediatr Anaesth* 1995; **5**: 223–7.

56. Rosenblatt R. Continuous femoral anesthesia for lower extremity surgery. *Anesth Analg* 1980; **59**: 631–2.

57. McNicol L. Lower limb blocks for children: lateral cutaneous and femoral nerve blocks for postoperative pain relief in paediatric patients. *Anaesthesia* 1986; **41**: 27–31.

58. Johnson C. Continuous femoral nerve blockade for analgesia in children with femoral fractures. *Anaesth Intensive Care* 1994; **22**: 281–283.

59. Tobias JD. Continuous femoral nerve block to provide analgesia following femus fracture in a paediatric ICU population. *Anaesth Intensive Care* 1994; **22**: 616–18.

60. Bösenberg A. Lower limb nerve blocks in children using unsheathed needles and a nerve stimulator. *Anaesthesia* 1995; **50**: 206–210.

61. Markham SJ, Tomlinson J, Hain WR. Ilioinguinal nerve block in children. A comparison with caudal block for intra and postoperative analgesia. *Anaesthesia* 1986; **41**: 1098–103.

62. Dalens B. Regional anesthetic techniques. In: Bissonnette B, ed. *Pediatric anesthesia – principles and techniques.* New York: McGraw Hill, 2002: 563–5.

63. Lim SL, Ng Sb A, Tan GM. Ilioinguinal and iliohypogastric nerve block revisited: single shot versus double shot technique for hernia repair in children. *Paediatr Anaesth* 2002; **12**: 255–60.

64. Jöhr M, Sossai R. Colonic puncture during ilioinguinal nerve block in a child. *Anesth Analg* 1999; **88**: 1051–2.

65. Vaisman J. Pelvic hematoma after an ilioinguinal nerve block for orchialgia. *Anesth Analg* 2001; **92**: 1048–9.

66. Amory C, Mariscal A, Guyot E. Is ilioinguinal/iliohypogastric nerve block always totally safe in children? *Paediatr Anaesth* 2003; **13**: 164–6.

67. Jamieson RW, Swigart LL, Anson BJ. Points of parietal perforation of the ilioinguinal and iliohypogastric nerves in relation to optimal sites for local anaesthesia. *Q Bull Northwest Univ Med Sch* 1952; **26**: 22–6.

68. Schoor AN, Boon JM, Bösenberg AT. Anatomical considerations of the pediatric ilioinguinal/iliohypogastric nerve block. *Paediatr Anaesth* 2005; **15**: 371–7.

69. Smith T, Moratin P, Wulf H. Smaller children have greater bupivacaine plasma concentrations after ilioinguinal block. *Br J Anaesth* 1996; **76**: 452–5.

70. Notaras MJ. Transient femoral nerve palsy complicating preoperative ilioinguinal nerve blockade inguinal for herniorrhaphy. *Br J Surg* 1995; **82**: 854.

71. Ferguson S, Thomas V, Lewis I. The rectus sheath block in paediatric anaesthesia: new indications for an old technique. *Paediatr Anaesth* 1996; **6**: 463–6.

72. Courreges P, Poddevin F, Lecoutre D. Para-umbilical block: a new concept for regional anaesthesia in children. *Paediatr Anaesth* 1997; **7**: 211–4.

73. Williamson PS, Williamson ML. Physiologic stress reduction by a local anesthetic during newborn circumcision. *Pediatrics* 1983; **71**: 36–40.

74. Fontaine P, Dittberner D, Scheltema KE. The safety of dorsal penile nerve block for neonatal circumcision. *J Fam Pract* 1994; **39**: 243–8.

75. Weksler N, Atias I, Klein M, *et al.* Is penile block better than caudal epidural block for postcircumcision analgesia? *J Anesth* 2005; **19**: 36–9.

76. Retik AB, Bauer SB, Mandell J *et al.* Management of severe hypospadias with a 2-stage repair. *J Urol* 1994; **152**: 749–51.

77. Schuepfer G, Jöhr M. Generating a learning curve for penile block in neonates, infants and children: an empirical evaluation of technical skills in novice and experienced anaesthetists. *Paediatr Anaesth* 2004; **14**: 574–8.

78. Berens R, Pontus SP, Jr. A complication associated with dorsal penile nerve block. *Reg Anesth* 1990; **15**: 309–10.

79. Burke D, Joypaul V, Thomson MF. Circumcision supplemented by dorsal penile nerve block with 0.75 per cent ropivacaine: a complication. *Reg Anesth Pain Med* 2000; **25**: 424–7.

80. Bösenberg AT, Kimble FW. Infraorbital nerve block in neonates for cleft lip repair: anatomical study and clinical application. *Br J Anaesth* 1995; **74**: 506–8.

81. Molliex S, Navez M, Baylot D *et al.* Regional anaesthesia for outpatient nasal surgery. *Br J Anaesth* 1996; **76**: 151–3.

82. Prabhu KP, Wig J, Grewal S. Bilateral infraorbital nerve block is superior to peri-incisional infiltration for analgesia after repair of cleft lip. *Scand J Plast Reconstr Surg Hand Surg* 1999; **33**: 83–7.

83. Bösenberg AT, kimble FW. Infraorbital nerve block in neonates for cleft lip repair: anatomical study and clinical application. *Br J Anaesth* 1995; **74**: 506–8.

84. Tobias JD, Martin LD, Oakes L *et al.* Postoperative analgesia following thoracotomy in children: interpleural catheters. *J Pediatr Surg* 1993; **28**: 1466–70.

ADDENDUM 26.1

Recommendations for local anaesthetics and additives for central blocks. Note that the specified block durations are only approximations and may vary widely with age.

Caudal anaesthesia with ropivacaine

- Local anaesthetic: ropivacaine 0.2 per cent
- Dose recommendation: 0.8–1.3 mL/kg
- Useful additives: clonidine 1–2µg/kg; S(+)-ketamine 0.25–0.5 mg/kg
- Onset time: 9 minutes
- Sensory block duration: 4 hours without additives, 24 hours with additives.

Caudal anaesthesia with levobupivacaine

- Local anaesthetic: levobupivacaine 0.2 per cent
- Dose recommendation: 0.5–1.0 mL/kg

- Useful additives: clonidine 1–2 µg/kg; S(+)-ketamine 0.25–0.5 mg/kg
- Onset time: 9 minutes
- Sensory block duration: 3–6 hours without additives, 24 hours with additives.

Awake caudal anaesthesia

- Local anaesthetic: levobupivacaine 0.25 per cent
- Dose recommendation: 1 mL/kg
- Onset time: 9 minutes
- Sensory and motor block duration (surgical anaesthesia): 1.5–3 hours.

Continuous epidural anaesthesia (for opioid additives and neonatal doses see Table 27.7)

LUMBAR LEVELS

- Initial bolus: levobupivacaine 0.7 mL/kg of 0.25 per cent solution
- Continuous infusion: levobupivacaine 0.1–0.4 ml/kg/h of 0.125 per cent solution
- Useful additives: clonidine 1 µg/kg/h.

THORACIC LEVELS

- Initial bolus: levobupivacaine 0.5 ml/kg of 0.25 per cent solution
- Continuous infusion: levobupivacaine 0.1–0.4 mL/kg/h of 0.125 per cent solution
- Useful additives: clonidine 1 µg/kg/h.

Spinal anaesthesia

- Local anaesthetic: levobupivacaine 0.5 per cent
- Dose recommendation: 0.3 mL basic dose plus 0.1 mL/kg body weight exceeding 2 kg
- Useful additives: none
- Onset time: 2 minutes
- Block duration: 50 minutes.

ADDENDUM 26.2

Detailed neural anatomy.

Musculocutaneous nerve (C5–7)

Selective block techniques are not used on this nerve.
Sensory distribution: radial side of forearm (lateral antebrachial cutaneous nerve).
Motor feedback: flexion at elbow (biceps brachial muscle).

Radial nerve (C5–T1)

Includes part of all three trunks of the brachial plexus. Starts at the posterior fascicle and is located behind the artery in the axillary region. Then crosses the humeral sulcus, approaching the humerus laterally halfway down the shaft. Then continues radially (lateral to the biceps tendon) to the elbow and divides there into a superficial and a deep branch.
Sensory distribution: radial side of back of hand, radial 2½ fingers.
Motor feedback: flexion at elbow, flexion/radial abduction of wrist, supination of forearm/hand, extension of fingers.

Ulnar nerve (C8–T1)

Formed by parts of the medial fascicle originating from the inferior trunk. Located medial and dorsal to the artery in the axillary region. Enters the forearm through the ulnar nerve sulcus.
Sensory distribution: ulnar palm and back of hand, ulnar 2½ fingers (dorsal) and 1½ fingers (palmar).
Motor feedback: ulnar flexion of wrist, flexion of third to fifth fingers, adduction of thumb.

Median nerve (C6–T1)

Formed by the ventral parts of all three trunks joining via the lateral and medial fascicles. Always close to the axillary/brachial artery. Usually ventral to the artery in the axillary region and medial (hence ulnar) to the artery in the cubital region. Close to the surface in the cubital region. Sometimes has a larger diameter than the artery itself.
Sensory distribution: palmar side radial 3½ fingers and corresponding palm, dorsal distal parts of radial 3 fingers.
Motor feedback: flexion at elbow, flexion and radial abduction of wrist, supination of forearm and hand, extension of fingers.

Suprascapular nerve (C5–6)

Selective block techniques are not used on this nerve.
Sensory distribution: shoulder areas.
Motor feedback: abduction and outside rotation of shoulder (supraspinatus and infraspinatus muscles).

Medial brachial cutaneous nerve (C8–T1)

Selective block techniques are not used on this nerve.
Sensory distribution: medial area of upper arm.

Medial antebrachial cutaneous nerve (C8–T1)

Selective block techniques are not used on this nerve.
Sensory distribution: ulnar side of forearm.

Iliohypogastric nerve (T12–L1)

Passes laterally from the psoas muscle through the abdominal transverse muscle.
Sensory distribution: suprapubic and ventral region of hip.

Ilioinguinal nerve (L1)

Passes through the inguinal canal and communicates with the genitofemoral nerve in one-third of cases.
Sensory distribution: proximal thigh, anterior parts of scrotum or labium.

Genitofemoral nerve (L1–2)

Divides into a genital and femoral branch. The genital nerve passes to the skin, scrotum (or labium) and adjacent thigh region.
Sensory distribution: inguinal area (femoral branch) and scrotum/labium (genital branch).

Lateral femoral cutaneous nerve (L2–3)

Above the iliac muscle. Enters the lateral thigh medial to the anterosuperior iliac spine. Continues below the inguinal ligament.
Sensory distribution: lateral thigh areas.

Obturator nerve (L2–4)

Divides from the plexus medial to the psoas muscle. Joins the obturator artery and vein in passing through the obturator canal. Separates in medial thigh to form an anterior branch (above and between the short/long adductor muscles) and a posterior branch (below the short adductor muscle).
Sensory distribution: hip joint, some medial thigh areas (anterior branch) and knee joint (posterior branch).
Motor feedback: adductor muscles.

Femoral nerve (L2–4)

Largest nerve of lumbar plexus. Arrives at anterior thigh on a route ventral to the psoas muscle, below the inguinal ligament and medial to the inguinal vessels. Then divides into several motor and sensory fibres. Its sensory end branch is the saphenous nerve. This nerve joins the artery in a distal route below the sartorius muscle. Pierces tendon of this muscle at patellar level. Joins great saphenous vein on a superficial skin route down to medial ankle and medial back of foot.
Sensory distribution: anterior thigh area, medial leg to ankle joint.
Motor feedback: quadriceps femoris muscle (patellar bounce), sartorious/pectineus muscles.

Sciatic nerve (L4–S3)

Largest nerve, has a tibial and a peroneal component. The dividing point is usually in the popliteal fossa. Leaves the small pelvis through the infrapiriformic foramen. Then takes a caudal route above the obturator, gemelli, quadratus femoral and great adductor muscles. Continues to the popliteal fossa below the long head of the biceps femoral muscle and between the adductor and flexor muscles. Arrives at the popliteal fossa between the medial and lateral flexor muscles and lateroposterior to the popliteal vessels. Separates into the tibial and peroneal nerves.

Sensory distribution of tibial nerve: lateral leg; sole; lateral heel and foot after anastomosis with communicant branch of peroneal (suralis) nerve.

Motor response of tibial nerve: toe and foot flexor muscles.

Sensory distribution of peroneal nerve: toes I and II; superficial part: dorsum of foot (except toes I and II).

Motor response of peroneal nerve: toe and foot extensor muscles.

Posterior femoral cutaneous nerve (S1–3)

Leaves pelvis through the infrapiriformic foramen together with the sciatic and gluteal inferior nerves. Has a medial position to the sciatic nerve and arrives at dorsal thigh below the greater gluteal muscle.

Sensory distribution: dorsal thigh areas.

27

Complex pain management

RICHARD F HOWARD

KEY LEARNING POINTS

- Nociception is present in children of all ages.
- Maturation of the nervous system alters the physiological response to pain in the very young.
- There may be long-term changes in nociception consequent upon untreated pain in early life.
- Pain assessment is central to improved therapy.
- Multimodal analgesia is key to effective pain control.

- A designated pain control service facilitates optimal pain management.
- Chronic pain in children most commonly follows surgery, trauma or the development of complex regional pain syndrome.
- A multidisciplinary approach is required to manage chronic pain.

INTRODUCTION

Adequate treatment of pain is an acknowledged basic human right. However, many children, especially the youngest and most immature, are potentially denied the best available treatment due to inadequate education of their caregivers. Safe pain management in children can be difficult, as significant background knowledge is required, and developmental age has a profound effect on both the processing of nociceptive information and the response to analgesia. In addition, changing body size, body composition and immaturity of excretory systems alters drug disposition, requires dosage adjustments for both size and age, and can predispose to toxicity and side-effects. Communication difficulties due to immaturity or developmental delay also influence our ability to assess pain and the response to treatment, thereby further complicating management, particularly in the very young. These factors have contributed to the frequently documented relative under-treatment of pain in children,

and have led to misunderstandings about the ability of newborn infants to feel pain.

PAIN NEUROPHYSIOLOGY

Physiologically pain is described as nociceptive, inflammatory or neuropathic, according to the underlying mechanisms involved. Nociception is the process by which the somatosensory system detects noxious, potentially tissue-damaging stimuli. If the stimulus is brief and causes little damage, then, following an initial 'alerting' painful sensation and withdrawal from the stimulus, the system resumes its resting state until further inputs provoke a response. This is known as nociception or nociceptive pain. In contrast, if the stimulus is sufficiently intense, prolonged and tissue damaging, then inflammation, a series of neurophysiological events, leads to changes in the sensitivity and functioning of the system, whereby sensory thresholds are temporarily reduced such that there is pain and tenderness both at the site of injury and in surrounding tissue.

Inflammatory pain is characterised by:

- allodynia – the sensation of pain in response to what would normally be a non-painful stimulus
- hyperalgesia – the increased pain in response to an input that would normally be painful.

Primary hyperalgesia is the term used to describe sensitivity at the site of injury which is thought to be primarily due to local events causing sensitisation of nociceptors, while secondary hyperalgesia describes increased sensitivity in the surrounding area or distant from the injury that is due to events occurring in the central nervous system (CNS).

Inflammatory pain is a normal physiological response to injury and it resolves as part of the normal healing process. In contrast, neuropathic pain, the third mechanism, is an abnormal response persisting beyond the normal expected period of healing and serving no obvious useful purpose. Both inflammatory pain and neuropathic pain share some clinical features, including spontaneous pain, allodynia and hyperalgesia, which can confound clinical differentiation. Neuropathic pain, however, usually follows direct nerve damage or damage to pain-processing areas of the spinal cord or brain. It is mechanistically distinct from inflammatory pain and is characterised by spontaneous pain, dysaesthesias, sensory deficits and involvement of the sympathetic nervous system.

Once established, neuropathic pain can be difficult to treat. It does not respond well to conventional analgesic drugs such as opioids or non-steroidal anti-inflammatory drugs (NSAIDs) and it also has an unpredictable time course and outcome. Inflammatory and neuropathic pain can coexist, particularly after extensive surgery or trauma [1]. Persistent neuropathic pain is treated with non-conventional analgesic drugs, such as anticonvulsants or antidepressants, physiotherapy and other non-pharmacological approaches, and requires specialised multidisciplinary management.

Nociceptive and inflammatory pain

Pain is detected by nociceptors which transduce mechanical, thermal or chemical inputs into electrical impulses in primary afferent nerves. Nociceptive afferents comprise low-threshold, fast-conducting, large-diameter A δ myelinated fibres and high-threshold, slower, small-diameter, unmyelinated C-fibres. Information is conveyed centrally to nociceptive-specific areas of the spinal cord within laminae I and II of the superficial dorsal horn, and to wide dynamic range neurons in lamina V. From the spinal cord it is carried to the brain in a number of parallel pathways, the principal ones being the spinothalamic and spinoparabrachial tracts. The spinothalamic pathway carries information from the superficial dorsal horn to the thalamus and somatosensory cortex, providing information contributing to the discriminatory aspects of pain.

The spinoparabrachial pathway carries information from lamina I neurons to the ventromedial thalamus, amygdala and cortical areas involved in the affective and motivational components of pain, with projections to the areas of the brain concerned with arousal and the regulation of descending pathways [2]. Descending pathways from higher centres are known to modulate pain transmission in the spinal cord by presynaptic action on primary afferents, postsynaptically on projection neurons and by effects on dorsal horn interneurons. Activity in these pathways can be facilitatory or inhibitory, depending on the circumstances, and changes in the normal balance of descending control have been implicated in a number of persistent pain states [3].

Tissue damage leads to the local release of a number of substances, such as bradykinin and other inflammatory mediators, that cause A- and C-fibre nociceptors to be sensitised. Peripheral sensitisation leads to a reduction in firing thresholds and spontaneous discharge of impulses in nociceptors, and is one of the key events of inflammatory pain and the principal mechanism of primary hyperalgesia. Sustained C-fibre inputs to the CNS following peripheral sensitisation lead to amplification of the signal in the spinal cord due to activation of N-methyl-D-aspartate (NMDA) and other receptors. Enhanced synaptic transmission, changes in gene expression and changes in modulating systems further reduce thresholds and increase neuronal activity in the spinal cord, a state known as 'central sensitisation', which will also lead to increased sensitivity peripherally at sites beyond that of the original injury (i.e. secondary hyperalgesia) [4]. As long as the injury persists, this sensitised state is maintained until healing takes place, following which activity returns to resting levels.

Nociception, and primary and secondary hyperalgesia have all been described in children, but during development there are important differences in the mechanisms and time course of many of these processes that profoundly affect the immature response to pain.

Neuropathic pain

In some circumstances, usually related to direct nerve or CNS damage, enhancement or maintenance of neuronal sensitisation can occur in the absence of ongoing inflammation. Pain generated in this way is known as neuropathic pain, and is characterised clinically as both spontaneous and stimulus-evoked pain, including mechanical or thermal allodynia, frequently accompanied by paraesthesia, painful dysaesthesias and sensory deficits. The mechanisms of neuropathic pain, although incompletely understood, are known to differ in many important respects from those in inflammatory pain, although crucially both may operate at the same time in a single patient [5]. When nerves are damaged, peripheral nociceptor sensitisation is characterised by reduced thresholds and spontaneous firing due to over-expression and transport of sodium channels in the primary afferent and dorsal horn neurons. Centrally, increased input from the periphery and release of mediator substances from spinal microglia lead to a prolonged central sensitisation, there is a reduction in inhibitory control mechanisms, and an abnormal and characteristic hypersensitive state occurs. Pathological neuroanatomical changes in neuropathic pain, including 'coupling' of sympathetic fibres with somatic afferents and 'sprouting' of non-nociceptive sensory fibres into nociceptive specific laminae of the spinal cord, contribute to this complex clinical syndrome. Although many of the functional and anatomical changes in neuropathic pain have been described, it is still not clear why some individuals develop a persistent pain state after injury whilst others do not. Again, neuropathic pain can occur in childhood, but differing epidemiology and clinical findings have shown that important age-related differences in the mechanisms, clinical picture and prognosis occur during development (see Management of chronic and long-term pain, page 413).

DEVELOPMENT OF NOCICEPTION AND THE RESPONSE TO INJURY

Nociceptive pathways are present from birth and even the most premature infant is born with the capacity to detect and respond to painful stimulation [6]. Nevertheless, CNS reorganisation and fine-tuning occur after birth and the expression of many important molecules and receptors may vary during the developmental period [7]. Structural and functional changes take place at this time, which not only affect the immediate and short-term response to pain, but may also predispose to long-term changes not seen in adulthood because the developing nervous system uses sensory inputs as 'cues' to drive normal development [8,9].

Activity in peripheral nociceptors is important for the generation of nociceptive pain, and primary and secondary hyperalgesia. The C-fibre nociceptors, although present and functional at birth, are initially incapable of evoking activity in the spinal cord or of sensitising dorsal horn neurons by repeated or sustained depolarisations. Conversely, low-threshold A β fibres, which are not nociceptive in the adult, project to nociceptive areas of the spinal cord during early postnatal development only to withdraw later as C-fibres mature. A-fibres at this stage of development are able to activate and induce 'wind-up' in secondary neurons with projections to higher centres. Probably as a result of this overlap in the termination of A- and C-fibre primary afferents in the nociceptive specific superficial dorsal horn of the spinal cord, the peripheral receptive field size of individual dorsal horn neurons is relatively larger and fields are more overlapping in the infant. This means that a given peripheral stimulus will activate many more neurons at this time and is therefore more likely to activate downstream processes.

Descending inhibitory controls and local inhibitory mechanisms in the spinal cord are also immature at birth, with the implication that normal mechanisms for modulating responses from higher centres are less effective and

therefore inputs will be transmitted with little modification in the spinal cord. Consequent upon A-fibre dominance, overlap of receptive fields and lack of descending inhibition, thresholds to sensory stimulation are lower in infancy, and this increased sensitivity is an important characteristic of the developing nociceptive system [10].

Hyperalgesia, and mechanical and thermal allodynia have been observed at all ages, although the magnitude of increased sensitivity may not always be equivalent to that seen in the adult, possibly because the system is already relatively more sensitive [9]. Using chemical models of inflammatory pain in rodents it has been found that the pattern of response differs in neonates from that in the adult, the precise mechanisms of which have been studied but as yet are not fully determined. Nevertheless, studies in humans have demonstrated that postoperative local hyperalgesia and referred visceral hyperalgesia can occur in very young infants [11], apparently responding to simple analgesics, e.g. paracetamol [12]. Sensitivity to analgesics may actually be different at this time; for example, lower doses of epidural bupivacaine and dexmedetomidine (an α_2 agonist) were able to abolish inflammatory hypersensitivity in younger neonatal rats in comparison to more mature animals [12,13]. In contrast, cyclo-oxygenase 1 (COX-1) inhibitors appear to be less effective in such models in the immature, paralleling developmental changes in expression of the enzyme after injury-induced hypersensitivity [14,15]. As A-fibre-induced 'wind-up' seems to be much more important than C-fibre effects in producing central sensitisation in young rats, and as μ-opioid receptors have been found to be expressed in far greater numbers on A-fibres early in development, this may explain why epidural morphine also showed more potent effects in infant models [16,17]. For a more detailed review, see Fitzgerald and Howard [6] and Fitzgerald [9].

Long-term consequences of early pain

Normal maturation of the somatosensory system is dependent on 'normal' sensory inputs during the developmental period which promote and sustain appropriate synaptic connections and sensory pathways [8]. Importantly, it is possible that if sensory inputs are 'abnormal', e.g. there is severe pain or nerve damage, during the developmental period or during an important stage of development then there may be persistent or long-term consequences affecting the functioning of the somatosensory system in later life [9,18].

It has been clear for some time that pain and its management in infancy may have consequences for later pain behaviour and perception, but precise effects and mechanisms have not been elucidated [18]. Studies in boys who were circumcised as neonates, with and without analgesia, have shown that the response to vaccination pain 3 months later was greater in those who did not receive analgesia [19]. Following abdominal surgery with 'effective' postoperative analgesia in the neonatal period, no such difference in response to subsequent vaccination was found in another study [20].

Premature neonates who spent time in intensive care have also been found to have altered pain responses later [21].

In the laboratory, it has also been shown that it is possible to induce long-term physical and behavioural changes following early injury. In the rat, skin wounding at birth leads to events not seen when similar wounds occur in the adult, which include local hyperinnervation and prolonged mechanical hypersensitivity for some time after the wound has apparently healed [22]. Chronic inflammation and nerve injury in the first postnatal week can permanently alter the spinal projection of peripheral nerve terminals, whereas less severe inflammation leads to temporary changes that are also not seen in the adult [23]. At the present time, the degree of injury and the extent to which analgesia can influence sensory development in human infants are not known, but it is of the utmost importance that clinicians who must manage pain in this group of patients are aware of the potential impact of untreated pain.

ASSESSMENT OF PAIN

The clinical assessment of pain is obviously central to good pain management, both for the prompt administration of analgesia and in the monitoring of treatment. As pain is fundamentally subjective in nature, self-reporting of pain, often using a scale or measurement tool such as the linear visual analogue scale (VAS, Fig. 27.1), is generally regarded as the nearest thing to a gold standard measure. Self-report tools have been adapted in order to make them easier to understand and use by children; however, using such tools still requires a degree of understanding, memory and physical capability not normally attained before 5 or 6 years of age or later. Clearly, therefore, this approach is unsuitable for younger, and especially non-verbal, children and for those with neurological deficits causing impaired cognition or communication difficulties. Pain assessment scales have been developed for use with children who are unable to self-report; generally based on observations of behaviour, physiological measurements or combinations of the two, none has emerged as clearly superior or universally applicable and consequently the most appropriate must be selected according to its characteristics, the requirements of the individual and circumstances (for a fuller discussion, see Franck *et al.* [24]).

Choosing a pain assessment tool

The vast majority of scales have been developed for use in acute pain settings. There are few that are suitable for the assessment of more long-term pain at any age, and scales reflecting modalities other than pain intensity or location, such as tools to measure the functional consequences of pain, are not widely available. Tools for routine clinical use should be practical, valid for the clinical setting for which

they are to be used and acceptable to patients, clinical staff and parents. Many of the most popular tools have been validated for specific circumstances and age groups. They should not generally be used for purposes or situations other than those for which they were developed, unless scientific validity testing has been undertaken. The UK Royal College of Nursing has produced an evidence-based guideline on the selection of assessment tools for children and it is available together with supporting documentation and an implementation guide [25]. Great Ormond Street Hospital provides a web-based guide, the 'Children's Pain Assessment Project' (available at http://www.ich.ucl.ac.uk/cpap/index.html), which includes advice and links to many relevant resources.

Acute pain assessment: self-report

Self-report using a linear VAS is generally accepted to be possible in children older than 7 or 8 years. Cognitive development sufficient to allow the reporting of the degree of pain is adequate by about 4 years. 'Child-friendly', easier-to-understand adaptations have been designed for younger children, e.g. face-type scales using easy-to-understand graphics (Fig. 27.1) or the 'oucher', which uses photographs of a child showing facial expressions of increasing pain [26–28]. These scales are generally easy to use but it is important to recognise that they may not be truly 'linear' and therefore not interchangeable or numerically directly comparable to other scales. It has been reported that affective factors determined by facial expressions chosen as 'no pain' and 'worst pain', when used as anchors in these scales, can influence their reliability; cultural factors may also influence the accuracy and use of such scales [29,30].

Behavioural and physiological measures

Observations of pain-related behaviours are considered to be one of the most reliable indirect methods of pain assessment. Combined observations coded for severity frequently include facial expression, cry, posture of body or limbs, and muscle tone. It is important to remember that behaviour changes with age and can be influenced by other factors, including hunger, anxiety, distress and the effects of drug treatments. Observers may differ in their interpretation of behaviours and, in comparison with self-report by patients, health-care workers have been shown to underestimate pain [31]. Table 27.1 shows those behaviours most closely correlated with the need for analgesia at a wide range of ages [32], while an example of a popular measurement tool, the FLACC, is shown in Fig. 27.1 [33].

Physiological observations, such as heart rate, blood pressure, sweating and hormonal responses, have all been used to assess pain, alone or in conjunction with behavioural observations. This approach is limited by the lack of

Behavioural and self-report pain measurement tools.

- ■ **Assess pain**   Using one of the following scoring systems
- ■ **Plan**   Is an intervention required if so what?
- ■ **Implement**   Implement intervention(s)
- ■ **Evaluate**   Re-score at an appropriate interval to evaluate effectiveness

FLACC   Behavioural Pain Assessment

CATEGORIES	SCORING		
	0	1	2
Face	No particular expression or smile	Occasional grimace or frown, withdrawn, disinterested	Frequent to constant quivering chin, clenched jaw
Legs	Normal position or relaxed	Uneasy, restless, tense	Kicking, or legs drawn up
Activity	Lying quietly, normal position, moves easily	Squirming, shifting back and forth, tense	Arched, rigid or jerking
Cry	No cry (awake or asleep)	Moans or whimpers, occasional complaint	Crying steadily, screams or sobs, frequent complaints
Consolability	Content, relaxed	Reassured by occasional touching, hugging or being talked to, distractible	Difficult to console or comfort

Each of the five categories: (F) Face; (L) Legs; (A) Activity; (C) Cry; (C) Consolability; is scored from 0 to 2 which results in a total score between 0 and 10

Wong & Baker   Self-report pain assessment

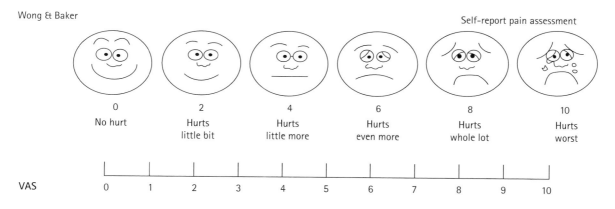

0	2	4	6	8	10
No hurt	Hurts little bit	Hurts little more	Hurts even more	Hurts whole lot	Hurts worst

VAS   0   1   2   3   4   5   6   7   8   9   10

Figure 27.1   Behavioural and self-report pain measurement tools. Adapted from Wong and Baker [26], and Merkel *et al.* [33] with permission.

sensitivity and specificity of these responses and internal homeostatic mechanisms, which tend to oppose change over time. Generally cardiorespiratory and other rapidly changing physiological variables have been used to assess brief painful episodes, such as medical procedures. Plasma and tissue levels of several hormones or their metabolites do change with pain, but, once again, often in a rather non-specific way, and fast, quantifiable, clinically useful relationships and tests have been difficult to achieve [24]. A validated measure for procedural pain in premature neonates, the PIPP (premature infant pain profile), uses a combined or 'multidimensional' approach with observations

of behaviour and simple physiological measurements in order to improve accuracy [34].

Assessment in children with neurodisability

Children with severe physical or cognitive impairment are a relatively neglected group in the field of pain assessment. Pain measurement in these children is often dependent on observational methods, and few suitable tools have been designed or validated. The PPP (Paediatric Pain Profile) has been specifically developed to assess postoperative pain in

Table 27.1 Behaviours with the highest specificity and validity for pain in children

Behavioural observation	Structure
1 Cry	None
	Moaning
	Screaming
2 Facial expression	Relaxed/smiling
	Wry mouth
	Grimace
3 Posture of the trunk	Neutral
	Variable
	Rears up
4 Posture of the legs	Neutral/relaxed
	Kicking
	Tightened
5 Motor restlessness	None
	Moderate
	Restless

Adapted from: Buttner and Fincke [32].

communication-impaired children using individual pain behaviours identified by their parents [35]. The Non-communicating Patients Pain Checklist has also been developed using a similar approach [36]. The FLACC (see Fig. 27.1) has also been validated for use in the cognitively impaired [36].

Chronic pain assessment

Assessment of long-term pain must focus not only on pain and its characteristics and intensity, but also on the effects of pain on daily activities, school attendance and relationships within and outside the family. Multidisciplinary assessment (physician, specialist physiotherapist, paediatric clinical psychologist) is frequently indicated and a full neurological examination may be required. A pain 'history' is required which should include documentation of the site or sites of pain, frequency, duration, severity, precipitating and relieving factors and functional effects. A pain diary can be helpful in evaluating pain and it should include a measure of pain intensity, such as a VAS score.

The impact of pain on daily life can be ascertained by direct questioning or, better, by the use of a validated questionnaire-type assessment that can be repeated at intervals to monitor progress; examples include the CALI interview and the Varni-Thompson questionnaire, which was originally designed for children with juvenile rheumatoid arthritis [37,38]. When neuropathic pain is present, or suspected, sensory testing should be included in the examination, while more formal quantitative sensory testing (QST) can be helpful in some cases by accurately determining the nature of sensory changes and the response to therapy [39].

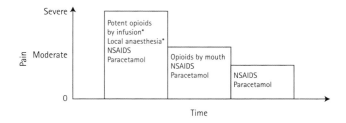

Figure 27.2 Stepwise multimodal approach to acute pain management.

PRINCIPLES OF PAIN MANAGEMENT

A multimodal approach to pain management is generally the most successful. Analgesics acting independently and synchronously on pain mechanisms at different stages of the pain pathway are likely to be more effective than a single drug and, in addition, lower doses of each agent may be necessary when combinations are used, thereby reducing side-effects and possibly accelerating recovery [40,41]. Figure 27.2 shows a stepwise multimodal approach to acute pain management; in addition, non-pharmacological pain control strategies, such as comfort measures and psychological techniques, should be incorporated whenever possible.

Analgesic plan

An analgesic plan should be formulated and discussed with children and their families prior to implementation in order to answer their questions, discuss preferences and take into account previous experience such as excessive postoperative nausea and vomiting (PONV) with opioids, acceptability of certain routes of administration or drug idiosyncrasy [42].

The following should be considered when formulating a pain management plan:

1. Availability:
   (a) Route of administration, e.g. the oral route is unlikely to be available immediately after surgery and in some cases oral intake is delayed for many hours or days
   (b) Certain analgesics or formulations are not readily available in some institutions or countries
   (c) Specialised equipment, e.g. patient-controlled analgesia (PCA) devices or monitors, must be available and suitable for use by children
2. Acceptability:
   (a) Routes of administration:
      - for example, some children will not take tablets or certain liquids; older children and teenagers may not accept rectal drug administration
      - although they may be physically capable, some children do not wish to operate a PCA device

- children or their families may have preconceptions regarding certain techniques, e.g. epidural analgesia, which should be discussed and addressed
  (b) Responsibility
    - if the plan includes out-of-hospital care, parents and children must understand their roles and be willing to undertake necessary tasks, e.g. completion of diaries, carrying out pain assessments or making dosage adjustments
3. Practicability:
  (a) Hospital facilities, staff training and skills should be adequate for safe and effective implementation of complex techniques
  (b) Developmental age influences analgesic regimens, especially during the neonatal period, and doses and frequency of administration need to be suitably modified accordingly
  (c) Treatment will have to be titrated to effect.

If these factors are taken into account, a successful, individualised plan can be developed.

Routes of administration

Decisions concerning route of administration can have an important impact on the effectiveness of pain management. Early reports highlighting inadequate pain control in children identified that the prescribing of intramuscular analgesics was a major cause of under-administration of analgesia. Because they were so disliked by children and nurses, intramuscular doses of strong analgesics were often refused or omitted. Today, intramuscular injections, because they are unpleasant, are relatively contraindicated in paediatric practice if other alternatives are suitable, even though they are clinically effective. Whenever possible, prescriptions should allow for several choices of route (e.g. paracetamol can be given orally, per rectum or intravenously).

ORAL

The oral route is always preferred over other methods. Special attention should be paid to the palatability of formulations; children can be capricious regarding the acceptability of certain flavours or may have preferences for liquid or tablet form. Analgesics may be rejected by patients and omitted by parents or nurses if alternatives are not available. Close liaison with families, a hospital pharmacist or primary care physician, together with provision of choices of analgesic formulation, will help to reduce unanticipated difficulties.

RECTAL

The rectal route is popular in paediatric acute pain practice. Advantages include ease and convenience of formulation and administration, availability when the oral route is impractical and, for paracetamol at least, relatively well investigated pharmacokinetics. Disadvantages include slow, erratic and unreliable absorption; moreover, some may find rectal administration unpleasant or unacceptable (often teenagers). It is common practice to administer rectal analgesia under general anaesthesia prior to surgery: this is usually acceptable to patients if it has been discussed beforehand.

INTRAVENOUS

Rapid onset and high efficacy have made intravenous (IV) administration of potent analgesics, especially morphine, the mainstay of the management of severe acute pain. Patient-controlled analgesia and nurse-controlled analgesia (NCA) are most commonly prescribed intravenously. More recently, IV formulations of NSAIDs and paracetamol have also become available and these are also convenient for perioperative use. Disadvantages are that it is sometimes difficult to obtain and maintain IV access in children, although this is often conveniently done under general anaesthesia prior to surgery. Special equipment and monitoring are also required and patients must be cared for in a suitable area by staff trained to manage potentially dangerous side-effects and complications.

SUBCUTANEOUS

The subcutaneous route is convenient to use and is suitable for both intermittent and continuous infusion of low volumes; subcutaneous PCA and NCA have also been described. Advantages are that subcutaneous access is much easier to establish and maintain than IV access and can last about 7–10 days before replacement is necessary. However, the pharmacokinetics of subcutaneous analgesics have not been well studied in children. Absorption seems to be rapid and predictable provided that peripheral tissue perfusion is normal at the injection site. Local anaesthetics can also be injected or infused subcutaneously close to surgical wounds, providing effective postoperative analgesia for many hours.

EPIDURAL

The epidural route has the advantage of segmental analgesia due to proximity to spinal cord pain-processing areas, extensive and profound analgesia with few systemic effects, and the possibility of long-term infusion. Postoperative epidural analgesia using local anaesthetics with or without other agents such as opioids, ketamine and clonidine is quite common practice. Limitations include impracticability of epidural placement in awake patients, failure rates of equipment, especially small catheters, and the need for special skills and training in epidural placement and subsequent management. Epidural local anaesthetics (LAs) and steroids are also used in children for nerve root compression and other neuropathic pain syndromes, such as complex regional pain syndrome (CRPS).

TRANSDERMAL AND TRANSMUCOSAL

Lipid-soluble opioids such as fentanyl and diamorphine are suitable for novel methods of administration. Oral transmucosal fentanyl citrate (OTFC) 10–20 μg/kg has been used for procedural pain, preanaesthetic medication and sedation; it is acceptable to children and effective, but side-effects of respiratory depression and nausea and vomiting can be troublesome. Transdermal fentanyl, commonly used in opioid-tolerant patients for cancer pain and long-term pain, may also be useful in acute sickle cell pain and other types of acute pain, although it has been little studied [43]. Variations in patch design from different pharmaceutical companies mean that they are not interchangeable. Intranasal diamorphine is used in the emergency room and for procedural pain in children. Topical local anaesthetics are frequently used for the pain of minor procedures, such as venepuncture or lumbar puncture, or to improve tolerability of LA nerve-blocking procedures in awake children. Recently a 5 per cent lidocaine patch, with a long duration of action, has been introduced for local neuropathic pain.

INHALATION

Nitrous oxide inhalation, usually delivered pre-mixed with oxygen (Entonox) using a demand flow system, is used extensively for the management of brief painful procedures, such as dental extraction, change of dressings after surgery or following burns, and for removal of chest drains. A free-flow system is in common use in France (Kalinox) [44]. Acceptability is good but staff training, special apparatus and a suitable environment with a means of gas scavenging are required.

NON-PHARMACOLOGICAL APPROACHES TO PAIN MANAGEMENT

There has been increasing interest in the use of psychological, complementary or alternative methods of pain management [45]. These techniques can sometimes be used alone or more commonly as part of a multimodal strategy or programme of pain management. A recent survey showed that 86 per cent of pain management programmes in tertiary paediatric centres in the USA offered some kind of complementary or alternative approach [46].

Children respond well to psychological and behavioural techniques of management for both acute and long-term pain. Distraction, hypnosis, relaxation, biofeedback, guided imagery and types of cognitive–behavioural therapy (CBT) are used extensively. Health professionals can easily learn some of these techniques, and training courses are available in many paediatric pain centres.

Physical methods of pain management include massage, the use of hot or cold thermal packs, transcutaneous electrical nerve stimulation (TENS) and desensitisation. Physiotherapy and exercise therapy are important in the treatment of long-term neuropathic pain in CRPS and other conditions. Acupuncture by specialist practitioners is offered in some centres with success, particularly in the area of long-term pain management, despite the common preconception that children will not tolerate the use of needles [47].

PAIN MANAGEMENT TEAMS

Teams of professionals, including paediatric anaesthetists, nurses and pharmacists with special responsibility for postoperative pain management, were extensively developed in the late 1980s and early 1990s in the UK and elsewhere [48]. These services established the use of complex methods of pain management such as PCA, NCA and continuous epidural analgesia in young children. The advantages of such teams in coordinating care, staff education and maintenance of high standards of clinical practice for postoperative pain have become self-evident. More recently, the role of pain management teams has been expanded to include assisting in the care of children with other kinds of acute and chronic pain. Pain management has become of professional interest in its own right, with anaesthetists, nurses, pharmacists, psychologists, physiotherapists and other practitioners with relevant sub-specialist skills and qualifications as members of the multidisciplinary team.

ACUTE POSTOPERATIVE PAIN

Acute pain is of limited duration and it is expected that, as the acute injury heals, pain will decrease. In the case of postoperative pain, pain intensity and duration are often quite predictable, with full recovery taking place after a few days or weeks. Because of this predictability, it is relatively easy to plan effective treatment from the outset, anticipate changing analgesic requirements, monitor and treat side-effects and plan hospital discharge. Responsibility for the planning and implementation of pain management after surgery resides with the anaesthetist unless it is formally delegated elsewhere (e.g. to a postoperative pain management service). The aim of a postoperative pain management plan is to ensure that sufficiently potent and acceptable analgesia is administered on a regular basis when pain is present and that more is available if and when it is needed due to individual differences in analgesic requirement or changing levels of activity. A cycle of regular pain assessments coupled with timely analgesic administration and frequent reassessment should be established. Analgesia should therefore be flexible, safe and acceptable to children and families, and side-effects must be promptly diagnosed and treated. As pain decreases, transition from parenteral to oral analgesia can be planned, and preferably initiated as soon as it is feasible to do so, as this will promote mobility, recovery and early hospital discharge.

Suitable follow-up, including prescription of 'take home' analgesia and advice about pain management outside the hospital environment and who to contact for further advice should also be included.

Analgesia

As part of a multimodal strategy, opioids, NSAIDs and paracetamol are administered routinely 'by the clock' for the first few postoperative days. Local anaesthesia can be used in the form of a 'single-shot' technique at the time of surgery or as a postoperative infusion, e.g. centrally in the epidural space or peripherally to a nerve plexus. Figure 27.2 (page 406) shows a stepwise approach to acute pain management with potent analgesic combinations used initially, with a gradual reduction over time such that, as healing occurs, pain is managed by simple, readily available analgesics. Newer agents, such as ketamine (an NMDA antagonist) and clonidine (an α_2-adrenergic agonist),

can be used as supplements when pain relief is inadequate or opioid side-effects necessitate a dose reduction, or in order to prolong single-shot caudal analgesia. Many combinations of techniques are possible, depending on the expected time course of postoperative pain. Recommended doses of analgesics in common use are given in Table 27.2, and are discussed further in Chapters 12 and 13).

'Single-shot' LA techniques

Local anaesthesia has become very important in recent years as a component of multimodal analgesia, especially in the perioperative period. Advantages include site-specific analgesia, lack of sedative or respiratory side-effects, reduction in intraoperative and postoperative systemic analgesic requirements (and therefore their side-effects) and an excellent safety record [49]. There are few procedures in which LAs cannot be used in some form, and it should always be considered. Although numerous techniques have been

Table 27.2   Analgesics commonly used as part of a multimodal strategy

Drug	Class of analgesic	Routes of administration	Doses
Paracetamol	Antipyretic–analgesic	Oral/rectal	15–20 mg/kg qds, max. 90 mg/kg/day (60 mg/kg/day term neonate) (45 mg/kg/day preterm)
		Intravenous	15 mg/kg qds (60 mg/kg/day <50 kg body weight, 4 g daily >50 kg)
Ibuprofen	NSAID	Oral	5 mg/kg qds (20 mg/kg/day) <6 months 10 mg/kg tds (30 mg/kg/day) >6 months (max. 2.4 g/day)
Diclofenac	NSAID	Oral	1 mg/kg (3 mg/kg/day)
		Rectal	1 mg/kg (3 mg/kg/day)
Ketorolac	NSAID	Oral	0.5–1 mg/kg qds (max. 10 mg/dose)
		Intravenous	0.5 mg/kg qds (max. 10 mg/dose)
Codeine	Opioid	Oral	1 mg/kg qds
		Rectal	1 mg/kg qds
		Intravenous	Not recommended
Tramadol	Opioid/5HT antagonist	Oral	1 mg/kg qds
		Intravenous	1 mg/kg qds
Oxycodone	Opioid	Oral	0.2 mg/kg qds
Morphine	Opioid	Oral	0.1 mg/kg qds (<1 month) 0.2 mg/kg qds (>1 month)
		Intravenous	0.02–0.05 mg/kg qds (<1 month) 0.05–0.1 mg/kg qds (>1 month)
Clonidine	α_2-Adrenergic agonist	Oral	0.001–0.002 mg/kg tds
		Intravenous	0.001–0.002 mg/kg tds
		Epidural (caudal)	0.001–0.002 mg/kg ± local anaesthetic
Ketamine	NMDA receptor antagonist	Oral	0.5–1 mg/kg qds
		Intravenous	0.1 mg/kg qds
Ketamine (pre-servative free)	NMDA receptor antagonist	Epidural (caudal)	0.25–0.5 mg/kg ± local anaesthetic

5HT, 5-hydroxytryptamine; NMDA, N-methyl-D-aspartate; NSAID, non-steroidal anti-inflammatory drugs. qds, 6-hourly; tds, 8-hourly.

described, only a small number are common and they are generally easy to learn (see below). Wound infiltration and local nerve blocks can improve early postoperative analgesia and catheter techniques can extend analgesia for days if necessary. Epidural analgesia has a long history in paediatric pain management, and recently the addition of adjuvants, such as ketamine and clonidine, to the LA solution can extend the quality and duration of analgesia. The pharmacology of LAs and the practicalities of LA techniques are discussed in detail in Chapter 14.

WOUND INFILTRATION

Infiltration of the surgical incision with LA has been shown to contribute significantly to postoperative analgesia. Infiltration with bupivacaine after inguinal hernia repair has been found to give comparable postoperative analgesia to more complicated procedures such as caudal block [50]. Good relative efficacy has also been shown for strabismus surgery and otoplasty [51,52]. A systematic review of local anaesthetic infiltration after tonsillectomy did not unequivocally show benefit, but concluded that further trials were required to evaluate the technique properly [53].

NERVE BLOCKS, CAUDAL ANALGESIA AND INTRATHECAL OPIOIDS

Some of the most useful nerve blocks are listed in Table 27.3, which also summarises levels of evidence for their efficacy in the more frequently encountered procedures. The safety and effectiveness of peripheral nerve blocks have been established in large published series [49,54]. Ilioinguinal block, dorsal nerve block and caudal epidural block are by far the three most common in practice; they are simple and easy to learn with few serious adverse effects [55]. Success in peripheral nerve blockade may be increased by the use of techniques such as ultrasound and electrical 'surface mapping' in order to identify nerve location and therefore improve the accuracy of LA injection [56,57]. Caudal analgesia is a particularly popular and versatile technique, and the addition of adjuvant drugs such as opioids, clonidine and ketamine to the local anaesthetic solution can improve and prolong analgesia, although with additional risk of adverse effects. Caudal opioids, although they reduce analgesic requirements, have become less popular in recent years, because of significant incidences of PONV, itching and urinary retention [58]. Respiratory depression, sometimes delayed for several hours following administration, has also been reported [59]. Ketamine and clonidine are potentially more useful; both prolong analgesia, but sedation and hypotension can occur with clonidine and neurobehavioural disturbance has been reported at higher doses with ketamine [60].

Intrathecal morphine 0.02 mg/kg decreases postoperative systemic morphine requirements after cardiac surgery, and lower doses, 0.002 and 0.005 mg/kg, have also been shown to improve analgesia after spinal surgery in another study [61,62].

Infusion techniques

Analgesic infusions should always be supported in practice by clear protocols covering:

- appropriate infusion rates and dose limits
- mandatory minimum monitoring standards
- identification and treatment of adverse effects
- procedures to follow in the event of an emergency.

Medical and nursing staff will be primarily responsible for the care of patients receiving analgesic infusions and they should receive appropriate training in safe management practice. Suggested minimum standards of monitoring for patients receiving analgesic infusions, including NCA, PCA and epidural, are given in Table 27.4. In addition,

Table 27.3 Postoperative efficacy of local anaesthetic blocks after surgery

Block	Procedure	Evidence level[a]
Ilioinguinal nerve	Inguinal hernia	**
	Orchidopexy	**
Penile dorsal nerve	Circumcision	**
Infraorbital nerve	Cleft lip:	
	– child	**
	– infant	**
	– neonate	*
Axillary	Hand surgery	**
Fascia iliaca nerve	Surgery to thigh/femur	*
Intercostal nerve	Thoracotomy	*
Paravertebral	Abdominal	*
	Thoracotomy	*
Epidural (caudal, thoracic or lumbar)	Circumcision	***
	Abdominal/genitourinary	**
	Orthopaedics/spinal	**
	Thoracotomy	*
	Cardiac surgery	*

[a]Evidence level: *, cohort study or non-randomised trials; **, one or more randomised controlled trials; ***, systematic review.

Table 27.4 Suggested monitoring for children receiving parenteral opioids

Parameter	Method
Analgesia	Validated pain score
Sedation	Sedation scale*
Respiration	Respiratory rate, pulse oximetry (in air)
Cardiovascular	Heart rate/blood pressure
Nausea and vomiting	Nausea scale

*For example, University of Michigan Sedation Score (Malviya et al. [82]).

antiemetics, antipruritics and naloxone (in case of severe respiratory depression) must be available when opioids are used.

OPIOIDS

Morphine infusion is one of the simplest approaches; most postoperative pain can be managed within the dose range 10–40 μg/kg/h, with lower infusion rates needed in the neonate [63]. Suggested regimens are given in Table 27.5; lower doses are required in the neonate for pharmacokinetic reasons, and therefore infusion protocols are adapted accordingly. Subcutaneous morphine is also satisfactory provided that peripheral perfusion is not compromised. Fentanyl is a useful alternative to morphine, particularly if pulmonary hypertension is present or a risk.

Continuous infusion techniques can provide excellent analgesia, even in comparison with more flexible approaches such as PCA and NCA (see below), but it is important to remember that changes in infusion rate will increase plasma levels slowly in comparison with supplemental boluses, and for this reason more complicated techniques are often preferred [64,65].

NURSE-CONTROLLED ANALGESIA

A continuous opioid infusion may be made more flexible by allowing supplementary doses of analgesia to be given using a programmable infusion device. Commonly known as nurse-controlled analgesia, the technique of using a moderate continuous or background infusion with two or three extra 'bolus' doses allowed per hour is a simple form of demand-led analgesia which allows an individualised regimen and also facilitates transition from parenteral to other routes [48] (Table 27.6). To be effective, NCA must be used with a reliable method of pain assessment linked to a clear action plan.

PATIENT-CONTROLLED ANALGESIA

Children as young as 5 years may be capable of using PCA, provided that suitable and sufficient supervision and monitoring are available. Morphine has been used most commonly for PCA, but fentanyl, tramadol and other opioids may be useful alternatives for certain patient groups or circumstances. In contrast to 'traditional' PCA in the adult, a small background infusion is often included in paediatric practice: 4 μg/kg/h has been shown to improve night-time sleep patterns without increasing side-effects such as nausea and vomiting [66] (Table 27.6).

Management of opioid side-effects

Opioids can cause unwanted effects that can limit their safety and efficacy. Nausea, vomiting, itching and depression of respiration can occur in a dose-dependent fashion.

Table 27.5 The composition and doses of common opioids given by infusion

Infusion	Preparation (0.9% saline)	Concentration (μg/kg/mL)	Initial dose (mL)/(μg/kg)	Infusion (mL)/(μg/kg/h)
Intravenous morphine	1 mg/kg in 50 mL	20	2.5–5.0/50–100	0.1–2.0/2–40
Intravenous morphine – neonate	1 mg/kg in 50 mL	20	0.5–2.5/10–50	0.1–0.6/2–12
Subcutaneous morphine	1 mg/kg in 20 mL	50	1.0–2.0/50–100	0.2–0.8/10–40
Intravenous fentanyl	1 μg/kg in 50 mL	0.2	1.0–2.0/0.2–0.4	0.5–2.0/0.1–0.4

Table 27.6 Nurse-controlled analgesia (NCA) and patient-controlled analgesia (PCA) using standard morphine infusions (see Table 27.5). A 4-hour limit of 400 μg/kg is programmed into the patient-controlled infusion device

Technique	Background infusion (mL/h)/(μg/kg/h)	Bolus dose (mL)/(μg/kg)	Lockout interval (mins)
NCA	0–0.5/0–10	0.5–1.0/10–20	20
NNCA	0–0.5/0–10	0–1.0/0–20	20*
PCA	0–0.2/0–4	0.5–1.0/10–20	5

NNCA, neonatal nurse-controlled analgesia.
* High-dependency unit/intensive care unit cardiorespirotory observation is mandatory for NNCA.

POSTOPERATIVE NAUSEA AND VOMITING

Children at high risk of PONV should receive prophylactic antiemetic treatment with dexamethasone or a 5-hydroxy-tryptamine (5HT) antagonist [67]. If PONV occurs, it should be treated with one or a combination of the following unless previously used for prophylaxis: a 5HT antagonist, an antihistamine (e.g. cyclizine) or a phenothiazine (e.g. perphenazine).

ITCHING

This frequent side-effect is particularly common after epidural or intrathecal opioids. The most effective therapy is reduction in opioid dosage and substitution of alternative analgesia. If this is not possible, a small dose of naloxone or chlorphenamine (chlorpheniramine) may be effective.

RESPIRATORY DEPRESSION

Respiratory depression is potentially a disastrous complication, but thankfully anxiety that it would be a high risk when using opioids in young children has proven to be unfounded, provided that standard age-related dose restrictions are followed. Prevention of respiratory depression is largely a matter of good monitoring and protection against overdose. Some authorities recommend that pulse oximetry should be used for all children receiving parenteral opioids (see Table 27.4). Naloxone is an effective opioid antagonist, but supplementary oxygen and respiratory support may still be required in emergency situations. If respiration is depressed, the opioid infusion should be stopped, oxygen given, the airway assessed and respiration supported as required. A minimum acceptable respiration rate should be part of the patient's analgesic plan.

OPIOID WITHDRAWAL

On occasion, patients may require opioid analgesia for long periods, for example those in intensive care or those needing analgesia during chemotherapy. Precipitate cessation of opioid therapy can result in unwanted symptoms and signs, e.g. tremors, movement disorders, hallucinations, crying or agitation, pupillary dilatation, sweating and diarrhoea. Moreover, when exposed to chronic opioid use *in utero*, the neonate may manifest withdrawal, the 'neonatal abstinence syndrome' [68].

Where this occurs, patients should be scored for withdrawal symptoms using a designated chart (http://www.ich.ucl.ac.uk/paincontrol/). Opioid therapy should be stabilised and thereafter reduced at a rate of 10 or 20 per cent of the original highest dose either daily or on alternate days. When convenient, IV morphine therapy can be converted to oral dosing by calculating the total IV dose given in 24 hours and multiplying this by three to give a total daily oral dose. Oral dosing is commenced on a 4-hourly basis. In the neonatal abstinence syndrome, opioid administration is superior to phenobarbital, benzodiazepines or supportive care in minimising symptoms and facilitating weight gain [68].

In all patients being slowly withdrawn from opioids, IV or oral clonidine (1–4 µg/kg 8-hourly) can be used for symptomatic relief; hypotension is a potential side-effect.

Local anaesthetic infusions

The longer-acting LAs, bupivacaine, levobupivacaine and ropivacaine are suitable for continuous infusion techniques over periods of several days or even weeks in some cases. The efficacy and duration of such techniques are limited by LA accumulation, leading to toxicity, and by the incidence of local infection at the site of infusion. Technical problems such as occlusion or dislodgement of catheters can also be a problem, especially during epidural analgesia in very small patients. Because of the slow elimination of LAs, it is usual to limit the total dose administered in any 4-hour period to 2.5 mg/kg in infants and older children, and to 2.0 mg/kg in neonates. Therefore suggested doses for infusion of all three drugs are:

- Neonates: 0.1–0.25 mg/kg/h
- Infants and children: 0.1–0.5 mg/kg/h.

Local anaesthetic can be infused into the site of surgery through an indwelling catheter. This technique has been used at iliac crest bone graft donor sites and for median sternotomy in adults, but the technique has been little studied in children. Continuous techniques for intrapleural, paravertebral, brachial plexus blocks, sciatic nerve blocks, fascia iliaca compartment block, popliteal and others have also been reported, but again there are few comparative studies of efficacy.

CENTRAL (EPIDURAL) LA INFUSION

Lumbar and thoracic epidural infusions have an established place in severe acute pain management in children. In the neonate, catheters can be threaded to the required height from lower, and therefore safer and technically easier to access, intervertebral or sacral (caudal) spinal levels. Catheters for thoracic epidural analgesia inserted at the caudal level have been described for neonatal surgery such as repair of tracheo-oesophageal fistula. Dosage guidance and restrictions given above apply equally to epidural infusion as to other LA infusions and, partly because of this, opioids are frequently combined with LA to improve efficacy while limiting LA dosage. Morphine, fentanyl, diamorphine, hydromorphone and other opioids in preservative-free formulations have all been used with apparent success, but again there have been few controlled comparisons. Clonidine 0.0008–0.0012 mg/kg/h has also been combined with LA and shown to improve analgesia in comparison with LA alone

[69]. Some suggested regimens for epidural analgesia are given in Table 27.7. Patient-controlled epidural analgesia (PCEA) has been reported as feasible in children, and analgesia equivalent to continuous infusion has been demonstrated, at a lower total dose of LA [70,71].

Epidural analgesia is indicated for thoracic, thoracoabdominal and major abdominal surgery, particularly if there is pre-existing respiratory compromise. The need for postoperative ventilation is reduced after tracheo-oesophageal surgery in neonates, and benefits following Nissen fundoplication have also been reported [72,73].

Epidural insertion

Epidural catheters are almost invariably inserted under general anaesthesia prior to surgery in children. Most practitioners favour a loss-of-resistance (LOR) technique using saline, as this avoids inadvertent IV air injection, and dural puncture may also be less frequent using this method. Additionally, injection of air into the epidural space may lead to the formation of air loculi, preventing spread of LA solution and consequent 'missed segments' or incomplete blockade. Several methods have been advocated to improve the accuracy of catheter tip location, including electrical stimulation, ECG signal and ultrasound [74–76]. The technique of insertion of epidural catheters is described in detail in Chapter 26.

Table 27.7   Drug doses and infusion rates for epidural analgesia

Levobupivacaine–morphine	
Initial dose:	levobupivacaine 0.25%, 0.5–0.75 mL/kg
Infusion:	levobupivacaine 0.125% with preservative-free morphine 0.001%
Rate:	0.1–0.4 mL/h* (max. 15 mL/h)
Levobupivacaine–fentanyl	
Initial dose:	levobupivacaine 0.25% 0.5–0.75 mL/kg
Infusion:	levobupivacaine 0.125% with fentanyl 1–2 μg/mL
Rate:	0.1–0.4 mL/h* (max. 15 mL/h)
Ropivacaine	
Initial dose:	ropivacaine 0.2% 0.5–0.75 mL/kg
Infusion:	ropivacaine 0.2%
Rate:	0.1–0.4 mL/h*

*Maximum rate 0.2 mL/h in neonates (max. 15 mL/h).

Epidural management

Children with epidural infusions in progress can be nursed in general ward areas provided that there is adequate supervision and monitoring by suitably trained staff. Complications include catheter failure due to migration or disconnection, excessive or unwanted motor block, retention of urine and local infection at the catheter entry site. If opioids are included in the infusate, retention of urine is more common and itching and respiratory depression can also occur. If it is planned to continue an epidural infusion using opioids in the postoperative period, urethral catheterisation at the time of surgery is recommended. In the absence of a catheter, proven retention should be treated by reducing the rate of opioid infusion, giving naloxone 0.0005 mg/kg as IV boluses every 10 minutes (Table 27.8), or urethral catheterisation. Less commonly, drug toxicity due to overdose or plasma accumulation during prolonged infusion occurs. Staff who are caring for patients with epidural infusions are required to be vigilant for such complications, and to be acquainted with strategies for prevention and treatment.

MANAGEMENT OF CHRONIC AND LONG-TERM PAIN

Background

Chronic pain in children is increasingly recognised as a clinical problem, yet health-care provision is often poor for this group. As the underlying causes and mechanisms of chronic pain are not well understood, and the effects are often profound and complex, specialist multidisciplinary management is needed, preferably coordinated by a dedicated children's pain management service. Typically, such a service would include clinicians in possession of paediatric experience and pain management skills, specialist nurses, psychologists, physiotherapists, occupational therapists and pharmacists. It is important to recognise that often the treatment of long-term pain does not necessarily or primarily focus on pharmacological reduction in pain intensity (which is often difficult to achieve) but on restoration of normal function and rehabilitation. Assessment of such patients will therefore include not only an account of the

Table 27.8   Supplementary drugs with opioid infusions

Drug	Indication	Dose	Route	Frequency
Ondansetron	PONV	0.1 mg/kg, max. 4 mg per dose	Oral/IV	tds
Cyclizine	PONV	1 mL/kg, max. 50 mg per dose	Oral/IV	tds
Chlorphenamine	Itching	0.025–0.1 mg/kg, max. 24 mg/day	Oral/IV	qds
Naloxone	Itching	0.0005 mg/kg	IV	qds
Naloxone	Respiratory depression	0.004 mg/kg	IV	prn

IV, intravenous; PONV, postoperative nausea and vomiting.
prn, as required; qds, 6-hourly; tds, 8-hourly.

pain history but also specific inquiries regarding the impact of pain on daily life, including the family, peer group and schooling. Although treatment involves significant specialist input, the majority of patients can be managed on an outpatient basis. Some patients require inpatient admission and this is best organised in the form of an intensive pain management programme in a specialist centre able to combine psychological, physical and pharmacological assessments and treatments in a coordinated manner.

Assessment

The objectives of assessment in chronic pain conditions are not only to establish the site, severity and other characteristics of the pain but also to document the physical and emotional impact, as well as any related physical disease, to determine the underlying pathophysiological mechanisms, and to formulate a treatment plan (see Chronic pain assessment on page 412).

General principles of chronic pain management

Treatment should include specific therapy directed at the underlying cause or pain mechanisms and associated symptoms such as muscle spasms, sleep disturbance, anxiety or depression. Pharmacological management not only includes the use of 'standard' analgesics such as opioids and NSAIDs, if they are effective, but also novel treatments directed at neuropathic pain mechanisms (see later), and treatments for pain-related symptoms such as antiemetics, antispasmodics and muscle relaxants. In addition, non-drug management may include TENS, massage, acupuncture and thermal treatment with hot or cold packs. Teaching of self-management skills may include the use of formal CBT or related strategies such as guided imagery, hypnosis and biofeedback. Physiotherapy has an important therapeutic and rehabilitative role in many pain conditions, and occupational therapy is frequently helpful as well. Information-giving and education about pain and the consequences of pain are also components of successful management. Measures extending beyond the patients and their immediate symptoms are also useful and may include family therapy and involvement of community services such as education, mental heath and social welfare. Improvements in school attendance, social interaction with peers and participation in appropriate physical activity are key objectives of therapy.

Management of pain related to a known underlying pathological process or disease

Frequently, pain in this group of patients is closely related to the progress or state of activity or remission of the underlying condition. It is important to ensure that such patients are receiving appropriate specialist management, because treatment of the underlying condition often influences pain intensity and consequently these patients should always be managed in close cooperation with a paediatric specialist, e.g. rheumatologist, oncologist or immunologist. The pathophysiology of the condition and pain mechanisms involved may be relatively well established, allowing a rational selection of analgesics, anticipation of potential exacerbating or alleviating factors, and a meaningful discussion of disease progression and prognosis. Examples include pain from sickle cell crises, rheumatoid arthritis and cancer. Pharmacological pain management should be directed towards the probable mechanisms involved, i.e. inflammatory or neuropathic, and a regimen that includes the treatment of 'background' pain, and measures for dealing with acute exacerbations and 'breakthrough', should be constructed. In most cases, there is a detailed literature available for consultation and often there are numerous sources of help and support from professional and patient groups towards which patients and their families can be directed.

Neuropathic pain

Complex regional pan syndrome and post-surgical or post-traumatic neuropathic pain are the commonest diagnoses encountered in children seen in chronic pain clinics, accounting for up to 40 per cent of patients [77,78]. Nevertheless, neuropathic pain syndromes appear to be rather less common in children than adults, and are rare below the age of 6 years. The mechanisms of neuropathic pain are distinct from inflammatory pain, and therefore pharmacological management is likely to require the use of alternative analgesics, such as gabapentin, anticonvulsant and antidepressant compounds. Localised neuropathic pain, e.g. at the site of a surgical wound or where there has been nerve damage, sometimes responds to local treatment, e.g. 5 per cent lidocaine patches or lidocaine infiltration with or without a long-acting corticosteroid. Because neuropathic pain is rare in children and is frequently difficult to treat, and because many therapies are not supported by good research evidence, management by skilled specialist practitioners is strongly recommended.

COMPLEX REGIONAL PAN SYNDROME

Complex regional pain syndrome is severe and prolonged limb pain accompanied by sensory changes and autonomic disturbance. It has been reported in adults and children (mostly adolescents) for many years. The condition is incompletely understood and it is commonly classified into two subtypes, depending upon whether nerve damage can be shown to be present. Originally known as reflex sympathetic dystrophy (RSD) and causalgia, they are currently called CRPS types I and II, respectively. Confusingly, a number of other terms have been applied to these conditions, including Sudek's atrophy, reflex neurovascular dystrophy and shoulder–hand syndrome, among others. Complex regional pan syndrome is characterised by spontaneous pain, allodynia (mechanical and thermal), swelling, temperature change, sudomotor dysfunction and atrophic changes of skin in the distal part of the affected limb and nails. Girls are affected five or six times more commonly than boys and, in contrast to presentations in the adult, the lower limb is the usual site in children.

Early diagnosis and mobilisation of the affected area are thought to improve the prognosis, but this is frequently not achieved in children due to delays in diagnosis and failure to implement suitable therapy. Physiotherapy is considered to be the mainstay of treatment; a programme of moderately intensive exercises, including desensitising strategies, has been show to be effective [79–81]. Strategies to alleviate the pain and allodynia have included systemic medication, intravenous regional analgesia, local nerve blocks, sympathetic nerve blocks, epidural infusions and even spinal cord stimulation, sympatholysis and amputation. In fact, there is little evidence to support the use of invasive therapy and it is rarely indicated. Systemic analgesia using a combination of conventional analgesics and specific treatments for neuropathic pain (see above), physical treatments (e.g. TENS) and psychological and behavioural methods should be used first.

REFERENCES

Key references

Chalkiadis GA. Management of chronic pain in children. *Med J Aust* 2001; **175**: 476–9.

Fitzgerald M, Howard RF. The neurobiologic basis of paediatric pain. In: Schechter NL, Berde CB, Yaster M, eds. *Pain in infants, children and adolescents*. Balitmore, MA: Lippincott, Williams & Wilkins, 2003: 19–42.

Franck LS, Greenberg CS, Stevens B. Pain assessment in infants and children. *Pediatr Clin North Am* 2000; **47**(3): 487–512.

Howard RF. Current status of pain management in children. *JAMA* 2003; **290**: 2464–9.

Lloyd-Thomas AR, Howard RF. A pain service for children. *Paediatr Anaesth* 1994; **4**: 3–15.

References

1. Kehlet H, Jensen TS, Woolf CJ. Persistent postsurgical pain: risk factors and prevention. *Lancet* 2006; **367**(9522): 1618–25.
2. Hunt SP, Mantyh PW. The molecular dynamics of pain control. *Nat Rev Neurosci* 2001; **2**(2): 83–91.
3. Millan MJ. Descending control of pain. *Prog Neurobiol* 2002; **66**(6): 355–474.
4. Woolf CJ, Salter MW. Neuronal plasticity: increasing the gain in pain. *Science* 2000; **288**(5472): 1765–69.
5. Bridges D, Thompson SW, Rice AS. Mechanisms of neuropathic pain. *Br J Anaesth* 2001; **87**(1): 12–26.
6. Fitzgerald M, Howard RF. The neurobiologic basis of paediatric pain. In: Schechter NL, Berde CB, Yaster M, eds. *Pain in infants, children and adolescents*. Balitmore, MA: Lippincott, Williams & Wilkins, 2003: 19–42.
7. Alvares D, Fitzgerald M. Building blocks of pain: the regulation of key molecules in spinal sensory neurones during development and following peripheral axotomy. *Pain* 1999; **6**: S71–85.
8. Fitzgerald M, Walker SE. The role of activity in developing pain pathways. In Dostrovsky J, Carr D, Koltzenburg M, eds. *Proceedings of the 10th World Congress on Pain, Progress in Pain Research and Management, Vol. 24*. Seattle: IASP Press, 2003: 185–96.
9. Fitzgerald M. The development of nociceptive circuits. *Nat Rev Neurosci* 2005; **6**(7): 507–20.
10. Andrews K, Fitzgerald M. The cutaneous withdrawal reflex in human neonates: sensitization, receptive fields, and the effects of contralateral stimulation. *Pain* 1994; **56**(1): 95–101.
11. Andrews K, Fitzgerald M. Wound sensitity as a measure of analgesic effects following surgery in human neonates and infants. *Pain* 2002; **99**: 185–95.
12. Howard RF, Hatch DJ, Cole TJ, Fitzgerald M. Inflammatory pain and hypersensitivity are selectively reversed by epidural bupivacaine and are developmentally regulated. *Anesthesiology* 2001; **95**: 421–7.
13. Walker SM, Howard RF, Keay KA, Fitzgerald M. Developmental age influences the effect of epidural dexmedetomidine on inflammatory hyperalgesia in rat pups. *Anesthesiology* 2005; **102**(6): 1226–34.
14. Ririe DG, Prout HM, Eisenach JC. Effect of cyclooxygenase-1 inhibition in postoperative pain is developmentally regulated. *Anesthesiology* 2004; **101**(4): 1031–5.
15. Ririe DG, Prout HD, Barclay D *et al*. Developmental differences in spinal cyclooxygenase 1 expression after surgical incision. *Anesthesiology* 2006; **104**(3): 426–31.
16. Marsh D, Dickenson A, Hatch D, Fitzgerald M. Epidural opioid analgesia in infant rats II: responses to carrageenan and capsaicin. *Pain* 1999; **82**(1): 33–8.
17. Nandi R, Beacham D, Middleton J *et al*. The functional expression of mu opioid receptors on sensory neurons is developmentally regulated: morphine analgesia is less selective in the neonate. *Pain* 2004; **111**(1–2): 38–50.
18. Howard RF. Current status of pain management in children. *JAMA* 2003; **290**: 2464–9.
19. Taddio A, Goldbach M, Ipp M *et al*. Effect of neonatal circumcision on pain responses during vaccination in boys. *Lancet* 1995; **345**(8945): 291–2.
20. Peters JW, Koot HM, de BJ. *et al*. Major surgery within the first 3 months of life and subsequent biobehavioral pain responses to immunization at later age: a case comparison study. *Pediatrics* 2003; **111**: 129–35.
21. Grunau R. Early pain in preterm infants. A model of long-term effects. *Clin Perinatol* 2002; **29**: 373–94, vii–viii.

22. Reynolds ML, Fitzgerald M. Long-term sensory hyperinnervation following neonatal skin wounds. *J Comp Neurol* 1995; **358**(4): 487–98.

23. Walker SM, Meredith-Middleton J, Cooke-Yarborough C, Fitzgerald M. Neonatal inflammation and primary afferent terminal plasticity in the rat dorsal horn. *Pain* 2003; **105**(1–2): 185–95.

24. Franck LS, Greenberg CS, Stevens B. Pain assessment in infants and children. *Pediatr Clin North Am* 2000; **47**(3): 487–512.

25. Royal College of Nursing. *Clinical guidelines for the recognition and assessment of acute pain in children.* London: Royal College of Nursing Institute, 1999.

26. Wong DL, Baker CM. Pain in children: comparison of assessment scales. *Pediatr Nurs* 1988; **14**: 9–17.

27. Bieri D, Reeve RA, Champion GD *et al.* The Faces Pain Scale for the self-assessment of the severity of pain experienced by children: development, initial validation, and preliminary investigation for ratio scale properties. *Pain* 1990; **41**(2): 139–50.

28. Beyer JE, Denyes MJ, Villaruel AM. The creation, validation and continuing develpment of the oucher: a measure of pain intensity in children. *J Paediatr Nurs* 1992; **7**, 335.

29. Chambers CT, Craig KD. An intrusive impact of anchors in children's faces pain scales. *Pain* 1998; **78**: 27–37.

30. Luffy R, Grove SK. Examining the validity, reliability, and preference of three pediatric pain measurement tools in African-American children. *Pediatr Nurs* 2003; **29**: 54–9.

31. Romsing J, Moller-Sonnergaard J, Hertel S, Rasmussen M. Postoperative pain in children: comparison between ratings of children and nurses. *J Pain Symptom Manag* 1996; **11**(1): 42–6.

32. Buttner W, Fincke W. Analysis of behavioural and physiological parameters for the assessment of postoperative analgesic demand in newborns, infants and young children. *Paediatr Anaesth* 2000; **10**: 303–18.

33. Merkel SI, Voepel-Lewis T, Shayevitz JR, Malviya S. The FLACC: a behavioral scale for scoring postoperative pain in young children. *Pediatr Nurs* 1997; **23**(3): 293–7.

34. Ballantyne M, Stevens B, McAllister M *et al.* Validation of the premature infant pain profile in the clinical setting. *Clin J Pain* 1999; **15**(4): 297–303.

35. Hunt A, Goldman A, Seers K *et al.* Clinical validation of the paediatric pain profile. *Dev Med Child Neurol* 2004; **46**(1): 9–18.

36. Breau LM, McGrath PJ, Camfield C *et al.* Preliminary validation of an observational pain checklist for persons with cognitive impairments and inability to communicate verbally. *Dev Med Child Neurol* 2000; **42**: 609–16.

37. Varni JW, Thompson KL, Hanson V. The Varni/Thompson Pediatric Pain Questionnaire. I. Chronic musculoskeletal pain in juvenile rheumatoid arthritis. *Pain* 1987; **28**: 27–38.

38. Palermo TM, Witherspoon D, Valenzuela D, Drotar DD. Development and validation of the Child Activity Limitations Interview: a measure of pain-related functional impairment in school-age children and adolescents. *Pain* 2004; **109**(3): 461–70.

39. Siao P, Cros DP. Quantitative sensory testing. *Phys Med Rehabil Clin North Am* 2003; **14**(2): 261–86.

40. Kehlet H. Multimodal approach to control postoperative pathophysiology and rehabilitation. *Br J Anaesth* 1997; **78**(5): 606–17.

41. Morton NS, O'Brien K. Analgesic efficacy of paracetamol and diclofenac in children receiving PCA morphine. *Br J Anaesth* 1999; **82**(5): 715–17.

42. Seth N, Llewellyn NE, Howard RF. Parental opinions regarding the route of administration of analgesic medication in children. *Paediatr Anaesth* 2000; **10**(5): 537–44.

43. Finkel JC, Finley A, Greco C *et al.* Transdermal fentanyl in the management of children with chronic severe pain: results from an international study. *Cancer* 2005; **104**(12): 2847–57.

44. Gall O, Annequin D, Benoit G *et al.* Adverse events of premixed nitrous oxide and oxygen for procedural sedation in children. *Lancet* 2001; **358**(9292): 1514–5.

45. Rusy LM, Weisman SJ. Complementary therapies for acute pediatric pain management. *Pediatr Clin North Am* 2000; **47**: 589–99.

46. Lin YC, Lee AC, Kemper KJ, Berde CB. Use of complementary and alternative medicine in pediatric pain management service: a survey. *Pain Med* 2005; **6**(6): 452–58.

47. Kemper KJ, Sarah R, Silver-Highfield E *et al.* On pins and needles? Pediatric pain patients' experience with acupuncture. *Pediatrics* 2000; **105**(4 Pt 2): 941–7.

48. Lloyd-Thomas AR, Howard RF. A pain service for children. *Paediatr Anaesth* 1994; **4**: 3–15.

49. Giaufre E, Dalens B, Gombert A. Epidemiology and morbidity of regional anesthesia in children: a one-year prospective survey of the French-Language Society of Pediatric Anesthesiologists. *Anesth Analg* 1996; **83**(5): 904–12.

50. Machotta A, Risse A, Bercker S *et al.* Comparison between instillation of bupivacaine versus caudal analgesia for postoperative analgesia following inguinal herniotomy in children. *Paediatr Anaesth* 2003; **13**(5): 397–402.

51. Cregg N, Conway F, Casey W. Analgesia after otoplasty: regional nerve blockade vs local anaesthetic infiltration of the ear. *Can J Anaesth* 1996; **43**(2): 141–7.

52. Ates Y, Unal N, Cuhruk H, Erkan N. Postoperative analgesia in children using preemptive retrobulbar block and local anesthetic infiltration in strabismus surgery. *Reg Anesth Pain Med* 1998; **23**(6): 569–74.

53. Hollis LJ, Burton MJ, Millar JM. *Perioperative local anaesthesia for reducing pain following tonsillectomy (Cochrane review).* Oxford: Update Software, 2000.

54. Auroy Y, Narchi P, Messiah A *et al.* Serious complications related to regional anesthesia: results of a prospective survey in France. *Anesthesiology* 1997; **87**: 479–86.

55. Markakis DA. Regional anesthesia in pediatrics. *Anesthesiol Clin North Am* 2000; **18**(2): 355–81, vii.

56. Bosenberg AT, Raw R, Boezaart AP. Surface mapping of peripheral nerves in children with a nerve stimulator. *Paediatr Anaesth* 2002; **12**(5): 398–403.

57. Willschke H, Marhofer P, Bosenberg A *et al.* Ultrasonography for ilioinguinal/iliohypogastric nerve blocks in children. *Br J Anaesth* 2005; **95**(2): 226–30.

58. de Beer DA, Thomas ML. Caudal additives in children – solutions or problems. *Br J Anaesth* 2003; **90**(4): 487–98.

59. Krane EJ. Delayed respiratory depression in a child after caudal epidural morphine. *Anesth Analg* 1988; **67**(1): 79–82.

60. Ansermino M, Basu R, Vandebeek C, Montgomery C. Nonopioid additives to local anaesthetics for caudal blockade in children: a systematic review. *Paediatr Anaesth* 2003; **13**(7): 561–73.

61. Gall O, Aubineau JV, Berniere J *et al.* Analgesic effect of low-dose intrathecal morphine after spinal fusion in children. *Anesthesiology* 2001; **94**(3): 447–52.

62. Suominen PK, Ragg PG, McKinley DF *et al.* Intrathecal morphine provides effective and safe analgesia in children after cardiac surgery. *Acta Anaesthesiol Scand* 2004; **48**(7): 875–82.

63. Kart T, Christrup LL, Rasmussen M. Recommended use of morphine in neonates, infants and children based on a literature review: Part 2 – Clinical use. *Paediatr Anaesth* 1997; **7**(2): 93–101.

64. Berde CB, Lehn BM, Yee JD *et al.* Patient-controlled analgesia in children and adolescents: a randomized, prospective comparison with intramuscular administration of morphine for postoperative analgesia. *J Pediatr* 1991; **118**(3): 460–6.

65. Bray RJ, Woodhams AM, Vallis CJ *et al.* A double-blind comparison of morphine infusion and patient controlled analgesia in children. *Paediatr Anaesth* 1996; **6**(2): 121–7.

66. Doyle E, Robinson D, Morton NS. Comparison of patient-controlled analgesia with and without a background infusion after lower abdominal surgery in children. *Br J Anaesth* 1993; **71**(5): 670–73.

67. Gan TJ, Meyer T, Apfel CC *et al.* Consensus guidelines for managing postoperative nausea and vomiting. *Anesth Analg* 2003; **97**: 62–71.

68. Osborn DA, Jeffery HE, Cole M. Opiate treatment for opiate withdrawal in newborn infants (Review). Cochrane Library 2007; **1**: 1–24.

69. De Negri P, Ivani G, Visconti C *et al.* The dose–response relationship for clonidine added to a postoperative continuous epidural infusion of ropivacaine in children. *Anesth Analg* 2001; **93**(1): 71–6.

70. Antok E, Bordet F, Duflo F *et al.* Patient-controlled epidural analgesia versus continuous epidural infusion with ropivacaine for postoperative analgesia in children. *Anesth Analg* 2003; **97**(6): 1608–11.

71. Birmingham PK, Wheeler M, Suresh S *et al.* Patient-controlled epidural analgesia in children: can they do it. *Anesth Analg* 2003; **96**: 686–91.

72. McNeely JK, Farber NE, Rusy LM, Hoffman GM. Epidural analgesia improves outcome following pediatric fundoplication. A retrospective analysis. *Reg Anesth* 1997; **22**(1): 16–23.

73. Hodgson RE, Bosenberg AT, Hadley LG. Congenital diaphragmatic hernia repair – impact of delayed surgery and epidural analgesia. *S Afr J Surg* 2000; **38**(2): 31–4; discussion 34–5.

74. Tsui BC, Seal R, Koller J *et al.* Thoracic epidural analgesia via the caudal approach in pediatric patients undergoing fundoplication using nerve stimulation guidance. *Anesth Analg* 2001; **93**(5): 1152–5.

75. Tsui BC, Seal R, Koller J. Thoracic epidural catheter placement via the caudal approach in infants by using electrocardiographic guidance. *Anesth Analg* 2002; **95**(2): 326–30.

76. Willschke H, Marhofer P, Bosenberg A *et al.* Epidural catheter placement in children: comparing a novel approach using ultrasound guidance and a standard loss-of-resistance technique. *Br J Anaesth* 2006; **97**(2): 200–7.

77. Chalkiadis GA. Management of chronic pain in children. *Med J Aust* 2001; **175**: 476–9.

78. Berde CB, Lebel AA, Olsson, G. Neuropathic pain in children. In: Schechter NL, Berde CB, Yaster M, eds. *Pain in infants, children and adolescents.* Balitmore, MA: Lippincott, Williams & Wilkins, 2003; 620–38.

79. Wesdock KA, Stanton RP, Singsen BH. Reflex sympathetic dystrophy in children. A physical therapy approach. *Arthritis Care Res* 1991; **4**: 32–38.

80. Maillard SM, Davies K, Khubchandani R *et al.* Reflex sympathetic dystrophy: a multidisciplinary approach. *Arthritis Rheum* 2004; **51**: 284–90.

81. Lee BH, Scharff L, Sethna NF *et al.* Physical therapy and cognitive-behavioral treatment for complex regional pain syndromes. *J Pediatr* 2002; **141**: 135–40.

82. Malviya S, Voepel-Lewis T, Tait AR *et al.* Depth of sedation in children undergoing computed tomography: validity and reliability of the University of Michigan Sedation Scale (UMSS). *Br J Anaesth* 2002; **88**: 241–5.

28

Congenital and inherited disease

SALLY E RAMPERSAD, ANNE M LYNN

KEY LEARNING POINTS

- Congenital anomalies may have significant implications for anaesthesia.
- Meticulous preoperative evaluation is mandatory because many abnormalities involve multiple organ system.
- Patients with congenital abnormalities may undergo multiple operations; parents (or carers) will be familiar with the child's condition and often a useful source of advice.

- Difficult airway management is a feature of many anomalies.
- Congenital cardiac disease is associated with many anomalies.
- Hypotonia and weakness may be the presenting sign of several neuromuscular diseases with significant anaesthetic implications.

INTRODUCTION

Since it is impossible to write comprehensively of every congenital syndrome that might affect anaesthetic management, this chapter will present an approach to the evaluation of children with congenital syndromes. It will include a discussion of those anomalies with obvious implications for anaesthesia management or monitoring, and some syndromes with subtle or hidden potential problems. A more complete list of syndromes grouped by area of potential anaesthetic impact appears in Table 28.1, which expands and reorganises the indices of Jones and Pelton [1] and Steward and Lerman [2]. Roizen and Fleisher [3], and Baum and O'Flaherty [4] are recommended further reading.

PREOPERATIVE EVALUATION

Thorough preoperative evaluation is essential to ensure optimum perioperative monitoring and care, and to identify the patient needing sub-specialty consultation before surgery. Past anaesthetic records can provide a wealth of information concerning airway, respiratory, cardiovascular and metabolic function.

The general health of the child may be assessed by reviewing height and weight, including percentiles obtained from growth charts. Many syndromes cause alterations in overall growth. Most will be associated with growth failure, as in the syndromes associated with dwarfing [5], but several are distinctive for excessive size or weight such as the multiple X or multiple Y syndromes, Beckwith–Wiedeman, Prader–Willi or Soto syndromes [6].

Evaluation of the upper airway seeks to identify conditions that will modify anaesthesia planning. If abnormalities are found, parents may be informed of potential problems and therapeutic plans. A history of snoring that awakens the child or causes daytime somnolence reveals significant airway obstruction. The child with micrognathia who may present difficulties during induction and intubation can be identified if the child's face, especially in

Table 28.1 Congenital syndromes affecting anaesthesia[†]

(a) Airway (difficult intubation or mask fit): J, micrognathia; C, cervical spine instability or limited motion; M, soft tissue mass or macroglossia; L, small larynx; S, increased secretions; F, facial configuration hinders mask fit

Aaskog–Scott C	Crouzon J, occasionally	Juvenile rheumatoid arthritis C	Pierre Robin J, cleft, F
*Achondroplasia C, F	Cystic hygroma M	Kabuki cleft, J	*Pompe disease M
Aglossia–adactylia J	Diastrophic dwarfism C, J	Klippel–Feil C	*Prader–Willi F, J
Anderson's midface hypoplasia, F	*Down (trisomy 21) C, M	Kniest C	Rieger abnormal teeth
Angioneurotic odema L (swelling)	Dyggue–Melchoir–Clausen C	Larsen C	Russell–Silver dwarf J
	*Edwards (trisomy 18) J	*Meckel J	*Scleroderma–small mouth
*Apert J, F	Epidemolysis bullosa see text, L	Median cleft face J, cleft	*Smith–Lemli–Opitz J
Arthrogryposis multiplex C, J	*Farber disease L	Miller J, F	Spondylometaphyseal dysplasia C
Beckwith–Wiedemann M	Freeman–Sheldon small mouth	Möbius J	
*Behçet's ulcers of pharynx	*Goldenhar (hemifacial microsomia) J, F	*Morquio C	Spondyloepiphyseal dysplasia C
Carpenter J		*Multiple mucosal neuroma M	
*CHARGE association J; choanal atresia	Goltz–Gorlin abnormal teeth, C	*Myositis ossificans C	Sprengel C
	Hallermann–Strief J, small mouth	Najjars J, F	Treacher Collins J small mouth, F
*Cherubism M, F		Noack J	
*Christ–Siemens–Touraine J, F	Hallervorden–Spatz torticollis, trismus	*Noonan C	*Turner C, J
Chotzen J, F		*Opitz–Frias J, L, cleft	Urbach–Wiethe disease L
Cornelia de Lange C, J	*Hand–Schüller–Christian L	*Orofacial-digital cleft	*Velocardiofacials F, cleft, J
*Cretinism M	*Hunter S, M	Pallister Hall J	*von Recklinghausen's disease M
*Cri-du-chat M, J, F	*Hurler S, M	*Patau (trisomy 13) J, cleft	
	*I-cell disease C, J	Pendred M	Weaver J

(b) Ventilation problems (L, intrinsic lung disease; W, muscle weakness; C, chest wall deformity)

Achondroplasia C	Gaucher disease L (aspiration)	*Marfan L, C	*Polycystic kidneys L (cysts in 33%)
Amyotonia congenita W, see text	*Guillain–Barré W	*Maroteaux–Lamy C	
	*Hand–Schüller–Christian L	*Morquio C	*Pompe disease W
Central core myopathy W	*I-cell disease L, C (stiff)	Myasthenia congenita W	*Prader–Willi W (in infancy)
Chronic granulomatous disease L	Jeune C	Myasthenia gravis W	*Prune belly W
*Cretinism W	Kartagener L	*Myositis ossificans C (stiff)	*Riley–Day L
*Cutis laxa L	*Kearnes–Sayre W	*Myotonic dystrophy, see text	*Rubinstein L
*Cystic fibrosis L	Kugelberg–Welander muscular atrophy W	*Niemann–Pick disease L	*Scleroderma L
*Duchenne muscular dystrophy W		*Opitz–Frias L	*Smith–Lemli–Opitz L
	*Leigh W	*Osler–Weber–Rendu pulmonary AVMs	*VATER L
*Ehlers–Danlos L (pneumothorax	*Letterer–Siwe disease L		Werdnig–Hoffman disease W
*Familial periodic paralysis W	*McArdle disease W	*Osteogenesis imperfecta C	Wilson–Mikity L

(c) Cardiovascular (C, congenital heart disease; M, cardiomyopathy; A, autonomic or arrhythmias; I, ischaemic; T, thrombotic risk)

Albright osteodystrophy A	Fabry disease I	*Leigh M	Sebaceous naevi C
*Apert C	*Farber disease M	Leopard C	Shy–Drager A
Asplenia (Ivemark) C	Friedreich ataxia M	*McArdle disease M	Sipple A
*CHARGE association C	*Guillain–Barré A	*Marfan C	*Stevens–Johnson M
*Cherubism C	*Goldenhar C	*Maroteaux–Lamy M	Tangier disease I
Conradi C	*Grönblad–Strandberg T	*Meckel C	*TAR C
*Cretinism M	Holt–Oram C	*Myotonic dystrophy M	*Turner C
*Cri-du-chat C	*Homocystinuria T	*Noonan C	*VATER C
*DiGeorge C	*Hunter M	*Opitz–Frias C	*Velocardiofacial (Shprintzen) C
*Down (trisomy 21) C	*Hurler M	*Patau (trisomy 13) C	
*Duchenne muscular dystrophy M	*I-cell disease C (valvular)	Polysplenia C	*Werner I
	Ivemark C	*Pompe disease M	*Williams C
*Edward (trisomy 18) C	Jervell–Nielson A	Progeria I	Wolff–Parkinson–White A
*Ehlers–Danlos T	*Kearns–Sayre A	*Riley–Day A	
Ellis–van Creveld C	*Laurence–Moon–Biedl C	*Rubinstein C	

(*Continued*)

Table 28.1 (Continued)

(d) Endocrine (S, steroid coverage perioperatively; P, phaeochromocytoma; T, thyroid)

*Adrenogenital S	Dermatomyositis S	Lupus S	Sipple T, P
*Behçet S (often)	*Down T	Multiple mucosal neuroma	*Scleroderma S
*Blackfan–Diamond S	Epidermolysis bullosa	(multiple endocrine	*von Hippel–Lindau P
*Chédiak–Higashi S	S (often)	adenomatosis type IIb) P	*von Recklinghausen's disease P
Collagen vascular diseases	*Hand–Schüller–Christian S	Myositis ossificans S (often)	
S (often)	Juvenile rheumatoid arthritis S	Pendred T	
*Cretinism T	*Kasbach–Merrit S	Periarteritis nodosa	

(e) Metabolic (A, acid–base; G, glucose; E, electrolyte; C, calcium abnormalities)

*Adrenogenital E	*DiGeorge C	Lowe C	Von Gierke's disease G
*Albers–Schönberg C	*Down G	*McArdle disease G	*Wermer (multiple endocrine
Albright osteodystrophy C	*Familial periodic paralysis E	Maple syrup urine disease E, G	adenomatosis I) G, C
Albright–Butler E	*Fanconi E	*Mitochondrial disorders	*Werner G, C
Alström G	Hand–Schüller–Christian E	A, C, E, G	*Williams C
Andersen disease G	Homocystinuria G	*Paramyotonia congenita E	
Bartter E	*Laurence–Moon–Biedl	Phenylketonuria A, G	
*Beckwith–Wiedemann G	E (diabetes insipidus)	Prematurity G, E, C	
*Cretinism G, E	Leprechaunism G	*Prader–Willi G	
*Cystic fibrosis E (in hot	*Lesch–Nyhan uric acid	Seizure disorders (on	
climates)	*Lipodystrophy G	ketogenic diet); A, E, G	

(f) Skin problems (careful positioning, intravenous access may be difficult and/or temperature regulation may be problematic)

*Behçet ulcers in mouth	*Ehler–Danlos	*Grönblad–Strandberg	*Stevens–Johnson
*Christ–Siemens–Touraine	*Epidermolysis bullosa	*Osler–Weber–Rendu	
*Cutis laxa	mucosal	Ritter's disease	
*Down	and skin ulcers	*Scleroderma	

(g) Orthopaedic (limited joint mobility or fragile bones)

*Albers–Schönberg	*Marfan	*Osteogenesis	Scheie disease
disease	Ollier	imperfecta	

(h) Haematological (anaemia, platelet decrease or dysfunction, or clotting disturbance)

*Albers–Schönberg	*Hand–Schüller–Christian	*Maroteaux–Lamy	von Willebrand's disease
*Blackfan–Diamond	Hermansky	Moschkowitz disease	Wiskott–Aldrich
*Chédiak–Higashi	*Homocystinuria	*Niemann–Pick disease	Wolman's disease
Christmas disease	*Kasabach–Merrit	Sickle cell disease avoid	
Collagen vascular diseases	Klippel–Trenauney	pneumatic tourniquets	
Favism	*Letterer–Siwe disease	Tangier disease	
Gaucher disease	*Lipodystrophy	*TAR	

(i) Renal (renal dysfunction affects use of drugs such as muscle relaxants, morphine, pethidine)

Alport	*Edwards (trisomy 18)	Lowe	*VATER
Alström	Fabry disease	*Meckel	*von Hippel–Lindau
Bowen (cerebrohepatorenal)	*Fanconi	Orofacial–digital	*Wermer
Chotzen	*Farber disease	Polycystic kidneys	*Wilson disease
Conradi	*Laurence–Moon–Biedl	*Prune belly	
Denys Drash	*Lesch–Nyhan	Tuberous sclerosis	

(j) Pharmacology (S, avoid suxamethonium; M, careful use of muscle relaxants or barbiturates; H, avoid halothane; B, avoid barbiturates)

Amyotonia congenita M	*Familial periodic paralysis M	*McArdle disease S	Phenylketonuria M
*Arthrogryposis multiplex M	*Guillain–Barré S	*Mitochondrial disorders M,S	Porphyria B
Bowen M	Hallervorden–Spatz disease S	*Mytonia congenita M, S	*Wilson disease M
*Central core myopathy M, S, H	King S, H	*Myotonic dystrophy S, H, M	
*Duchenne muscular	Lesch–Nyhan S	*Paramyotonia congenital	
dystrophy M, S, H	*Lipodystrophy H	S, H, M	

†Listed by system; *These syndromes are listed in several sections.
AVM, arteriovenous malformation.

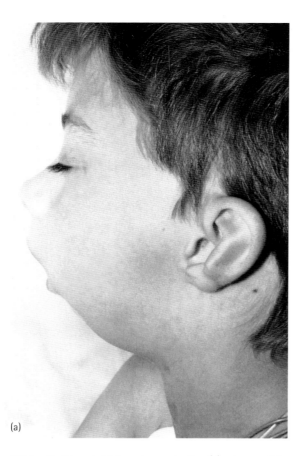
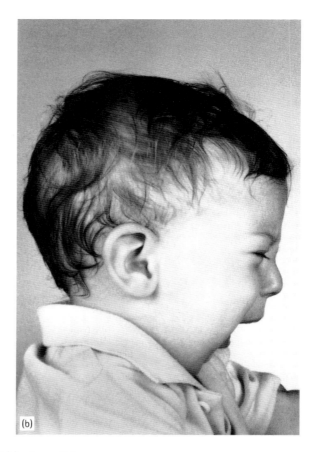

(a)
(b)

Figure 28.1 Profiles of children demonstrating (a) micrognathia and (b) retrognathia.

profile, is examined (Fig. 28.1). Stehling reported in adults that if the distance from the lower border of the mandible to the thyroid notch, measured with the neck extended, is less than 6 cm, visualisation of the larynx by conventional direct laryngoscopy will be impossible [7]. A distance of 6.5 cm, if associated with prominent upper teeth or limited cervical or temporomandibular motion, will also lead to difficult direct laryngoscopy. The equivalent distance in paediatric patients has not been reported. The child should also be assessed for facial asymmetry that may make mask fit problematic.

A complete history and physical examination of the respiratory system will identify patients with poor pulmonary reserve and may guide perioperative care and family counselling. A history of infant respiratory distress syndrome requiring mechanical ventilation, cystic fibrosis, recurrent pneumonia, asthma or muscular dystrophy will identify patients at risk for intraoperative or postoperative respiratory problems. Pulmonary function testing in older children with a progressive disease course such as Duchenne muscular dystrophy can quantify pulmonary reserve and guide anaesthesia and perioperative management.

The cardiovascular assessment should include enquiries about congenital heart disease, the use of cardiac medications (digoxin, diuretics, afterload reduction agents,

β blockers or antiarrhythmics), the exercise tolerance of the child or a history consistent with arrhythmias (syncopal episodes or paroxysmal tachycardia). The signs and symptoms of congestive heart failure in infants are non-specific and may be subtle. Tachypnoea, nasal flaring or grunting respirations are often present. The infant may feed slowly, tire during feeding or sweat profusely, and weight gain is often poor. The older child may tire more quickly than playmates. Physical examination may reveal a cardiac murmur, tachycardia at rest or arrhythmias, hepatomegaly, cyanosis or clubbing of the fingers. Recent cardiological evaluations should be reviewed or obtained to aid perioperative care. Cardiac evaluation should be considered when major anomalies are present in other systems, such as gastrointestinal (e.g. omphalocele, duodenal atresia), or with extremity malformations (Holt–Oram syndrome, VATER syndrome; Table 28.2), since cardiac development occurs concurrently with gastrointestinal and extremity formation, and anomalies may be present in both.

In congenital syndromes known to include metabolic abnormalities (Table 28.1), laboratory studies are needed and should include evaluation of glucose levels, acid–base status, electrolytes and calcium concentrations. General neurological development needs to be assessed in more detail in children with congenital anomalies than in the normal population, since it affects anaesthetic plans. Focal

Table 28.2   Congenital syndromes frequently found to have associated congenital heart defects

Syndrome	Findings	Congenital cardiac lesion	Incidence (%)
Alagille	Intrahepatic cirrhosis, vertebral anomalies,	Peripheral pulmonary stenosis	
Apert	Craniosynostosis, midfacial hypoplasia, syndactyly of extremities	VSD, ToF	
Blackfan–Diamond	Anaemia in infancy	VSD	
Carpenter	Synostosis of coronal, sagittal or lamboid sutures, brachydactyly and partial syndactyly of hands and feet, polydactyly of feet	PDA, VSD	
CHARGE association	Coloboma, choanal atresia, slow growth, developmental delay, microphallus, cryptorchidism, micrognathia/cleft palate, ear anomalies/deafness	Vascular ring or interrupted aortic arch, AV canal, ToF, truncus arteriosus, DORV with AV canal, VSD, PDA	60–70
Cri-du-chat	Slow growth, developmental delay, microcephaly, hypertelorism, strabismus, simian crease	VSD, ASD	25
Crouzon	Craniostenosis, shallow orbits	Coarctation of aorta	
DiGeorge	Hypoparathyroidism, hypocalcaemia, deficient T-cell-mediated immunity, thymic hypoplasia, micrognathia, cleft palate, hypertelorism	Truncus arteriosus, double aortic arch (vascular ring), right aortic arch, ToF, interrupted aortic arch, VSD	13–30 TA, 8–25 VSD 14–26 R Ao arch 20–30 ToF, 30–56 IAA
Down syndrome	(See trisomy 21)		
Duchenne muscular dystrophy	Myopathy with progressive weakness, scoliosis, at risk for aspiration, malignant hyperthermia risk, progressive respiratory insufficiency	Cardiomyopathy Mitral valve prolapse	Eventual 100 25
Ehlers–Danlos	Hyperextensible joints, blue sclerae, easy bruising, parchment scars, scoliosis, hernias, pes planus	Mitral insufficiency	50
Ellis–van Creveld	Short distal extremities, polydactyly, hypoplastic nails, dysplastic teeth, small thorax	ASD	50
Foetal alcohol	Microphthalmos, microcephaly, developmental delay, growth failure	VSD, PDA	
Goldenhar	See text	ToF, VSD	33
Holt–Oram	Radial club hand or hypoplasia, proximal thumb placement	ASD, VSD	
Homocystinuria	Lens dislocation (downward), slender, pectus excavatum, osteoporosis, malar flush	Thrombotic events	
Hurler	See text	Aortic insufficiency, mitral insufficiency	
Ivemark (asplenia)	Absent spleen, infection risk increased, situs inversus of abdominal viscera	Dextrocardia, complex cyanotic heart disease (e.g. TGA, single ventricle), AV canal defects	100
Kartagener	Ciliary dyskinesis with sinusitis, male infertility	Dextrocardia, situs inversus	
Marfan	Long thin limbs and fingers, joint laxity with scoliosis, pectus excavatum, tall stature, lens dislocation (upward), high arched palate	Aortic aneurysm, aortic regurgitation, mitral valve prolapse	60

(Continued)

Table 28.2   (*Continued*)

Syndrome	Findings	Congenital cardiac lesion	Incidence (%)
Multiple lentigines (Leopard)	Hypertelorism, dark lentigenes especially on face or trunk, prominent ears, sensorineural deafness, developmental delay	PS	95
Noonan	See text	PS, ASD	62 (PS)
	Cardiomyopathy	Hypertrophic cardiomyopathy	20
Rubella	Cataract, deafness, developmental delay, cryptorchidism	PDA, PS (peripheral), VSD	
Scimitar	Hypoplasia right lung and right pulmonary artery	Right pulmonary veins into IVC	
Smith–Lemli–Opitz	Developmental delay, microcephaly, ptosis, strabismus, micrognathia, hypospadias, cryptorchidism	ASD, VSD, ToF	
TAR (thrombocytopenia, absent radius)	Decreased platelets and megakaryocytes, bilateral radial hypoplasia/aplasia	ToF	
Trisomy 13	Small-for-age, severe developmental delay, deafness, microcephaly, retinal dysplasia, cleft lip/palate (80%), polydactlyly, parieto-occipital scalp skin defects	VSD, dextroversion	90
Trisomy 18	Growth deficiency, developmental delay, low-set ears, micrognathia, short sternum, clenched hand	VSD, PDA, PS	99
Trisomy 21	See text	AV canal, ASD, VSD	50
		ToF	8
Tuberous sclerosis	Adenoma sebaceum, ash-leaf spots, café-au-lait spots, hamartoma of brain, seizures, developmental delay	Rhabdomyomas	
Turner	Pterygium colli, infantile lymphoedema, short stature, webbed neck, low hairline	Coarctation of aorta, AS	35
VATER	Vertebral anomalies, anal atresia, T-O fistula, radial dysplasia	VSD	20-30
Velocardiofacial syndrome (overlap with Di George syndrome)	Hypotonia, slender fingers, high arch or cleft palate, variable developmental delay, long face with deficient malar area, micrognathia	VSD	75
		ToF	20
		Right aortic arch	50
Williams	See text	AS, PS	

AS, aortic stenosis; ASD, atrial septal defect, AV, arteriovenous; DORV with AV canal double outlet right ventricle with atrioventricular canal; IAA, interrupted aortic arch. PDA patent ductus arteriosus; PS, pulmonary stenosis; TGA, transposition of great arteries; ToF, tetralogy of Fallot; T-O, tracheo-oesophageal; VSD, ventricular septal defect.

findings such as spastic diplegia or hemiparesis may affect the placement of intravenous or arterial catheters or choice of anaesthesia (general compared with regional techniques). Positioning of these children to avoid pressure areas can be more challenging. The infant with hydrocephalus requires a smooth induction and intubation to avoid potential problems from increases in intracranial pressure.

Musculoskeletal abnormalities may also affect anaesthesia choices. In the myotonia syndromes, suxamethonium should be avoided. Duchenne muscular dystrophy may be associated with malignant hyperthermia (MH) and a non-triggering anaesthetic technique that avoids suxamethonium and inhalational agents should be strongly considered with careful monitoring of vital signs, including temperature. Cardiac arrests in infants and children, especially those where hyperkalaemia was a factor during the arrest, have been shown to have occurred in patients with occult myopathies [8]. It is essential that the possibility of an occult myopathy is considered preoperatively, particularly in male infants and that hyperkalaemia is considered in the differential diagnosis of any pulseless rhythms seen in the operating theatre. The differential diagnosis for infants who are hypotonic and weak is extensive and includes several diseases with anaesthetic implications [9].

Children with unusual facies or defects in multiple systems can be identified and seen by genetic or dysmorphology consultants to aid preoperative diagnosis before elective surgical procedures.

SYNDROMES AFFECTING AIRWAY MANAGEMENT

The infant or child with a congenital syndrome, which includes compromise of the airway, can be identified at the preoperative examination by symptoms such as stridor, by the presence of an obstructing mass (e.g. cystic hygroma or a large tongue), micrognathia, limited mouth opening or neck mobility. Pratical guidance on airway management is given in Chapter 21. Perkins *et al.* [10] reviewed over 100 patients with bilateral craniofacial abnormalities and separated them into three groups: those with only mandibular hypoplasia (such as Pierre Robin syndrome); those with only mid-face hypoplasia (such as Apert syndrome); and those with a combination of mid-face and mandibular hypoplasia (such as Treacher Collins syndrome). Sixty-five per cent required

airway intervention, ranging from positioning (during natural sleep) to tracheostomy and airway intervention was most commonly needed in the first month of life, with a few older patients requiring intervention for sleep apnoea or post-surgical obstructive symptoms. Tracheostomy was most commonly needed in the patients with both mid-face and mandibular abnormalities [10].

Pierre Robin syndrome

Pierre Robin syndrome or the Robin anomalad includes micrognathia, glossoptosis and a U-shaped cleft palate (Fig. 28.2). *In utero* mandibular hypoplasia displaces the tongue posteriorly, interfering with closure of the soft palate. These children may present in infancy for glossopexy or tracheostomy if the tongue and small mandible cause severe airway obstruction with cyanosis and apnoea. This condition is seen in otherwise normal children, and growth of the mandible in the first year of life is possible, resulting in a normal jaw in later childhood. However, the Robin anomalad may be seen as a part of other syndromes, including Stickler, Cornelia de Lange, Hallerman–Streiff or femoral hypoplasia syndromes. Most of these infants used to be cared for with prone positioning for their first weeks or months of life, but many feel that the use of nasopharyngeal airways is safer. Severe airway compromise may necessitate surgery to improve airway patency (Fig. 28.2).

Goldenhar syndrome

Goldenhar syndrome (hemifacial microsomia) occurs as a unilateral defect in development of the first and second branchial arches (Fig. 28.3). These children show asymmetrical hypoplasia of malar, maxillary and mandibular

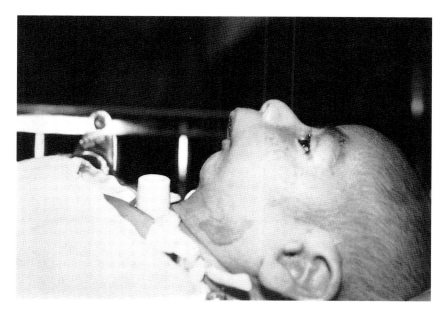

Figure 28.2 Pierre Robin anomalad; severe airway obstruction necessitated tracheostomy.

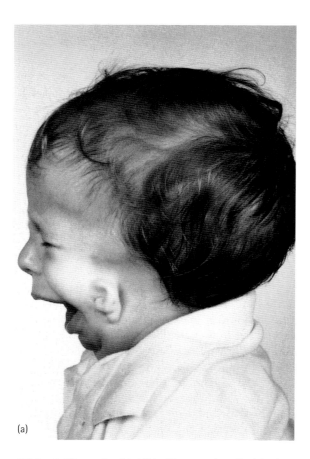
(a)

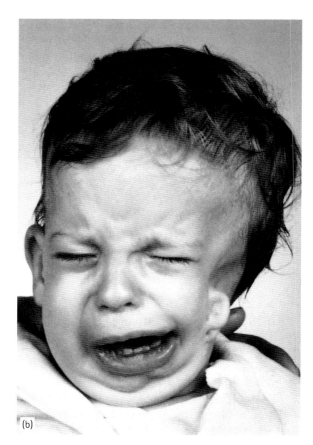
(b)

Figure 28.3   A 16-month-old child with severe hemifacial microsomia. His profile from the unaffected side is shown in Fig. 28.1b.

development, which may include soft tissues and the tongue. Goldenhar syndrome is the diagnosis if epibulbar dermoids, congenital heart disease or cervical vertebral defects accompany the facial defects. If involvement is primarily facial, then hemifacial microsomia is the diagnosis given, but these probably represent gradations of the same defect in morphogenesis [11]. The mouth often has a cleft-like extension on the affected side, making mask fit during anaesthesia a problem. A deformed to absent external pinna or a preauricular skin tag is often associated with unilateral deafness. Cardiac defects, especially ventricular septal defect (VSD) or tetralogy of Fallot (ToF), are associated conditions in Goldenhar syndrome. These children present for reconstructive surgery of their mandibles or external ear. Induction of general anaesthesia may present difficulties in maintaining a patent airway and in laryngoscopy and intubation, particularly if the right side is affected. The facial asymmetry may worsen as the child ages increasing airway problems during anaesthetic induction.

Treacher Collins syndrome

This is an autosomal dominant mandibulofacial dysostosis with down-slanting palpebral fissures, eyelid colobomas, bilateral malar and mandibular hypoplasia, and

malformation of the external pinna and ear canal (Fig. 28.4). Conductive deafness is seen in 40 per cent of these children. Mandibular and pharyngeal hypoplasia in these children are significant contributors to apnoea during awake and sleep states, as well as to difficult intubations during anaesthesia [12]. Unlike most other craniofacial syndromes that often improve with age, the risk of apnoea does not improve and may even worsen. Mandibular and maxillary advancement osteotomies, which reorientate growth in a more normal direction, provide functional as well as aesthetic benefits [13]. Mental development is normal. Miller and Nager syndromes share the facial features of Treacher Collins syndrome, in association with limb defects.

Kabuki syndrome

This was first described in Japan in 1981 and consists of five characteristics including a peculiar face resembling the make-up used in Kabuki theatre, skeletal anomaly, dermatoglyphic abnormality, moderate learning disability and short stature [14]. Other manifestations of anaesthetic importance include retrognathia (36 per cent), cardiac defects such as VSD and atrial septal defect (ASD) (32 per cent) and, in non-Japanese patients, neonatal hypotonia (33 per cent) and seizures (29 per cent).

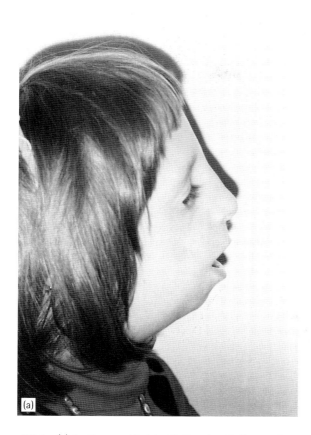 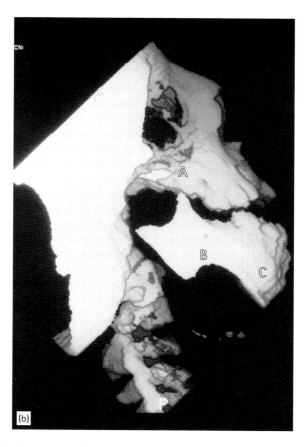

Figure 28.4   (a) An 8-year-old girl with Treacher Collins syndrome, with (b) corresponding three-dimensional computed tomographic scan showing complete absence of zygoma (A), characteristic mandibular deformity with prominent antigonial notch (B) and severe mandibular retrusion (C). (Photographs courtesy of Dr Joseph Gruss.)

Möbius syndrome

This rare defect results from agenesis or hypoplasia of cranial nerve nuclei, in particular cranial nerves VI and VII. The facial nerve palsies can be associated with poor mandibular growth and secondary micrognathia; twelfth nerve involvement may limit tongue movement. A small number (approximately 10 per cent) of affected children have other brain anomalies. Difficulties in intubation in these children relate mainly to the degree of micrognathia or limited mouth opening. [15]

Klippel–Feil anomalad

In the Klippel–Feil anomalad there is fusion of cervical vertebrae causing a short neck with limited mobility owing to a congenital defect in the formation or segmentation of the cervical spine [16]. This may interfere with positioning for intubation, making visualisation of the larynx difficult. Frequently associated findings in these children include neurological deficits, deafness, congenital heart disease (VSD) and scoliosis. The limited neck motion can be easily missed, resulting in unanticipated intubation difficulties.

Arthogryposis multiplex congenita

This diagnostic complex results from a number of neuro-pathic or myopathic problems active *in utero*, which lead to limited foetal joint mobility and cause congenital joint contractures. The immobile joints are most obvious in the extremities, but these children cause most concern to anaesthetists when limited temporomandibular and cervical spine movement make intubation difficult. These patients are discussed in detail by Hall [17]; two-thirds have a good prognosis for mental development, but one-third will have severe central nervous system abnormalities and most of the latter group die in infancy. Whether these patients are at risk for MH continues to be an area of dispute [18–20]. Venous access can often be difficult to obtain in this patient group.

Similar limitations in joint mobility in the jaw and neck may be seen in children with juvenile rheumatoid arthritis.

Mucopolysaccharidoses

The mucopolysaccharidoses are lysosomal storage disorders characterised by the progressive diffuse accumulation of mucopolysaccharides in lysosomes in bone, muscle and visceral organs and in the soft tissues of the mouth and pharynx. Classification of these disorders is based on clinical, biochemical and/or genetic differences.

Hurler syndrome (mucopolysaccharidosis type I) shows the most severe involvement with coarse facies, macroglossia, infiltration of pharyngeal and laryngeal soft tissues, short neck, kyphosis, corneal opacities, claw hand and limited cardiac function as distinctive features (Fig. 28.5). Profuse secretions from upper and lower airways are usual, and severe learning disability is obvious by 3 years of age. Hunter syndrome (mucopolysaccharidosis type II) differs only in the more gradual onset of symptoms, lack of corneal opacities and presentation only in males. The combination of learning disability with limited ability to cooperate, profuse airway secretions and increasing soft-tissue infiltration with the mucopolysaccharide tissue make airway management and intubation a major anaesthetic problem, particularly in the child past infancy.

Baines and Keneally reported their experience with these children: some 50 per cent of their patients had difficulties with airway management during anaesthesia [21]. Profuse secretions occluding a tracheostomy, coughing spasms, difficulty maintaining a patent airway during mask anaesthesia and failed intubation were the main problems. Inhalational inductions were used in the majority, with small amounts of intravenous agents to aid induction in uncooperative children. Recommendations included maintaining spontaneous ventilation until airway control is secured and preoperative atropine. Moores and coworkers summarized experience with these patients, including cardiac and ventilatory difficulties [22].

Morquio syndrome (mucopolysaccharidosis type IV) presents fewer problems with soft-tissue infiltration of the upper airway and mental development is usually normal (Fig. 28.6). Chest-wall deformities result in limited ventilatory reserve. These children also have odontoid hypoplasia,

putting them at risk of anterior dislocation of the C1 vertebra with resultant spinal cord compression. This can occur during head positioning for tracheal intubation, so extreme flexion should be avoided by having an assistant

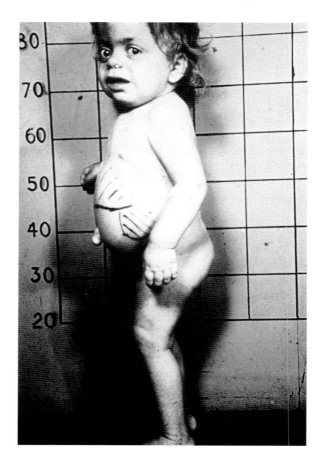

Figure 28.5 Hurler syndrome (mucopolysaccharidosis type I). Note thickened facial features, short neck and nasal secretions. (Photograph courtesy of Dr VA McKusick.)

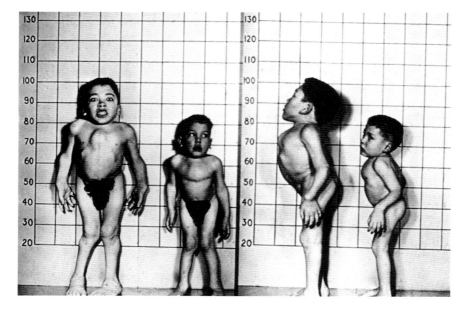

Figure 28.6 Morquio syndrome in two brothers. (Photograph courtesy of Dr VA McKusick.)

hold the head in the neutral position during laryngoscopy. Several other congenital syndromes associated with odontoid hypoplasia have been included in Table 28.1.

Cleft lip and/or palate

Cleft lip and/or palate may be seen as part of many syndromes, including the CHARGE association (*c*oloboma of the eye, *h*eart defects, *a*tresia of the choanae, *r*etardation of growth and/or development, *g*enital and/or urinary abnormalities, and *e*ar abnormalities and deafness), foetal hydantoin and trimethadione, Robert's 4P⁻, Mohr, orofacial–digital and velocardiofacial syndromes and trisomy 18. It is an isolated defect in 90–95 per cent of affected children. Isolated cleft palate is more commonly associated with other congenital anomalies than is cleft lip/palate. Airway management and intubation are usually straightforward, but on occasion a modified approach to intubation may be needed (see Chapters 21 and 35) Following palate closure, the tongue may cause airway obstruction, so these children should be extubated when they are fully awake after removal of pharyngeal packs and inspection for tongue swelling from the mouth gag used intraoperatively (further details can be found in Chapter 35).

Haemangiomas and lymphangiomas

Haemangiomas and lymphangiomas (cystic hygromas) are congenital benign tumours but can cause significant airway problems, particularly if intraoral extension limits airway access or their large size causes extrinsic tracheal compression (Fig. 28.7). Haemangiomas, if present elsewhere, can provide a clue to their presence in the trachea and, like laryngeal webs or cysts, may present with stridor or other symptoms of airway obstruction.

Beckwith–Wiedemann syndrome

This syndrome includes omphalocele, macroglossia, large size and neonatal hypoglycaemia (Fig. 28.8). Because

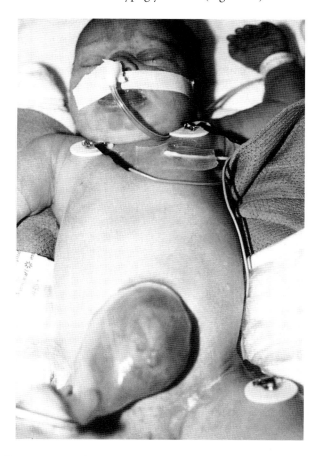

Figure 28.8 Infant with Beckwith–Wiedemann syndrome showing omphalocele, macroglossia and large size (birth weight 4.1 kg). Hypoglycaemia responded to intravenous 10 per cent dextrose solution.

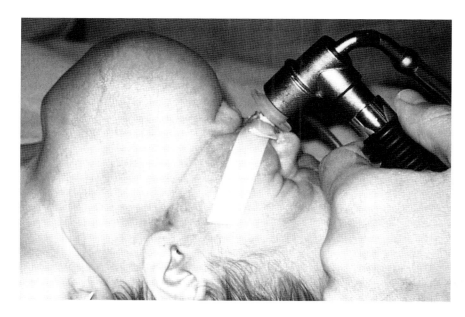

Figure 28.7 Infant with large cystic hygroma.

omphaloceles are also seen in 10–50 per cent of infants with trisomy 13 or 18, chromosomal studies are indicated in all infants with omphaloceles [11]. Congenital heart disease is seen in 20 per cent of infants with omphaloceles and genitourinary defects, including exstrophy of the bladder, have been reported frequently [23]. These infants should have frequent blood sugar determinations while under anaesthesia because hypoglycaemia may occur [24]. Extubation following omphalocele repair is attempted only when the infant has demonstrated adequate spontaneous ventilation, because limitations of diaphragmatic excursion often necessitate a period of postoperative mechanical ventilation.

SYNDROMES AT RISK FOR RAPID INTRAOPERATIVE BLOOD LOSS

Craniosynostosis, is premature fusion of one or more of the skull sutures, and is a major component of several congenital syndromes, including Crouzon (Fig. 28.9), Saethre–Chotzen, Pfeiffer, Carpenter and Apert syndromes (Fig. 28.10). All but Crouzon syndrome have associated syndactyly. Most patients

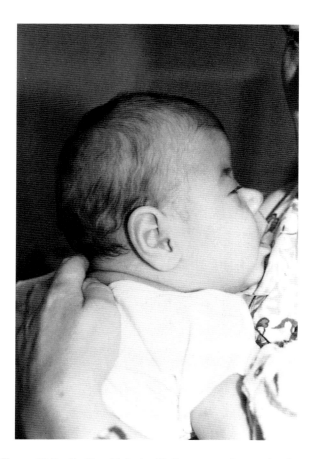

Figure 28.9 Profile of infant with Crouzon syndrome, showing small cranial vault in relation to normal size of facial features. Craniectomy is performed to prevent intracranial pressure problems during the infant's period of rapid brain growth.

with these disorders are of normal intellect or mildly delayed. These children present at several months of age for craniectomy or for more extensive revision of the skull and orbital area. The anaesthetic management of these syndromes is discussed in Chapter 38.

Many other congenital anomalies carry a high risk of blood loss, including separation of conjoined twins [25] correction of kyphoscoliosis in a child with Morquio syndrome or resection of a sacrococcygeal teratoma. Adequate intravenous access is necessary to allow rapid transfusion, and cross-matched blood must be present in the operating theatre or immediate environment and checked so that transfusion can be given immediately with warming equipment for blood products. Intra-arterial catheters (for continuous blood pressure monitoring) aid recognition of occult blood loss into the surgical drapes. Urinary catheters are a helpful adjunct to assess the adequacy of fluid resuscitation. Doppler monitoring for recognition of entrainment of air through bony venous channels has been reported to be useful but may not be possible in operations undertaken in the prone position.

SYNDROMES ASSOCIATED WITH VENTILATORY PROBLEMS

Ventilation difficulties may be present before surgery, or may develop intraoperatively or in the postoperative period. They may be caused by intrinsic lung disease, chest-wall deformities or muscular weakness (see Table 28.1). Pratical advice on ventilatory management can be found in Chapter 31.

Myotonic dystrophy

This autosomal dominant disorder is characterised by myotonia (persistent contracture of skeletal muscle following stimulation), cataracts, frontal baldness, testicular atrophy in males and expressionless 'myopathic' facies [26]. Presentation in late adolescence is most common, with progressive muscle weakness and swallowing difficulties, but subtle symptoms have been reported in childhood. Cardiac conduction abnormalities are present in over 50 per cent of patients.

Myotonia congenita, another autosomal dominant disorder, shows hypertrophied muscle and more severe myo-tonia but no weakness or cardiac involvement. Paramyotonia presents as myotonia and weakness induced by exposure to cold; potassium levels should be evaluated in these patients since myotonia may be seen in patients with familial periodic paralysis where episodes of weakness may be seen in association with abnormal serum potassium. Hypokalaemia-related episodes tend to be longer (up to 36 hours), while in the hyperkalaemia type duration is several hours.

Anaesthetic management in the myotonia syndromes is influenced by several special considerations. Since cold or shivering increases myotonia, a warm environment is

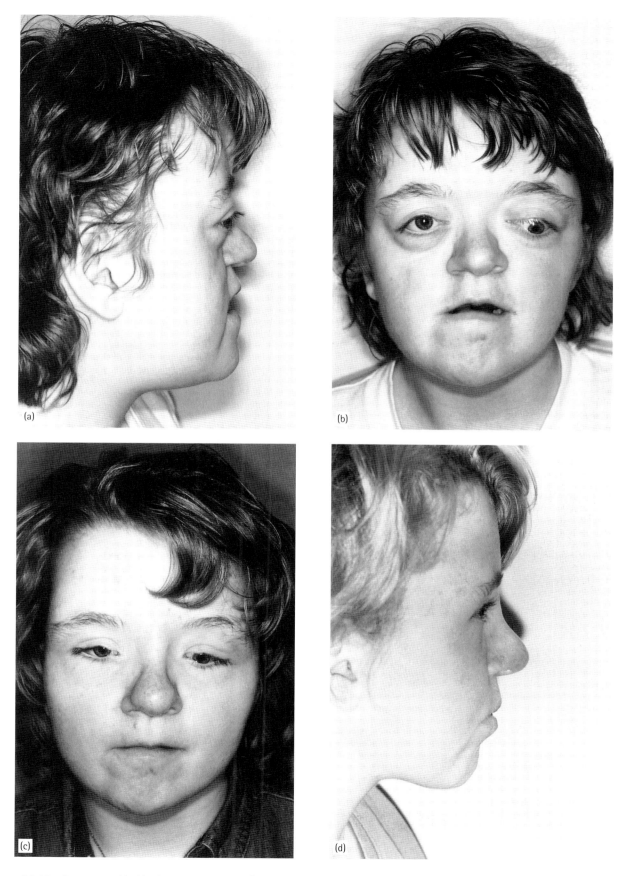

Figure 28.10 A 14-year-old girl with Apert syndrome (craniosynostosis, midface hypoplasia): (a,b) preoperative and (c,d) post-Lefort III mid-face advancement. (Photographs courtesy of Dr Joseph Gruss.)

essential. Depolarising muscle relaxants are absolutely contraindicated, since generalised myotonia has been seen following suxamethonium, making ventilation difficult or even impossible for several minutes. Non-depolarising muscle relaxants may be used safely with a transcutaneous nerve stimulator to titrate dosage, but are ineffective if local manipulation causes myotonia. In fact, if rigidity persists after a full paralysing dose of relaxant, this indicates that the problem is more distal than the neuromuscular junction, myotonia being an example of this [27]. Muscle relaxants should be avoided if possible, especially in familial periodic paralysis. Minimal fasting and avoiding hypoglycaemia are important in the hyperkalaemic variant, while glucose loading can precipitate weakness in the hypokalaemic type. Direct injection of local anaesthetic into the affected muscle has been suggested to treat local myotonia [28]. Demonstration of adequate spontaneous ventilation prior to extubation should include an inspiratory effort greater than $-30\,cmH_2O$ and a tidal volume greater than 5 mL/kg. Postoperative monitoring should last for several hours or overnight to observe for delayed episodes of weakness.

Inadequate ventilation may be seen in congenital neuromuscular syndromes associated with weakness or inadequate cough, such as Werdnig–Hoffmann syndrome, myasthenia gravis, nemaline myopathy, central core disease or the muscular dystrophies of which Duchenne is the most common and the most severe. Careful titration of muscle relaxants, if any are used, and assisted or controlled ventilation intraoperatively guide care. Assessment of chest-wall and diaphragmatic function should include inspiratory effort (normal > $-30\,cmH_2O$) and tidal volume (>5 mL/kg) prior to extubation. Children with central core disease and nemaline myopathy are at risk for MH and many anaesthetists would also choose a non-triggering technique for patients with Duchenne muscular dystrophy (see Chapters11 and 29).

Cystic fibrosis

This autosomal recessive disorder, in which the gene locus on chromosome 7 has been isolated, involves abnormal sweat and mucus production and pancreatic insufficiency with diffuse effects, but it is the pulmonary involvement that impinges most directly on anaesthetic management. The ventilatory problems include inspissated secretions, ventilation–perfusion mismatching with resultant hypoxaemia and infection of large and small airways with mul-tiple organisms, often including *Pseudomonas* species. Advanced pulmonary disease results in cor pulmonale. The use of chest percussion, postural drainage and antibiotics preoperatively to optimise pulmonary function has been generally recommended [28]. Atropine will cause drying of secretions and is usually omitted. Ketamine is best avoided because of its stimulation of airway reflexes, with exacerbation of coughing. General anaesthesia with tracheal intub-ation allows intraoperative suctioning of secretions as needed, and controlled or assisted ventilation is used to minimise atelectasis.

Inhalational anaesthesia with halothane or sevoflurane is well tolerated, but induction may be prolonged owing to ventilation–perfusion mismatching. Intra-arterial monitoring for serial blood gases is indicated in the presence of severe lung disease or cor pulmonale. Adequacy of ventilation must be demonstrated before extubation, as detailed above, with inspiratory effort and tidal volume and, in the severely affected child, by blood-gas measurement during spontaneous ventilation. Postoperative chest physiotherapy and close observation remain necessary, since deterioration in lung function has been reported following general anaesthesia [29]. Information on post-operative analgesia is limited but regional techniques have been used with good results [30].

Prune–belly syndrome

This syndrome results from a congenital deficiency of the abdominal musculature, associated with genitourinary anomalies (Fig. 28.11) [31]. The long-term prognosis in these children is determined by the degree of compromise of their renal function. The abdominal musculature deficiency raises the potential problem of inadequate cough and breathing before, during or after anaesthesia.

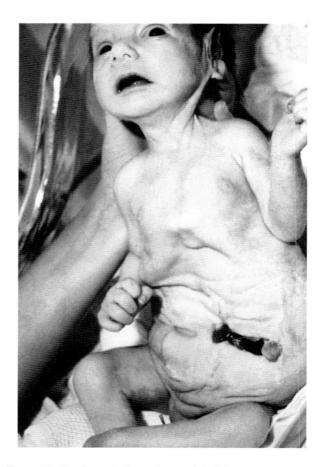

Figure 28.11   Prune-belly syndrome with air hunger.

SYNDROMES ASSOCIATED WITH CARDIOVASCULAR PROBLEMS

Congenital heart disease and its implications for anaesthesia are addressed in Chapters 3, 30 and 39, but Table 28.2 lists syndromes frequently associated with congenital heart disease [28,32,33].

Trisomy 21 (Down syndrome)

Down syndrome is a chromosomal disorder involving all body systems. The characteristic flat facies, protruding tongue, inner canthal folds, up-slanting palpebral fissures, hypotonia and hyperflexible joints, learning disability and short, broad hands with simian creases are easily recognised. Some 50 per cent of these children have congenital heart disease, most commonly endocardial cushion defects or ventricular septal defect. The hyperflexible joints necessitate careful intubation, since cervical dislocation with spinal cord damage has been reported [34,35].

Turner syndrome

This should be suspected in any female with short stature. Ovarian dysgenesis with failure of sexual maturation at puberty and infertility, as well as short neck, low hairline with posterior webbing or pterygium and widely spaced nipples, are additional findings (Fig. 28.12). Thirty per cent of these children have cardiac defects, usually coarctation of the aorta. Chromosome studies demonstrate the XO karyotype.

Noonan syndrome represents the phenotype of Turner syndrome but with normal chromosomes. Short stature, webbed neck and cryptorchidism in males are findings similar to Turner syndrome; learning disability and pectus excavatum are more common in Noonan syndrome and the congenital heart disease seen is commonly pulmonary stenosis rather than coarctation of the aorta [36].

Williams syndrome

This sporadic disorder includes prominent lips, wide mouth, elfin facies, mild growth retardation and learning disability, hypercalcaemia in infancy (20 per cent), and valvular and supravalvular aortic and/or pulmonary stenosis. These children have a distinctive hoarse voice and most have a talkative manner but 10 per cent have severe behavioural problems.

Arrhythmias

Arrhythmias are the major feature in Romano–Ward syndrome (prolonged QT), Jervell–Lange–Nielsen syndrome (prolonged QT and deafness) and Wolff–Parkinson–White syndrome (aberrant arteriovenous conduction, with a short PR interval and delta waves on the ECG). Placement of a transvenous pacemaker for perioperative care is the safest course for the prolonged QT syndromes, but left stellate ganglion block has also been used with success [37,38]. In patients with Wolff–Parkinson–White syndrome, avoidance of tachycardia and excitation is recommended. If supraventricular tachycardia appears, the use of esmolol 0.01 mg/kg increments given intravenously or intravenous adenosine 0.05 mg/kg, with doubling of the dose if no effect is seen, has been successful in converting the rhythm to normal sinus rhythm. The use of verapamil (0.1 mg/kg) is suggested by some, but discouraged by others. In recalcitrant cases, synchronised DC cardioversion should be available for intraoperative use.

Tuberous sclerosis

Tuberous sclerosis is characterised by hamartomatous lesions that may involve multiple systems. It is dominantly inherited, with many cases representing fresh mutations. The skin changes appear in early to mid-childhood, have been called adenoma sebaceum (a misnomer) and prominently affect nasolabial folds. Affected children have

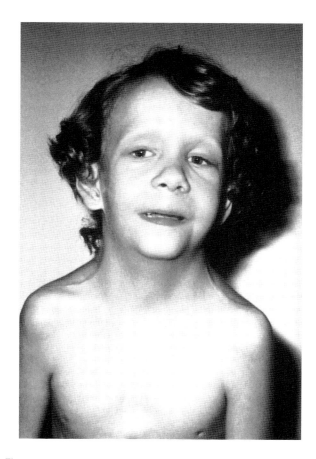

Figure 28.12 Female child with Turner syndrome. Past surgical scars from resection of nuchal lymphoedema can be seen.

ash-leaf spots (hypopigmented areas) and café-au-lait spots are visible from infancy. Seizures and learning disability are seen in most affected children; intracranial hamartomas can present in some. Cardiac involvement with rhabdomyomas may present with arrhythmias or signs of obstruction to blood flow. Anaesthetic management should avoid possible arrhythmogenic agents (e.g. halothane) and should maintain normal intravascular volume to minimise ventricular outflow obstruction.

VATER association

Children with congenital heart disease should be examined for other anomalies. If abnormalities of the vertebrae, anus (imperforate) or arms (radial dysplasia) are found, careful evaluation for the presence of tracheo-oesophageal fistula is mandatory; this symptom complex represents the VATER association (**v**ertebral anomalies, imperforate **a**nus, **t**racheo-oesophageal fistula, **r**adial or **r**enal anomalies) [39]. Congenital heart disease is seen in 20–30 per cent of these children.

Familial dysautonomia (Riley–Day syndrome)

Disturbances of autonomic function with this condition have profound anaesthetic implications. There may be a defect in the formation of noradrenaline from levo-dopa, which is manifest clinically by cardiovascular and temperature instability, hypotonia, no tear production and insensitivity to pain. Recurrent pulmonary aspiration after gastro-oesophageal reflux is common, so that lung function deteriorates as the child ages and is usually the eventual cause of death. Nissen fundoplication and feeding jejunostomy are frequently required [40].

The absence of compensatory cardiovascular reflexes may make anaesthesia hazardous. Respiratory-depressant analgesics should be used with great care and in reduced doses. Premedication with a benzodiazepine is satisfactory, but atropine should be avoided where possible. There is no contraindication to the use of muscle relaxants, but inhalational agents must also be used with care. Hypovolaemia is poorly tolerated. Hypotension may be controlled by fluid administration and hypertension by increasing the dose of inhalational agent. Where appropriate, epidural anaesthesia is recommended [41]. Postoperative respiratory support may be necessary.

SYNDROMES THAT REQUIRE SPECIAL CARE WITH MOVEMENT OR POSITIONING

Difficulties with positioning occur in the infant with meningomyelocele or in thoracopagus conjoined twins. Intubation is usually possible with such infants in a lateral position.

Epidermolysis bullosa

Epidermolysis bullosa is a genetically inherited group of skin disorders that result in vesicles and bullae, occurring either spontaneously or with minimal trauma or friction. Both dominant and recessively inherited forms of the disorder have been described. The most severely involved are the recessive forms, where bullae heal with scarring that can result in significant contractures and syndactyly. Involvement of oral mucosa in these patients can result in microstomia and involvement of mucosa in the larynx and pharynx has been reported [42]. James and Wark reported no tracheal or laryngeal problems after anaesthesia with tracheal intubation in 131 patients with epidermolysis bullosa dystrophica [43]. Stomal ulcers, strictures, reduced mouth opening and limited neck movement can contribute to difficult laryngoscopy as well as acquired microstomia and poor dentition [44]. Special care is essential to prevent trauma to skin or mucosa; recommendations for management are given in Table 28.3. If using a tracheal tube, one of 0.5–1 mm internal diameter smaller than predicted has been recommended [28]. Ketamine and halothane have both been used successfully. When tracheal tubes have been used the pharynx and vocal cords should be visualised prior to extubation to look for bullae formation. A carefully inserted, well-lubricated laryngeal mask airway has proved satisfactory in many cases.

No problems have been reported with the use of suxamethonium but unpredictable sensitivity to non-polarising neuromuscular relaxants demands strict monitoring if these drugs are used.

Regional anaesthesia is gaining in popularity [45] despite theoretical risks of sepsis and infective complications. Skin condition needs careful assessment before percutaneous needle placement as typical landmarks and 'tissue feel' are often altered.

Children with ectodermal dysplasis (Christ–Siemens–Touraine syndrome) have no sebaceous or sweat glands, absent hair and absent teeth (partial or complete). Full expression of this sex-linked recessive disorder is seen in males and the facial features include depressed nasal bridge, deformed external ears, thick lips and underdeveloped maxilla and mandible. Airway management may be a problem in these children. Thermoregulation is defective because of the lack of sweat glands; therefore, cooling measures should be available (cooling mattress, cool intravenous solutions) and temperature should be closely monitored. Anticholinergic medication is avoided because of its effect on temperature.

Osteogenesis imperfecta

Patients with osteogenesis imperfecta or with osteopetrosis are at risk of fractures and joint dislocations with minimal trauma. Care in moving and positioning these patients extends to intubation, since their teeth are more fragile than normal (see also Chapter 36).

Table 28.3 Guidelines for the care of children with epidermolysis bullosa. These patients must be handled with great care during anaesthesia

Monitoring
  Pulse oximeter
    Should be secured over Clingfilm placed directly over a digit
  Neonatal ECG dots
    Can be stuck onto defibrillator pads cut to an appropriate size, with a further piece of defibrillator pad on top to secure them
  Blood pressure cuffs
    Should have a protective layer of vellband underneath
Airway
  Lubrication
    The facemask, laryngoscope and airway should be lubricated with white soft paraffin jelly or Vaseline petroleum gauze
  Intubation
    If patient is to be intubated Vaseline gauze should be put behind the neck
  ET tube
    Rolled Clingfilm can be used to secure the ET tube
    Pink plaster stuck directly onto the ET tube aids, securing it with Clingfilm
  Airway insertion
    Avoid if possible
  LMAs
    Well-lubricated LMAs can be used with caution
  Prior to extubation
    Clear oropharyngeal secretions with lubricated soft suction catheters under low pressure and avoid touching the oral mucosa
  IV access
    Secured with Mepitel
Miscellaneous
  PR drugs
    Can be used while anaesthetised, but not awake
  Pat slide
    Must not be used for transfer

ECG, electrocardiogram; ET, endotracheal; IV, intravenous; LMA, laryngeal mask airway; PR, per rectum.

PATIENTS ON KETOGENIC DIETS

The ketogenic diet is a high-fat, low-carbohydrate, low-protein diet that has been used since the 1920s for the treatment of medically intractable seizures. There has been a recent resurgence of interest in this treatment and so now an increasing number of children on the diet are presenting for surgery. The exact mechanism of action of the diet is unknown but it effectively induces a state of fasting (ketosis) while simultaneously providing the fat needed for energy production. Children are better able than adults to produce ketone bodies and to use them for energy production in the brain. The state of ketosis causes changes in intracellular and extracellular membrane excitability that may be responsible for the effectiveness of the diet in improving seizure control in children with responsive seizure disorders.

Patients typically eat a ratio of fat to carbohydrate + protein of 2.5:1 to 4:1. Total calories are controlled to prevent excessive weight gain and fluids are restricted to an intake of 30–50 mL/kg/day so that the ketone bodies are not excessively diluted. Supplements of calcium, magnesium, vitamins and iron are needed.

Typical blood chemistry for a child on this treatment may include low serum albumin and plasma proteins, and low serum calcium and magnesium. Urine ketones are usually maintained in the range 40–160 mg/dL. Blood glucose is typically within the normal range and is maintained even during prolonged fasting [46]. Longer-term complications of the ketogenic diet include renal stones, elevated serum lipids, constipation, deficiencies of water-soluble vitamins, recurrent infections and hyperuricaemia.

Having knowledge of the usual blood chemistry derangements allows the anaesthetist to predict some of the perioperative problems that are likely to occur. For elective surgery, particularly if it is major or prolonged, there should be a consultation with the patient's dietician. An increase in caloric intake may be recommended to increase the patient's adipose stores. Blood glucose, pH, serum bicarbonate and urine ketones should be measured at baseline, during surgery and then postoperatively until the diet is re-established. Excessive ketosis may present as nausea and vomiting, decreased urine output, acidosis, tachypnoea and lethargy. These are common postoperative symptoms in patients not on the ketogenic diet and so measurement of urine ketones may be helpful in the differential diagnosis. If urine ketones are elevated treatment with carbohydrate may be needed. If there is not excessive ketosis then perioperative clear fluids and intravenous fluids should be free of carbohydrate. Caffeine is avoided as it can inhibit ketosis. Many oral medications contain carbohydrate in an amount that is significant for these patients. Consultation with a pharmacist will be helpful to determine which medications are required in a different formulation. Sometimes it is necessary to use the intravenous form of a medication, such as midazolam, and to give that by mouth instead of the usual syrup-based oral formulation.

The use of the ketogenic diet is increasing and so it will become important for those who anaesthetise children to become familiar with its management in the perioperative period. At present, the guidelines available are based on case reports [47] and small case series [46]. These reports do indicate that patients can be successfully maintained on this diet throughout the perioperative period without an increase in seizures or other postoperative implications [46].

MITOCHONDRIAL DEFECTS AND METABOLIC DISORDERS

Mitochondrial defects

CLINICAL AND BIOCHEMICAL FEATURES OF MITOCHONDRIAL DISEASE

Structural and functional defects in mitochondrial function result in a group of disorders that are genetically and phenotypically heterogeneous. Tissues that are metabolically most active such as the nervous system and muscles are most affected but there is also involvement of other organ systems. Most commonly mitochondrial defects result in myopathies, cardiomyopathies and encephalopathies (including seizures and cerebral ataxia). Clinically, these patients may present with proximal muscle weakness, fatigue, poor stamina, movement disorders, abnormal respiratory function, impaired swallowing or bulbar function, abnormal cardiac conduction or hypertension. Serum lactate and creatinine kinase may also be elevated and muscle biopsy shows mitochondrial dysfunction. There is an increased incidence of diabetes in these patients. Newborns with mitochondrial disease are particularly at risk for hypoglycaemia, which can have serious consequences as they are dependent upon carbohydrate as an energy source for cardiac muscle.

The citrate cycle, fatty acid oxidation and oxidative phosphorylation all occur in the mitochondria and result in the production of ATP for energy. The oxidative phosphorylation pathway comprises five protein complexes that use different substrates to produce energy. Complex I can use several carbon sources to transfer electrons to coenzyme Q and then sequentially to complexes III–V. Complex II must use succinate as its energy source. Mutations in mitochondrial DNA result in defects in the respiratory chain enzymes and a reduction in the capacity for oxidative phosphorylation.

There is no specific treatment for the mitochondrial disorders although various vitamins and cofactors are sometimes given. Steroids and high-carbohydrate diets have also been advocated. Nearly all organ systems use oxidative metabolism but the precise symptomatology in mitochondrial disease will vary with the different mutations that occur in the mitochondrial DNA.

ANAESTHESIA AND MITOCHONDRIAL DISEASE

The extent of the preoperative work-up for these patients will be determined by their clinical condition, but should include a 12-lead electrocardiogram and respiratory function assessment (chest radiograph, arterial blood gases and pulmonary flow–volume loops). A full blood count, electrolytes (including calcium and magnesium), erythrocyte sedimentation rate, glucose, lactate, pyruvate, creatinine kinase, liver and renal function, thyroid function, urinalysis and glycated haemoglobin may all be needed for full evaluation of functional organ system reserve before surgery.

A subset of patients – those with defects involving complex I – may be particularly sensitive to volatile anaesthetics [48]. Morgan et al. [48] used a Bispectral Index (BIS) monitor to guide their dosage of volatile anaesthetic in a group of patients that were suspected of having mitochondrial disease and who presented for muscle biopsies. However, although there is no proven link between MH and mitochondrial disease, some have advocated the use of a total intravenous technique to avoid volatile agents altogether, particularly when the diagnosis of mitochondrial disease is not yet established and other causes of abnormal motor tone and/or developmental delay remain in the differential diagnosis. A single case of MH has been reported in this group of patients, associated with the use of suxamethonium. In general, patients with mitochondrial disease are sensitive to non-depolarising muscle relaxants.

Local anaesthetics uncouple oxidative phosphorylation and inhibit enzymatic complexes, reducing the efficiency of ATP synthesis, which would augment the depressant effects of bupivacaine on the heart in hypoxic conditions. However, local anaesthetics have been used successfully in patients with mitochondrial disease and have the advantage that their use may allow the avoidance of the use of general anaesthesia and muscle relaxants. Epidural analgesia is recommended to reduce the oxygen demand during labour. In some patients an elective caesarean section is performed to prevent life-threatening lactic acidosis from occurring in labour.

Rather than recommending any one particular drug or technique, the most important consideration for patients with mitochondrial disease is to try to minimise their physiological stress and thus try to prevent the development of lactic acidosis. Lactated Ringer's should be avoided as an intravenous fluid. Maintaining normothermia, normoglycaemia and providing adequate analgesia are vital in these patients. Cardiostability is important, with prevention of postoperative shivering and adequate treatment of pain. Shipton and Prosser have provided a summary of the considerations for anaesthesia in patients with mitochondrial myopathies [49].

Propofol

In 1992 Parke et al. reported a case series of five deaths in a paediatric intensive care unit (PICU) of previously healthy children who were sedated with propofol while they required intubation for respiratory disease [50]. Each child developed increasing metabolic acidosis, bradyarrhythmia and progressive myocardial failure, with lipaemic serum. The name 'propofol infusion syndrome' has subsequently been used to describe children affected in this way. Since then propofol has been used with caution for prolonged paediatric sedation and in most hospitals is limited to use for 24 hours or less. In 2003 Felmet et al. concluded that the FDA (Food and Drug Administration of the USA) warning against prolonged sedation with propofol in children remains warranted [51]; this recommendation is also outlined in the *British National Formulary* (BNF: http://www.bnf.org).

In states of physiological stress children generally have lower carbohydrate stores than adults and so are more dependent on fatty acids as fuel substrates. Children usually require a higher dose of propofol for sedation than adults and this, combined with their use of fatty acids for fuel, may account for their greater susceptibility to propofol infusion syndrome. Propofol can impair mitochondrial electron transport and so the propofol infusion syndrome may mimic mitochondrial defects. Propofol infusion syndrome has been successfully treated with haemofiltration [52]. Propofol has not been considered contraindicated in patients with mito-chondrial disease but given the similar-ities in the biochemical abnormalities seen in the propofol infusion syndrome and in mitochondrial disease it seems logical to conclude that these patients would be unduly susceptible to the infusion syndrome. Therefore, propofol should be used cautiously, if at all, for sedation in this vulnerable group.

Genetic metabolic disease

It is beyond the scope of this chapter to review all of the many disorders of carbohydrate, amino acid, organic acid, lipid and lipoprotein, purine, bilirubin metabolism and lysosomal enzyme disorders. The reader is referred to an excellent review by Linda Stehling in Katz and Steward's *Anesthesia and Uncommon Pediatric Diseases* [53].

The acute porphyrias are a rare but important group of disorders relating to haem metabolism. Because a wide range of agents can trigger an acute crisis the recognition of these disorders is important preoperatively. As is the case for the mitochondrial disorders, avoidance of physiological stress is important, in particular, adequate hydration and carbohydrate supply are helpful. Thiopental is contra indicated because it induces δ-aminolaevulinic acid synthetase. Propofol is considered safe and ketamine has also been used safely. The inhalational agents, muscle relaxants and analgesics are generally safe but the anaesthetist should refer to a recent reference for specific agents [54].

REFERENCES

Key references

Baum VC, O' Flaherty JE, eds. *Anesthesia for genetic, metabolic and dysmorphic syndromes of childhood*, 2nd edn. Baltimore, MA: Lippincott, Williams & Wilkins 2007.

Bissonette &, Luginbuchl I, Marciniak B, Dalers &J. *Syndrome: rapid recognition and perioperative complications.* New York: Mcgraw Hill, 2006.

Jones K. *Smith's recognizable patterns of human malformation*, 5th edn. Philadelphia: WB Saunders, 2005.

Katz J, Steward DJ. *Anesthesia and uncommon pediatric diseases*, 2nd edn. Philadelphia: WB Saunders, 1993.

References

1. Jones AE, Pelton DA. An index of syndromes and their anaesthetic implications. *Can Anaesth Soc J* 1976; **23**: 207–26.
2. Steward DJ, Lerman J. *Manual of pediatric anesthesia*, 5th edn. Philadelphia: Churchill Livingstone, 2001.
3. Roizen MF, Fleisher LA, eds. *Essence of anesthesia practice*, 2nd edn. Philadelphia: WB Saunders, 2002.
4. Baum VC, O'Flaherty JE, eds. *Anesthesia for genetic, metabolic and dysmorphic syndromes of childhood.* Philadelphia: Lippincott, Williams & Wilkins, 1999.
5. Berkowitz ID, Raja SN, Bender KS, Kopits SE. Dwarfs. Pathophysiology and anesthetic implications. *Anesthesiology* 1990; **73**: 739–59.
6. Adhami EJ, Cancio-Babu CV. Anaesthesia in a child with Sotos syndrome. *Paediatr Anaesth* 2003; **13**: 835–40.
7. Stehling LC. The difficult intubation and fiberoptic techniques. In: *ASA annual refresher course lectures.* Park Ridge: American Society of Anesthesiologists, 1984: 230.
8. Larach MG, Rosenberg H, Gronert GA, Allen GC. Hyperkalemic cardiac arrest during anesthesia in infants and children with occult myopathies. *Clin Pediatr* 1997; **36**: 9–16.
9. Johnston HM. The floppy weak infant revisited. *Brain Dev* 2003; **25**: 155–8.
10. Perkins JA, Sie KC, Milczuk H, Richardson MA. Airway management in children with craniofacial anomalies. *Cleft Palate-Craniofac J* 1997; **34**: 135–40.
11. Jones KL. *Smith's recognizable patterns of human malformation*, 5th edn. Philadelphia: WB Saunders, 2005.
12. Roa NL, Moss KS. Treacher Collins syndrome with sleep apnea: anesthetic considerations. *Anesthesiology* 1984; **60**: 71–3.
13. Arvystas M, Shprintzen RJ. Craniofacial morphology in Treacher Collins syndrome. *Cleft Palate-Craniofac J* 1991; **28**: 226–31.
14. Matsumoto N, Niikawa N.Kabuki make-up syndrome: a review. *Am J Med Genet* 2003; **117**: 57–65.
15. Ferguson S. Moebius syndrome. a review of the anaesthetic implications. *Paediatr Anaesth* 1996; **6**: 51–6.
16. Tracy MR, Dormans JP, Kusumi K. Klippel–Feil syndrome. clinical features and current understanding of etiology. *Clin Orthopaed Rel Res* 2004; **424**: 183–90.
17. Hall JG. Arthrogryposes. In: *Emery and Rimoin's principles and practice of medical genetics*, 4th edn. London: Churchill Livingstone, 2002.
18. Hopkins PM, Ellis FR, Halsall PJ. Hypermetabolism in arthrogryposis multiplex congenita. *Anaesthesia* 1991; **46**: 374–5.
19. Froster-Iskenius UG, Waterson JR, Hall JG. A recessive form of congenital contractures and torticollis associated with malignant hyperthermia. *J Med Genet* 1988; **25**: 104–12.
20. Baines DB, Douglas ID, Overton JH. Anaesthesia for patients with arthrogryposis multiplex congenita: what is the risk of malignant hyperthermia? *Anaesth Intensive Care* 1986; **14**: 370–2.

21. Baines D, Keneally J. Anaesthetic implications of the mucopolysaccharidoses. a fifteen year experience in a children's hospital. *Anaesth Intensive Care* 1983; **11**: 198–202.

22. Moores C, Rogers JG, McKenzie IM, Brown TC. Anaesthesia for children with mucopolysaccharidoses. *Anaesth Intensive Care* 1996; **4**: 459–463.

23. Stehling LC, Zauder HL. *Anesthetic implications of congenital anomalies in children*. New York: Appleton-Century-Crofts, 1980.

24. Tobias JD, Lowe S, Holcomb GW. Anesthetic Considerations of an Infant with Beckwith–Wiedemann syndrome. *J Clin Anesth* 1992; **4**: 484–6.

25. Thomas JM, Lopez JT. Conjoined twins – the anaesthetic management of 15 sets from 1991 to 2002. *Paediatr Anaesth* 2004; **14**: 117–29.

26. White RJ, Bass SP. Myotonic dystrophy and paediatric anaesthesia. *Paediatr Anaesth* 2003; **13**: 94–102.

27. Rosenbaum HK, Miller JD. Malignant hyperthermia and myotonic disorders. *Anesthesiol Clin North Am* 2002; **20**: 623–64.

28. Gregory GA, ed. *Pediatric anesthesia*, 4th edn. Philadelphia: Churchill Livingstone, 2002.

29. Richardson VF, Robertson CR, Mowat AP *et al*. Deterioration in lung function after general anaesthesia in patients with cystic fibrosis. *Acta Paediatr Scand* 1984; **73**: 75–79.

30. Cain JC, Lish MC, Passannante AN. Epidural fentanyl in a cystic fibrosis patient with pleuritic chest pain. *Anesth Analg* 1994; **78**: 793–4.

31. Henderson AM, Vallis CJ, Sumner E. Anaesthesia in the prune belly syndrome. *Anaesthesia* 1987; **42**: 54–60.

32. Lake CL, Booker PD, eds. *Pediatric cardiac anesthesia*, 4th edn. Philadelphia: Lippincott, Williams & Wilkins, 2005.

33. Nichols DG, Cameron DE, Greeley WJ *et al*., eds. *Critical heart disease in infants and children*. St Louis, Mo: Mosby Year-Book, 1995.

34. Kobel M, Creighton RE, Steward DJ. Anaesthetic considerations in Down's syndrome: experience with 100 patients and a review of the literature. *Can Anaesth Soc J* 1982; **29**: 593–9.

35. Mitchell V, Howard R, Facer EK. Down's syndrome and anaesthesia. *Paediatr Anaesth* 1995; **5**: 379–84.

36. Noonan JA. Noonan syndrome: an update and review for the primary pediatrician. *Clin Pediatr* 1994; **33**: 548–55.

37. Callaghan ML, Nichols AB, Sweet RB. Anesthetic management of prolonged QT interval syndrome. *Anesthesiology* 1977; **47**: 67–9.

38. Joseph-Reynolds AM, Auden SM, Sobczyzk WL. Perioperative considerations in a newly described subtype of congenital long QT syndrome. *Paediatr Anaesth* 1997; **7**: 237–41.

39. Quan L, Smith DW. The VATER association. Vertebral defects, anal atresia, T-E- fistula with esophageal atresia, radial and renal dysplasia: a spectrum of associate defects. *J Pediatr* 1973; **82**: 104–7.

40. Cox RG, Sumner E. Familial dysautonomia. *Anaesthesia* 1983; **38**: 293.

41. Challands JF, Facer EK. Epidural anaesthesia and familial dysautonomia (the Riley–Day syndrome). Three case reports. *Paediatr Anaesth* 1998; **8**: 83–8.

42. Stehling LC. *Common problems in pediatric anesthesia*, 2nd edn. New York: CV Mosby, 1992.

43. James I, Wark H. Airway management during anesthesia in patients with epidermolysis bullosa dystrophica. *Anesthesiology* 1982; **56**: 323–6.

44. Griffin RP, Mayou BJ. The anaesthetic management of patients with dystrophic epidermolysis bullosa. A review of 44 patients over a 10-year period. *Anaesthesia* 1993; **48**: 810–15.

45. Farber NE, Troshynski TJ, Turco G. Spinal anesthesia in an infant with epidermolysis bullosa. *Anesthesiology* 1995; **83**: 1364–7.

46. Valencia I, Pfeifer H, Thiele EA. General anesthesia and the ketogenic diet: clinical experience in nine patients. *Epilepsia* 2002; **43**: 525–9.

47. McNeely JK. Perioperative management of a paediatric patient on the ketogenic diet. *Paediatr Anaesth* 2000; **10**: 103–6.

48. Morgan PG, Hoppel CL, Sedensky MM. Mitochondrial defects and anesthetic sensitivity. *Anesthesiology* 2002; **96**: 1268–70.

49. Shipton EA, Prosser DO. Mitochondrial myopathies and anaesthesia. *Eur J Anaesthesiol* 2004; **1**: 173–8.

50. Parke TJ, Stevens JE, Rice AS *et al*. Metabolic acidosis and fatal myocardial failure after propofol infusion in children. five case reports. *BMJ* 1992; **305**: 613–16.

51. Felmet K, Nguyen T, Clark RS *et al*. The FDA warning against prolonged sedation with propofol in children remains warranted. *Pediatrics* 2003; **112**: 1002–3.

52. Wolf A, Weir P, Segar P *et al*. Impaired fatty acid oxidation in propofol infusion syndrome. *Lancet* 2001; **357**: 606–7.

53. Stehling LC. Genetic metabolic diseases. In: Katz J, Steward DJ, eds. *Anesthesia and uncommon pediatric diseases*, 2nd edn. Philadelphia: WB Saunders, 1993: 461–80.

54. James MFM, Hift RJ. Porphyrias. *Br J Anaesth* 2000; **85**: 143–53.

29

Anaphylaxis and malignant hyperthermia

JANE E HEROD

KEY LEARNING POINTS

Anaphylaxis

- One in 13 000 general anaesthetics is complicated by an anaphylactic reaction. This rises to 1:6000 if muscle relaxants are used.
- Anaphylactic reactions occur soon after drug administration (90 per cent), the exception being latex allergy, which usually presents 30–40 minutes after exposure.
- Adrenaline is the mainstay of treatment, supplemented by the administration of steroids and histamine antagonists.
- Where the clinical environment is virtually latex free, pretreatment may no longer be required for latex-allergic patients.

Malignant hyperthermia

- One in 10 000–15 000 paediatric and 1:50 000 adult anaesthetics are complicated by a malignant hyperthermia (MH) reaction.
- Fifty per cent of all MH reactions are seen in children under 15 years old.
- Fifty per cent of MH patients have a family history where the genetic inheritance is autosomal dominant; 20 per cent are polygenic and 30 per cent are sporadic cases.
- Patients can have several uneventful exposures to trigger agents without a full-blown reaction.
- Dantrolene is the mainstay of treatment, supplemented by supportive measures.
- Muscle testing is only done in postpubertal patients or those weighing at least 20 kg.

INTRODUCTION

Two of the most challenging situations that can be encountered during the administration of general anaesthesia are anaphylaxis and malignant hyperthermia (MH). Both are life threatening, especially if not diagnosed or if inadequately treated. Recognition of and management of susceptible patients are also important.

ANAPHYLAXIS

Definition and pathogenesis

ANAPHYLAXIS

The word anaphylaxis comes from the Greek *phylaxis* for protection and *ana-* for backwards. It is a disorder of the immune system, leading to an exaggerated allergic response to a trigger substance. A second exposure to the trigger agent causes a severe and systemic response, resulting from the release of histamine, serotonin, slow-reacting substance-A (SRS-A) leukotrienes, prostaglandins, thromboxanes and bradykinins. These vasoactive mediators are released in an IgE-mediated (or type 1) degranulation of sensitised mast cells and basophils. Occasionally, this reaction may be mediated by the IgG4 subclass of antibodies rather than IgE. The signs and symptoms of such a reaction usually occur rapidly after re-exposure to a sensitising antigen, sometimes within minutes [1–4].

ANAPHYLACTOID REACTIONS

These responses differ from anaphylaxis in that the degranulation of mast cells is not IgE mediated but is due to either direct mast cell histamine release or complement activation by the classic or alternative pathways. They do not necessarily require previous exposure to the trigger agent. Anaphylactoid reactions are most commonly seen in reactions to blood products and contrast media. When they are severe, they are clinically indistinguishable from anaphylaxis.

Some frequently used drugs in anaesthesia, such as atracurium, mivacurium and morphine, may cause direct histamine release from mast cells. The clinical manifestations of these mild anaphylactoid reactions are usually confined to the skin, such as cutaneous flushing and pruritus, and may be present in up to 30 per cent of patients receiving these medicines [1,2].

The exact incidence of all anaphylactic reactions occurring under anaesthesia is unknown, but it is thought to be in the region of 1 in 13 000 anaesthetics, rising to an incidence of 1 in 6000 if neuromuscular blocking agents are used. Up to 70 per cent of patients who have an allergy to one neuromuscular blocking drug may exhibit cross-reactivity to others. The female to male ratio of anaphylactic reactions is 2.5:1 [2,5,6]. Thus, on average, most anaesthetists will encounter a patient who has an anaphylactic episode during their professional lifetime and must be able to recognise and treat such an event.

Clinical history and diagnosis

There is no universally accepted and all-inclusive definition for anaphylaxis due to differing severity and presenting symptoms. A diagnosis of anaphylaxis requires that the patient exhibit, in response to a trigger agent, a severe allergic reaction of sudden onset, which generally lasts less than 24 hours. It may be multisystem and include cardiovascular collapse, bronchospasm and stridor, erythema, urticaria and rash, and gastrointestinal upset such as diarrhoea and vomiting [7,8]. Under anaesthesia, cardiovascular symptoms are the most common, with cardiovascular collapse being the only presenting sign in approximately 10 per cent of patients (Table 29.1) [8]. This may be misdiagnosed and attributed to other causes [8].

Cardiovascular collapse is the dominant finding in over 80 per cent of patients with anaphylaxis, whereas bronchospasm

Table 29.1　Presenting features of anaphylaxis [8]*

Cough
Flushing
Rash
Urticaria
Subjective feelings (if not unconscious)
Electrocardiogram (ECG) abnormality
Desaturation
Difficulty in lung inflation
No pulse
No bleeding at operative site

*Adapted with permission from Elsevier.

is the most severe in just under 10 per cent. Asthmatics who develop anaphylaxis are much more likely to have bronchospasm, and this may be severe and resistant to treatment. Furthermore, patients concurrently using β-adrenoceptor blockers and those who have had a central neuraxial block may have a severe cardiovascular collapse due to a decreased compensatory catecholamine response. Circulatory compromise from central local anaesthetic blocks may mask the physical signs and delay diagnosis and treatment. Cardiovascular collapse or bronchospasm, or a combination of both, is responsible for most deaths [7,8].

Anaphylactic reactions may occur at any time during the administration of general anaesthesia, although most (>90 per cent) occur during or soon after induction; the more rapid the onset of symptoms, the more severe the reaction [7]. The main exception to this is latex hypersensitivity, which tends to cause an anaphylactic reaction 30–60 minutes into the procedure [4].

About 80 per cent of all anaphylactic reactions resolve within hours of treatment, however; approximately 20 per cent follow a biphasic, course. The second peak of symptoms and signs follows a quiescent phase and may occur up to 38 hours after initial exposure, although a more usual time interval is in the region of 8–10 hours. If an anaphylactic reaction is biphasic then a rule of thirds tends to apply: a third being more severe, a third being as severe and a third being less severe than the initial presentation [7,9].

The administration of corticosteroids may be beneficial in decreasing, or even preventing, the severity of this second anaphylactic phase, although patients who have received corticosteroids can still have a severe biphasic reaction. A prolonged anaphylactic episode is often associated with a protracted and profound hypotensive reaction and has a poor prognosis [7,9,10].

Differential diagnosis

As the treatment for both anaphylactic and anaphylactoid reactions is the same, it is not necessary to distinguish between the two at the time of presentation. However, it is important to differentiate between these reactions and other causes of cardiovascular and respiratory collapse.

Probably the most common condition that can mimic an anaphylactic event is vasovagal collapse. Here, profound hypotension and collapse may be seen accompanied by bradycardia, pallor, nausea, vomiting and sweating, but urticaria and other symptoms of histamine release, such as tachycardia, pruritus, oedema and bronchospasm, are not seen. Other causes of sudden respiratory compromise, such as bronchospasm secondary to an acute exacerbation of asthma, pulmonary aspiration or even pulmonary embolism may also mimic an anaphylactic event but are not accompanied by signs of histamine release. Hereditary angioedema secondary to C1-esterase deficiency results in complement activation and usually presents with orofacial swelling, including upper airway mucosal swelling and bronchospasm, as well as gastrointestinal symptoms such as abdominal cramps and diarrhoea. It may easily be confused with anaphylaxis, but as this is an autosomal dominant condition, there will usually be a family history of recurrent episodes that are triggered by a combination of non-specific environmental factors, including psychological stress alone.

Management of suspected anaphylaxis reactions

Anaphylaxis is a medical emergency. Under general anaesthesia patients are unable to report prodromal symptoms before manifesting anaphylactic shock. Despite later detection, even severe cases occurring under anaesthesia can have a prompt and successful response to appropriate treatment. An anaphylaxis guideline should be clearly displayed in all areas where anaesthesia is administered (Fig. 29.1).

IMMEDIATE MANAGEMENT

The suspected causative agent should be discontinued, 100 per cent oxygen should be given and help summoned. The patient should be laid flat with the legs elevated above the level of the heart to aid venous return and thus help maintain an adequate cardiac output. Intramuscular adrenaline 1:1000, is the drug of choice for the initial treatment of both anaphylactic and anaphylactoid reactions [1,11,12]. Subcutaneous administration has no place due to its unpredictable absorption [13]. For simplicity, the dose of adrenaline can be stratified according to the age of the patient, although, if the weight is known, the dose is 5–10 µg/kg (Table 29.2) [13,14]. Intramuscular adrenaline may be given every 10 minutes to treat persistent hypotension or bronchospasm.

During anaesthesia or if there is severe cardiovascular collapse, the intravenous (IV) route is best, but only using 1:10 000 adrenaline. Undiluted 1:1 000 adrenaline should never be administered intravenously in the treatment of anaphylaxis. If IV adrenaline is used, it should be given in divided doses of 1 µg/kg and titrated until there is a response [2]. A continuous IV infusion (300 µg/kg of adrenaline diluted to 50 mL; 1 mL/hour = 0.1 µg/kg/minute) may be required, starting at 0.1 µg/kg/minute and titrated to achieve an effect [2,14].

There have been several reports, in adults, of the α agonist metaraminol being used successfully in cases of adrenaline-resistant hypotension [15]. These drugs have not been validated for first-line treatment in either adults or children.

Resuscitation should also include the rapid administration of IV fluids, in boluses of 10–20 mL/kg. Large volumes may be required – large children and adults may require up to 2–4 L of fluid [2,14]. If the degree of cardiovascular collapse is so great that there are no palpable pulses then external cardiac compressions should commence and the patient should be treated as a full cardiac arrest (see Chapter 23).

SECONDARY MANAGEMENT

A bronchodilator may be required for adrenaline-resistant bronchospasm. A loading dose of either salbutamol or aminophylline, followed by a continuous infusion, should be considered (Fig. 29.1).

In order to try to prevent or diminish the secondary peak of activity [7,9], both steroids, such as hydrocortisone 4 mg/kg, and antihistamines (H_1-receptor antagonists), such as chlorphenamine (chlorpheniramine), should be given [2,14] (Fig. 29.1). The dose of chlorpheniramine is age dependent and it should not be given to neonates due to its antimuscarinic properties [14,16] (Table 29.3). The H_2-receptor antagonist ranitidine (1 mg/kg, maximum 50 mg) may also be given. In experimental models, blocking both H_1- and H_2-receptors reduces the severity of anaphylaxis [7,17].

If resuscitation has been prolonged arterial blood gas tensions should be measured to determine both the oxygenation status and the degree of acidosis. Acidosis may require treatment with sodium bicarbonate [14]. Once the patient has been stabilised, blood samples should be taken for analysis [14] (Fig. 29.1).

Anaphylaxis from drugs used in anaesthesia

Neuromuscular blockers are thought to account for between 60 and 70 per cent of all anaphylactic reactions seen during general anaesthesia [1,2]. Vecuronium is the most common drug to cause anaphylaxis and the others, in

Table 29.2 Dose of intramuscular adrenaline (1:1000) used in the treatment of anaphylaxis*

Age	Dose of 1:1000 adrenaline
<6 months	50 µg IM (0.05 mL)
>6 months to 6 years	120 µg IM (0.12 mL)
6–12 years	250 µg IM (0.25 mL)
>12 years	500 µg IM (0.5 mL)

*Undiluted 1:1000 adrenaline must NOT be used intravenously.

Table 29.3 Dose of chlorpheniramine used to reduce or prevent the secondary peak of activity in the treatment of anaphylaxis

Age	Dose
1 month to 1 year	250 µg/kg IV
1–5 years	2.5–5 mg IV
6–12 years	5–10 mg IV
>12 years	10–20 mg IV

Basic monitoring assumed
Exercise CAUTION if diagnosis is not certain

IMMEDIATE MANAGEMENT	SECONDARY MANAGEMENT

Discontinue administration of suspect drug

Summon help

Maintain airway with 100% oxygen
(consider tracheal intubation and IPPV)
Lie patient flat with legs elevated

Give ADRENALINE

- 0.05–0.1 mL/kg of 1:1000 IM (max. 0.5 mL)
  i.e. 5–10 μg/kg especially if bronchospasm present

- Can give Intravenously but use 1:10 000 (1 μg/kg)
  and titrate to effect

- Titration of further similar doses may be
  necessary for persistent hypotension and bronchospasm

- Continuous infusion of adrenaline may be
  necessary 0.1–0.5 μg/kg/min

- To make solution   300 μg/kg in 50 mLs
  and start at   1 mL/h – 0.1 μg/kg/min

Start intravascular volume expansion

- With Hartmann's or saline solution

- Initially   10–20 mL/kg bolus – rapidly

- Repeat as necessary

Consider external chest compressions

When patient has stabilised

- Blood samples (5–10 mL) for mast cell tryptase should be
  taken and placed in plain tubes as soon as possible after
  the event at 1 hour and 6 hours and put in a fridge
  until analysed

- Immunology should be contacted when feasible
  to arrange the investigations

- The drug, fluid or blood thought to be responsible for
  the reaction should also be kept for investigation

Adrenaline-resistant bronchospasm

Consider
Salbutamol
Loading dose   5 μg/kg IV

Then   0.2–4 μg/kg/min
(3 mg/kg in 50 mL   1 mL/h = 1 μg/kg/min)

OR
Aminophylline
Bolus over 20 min   5 mg/kg IV

Then   800 μg/kg/h
(40 mg/kg in 50 mL 1 mL/h = 800 μg/kg/min)

Consider

1. Steroids
Hydrocortisone 4 mg/kg IV *OR*

Methylprednisolone
500 μg–1 mg/kg IV up to **max dose:** 4 mg/kg

and

2. Antihistamines
Chlorpheniramine
(diluted and given slowly over one minute)

<1 year   250 μg/kg IV
1–5 years   2.5–5 mg IV
6–12 years   5–10 mg IV
>12 years   10–20 mg IV

ACIDOSIS
If severe after 20 min:
Sodium bicarbonate 0.5–1 mmol/kg

Catecholamine infusions
Adrenaline   **Dose range**
Noradrenaline   0.1–0.5 μg/kg/min

To make solution 300 μg/kg in 50 mL
Start at   1 mL/h = 0.1 μg/kg/min

Clotting screen
Consider possibility of coagulopathy

Measure arterial blood gas tensions

Figure 29.1   Suggested guideline for the management of acute anaphylaxis occurring under general anaesthesia.

decreasing order of frequency of reactions, are atracurium, suxamethonium, pancuronium, rocuronium and mivacurium, although this may partially reflect usage [1,2]. Cross-reactivity occurs, as up to 70 per cent of previously allergic patients can be shown, on testing, to react to other relaxants. Interestingly, the steroid-based drugs, such as vecuronium and pancuronium, tend to cause anaphylactic reactions, whereas the benzylisoquinoliniums, such as atracurium and mivacurium, tend to cause anaphylactoid reactions. More than 50 per cent of these reactions occur upon first exposure. The quaternary ammonium group found in relaxants is also present in many other drugs, foods and cosmetics so that prior exposure may have occurred. The latter may explain why females are more likely to have a drug anaphylaxis than males [1].

The second most frequent cause of anaphylaxis under anaesthesia is latex and this is responsible for between 12 and 17 per cent of reactions. After relaxants, other drugs causing anaphylaxis are, in decreasing order of frequency: antibiotics (3–8 per cent); induction agents (4–5 per cent); colloids, especially gelatins (3–5 per cent); and opioids (2–3 per cent).

Of the induction agents thiopental is most frequently implicated in anaphylaxis, with an incidence of approximately 1:14 000, although reactions to propofol and rarely etomidate have also been reported. Reactions to synthetic opioids such as fentanyl and its derivatives are rare and the most frequently implicated opioid is morphine [1,2].

Penicillins, especially β-lactams, are responsible for most antibiotic reactions. In considering substitutes it should be remembered that 8 per cent of sensitive patients show cross-reactivity with cephalosporins. Anaphylaxis to protamine, aprotinin, atropine, benzodiazepines, bone cement and iodine-containing radio-contrast dye have been reported during anaesthesia.

Latex allergy

Latex hypersensitivity is responsible for between 12 and 17 per cent of anaphylactic reactions seen during anaesthesia [1,2], with the peak response characteristically seen 30–60 minutes after exposure [4]. It appears to be increasing in frequency [18,19], especially in children who have had repeated latex exposure as a result of multiple surgical procedures, usually for either urological problems or spinal dysraphism [18–21]. The latter has a 500-fold increase in incidence of latex allergy than the general population [18]. Latex allergy should decrease as hospitals become latex-free environments.

Patients at risk of latex allergy fall into three groups (Fig. 29.2). Children may undergo preoperative screening for sensitivity utilising the radioallergosorbent test (RAST) or the enzyme-linked immunosorbent assay (ELISA) test for latex-specific IgE antibodies. Skin-prick testing has been suggested for high-risk patients. However, all these

tests lack the specificity to predict the likely occurrence of an anaphylactic reaction. The elevation of IgE levels in conjunction with a positive clinical history is a better predictor of the likelihood of an anaphylactic reaction occurring during surgery [22].

Patients who have a clinical history of either anaphylaxis or allergy to latex or rubber should be regarded as 'high risk' and should be treated according to local latex allergy guidelines (Fig. 29.2). In the recent past, this has included pretreatment with a combination of corticosteroids and histamine (H_1 and H_2) antagonists. This is now no longer thought to be necessary [23–25]. Instead the theatre department should be made aware of patients with a history of latex allergy (with or without positive blood tests) or those who have a positive RAST to latex allergens. Any latex should be removed from the theatre and patients should be scheduled first on the operating list, so that the level of circulating latex particles in the environment is kept to a minimum [14]. Most disposable items used in the operating suite are now latex free and are clearly labelled . The injection ports of most fluid-giving sets still contain latex and so injections should not be given through these ports. Most of the bungs on antibiotic and other ampoules are also now latex free; however, this should be checked beforehand – if there is uncertainty, the bung should be removed before mixing. All non-disposable latex-containing items such as the operating table and monitoring leads can be made safe by covering with a sheet and paper tape, respectively.

Patients who do not have a history of latex allergy but have a positive RAST should be classed as latex sensitive, rather than allergic, but do fall into a high-risk group for developing latex allergy. Extra vigilance for an allergic reaction should be maintained in patients with certain food allergies, e.g. avocados, bananas, kiwi fruit, chestnuts, melons, strawberries, mangoes, guavas, peaches, cherries, tomatoes, papains and even potatoes, as there is cross-sensitisation with the latex allergen. The list of potential allergens is growing. Patients who are allergic to fruit have an 11 per cent risk of latex allergy, and those who are allergic to latex have a 35 per cent risk of a fruit allergy [20,21,23].

Investigation and follow-up of anaphylaxis

Once the patient is stable, blood should be taken for measurement of serum tryptase, which is the marker for mast cell activation and degranulation, and is present in both anaphylactic and anaphylactoid reactions. Three blood tests are needed: one immediately after treatment of the reaction, the second 1 hour after the reaction and the third at 6 hours. The timing of the blood samples is important because the rise in tryptase is transient. The peak rise is thought to be at about 1 hour after the onset of the reaction, although it may be earlier in reactions where hypotension is prominent. A negative test does not exclude an anaphylactic reaction, and tryptase is unlikely to be grossly elevated in mild reactions.

Three groups of patients exist

Group 1   History of anaphylaxis to latex
Group 2   History of allergy to latex or rubber,
           e.g. urticaria, central dermatitis, eye swelling,
           bronchospasm
Group 3   High-risk group:
           No previous reaction but have:
           Spina bifida
           Genitourinary anomalies
           Multiple surgical procedures
           Documented reactions to IV drugs

Groups 1 and 2 should be treated identically

Pretreatment*

IV medication
(1) Methylprednisolone   1 mg/kg 6-hourly IV
                          maximum dose 50 mg/dose
(2) Ranitidine   1 mg/kg 6-hourly IV over 2 minutes
(3) Chlorpheniramine   1 month–1 year   250 mcg/kg
                          1–5 years   2.5–5 mg
                          6–12 years   5–10 mg
                          All doses 6-hourly GIVEN SLOWLY
Notes: (1) At least two doses must be given preoperatively and
             continued postoperatively
         (2) Diluents must not be added to vials through rubber bungs.
             The bung must be removed or dispensing pin with filter
             to be used

PATIENTS WITH ASTHMA
Salbutamol inhaler 6-hourly two doses preoperatively

Group 3 High-risk patients
         No special precautions; maintain high index of suspicion
         during and after case

Treatment of anaphylaxis to latex

As per anaphylaxis protocol
Anaphylaxis may be slow in onset and difficult to diagnose
A smaller dose of adrenaline may be used if reaction is not severe

In addition give:
(1) Methylprednisolone   1 mg/kg IV
(2) Chlorpheniramine   1 month–1 year   250 mcg/kg
                          1–5 years   2.5–5 mg
                          6–12 years 5–10 mg
(3) Ranitidine   1 mg/kg slowly IV

Other points

Patient must be first on operating list
Avoid touching latex product and then touching patient
All staff in department made aware of status
Reduction of numbers in theatres where possible
Notices in theatre involved

Figure 29.2 Suggested guideline for the management of patients with latex allergy. *Pretreatment is no longer necessary where minimal latex exposure can be guaranteed.

A rise in tryptase proves that a reaction has occurred but does not identify the causative agent. Further testing and follow-up are required and the patient should be referred to an allergy specialist who will need copies of all the relevant notes (anaesthetic chart, drug chart) and tryptase results. The allergist may recommend a series of intradermal skin-prick tests with anaesthetic drugs – these test the presence of IgE-specific antibodies. This is usually done 4–6 weeks after the reaction. Currently there is only one commercially available drug-specific IgE assay: to suxamethonium. As well as drug testing, latex allergy can also be tested for by measuring the specific IgE in plasma using the RAST. Baseline tryptase is also measured.

Once all the results are available, an anaesthetist must ensure that the child's parents are given suitable advice for further anaesthetics. A written record of their reaction should be kept by the parents. A MedicAlert bracelet can be worn by the child. In the UK, all drug reactions require reporting to the Committee on Safety of Medicines via the 'yellow card' scheme [1].

MALIGNANT HYPERTHERMIA

Introduction, pathogenesis and clinical history

Malignant hyperthermia is a rare and potentially lethal disorder causing a hypermetabolic state usually triggered by certain anaesthetic agents. It was first described in 1960 in Melbourne, Australia, in a patient who had had 10 close relatives die either during or soon after anaesthesia [26]. Since then it been described throughout the world and in all racial groups, although it is more common in Caucasians of northern European descent [27]. Approximately 50 per cent of cases are due to an inherited autosomal dominant trait, approximately 20 per cent have autosomal recessive inheritance (or polygenic) and the remaining 30 per cent are sporadic [28].

The genetics of MH give rise to a defect in skeletal muscle calcium metabolism and the precise chromosomal defects are complex. The gene mutations identified at loci on chromosomes 1q, 3q, 5p, 7q and 19q (ryanodine receptor) are thought to account for the majority of all MH susceptibility in humans [28,29]. Currently more than 25 different genetic mutations causing MH have been described [30].

When a susceptible individual is exposed to a trigger agent (suxamethonium, halothane, isoflurane, desflurane or sevoflurane), an MH reaction may be initiated. Defective calcium channels, usually at the ryanodine receptor in the sarcoplasmic reticulum, release Ca^{2+} at an abnormally high rate, thereby causing excessive activation of actin and myosin muscle filaments, which results in sustained contractions and a hypermetabolic state. In normal muscle filaments, relaxation is brought about by adenosine triphosphatase (ATPase) membrane pumps, which restore calcium homeostasis by returning the myoplasmic calcium to the sarcoplasmic reticulum. In an MH reaction, such large amounts of Ca^{2+} are released that normal homeostatic mechanisms are overwhelmed. Sustained filament contraction causes high consumption of ATP, which in turn increases oxygen demand

Table 29.4 Clinical signs of a malignant hyperthermia reaction*†

Clinical sign	Early	Late
Masseter muscle spasm (after suxamethonium)	+	
Hypercapnia	+	
Tachypnoea (if not ventilated)	+	
Tachycardia	+	
Arrhythmias	+ +	
Hyperthermia	+	+
Hypoxia and cyanosis	+	+
Rapid soda lime consumption		+
Generalised muscle rigidity		+
Disseminated intravascular coagulation		+
Myoglobinuria		+
Oligo-anuria		+
Death		+

*These signs are not sequential but are shown as either early or late presentation.
†Adapted by permission of Oxford University Press.

and elevates carbon dioxide production. This causes tachypnoea in the unventilated patient and hypercapnia in the ventilated one. Rises in the end-tidal carbon dioxide, followed by a tachycardia, are usually the first presenting symptoms of an MH reaction (Table 29.4).

High ATP consumption and consequent hypermetabolic state results in heat production (Table 29.4); indeed the basal metabolic rate may increase by up to 500 per cent. Small infants and children, who already have a higher resting metabolic rate and less well-controlled thermoregulation than adults, may have a rise in body temperature that is twice as rapid as in adults [31]. When the oxygen demand exceeds supply, anaerobic metabolism causes a lactic acidosis. The combination of respiratory and metabolic acidosis increases sympathetic outflow, producing a tachycardia. Once myoplasmic ATP is depleted, the muscle cell membrane pumps fail, resulting in rhabdomyolysis and leakage of intracellular elements, including K^+, Ca^{2+}, creatine phosphokinase (CPK) and myoglobin. Plasma CPK may be up to 1000 times higher than normal and this usually peaks 2–3 days after the reaction and may return to normal in 10–15 days. Myoglobinaemia, and consequent myoglobinuria, can cause acute renal failure. Acute hyperkalaemia combined with sympathetic hyperstimulation can cause death from cardiac arrhythmias [30,32,33]. Other late complications of a MH reaction include disturbed clotting and disseminated intravascular coagulation [34].

Malignant hyperthermia usually occurs 10–20 minutes after exposure to a triggering agent, but occasionally it may not manifest until several hours later. Sometimes a mild reaction may be unnoticed but present 2–3 days later with myoglobinuria.

The exact prevalence of MH susceptibility (MHS) in the general population is unknown. An MH-susceptible individual may have several uneventful anaesthetics prior to a full-blown reaction. The occurrence of an unanticipated MH reaction under anaesthesia is approximately 1:10 000–1:15 000 for children and 1:50 000 for adults; most paediatric anaesthetists are likely to meet one new presentation of MH in their career. Furthermore, half of all MH cases are in children younger than 15 years and it may be more common in males [27,29,31,35,36]. Of the triad of symptoms of metabolic acidosis, hyperthermia and muscle rigidity, the last may not always be present, as the threshold for calcium-induced hypermetabolism is lower than that required for inducing muscle contraction [28,31].

Features of MH occur in up to 1:16 000 people under anaesthesia but this does include isolated masseter muscle spasm (MMS). Indeed, MMS is observed in up to 1 per cent of all paediatric patients who have been given suxamethonium after a halothane induction, and 60 per cent of these were later found to be MHS, although only 7 per cent of them had shown typical signs of MH [27,30,36,37].

Associated syndromes

Many neurological and neuromuscular clinical syndromes have been postulated to be linked to a state of MHS. Currently the only known syndrome that is linked with MH is central core disease, although this link is not always consistent. Nevertheless a link is suspected in Evans myopathy and King–Denborough syndrome, and patients who have either of these diseases should be assumed to be MHS and given a non-triggering anaesthetic [33,34,36,38].

Duchenne and other muscular dystrophies, myotonica congenita, osteogenesis imperfecta and other myopathies have been associated with MHS, but evidence is lacking. Extra vigilance is required in patients with these conditions.

Rarely, MH may present without anaesthesia. Strenuous exercise in hot climates has precipitated MH reactions, and MHS has been found in patients who have had episodes of virus-induced rhabdomyolysis. An increased incidence of MHS has also been described in epidemiological studies of the parents of children who have died from the sudden infant death syndrome (SIDS). There may be an excess of deaths related to anaesthesia in families with SIDS [34].

Differential diagnosis

Unfortunately, none of the clinical signs is specific to MH and a list of the most common differential diagnoses is shown in Table 29.5.

Management of suspected MH reaction under anaesthesia

Anaesthetic departments should have a local treatment protocol displayed in all areas where general anaesthesia

Table 29.5 Conditions that may present with clinical signs suggestive of a malignant hyperthermia reaction*†

'Light' level of anaesthesia
Anaesthetic circuit rebreathing
Over-zealous patient warming
Hypercapnia due to laparoscopy
Impaired ventilation due to respiratory disease
Impending sepsis
Tourniquet release
Phaeochromocytoma
Thyroid storm
Anaphylaxis
Other muscle diseases

*Rapid clinical assessment should be undertaken to determine the origin of the unexpected reaction.
†Adapted by permission of Oxford University Press.

is given (Fig. 29.3). Once an MH reaction is suspected, all triggering agents should be discontinued and the patient ventilated with 100 per cent oxygen through a vapour-free circuit. This is an emergency and help must be obtained straight away. Surgery should be discontinued as rapidly as possible and anaesthesia maintained with IV agents while this is happening. Cooling of the patient should be started while dantrolene is being prepared (Fig. 29.3).

Dantrolene, first manufactured in 1967, is a skeletal muscle relaxant and acts by inhibiting excitation–contraction coupling [1,32]. It was initially used as a treatment for long-term muscle spasticity and has been used as the treatment of MH since the late 1970s. It has helped to reduce the mortality from over 80 per cent in untreated reactions in the 1960s to 5–10 per cent today. It works by directly blocking calcium release from the sarcoplasmic reticulum of skeletal muscle and binds to a site at amino acid area 590–609 on the ryanodine receptor of skeletal muscle (RYR1). Calcium release from the sarcoplasmic reticulum of either cardiac muscle (RYR2) or brain tissue (RYR3) is not inhibited by dantrolene [32].

Dantrolene is a highly lipophilic drug and thus is poorly soluble in water. To improve water solubility it is presented in vials containing 20 mg of the sodium salt plus 3 g mannitol and sodium hydroxide. It should be dissolved in 60 mL water to give a final solution of 0.33 mg/mL dantrolene at pH 9.5 and must be used within 6 hours of preparation. Dantrolene is highly irritant to small peripheral veins due to its high pH and so should be injected only into a large or central vein or a fast-running infusion; an extravasation injury results in severe tissue necrosis. An MH reaction may be terminated by incremental doses starting at 1 mg/kg and increasing up to a maximum of up to 10 mg/kg (Fig. 29.3). Plasma levels are sustained for approximately 5 hours after injection because the elimination half-life is approximately 10 hours in children and 12 hours in adults. It undergoes hepatic metabolisation to the active metabolite 5-hydroxydantrolene before being finally excreted via bile and urine.

Side-effects of dantrolene administration, in addition to local phlebitis, include nausea and vomiting, drowsiness, dizziness and confusion. If it is required during a caesarean section then the neonate may have 'floppy baby syndrome' because neonatal plasma levels become approximately 65 per cent of those of the mother. There is also a risk of maternal uterine atony. The concurrent use of verapamil should be avoided because, in pigs, it is associated with ventricular fibrillation in the presence of hyperkalaemia. There also appears to be a marked attenuation of vecuronium after dantrolene administration [32,39].

In addition to dantrolene, supportive measures such as active cooling of the patient to a body temperature of between 38 and 39°C should be initiated. Hypothermia should be avoided and, if shivering does occur, benzodiazepines or even non-depolarising muscle relaxants may be needed [31]. Sodium bicarbonate (0.5–1.0 mmol/kg) may be used to treat the profound metabolic acidosis, and an infusion of glucose and insulin used to control hyperkalaemia. Cardiac arrhythmias should be treated appropriately A urinary catheter should be inserted to quantify output (>2 mL/kg/hour is required), to manage the osmotic diuresis caused by the mannitol (present in IV dantrolene) and to assess the degree of myoglobinuria. Intravascular volume replacement is often needed, after which furosemide may be needed to enhance urinary output.

After successful treatment, the patient should be transferred to an intensive care unit for continuing treatment and ongoing observation. Further doses of dantrolene at 1 mg/kg should be given every 6 hours for the next 24–48 hours to prevent recurrence [27].

Patients with known MHS do not require dantrolene prophylaxis and may safely have day-care procedures. Obviously a trigger-free anaesthetic must be used, and once IV access is established, propofol TIVA (total IV anaesthesia) with or without opioids and non-depolarising muscle relaxants is safe [33].

Investigation and follow-up

Patients who have had a suspected MH reaction or an episode of MMS under anaesthesia may be offered a muscle biopsy to check for MH. This is usually done at a regional MH testing centre under local anaesthesia. A femoral nerve block with prilocaine 5 mg/kg can be used and approximately 500 mg of muscle is required, taken from the vastus lateralis muscle. This is done only after a time interval of at least 6 months after the reaction. The muscle testing has only been validated in postpubertal patients or those who weigh over 20 kg [27,30]. Anaesthesia in susceptible children should always be trigger free until they are old enough.

In vitro contracture testing (IVCT) is currently the gold standard. In Europe the fresh muscle biopsy is exposed to incremental halothane concentrations up to 2 per cent and also incremental doses of caffeine up to 2 mmol/L. A positive

Signs and symptoms

Early signs

- ↑ End-tidal CO_2
- Tachycardia
- Tachypnoea
- ↓ SpO_2
- Labile blood pressure
- Intense masseter spasm after suxamethonium

Later signs

- Fever –↑ 2°C per hour
- Sweating
- Rigidity
- Arrhythmias
- ↑ Plasma CK
- Myoglobinuria
- Hyperkalaemia

COOLING to include

Simple measures

- Remove excess drapes
- Cold intravenous fluids
- Ice packs – groin and axillae (avoid peripheral vasoconstriction)
- Cooling blankets
- Fans

Extreme cases

- Intragastric cooling
- Peritoneal dialysis using cold diasylate
- Extracorporeal cooling (contact perfusion team)

MONITORING to include

- Core and peripheral temperature
- Arterial line and CVP line
- Urinary catheter
- ECG
- Pulse oximetry and capnography
- Blood gases
- Serum glucose
- Serum potassium
- Blood for CPK
- Urine for myoglobin

Early diagnosis is the key to successful management

IMMEDIATE MANAGEMENT

Terminate anaesthesia and surgery
as soon as possible

▼

SUMMON HELP

▼

Hyperventilate with 100% oxygen through vapour-free circuit
and convert to an intravenous technique during termination of surgery

▼

Start active cooling

▼

DANTROLENE 1 mg/kg IV

 Assign one member of staff to prepare the dantrolene
 Repeat as required at 5–10 min intervals
to a **maximum cumulative dose** of 10 mg/kg
 Favourable response indicated by

              (a) decrease in heart rate
              (b) decrease in end-tidal CO_2
              (c) decline in body temperature
              (d) reduced muscle tone

▼

 ARRHYTHMIAS — If these persist despite dantrolene treat as clinically indicated

 HYPERKALAEMIA — Control with 100 ml **25% GLUCOSE** + 12 units **INSULIN** given at 5 ml/kg over 30 minutes

ACIDOSIS — Correction with **SODIUM BICARBONATE** 0.5–1.0 mmol/kg/dose IV – repeated as necessary

URINE OUTPUT — Need to maintain urine output at least 2 ml/kg/h
If required use: **MANNITOL** 0.5–1.0 g/kg
(2.5–5 ml/kg of 20% solution)
and/or FUROSEMIDE 1 mg/kg IV

▼

TRANSFER TO ICU as soon as possible

▼

Recurrence of hyperthermia may occur during first 24 hours

WHEN PATIENT IS STABILISED
arrange investigation of patient and relatives

Figure 29.3 Suggested guideline for the management of malignant hyperthermia. CVP, central venous pressure, CPK, creatine phosphokinase.

test is where there is an increase in fascicular contracture of at least 0.2 g [30,40,41]. Investigation of the *RYR1* gene, in families known to be MH susceptible, may be a useful blood test and obviate the need for muscle biopsies. If muscle taken from the patient proves to be MHS on IVCT, family screening is offered to first-degree relatives (parents and siblings). People with MHS are encouraged to wear a MedicAlert bracelet. Public advice can be obtained from the British Malignant Hyperthermia Association (http://www.bmha.co.uk/index.html).

REFERENCES

Key references

Association of Anaesthetists of Great Britain and Ireland. Anaphylaxis under anaesthesia. *Association of Anaesthetists of Great Britain and Ireland Guidelines.* London, UK: AAGBI, 2003 (http://www.aagbi.org).

Denborough M. Malignant hyperthermia. *Lancet* 1998; **352**: 1131–6.

Ellis AK, Day JH. Diagnosis and management of anaphylaxis. *Can Med Assoc J* 2003; **169**(4): 307–12.

Hepner DL, Castellis MC. Latex allergy: an update. *Anesth Analg* 2003; **96**(4): 1219–29.

Hopkins PM. Malignant hyperthermia: advances in clinical management and diagnosis. *Br J Anaesth* 2000; **85**(1): 118–28.

References

1. Ryder S, Waldmann C. Anaphylaxis: continuing education in anaesthesia. *Crit Care Pain* 2004; **4**: 111–13.
2. Association of Anaesthetists of Great Britain and Ireland. Anaphylaxis under anaesthesia. *Association of Anaesthetists of Great Britain and Ireland Guidelines.* London, UK: AAGBI, 2003 (http://www.aagbi.org).
3. Anonymous. Part 8: Advanced challenges in resuscitation; section 3: special challenges in ECC 3D: Anaphylaxis. *Resuscitation* 2000; **46**: 285–8.
4. McLean-Tooke AP, Bethune CA, Fay AC, Spickett GP. Adrenaline in the treatment of anaphylaxis: what is the evidence? *BMJ* 2003; **327**: 1332–5.
5. Mertes PM, Laxenaire MC, Alla F. Anaphylactic and anaphylactoid reactions occurring during anaesthesia in France 1999–2000. *Anesthesiology* 2003: **99**: 536–45.
6. Laxenaire MC, Mertes PM. Anaphylaxis during anaesthesia. resulsts of a two-year survey in France. *Br J Anaesth* 2001; **87**: 549–58.
7. Ellis AK, Day JH. Diagnosis and management of anaphylaxis. *Can Med Assoc J* 2003; **169**(4): 307–12.
8. Whittington T, Fisher MM. Anaphylactic and anaphylactoid reactions. *Baillière's Clin Anesthesiol* 1998; **12**: 301–21.
9. Stark BJ, Sullivan TJ. Biphasic and protracted anaphylaxis. *J Allergy Clin Immunol* 1986; **78**(1 pt 1): 76–83.
10. Sheffer AL. Anaphylaxis. *J Allergy Clin Immunol* 1985; **75**(2): 227–33.
11. McLean-Tooke APC, Bethune CA, Fay AC, Spickett GP. Adrenaline in the treatment of anaphylaxis: what is the evidence? *BMJ* 2003; **327**(7427): 1332–5.
12. Hughes G, Fitzharris P. Managing acute anaphylaxis: new guidelines emphasise importance of intramuscular adrenaline. *BMJ* 1999; **319**(7201): 1–2.
13. Resuscitation Council (UK). *The emergency medical treatment of anaphylactic reactions for first medical responders and for community nurses.* London: Resuscitation Council (UK), 2002.
14. Great Ormond Street Hospital. *Department of Anaesthesia drug administration guidelines*, 9th edn. London: GOSH, 2004.
15. Advanced Paediatric Life Support Group. *Advanced Paediatric Life Support: The Practical Approach course manual*, 4th edn. London: BMJ Books, 2005: 107–9.
16. Heytman M, Rianbird A. Use of alpha-agonists for management of anaphylaxis occuring under anaesthesia: case studies and review. *Anaesthesia* 2004; **59**: 1210–15.
17. Lieberman P. The use of antihistamines in the prevention and treatment of anaphylaxis and anaphylactoid reactions. *J Allerg Clin Immunol* 1990; **86**(4 pt 2): 684–6.
18. Ziylan HO, Ander AH, Alp T et al. Latex allergy in patients with spinal dysraphism: the role of multiple surgery. *Br J Urol* 1996; **78**(5): 777–9.
19. Ricci G, Gentili A, Di Lorenzo F et al. Latex allergy in subjects who had undergone multiple surgicla procedures for bladder extrophy: relationship with clinical intervention and atopic diseases. *BJU Int* 1999; **84**(9): 1058–62.
20. Sussman GL, Beexhold DH. Allergy to latex rubber. *Ann Intern Med* 1995; **122**(1): 43–6.
21. Holme SA, Lever RS. Latex allergy in atopic children. *Br J Dermatol* 1999; **140**(5): 919–21.
22. Kelly KJ, Pearson MI, Kurup VP et al. A cluster of anaphylactic reactions in children with spina bifida during general anaesthesia: epidemiologic features, risk factors and latex hypersensitivity. *J Allerg Clin Immunol* 1994; **94**: 53–61.
23. Hepner DL, Castellis MC. Latex allergy: an update. *Anesth Analg* 2003; **96**(4): 1219–29.
24. Hepner DL, Castellis MC. Anaphylaxis during the perioperative period. *Anesth Analg* 2003: **97**(5): 1381–95.
25. Holzman RS. Clinical management of latex-allergic children. *Anesth Analg* 1997; **85**: 529–33.
26. Denborough MA, Lovell RRH. Anaesthetic deaths in a family. *Lancet* 1960; **ii**: 45.
27. McCarthy EJ. Malignant hyperthermia: pathophysiology, clinical presentation and treatment. *Adv Pract Acute Clin Care* 2004; **15**(2): 231–7.
28. Gurrera RJ. Is neuroleptic malignant syndrome a neurogenic form of malignant hyperthermia? *Clin Neuropharmacol* 2002; **25**(4): 183–93.
29. Hogan K. The anesthetic myopathies and malignant hyperthermias. *Curr Opin Neurol* 1998; **11**(5): 469–76.
30. Hopkins PM. Malignant hyperthermia: advances in clinical management and diagnosis. *Br J Anaesth* 2000; **85**(1): 118–28.

31. Halloran LL, Bernard DW. Management of drug induced hyperthermia. *Curr Opin Pediatr* 2004; **16**(2): 211–15.

32. Krause T, Gerbershagen MU, Fiege M *et al.* Dantrolene – a review of its pharmacology, therapeutic use and new developments. *Anaesthesia* 2004; **59**(4): 364–73.

33. Jurkat-Rott K, Lerche H, Lehmann-Horn F. Skeletal muscle channelopathies. *J Neurol* 2002; **249**: 1493–502.

34. Denborough M. Malignant hyperthermia. *Lancet* 1998; **352**: 1131–6.

35. Bryson GL, Chung F, Cox RG *et al.* Patient selection in ambulatory anesthesia – an evidence-based review: part II. *Can J Anaesth* 2004; **51**: 782–94.

36. Rosenberg H, Shutack JG. Variants of malignt hyperthermia. Special problems for the paediatric anaesthesiologist. *Paediatr Anaesth* 1996; **6**: 87–93.

37. Littleford JA, Patel L, Bose D *et al.* Masseter muscle spasm in children: implications of continuing the triggering anesthetic. *Anesth Analg* 1991; **72**: 151–60.

38. Shepherd S, Ellis F, Hopkins P, Robinson R. RYR1 mutations in UK central core disease: more than just the C-terminal transmembrane region of the RYR1 gene. *J Med Genet* 2004; **41**(3): e33.

39. Costello I, ed. *British national formulary for children.* London: BMJ Books/Pharmaceutical Press, 2005 (http:\\www.bnfc.org).

40. European Malignant Hypepyrexia Group. A protocol for the investifgation on malignant hyperpyrexia (MH) susceptibility. *Br J Anaesth* 1984; **56**: 1267–71.

41. Robinson RL, Hopkins PM. A breakthrough in the genetic diagnosis of malignant hyperthermia. *Br J Anaesth* 2001; **86**: 166–8.

Difficult circulations

SALLY WILMSHURST

KEY LEARNING POINTS

- Most children with congenital heart disease are surviving into adulthood and may present for non-cardiac surgery.
- Stable children with repaired congenital heart disease can usually be safely managed outside a paediatric cardiac centre.
- Children with unstable disease or unrepaired defects should be transferred to a specialist centre where possible.

- Antibiotic prophylaxis against bacterial endocarditis will be required for any major surgery or surgery causing bacteraemia.
- For most children with congenital heart disease a balanced anaesthetic technique involving controlled ventilation is preferable for all but the briefest procedures.

INTRODUCTION

Children with difficult circulations often present for non-cardiac surgery. The incidence of congenital heart disease is increasing and affects 1 in 145 children in the UK [1]. Advances in diagnosis, surgical and medical management have improved survival. Previously only one in five children with complex cardiac disease survived into adulthood and now the figure is well over 80 per cent [2]. It is therefore increasingly likely that a paediatric anaesthetist will be faced with a child with heart disease.

The more common congenital cardiac abnormalities along with their prevalence are listed in Table 30.1.

This chapter reviews the general principles of managing a child with cardiovascular disease and includes discussion of the common and important specific difficult circulations. In many cases, especially those with functional limitation, anaesthesia techniques need to be modified. Sometimes referral to a specialist centre is indicated [3] (Table 30.2,

extrapolated from adults). As a general rule, all except essential surgery is best deferred in children with major *limiting* cardiac disease until after their status has been optimised by either medical treatment or cardiac surgery.

RISK

In a North American study, congenital cardiac disease was found to increase significantly 1-, 3- and 30-day mortality in children undergoing inpatient non-cardiac surgery. The 30-day mortality rate was 6 per cent in these children versus 3.8 per cent in children without cardiac disease. Mortality was greatest in neonates and in more complex cardiac defects [4]. In another study, the complication rate was 5.8 per cent and major risk factors were cyanosis, current treatment for cardiac failure, poor general health and younger age. Procedures on the respiratory and neurological systems were associated with the worst outcome [5].

Table 30.1 Prevalence of lesions, expressed as a percentage of total congenital heart disease (CHD) [6]

Condition	Prevalence (%)
Ventricular septal defect (VSD)	20
Tetralogy of Fallot (ToF)	11
Atrial septal defect	6–10
Aortic stenosis	5–10
Transposition of the great arteries (TGA)	5–7
Coarctation of the aorta	5
Atrioventricular septal defect (AVSD)	3
Pulmonary atresia with intact ventricular septum (PA/IVS)	3
Total anomalous pulmonary venous connections (TAPVC)	2
Tricuspid atresia	1–3
Ebstein's anomaly	0.5
Coronary artery anomalies	0.25–0.5
Hypoplastic left heart syndrome (HLHS)	0.02
Double-outlet right ventricle (DORV)	0.01

Table 30.2 Factors requiring referral to a specialist centre [3]

Significant intracardiac shunting
More than mildly elevated pulmonary vascular resistance
More than moderate left-ventricular dysfunction or failure
More than mild right-ventricular dysfunction or failure
Systemic pressures in the right ventricle
Functional univentricular heart (possible exception of stable Fontan circulation)
More than mild obstructive valvular disease
Coronary artery anomalies
New-onset arrhythmias

PREOPERATIVE ASSESSMENT

History

A detailed history of the child's cardiac disease and any prior surgery or catheter treatments must be taken. In particular, a history of decompensated cardiac or respiratory function must be sought. In neonates and infants, failure to thrive and difficulty with feeding due to tachypnoea and sweating indicate cardiac failure. Older children may have limited exercise tolerance and be unable to keep up with their peers. The functional status can be recorded using the New York Heart Association (NYHA) system:

1 = No limitation in physical activity
2 = Mild impairment of physical activity
3 = Marked impairment of activity, dyspnoea on mild exertion
4 = Breathlessness at rest.

Table 30.3 Classification of heart murmurs [6]

Systolic	Aortic stenosis
	Pulmonary stenosis
	Atrial septal defect
	Tricuspid regurgitation
	Mitral regurgitation
	Ventricular septal defect
	Coarctation
Diastolic	Pulmonary regurgitation
	Aortic regurgitation
	Mitral stenosis
	Tricuspid stenosis
Continuous	Patent ductus arteriosus
	Venous hum
	Surgical shunt
	Aortopulmonary window
	Arteriovenous fistula
	Bronchial collaterals

A history of arrhythmias, cardiac pacing or chest discomfort must be sought. A detailed drug history is important as it yields useful information about the progress of the child's clinical condition as well as warning of potential perioperative problems such as bleeding secondary to aspirin or anticoagulants, or any history of allergy. Evidence of any intercurrent illness should be sought, as well as any history of complications occurring with previous anaesthetics.

Examination

The child's overall nutritional status should be assessed and the heart and lungs auscultated, in particular looking for evidence of heart failure. In neonates and infants right heart failure is evident by hepatic enlargement rather than peripheral oedema whereas in older children peripheral oedema and an elevated jugular venous pulsation are clinically relevant. Left heart failure manifests with pulmonary oedema which may cause crepitations in the lung bases. The baseline blood pressure should be recorded and the peripheral pulse volume, character, rate and rhythm noted. The child should be examined for the presence of cyanosis or clubbing. Congenital heart defects associated with right heart volume overload, such as septal defects, may have an audible pansystolic murmur of tricuspid regurgitation due to enlargement of the right heart. Some defects have pathognomic murmurs (Table 30.3).

In addition to cardiorespiratory examination it is vital to assess the airway. Congenital heart disease is strongly associated with syndromes affecting the airway and other midline structures (e.g. Goldenhar syndrome, Treacher Collins syndrome and trisomy 21). Heart disease may also complicate other conditions known to be associated with a difficult airway such as Hunter or Hurler syndrome. Prolonged intubation following cardiac surgery may predispose to subglottic stenosis. Children with cyanotic defects or hyperreactive pulmonary vasculature will tolerate difficulties with airway management very poorly.

Investigations

The electrocardiogram (ECG) is subject to a large degree of normal variation depending on the age (see Chapter 20). For example, in the neonate the right and left ventricles are more equal in size and therefore right-ventricular dominance may be normal in a neonate, whereas this would be a pathological finding in the older child with right heart volume overload secondary to an atrial septal defect (ASD), for example. Therefore an ECG is most useful in establishing a baseline for intraoperative and post-operative comparison. Arrhythmias and paced rhythms may also be visible on a standard 12-lead ECG.

ECHOCARDIOGRAPHY

A recent echocardiographic examination (echo) is most useful in evaluating the cardiac functional status and anatomy. A standard transthoracic examination will assess the heart via six acoustic 'windows' using two-dimensional echocardiography supplemented by Doppler ultrasound and M-mode echo. Specific terminology is used in paediatric echocardiography [6]. Acronyms are common in congenital heart disease and echo reports and common ones are detailed in Table 30.4. The echo is reported as a morphological, positional and segmental analysis of the heart. The heart has three 'segments' (atria, ventricles and great vessels) with two connections (atrioventricular [AV] and ventriculoarterial [VA]). The connections are concordant if normally connected and discordant if reversed, e.g. in transposition of the great arteries where there is VA discordance. Other abnormal connections include double-inlet and double-outlet ventricles. Situs refers to the anatomical position of the heart. Situs solitus is normally positioned. The heart may be morphologically normal but abnormally positioned, e.g. mirror-image dextrocardia (or situs inversus) or segments may be absent or duplicated as they are in isomerism. In these cases,

the segments are described by their morphological appearance as well as their relationship to each other. Finally, the aortic arch may be abnormally positioned on the right side in congenital heart disease. If an echo is reported as SCCL, this refers to situs **s**olitus, **c**oncordant AV and VA **c**onnections and a **l**eft-sided aortic arch. Simple transposition of the great arteries would be reported as SCDL.

An echo can provide a detailed assessment of ventricular function. The stroke volume can be measured and an indication of cardiac output and index made. Fractional shortening and ejection fraction can be assessed, as can regional wall motion abnormalities. As with ECGs a wide variety of normal values exist and tables of age-specific values are available. Valvular disease, surgical shunt patency, and vessel sizes can be assessed. Pulmonary hypertension can be estimated in the presence of tricuspid regurgitation using the modified Bernoulli equation (pressure gradient $(mmHg) = 4 \times (max.$ velocity of tricuspid regurgitant jet$)^2$, which gives the gradient across the valve and thus the right ventricular pressure less the right atrial pressure.

CHEST X-RAY

A preoperative chest X-ray (CXR) can provide information about the size of the heart in relation to the thoracic diameter and show the presence of clips, coils or pacemaker wires from previous interventions. Prominent pulmonary vascular markings may indicate increased pulmonary blood flow as in left-to-right shunts whereas absent pulmonary markings or pulmonary pruning may indicate pulmonary hypertension or pulmonary artery stenosis. Increased lung markings in the upper lobes and Kerley B lines are signs of left-ventricular failure and pulmonary congestion. The CXR may also demonstrate signs of intercurrent infection or atelectasis.

BLOOD TESTS

Children with cyanotic heart defects (Table 30.5) respond to chronic hypoxaemia by elevating their haemoglobin concentration. Polycythaemia occurs and causes increased blood viscosity (haematocrits can be over 70 per cent), this results in impaired peripheral perfusion and can lead to a relative iron deficiency. In addition to causing symptoms of hyperviscosity (Table 30.6) the iron-deficient, sluggish red cells can become damaged and trigger a low-grade disseminated intravascular coagulation, therefore depleting clotting factors and causing abnormal coagulation. Reduced platelet numbers and dysfunction is common. Children with a

Table 30.4 Congenital heart disease acronyms

RAI	Right atrial isomerism (both atrial appendages morphologically right sided)
LAI	Left atrial isomerism (both atrial appendages morphologically left sided)
DORV	Double-outlet right ventricle
DILV	Double-inlet left ventricle
MAPCA	Major aortopulmonary collateral artery
RVOTO	Right-ventricular outflow tract obstruction
LVOTO	Left-ventricular outflow tract obstruction
R(L)MBTS	Right (left) modified Blalock–Taussig shunt
T(P)APVD	Total (partial) anomalous pulmonary venous drainage

Table 30.5 Common causes of cyanotic heart disease

Tetralogy of Fallot
Transposition of the great arteries
Anomalous pulmonary venous drainage
Tricuspid atresia
Pulmonary atresia with ventricular septal defect
Eisenmenger syndrome

Table 30.6   Hyperviscosity syndrome

Central nervous system	Headache
	Faintness
	Amaurosis fugax
	Dizziness
	Blurred vision
General	Fatigue
	Lethargy
	Muscle weakness
	Myalgia
	Paraesthesiae

haematocrit greater than 65 per cent or with symptoms of hyperviscosity should be intravenously hydrated prior to surgery and venesection considered.

Clotting studies are important in children who are anti-coagulated or with cyanotic heart disease for the reasons given above. In addition, hepatic dysfunction secondary to congestion can impair clotting factor production. In children taking certain medications, including diuretics, angiotensin-converting enzyme inhibitors and anti-rejection drugs, baseline urea, electrolyte and creatinine levels should be measured. Finally, children who have had cardiac surgery in the past are likely to have received blood transfusions or blood products and may have cross-matching difficulties. An early group and save or crossmatch is indicated. Children with DiGeorge syndrome, a chromosomal abnormality strongly associated with congenital cardiac malformations, may require irradiated blood because of thymus dysfunction and the risk of graft-versus-host reaction [7].

ANAESTHESIA

Monitoring

Standard anaesthetic monitoring is required as recommended by the Association of Anaesthetists of Great Britain and Ireland (AAGBI) [8]. Intra-arterial blood pressure measurement should be considered in unstable patients or where clinically indicated for the planned surgery. It is particularly useful where large fluctuations in blood pressure or large blood loss are anticipated and for monitoring blood gases and acid–base status. Central venous access may be indicated for vasoactive drug administration. Arterial pressure and saturation monitoring will be more accurate on the opposite side to any surgical subclavian artery to pulmonary artery shunt (modified Blalock–Taussig, BT). Central venous access via jugular or subclavian routes should be avoided in children with Glenn or Fontan circulations (or total cavopulmonary connection, TCPC) because of the risk of infection or thrombosis and because the superior vena cava connects directly to the pulmonary artery. Any invasive lines must be

free of air to avoid air entering the cerebral circulation (paradoxical air embolism) via shunts. Transoesophageal echocardiography can be useful in assessing cardiac function perioperatively but complex cardiac lesions will need expert interpretation.

Premedication and endocarditis prophylaxis

Oxygen consumption secondary to sympathetic stimulation can be reduced with the use of anxiolytic or sedative premedication (e.g. midazolam 0.5 mg/kg orally) [9]. Premedication with antimuscarinics, antacids, analgesics and antihistamines can be used where indicated.

Congenital heart disease was responsible for 9 per cent of all endocarditis cases in a Japanese study [10]. A recent review of the guidelines for prophylaxis against endocarditis from the British Society for Antimicrobial Chemotherapy [11] examined the current evidence, a substantial amount of which is animal based. In rabbits, the use of antibiotics substantially reduced the development of endocarditis on damaged heart valves exposed to very high bacterial loads but this may not be directly applicable to humans. Anecdotal evidence suggests that some procedures are causally linked to bacteraemia, or to endocarditis, but there are no double-blind studies evaluating the efficacy of antibiotics in humans. Prophylaxis is usually administered prior to dental procedures although a case–control trial of 273 patients found no link between dental treatment and endocarditis [12] and a transient bacteraemia can be demonstrated after tooth-brushing or chewing. Despite the lack of evidence in dental procedures, but in view of the serious nature of endocarditis, the current guidelines recommend prophylaxis in high-risk children, which include those with a previous history of endocarditis, a valve prosthesis or a surgically placed shunt.

In gastrointestinal or genitourinary procedures, the indications for prophylaxis are wider and include all congenital lesions except simple patent ductus arteriosus (PDA) and secundum ASD. Highly virulent organisms such as enterococci, streptococci and staphylococci are often implicated. Recommended regimens are listed in Table 30.7.

Common paediatric procedures associated with endocarditis or bacteraemia and therefore requiring prophylaxis include urethral catheterisation, cystoscopy, tonsillectomy or other upper respiratory tract surgery and surgery involving the gastrointestinal mucosa.

Anaesthesia technique

The effects of commonly used intravenous and volatile anaesthetic drugs on the cardiovascular system are summarised in Table 30.8. Prolonged spontaneous ventilation with high-dose volatile anaesthesia is potentially hazardous in the child with cardiac disease. The goal is balanced anaesthesia using hypnotic agents, relaxants and analgesia usually

Table 30.7 Antibiotics for endocarditis prophylaxis

Dental

Amoxicillin orally 1 hour before
<5 years	750 mg
5–10 years	1.5 g
>10 years	3.0 g

Penicillin allergy use clindamycin
<5 years	150 mg
5–10 years	300 mg
>10 years	600 mg

OR

Amoxicillin intravenously at induction
<5 years	250 mg
5–10 years	500 mg
>10 years	1.0 g
Penicillin allergy use clindamycin half oral dose	

Genitourinary or gastrointestinal procedures

Ampicillin/amoxicillin at induction / plus aminoglycoside (gentamicin 2 mg/kg or amikacin 10 mg/kg)
<5 years	250 mg
5–10 years	500 mg
>10 years	1.0 g
Penicillin allergy or penicillin in last month use teicoplanin at induction	
<14 years	6 mg/kg
>14 years	400 mg

OR

Vancomycin 1–2 hours pre-procedure by slow intravenous infusion (1 hour)
<10 years	20 mg/kg
>10 years	1.0 g
Plus gentamicin	2 mg/kg

Condensed from the *British National Formulary for Children* (http://www.bnfc.org).

with controlled ventilation. Regional anaesthesia may be indicated but care should be taken with those on anti-coagulant therapy and the risk of dropping the systemic vascular resistance should be considered in children with right-to-left shunts or left-ventricular outflow tract obstruction.

Postoperative care

A well child having simple surgery may be suitable for a day-case procedure. Conversely, unstable children or those having complex surgery may require observation in a high-dependency or intensive care setting postoperatively.

SPECIFIC 'CIRCULATIONS'

Intracardiac shunting

Shunting is the movement of blood from one side of the heart to the other and its presence is pathological. Shunts can be defined as left to right, right to left or complex (see Chapter 40). All patients are at risk of endocarditis and paradoxical air embolus. Otherwise a spectrum of significance exists varying from the asymptomatic finding through to lesions complicated by severe cardiac failure or pulmonary hypertension.

Left-to-right shunts

These are common defects and include ASDs, ventricular septal defects (VSDs), PDA, atrioventricular septal defects (AVSDs) and partial anomalous pulmonary venous drainage (PAPVD). These patients will have normal arterial saturations but a long-term risk of right heart volume overload and the development of heart failure and pulmonary hypertension. If pulmonary hypertension develops the shunt can 'reverse', resulting in cyanosis. Over a long period of time Eisenmenger syndrome can develop where the right heart pressure is suprasystemic, right-to-left

Table 30.8 Cardiovascular properties of anaesthetics [13–15]

Agent	Contract	MAP	HR	SVR	PVR	L–R shunt	R–L shunt
Sevoflurane	↓	↓	↔	↓		↔	↑
Isoflurane	↓	↓	↑	↓ ↓		↔	↑
Halothane	↓	↓	↓	↓		↔	↑
NO₂	↓		↓		↑		↑
Propofol		↓	↔	↓ ↓	↔	↓	↑
Thiopental	↓			↓			↑
Etomidate		Mild ↓	↑	Mild ↓			
Ketamine		↑		↔	↔	↔	↔
Fentanyl	↔	↔	↓	↔	↔	↔	↔

HR, heart rate; L–R shunt, left-to-right shunt; MAP, mean arterial pressure; PVR, pulmonary vascular resistance; R–L shunt, right-to-left shunt; SVR, systemic vascular resistance.

Table 30.9 Goals of anaesthesia for left-to-right shunts

Assessment	Check recent echo
	Anticipate pulmonary hypertension in larger shunts:
	Improving failure symptoms sometimes means increasing PVR
	Cyanotic spells imply shunt reversal
Considerations	Avoid air bubbles
	Endocarditis prophylaxis
Anaesthesia	Avoid spontaneous ventilation – plethoric lungs have poor compliance
	Decrease shunt:
	Maintain PVR – avoid excessive O_2 and hyperventilation
	Normal or low SVR
	Balanced anaesthesia

PVR, pulmonary vascular resistance; SVR, systemic vascular resistance.

shunting occurs and severe pulmonary hypertension exists. This is inoperable and the only treatment is cardiac transplantation. Although all the above may be associated with other congenital abnormal-ities there is a particularly strong link between AVSD and trisomy 21. For a detailed description of the lesions associated with left-to-right shunts see Chapter 40.

ANAESTHESIA FOR LEFT-TO-RIGHT SHUNTS (Table 30.9)

The goal is to decrease shunt and maintain adequate perfusion and oxygenation [16]. Cardiac failure should be optimised preoperatively and antifailure medication continued. Pulmonary hypertension should be anticipated in children with large unrepaired shunts. Excessive pulmonary blood flow can decrease lung compliance and positive pressure ventilation should be employed for all but the very shortest procedures.

Right-to-left shunts

Cardiac lesions resulting in right-to-left shunts include common conditions such as tetralogy of Fallot (ToF) and rarer conditions such as tricuspid atresia and pulmonary atresia.

TETRALOGY OF FALLOT

This is a common cardiac lesion with a prevalence of 1 in 2000 live births [1]. The tetralogy consists of VSD, right-ventricular outflow tract obstruction (RVOTO), right-ventricular hypertrophy and an overriding aorta (Fig. 30.1). It can occur in association with other congenital defects requiring more urgent surgery (e.g. congenital diaphragmatic hernia and tracheo-oesophageal fistula). Repair usually takes place in infancy and consists of closure of the

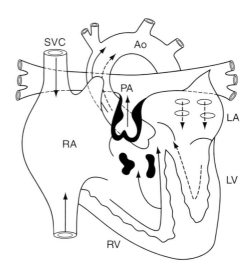

Figure 30.1 Tetralogy of Fallot. The right-ventricular outflow obstruction can be subvalvular, valvular or supravalvular. The aorta is overriding both ventricles and there is a ventricular septal defect (VSD). Ao, aorta; LA, left atrium; LV, left ventricle; PA, pulmonary artery; RA, right atrium; RV, right ventricle; SVC, superior vena cava. From May [52] with kind permission.

VSD redirecting blood from the left ventricle (LV) to the aorta and relief of RVOTO. Occasionally a systemic-to-pulmonary shunt is required in the neonatal period if RVOTO is severe (see page 467).

UNREPAIRED ToF

Children may be chronically cyanosed or have normal saturations. A spectrum of severity occurs and variants include pulmonary stenosis (ToF-PS), pulmonary atresia (ToF-PA) and absent pulmonary valve (ToF-APV). Presentation may be with an asymptomatic murmur at the milder end or with duct-dependent cyanosis in the more severe forms. Severe disease may be managed with a BT (subclavian to pulmonary artery) shunt as a neonate prior to complete repair at a later stage, usually between 6 months and 2 years. A history of hypercyanotic or 'tet' spells should be sought. This is caused by right-ventricular infundibular spasm increasing RVOTO and increases the right-to-left shunt, leading to cyanosis and systemic acidosis. This acidosis, in turn, worsens the shunt and a vicious circle can develop. Management aims to alleviate the RVOTO and to increase SVR. Spells are managed prophylactically with oral propranolol and it is important to check that this medication is up to date before surgery. Acute management of a spell during anaesthesia includes intermittent positive pressure ventilation (IPPV) with 100 per cent O_2, fluid boluses (10 mL/kg), opioid administration, vasopressors such as phenylephrine, metaraminol or noradrenaline, and β blockade with intravenous propranolol (0.1 mg/kg if not adequately β blocked). Spells can be triggered by surgical stimuli or by pain and anxiety and these precipitants should be minimised as far as possible.

REPAIRED ToF

Long-term follow-up of adults and children with repaired ToF shows a high incidence of pulmonary regurgitation leading to cardiomegaly and exercise intolerance [17] and restrictive right-ventricular physiology (52–57 per cent) [18,19]. Pulmonary regurgitation has been shown to increase with high airway pressures [20]. Left ventricular function is usually preserved [21]. Late sudden cardiac death occurs in 2 per cent, usually more than two decades post-repair [22], and is associated with severe pulmonary regurgitation, ventricular tachyarrhythmias, QRS duration of >180 ms on the ECG and left-ventricular dysfunction [23]. Restrictive physiology reduces the amount of pulmonary regurgitation and hence improves exercise tolerance and the development of cardiomegaly and arrhythmias. Anaesthetic agents, particularly volatile agents, are negatively inotropic [24] and should be used with caution in the setting of right-ventricular dysfunction.

ANAESTHESIA FOR RIGHT-TO-LEFT SHUNTS (Table 30.10)

The goal in these children is to maintain oxygenation and cardiac output and to minimise the right-to-left shunt [25]. Decreases in SVR will worsen the shunt and therefore anaesthetic agents need to be used cautiously. Induction using volatile agents can theoretically be slow owing to impaired uptake, although this is rarely clinically apparent. Systemic vascular resistance can be maintained with fluid therapy and occasionally vasopressors. In the presence of desaturation, arterial blood gas measurement can be useful to monitor acid–base balance, which may give an early indication of poor perfusion. Muscle relaxation and gentle positive pressure ventilation are helpful as muscular work is minimised and mixed venous saturations increased. Chronic cyanosis causes polycythaemia and these children tolerate acute reductions in haematocrit poorly, so blood volume must be maintained in surgery involving large blood loss.

Complex shunts: transposition of the great arteries (see Figure 40.2 Chapter 40)

Transposition of the great arteries (TGA) is a common defect accounting for 5–7 per cent of cardiac malformations. In TGA the aorta arises from the right ventricle and pulmonary artery from the left ventricle. The arterial switch operation, in which the great arteries and coronary arteries are surgically returned to the normal position, is the definitive corrective procedure for TGA. Short-term complications include left-ventricular dysfunction, pulmonary hypertension and rhythm disturbances. Mortality rate varies from 4 per cent in complex cases to 0 per cent in simple TGA [26]. Long-term follow-up shows that 96 per cent are in NYHA class I and 2 per cent in class II. Pulmonary stenosis is common, occurring in 17 per cent, often necessitating intervention. Symptomatic left-ventricular dysfunction is rare, although impaired contractility and wall motion abnormalities are commonly present [27]. Well children presenting after an arterial switch operation for non-cardiac surgery should be fit for anaesthesia although knowledge of the complications is helpful. Infants with TGA presenting prior to surgical correction should be managed in a specialist centre.

PACEMAKERS (Table 30.11)

Children with cardiac disease presenting for non-cardiac surgery may have an implanted pacemaker for postsurgical or congenital heart rhythm disturbances. Pacemakers are given a four-letter code. The first letter refers to the chamber being paced (atria = A, ventricle = V, both = D) and the second to the chamber being sensed (A, V or D). The third

Table 30.10 Goals of anaesthesia for right-to-left shunts

Assessment	Check recent echo
	Ascertain SpO$_2$ (usual)
	Check for hypercyanotic spells
	Check haematocrit
Considerations	Avoid excessive fasting and dehydration
	Endocarditis prophylaxis
	Avoid air bubbles
Anaesthesia	Use IPPV; neuromuscular blockade will increase SvO$_2$ and therefore SaO$_2$
	In ToF particularly avoid sympathetic stimulation
	Reduce shunt – maintain SVR and minimise PVR
	Avoid anaemia

IPPV, intermittent positive pressure ventilation; PVR, pulmonary vascular resistance; SaO$_2$, arterial oxygen saturation; SpO$_2$, peripheral oxygen saturation; SvO$_2$, venous oxygen saturation; SVR, systemic vascular resistance;.ToF, tetralogy of Fallot.

Table 30.11 Goals of anaesthesia for a child with a pacemaker

Assessment	Indication for pacing
	Recent check
	Back-up mode
	Underlying rhythm
Considerations	Bipolar or remote diathermy
	Reprogram pacemaker to back-up mode
	Alternatively use pacemaker magnet
	Consider alternative pacing source if underlying rhythm is life threatening
Anaesthesia	Child will be intolerant of hypovolaemia and vasodilatation
	No heart rate response to stimuli – awareness risk
	Postoperative pacemaker check

letter is the response of the generator to sensing of natural electrical activity (inhibition = I, trigger = T, dual response = D) and the fourth letter refers to any rate modulation (e.g. increasing the pacemaker output with exercise) [28]. Many methods of signalling a rate response are in use, including detection of elevated minute ventilation or sensing muscle activity [29]. A fifth letter is used for antitachycardia capabilities [28]. Examples of common pacemaker codes are DDDR, VOO, AAI. In children, increasingly sophisticated and physiological pacemaker functions are used.

When preoperatively assessing the child with a pacemaker, if possible, determine the reason for pacemaker insertion and date, site of generator and the underlying rhythm from the case notes and history. From the pacemaker paperwork determine the type of pacemaker, the back-up program that the pacemaker defaults to, the date of the last pacemaker check, battery status and lead thresholds. Some evidence of satisfactory function may be evident on a 12-lead ECG. In all but emergency situations in hospitals without pacemaker support, it is advisable to have a pacemaker check before surgery or anaesthesia. The pacemaker may require remote reprogramming by a pacemaker technician to ensure safe surgery, e.g. where diathermy interference is likely near to the generator or where rate response programs may malfunction because of artificial ventilation or movement.

Perioperatively the biggest risk to a pacemaker is interference from diathermy. Bipolar is preferred where possible and avoid diathermy near to the pacemaker site. In an extreme situation where loss of pacemaker activity would result in electrical activity incompatible with life, it may be necessary to consider temporary trans-venous or transthoracic pacing. Where preoperative reprogramming is not possible, use of a pacemaker magnet over the generator will revert the pacemaker to its back-up mode (usually asynchronous VOO) and inactivate any demand modes. Postoperatively the pacemaker will require a check and restoration of its original functions.

Rarely, children may present for surgery with an implantable defibrillation device inserted for conditions such as long-QT syndrome, cardiomyopathies or in children who have suffered an 'out-of-hospital' cardiac arrest. The management of these devices should always be guided by a specialist but the principles are similar to those of pacemakers. The antitachycardia function should be disabled before surgery and an alternative means of defibrillating should be readily available.

THE TRANSPLANTED HEART (Table 30.12)

The first successful adult heart transplantation took place in 1967 but the procedure was not performed in children until 1982. The International Heart and Lung Transplant Registry [30] has reported paediatric heart and heart–lung transplantations world-wide since that time. Children may present for anaesthesia in connection with their transplant, such as for regular cardiac catheterisation procedures or

Table 30.12 Goals of anaesthesia after heart transplantation

Assessment	Check recent echo/transplant assessment
	Exercise tolerance
	Beware asymptomatic myocardial ischaemia – electrocardiogram (ECG)
	Continue immunosuppression – steroids may require intravenous supplementation
Considerations	Infection risk – strict asepsis
	Complications:
	Vasculopathy
	Hypertension
	Malignancies
Anaesthesia	Denervated heart:
	Unresponsive to atropine
	Poor tolerance of hypovolaemia and vasodilatation
	Delayed heart rate response to stimuli

endomyocardial biopsies to look for evidence of rejection, for procedures related to malignancy (which is increased post-transplantation) or they may present for incidental procedures. In one American centre, 13 per cent of transplanted children presented for non-cardiac surgery [31]. Important considerations include the presence of a 'denervated' heart, complications related to rejection, complex drug therapy, immunosuppression, infection risk and hypertension.

The denervated heart

Because the heart receives no extracardiac nerve supply, it loses many of its reflex mechanisms for increasing cardiac output at times of need. The transplanted heart shows a twofold and delayed response to stress. First, the Frank–Starling mechanism of increased preload enhances left-ventricular end-diastolic volume and cardiac output. Later the heart is able to increase rate and contractility in response to circulating catecholamines. A similar delayed response occurs with exercise and the effects persist for longer.

Because of denervation, the response to cardioactive drugs is changed. Directly acting agents will be required. There is enhanced responsiveness to adrenergic drugs via a presynaptic effect. Drugs acting indirectly through the parasympathetic nervous system, such as atropine, will have no effect [32]. Antiarrhythmic drugs have been studied [33]. Class 1B drugs such as lidocaine retain their effects as do β blockers and calcium-channel antagonists. Digoxin partially acts indirectly via the vagus nerve and loses this activity; however, it also has a direct action on atrioventricular conduction and may be used for arrhythmia management.

Recent research suggests that unpredictable sympathetic reinnervation may occur following heart transplantation [34]. Histological evidence of nerves travelling across suture lines has been found as well as appropriate pharmacological responses. This is more likely in the absence of rejection and in young donor age.

Complications of cardiac transplantation

A child may present for anaesthesia for an indication related to a complication or the risk of the anaesthetic itself may relate to the presence of complications. Graft rejection is the cause of 30 per cent of deaths. It is most likely to occur in the first 3 months after transplantation with a peak incidence at 4–6 weeks [30]. Patients may present for anaesthesia to assess the severity and incidence of rejection. Management includes increasing immunosuppressive therapy such as steroids. The cardiac function may deteriorate during an episode of rejection and arrhythmias are common.

Coronary vasculopathy is the accelerated development of diffuse coronary artery disease following heart transplantation. It may present as congestive cardiac failure, silent myocardial infarction – owing to absent pain pathways – and sudden death. The disease is related to the presence of rejection and is limited to the coronary vessels, suggesting an inflammatory cause. A recent study of 337 paediatric transplant recipients showed that 18 per cent developed vasculopathy at a mean time of 6.5 ± 3 years post-transplantation [35]. Risk factors included rejection occurring within the first post-transplantation year, haemodynamically compromising rejection outside of the first year and multiple rejection episodes [35,36].

Diagnosis is made using conventional coronary angiography and intravascular ultrasound, which is more sensitive at detecting early diffuse intimal thickening. Dobutamine stress echocardiography has also been used.

The presence of coronary vasculopathy is an indication for retransplantation because of the risk of sudden death, although revascularisation may be attempted in the presence of discrete lesions. Anaesthetic management is similar to that in conventional coronary artery disease. Electrocardiographic monitoring to detect ischaemia or transoesophageal echocardiography should be considered and an anaesthetic technique to balance myocardial oxygen supply and demand should be used.

Arrhythmias occur in 40 per cent of paediatric cardiac transplant recipients [37] and management should take into account the action of drugs on the denervated heart as previously discussed. Three per cent will require a pacemaker.

IMMUNOSUPPRESSION

Immunosuppressive drugs are continued indefinitely after transplantation and must be continued perioperatively including during prolonged 'nil-by-mouth' periods. A number of different regimens are used, tailored to the individual patient. Drugs of particular importance to the anaesthetist include steroids and ciclosporin. Steroids are given in the initial period or in the management of

rejection episodes. High-dose and chronically administered steroids suppress the hypothalamic–pituitary axis and patients will require supplemental steroids during anaesthesia and surgery.

Ciclosporin is commonly used as a steroid-sparing agent. Its most common side-effect is nephrotoxicity which is dose related and partly reversible. Hypertension, vascular disease and hepatotoxicity also occur.

Because the patients are chronically immunosuppressed, infection remains a serious risk and is a major cause of death. Avoidance of unnecessary invasive procedures and strict asepsis are therefore essential. A further complication of immunosuppression, which may require anaesthetic involvement, is lymphoproliferative disease.

PULMONARY HYPERTENSION (Table 30.13)

Pulmonary hypertension is defined as a resting pulmonary arterial pressure (PAP) of greater than 25 mmHg or greater than 30 mmHg on exercise. Children may present for anaesthesia for procedures related to the disease or to its therapy, such as for Hickman line insertion or cardiac catheterisation, procedures to limit the pulmonary hypertension, such as adenotonsillectomy in those with obstructive symptoms, or unrelated incidental procedures.

Table 30.13 Goals of anaesthesia in pulmonary hypertension (transfer to specialist centre if possible)

Assessment	Aetiology
	Exercise tolerance
	Electrocardiogram
	Echocardiogram – particularly high risk if:
	TR jet > 4 m/s
	Right ventricle dilatation
	Left ventricle compression
Considerations	Maintain drug therapy
	Consider postoperative intensive care unit
	Have NO available
Anaesthesia	Use IPPV
	Avoid precipitating ↑ PVR (see Table 30.15)
	High FiO$_2$
	Hypo- or normocapnia
	Avoid N$_2$O
	Low intrathoracic pressure and PEEP (but avoid atelectasis)
	Smooth wakening (or consider postoperative IPPV)
	Pharmacological therapy
	NO
	Glyceryl trinitrate
	Milrinone

FiO$_2$, inspired oxygen concentration; IPPV, intermittent positive pressure ventilation; PEEP, positive end-expiratory pressure; PVR, pulmonary vascular resistance; TR, tricuspid regurgitation.

Table 30.14 Evian classification of pulmonary hypertension

Pulmonary arterial hypertension	Idiopathic Systemic-to-pulmonary shunts Collagen vascular disease Human immunodeficiency virus Drugs Portal hypertension Persistent pulmonary hypertension of the newborn
Pulmonary venous hypertension	Left-sided heart disease Compression of the pulmonary veins Veno-occlusive disease
Secondary to disorders of the respiratory system	Thrombotic or thromboembolic disease Pulmonary emboli Sickle cell disease
Disorders of the pulmonary vasculature	Sarcoidosis Pulmonary haemangiomas

Table 30.15 Factors affecting pulmonary vascular resistance (PVR)

Decrease PVR	Increase PVR

↑ PaO_2
Hypocapnia
Alkalosis
Minimising intra-alveolar pressure:
  Spontaneous ventilation
  Normal lung volumes
  Avoid PEEP
Avoidance of excess sympathetic stimulation:
  Anaesthesia
  Pain management
Pharmacological:
  Isoprenaline
  Phosphodiesterase III inhibitors (e.g. milrinone)
  Prostacyclin
  Inhaled NO
	Sympathetic stimulation:
	  Light anaesthesia
	  Pain
	  Anxiety
	  Acidosis
	  Hypoxia
	  Hypercapnia
	  Hypothermia
	
	Increased intrathoracic pressure:
	  PEEP
	  IPPV
	  Atelectasis

IPPV, intermittent positive pressure ventilation; PaO_2, partial pressure of arterial oxygen; PEEP, positive end-expiratory pressure.

These patients should be managed in a specialist centre with experience in pulmonary hypertension. The perioperative mortality is three times that of other congenital cardiac diseases [38] and has been reported as between 2 per cent and 7 per cent at two specialist centres [39,40]. Serious complications occur in up to 42 per cent of patients undergoing non-cardiac surgery [40]. Pulmonary hypertension was recently reclassified [41] as shown in Table 30.14.

Idiopathic pulmonary hypertension has shown improved survival in recent years owing to advances in drug treatment. In 1991 median survival from diagnosis was 2.8 years with 1-, 3- and 5-year survival rates at 68 per cent, 48 per cent and 34 per cent, respectively [42]. The 3-year survival rate is now almost 100 per cent.

Significant factors in anaesthetic assessment

Assessment includes history, examination and investigations which should include ECG, CXR and echocardiography. In the presence of pulmonary hypertension an estimate of pulmonary arterial pressure can be made on echo using the measured maximum velocity of tricuspid regurgitation and the modified Bernoulli equation (pressure = $4V_{max}^2$). Assessment may also include data from cardiac catheterisation such as pulmonary vascular resistance, direct pulmonary artery pressure and reversibility in oxygen and with NO.

A paper examining 30-day morbidity and mortality in adult pulmonary hypertension patients undergoing non-cardiac surgery found a 42 per cent morbidity rate and a 7 per cent incidence of death. Factors independently associated with morbidity included NYHA class 2 or higher

symptoms, a history of pulmonary embolic disease, high-risk surgery and a duration of anaesthesia greater than 3 hours. Right axis deviation and right-ventricular hypertrophy on the ECG and a ratio of right-ventricular to systemic pressure of greater than 0.66 correlated with mortality in these patients [40]. In a paper investigating children undergoing cardiac catheterisation, major morbidity occurred in 6 per cent of children and death in 2 per cent. Variables strongly linked to these outcomes included a history of idiopathic aetiology, symptoms of syncope and dizziness and a tricuspid regurgitant jet of >4 m/s on echocardiography [39].

Factors affecting pulmonary vascular resistance (Table 30.15)

Healthy volunteers show no response to inhaled nitric oxide, confirming that the pulmonary vasculature has no resting vasoconstrictor tone. In physiology the pulmonary vascular resistance (PVR) can be modified by a number of factors:

- acidosis
- lung volumes
- hypoxia
- nitric oxide
- endothelins.

Acidosis and hypercapnia are potent stimulators of increased PVR; acidosis acts independently of CO_2

Hypoxia also stimulates vasoconstriction (hypoxic pulmonary vasoconstriction). Both mechanisms are protective and aim to prevent ventilation–perfusion mismatching in physiologically challenging conditions. Pulmonary vascular resistance varies with lung volumes and is at its lowest at functional residual capacity (FRC) and decreases at either extreme of volume. Pulmonary vascular resistance is controlled *in vivo* by nitric oxide (NO) via cyclic GMP.

Endothelins are endogenous substances that also produce vasomotor changes in the lung.

Medical treatment of pulmonary hypertension [42]

Drug treatment has advanced over recent years and is based on vasodilator therapy in responsive patients. Inhaled nitric oxide is used as an acute therapy and aids in assessing an individual patient's likely response to treatment. Chronic therapy includes intravenous prostacyclin administered through long-term central access or by subcutaneous analogues, oral drugs such as sildenafil (a phosphodiesterase V inhibitor that prolongs the action of cyclic GMP) and bosentan, an endothelin antagonist. In advanced cases, atrial septostomy is performed to allow right-to-left shunting and prevent acute right-ventricular failure.

Impact of anaesthesia on PVR

General anaesthesia affects PVR directly through a number of mechanisms including drugs, positioning, ventilation and blood gases, and indirectly by altering SVR and ventricular function. In addition the pulmonary ventricle can be directly impaired by general anaesthetic agents. Patients with pulmonary hypertension should be anaesthetised in specialist centres wherever possible, with invasive monitoring and intensive care support available.

THE PARALLEL CIRCULATION (Table 30.16)

A parallel circulation is one in which both the pulmonary and the systemic circulations are supplied by the same ventricle. Therefore, the circulations exist in parallel rather than in series as in the normal heart. Examples of parallel circulations include systemic-to-pulmonary shunts such as BT shunts, the hypoplastic left heart, double-outlet right ventricle, tricuspid atresia, complete AVSD and pulmonary atresia.

Regardless of the aetiology of the cardiac defect, in a parallel circulation blood flow to the lungs or the systemic circulation is dependent on the cardiac output from the pumping ventricle and the magnitude of the pulmonary and systemic vascular resistances. Preload is from both systemic and pulmonary venous drainage as the atria are usually connected by an ASD, a patent foramen ovale or a surgically created connection. A parallel circulation is inherently

Table 30.16 Goals of anaesthesia in the parallel circulation (transfer to specialist centre if possible)

Assessment	Check recent echo
	Ascertain usual SpO_2
Considerations	Antibiotic prophylaxis
	Avoid air bubbles
Anaesthesia	Use IPPV (neuromuscular blockade will increase SaO_2 with same $\dot{Q}p/\dot{Q}s$)
	Place monitors on opposite limb to shunt
	Maintain preload
	Aim for $\dot{Q}p = \dot{Q}s$ (SaO_2 in the 70s to 80s) by manipulating SVR and PVR
	If high SpO_2, ↑ lactate – ↑ PVR (reduce FiO_2 and minute ventilation)
	If low SpO_2, ↑ lactate – increase FiO_2 and minute ventilation and consider vasoconstrictors
	If low SpO_2 and normal lactate – cautious increase in FiO_2

FiO_2, inspired oxygen concentration; PVR, pulmonary vascular resistance; SaO_2, arterial oxygen saturation; SpO_2, peripheral oxygen saturation; SVR, systemic vascular resistance.

inefficient as volume overload and recirculation of blood occur. This leads to ventricular dysfunction. Pulmonary blood flow can exceed systemic blood flow ($\dot{Q}_p > \dot{Q}_s$), leading to poor tissue perfusion and increased myocardial work for a given $\dot{Q}_s$. Lactate is the best maker of tissue perfusion. The situation is compounded when the pumping ventricle is originally of right-ventricular origin, as in the hypoplastic left heart syndrome, because this ventricle adapts less well to the systemic vasculature. Any valvar stenosis or regurgitation, outflow tract obstruction or arrhythmias are poorly tolerated. Excessive pulmonary blood flow can cause 'steal' from the coronary arteries, which further impairs ventricular function.

Systemic–to–pulmonary shunts

These are surgically placed shunts used to provide pulmonary blood flow or to augment it where inadequate. The most common shunt is the BT shunt which joins the subclavian artery to the pulmonary artery on one, or both, sides. Occasionally, a central shunt is formed from the aorta to the central pulmonary artery. Excessive pulmonary blood flow leading to pulmonary vascular occlusive disease is a risk, especially from a central shunt. Conversely, an inadequately sized shunt or one that becomes blocked or kinked can severely restrict pulmonary blood flow.

Blalock–Taussig shunts were first described in 1944 [43] for the treatment of blue babies with tetralogy of Fallot. Initially the subclavian artery was anastomosed directly to the pulmonary artery but the technique was modified as this compromised the arterial supply to the upper limb. The modified technique uses an interposed synthetic tube graft.

Anaesthesia in a child with a BT or central shunt must proceed cautiously. Flow through the shunt is dependent on shunt width and length, which is not controllable, and on the pulmonary and systemic vascular resistances, which can be manipulated. Myocardial depression is a side-effect of anaesthetic drugs as previously discussed and maintenance of systemic blood pressure is essential. If shunt flow is precarious, allowing the SVR to fall can prove disastrous whereas a low SVR will help limit excessive pulmonary blood flow. Pulmonary vascular resistance is more sensitive to changes in inspired oxygen, hypercarpnia and acidosis than SVR. In addition, children who are shunt dependent may be taking aspirin or other anticoagulants. If dehydrated the shunt may thrombose. Blood pressure and saturation monitoring are more reliably measured from a different limb to the shunt.

Hypoplastic left heart syndrome (see Figure 40.4, Chapter 40)

In hypoplastic left heart syndrome (HLHS) the mitral valve, aortic apparatus and/or left ventricle are underdeveloped or atretic. Repair is attempted by a three-stage procedure eventually resulting in a Fontan circulation based on the right ventricle.

Non-cardiac surgery would be extremely unusual in a neonate pre-stage 1 (Norwood) and very high risk up to the time of the third stage of surgery. Although the principles are as for other parallel circulations, the presence of a right-sided pumping ventricle increases risk and any anaesthesia would be best carried out at a specialist centre.

THE UNIVENTRICULAR HEART AND THE FONTAN CIRCULATION

The normal heart has a pulmonary (right) ventricle and a systemic (left) ventricle operating 'in series'. In univentricular hearts there is only one anatomical or functional ventricle either as a result of a congenital anomaly or as a result of surgery that restores an in-series circulation – the single ventricle supplies the systemic circulation and pulmonary blood flow is supplied by systemic venous return. The total cavopulmonary circulation (TCPC) is the common palliative surgical pathway for a number of congenital 'univentricular' cardiac anomalies (Table 30.17), although it was first described for the management of tricuspid atresia. It is often, but not always, reached through a series of stages including BT shunts and the Glenn (bidirectional cavopulmonary anastomosis). The single ventricle can be from left (e.g. pulmonary atresia) or right (e.g. hypoplastic left heart syndrome) origin.

A successful Fontan circulation demands good ventricular function, unobstructed ventricular inflow, absent atrioventricular valve regurgitation, unobstructed outflow, good-sized unobstructed pulmonary arteries, low or normal

Table 30.17 Cardiac malformations suitable for Fontan-type repair

Hypoplastic left heart
Tricuspid atresia
Pulmonary atresia with intact ventricular septum
Double-inlet left ventricle
Double-inlet right ventricle
Severe complete unbalanced AVSD

AVSD, atrioventricular canal defect.

PVR, unobstructed pulmonary venous drainage and a low transpulmonary gradient. Consequently, it is not possible to construct a Fontan circuit in the neonate who will have a persistently elevated PVR and small vessels. Staged palliative procedures are often required to ensure optimal conditions for a Fontan circulation later on. The infant will be cyanosed during this time. The staged approach to a Fontan circulation has shown reduced operative morbidity and mortality. After the neonatal period (with any required palliative surgery), usually at 4–12 months of age, a bidirectional cavopulmonary connection is made (Glenn shunt) (see Chapter 40, Fig. 40.6) where the superior vena cava is anastomosed to the proximal pulmonary arteries. At this stage the infant will remain cyanosed because of right-to-left shunting of IVC (inferior venacava) blood to the aorta. At 1–5 years of age the TCPC is completed by anastomosis of the IVC to the pulmonary circulation. The original Fontan operation directly connected the right atrium to the pulmonary artery, but now the IVC is connected using a lateral tunnel in the atrial wall or an extracardiac conduit, depending on the age. Sometimes a fenestration is left in the atrial wall between the tunnel or conduit and the atrium to allow some right-to-left shunt. As ventricular preload and therefore cardiac output is dependent on pulmonary venous return, a fenestration protects the cardiac output if pulmonary perfusion should fall by allowing desaturated blood to enter the atrium and maintain preload at the expense of cyanosis. This fenestration may be closed at a later date.

COMPLICATIONS OF A FONTAN CIRCULATION

When facing a child with a Fontan circulation presenting for non-cardiac surgery, consideration should be made of any existing complications. These relate to chronically elevated systemic venous pressure and low cardiac output and include arrhythmias (10–40 per cent), ventricular dysfunction, thromboembolic disease (3–20 per cent) [45], protein-losing enteropathy (13 per cent) [46], ascites and peripheral oedema, and reduced exercise tolerance. In addition, chronic cyanosis may be present if a fenestrated circuit exists. Most patients with a Fontan circulation are able to lead a normal life and 90 per cent are in NYHA functional class 1 or 2. However, the procedure is palliative and reduction in function occurs with time.

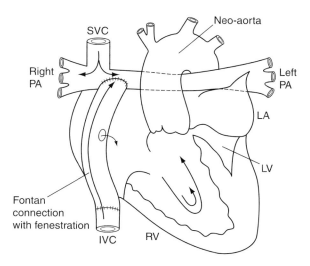

Figure 30.2 'Fontan' circulation. The pulmonary blood flow is provided by direct connection of the great veins to the pulmonary artery. IVC, inferior vena cava; LA, left atrium; LV, left ventricle; PA, pulmonary artery; RV, right ventricle; SVC, superior vena cava.

Table 30.18 Goals of anaesthesia in the Fontan circulation

Assessment	Check recent echo
	Assess venous pressures – JVP and liver size
	Check for fenestration:
	If fenestrated, what is usual SpO$_2$?
Considerations	Avoid prolonged fasting and dehydration
	Antibiotic prophylaxis
	Avoid air bubbles, particularly if fenestrated
	Consider postoperative HDU or ICU
Anaesthesia	Minimise SVR and PVR
	Maintain circulating volume
	Maintain sinus rhythm
	Use spontaneous ventilation if possible but gentle IPPV is better than respiratory compromise
	If IPPV used, minimise intrathoracic pressure:
	Minimise PIP
	Low or no PEEP but avoid atelectasis
	Short inspiratory times
	Rapid return to spontaneous ventilation

HDU, high-dependency unit; ICU, intensive care unit; IPPV, intermittent positive pressure ventilation; JVP, jugular venous pressure; PEEP, positive end-expiratory pressure; PIP, peak inspiratory pressure; PVR, pulmonary vascular resistance; SpO$_2$, peripheral oxygen saturation; SVR, systemic vascular resistance.

Ventricular dysfunction is multifactorial. It can be secondary to the original anomaly, result from previous surgical damage or be a consequence of the Fontan circulation itself. In the early staged repair the ventricle is volume overloaded and becomes spherical, dilated and hypertrophied. When the final stage offloads the ventricle some of these changes regress. It is hoped that earlier completion helps to normalise the ventricle. In addition, the overloaded ventricle becomes significantly underloaded at the time of the Fontan operation and reduced preload can lead to systolic and diastolic dysfunction. Furthermore, ventricular dysfunction post-Fontan does not respond to the usual pharmacological treatments as it is the reduced preload that is the most limiting factor. Patients with a Fontan circulation are predisposed to atrial arrhythmias, especially older circuits or the lateral tunnel that incorporates some of the atrial wall. This is increased where the PVR and transpulmonary gradient are high. The incidence of arrhythmias is 40 per cent after 10 years [44]. The safest treatment of an acute arrhythmia is DC cardioversion as antiarrhythmic drugs can significantly alter pulmonary and systemic vascular resistances and reduce cardiac output further. The patient should be anticoagulated. Symptomatic bradycardia occurs in 13–16 per cent of patients due to sinus node dysfunction [47].

Protein-losing eneteropathy is a severe disorder characterised by pleural effusions, ascites, oedema and chronic diarrhoea. It can lead to an acquired immunodeficiency and loss of coagulation factors. The aetiology is not fully understood and treatment includes diuretics, dietary modification, low-molecular-weight heparin and steroids. The only cure is heart transplantation and the 10-year mortality exceeds 50 per cent [46].

ANAESTHESIA AND THE FONTAN CIRCULATION (Table 30.18)

As survival from congenital heart disease improves an increasing number of children and adults with 'Fontan' physiology may present for anaesthesia for unrelated procedures, often outside a specialist centre. There are case reports from adults and children [48,49]. Safe anaesthesia depends on maintaining pulmonary blood flow which is passive and depends on the transpulmonary gradient (central venous pressure [CVP] − left atrial pressure [LAP]) and the PVR. Many aspects of general anaesthesia can disturb this, including preoperative fasting, IPPV, blood gas abnormalities, administered drugs, positioning and surgical technique. Children with Glenn physiology and some fenestrated Fontan circuits may be chronically cyanosed and polycythaemic. In addition, pulmonary blood flow will be sluggish in a dehydrated child. For these reasons long periods of fasting or dehydration must be avoided.

Positive pressure ventilation has been shown to reduce pulmonary blood flow [50], or even to reverse it. In short procedures spontaneous ventilation may be preferable; however, during longer cases, spontaneous ventilation, especially through long and narrow high-resistance breathing circuits, may lead to atelectasis and increased work of breathing and consequently may increase PVR and reduce pulmonary blood flow. Careful IPPV should therefore be used in these situations. Some surgical positions or techniques (e.g. prone position, laparoscopic procedures) [48] put additional stress on pulmonary blood flow and venous return. If a child presents for surgery with a Glenn anastomosis the goals are very similar to that of a Fontan. The child will remain desaturated, however, owing to intracardiac shunting of IVC blood. Intrapulmonary arteriovenous malformations have been reported in these children due to exclusion of the hepatic venous blood from the pulmonary circulation [51].

REFERENCES

Key references

Baum VC, Barton DM, Gutgesell HP. Influence of congenital heart disease on mortality after noncardiac surgery in hospitalized children. *Pediatrics* 2000; **105**(2): 332–5.

Gould FK, Elliott TS, Foweraker J *et al*. Guidelines for the prevention of endocarditis. A report of the working party of the British Society for Antimicrobial Chemotherapy. *J Antimicrob Chemother* 2006; **57**(6): 1035–42.

Laird TH, Stayer SA, Riveres SM *et al*. Pulmonary-to-systemic blood flow ratio effects of sevoflurane, isoflurane, halothane and fentanyl/midazolam with 100 per cent oxygen in children with congenital heart disease. *Anesth Analg* 2002; **95**(5): 1200–6.

Penny DJ, Redington AN. Doppler echocardiographic evaluation of pulmonary blood flow after the Fontan operation: the role of the lungs. *Br Heart J* 1991; **66**(5): 372–4.

References

1. Peterson S, Peto V, Rayner M *et al*. *Congenital heart disease statistics. British Heart Foundation Statistics Database.* London: British Heart Foundation, 2003.

2. Lovell AT. Anaesthetic implications of grown-up congenital heart disease. *Br J Anaesth* 2004; **93**: 129–39 .

3. Landzberg MJ, Murphy DJ Jr, Davidson WR Jr *et al*. Task force 4: organization of delivery systems for adults with congenital heart disease. *J Am Coll Cardiol* 2001; **37**: 1187–93.

4. Baum VC, Barton DM, Gutgesell HP. Influence of congenital heart disease on mortality after noncardiac surgery in hospitalized children. *Pediatrics* 2000; **105**(2): 332–5.

5. Warner MA, Lunn RJ, O'Leary PW, Schroeder DR. Outcomes of noncardiac surgical procedures in children and adults with congenital heart disease. Mayo Postoperative Outcomes Group. *Mayo Clin Proc* 1998; **73**(8): 728–34.

6. Lake C, Booker P. *Pediatric cardiac anesthesia*, 4th edn. London: Lippincott, Williams & Wilkins, 2005.

7. Brouard J, Morin M, Borel B *et al*. DiGeorge's syndrome complicated by graft versus host reaction. *Arch Fr Pediatr* 1985; **42**(10): 853–5.

8. Association of Anaesthetists of Great Britain and Ireland. *Recommendations for standards of monitoring of anaesthesia and recovery*, 3rd edn. London: AAGBI, 2000.

9. Rautakorpi P, Manner T, Kanto J, Lertola K. Metabolic and clinical responses to different types of premedication in children. *Paediatr Anaesth* 1999; **9**(5): 387–92.

10. Nakatani S, Mitsutake K, Hozumi T *et al*. Current characteristics of infective endocarditis in Japan – an analysis of 848 cases in 2000 and 2001. *Circ J* 2003; **67**: 901–5.

11. Gould FK, Elliott TS, Foweraker J *et al*. Guidelines for the prevention of endocarditis. A report of the working party of the British Society for Antimicrobial Chemotherapy. *J Antimicrob Chemother* 2006 June; **57**(6): 1035–42.

12. Roberts GJ, Holzel H, Sury MRJ *et al*. Dental bacteraemia in children. *Pediatr Cardiol* 1997; **18**; 24–7.

13. Sasada M, Smith S. *Drugs in anaesthesia and intensive care*, 2nd edn. Oxford: Oxford University Press, 1997.

14. Laird TH, Stayer SA, Rivenes SM *et al*. Pulmonary-to-systemic blood flow ratio effects of sevoflurane, isoflurane, halothane and fentanyl/midazolam with 100 per cent oxygen in children with congenital heart disease. *Anesth Analg* 2002; **95**(5): 1200–6.

15. Oklu E, Bulutcu FS, Yalcin Y *et al*. Which anaesthetic agent alters the haemodynamic status during pediatric catheterization? Comparison of propofol versus ketamine. *J Cardiothorac Vasc Anesth* 2003; **17**(6): 686–90.

16. Mann D, Ouj Z, Mehta V. Congenital heart diseases with left-to-right shunts. *Int Anesth Clin* 2004; **42**(4): 45–58.

17. Helbing WA, Niezen RA, Le Cessie S *et al*. Right ventricular diastolic function in children with pulmonary regurgitation after repair of tetralogy of Fallot: volumetric evaluation by magnetic resonance velocity mapping. *J Am Coll Cardiol* 1996; **28**(7): 1827–35.

18. Gatzoulis MA, Clark AL, Cullen S *et al*. Right ventricular diastolic function 15–35 years after repair of tetralogy of Fallot. Restrictive physiology predicts superior exercise performance. *Circulation* 1995; **91**(6): 1775–81.

19. Eroglu AG, Sarioglu A, Sarioglu T. Right ventricular diastolic function after repair of tetralogy of Fallot: its relationship to the insertion of a 'transannular' patch. *Cardiol Young* 1999; **9**(4): 384–91.

20. Chaturvedi RR, Kilner PJ, White PA *et al*. Increased airway pressure and simulated branch pulmonary artery stenosis increase pulmonary regurgitation after repair of tetralogy of Fallot. Real-time analysis with a conductance catheter technique. *Circulation* 1997; **95**(3): 643–9.

21. Kondo C, Nakazawa M, Kusakabe K *et al*. Left ventricular dysfunction on exercise long-term after total repair of tetralogy of Fallot. *Circulation* 1995; **92**(9 suppl II): 250–5.

22. Gatzoulis MA, Balaji S, Webber SA *et al*. Risk factors for arrhythmia and sudden cardiac death late after repair of tetralogy of Fallot: a multicentre study. *Lancet* 2000; **356**(9234): 975–81.

23. Ghai A, Silversides C, Harris *et al*. Left ventricular dysfunction is a risk factor for sudden cardiac death in adults late after repair of tetralogy of Fallot. *J Am Coll Cardiol* 2002; **40**(9): 1675–80.

24. Housmans PR, Murat I. Comparative effects of halothane, enflurane and isoflurane at equipotent anesthetic concentrations on isolated ventricular myocardium of the ferret. *Anesthesiology* 1988; **69**(4): 451–63.

25. Qu J. Congenital heart diseases with right-to-left shunts. *Int Anesth Clin* 2004; **42**(4): 59–72.

26. Hutter PA, Kreb DL, Mantel SF *et al.* Twenty-five years' experience with the arterial switch operation. *J Thorac Cardiovasc Surg* 2002; **124**(4): 790–7.

27. Hui L, Chau AK, Fang CH *et al.* Assessment of left ventricular function long term after arterial switch operation for transposition of the great arteries by dobutamine stress echocardiography. *Heart* 2005; **91**(1): 68–72.

28. Bernstein AD, Camm AJ, Fletcher RD. The NASPE/BPEG Generic Pacemaker Code for anti-bradycardia and adaptive-rate and anti-tachyarrhythmia devices. *PACE* 1987; **10**: 794–9.

29. Salukhe TV, Dob D, Sutton R *et al.* Pacemakers and defibrillators: anaesthetic implications. *Br J Anaesth* 2004; **93**: 95–104.

30. Waltz DA, Boucek MM, Edwards LB *et al.* Registry of the International Society for Heart and Lung Transplantation: ninth official pediatric lung and heart-lung transplantation report – 2006. *J Heart Lung Transpl* 2006; **25**(8): 904–11.

31. Mason L, Applegate R, Thompson T. Anesthesia for non-cardiac surgery in pediatric patients following cardiac transplantation. *Semin Cardiothorac Vasc Anesth* 2001; **5**: 62–66.

32. Cannom D, Graham AF, Harrison DC. Electrophysiological studies in the denervated transplanted human heart. Response to atrial pacing and atropine. *Circ Res* 1973; **32**: 268–78.

33. Stein KL, Darby JM, Grenvik A. Intensive care of the cardiac transplant recipient. *J Cardiothorac Anesth* 1988; **2**: 543–553.

34. Murphy DA, Thompson GW, Ardell JL *et al.* The heart reinnervates after transplantation. *Ann Thorac Surg* 2000; **69**(6): 1769–81.

35. Hathout E, Beeson WL, Kuhn M *et al.* Cardiac allograft vasculopathy in pediatric heart transplant recipients. *Transpl Int* 2006; **19**(3): 184–9.

36. Mulla NF, Johnston JK, Vander Dussen L *et al.* Late rejection is a predictor of transplant coronary artery disease in children. *J Am Coll Cardiol* 2001; **37**: 243–50.

37. Kertesz NJ, Towbin JA, Clunie S *et al.* Long-term follow-up of arrhythmias in pediatric orthotopic heart transplant recipients: incidence and correlation with rejection. *J Heart Lung Transpl* 2002; **22**: 889–93.

38. Warner MA, Lunn RJ, O'Leary PW, Schroeder DR. Outcomes of non-cardiac surgical procedures in children and adults with congenital heart disease. *Mayo Clin Proc* 1998; **73**: 728–34.

39. Taylor C, Derrick G, Haworth S, Sury M. Risk of cardiac catheterisation under anaesthesia in children with pulmonary hypertension. *Br J Anaesth* 2007; **98**(5): 657–61.

40. Ramakrishna G, Sprung J, Raui BS *et al.* Impact of pulmonary hypertension on the outcomes of noncardiac surgery. *J Am Coll Cardiol* 2005; **45**: 1691–9.

41. Simonneau G, Galie N, Rubin LJ *et al.* Clinical classification of pulmonary hypertension. *J Am Coll Cardiol* 2004; **43**: 5–12.

42. Humbert M, Sitbon O, Simonneau G. Treatment of pulmonary hypertension. *N Engl J Med* 2004; **351**(14): 1425–37.

43. Blalock A, Taussig H. The surgical treatment of malformations of the heart in which there is pulmonary stenosis or pulmonary atresia. *JAMA* 1945; **128**: 189–202.

44. Gewillig M. The Fontan circulation. *Heart* 2005; **91**: 839–46.

45. Kaulitz R, Ziemer G, Rauch R. *et al.* Prophylaxis of thromboembolic complications after the Fontan operation. *J Thorac Cardiovasc Surg* 2005; **129**: 569–75.

46. Kim SJ, Park IS, Song JU *et al.* Reversal of protein-losing enteropathy with calcium replacement in a patient after the Fontan operation. *Ann Thorac Surg* 2004; **77**: 1456–7.

47. Dilawar M, Bradley SM, Saul JP *et al.* Sinus node dysfunction after intra-atrial lateral tunnel and extracardiac conduit Fontan procedures. *Pediatr Cardiol* 2003; **24**: 284–8.

48. Taylor K, Holtby H, Macpherson B. Laparoscopic surgery in the pediatric patient post Fontan procedure. *Paediatr Anasth* 2006; **16**: 591–95.

49. Cohen AM, Mulvein J. Obstetric anaesthetic management in a patient with the Fontan circulation. *Br J Anaesth* 1994; **73**: 252–5.

50. Penny DJ, Redington AN. Doppler echocardiographic evaluation of pulmonary blood flow after the Fontan operation: the role of the lungs. *Br Heart J* 1991; **66**(5): 372–4.

51. Ashrafian H, Swan L. The mechanisms of formation of pulmonary arteriovenous malformations associated with the classic Glenn shunt. *Heart* 2002; **88**(6): 639.

52. May L Eliot. *Paediatric heart Surgery: a ready reference for professionals*, 3rd edn. Milwaukee, TN: Maxishane, 2005.

Difficult ventilation

DUNCAN MACRAE, ROBERT BINGHAM, ADRIAN R LLOYD-THOMAS, MICHAEL RJ SURY

KEY LEARNING POINTS

- Pulmonary damage must be avoided by limiting pressure and volume – permissive hypercapnia is preferable in some circumstances.
- Expiratory phase should be monitored in bronchospasm to prevent gas trapping.
- Positive end-expiratory pressure (PEEP) is useful for alveolar recruitment, and can be adjusted to optimise compliance.

- High-frequency oscillation and extracorporeal membrane oxygenation (ECMO) can be life saving.
- Preoperative assessment may predict long-term ventilation problems.
- Tension pneumothorax must be treated promptly to achieve a good outcome.

INTRODUCTION

Pulmonary ventilation can occasionally and unexpectedly become difficult during anaesthesia. Children with chronic disease may have contributory problems that can be detected and assessed beforehand. There are also conditions that prevent effective breathing afterwards. This chapter discusses the mechanisms of difficult or problematic ventilation together with the common causative diseases, important pharmacological treatment and mechanical support. The management of specific and important problems are covered and the reader will find several links with related subjects such as the respiratory system (Chapter 2) and thoracic surgery (Chapter 39). Further information can be found in texts and reviews of intensive care [1,2]. Rather than a review of the intensive care of pulmonary disease this chapter brings together information that an anaesthetist must understand in order to manage a ventilation problem successfully before, during or after anaesthesia.

GENERAL CONSIDERATIONS

Compliance

Low compliance (low tidal volume per unit of inflation pressure) may be caused by both pulmonary disease and compression of the lungs from the chest wall or by abdominal distension. Such a situation is common in intensive care patients who may require abdominal surgery. Usually a combination of high inflation pressure, positive end-expiratory pressure (PEEP) and high inspired oxygen concentrations improves oxygen saturations and controls carbon dioxide tension. This is especially important and its value is discussed in Chapters 2 and 20. Occasionally, however, these measures are insufficient and more advanced techniques are necessary. The major benefit of PEEP is to recruit (open and expand) airways and alveoli so that compliance is maximised [3] but it is important to appreciate that damage can be caused by over-distension of alveoli by either excessive pressure (barotrauma) or excessive volume (volutrauma) and that reducing this damage by accepting hypercapnia, and rarely hypoxia, may be less harmful. Useful pressure and volume limits are suggested in Table 31.1.

Advanced techniques involve, in the main, increasing the respiratory rate, decreasing tidal volume and applying PEEP [1]. Decreasing expired time prevents full expiration and causes dynamic hyperinflation (auto-PEEP) (see Chapter 2). Increasing inspired time may reduce peak inspired pressures yet encourage recruitment. Such measures are designed both to optimise oxygenation and to protect the lungs from iatrogenic damage [4]. Other therapy may be able to resolve the lung pathology and improve gas exchange. For example, surfactant improves the outcome of respiratory distress of prematurity, diuretics reduce pulmonary oedema and antibiotics are crucial in the treatment of bacterial pneumonia.

Faced with a compliance problem, attention to detail is important. First the tracheal tube should have little if any leak, and this is a scenario in which a cuffed tube may be particularly useful. The tracheal tube should be checked to ensure that it is sited in the mid-trachea and not abutted against the tracheal wall or the carina or within a main bronchus. If necessary fibre-optic bronchoscopy should be considered and this will also check that all bronchi are unobstructed. Secretions, especially blood, must be removed by suctioning. A chest X-ray should help assess the problem and may determine its cause. Air, fluid or blood within the pleural space will reduce compliance and may need to be drained promptly. If abdominal distension is contributing a gastric tube may help to decompress it but other specific measures may be necessary (e.g. a laparotomy).

Collapsed and consolidated lung tissue may continue to be perfused and cause intrapulmonary shunting (ventilation–perfusion mismatch). The effect of such shunting can be minimised by increasing cardiac output because this will improve oxygen transport to the tissues and increase mixed venous oxygenation. Consequently, poor venous return should be considered as a contributing factor in persistent hypoxia, and intravenous volume loading, inotrope infusion and relieving intra-abdominal pressure may all be helpful.

Single lung ventilation, used for some thoracic procedures, is a situation of intentional reduction in pulmonary compliance and is discussed in Chapter 39.

Airway resistance

BRONCHOSPASM

Two situations are discussed: the management of a child with acute asthma who requires emergency anaesthesia, and the more common situation of a child who has unexpected bronchospasm during anaesthesia.

Bronchospasm, caused by asthma, should, if possible, be treated before any anaesthetic intervention. Inhaled or intravenous β-adrenergic stimulants and corticosteroids are the first line of management (Table 31.2). The severity of bronchospasm is assessed by a combination of simple behavioural observations and measurement of blood oxygen and carbon dioxide tensions. Measurement of expiratory flow may be possible in cooperative children. Non-invasive pulse oximetry and capnography (microstream technology) are extremely useful. Capnography assesses bronchospasm both by the degree of end-tidal slope and as a trend monitor of end-tidal carbon dioxide. If anaesthesia is necessary, such as for uncontrolled bleeding, ketamine may be the ideal hypnotic drug and, in almost all cases, tracheal intubation is advised using either suxamethonium for rapid paralysis or pancuronium because, of all the muscle relaxants, it may cause the least histamine release. After tracheal intubation, volatile anaesthetic agents may be successful in reducing bronchospasm because of their smooth-muscle relaxant effects. Care must be taken to not over-ventilate and not to reduce carbon dioxide levels too quickly because this is associated with hypotension.

Sudden bronchospasm during surgery can be triggered in asthmatic children by the mechanical stimulation of the carina. The tracheal tube position should be checked. In otherwise normal children, bronchospasm can also be caused by anaphylaxis or by aspiration of gastric contents. The management of anaphylaxis is covered in detail in Chapter 29.

Aspiration should be managed by suction of the airways to remove all inhaled debris either by simple 'blind' suctioning or, if solid matter is involved and difficult to remove, by using bronchoscopic methods appropriately. If the patient is breathing spontaneously it may be better, if the planned procedure is not urgent, to stop the anaesthetic and to allow prompt recovery so that the child can cough

Table 31.1 Limits of ventilation pressures, volumes and times to prevent pulmonary damage during the management of low pulmonary compliance

	Working maximum	Trigger for further management
Inspiratory pressure	30 cmH$_2$O	MAP > 16 cmH$_2$O, FiO$_2$ > 0.6 consider high-frequency oscillation
PEEP	Depends on clinical scenario typically start at 8 cmH$_2$O in low compliance	MAP > 16 cmH$_2$O, FiO$_2$ > 0.6 consider high-frequency oscillation
Tidal volume	*6 mL/kg	If severe respiratory acidosis (pH < 7.25) consider reducing expired time to cause dynamic hyperinflation

FiO$_2$, inspired oxygen concentration; MAP, mean airway pressure; PEEP, positive end-expiratory pressure.
*6 mL/kg is appropriate for acute lung injury and the acute respiratory distress syndrome but normal lungs can tolerate 10 mL/kg [9].

Table 31.2 Drug treatment of asthma

Drug	Method of delivery	Dose	Frequency
Salbutamol	Nebuliser	<2 years: 2.5 mg	20–30 minutes
		>2 years: 2.5–5 mg	20–30 minutes
Salbutamol	Intravenous	>1 month <2 years: 5 μg/kg	1 dose
	>2 years: 15 μg/kg	1 dose	
	(max. 250 μg)		
Ipratropium	Nebuliser	<2 years:125–250 μg	20–30 minutes
	>2 years: 250 μg	20–30 minutes	
Aminophylline	Intravenous	>1 month: 5 mg/kg	Over 20 minutes
Hydrocortisone	Intravenous	1 month–1 year: 25 mg	× 3 daily
	1–6 years: 50 mg	× 3 daily	
	6–12 years: 100 mg	× 3 daily	
	12–18 years: 100–500 mg	× 3 daily	
Magnesium	Intravenous	40 mg/kg (max. 2 g)	Over 20 minutes

up aspirated material. There is no evidence that steroids or antibiotics prevent pulmonary sequelae from aspiration.

Bronchodilators can be administered intravenously or by inhalation (by nebulisation during manual assisted ventilation). Salbutamol is the standard drug and, if this is not effective, ipratropium can be added. Intravenous aminophylline can also be considered in severe cases but care must be taken to avoid toxicity (some children may already have received theophylline). Volatile anaesthetic drugs and ketamine are bronchodilators and can be used if they are appropriate. In resistant cases intravenous hydrocortisone should also be administered. Although evidence of benefit is limited, magnesium may be helpful.

Positive pressure ventilation in bronchospasm is potentially problematic because of gas trapping during expiration. Consequently, expiration should be carefully monitored, by measuring inspired and expired tidal volumes, or by auscultating the chest, or by capnography, and the expiratory time should be adjusted to ensure that emptying is complete; this may necessitate toleration of hypercapnia.

GAS TRAPPING

Aside from bronchospasm, diseased bronchial walls may collapse during expiration, before their lung segments have emptied. In congenital lobar emphysema and bronchial cysts (see below and Chapter 39) gas enters during inspiration but obstruction during expiration causes gas retention that expands them further. The problem may be intractable and will then require prompt surgical excision.

There is a similar but less severe problem with tracheomalacia and bronchomalacia although in these conditions, conversely, positive pressure maintains the patency of the airways and problems during anaesthesia itself are unusual. During spontaneous breaths, however, such as after tracheal extubation, coughing may cause large swings in airway and pulmonary pressures that can provoke gas trapping and cause hypoxia; pneumothorax may occur. Oesophageal reflux can be caused by the excessive negative intrathoracic pressure of inspiration and may be responsible for provoking near-death spells that are a feature of infants and small children with this disease.

Tracheal stenosis is a dangerous condition in which the unfortunate infant is likely succumb to any respiratory provocation. Tracheal intubation may help briefly but gas trapping beyond the stenosis is a major problem. Intravenous dexamethasone and inhaled adrenaline may help temporarily. Long expiratory times may increase carbon dioxide clearance but, *in extremis*, extracorporeal membrane oxygenation (ECMO) may be required.

SECRETIONS

Children with cystic fibrosis, alveolar proteinosis and bronchopulmonary infections or abscesses may have copious or viscid secretions that can cause sudden obstruction of the airway. Blood within the airway can clot and be extremely difficult to remove by suctioning through conventional plastic catheters. Injection of warm saline into the trachea and vigorous shaking of the chest may help to dislodge inspissated secretions or clots. Obstruction of the tracheal tube is possible and if this occurs the tube must either be cleared by suction with the largest suction catheter or be removed altogether and replaced promptly.

Pulmonary blood flow

Although compromise to pulmonary blood flow is strictly a circulation problem, ventilation strategies can adversely affect pulmonary blood flow and exacerbate pulmonary disease.

SHUNTING AND $\dot{V}/\dot{Q}$ MISMATCH

A ventilation–perfusion ($\dot{V}/\dot{Q}$) mismatch (or intrapulmonary shunting) can be reduced by recruitment of alveoli or lung segments. Further, oxygenation can be improved by increasing inspired oxygen. Nitric oxide may also be used in some circumstances to optimise local blood flow to aerated alveoli (see page 479).

In pure shunting, however, whether it is intracardiac (or other extrapulmonary) or intrapulmonary, arterial oxygenation cannot be improved by the use of ventilation measures alone. Indeed, attempts to increase oxygenation may be futile and unnecessary since children with cyanotic heart disease usually have effective physiological compensation. The degree of theoretical pure shunt can be estimated non-invasively by using a series of iso-shunt graphic plots (oxyhaemoglobin saturation versus inspired oxygen pressure) and by matching the rise in oxygenation in response to an increase in inspired oxygen [5].

Whenever the pulmonary blood flow is dependent upon a systemic-to-pulmonary shunt (such as a Blalock–Taussig shunt) oxygen saturation is related to systemic blood pressure (see Chapter 30).

EXCESS (HIGH FLOW THROUGH SURGICAL SHUNTS)

When a surgical systemic to pulmonary shunt has been created, pulmonary blood flow can become excessive. If so, the lungs become 'flooded', pulmonary oedema develops, and blood is diverted away from the systemic circulation and into the pulmonary circulation. Not only is gas exchange reduced but cardiac output to the tissues may also be severely decreased and therefore compromise organ perfusion. This is common after a stage 1 Norwood repair for hypoplastic left heart and occasionally after an excessively large systemic-to-pulmonary shunt. It is crucial that it is understood that high inspired oxygen concentrations will cause pulmonary vasodilatation and thereby increase pulmonary blood flow further. Inspired oxygen should be reduced to control pulmonary blood flow and maintain adequate systemic oxygen delivery.

REDUCED (FONTAN AND PULMONARY HYPERTENSION)

In the Fontan operation (or cavopulmonary anastomosis) pulmonary blood flow is dependent upon the systemic venous pressure alone. Consequently, high pulmonary inflation pressures may reduce pulmonary blood flow and cause raised venous pressure and a significant fall in cardiac output. Nevertheless, in almost all situations requiring tracheal intubation, gentle positive pressure ventilation does not adversely affect pulmonary blood flow. Although spontaneous ventilation is better in theory, because the thoracic pump effect ought to improve pulmonary blood flow, positive pressure ventilation has the advantage of maintaining lung expansion and recruitment. In any intubated patient coughing and struggling markedly increase intrathoracic

pressure and can obstruct pulmonary blood flow. In the Fontan circulation pulmonary inflation pressures should be minimised.

Pulmonary hypertension is a potentially dangerous condition in which either the child can have constant high pulmonary artery pressures or have 'crises' in which the heart is unable to pump sufficient blood into the high-resistance pulmonary arteries. Crises are managed by high inspired oxygen concentrations, minimisation of pulmonary artery carbon dioxide tension (by hyperventilation) and maximisation of cardiac performance (see Chapter 30).

NEUROMUSCULAR DISEASE

Patients with neuromuscular disorders may experience type II respiratory failure (ventilatory failure with hypercapnia) as a result of their preoperative condition or as a consequence of the surgery and anaesthesia. Both primary neurological and myopathic pathology may be seen (Table 31.3).

Preoperative assessment requires a review of symptoms and simple exercise testing. Basic respiratory function can be tested with peak expiratory flow rate (PEFR) and forced expiratory volume in 1 second (FEV_1); both are expressed as a percentage of the predicted value from a nomogram. Parents should be made aware of the possible need for post-operative respiratory support.

General anaesthesia using short-acting agents should be supplemented, where possible, with regional anaesthesia. Neuromuscular blocking drugs are generally avoided; depolarising relaxants are contraindicated in myotonic syndromes and in those conditions associated with susceptibility to malignant hyperpyrexia (definitely in central core disease and nemaline myopathy, and possibly in Duchenne muscular dystrophy). Where non-depolarising relaxants are needed, transcutaneous neuro-muscular monitoring should be used to titrate dosage and establish recovery.

Before extubation ventilatory performance should be assessed and the patient should be able to generate a negative airway pressure of at least $30\,cmH_2O$ and a tidal volume of greater than 5 mL/kg. In the event that these criteria cannot be met, admission to a paediatric intensive care unit (PICU) and respiratory support are indicated, until recovery has been achieved. Subsequent weaning may be difficult and may require support patterns of ventilation such as bi-level positive airway pressure (CPAP) (see page 479).

Myasthesia gravis

Patients with myasthenia gravis (MG) have autoimmune antibodies directed against acetylcholine receptors; it is the most common disorder to affect the neuromuscular junction (2–7 patients per 10 000 UK population). Presentation can be neonatal, owing to transfer of antibodies from the mother to the baby, and treatment may be needed for up to 3 weeks after

Table 31.3 Neuromuscular diseases that may be associated with ventilatory failure*

System	Area	Aetiology	Examples
Central	Central nervous system	Acquired	Encephalopathy
			Injury
		Congenital	Progressive ataxias
			Basal ganglia diseases
		Dementias	Progressive
	Spinal	Acquired	Infective: poliomyelitis
			Non-infective: acute myelitis
		Chronic degenerative	Ataxias
			Spinal muscular atrophies
			Amyotrophic lateral sclerosis
Peripheral	Neuropathies	Parainfectious	Guillain–Barré syndrome
			Diphtheria
	Myopathies	Myasthenia	Myasthenia gravis
			Neonatal myasthenia
		Congenital	Central core disease
			Nemaline myopathy
			X-linked myotubular myopathy
		Metabolic	Type II glycogen storage disease (Pompe's disease)
	Congenital absence of muscles		Prune-belly syndrome

*For further information the reader is directed to a standard text of paediatric medicine.

which the infant is normal. Children commonly present with ocular symptoms and signs (strabismus, diplopia and ptosis) but they may also present with weakness and fatigue after exercise. Rarely, they may have a myasthenic crisis with ventilatory failure secondary to involvement of the diaphragm and respiratory muscles. The American Myasthenia Gravis Foundation has developed a standardised international classification of severity (I–V) [6].

The neuromuscular junction is abnormal in several ways [7]. There is: (1) an increased synaptic gap size; (2) flattening of the folds in the post-synaptic membrane; and (3) an absolute reduction in the number of acetylcholine receptors. The majority of peri and post-pubertal patients (85 per cent) are seropostive for antiacetylcholine receptor antibodies (anti-AChR), whereas only 55 per cent of prepubertal patients are seropositive [8]. Antibodies to muscle specific tyrosine kerase (MuSK – a surface membrane enzyme that is essential in aggregating AChR during the development of the neuromuscular junction) have been found in seronegative patients with MG [9]. Edrophonium is used as a diagnostic test.

The mainstays of treatment are acetylcholinesterase inhibitors (pyridostigmine), corticosteroids and immunosuppressants (azathioprine). In severe cases plasmapheresis and intravenous immunoglobulin are necessary. Thymectomy is commonly recommended as 10 per cent of MG patients have thymic tumours and 80–85 per cent experience improvement in symptoms after excision, though this can

take months or years to manifest [9]. Thymectomy may not be as effective in young patients so delaying the operation until 10 years of age is recommended [8].

ANAESTHESIA FOR THYMECTOMY

Thymectomy is performed via a midline sternotomy or by thoracoscopy. Preoperative therapy including anticholinesterases should have been optimised beforehand. Unless the child has severe disease, the last dose of anticholinesterase is given the night before surgery and the operation done as the first morning case.

Neuromuscular blocking drugs have a faster onset and a longer duration of action in MG patients even if given in low doses (10–15 per cent of the standard dose is recommended) [8]. Furthermore reversal using anticholinesterases can confuse postoperative therapy. Volatile agents depress neuromuscular function and these effects are exaggerated in patients with MG. Where possible, neuromuscular blockers should be avoided and in most cases intubation using a combination of propofol and remifentanil is satisfactory. Indeed a total intravenous anaesthesia (TIVA) technique may be optimal in these patients [10] and recommended regimens for children are given in Chapter 11. If neuromuscular blockers have to be used, monitoring is essential.

High temperatures and hypokalaemia both worsen the symptoms of MG and should be avoided in the course of anaesthesia [9].

Extubation at the end of surgery or within a short period afterwards should be possible and patients should be managed in a PICU afterwards. Morphine by patient-controlled analgesia (PCA)/nurse-controlled analgesia (NCA) is used for postoperative analgesia, while thoracic extradural analgesia has been described in adults, there is no published experience in children. Non-invasive ventilation may be appropriate in some cases [11].

ADVANCED ACUTE PULMONARY SUPPORT

The following sections summarise the important support strategies available in the intensive care management of children with acute pulmonary failure. Not all of these will be applicable in the operating theatre, but the anaesthetist should understand the principles behind all of the methods below so that appropriate care can be given during surgery and, if pulmonary function should deteriorate, post-operative management can be discussed, planned and started without delay. Mehta and Arnold have recently reviewed the evidence for the interventions discussed below [12].

Conventional pulmonary ventilation

Acute hypoxic respiratory failure, such as acute respiratory distress syndrome (ARDS), is characterised by impaired oxygenation, reduced respiratory compliance and loss of functional lung volume. In comparison with standard ventilation strategies advanced conventional pulmonary ventilation minimises lung damage by using a combination of higher PEEP and lower tidal volume ventilation because these are associated with better outcomes in ARDS [13]. A large multicentre trial has demonstrated this advantage clearly in adults [14].

Non-compliant lungs should be inflated 'gently' and long inspired times may have an advantage in this respect. Nevertheless, it is PEEP that maintains alveolar expansion or 'recruitment' (PEEP levels typically of 8–12 cm H_2O) and low tidal volume ventilation (typically 6 mL/kg) is accepted and the arterial partial pressure of CO_2 ($PaCO_2$) is allowed to rise; respiratory acidosis to a pH of 7.20–7.25 is acceptable. Systemic oxygen delivery can be impaired by high PEEP, so that it may be reasonable not to strive too hard to achieve a high value for partial pressure of arterial oxygen (PaO_2), but instead to accept a mid-level PaO_2 sufficient to maintain arter-ial oxygen saturation (SaO_2) values of 90–92 per cent.

There have been reports to suggest that the prone position can reduce $\dot{V}/\dot{Q}$ mismatch but a recent randomised controlled trial (RCT) failed to demonstrate any beneficial effect on outcome [15].

If a child requires transport to the operating theatre or scanning departments, it is important to avoid multiple disconnections that cause loss of PEEP. Fortunately most modern conventional ventilators have battery power.

High–frequency ventilation

An alternative to conventional ventilation for children with severe lung disease is high-frequency oscillatory ventilation (HFOV) [16,17]. High levels of PEEP and small tidal volumes are delivered by a ventilator that applies sine wave oscillation via an oscillating diaphragm. Lung inflation and recruitment are achieved while avoiding damaging 'volu-trauma' and 'barotrauma'. Disadvantages may include the need to increase sedation or muscle relaxation in comparison with other ventilation methods because HFOV may be uncomfortable. Nevertheless, all children with severe acute respiratory failure will need to be immobile and sedated in order to reduce metabolic rate and unwanted pulmonary pressure effects of coughing or straining. Reduced venous return may cause a fall in cardiac output so that it may be necessary to expand circulating volume and to use inotropic support. There are no portable HFO ventilators and transport involves changing to conventional ventilation.

Extracorporeal membrane oxygenation

The ultimate means of respiratory support is ECMO. It is indicated when all other treatments are ineffective. By using ECMO, pulmonary ventilation can cease, or be markedly reduced, and so avoid potentially damaging high inflation pressures. The aim is to facilitate lung recovery, under optimal 'rest' conditions, and to effect adequate oxygen delivery to prevent hypoxic injury to other organs. The benefit of ECMO in supporting mature neonates with severe respiratory failure has been demonstrated by the UK Collaborative ECMO Trial Group [18]. In their series, the criteria for entry into the trial was severe respiratory failure defined as an oxygenation index (oxygenation index = (FiO_2 × mean airway pressure × 100)/PaO_2) of $\geq$ 40 and arterial $PaCO_2$ > 12 kPa for more than 3 hours; infants were more than 35 weeks' gestation at birth, weighing at least 2 kg, had less than 10 days of high-pressure ventilation and were younger than 28 days. There have been no randomised trials of ECMO in other paediatric diseases, but its use is widely believed to be successful in selected children with severe, but recoverable, respiratory failure. The Extracorporeal Life Support Organisation (ELSO) reports that overall 76 per cent of neonates and 56 per cent of children receiving 'respiratory' ECMO survive to hospital discharge.

Liquid ventilation

Liquid ventilation (LV), using oxygen-carrying perflurocarbons, remains experimental, but is an alternative method of ensuring pulmonary gas exchange that may reduce ventilator-induced lung injury [19–22]. An important practical point is that perflurocarbons are radio-opaque and clear slowly from the lung even after LV is discontinued – the appearance of chest X-rays during and after LV are therefore striking.

Special inhalational therapy

NITRIC OXIDE

Nitric oxide is a small reactive molecule that has important biological roles in the regulation of vascular tone, neurotransmitter release and leukocyte function. Nitric oxide, which is a gas at room temperature, has two important physiological effects when inhaled at low concentrations (1–20 p.p.m.). First, inhaled NO (iNO) has a direct effect on the pulmonary vascular bed and causes pulmonary vasodilatation. Second, by lowering PVR in areas of ventilated lung, and not in unventilated lung (such as atelectatic areas), iNO tends to improve the matching of ventilation to perfusion and thereby improves oxygenation. The therapeutic role for iNO has been established in neonatal respiratory failure associated with pulmonary hypertension (primary or secondary persistent pulmonary hypertension of the newborn); iNO is associated with a slightly lower need for ECMO. Although it is used widely to treat hypoxic respiratory failure, studies have shown that the early beneficial effect is not sustained and there is no change in outcome. Nevertheless, in recent consensus meetings [23,24], it has been agreed that iNO is beneficial in a variety of diseases associated with reversibly raised PVR such as in some congenital heart diseases and in right-ventricular failure following cardiac transplantation.

Occasionally, iNO may be required during anaesthesia. Delivery devices are available that ensure safe and accurate delivery, as NO and its oxidative metabolite NO_2 are potentially toxic. Anaesthetists must be aware that iNO cannot be administered if soda lime is in use and that iNO should never be discontinued abruptly because this can trigger a rebound pulmonary hypertensive crisis. If a child is receiving iNO in intensive care and they require transport, iNO should continue throughout their journey. Although iNO therapy has a small effect on platelet function, this effect is thought to be clinically unimportant and a haemostasis disorder is not a contraindication.

SURFACTANT

Artificial and natural inhaled lung surfactants are of proven benefit in the management of respiratory distress syndrome in preterm neonates. In addition, surfactant therapy may benefit some children who have ARDS and infections such as with *Pneumocystis carinii* [25]. However, a recent meta-analysis of the use of surfactant therapy in adults with ARDS and acute lung injury showed that, while surfactant improved oxygenation, it did not reduce mortality [26] perhaps because the cause of death in patients with ARDS is often multisystem failure, over which surfactant

therapy has limited impact. Further studies are required to define the role of surfactant therapy in adults and older children with respiratory failure.

LONG-TERM VENTILATION

There is an increasing number of children in the community who depend on ventilators for partial or total respiratory support. Many of these children have severe lung disease, including bronchopulmonary dysplasia, and congenital neuromuscular conditions such as spinal muscular atrophy, a mitochondrial myopathy or a muscular dystrophy [27]. Some have muscle paralysis following spinal cord damage. Rare problems include skeletal abnormalities such as asphyxiating thoracic dystrophy or severe kyphoscoliosis. Whether ventilated or not, any child with neuromuscular or other disease that potentially compromises the respiratory system must be assessed before anaesthesia. The limits of their respiratory reserve, any limitations to upper airway function and the child's ability to cough and clear airway secretions adequately are particularly important. The effect of anaesthesia is likely to be deleterious unless the secretions, which can be aspirated, are a major component of the disease. Some children may require ventilation only at night or for rest periods during the day, but usually they need to recover on their long-term ventilator and under supervision of 'long-term' ventilation team.

Non-invasive ventilation

Nasal CPAP and mask-delivered bi-level positive pressure ventilation (BiPAP) are increasingly being advocated as modes of 'step-up' or 'step-down' respiratory care with the aim of shortening the period of tracheal intubation (step-down) or preventing intubation (step-up) [28]. Although perhaps more pleasant for patients and parents, there is as yet no unequivocal evidence that non-invasive strategies are clinically beneficial.

SPECIFIC INTRAOPERATIVE PROBLEMS

Pneumothorax

Pneumothorax may occur in any patient but is more likely in children with asthma or congenital pulmonary abnormalities such as lobar emphysema or congenital cystic adenomatoid malformation (CCAM). In some otherwise normal children spontaneous pneumothorax may develop owing to lung surface blebs. Irrespective of the presence or absence of an underlying condition, pneumothorax is more likely at times of surges in intrapulmonary pressure such as may occur during anaesthesia. Particular risks are coughing against an obstructed airway and asynchrony with mechanical ventilators.

Diagnosis depends on detecting the increasing oxygen requirements and the classic signs of reduction in breath sounds over one lung field combined with a resonance to percussion. In small pneumothoraces, these signs may be subtle and a chest X-ray is required for confirmation. In the standard anteroposterior (AP) supine X-ray, usually obtained in theatre and recovery, the intrapleural air will collect anteriorly and small volume pneumothoraces may not be visible. Lateral decubitus views may be necessary. Treatment is by chest drain insertion (see Chapter 39) but this is not always necessary for small pneumothoraces in which further expansion is unlikely. The standard insertion site for chest drains is the fifth intercostal space in the mid-axillary line. The drain itself is mounted over a rigid, sharp-ened trochar and, in order to avoid damage to intrathoracic structures, it is preferable to remove this and insert the drain alone through a passage created by blunt dissection down to the pleural space. 'Pig-tail' chest drains, which are inserted by the Seldinger technique, are suitable for draining air but the small lumen is usually too small for draining blood or viscous fluid such as in empyema.

In large or continuing air leaks the intrapleural pressure may be greater than that within the alveoli, resulting in compression of lung tissue and distortion of other intra-thoracic structures – this causes a tension pneumothorax. The air may be trapped because of a flap-valve effect at the pulmonary or pleural leak site. As well as impairing venti-lation and gas exchange, tension pneumothorax usually results in a severe fall in cardiac output because of distortion of the heart and great vessels and a reduction in venous return due to raised intrathoracic pressure. The diagnosis is usually simple because, in addition to the signs listed above, there is over-expansion of the chest wall on the affected side, a hyper-resonant percussion note and shift of mediastinal structures (trachea and apex beat) to the con-tralateral side. This is a medical emergency because cardiac arrest is likely. Treatment should not be delayed to obtain a chest X-ray. The immediate management is needle thora-cotomy with a cannula inserted into the second intercostal space in the mid-clavicular line. In a spontaneously breath-ing patient this should be occluded once the initial tension has been released. It can remain *in situ* to allow intermit-tent further decompression until a definitive chest drain has been inserted. In a patient receiving IPPV the cannula can remain open to the air until the chest drain is inserted.

Bilateral tension pneumothoraces are possible, particularly following barotrauma. This can be an extremely difficult diagnosis to make because the classic lateralising signs are absent. The main features are extremely poor pulmonary compliance, cardiovascular collapse and bilaterally dimin-ished breath sounds with hyper-resonance. If there is any doubt, needle thoracocentesis should be performed imme-diately and is diagnostic. There may be leakage of air, under pressure, into the skin of the neck and face (surgical emphy-sema) and into the mediastinum to cause cardiac tamponade.

Fistulae

A bronchopleural fistula occurs when there is a communica-tion between the bronchi and the pleura, usually the result of infection such as empyema. There may be a valve-like effect at the leak site so that rises in airway pressure will trap gas in the pleural space, which will eventually result in a tension pneumothorax. With a chest drain in place, IPPV will result in gas leaking through the fistula into the pleura and thence through the drain into the outside world. If the leak is small this is easily managed by increasing the fresh gas flow rate to the circuit or ventilator to compensate for the lost gas. However, if the leak is large this strategy is inadequate and effective conventional ventilation may be impossible irre-spective of the fresh gas flow. Anaesthesia in this circum-stance can be extremely difficult as controlled ventilation is usually necessary since surgical management of bron-chopleural fistulae is either by pleurodesis, oversewing of the fistula or, in severe or recurrent cases, excision of the lobe.

For simple, short procedures, such as computed tomo-graphy (CT), spontaneous ventilation avoids the problem although it would be difficult to manage prolonged apnoea by conventional means and care should be taken with the administration of respiratory depressants. Anaesthesia involving IPPV, such as for a thoracotomy, requires careful preparation. It may be possible to manage patients with a small fistula using conventional techniques but it is too dif-ficult to predict in which patients this is safe. There are two possible alternative approaches: single lung ventilation (SLV) and alternative ventilation modes – particularly HFOV.

If an SLV technique is chosen (see Chapter 39) the aim is to maintain spontaneous ventilation until both the dis-eased lung is isolated and the ability to perform IPPV suc-cessfully has been confirmed (although temporary paralysis with suxamethonium may be acceptable). If techniques such as bronchial blockade or bronchial intubation are used, the lung with the fistula is isolated but not ventilated and there may be difficulty with oxygenation because of shunting of the pulmonary blood flow to the unventilated lung. A double-lumen tube avoids this problem as CPAP with oxygen or limited ventilation can also be provided to the side with the fistula. In children who are too small for a double-lumen tube, HFOV of both lungs via a tracheal tube may provide better oxygenation and is successful because gas exchange is achieved by augmented diffusion, rather than mass movement of gas. Surgery can be success-fully performed during HFOV as access to the lobe with the fistula can be achieved by lung retraction.

Congenital lobar emphysema and bronchogenic cysts

Gas trapping may be general as in bronchospasm or local as in congenital lobar emphysema or lung cysts. It has a deleterious effect on ventilation, gas exchange and cardiac output as venous drainage may be impaired owing to raised intrathoracic pressure; it causes a similar situation to tension pneumothorax. It is particularly relevant to anaesthesia as positive pressure ventilation has the potential to exacerbate the problem and cause acute cardiorespiratory deterioration.

In both congenital lobar emphysema and bronchogenic cysts, gas trapping is local. As its name implies, the former involves one (or occasionally more) lobe of the lung, which becomes hyperinflated because of a defect in a segment of bronchial wall. Bronchogenic lung cysts arise from the bronchial tree and there is usually an open connection. In both cases, there may be a one-way valve effect during positive pressure ventilation such that gas enters the lobe or cyst during inspiration and is trapped during expiration.

Since the treatment of both these conditions is surgical, there are obvious implications for the anaesthetist. It has been recommended that positive pressure ventilation should be avoided until the communication between the cyst or lobe and the bronchial tree has been ligated by the surgeon. However, since this can be achieved only following thoracotomy, this approach seems impractical. An alternative is to isolate the over-inflated lobe or cyst using SLV but as these conditions usually occur in neonates or small infants the possibilities are limited. Bronchial intubation with a small tracheal tube, either alone or in combination with a laryngeal mask airway (to allow ventilation of the unintubated bronchus), has been described [29]. An alternative is to place a bronchus blocker alongside a tracheal tube (3Fr Fogarty catheter or balloon-tipped angiography catheter or 5Fr paediatric bronchus blocker) under fibre-optic bronchoscope control [30].

In practice, however, there are few problems with careful and gentle positive pressure ventilation; high airway pressures (such as during coughing) must be avoided during IPPV and by ensuring neuromuscular blockade. Hypercapnia can be tolerated until the cyst or lobe is removed. Surgeons can usually gain satisfactory access to the lobe or cyst using lung retraction so that SLV techniques are seldom required.

Mediastinal mass

A large mediastinal mass, especially in the anterior mediastinum, is dangerous during anaesthesia because it can compress the trachea and bronchi (commonly at the carina) and may obstruct the pulmonary or caval veins. Management is discussed in detail in Chapter 39. Anaesthesia may lead to complete obstruction of the airway [31] while positive pressure ventilation may cause hypotension by compression of major vessels [32]. Airway symptoms and superior vena cava syndrome are both associated with the development of acute airway obstruction [33] but lack of symptoms does not ensure a safe anaesthetic [34]. Ideally, an anaesthetic technique should maintain spontaneous ventilation. The lateral or semi-prone position is

recommended – finding the optimum position may be life saving. Overcoming tracheal obstruction may be possible with a rigid bronchoscope and if this fails cardiopulmonary bypass may be the only option [32]. Postoperative airway obstruction must be anticipated because bronchial or tracheal oedema can be provoked.

REFERENCES

Key references

Macrae DJ, Field D, Mercier JC et al. Inhaled nitric oxide therapy in neonates and children: reaching a European consensus. Intensive Care Med 2004; **30**(3): 372–80.

Marraro GA. Protective lung strategies during artificial ventilation in children. Paediatr Anaesth 2005; **15**(8): 630–7.

Tobias JD, Burd RS. Anaesthetic management and high frequency oscillatory ventilation. Paediatr Anaesth 2001; **11**(4): 483–7.

UK Collaborative ECMO Trial Group. UK collaborative randomised trial of neonatal extracorporeal membrane oxygenation. Lancet 1996; **348**(9020): 75–82.

Willson DF, Thomas NJ, Markovitz BP et al. Effect of exogenous surfactant (calfactant) in pediatric acute lung injury: a randomized controlled trial. JAMA 2005; **293**(4): 470–6.

References

1. Wunsch H, Mapstone J, Takala J. High-frequency ventilation versus conventional ventilation for the treatment of acute lung injury and acute respiratory distress syndrome: a systematic review and Cochrane analysis. Anesth Analg 2005; **100**(6): 1765–72.

2. Slutsky AS, Tremblay LN. Multiple system organ failure. Is mechanical ventilation a contributing factor? Am J Respir Crit Care Med 1998; **157**(6 Pt 1): 1721–5.

3. Halbertsma FJ, van der Hoeven JG. Lung recruitment during mechanical positive pressure ventilation in the PICU: what can be learned from the literature? Anaesthesia 2005; **60**(8): 779–90.

4. Marraro GA. Protective lung strategies during artificial ventilation in children. Paediatr Anaesth 2005; **15**(8): 630–7.

5. Quine D, Wong CM, Boyle EM et al. Non-invasive measurement of reduced ventilation: perfusion ratio and shunt in infants with bronchopulmonary dysplasia: a physiological definition of the disease. Arch Dis Child Fetal Neonatal Ed 2006; **91**(6): F409–14.

6. Jaretzki A, Barohn RJ, Ernstoff RM et al. Myasthenia gravis: recommendations for clinical research standards. Task Force of the Medical Scientific Advisory Board of the Myasthenia Gravis Foundation of America. Neurology 2000; 12; **55**(1): 16–23.

7. Drachman DB. Medical progress: myasthenia gravis. N Engl J Med 1994; **330**: 1797–810.

8. White MC Stoddart PA. Anaesthesia for thymectomy in children with myasthenia gravis. Paediatr Anaesth 2004; **14**: 625–35.

9. Thanvi BR, Lo TCN. Update on myasthenia gravis. *Postgrad Med J* 2004; **80**: 690–700.

10. Lorimer M, Hall R. Remifantanil and propofol total intravenous anaesthesia for thymectomy in myasthenia gravis. *Anaesth Intensive Care* 1988; **26**: 210–12.

11. Piastra M, Conti G, Caresta E *et al.* Noninvasive ventilation options in pediatric myasthenia gravis. *Paediatr Anaesth* 2005; **15**(8): 699–702.

12. Mehta NM, Arnold JH. Mechanical ventilation in children with acute respiratory failure. *Curr Opin Crit Care* 2004; **10**(1): 7–12.

13. Amato MB, Barbas CS, Medeiros DM *et al.* Effect of a protective-ventilation strategy on mortality in the acute respiratory distress syndrome. *N Engl J Med* 1998; **338**(6): 347–54.

14. The Acute Respiratory Distress Syndrome Network. Ventilation with lower tidal volumes as compared with traditional tidal volumes for acute lung injury and the acute respiratory distress syndrome. *N Engl J Med* 2000; **342**(18): 1301–8.

15. Fineman LD, LaBrecque MA, Shih MC, Curley MA. Prone positioning can be safely performed in critically ill infants and children. *Pediatr Crit Care Med* 2006; **7**(5): 413–22.

16. Arnold JH. High frequency oscillatory ventilation: theory and practice in paediatric patients. *Paediatr Anaesth* 1996; **6**: 437–41.

17. Tobias JD, Burd RS. Anaesthetic management and high frequency oscillatory ventilation. *Paediatr Anaesth* 2001; **11**(4): 483–7.

18. UK Collaborative ECMO Trial Group. UK collaborative randomised trial of neonatal extracorporeal membrane oxygenation. *Lancet* 1996; **348**(9020): 75–82.

19. Kaisers U, Kelly KP, Busch T. Liquid ventilation. (Review.) *Br J Anaesth* 2003; **91**(1): 143–51.

20. Numa AH. Acute lung injury: outcomes and new therapies. *Paediatr Respir Rev* 2001; **2**(1): 22–31.

21. Davies MW, Sargent PH. Partial liquid ventilation for the prevention of mortality and morbidity in paediatric acute lung injury and acute respiratory distress syndrome. *Cochrane Database Syst Rev* 2004; (2): CD003845.

22. Wolfson MR, Shaffer TH. Liquid ventilation: an adjunct for respiratory management. *Paediatr Anaesth* 2004; **14**(1): 15–23.

23. Germann P, Braschi A, Della RG *et al.* Inhaled nitric oxide therapy in adults: European expert recommendations. *Intensive Care Med* 2005; **31**(8): 1029–41.

24. Macrae DJ, Field D, Mercier JC *et al.* Inhaled nitric oxide therapy in neonates and children: reaching a European consensus. *Intensive Care Med* 2004; **30**(3): 372–80.

25. Willson DF, Thomas NJ, Markovitz BP *et al.* Effect of exogenous surfactant (calfactant) in pediatric acute lung injury: a randomized controlled trial. *JAMA* 2005; **293**(4): 470–6.

26. Davidson WJ, Dorscheid D, Spragg R *et al.* Exogenous pulmonary surfactant for the treatment of adult patients with acute respiratory distress syndrome: results of a meta-analysis. *Crit Care* 2006; **10**(2): R41.

27. Young HK, Lowe A, Fitzgerald DA *et al.* Outcome of noninvasive ventilation in children with neuromuscular disease. *Neurology* 2007; **68**(3): 198–201.

28. Joshi G, Tobias JD. A five-year experience with the use of BiPAP in a pediatric intensive care unit population. *J Intensive Care Med* 2007; **22**(1): 38–43.

29. Arai T, Yamashita M. Differential lung ventilation in an infant using LMA and a long tracheal tube. *Paediatr Anaesth* 2003; **13**(5): 438–40.

30. Guruswamy V, Roberts S, Arnold P, Potter F. Anaesthetic management of a neonate with congenital cyst adenoid malformation. *Br J Anaesth* 2005; **95**(2): 240–2.

31. Hammer GB. Anaesthetic management for the child with a mediastinal mass. Paediatr Anaesth 2004; **14**(1): 95–7.

32. Luckhaupt-Koch K. Mediastinal mass syndrome. *Paediatr Anaesth* 2005; **15**(5): 437–8.

33. Lam JC, Chui CH, Jacobsen AS *et al.* When is a mediastinal mass critical in a child? An analysis of 29 patients. *Pediatr Surg Int* 2004; **20**(3): 180–4.

34. Viswanathan S, Campbell CE, Cork RC. Asymptomatic undetected mediastinal mass: a death during ambulatory anesthesia. *J Clin Anesth* 1995; **7**(2): 151–5.

PART IV

SPECIALISED ANAESTHESIA

General surgery and urology

PETER STODDART

KEY LEARNING POINTS

- Paediatric general surgery and urology covers a wide range of procedures, conditions and ages.
- Most children do not need overnight admission for elective surgery.
- Laparoscopy and other minimally invasive techniques are increasingly being used.
- Two major neonatal operations that require special knowledge and practical techniques are repair of tracheo-oesophageal fistula and diaphragmatic hernia.

- Ex-preterm infants, who commonly require repair of inguinal hernia, are at risk of apnoea and need overnight admission
- Repair of pyloric stenosis is not an emergency.
- Infant laparotomy for bowel obstruction is an emergency because early surgery may prevent catastrophic bowel ischaemia.
- Oncological surgery often involves multiple operations and procedures.

INTRODUCTION

There is an enormous diversity of children with surgical conditions, from the sick premature infant who needs resuscitation and laparotomy to the chronically ill adolescent undergoing colonic resection for inflammatory bowel disease. There is also a considerable caseload of normal children who require anaesthesia for very common surgery such as hernia repair, orchidopexy and circumcision. This chapter covers the practical aspects of neonatal and paediatric anaesthesia under the headings general principles for elective and emergency surgery (including laparoscopy), common operations in neonates and infants, abdominal surgery, urological surgery and oncological surgery.

GENERAL PRINCIPLES

Common elective procedures

DAY CASES AND SELECTION FOR OVERNIGHT ADMISSION

Most healthy children having simple surgery do not need to recover overnight in hospital. The indications for admission after surgery vary among hospitals but the main factors are significant medical disease or surgical co-morbidity, pain requiring opioids, previous anaesthesia problems including prolonged recovery or postoperative nausea and vomiting (PONV) and social issues such as home circumstances and the need for long-distance travel.

Day-case surgery has many advantages. It reduces cost and increases efficiency, minimises emotional upset of the child and is associated with reduced morbidity such as infection. To work well it requires careful patient selection and care by experienced staff in a purpose-built facility [1].

DAY-CASE ANAESTHESIA TECHNIQUE

Many simple general and urological conditions can be performed with the child breathing spontaneously via a laryngeal mask airway. If possible, a local anaesthetic block should be used to supplement general anaesthesia and provide early postoperative analgesia. For sub-umbilical surgery a caudal block is effective and simple to perform, and if adjuvants are added to local anaesthesia analgesia is prolonged appreciably, e.g. clonidine (1–2 μg/kg) doubles the duration and preservative-free ketamine (0.5 mg/kg) increases it fourfold [2]. Alternatively a specific peripheral nerve block may be just as effective but with less chance of complications [3]. The ilioinguinal and iliohypogastric nerve blocks are suitable for inguinal surgery including hernia repair and orchidopexy. A penile block is an effective alternative to caudal blockade for circumcision and minor hypospadias surgery (see Chapter 26). For other minor operations, such as lymph node biopsy, only local skin infiltration is necessary. Non-opioid analgesics should always be used to reduce not only the surgical pain but also headache and sore throat. Intraoperative rectal diclofenac (1–1.5 mg/kg) or postoperative oral ibuprofen (10 mg/kg) every 8 hours is recommended. Paracetamol is also important either administered orally before anaesthesia or intravenously during surgery. Opioids are occasionally needed to control the autonomic responses to surgery and to *rescue* children who may be in pain during recovery. Opioids are more likely to be necessary in umbilical hernia repair and in older boys having orchidopexy. Antiemetics are not usually necessary unless there is a history of PONV or opioids have been used.

DISCHARGE CRITERIA

Before children leave hospital they must have recovered their preoperative conscious state, be comfortable (usually playing) and not vomiting [1]. Passing urine before discharge is unnecessary, even after a caudal block. Similarly, leg weakness after caudal block or femoral nerve block is not a contraindication to discharge. Parents should be given written instructions and can either make contact with or return to the hospital in the unlikely event of a problem.

Emergency surgery

Over the last 10–15 years in the UK, practice has changed to concentrate emergency surgery into day-time services within specialist hospitals; in most hospitals only life- or organ-threatening surgery takes place late at night. This has followed reports by the National Confidential Enquiry into perioperative death [4] and the British Paediatric Association report on the transfer of infants and children for surgery [5] which have recommended that the care of children is supervised by senior clinicians who are not fatigued.

RAPID SEQUENCE TRACHEAL INTUBATION

Intravenous access and fluid resuscitation is standard for all emergency surgery, as is a nasogastric tube to empty the stomach for abdominal emergencies. Rapid sequence induction (RSI) is important if there is a risk of aspiration but, in uncooperative infants and children, it will need to be modified for practical reasons. Preoxygenation is difficult without compliance. Also, during apnoea, the combination of low functional residual capacity and high oxygen consumption results in rapid oxygen desaturation [6,7]. Excessive cricoid pressure by inexperienced assistants may distort the airway, making intubation more difficult. It has been suggested that cricoid pressure in children is valuable only because it ensures that an assistant is present [8]. Surveys have found that 50–60 per cent of experienced paediatric anaesthetists did not use cricoid pressure in children – even in those at risk of aspiration [9,10]. Nevertheless, gentle cricoid pressure with standard RSI drill is wise if the stomach is full; if there is regurgitation, cricoid pressure can be adjusted, pharyngeal suction applied promptly and the trolley tilted head down (see Chapter 19).

Fortunately, aspiration during paediatric anaesthesia is a rare event. In two large North American audits, where RSI was widely used, the incidence of aspiration ranged from 0.4 to 1 per 1000 cases, serious morbidity was rare and there were no deaths [11,12]. Some of the aspiration cases were related to gagging or coughing during airway manipulation when muscle relaxation was either not present or inadequate [11]. In contrast, in France where cricoid pressure was less frequently used, only 73 per cent in a series of appendectomies were intubated [13] and in a large survey the incidence of aspiration was 0.1 per 1000 [14]. A review of closed malpractice claims for children in the USA found 5 cases of aspiration compared with 47 of inadequate ventilation, 13 of oesophageal intubation and 9 of difficult intubation [15]. It seems reasonable, in view of the practical limitations of RSI, that it should be reserved for the cooperative or sick child with gross abdominal distension or active upper gastrointestinal bleeding. All other children can be intubated, if necessary, either by a technique of deep intravenous or inhalational anaesthesia or with a non-depolarising muscle relaxant.

Laparoscopic surgery

In adult practice, laparoscopic techniques have been performed for many years in gynaecology and more recently have become the standard method for cholecystectomy and fundoplication. Improvements in equipment and expertise have enabled paediatric surgeons to adapt laparoscopy. The potential advantages of laparoscopy over open surgery are better cosmetic results, less postoperative pain, less postoperative lung dysfunction, reduced need for intensive care and shorter hospital stay. Yet the equipment is expensive, not only because of the high initial capital outlay but also because of the replacement of disposable parts. More important, however, is the disadvantage of the longer time taken for surgery, especially if the surgeon is learning. Complications include pneumothorax, subcutaneous emphysema, haemorrhage and organ perforation.

The technique relies upon the abdominal cavity being distended by insufflating gas, to allow the visualisation of viscera and manipulation of surgical instruments. Carbon dioxide is the best gas because it limits the fire risk during diathermy and, being highly soluble, any effects of a gas embolism are minimised. 'Gasless' laparoscopy is possible where the anterior abdominal wall is lifted and suspended using subcutaneous wires.

The physiological consequences of pneumo-peritoneum vary with intra-abdominal pressure (IAP), age and position. Gas insufflation raises IAP and causes cephalad displacement of the diaphragm. This increases airway pressure and decreases thoracic compliance and functional residual capacity (FRC); these changes are greater in small infants. The 'head-down' position is worst whereas the head-up position tends to preserve the compliance and FRC [16]. The mechanical changes increase pulmonary ventilation/perfusion ($\dot{V}/\dot{Q}$) mismatch causing a fall in peripheral haemoglobin oxygen saturation (SpO_2) that can be avoided by increasing inspired oxygen concentration (FiO_2) and applying positive end-expiratory pressure (PEEP) [17].

Cardiovascular effects are dependent upon IAP; a rise of less than 5 mmHg increases venous return and cardiac output but above 12 mmHg there is compression of the inferior vena cava causing a fall in venous return and cardiac output. High IAP can increase intrathoracic pressure and afterload to cause left ventricular wall dysfunction, and this has been observed using transoesophageal echocardiography [18].

A predictable and rapid absorption of CO_2 across the peritoneum causes hypercapnia; the resultant neurohumoral response tends to counteract the cardiovascular depression of elevated IAP. Absorption of CO_2 reaches a plateau with reduced peritoneal capillary perfusion when IAP > 10 mmHg, though arterial partial pressure of CO_2 ($PaCO_2$) continues to rise owing to increased $\dot{V}/\dot{Q}$ mismatch [19]. Coexisting portal hypertension exacerbates the rise in $PaCO_2$ during laparoscopy [20], secondary to an increase in peritoneal vascularity and blood flow. Extra time and care is required at the end of surgery because the CO_2 load causes an additional respiratory burden, especially in children with poor respiratory reserve. Carbon monoxide is produced by diathermy but probably has little clinical significance.

The physiological effects of retroperitoneal insufflation of CO_2 used for renal and adrenal surgery are less marked, even though higher pressures may be required to create a working 'pocket'. In piglets [21], neither the airway pressure, nor the $P_{ET}CO_2$ (end-tidal carbon dioxide partial pressure) rose, probably because the gas was isolated by retroperitoneal tissues. If gas leaks out into the peritoneal cavity all the aforesaid changes take place and visibility within the retroperitoneal pocket reduces.

PRACTICAL CONDUCT OF ANAESTHESIA FOR LAPAROSCOPY

There may be a perception that the overall risk of laparoscopy is less than open surgery. However, the contraindications should be considered (Table 32.1) and harmful effects of pneumo-peritoneum should be balanced against the potential reduction in postoperative morbidity.

Children should be intubated and mechanically ventilated. Muscle relaxation prevents coughing or respiratory effort during surgery. Beware of the cephalad movement of the diaphragm which may cause accidental bronchial intubation. The tracheal tube should have either minimal leak or a cuff. In addition to routine monitoring, direct arterial pressure can detect critical cardiovascular depression in high-risk patients and transoesophageal echocardiography also detects gas embolism. Capnography is usually reliable though has a tendency to overestimate $PaCO_2$ [22]. During surgery, the stomach must be emptied using a nasogastric or orogastric tube. Nitrous oxide must be avoided because it reduces surgical access by expanding the gas within the bowel; it also increases the size of other potentially dangerous gas-filled spaces. Body temperature needs active management because either hypothermia can occur from insufflation of cold gas or hyperthermia can develop later because abdominal contents are not exposed.

Analgesia requirements are usually less than for major open surgery such as fundoplication or nephrectomy but this may not be true for appendectomy. Certainly, laparoscopic fundoplication has reduced the need for epidural

Table 32.1 Contraindications or cautions against laparoscopy

Cardiac	Risk of gas embolism across intracardiac shunts
	Poorly tolerated in aortic stenosis or low cardiac output states
Respiratory	Respiratory failure may be provoked by intraoperative lung compression and postoperative hypercapnia
Acute trauma	Excessive haemorrhage may limit surgical view
	Hypotension may occur from hypovolaemia and impaired cardiac function
	Open vessels may predispose to gas embolism
History of spontaneous pneumothorax	Gas may leak into the pleura or mediastinum

analgesia. Local analgesia infiltration covers pain from port sites. Shoulder pain caused by residual peritoneal gas is reduced by careful deflation and non-opioid analgesia. Small doses of systemic intraoperative opioids can be continued postoperatively.

COMMON OPERATIONS IN NEONATES AND SMALL INFANTS

Small infants require anaesthesia and surgery for the correction and management of congenital abnormalities or for the complications of prematurity. Anaesthesia in this age group has a higher risk than in older children and adults [23,24]. The definition of a neonate is an infant less than 28 days old (after birth) but, because many infants are preterm, it must be appreciated that gestational age is also important; age after birth and gestation are added together to give postconceptional age (PCA). Neonates are different because they are adapting to extrauterine life and preterm infants may have many other problems. Body weight is also a useful concept when considering risk and it may be simpler to abandon the term neonate and to describe the infant in terms of weight and age (gestation, at birth and PCA). Anaesthesia in all small infants requires special knowledge, technical skill and judgement, and in the UK services are centralised into specialised paediatric centres where clinical expertise can be maintained and training is provided [25,26].

General principles

PREOPERATIVE CONSIDERATIONS

After the assessment of a newborn, the plan is discussed with the parents. This is often a distressing time for new families, and the mother may not be present if she is recovering from an operative delivery elsewhere. An obstetric history is important to seek information about gestational age, maternal health, family history, details of antenatal problems, mode of delivery, intrapartum complications and the infant's Apgar scores. The age and weight of the baby help estimate tracheal tube size, drug doses, fluid and calorie requirements. If there is a congenital abnormality, there may be other defects perhaps as part of an important syndrome, e.g., cardiac lesions are associated with tracheo-oesophageal fistula or Down syndrome.

Intubated babies may have a tracheal tube that is unsuitable for surgery because it is too short, too long or the leak is too great. Oxygen requirement and ventilatory or cardiovascular support must be noted. Sick or unstable infants must have intravenous access through which fluid can be given in sufficient volume. Feeble pulses or inadequate capillary return usually means that more fluid is required. Any suggestion of a cardiac abnormality, either cyanosis or murmur, is an indication for an echocardiogram. Many regional

neonatal intensive care units routinely use cranial ultrasonography to exclude significant periventricular bleeds and other abnormalities. Abdominal distension should be decompressed as far as possible with a gastric tube. An orogastric rather than anasogastric tube may cause less respiratory difficulty because infants are usually obligate nasal breathers. Hepatomegaly is an important sign of cardiac failure. Extremely sick infants may have life-threatening bradycardia, desaturation and apnoea induced by handling. Transitional circulation and persistent pulmonary hypertension are extra major hazards.

ANAESTHESIA

A sick baby, with, for example, diaphragmatic hernia or necrotising enterocolitis (NEC), should already be receiving intensive care before surgery. Transport to theatre should be in an incubator in which therapy can be continued and temperature maintained. All babies should be induced on the operating table in a warm theatre with full monitoring attached as soon as practicable. Routine monitoring consists of electrocardiogram (ECG), automated non-invasive blood pressure (NIBP), inspired/expired gas analysis, SpO_2 and temperature (central and peripheral). Invasive arterial (femoral, radial or umbilical) and central venous pressure (umbilical, femoral or jugular) may be added if the child is, or expected to become, critically ill. Many methods are available to control body temperature within the normal range, including overhead radiant heater, warmed fluids, breathing system heat and moisture exchanger, impervious surgical drapes, warmed wrapping (especially around the head) and under-body warm air duvets. Care must be taken to avoid overheating.

Ideally, anaesthesia aims for the earliest return to stability and this is more likely with the use of modern evanescent drugs such as sevoflurane, desflurane and remifentanil combined with effective local anaesthesia [27–31].

For elective surgery in our hospital, infants are fasted for 2 hours after clear fluids, 3 hours for breast milk and 4 hours for formula milk (see Chapter 18). If the stomach is not empty, a gastric tube must be carefully aspirated before induction. If possible, intravenous (IV) access should be obtained before anaesthesia is induced. In sick infants, IV 10 per cent glucose is commonly needed to maintain blood glucose concentration.

The method of induction depends on the condition of the baby, and the preference and experience of the anaesthetist. Infants should be routinely intubated and ventilated for all major surgery because they have high oxygen consumption and reduced lung function. At the author's hospital the preferred method for stable infants is inhalation of sevoflurane in oxygen followed by IV atracurium. An inhalational induction reduces the risk of hypoxia, especially if anaesthetists are being trained [32]. Alternatively, an IV induction using thiopental 3–5 mg/kg or propofol 2–3 mg/kg is favoured by others. Suxamethonium is rarely required.

A straight-bladed laryngoscope is preferred and its tip is typically placed into the oesophagus and gently withdrawn until the laryngeal inlet is visualised. Gentle pressure on the thyroid cartilage using the little finger may help fix the larynx to obtain a good view. The laryngoscope tip can either press against the epiglottis or sit in the vallecula – either way the laryngeal inlet can be readily visualised. A 3.0 or 3.5 mm uncuffed tracheal tube (TT) is effective for most neonates, and occasionally a stylet or bougie may help to direct it into the trachea. The infant trachea is short, so observation of bilateral chest wall movement and air entry into both lungs must be confirmed by auscultation to ensure correct positioning above the carina. Ideally, there should be a small leak around the TT, but it is very important to make sure that the leak is minimal if lung compliance is expected to reduce, such as in the closure of gastroschisis. In this situation a leak is of secondary importance to the ability to control ventilation.

Anaesthesia is normally maintained with an inhalational agent in air enriched with oxygen. In the premature baby SpO_2 should probably not be allowed to rise above 95 per cent for a prolonged period [33]. The analgesic properties and anaesthesia effects of nitrous oxide may be of benefit in older infants, and it can replace air if there are no contraindications. Isoflurane may now be the standard hypnotic maintenance agent and has largely superseded halothane. However, desflurane has the lowest blood gas solubility and it may be particularly suited to neonatal anaesthesia because recovery is rapid even after prolonged anaesthesia [30,34].

The choice of analgesia depends upon the surgery and the need for postoperative ventilation. Fentanyl in large doses (10 μg/kg) can be used if postoperative ventilation is planned. Many infants can be extubated after surgery provided that analgesia with paracetamol and a regional technique is sufficient. A caudal is suitable for subumbilical surgery and an epidural infusion for laparotomy. In these cases additional intraoperative analgesia can be provided, if necessary, with either a small dose of fentanyl 1–2 μg/kg or a remifentanil infusion.

Term infants need little maintenance fluid on their first day of life, though after surgery they usually receive 40–60 mL/kg/day of 10 per cent dextrose to prevent hypoglycaemia: in subsequent days this can be increased by 30 mL/kg/day to a maximum of 120 mL/kg/day (other electrolytes must be added to prevent dangerous water overload). Small premature infants, however, need up to 180 mL/kg/day because of greater insensible losses. Sodium and potassium requirements also depend on the age and maturity of the baby and daily requirements should be calculated. During major surgery there are additional insensible losses of fluid from the wound and there is little consensus on either which fluid or what volume should be used (our practice is to add Hartmann's solution at 10 mL/kg/h for a laparotomy and half that amount for minor surgery such as inguinal herniotomy). Colloid may also be used but there is no convincing evidence to suggest that it is superior to crystalloid. Human albumin solution (HAS) 4.5 per cent has frequently been used in neonates because it maintains oncotic pressure and plasma albumin levels; these should retain fluid in the intravascular space and preserve drug-binding capacity, especially if plasma bilirubin levels are high [35]. However, HAS is less frequently used because it is expensive and could transmit disease.

Intraoperative blood loss in neonatal surgery should be minimal because of scrupulous haemostasis. This, and the high haemoglobin concentration of the newborn, means that blood transfusion is rare. Exceptions are sick premature infants with NEC or others with major tumours such as sacrococcygeal teratoma. In these cases haemorrhage can be brisk and clinical judgement of observed loss and careful monitoring of cardiovascular signs and variables must guide fluid replacement.

RECOVERY

At the end of surgery, full monitoring and warming should be maintained until the baby has been extubated, and is awake and comfortable. Neonates and small infants should recover quickly because their high alveolar ventilation to FRC ratio enables rapid washout of inhalational agents. However, they are a heterogeneous group and the experienced anaesthetist is patient and does not extubate until spontaneous regular breathing is established, muscle relaxants are reversed, and the baby is awake, with eyes open and limbs moving. Mild positive pressure should be applied to the breathing system and extubation should coincide with inspiration when the vocal cords are abducted. Oxygen should be administered until there is stability. The infant should be wrapped up and kept warm.

Routine postoperative monitoring for all neonates includes temperature, blood pressure, respiratory and pulse rates (checking for apnoeas and bradycardia), and oxygen saturations for at least 24 hours or until they have stopped receiving systemic analgesia.

Regular pain assessment should also be performed and the FLACC scoring tool is useful [36]. Our standard neonatal analgesia includes paracetamol and codeine phosphate (orally or rectally) and for more severe or prolonged pain we use intravenous morphine or an epidural local anaesthetic infusion. Fluids are continued postoperatively until oral feeding becomes normal.

Neonatal bowel obstruction

Acute bowel obstruction may present in the first few hours or days of life. Diagnosis and surgical intervention are urgent to prevent bowel infarction. Warning signs include maternal polyhydramnios and premature labour. Proximal small bowel obstruction is usually caused by an atresia and causes bilious vomiting and dehydration. Distal obstruction causes abdominal distension and failure to pass meconium: the most common causes are meconium ileus, meconium plug, Hirschsprung's disease and anorectal anomaly. Obstruction can be mid-bowel such as a volvulus, and signs can be mixed. In all cases intravenous fluid resuscitation and gastric decompression are essential while the diagnosis is confirmed by X-ray.

VOLVULUS

Neonatal volvulus, secondary to malrotation, is a life-threatening condition in which there is both bile-stained vomiting and abdominal distension. The infant is usually otherwise normal and urgent laparotomy is imperative to untwist the volvulus. Hypotension and shock may follow reperfusion of the ischaemic bowel, requiring treatment with large volumes of fluid and, sometimes, inotropes. Once the bowel has been examined, any peritoneal bands are divided to widen the mesentery base and then non-viable bowel is resected. Appendectomy is also performed. Many of these infants will need a period of stabilisation in an intensive care unit.

ATRESIA

Of various bowel atresias, duodenal atresia is the commonest and is associated with congenital heart disease, Down syndrome (in 30 per cent) and anorectal anomalies. Approximately 50 per cent of affected babies are preterm or have low birth weight. A 'double bubble' is seen on the abdominal X-ray representing gas in the stomach and duodenal cap – there is no distal gas. Surgery can wait until after fluid resuscitation and investigations. Standard anaesthesia and analgesia techniques can be used and early extubation is usual.

MECONIUM ILEUS

Meconium ileus (MI) is the second commonest cause of small bowel obstruction and is the result of thick, sticky meconium impacting within the ileum. In 80–90 per cent of babies with MI this is an early manifestation of cystic fibrosis (CF). Uncomplicated simple MI is treated by fluid resuscitation and Gastrograffin or acetylcysteine enemas to evacuate the viscid matter from the small bowel. However, if this is unsuccessful, or a perforation occurs, laparotomy is required to form a stoma or T-tube enterotomy. Approximately 10–15 per cent of CF children present with MI and this is associated with a poor long-term prognosis.

HIRSCHSPRUNG'S DISEASE

Hirschsprung's disease usually presents in the neonatal period with variable degrees of vomiting and abdominal distension. The passage of meconium is delayed. Diagnosis is confirmed by the absence of the intramural ganglia in a full-thickness biopsy of the rectal mucosa. The incidence is 1 in 5000 births and it is associated with Down syndrome. The disease is isolated to the rectosigmoid junction in 75 per cent of cases but can be in a long segment affecting the whole of the colon and extending into the small intestine. Occasionally, infants present in shock with toxaemia and enterocolitis due to *Clostridium difficile* infection. Surgical management has evolved. In recent years, a colostomy was formed first with biopsies taken to confirm the extent of the disease. A pull-through operation was performed months later in which normal ganglionic bowel was anastomosed to the anus. The stoma was reversed as a separate procedure. Various inventive surgeons have given their names to operations (Soave, Duhamel and Swenson), which have different rectum-like anastomoses.

Currently, a single-staged procedure is performed in the neonatal period for isolated rectosigmoid disease. In the older child, where the diagnosis has been made later, the extent of the disease can be determined by laparoscopic biopsies, resection and anastomosis. Most infants can be managed by standard anaesthesia and extubated at the end of surgery.

Anorectal anomaly

Anorectal anomalies occur in 1 in 5000 live births and are classified into 'high' or 'low' defects depending on the stage of the embryological development failure. High defects are more common in boys who usually have a rectourinary fistula. Girls may have a rectovaginal fistula or a cloacal anomaly, which will require several extensive operations to isolate the intestinal and urogenital systems. Primary treatment involves the formation of a colostomy and then, at 6–9 months, a pull-through procedure (usually known as posterior sagittal anorectoplasty or PSARP). Anorectal anomalies are associated with the VACTERL (*v*ertebrae, *a*nus, *c*ardiovascular tree, *t*rachea, *o*esophagus, *r*enal system and *l*imb buds) syndrome in which cardiac defects are common; a preoperative echocardiogram is important. Vertebral and sacral abnormalities may prevent the use of a caudal catheter. The PSARP procedure necessitates the baby lying prone with the pelvis raised. This requires careful positioning to ensure that the tracheal tube is not kinked, that there is no hyperextension of the neck or pressure on the eyes. A single caudal injection of bupivacaine 0.75 mL/kg and preservative-free ketamine 0.5 mg/kg provides excellent postoperative analgesia for a procedure without an abdominal incision. Alternatively, if abdominal exposure is required, an epidural infusion or IV morphine infusion will be needed. The stoma is reversed at a later date when the rectoperitoneal wound has healed and the bowel is demonstrably patent.

Low anorectal anomalies often require a simple anoplasty in which the surgeon must first identify the perineal muscles using an electrical stimulator. A single caudal injection is a useful adjunct to general anaesthesia or could be used alone for minimal surgery.

Exomphalos and gastroschisis

Both conditions result from an abdominal wall defect and are treated in a similar way. The bowel is totally exposed in gastroschisis and, as it is vulnerable to infection, surgery is necessary as soon as possible after birth. In exomphalos the bowel is covered and the defect can be closed the following day. Table 32.2 has further details.

Most of these babies have an antenatal diagnosis and can either be delivered near to a paediatric surgical unit or have a planned retrieval. Initial first aid involves covering the exposed viscera, with plastic wrap or damp gauze to reduce infection and loss of fluid and heat. Because there is protein and fluid loss, IV crystalloid or HAS 4.5 per cent is required. Preoperative care must be in a thermoneutral environment and systemic antibiotics are crucial. The stomach must be decompressed.

Management depends on the size of the defect. A small defect with only a small amount of bowel outside the abdomen can have a primary closure; early extubation is possible. Bigger defects, however, often have so much bowel externalised that closure can be achieved only in stages. A Silastic *silo* (a tower-shaped sack) is needed to cover the bowel and viscera in the interim until final closure. This silo can be squeezed and made smaller in stages and eventually removed for complete closure. At any stage of closure the lungs may become compressed as abdominal compliance falls. Elective postoperative ventilation is usually necessary until visceral oedema reduces and the abdominal wall stretches.

Before the first procedure, most babies are stable and are breathing air. Following aspiration of the gastric tube, anaesthesia can be induced intravenously or with sevoflurane in air and oxygen. Full muscle relaxation is needed while the bowel is compressed into the abdominal cavity. Nitrous oxide is contraindicated, as it increases intra-abdominal pressure. Analgesia is directed by the need for postoperative ventilation. Simple closure can be managed with a small dose of fentanyl, local anaesthetic infiltration and paracetamol.

As the surgeon squeezes the bowel and viscera into the abdomen the rise in IAP can be readily appreciated if ventilation is by hand [37]. If pressure-controlled mechanical ventilation is used, under-ventilation may not be appreciated. Excessive IAP compresses the vena cava and reduces venous return and cardiac output; this is often apparent as a fall in $P_{ET}CO_2$ (end-tidal CO_2 tension). If these changes persist there is bowel ischaemia, reduced renal perfusion and metabolic acidosis. Experienced teams know how much 'squeezing' is safe for the bowel and they achieve full closure as soon as possible to minimise infection risk. In some units gastroschisis is managed entirely in the neonatal intensive care unit (NICU). Provided that the infant is already intubated, an anaesthesia team may not be needed [38]. Postoperative urine output must be measured and a careful assessment of fluid balance made, especially while the infants are ventilated, to minimise the potential abdominal compartment syndrome (high IAP) and to reduce bowel and generalised oedema.

Prognosis depends on the viability of the returned bowel and the presence of coexisting abnormalities. With exomphalos major and gastroschisis a prolonged postoperative ileus is common and most babies will require temporary total parental nutrition via a peripheral IV line. Occasionally, a long-term feeding line is necessary if short bowel syndrome develops.

Congenital diaphragmatic hernia

Congenital diaphragmatic hernia (CDH) occurs in 1 in every 4000–5000 live births and is associated with cardiac and neurological anomalies. It is a potentially lethal combination

Table 32.2 Summary details of exomphalos and gastroschisis

	Exomphalos	Gastroschisis
Anatomy	Herniation of viscera into base of umbilical cord through a central defect Membranous sac covers and protects gut (sac may rupture)	Evisceration through 2–5 cm defect lateral to umbilicus No protective sac Viscera exposed to chemical inflammation from amniotic fluid and environment
Pathology	Failure of gut to migrate into abdominal cavity and thus failure of abdominal wall to develop	Intrauterine occlusion of omphalomesenteric artery resulting in defect in abdominal wall
Incidence	1:5000–1:10 000	1:5000–1:10 000 Increasing worldwide
Associations	Beckwith–Wiedemann syndrome Also chromosomal and congenital cardiac, genitourinary, craniofacial abnormalities	Intestinal atresias and malrotation Low risk for congenital abnormalities
Prematurity	Infrequent	Frequent

of diaphragmatic defect, herniation of abdominal organs into the thorax and pulmonary hypoplasia. The major problem is the degree of pulmonary hypoplasia. Although the lung is smallest on the side of the hernia (70–85 per cent are left sided), there is reduced and hyperactive vasculature in both lungs. The severity of disease varies and infants can be divided into three outcome groups according to the degree of pulmonary function.

In the good outcome group, CDH is an incidental finding. Infants or small children present when a chest X-ray (CXR) is taken for another reason such as a chest infection. These children do well because herniation of the bowel into the thoracic cavity probably occurred late *in utero*, or after birth, and lung development is near normal.

In the poor outcome group there is insufficient pulmonary function to sustain life and this is associated with large diaphragmatic defects or agensis [39]. Resuscitation is necessary immediately at birth and a best post-ductal partial pressure of oxygen (PO_2) 13 kPa (<100 mmHg) predicts poor outcome [40]. Early surgery is not helpful unless the poor clinical state has been induced by another pathology such as malrotation. Severe CDH can be diagnosed in the antenatal period and although intrauterine surgery is possible it is experimental.

In a middle outcome group, infants present within 24 hours of birth with respiratory distress. A 'honeymoon' period is typical when the baby is initially stable but then becomes hypoxic owing to pulmonary vasospasm causing right-to-left shunting. This transitional circulation and pulmonary hypertension leads to a downward spiral of increasing hypoxia and acidosis, which is soon fatal unless treatment is effective. Other typical signs are a barrel chest and a scaphoid abdomen. A CXR demonstrates dextrocardia and bowel in the thorax (typically the left) (Fig. 32.1). The diagnosis may be confused with pneumothorax or congenital lobar emphysema.

Congenital diaphragmatic hernia is not considered a surgical emergency and should be undertaken only after a period of stabilisation on NICU. Pulmonary mechanical ventilation aims to optimise oxygenation and reduce carbon dioxide tension without submitting the lungs to barotrauma and the risk of pneumothorax. If conventional ventilation is ineffective or requires high inflation pressures, high-frequency oscillatory ventilation may be better. Permissive hypercapnia may be sensible rather than excessive ventilatory pressures. An arterial line for blood gas analysis and blood pressure monitoring is essential. Control of pulmonary hypertension is mainly achieved by opioid analgesia, sedation and maintenance of metabolic alkalosis. Cardiovascular support by intravenous filling and inotrope infusions is often necessary. Pulmonary vasodilatation with tolazoline has been used in the past but is no longer considered helpful. Tolazoline is a histamine agonist and it causes systemic hypotension and gastric haemorrhage. Inhaled nitric oxide (iNO) may be beneficial. Extracorporeal membrane oxygenation is occasionally used, especially in North America, but the evidence for improved survival compared with conventional treatment is not clear.

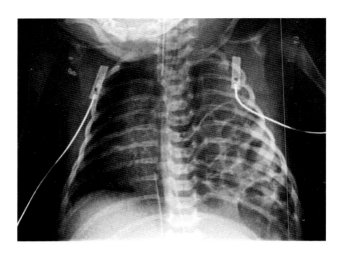

Figure 32.1 Chest X-ray of neonate with congenital diaphragmatic hernia.

Early surgery can cause deterioration and unnecessary morbidity and mortality. The criteria for safe surgery should be at least 24 hours of stability defined as conventional ventilation with inspired oxygen concentrations of less than 50 per cent and with minimal inotropic support. Anaesthesia in sick ventilated babies should be regarded as a continuation of their intensive care management. High-dose fentanyl 25–50 μg/kg, or a remifentanil infusion, with ventilation in 100 per cent O_2 may be required to maintain cardiovascular stability. Infants without significant pulmonary disease can have a standard anaesthetic, and may benefit from epidural analgesia. Surgery should be uneventful and involves primary repair of the defect or insertion of a synthetic patch.

The small lung on the side of the hernia appears collapsed but re-expansion is not possible and attempts to do so could cause a pneumothorax (on either side). All but the fittest of infants may have a difficult postoperative period of 24–48 hours and will need intensive care. Chest drains are not inserted routinely; however, pneumothorax is a common complication and prompt drainage may be necessary.

Oesophageal atresia and tracheo–oesophageal fistula

These occur in 1:3000–4000 live births. There are many anatomical variations and these are described in detail in a review by Kluth [41].

Nevertheless, there are five major types (Fig. 32.2), and the commonest (85 per cent) is a blind oesophageal pouch with distal oesophagus attached to the trachea by a fistula close to the carina. Up to 30 per cent of babies are premature or low birth weight. Between 30 and 50 per cent have additional congenital abnormalities of other midline structures including skeletal, anorectal anomalies and the heart (ventricular septal defect [VSD], tetralogy of Fallot); cardiac defects may significantly reduce survival [42].

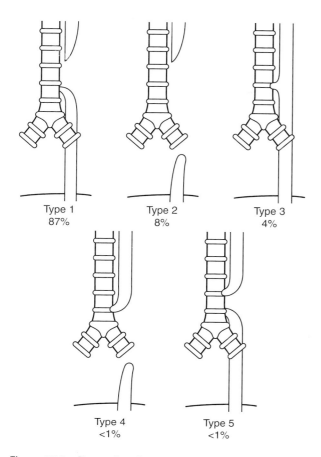

Figure 32.2 Types of tracheo-oesophageal fistula.

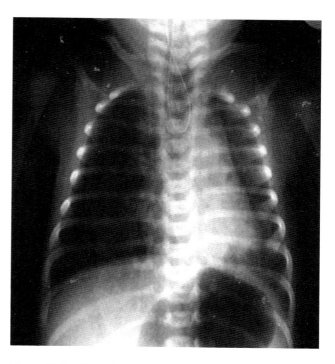

Figure 32.3 Chest X-ray of neonate with oesophageal atresia and tracheo-oesophageal fistula. Note the nasogastric tube coiled in the upper oesophageal pouch.

The diagnosis may be suspected in a 'mucusy' neonate with a history of maternal polyhydramnios. The baby coughs and chokes on the first feed and a gastric tube cannot be passed. A CXR (Fig. 32.3) demonstrates the level of obstruction where the upper pouch ends and the presence of gas in the stomach and small intestine indicates a tracheal fistula rather than an isolated oesophageal atresia. In rare instances of an 'H'-type fistula the diagnosis is often late and requires an experienced paediatric radiologist to demonstrate the fistula by Gastrograffin swallow. The baby should be kept fasted and nursed 'head up' or prone with regular suction of the upper pouch using a double-lumen Replogle orogastric tube. This tube is crucial because it removes secretions that cannot be swallowed and would otherwise cause airway obstruction. Surgery to ligate the fistula can usually be scheduled for daytime. A preoperative echocardiogram is essential. Some infants may require ventilation because of prematurity or pneumonitis, and this makes surgery urgent, because decreasing pulmonary compliance causes gastric distension; effective pulmonary support is difficult with a tracheal fistula. The anaesthetist's main task is to provide adequate intraoperative conditions for retropleural thoracotomy to close the fistula and anastomose the upper and lower parts of the oesophagus. The position of the aorta should be checked by echocardiography before the side is chosen for thoracotomy.

Various techniques have been described including awake intubation, intubation of the spontaneously breathing anaesthetised infant or a rapid sequence induction avoiding positive pressure mask ventilation until the TT has isolated the fistula. However, our practice is to induce with sevoflurane in oxygen, to use either atracurium or vecuronium and gently to hand ventilate until the TT is positioned such that both lungs can be ventilated without inflating the stomach too much – some gastric ventilation has to be tolerated. This is usually easily achieved with a TT of normal length. It is almost always unnecessary to pass the TT beyond the fistula, though occasionally the bevel of the TT needs to be rotated to direct airflow away from the fistula. If the stomach is distended it may be possible and worthwhile to occlude the fistula with a Fogarty catheter, using a bronchoscope [43]. The position of the TT must be checked by auscultation after placing the infant in the lateral position for surgery. The neck must not be extended because this causes the upper pouch to lie further away from the lower segment and will make the anastomosis more difficult. A nasal TT has the advantage of being ready for postoperative ventilation.

Some surgeons routinely perform an oesophagoscopy before the main operation to exclude an additional upper pouch fistula. Dissection of the upper pouch is facilitated by the anaesthetist manipulating the Replogle tube within it, and this should be made ready during positioning before surgery begins. Gentle ventilation by hand improves surgical access, so that some hypoxaemia is common, although this is usually well tolerated. Ligation of the fistula is a crucial stage and the surgeon and the anaesthetist must be certain that the fistula has been identified correctly for ligation and not the trachea or a main bronchus – both lungs should be expanded when the fistula is clamped before it is ligated. A nasogastric tube (NGT) may be directed across the anastomosis to decompress the stomach and enable postoperative enteral feeding (usually starting on the fifth postoperative day).

Babies that were in good condition preoperatively and with no surgical contraindications can be extubated once they are awake and pain free. Balanced anaesthesia with a combination of inhalational agent, desflurane, and fentanyl 2–3 µg/kg or remifentanil is standard. Postoperative analgesia can be provided with intercostal nerve block inserted by the surgeon, combined with intravenous morphine by nurse-controlled analgesia (NCA) and paracetamol or by thoracic epidural analgesia inserted by either the caudal or thoracic levels. All babies should be cared for in a high-dependency environment. Precipitous reintubation should be avoided because of the risk of both stretching the anastomosis and the fistula stump in the trachea.

In the sick premature infant, or if the anastomosis is at risk of breaking down, postoperative ventilation should be instituted for approximately 5 days or more. Overall survival has improved to around 90 per cent; however, oesophageal stricture, dysmotility reflux and tracheomalacia are common problems [44,45]. These may require further surgical intervention if symptomatic [46].

Pyloric stenosis

Congenital hypertrophic pyloric stenosis occurs in 1 in every 300–400 live births. It is caused by thickening of the circular muscle that develops from birth and gradually obstructs the pylorus. Infants are typically first-born males and present aged 4–6 weeks old. Sometimes there is a positive family history. Projectile non-bilious vomiting is the cardinal presenting feature in an otherwise healthy and hungry baby. There may be weight loss and dehydration and an olive-shaped 'tumour' can be palpated in the epigastrium after a feed. The diagnosis can be confirmed by ultrasound. Classically, because of the gastric loss of sodium, potassium and hydrochloric acid, there is hypochloraemic alkalosis, usually with hypokalaemia and mild uraemia. There may be hypoglycaemia and unconjugated hyperbilirubinaemia. Initially, the kidneys compensate by excreting bicarbonate ions (with sodium) to produce alkaline urine. However, with prolonged sodium and chloride loss, the kidneys conserve sodium ions and excrete hydrogen and potassium instead, thereby producing acid urine and making the hypokalaemia worse. Ketoacidosis and obvious dehydration are likely at this stage. In the most severe cases there may be compensatory hypoventilation and respiratory acidosis leading to hypoxia and apnoea.

Dehydration and alkalosis must be corrected over 48–72 hours with IV fluids using a combination of saline, dextrose and potassium supplementation. Physiological or 0.9 per cent saline can be used to correct hypovolaemia (may need up to 100 mL/kg) with additional maintenance fluid of 4 per cent dextrose/0.18 per cent saline (4 mL/kg/h). Biochemical correction should be monitored from repeated capillary blood gas samples until the plasma electrolyte concentrations are normal. A NGT tube must be inserted and regular washouts performed until the aspirate is clear and free of milk curds.

The surgical objective is to split the hypertrophic musculature without breaching the mucosa. Perforation can be tested during surgery by injecting air into the stomach via the NGT. The traditional Ramstedt's operation, with a horizontal hypogastric incision, has been replaced in some units by a peri-umbilical incision or even laparoscopic surgery. Prophylactic antibiotics are needed to reduce wound sepsis. Surgery is not an emergency and should be scheduled once the bicarbonate concentration is <28 mmol/L and the chloride >90 mmol/L; there is a risk of postoperative apnoea if electrolyte concentrations have not been corrected.

Before anaesthesia, the stomach is emptied by aspiration of the NGT; best stomach drainage may be achieved by aspirating while rotating the baby from the supine to the prone position. Rapid sequence induction may not be necessary if there is confidence that the stomach is empty. A survey in the UK showed that two-thirds of anaesthetists used an IV induction and only 50 per cent applied cricoid pressure [9]. Currently, in Bristol, we induce anaesthesia with sevoflurane and atracurium and the trachea is intubated after 1–2 minutes of gentle mask ventilation with the NGT in place. Anaesthesia is maintained with desflurane or sevoflurane in oxygen and NO [29]. In larger babies, especially in those having a peri-umbilical incision, 1 µg/kg of fentanyl is used along with paracetamol and wound local anaesthetic (LA) infiltration. The NGT is removed, but maintenance fluids continue until feeding begins at 12 hours. The baby should be monitored for apnoeas and may need additional paracetamol.

ABDOMINAL SURGERY IN OLDER CHILDREN

Intussusception

Idiopathic intussusception occurs in previously well infants and presents with acute colicky abdominal pain and the passing of 'redcurrant jelly' or bloody mucus stools. Typically, the child has had a recent gastroenteritis or upper respiratory tract infection. The intussusception is usually of the ileum at the ileocaecal junction. A sausage-shaped mass may be felt in the right upper quadrant or rectally. Occasionally, the intussusception may be secondary to a pathological lead point such as a Meckel's diverticulum, polyp, duplication cyst or tumour, and this should be suspected if it is a colo-colic or ileo-ileal intussusception. There is venous obstruction and traction on the mesentery as the lead point invaginates and progresses towards the rectum. This causes mucosal oedema and eventually ischaemia and necrosis. Ultrasound is diagnostic.

Reduction of the intussusception may be achieved without surgery by using rectal insufflation of air and a contrast enema – this is performed under fluoroscopic control [47]. Intravenous access is required to enable resuscitation and rehydration because of fluid loss from both the intussusception and reperfusion of the ischaemic bowel. The risk of perforation is low but is probably related to inexperience. Radiological reduction should be performed in a hospital with a paediatric surgical unit to enable an urgent laparotomy if necessary. Repeat radiological reduction can be performed but surgery is indicated if there are signs of sepsis or perforation, or if there is a pathological lead point. In this situation the child is usually ill with abdominal distension, sepsis and hypovolaemia. A NGT tube should be inserted.

Rapid sequence intubation is recommended using suxamethonium or rocuronium. Further fluid resuscitation with colloid is often required and a urinary catheter will simplify postoperative fluid management. Intravenous morphine will provide good analgesia supplemented by paracetamol. Non-steroidal anti-inflammatory drugs (NSAIDs) are probably best avoided in the acute phase until the child is recovering and taking oral fluids postoperatively. Although this is a serious condition, a mortality rate of 1–2 per cent is low if diagnosis and management occur early [48].

Fundoplication

Fundoplication for gastro-oesophageal reflux disease (GORD) is a common elective procedure performed on children with significant neurological and respiratory problems. Asymptomatic GOR is frequent in normal infants and children but in its severe form it causes failure to thrive, life-threatening apnoeas, oesophageal spasm with pain, recurrent pneumonia, chronic cough and bronchospasm. The diagnosis can be made by oesophageal biopsy or oesophageal pH probe monitoring. Laryngo-, tracheo- and bronchomalacia are associated and can be proven by laryngobronchoscopy. Treatment is initially medical, with combinations of antacids, feed thickening, motility stimulants, H_2-receptor antagonists and proton pump inhibitors. However, if the child does not improve surgery is indicated. This is likely in neurologically handicapped children who have impaired swallowing and require tube feeding. There are various types of anti-reflux procedures (Thal, Nissen and Watson), all of which involve wrapping the stomach around the oesophagus to create a valve.

If performed by an open operation the incision is upper abdominal and causes significant pain. Other common problems include poor seizure control and reduced respiratory reserve secondary to recurrent aspiration, cerebral palsy and scoliosis. Laparoscopic procedures are preferred because recovery is associated with less postoperative pain and minimal ileus. Most anaesthetists do not use a rapid sequence induction. Indeed some syndromic children (e.g. cri-du-chat or Cornelia de Lange syndrome) may be

difficult to intubate quickly. Many children are physically handicapped and need careful positioning and padding of their pressure points. Anti-reflux and anticonvulsant drugs should continue throughout the perioperative period and the latter need to be continued postoperatively, intravenously if necessary. Children having an open operation will benefit from postoperative epidural analgesia [49], whereas for laparoscopic surgery this rarely required.

Inflammatory bowel disease

Crohn's disease in children typically causes ileocaecal inflammatory granulomas leading to a mass in the right iliac fossa. Perianal ulcers, sinuses and fistulae are features of colorectal Crohn's disease and are particularly debilitating and difficult to heal. Children present with weight loss, abdominal pain, diarrhoea and general poor health, including an arthropathy. Treatment is primarily medical to control symptoms and modify disease progression. Standard treatment includes aminosalicylates, corticosteroids and azathioprine but in severe cases a monoclonal antibody to tumour necrosis factor is used (infliximab). Metronidazole is indicated for perianal disease but prolonged use can cause a peripheral neuropathy. Surgery is best avoided and is rarely curative, being reserved mainly to manage strictures, abscesses and fistulae.

Ulcerative colitis causes inflammation of the colon and rectum. It presents with diarrhoea (containing blood, mucus and pus), cramping lower abdominal pain and tenesmus. In extreme cases the child may present in shock with a toxic megacolon and this requires an urgent colectomy. Medical treatment is broadly similar to that used for Crohn's disease, though local rectal disease can be controlled with corticosteroid enemas. Failure of medical therapy is an indication for elective resection and ileoanal anastomosis – many are subsequently cured.

These children and adolescents can be debilitated, immunosuppressed and steroid dependent. For surgery they may need blood transfusion, additional steroid cover and parenteral nutrition. Antibiotic prophylaxis is required. They may have difficult peripheral venous access and therefore central venous access may be needed. An epidural infusion provides good postoperative analgesia, but must be inserted with scrupulous aseptic technique; immunosuppression may make epidural infection more likely and it must be removed if there are any signs of infection afterwards.

UROLOGY

Circumcision

Circumcision is one of the commonest operations performed in the world, principally for social and religious reasons. In the UK, however, it is becoming much less common and is mainly performed for phimosis [50]. This is a simple day-case procedure performed under general anaesthesia with a penile block, ring block or caudal for postoperative analgesia. Throughout the world religious circumcision in neonates is usually performed without anaesthesia and the use of analgesia is varied and controversial.

Hypospadias

In this condition the external urethral meatus is proximal to the tip of the penis. Surgical repair moves the meatus to the tip of the glans, covers the new urethra with skin and releases any coexisting chordee. Surgery is performed at around 12 months when there is sufficient penile tissue and nappies become unnecessary. General anaesthesia with a laryngeal mask airway and a spontaneous breathing technique is standard. Penile block is not ideal since analgesia may not be effective or last long enough and it may interfere with the surgical field, especially in more proximal hypospadias repairs. A caudal 0.5 mL/kg of 0.25 per cent bupivacaine with preservative-free ketamine 0.5 mg/kg (or clonidine 1 μg/kg) provides excellent postoperative analgesia and prevents intraoperative penile erection. A urinary catheter is inserted and the penis can be protected with a foam dressing. Recurrent fistula formation may require a buccal mucosal graft and this may necessitate tracheal intubation. Removal of the dressing can usually be achieved by skilled nurses on the ward using minimal analgesia and sedation; however, if a child is too distressed anaesthesia may be required.

Posterior urethral valve

Most posterior urethral valves (PUVs) are now diagnosed antenatally because secondary dilatation of the upper urinary tract with variable degrees of hydroureteronephrosis and bladder thickening can be seen on ultrasound. They occur in 1 in 5000–8000 male births. Severe obstruction is associated with oligohydramnios, renal parenchyma loss and pulmonary hypoplasia. This may require intrauterine bladder decompression with a stent to relieve the back pressure. Polyuria can occur after urethral catheterisation because of damaged urine-concentrating power of the distal tubules. Renal function and fluid balance should be monitored carefully. Definitive early ablation of the valves by direct incision is performed via a 10Fr cystoscope. This can be technically challenging and so tracheal intubation and ventilation are recommended. A caudal block will provide good postoperative analgesia even if the surgeon performs a cutaneous vesicostomy.

Bladder exstrophy

Bladder extrophy is a rare but important abnormality occurring in 1 in 30 000–50 000 live births (two-thirds are male). It is an abnormality in which the inside of the bladder is exposed on the lower abdominal wall and is caused by the failure of fusion of the midline structures, including the pubic symphysis, abdominal wall and genitourinary tract. It is the commonest of group of rare defects that range from simple epispadias to complete exstrophy of the cloaca exposing both the bladder and the rectum. Untreated children are incontinent of urine and changes in bladder mucosa result in an increased incidence of bladder tumours, especially adenocarcinoma. At birth the exposed bladder should be covered with a plastic film to keep the mucosa moist. As this is a rare condition the neonate should be managed in a national specialist centre. The repair is usually completed in three stages for boys, and two in girls, but other plastic and functional revisions may be necessary. The surgical aim is to close the bladder and abdominal wall as soon as possible. Surgery can be prolonged with significant blood loss, especially if a pelvic osteotomy is required. Intravenous cannulae should be sited in the upper body. Ideally, general anaesthesia is supplemented with an epidural infusion for postoperative analgesia because it may help to prevent straining and wound dehiscence. The baby may be nursed postoperatively with the legs in a supportive frame. Latex-containing materials must be excluded, particularly in this group, because of the risk of developing a subsequent latex allergy [51].

In boys the epispadias is repaired at around one year of age while the final stage to create a sphincter muscle for bladder control is done when the child is older and has developed a reasonable bladder capacity [52].

Ureteric reimplantation

Vesicoureteric reflux occurs in about 1 per cent of children but has a much higher incidence in children with urinary symptoms. These children are treated with prophylactic antibiotics to prevent renal damage. Reflux nephropathy accounts for 15–20 per cent of end-stage renal failure in children and young adults. Most reflux will resolve spontaneously as the child grows. However, if medical management fails, surgical intervention is indicated [53]. Various reimplantation procedures are described but they all involve a lower abdominal transverse incision and the creation of a sphincter mechanism in the bladder by increasing the intramural ureteric length. There may be a degree of renal impairment and associated hypertension. Prophylactic antibiotics and antihypertensive therapy should be continued perioperatively. Painful bladder spasms are a frequent postoperative complication and the pain can usually be lessened with a lumbar epidural infusion. Spasms may persist for several days and alternative techniques for this difficult problem include using antispasmodics, oxybutynin and diazepam or instillation of intravesical local anaesthetics [54]. More recently, endoscopic injection of a bulking agent under the ureteral orifice has been used to create an artificial flap–valve [55]. This technique is much less invasive, needing only cystoscopy, and therefore can be performed under a short general anaesthetic.

Pyeloplasty and nephrectomy

These procedures are performed for congenital abnormalities of the kidney or anomalies of the pelviureteric junction; the latter may cause pain and hydronephrosis. Renal tumours also require nephrectomy. In small children the kidney is approached retroperitoneally using a non-muscle-splitting incision. Minimally invasive techniques are increasingly being used [56] and this reduces the post-operative analgesia requirements to a low-dose morphine IV infusion with paracetamol supplementation Many babies recover and can be discharged home after 48 hours. An epidural is not usually required except for more complex reconstructions. Heminephrectomy requires division of the renal parenchyma and may cause brisk major haemorrhage.

ONCOLOGICAL SURGERY
(See also Chapters 7 and 44)

Malignancy is a major cause of death in childhood. Paediatric anaesthetists have an important role in the management of children with cancer because repeated anaesthesia may be necessary for procedures, including biopsy, scanning, insertion of long-term intravenous access, tumour resection, intrathecal chemotherapy and radiotherapy. Children may also need management of acute or prolonged pain. Families are stressed and frightened and appreciate an experienced and familiar anaesthetist. It should be remembered that many tumours can be cured provided that there are services for early diagnosis and aggressive treatment. For example, the combination of chemotherapy, surgery and adjuvant radiotherapy (if necessary) for nephroblastoma has increased overall survival from <10 per cent in 1935 to >85 per cent in 1996 [57,58]. Moreover the quality of care can be improved by early insertion of long-term venous access not only for blood sampling and IV therapy but also for the administration of effective sedation, analgesia and short-acting anaesthesia to cover painful and frightening procedures.

Problems caused by medical cancer treatment

There are important side-effects of chemotherapy and radiotherapy that have implications for anaesthesia [59]. Chemotherapeutic agents are classified into:

- alkylating agents (these alkylate nucleic acids)
- antimetabolites (interact with specific enzymes)
- hormones (e.g. steroids)
- plant alkaloids (cause arrest of mitosis)
- antibiotics (form complexes with DNA, thereby inhibiting DNA and RNA synthesis).

They all cause bone marrow suppression, especially the alkylating agents and antimetabolites. Platelet counts should be checked before surgery and a platelet transfusion may be required even for simple procedures such as lumbar puncture. Major surgery should be delayed until the marrow has recovered, and this may require recombinant human granulocyte colony-stimulating factor (G-CSF). Immunosuppre-ssion increases the chance of infection and paracetamol should be used carefully so that it does not mask pyrexia. Rectal medication may be contraindicated. All blood for transfusion should be irradiated to kill leukocytes that cause graft-versus-host disease. Mucositis is a particularly unpleasant condition associated with neutropenia following chemotherapy. Eating and swallowing can be so painful that even swallowing saliva is difficult. Treatment is supportive with mouth hygiene, intravenous paracetamol and morphine infusions. The dose of morphine may be as high as 40–50 µg/kg/h and sometimes analgesia is effective only if ketamine is added (it does not usually cause hallucinations). Rarely, neutropenia is associated with severe retroperitoneal inflammation that causes an acute abdomen with ileus and diarrhoea; laparotomy should be avoided unless there is a perforation.

Other important major side-effects from chemotherapy are:

- Cardiotoxicity from anthracyclines (doxorubicin and daunorubicin) is dose dependent and occurs more in females and in children receiving thoracic radiation. Toxicity can occur acutely during treatment or much later. About 65 per cent of children surviving acute lymphoblastic leukaemia may have abnormal cardiac function 6 years later [60]. Huettemann *et al.* demonstrated that even in asymptomatic children cardiac function can deteriorate by up to 50 per cent during one minimum alveolar concentration of isoflurane anaesthesia [61].
- Bleomycin damages the pulmonary endothelium causing interstitial oedema, necrosis of pneumocytes and, sometimes, pulmonary fibrosis. In animals oxygen increases pulmonary toxicity during bleomycin treatment, but not later [62]. Oxygen should not be given during treatment but may be given at other times. If there is lung dysfunction, more postoperative pulmonary complications occur following excessive fluid intake or blood transfusion [63].
- Vincristine is neurotoxic and is almost always lethal if it is accidentally injected intrathecally instead of methotrexate. Tragic cases in the UK have changed practice so that vincristine and methotrexate are administered in different clinical areas at different times [64]. Vincristine and cisplatin both cause a dose-related peripheral neuropathy.

All chemotherapy causes tumour lysis and the resultant metabolic debris causes renal failure. Urine output must be driven by high volumes of intravenous fluids to prevent renal necrosis.

Management of common abdominal tumours

The commonest abdominal tumours of childhood are neuroblastoma (NB) (approximate annual incidence 10 per million) and Wilms' tumour (approximate annual incidence 7 per million), and both present similar anaesthetic problems. Overall, NB has a worse prognosis especially in children over 1 year who often present with advanced disease; the overall cure rate is 55 per cent. Neuroblastomas are tumours of the sympathetic chain and mostly arise in the abdomen, principally in the adrenal gland or retroperitoneal sympathetic ganglia. Most (90 per cent) are diagnosed before the age of 5 years. Wilms' tumours arise in the kidney (bilateral in 5–10 per cent cases) and can be associated with other urological abnormalities. Microdeletions in chromosome 11 are associated. The median age of presentation is around 3 years.

Both the above usually present as a large abdominal mass. In 95 per cent of NBs high levels of catecholamines, homovanillic acid (HVA) and vanillylmandelic acid (VMA) are found in the urine. More marked hypertension occurs in phaeochromocytoma where urinary levels of HVA and VMA are much higher; these children tend to be older or have a multiple endocrine adenoma syndrome. Hypertension is a common feature present in 60 per cent of Wilms' tumours caused by renal ischaemia and high renin levels; VMA and HVA levels are normal.

Chemotherapy should shrink large tumours and allow resection. Wilms' tumour can spread along the vena cava even up to the right atrium, and resection of NBs can involve dissection around the major abdominal vessels. Consequently, in both, rapid blood transfusion may be necessary. The family will be very anxious and the anaesthesia and analgesia plan should be clearly and frankly explained to them, especially if the child is likely to need intensive care.

The children will have a long-term venous line (usually a Hickman line), so this can be used for an IV induction. Parents are usually helpful in comforting their child. If the child needs antihypertensive therapy this should be given on the morning of surgery as well; these drugs are often not required following successful tumour resection. Most families accept a thoracic epidural sited for postoperative analgesia and a urinary catheter is routinely inserted. An NGT is standard to check gastric emptying and because postoperative ileus is so common. Direct arterial pressure monitoring is necessary and the Hickman line can be used for central venous pressure. Periods of hypertension, even with a working epidural, are not infrequent and should be treated by deepening anaesthesia or adding opioid (either fentanyl or remifentanil). Except for phaeochromocytoma, it is unusual to require any specific hypotensive agents. A balanced anaesthetic of isoflurane in oxygen-enriched air, supplemented with fentanyl 3–7 µg/kg is suitable. During the retroperitoneal dissection the bowel should be placed inside a polythene bowel bag to reduce fluid and heat loss. Active body warming is important. Maintenance fluids of 10 mL/kg/h of Hartmann's solution are infused throughout. A large-bore peripheral cannula is ideal for blood and colloid infusion. If the tumour closely involves both renal vessels specific agents may improve urine output (dopamine, dopexamine, furosemide or mannitol), though there is no good evidence that they are any more effective than maintaining a positive fluid balance and cardiovascular stability [65].

At the end of surgery some children will need pulmonary ventilation until there is cardiovascular stability, adequate urine output and resolution of any metabolic acidosis. However, most can be extubated at the end of surgery if they are warm, well perfused with good arterial blood gases and comfortable with an effective epidural infusion (0.1–0.5 mL/kg/h of 0.1 per cent bupivacaine with 2 µg/mL fentanyl is effective). On the ward, they will require continued monitoring of their fluid balance and pain control.

CONJOINED TWINS

Separation of conjoined twins is a complex and rare operation and should be undertaken only in specialist centres. The anatomical variations and their surgical and anaesthesia management are reviewed in depth elsewhere [66]. The essential points are that two surgical and two anaesthesia teams are necessary and that major resources and careful planning are required for a successful outcome; often, many procedures are required and the children and their families need considerable support. In addition, there are further challenges of cardiac anomalies in thoracopagus twins [67] and technical difficulties separating intracranial circulations in craniopagus twins [68].

REFERENCES

Key references

Bannister CF, Brosius KK, Wulkan M. The effect of insufflation pressure on pulmonary mechanics in infants during laparoscopic surgical procedures. *Paediatr Anaesth* 2003; **13**(9): 785–9.

Diaz LK, Akpek EA, Dinavahi R, Andropoulos DB. Tracheoesophageal fistula and associated congenital heart disease: implications for anesthetic management and survival. *Paediatr Anaesth* 2005; **15**(10): 862–9.

Huettemann E, Sakka SG, Petrat G *et al.* Left ventricular regional wall motion abnormalities during pneumoperitoneum in children. *Br J Anaesth* 2003; **90**(6): 733–6.

Lally KP, Lally PA, van Meurs KP *et al.* Treatment evolution in high-risk congenital diaphragmatic hernia: ten years experience with diaphragmatic agenesis. *Ann Surg* 2006; **244**(4): 505–13.

Nordmann GR, Read JA, Sale SM *et al.* Emergence and recovery in children after desflurane and isoflurane anaesthesia: effect of anaesthetic duration. *Br J Anaesth* 2006; **96**(6): 779–85.

References

1. Brennan LJ. Modern day-case anaesthesia for children. *Br J Anaesth* 1999; **83**(1): 91–103.

2. Cook B, Grubb DJ, Aldridge LA, Doyle E. Comparison of the effects of adrenaline, clonidine and ketamine on the duration of caudal analgesia produced by bupivacaine in children. *Br J Anaesth* 1995; **75**(6): 698–701.

3. Giaufre E, Dalens B, Gombert A. Epidemiology and morbidity of regional anesthesia in children: a one-year prospective survey of the French-Language Society of Pediatric Anesthesiologists. *Anesth Analg* 1996; **83**(5): 904–12.

4. National Confidential Enquiry into Patient Outcome and Death. (http://www.ncepod.org.uk/pdf/NCEPODRecommendations.pdf).

5. British Paediatric Association. *The transfer of infants and children for surgery.* London: British Paediatric Association, 1993.

6. Morrison JE, Collier E, Friesen RH, Logan L. Preoxygenation before laryngoscopy in children: how long is enough? *Paediatr Anaesth* 1998; **8**(4): 293–8.

7. Xue FS, Luo LK, Tong SY *et al.* Study of the safe threshold of apneic period in children during anesthesia induction. *J Clin Anesth* 1996; **8**(7): 568–74.

8. Brock-Utne JG. Is cricoid pressure necessary? *Paediatr Anaesth* 2002; **12**(1): 1–4.

9. Stoddart PA, Brennan L, Hatch DJ, Bingham R. Postal survey of paediatric practice and training among consultant anaesthetists in the UK. *Br J Anaesth* 1994; **73**(4): 559–63.

10. Engelhardt T, Strachan L, Johnston G. Aspiration and regurgitation prophylaxis in paediatric anaesthesia. *Paediatr Anaesth* 2001; **11**(2): 147–50.

11. Warner MA, Warner ME, Warner DO *et al.* Perioperative pulmonary aspiration in infants and children. *Anesthesiology* 1999; **90**(1): 66–71.

12. Borland LM, Sereika SM, Woelfel SK *et al.* Pulmonary aspiration in pediatric patients during general anesthesia: incidence and outcome. *J Clin Anesth* 1998; **10**(2): 95–102.

13. Ecoffey C, Auroy Y, Pequignot F *et al.* A French survey of paediatric airway management use in tonsillectomy and appendicectomy. *Paediatr Anaesth* 2003; **13**(7): 584–8.

14. Tiret L, Nivoche Y, Hatton F *et al.* Complications related to anaesthesia in infants and children. A prospective survey of 40240 anaesthetics. *Br J Anaesth* 1988; **61**(3): 263–9.

15. Morray JP, Geiduschek JM, Caplan RA *et al.* A comparison of pediatric and adult anesthesia closed malpractice claims. *Anesthesiology* 1993; **78**(3): 461–7.

16. Manner T, Aantaa R, Alanen M. Lung compliance during laparoscopic surgery in paediatric patients. *Paediatr Anaesth* 1998; **8**(1): 25–9.

17. Bannister CF, Brosius KK, Wulkan M. The effect of insufflation pressure on pulmonary mechanics in infants during laparoscopic surgical procedures. *Paediatr Anaesth* 2003; **13**(9): 785–9.

18. Huettemann E, Sakka SG, Petrat G *et al.* Left ventricular regional wall motion abnormalities during pneumoperitoneum in children. *Br J Anaesth* 2003; **90**(6): 733–6.

19. Lister DR, Rudston-Brown B, Warriner CB *et al.* Carbon dioxide absorption is not linearly related to intraperitoneal carbon dioxide insufflation pressure in pigs. *Anesthesiology* 1994; **80**(1): 129–36.

20. Bozkurt P, Kaya G, Yeker Y *et al.* Arterial carbon dioxide markedly increases during diagnostic laparoscopy in portal hypertensive children. *Anesth Analg* 2002; **95**(5): 1236–40.

21. Diemunsch P, Becmeur F, Meyer P. Retroperitoneoscopy versus laparoscopy in piglets: ventilatory and thermic repercussions. *J Pediatr Surg* 1999; **34**(10): 1514–17.

22. Laffon M, Gouchet A, Sitbon P *et al.* Difference between arterial and end-tidal carbon dioxide pressures during laparoscopy in paediatric patients. *Can J Anaesth* 1998; **45**(6): 561–3.

23. Morray JP, Geiduschek JM, Ramamoorthy C *et al.* Anesthesia-related cardiac arrest in children: initial findings of the Pediatric Perioperative Cardiac Arrest (POCA) Registry. *Anesthesiology* 2000; **93**(1): 6–14.

24. Cohen MM, Cameron CB, Duncan PG. Pediatric anesthesia morbidity and mortality in the perioperative period. *Anesth Analg* 1990; **70**(2): 160–7.

25. Lunn JN. Implications of the national enquiry into perioperative deaths for paediatric anaesthesia. *Paediatr Anaesth* 1992; **2**: 69–72.

26. Arul GS, Spicer RD. Where should paediatric surgery be performed? *Arch Dis Child* 1998; **79**(1): 65–70; discussion 70–2.

27. Wee LH, Moriarty A, Cranston A, Bagshaw O. Remifentanil infusion for major abdominal surgery in small infants. *Paediatr Anaesth* 1999; **9**(5): 415–8.

28. Wolf AR, Stoddart P. Neonatal medicine. Awake spinal anaesthesia in ex-premature infants. *Lancet* 1995; **346**(suppl): s13.

29. Wolf AR, Lawson RA, Dryden CM, Davies FW. Recovery after desflurane anaesthesia in the infant: comparison with isoflurane. *Br J Anaesth* 1996; **76**(3): 362–4.

30. O'Brien K, Robinson DN, Morton NS. Induction and emergence in infants less than 60 weeks post-conceptual age: comparison of thiopental, halothane, sevoflurane and desflurane. *Br J Anaesth* 1998; **80**(4): 456–9.

31. Davis PJ, Galinkin J, McGowan FX *et al.* A randomized multicenter study of remifentanil compared with halothane in neonates and infants undergoing pyloromyotomy. I. Emergence and recovery profiles. *Anesth Analg* 2001; **93**(6): 1380–6.

32. Kong AS, Brennan L, Bingham R, Morgan-Hughes J. An audit of induction of anaesthesia in neonates and small infants using pulse oximetry. *Anaesthesia* 1992; **47**(10): 896–9.

33. Askie L, Henderson-Smart D. Restricted versus liberal oxygen exposure for preventing morbidity and mortality in preterm or low birth weight infants. *Cochrane Database Syst Rev* 2001 Iss 4 Art. No.: CD001077.

34. Nordmann GR, Read JA, Sale SM *et al.* Emergence and recovery in children after desflurane and isoflurane anaesthesia: effect of anaesthetic duration. *Br J Anaesth* 2006; **96**(6): 779–85.

35. Stoddart PA, Rich P, Sury MR. A comparison of 4.5 per cent human albumin solution and Haemaccel in neonates

undergoing major surgery. *Paediatr Anaesth* 1996; **6**(2): 103–6.

36. Merkel SI, Voepel-Lewis T, Shayevitz JR, Malviya S. The FLACC: a behavioral scale for scoring postoperative pain in young children. *Pediatr Nurs* 1997; **23**(3): 293–7.

37. Tan SSW, Sury MRJ, Hatch D. The 'educated hand' in paediatric anaesthesia – does it exist? *Paediatr Anaesth* 1993; **3**: 291–5.

38. Sandler A, Lawrence J, Meehan J *et al.* A 'plastic' sutureless abdominal wall closure in gastroschisis. *J Pediatr Surg* 2004; **39**(5): 738–41.

39. Lally KP, Lally PA, van Meurs KP *et al.* Treatment evolution in high-risk congenital diaphragmatic hernia: 10 years' experience with diaphragmatic agenesis. *Ann Surg* 2006; **244**(4): 505–13.

40. Wilson JM, Lund DP, Lillehei CW, Vacanti JP. Congenital diaphragmatic hernia: Predictors of severity in the ECMO era. *J Pediatr Surg* 1991; **26**(9): 1028–34.

41. Kluth D. Atlas of esophageal atresia. *J Pediatr Surg* 1976; **11**(6): 901–19.

42. Diaz LK, Akpek EA, Dinavahi R, Andropoulos DB. Tracheoesophageal fistula and associated congenital heart disease: implications for anesthetic management and survival. *Paediatr Anaesth* 2005; **15**(10): 862–9.

43. Andropoulos DB, Rowe RW, Betts JM. Anaesthetic and surgical airway management during tracheo-oesophageal fistula repair. *Paediatr Anaesth* 1998; **8**(4): 313–19.

44. Konkin DE, O'Hali W A, Webber EM, Blair GK. Outcomes in esophageal atresia and tracheoesophageal fistula. *J Pediatr Surg* 2003; **38**(12): 1726–9.

45. Tonz M, Kohli S, Kaiser G. Oesophageal atresia: what has changed in the last three decades? *Pediatr Surg Int* 2004; **20**(10): 768–72.

46. Nasr A, Ein SH, Gerstle JT. Infants with repaired esophageal atresia and distal tracheoesophageal fistula with severe respiratory distress: is it tracheomalacia, reflux, or both? *J Pediatr Surg* 2005; **40**(6): 901–3.

47. Bai YZ, Qu RB, Wang GD *et al.* Ultrasound-guided hydrostatic reduction of intussusceptions by saline enema: a review of 5218 cases in 17 years. *Am J Surg* 2006; **192**(3): 273–5.

48. Stringer MD, Pledger G, Drake DP. Childhood deaths from intussusception in England and Wales, 1984–9. *BMJ* 1992; **304**(6829): 737–9.

49. Wilson GA, Brown JL, Crabbe DG *et al.* Is epidural analgesia associated with an improved outcome following open Nissen fundoplication? *Paediatr Anaesth* 2001; **11**(1): 65–70.

50. Rickwood AMK, Kenny SE, Donnell SC. Towards evidence based circumcision of English boys: survey of trends in practice. *BMJ* 2000; **321**(7264): 792–3.

51. Holzman RS. Clinical management of latex-allergic children. *Anesth Analg* 1997; **85**(3): 529–33.

52. Gearhart JP. Editorial: Evolution of epispadias repair-timing, techniques and results. *J Urol* 1998; **160**: 177–8.

53. Elder JS, Peters CA, Arant BS Jr *et al.* Pediatric Vesicoureteral Reflux Guidelines Panel summary report on the management of primary vesicoureteral reflux in children. *J Urol* 1997; **157**(5): 1846–51.

54. Chiang D, Ben-Meir D, Pout K, Dewan PA. Management of post-operative bladder spasm. *J Paediatr Child Health* 2005; **41**(1–2): 56–8.

55. Kirsch A, Hensle T, Scherz H, Koyle M. Injection therapy: advancing the treatment of vesicoureteral reflux. *J Pediatr Urol* 2006; **2**(6): 539–44.

56. Valla JS, Breaud J, Carfagna L *et al.* Treatment of ureterocele on duplex ureter: upper pole nephrectomy by retroperitoneoscopy in children based on a series of 24 cases. *Eur Urol* 2003; **43**(4): 426–9.

57. Plesko I, Kramarova E, Stiller CA *et al.* Survival of children with Wilms' tumour in Europe. *Eur J Cancer* 2001; **37**(6): 736–43.

58. Gatta G, Capocaccia R, Coleman MP *et al.* Childhood cancer survival in Europe and the United States. *Cancer* 2002; **95**(8): 1767–72.

59. Huettemann E, Sakka SG. Anaesthesia and anti-cancer chemotherapeutic drugs. *Curr Opin Anesthesiol* 2005; **18**(3): 307–14.

60. Lipshultz SE, Colan SD, Gelber RD *et al.* Late cardiac effects of doxorubicin therapy for acute lymphoblastic leukemia in childhood. *N Engl J Med* 1991; **324**(12): 808–15.

61. Huettemann E, Junker T, Chatzinikolaou KP *et al.* The Influence of anthracycline therapy on cardiac function during anesthesia. *Anesth Analg* 2004; **98**(4): 941–7.

62. Veninga TS, Vriesendorp R, Blom-Muilwijk MC *et al.* Absence of an additional fibrotic response caused by oxygen in the lungs of rats after the intratracheal administration of bleomycin. *Br J Anaesth* 1988; **61**(4): 413–18.

63. Donat SM, Levy DA. Bleomycin associated pulmonary toxicity: is perioperative oxygen restriction necessary? *J Urol* 1998; **160**(4): 1347–52.

64. Dyer C. Doctors suspended after injecting wrong drug into spine. *BMJ* 2001; **322**(7281): 257.

65. O'Leary MJ, Bihari DJ. Preventing renal failure in the critically ill. *BMJ* 2001; **322**(7300): 1437–9.

66. Thomas JM, Lopez JT. Conjoined twins – the anaesthetic management of 15 sets from 1991 to 2002. *Paediatr Anaesth* 2004; **14**(2): 117–29.

67. Chen T-L, Lin C-J, Lai H-S *et al.* Anaesthetic managements for conjoined twins with complex cardiac anomalies. *Can J Anaesth* 1996; **43**: 1161–7.

68. Girshin M, Broderick C, Patel D *et al.* Anesthetic management of staged separation of craniopagus conjoined twins. *Paediatr Anaesth* 2006; **16**(3): 347–51.

Ear, nose and throat surgery

ADRIAN R LLOYD-THOMAS

KEY LEARNING POINTS

- Airway vigilance and smooth techniques of anaesthesia are essential in all ear, nose and throat (ENT) procedures.
- Comorbidity of anaesthetic significance is common in paediatric ENT patients.
- Postoperative nausea and vomiting is common in ENT surgery – prophylaxis should be given.
- A nasopharyngeal airway can help post-adenotonsillectomy management of patients with obstructive sleep apnoea.

- Preservation of spontaneous respiration is needed for diagnostic microlaryngoscopy and bronchoscopy; this is facilitated by good topical anaesthesia.
- A new tracheostomy needs meticulous care in the perioperative and postoperative period.
- Precise tracheal tube positioning is needed in laryngotracheal reconstruction.

INTRODUCTION

Ear, nose and throat (ENT) surgery presents the anaesthetist with significant challenges; patients may have life-threatening airway obstruction at one extreme or be otherwise healthy but in need of minor ear surgery. When the surgeon and anaesthetist share the airway, the potential for complications is great and considerable anaesthetic skill is needed to ensure patient safety [1].

GENERAL PATIENT ASSESSMENT AND PREOPERATIVE PREPARATION

Patient assessment should be undertaken as described in Chapter 17; many ENT operations can be performed on a day-stay basis and outpatient preassessment is common. Many older ENT patients have difficulty in communication (deafness or voice disturbance) and it is incumbent on the anaesthetist to recognise and adapt to their needs. Standard preoperative preparation (e.g. fasting) applies. Many children having ENT operations have airway abnormalities; a thorough preoperative airway assessment is mandatory. Associated anomalies are common and should be sought. A medication history is important as some patients with airway obstruction will have been given high-dose steroid therapy.

The airway

Many children presenting for ENT surgery, especially adenoidectomy, will have nasal obstruction, which must be distinguished from an acute upper respiratory tract infection (URTI). The latter is associated with an increased incidence of unwanted intraoperative airway events (e.g. laryngeal spasm) [2] and postponement of surgery is often advised. An algorithm to assist decision-making for the individual is given in Fig. 17.2 (Chapter 17).

Significant airway obstruction will often be a presenting symptom; common causes are given in Table 33.1. Stridor, sternal depression, and indrawing of the supraclavicular, intercostal and subdiaphragmatic areas are all signs of upper airway obstruction – seen when the airway is reduced by 70 per cent, especially in the compliant chest wall of infancy. Inspiratory stridor indicates obstruction at or above the thoracic inlet, while hoarseness suggests vocal cord involvement. Inspiratory and expiratory stridor (biphasic) is seen with obstruction above or below the vocal cords. Expiratory stridor alone is symptomatic of intrathoracic obstruction. Anticipation and preparation are central to minimising anaesthetic complications in cases with airway obstruction.

Syndromes associated with difficult intubation and airway management are commonly seen for ENT surgery (Table 33.1). Chapter 28 describes the conditions, while

Table 33.1 Common causes of upper airway obstruction in children presenting for ear, nose and throat (ENT) surgery*

Congenital	Acquired
Choanal atresia	Infections
Craniofacial malformations	Croup (laryngo-
Pierre Robin syndrome	tracheobronchitis)
Treacher Collins syndrome	Epiglottitis
Goldenhar syndrome	Quinsy
Mid-facial hypoplasia	Ludwig's angina
Macroglossia	Diphtheria
Down syndrome	Physical obstruction
Beckwith–Wiedemann	Foreign body
Mucopolysaccharidoses	Adenotonsillar hypertophy
Larynx	Trauma
Laryngomalacia	Thermal or chemical burns
Laryngeal web	Post-intubation
Laryngeal cleft	Postoperative
Vocal cord palsy	Angio-oedema
Subglottic stenosis	Acquired laryngeal or
Haemangioma	subglottic stenosis
Tracheal	Rheumatoid arthritis
Tracheomalacia	Tumours
Tracheal stenosis	Cysts
Vascular rings	Lymph nodes
	Neurogenic
	Depressed consciousness
	Nerve palsy

*Further conditions with significance for airway management are given in Chapter 28.

preparation for difficult airway management is explained in Chapter 21.

Associated anomalies

All ENT patients should be checked for other anomalies. Multisystem abnormalities, e.g. CHARGE syndrome (*c*oloboma of the eye, *h*eart defects, *a*tresia of the choanae, *r*etardation of growth and/or development, *g*enital and/or urinary abnormalities, and *e*ar abnormalities and deafness), are common in specialist ENT surgery and may require preoperative investigation (e.g. echocardiography). Cardiac lesions merit special consideration, as techniques of anaesthesia for airway assessment may result in myocardial depression [3]. Syndromes with cardiac defects are listed in Table 28.2 (Chapter 28).

Patients with sickle cell disease and obstructive sleep apnoea (OSA) commonly present for adenotonsillectomy and will require preoperative preparation according to local guidelines (see Chapter 7).

Bleeding in the airway (tonsillar fossa or nose) can result in serious morbidity in the perioperative period. Any history of a bleeding tendency in the child or family is an indication for preoperative investigation.

Pre-medication

Most children undergoing ENT surgery do not require preoperative sedation, although it may be offered to those with significant anxiety (oral midazolam 0.5 mg/kg, maximum 15 mg 30 minutes before induction). When intravenous induction is planned, topical anaesthetic cream is applied.

Sedation should be avoided in all patients with airway obstruction. An exception can be made for patients with a tracheostomy, where the risks of sedation-induced airway obstruction are circumvented. Many children with airway abnormalities require multiple procedures over many years (e.g. treatment of recurrent respiratory papillomatosis); consistent, empathetic psychological preparation can help smooth the perioperative course. They should be involved in anaesthesia planning, choosing, for example, their preferred method of induction.

Endoscopy for the assessment of airway abnormalities is facilitated when oropharyngeal secretions are minimised. Topical anaesthesia is more effective when mucous membranes are dry; however, systemic absorption of local anaesthetic may be increased [4]. Antimuscarinic medication also counteracts the vagotonic action of some volatile anaesthetics [5]. Atropine, by intramuscular injection, is the most effective (20 μg/kg, maximum 500 μg) but those undergoing repeat examinations may prefer oral administration (40 μg/kg, maximum 500 μg). The general use of antimuscarinics is in decline [6], but airway endoscopy remains an indication for their use.

GENERAL CONSIDERATIONS FOR ANAESTHESIA

For most ENT patients a standard approach to the induction of anaesthesia is employed (see Chapters 10 and 11). Those with significant airway obstruction are best managed by an inhalational technique.

Sharing the airway with the surgeon demands a smooth technique of anaesthesia; poor judgement of anaesthetic depth may result in coughing, breath-holding and laryngeal spasm at any stage of the operation. Close clinical observation is essential to gauge depth of anaesthesia, to check for adequacy of ventilation and to look for kinking, inadvertent displacement or disconnection of tracheal tubes or laryngeal mask airways (LMAs). Cooperation between the anaesthetist and surgeon is vital for a successful outcome.

Standard monitoring (pulse oximetry, electrocardiography, blood pressure measurement, inspired and expired gas analysis) are vital as access to the patient is often restricted. During insufflation anaesthesia, and during bronchoscopy iteslf, expired gas analysis is unreliable due to difficulties in sampling. If mechanical ventilation is used (intermittent positive pressure ventilation [IPPV]) airway pressure monitoring and a disconnect alarm are needed.

Minimising postoperative nausea and vomiting (PONV) is humane and assists the efficiency of day-care surgery. Ondansetron reduces postoperative vomiting (100 μg/kg, maximum 8 mg) [7] and has a synergistic effect when combined with dexamethasone (0.25 mg/kg maximum 8 mg) [8]. Dehydration may induce nausea and intraoperative intravenous rehydration (compound sodium lactate 20 mL/kg) should be given.

Multimodal analgesia is the key to effective pain relief for ENT surgery. Paracetamol (15 mg/kg intravenously [IV], maximum 1 g) is commonly combined with a non-steroidal anti-inflammatory drug (NSAID) (diclofenac suppository 1 mg/kg, maximum 50 mg) [9]. Peak analgesia from paracetamol, even intravenously, occurs between 1 h and 2 h after administration [10]. For short operations, oral paracetamol premedication [20 mg/kg 1 hour before operation, max. 1 g) may afford maximum postoperative analgesia at the time of recovery. Frequently, ENT surgeons infiltrate the operative site with adrenaline (epinephrine) (1:200 000) to reduce blood loss; this can be combined with a local anaesthetic (commonly lidocaine 1 per cent 3–5 mg/kg) to provide analgesia. Opioids are useful and are discussed in detail below.

As ENT operations commonly involve the airway, recovery in the post-anaesthesia care unit (PACU) demands continuing close clinical observation. In operations where there may be bleeding in the airway, patients should be positioned on their side and placed slightly head down so that blood can run out of the nose or mouth. Blood or secretions running onto the larynx may result in laryngeal spasm and obstruction.

EAR SURGERY

Myringotomy and tympanostomy tubes

Patients with recurrent otitis media and persistent middle-ear effusions (>3–6 months) are offered myringotomy and insertion of tympanostomy tubes [11]. Some patients present for repeat tube insertions, although the likelihood of this is reduced if adenoidectomy is performed [12]. Admission is on a day-case basis, unless intercurrent illness precludes this. Inhalational anaesthesia with spontaneous respiration, using an LMA, is indicated. A narrow external auditory canal (e.g. Down syndrome) can make surgical access difficult, increasing the duration of an otherwise brief operation. Paracetamol and an NSAID are given for postoperative analgesia. A short-acting opiate (fentanyl 0.5 μg/kg) may smooth the immediate recovery period, although its use increases the likelihood of PONV.

Open exploration of the middle ear, mastoidectomy, myringoplasty and cochlear implantation

Exploration of the middle ear and mastoid air cells may be needed for removal of infected material or clearance of cholesteatoma. Chronic perforation of the tympanic membrane may require reconstructive myringoplasty. Patients with profound sensorineural deafness, poorly managed with conventional hearing aids, are considered for cochlear implantation. An induction receiver–stimulator is implanted with an array of electrodes inserted in the cochlea; the latter stimulate spiral ganglion cells, giving auditory perception [13]. The child wears an external processor and must be able to cooperate with lengthy postoperative auditory training programmes. Unipolar diathermy is contraindicated in children with a cochlear implant.

Surgical and anaesthetic considerations for all middle-ear surgery are: (1) the control of bleeding, (2) the preservation of the facial nerve and (3) avoidance of graft displacement.

BLEEDING

All middle-ear surgery requires the use of an operating microscope; even trivial bleeding can impair the surgical view. Bleeding can be of arterial origin secondary to a hyperdynamic circulation with a high cardiac output, hypertension and tachycardia. Control of heart rate and cardiac output will minimise this loss. Venous ooze secondary to raised internal jugular venous pressure may be caused by poor patient positioning, partial airway obstruction during spontaneous respiration, abdominal compression, or raised mean intrathoracic pressure with IPPV or positive endexpiratory pressure (PEEP).

Strategies to minimise blood loss during middle-ear surgery are presented in Table 33.2. These involve controlled hypotension, which may be defined as a reduction

Table 33.2 Strategies to minimise blood loss during middle-ear surgery

Strategy	Method	Comment
Smooth induction of anaesthesia avoiding tachycardia or hypertension		
Calm, relaxed patient	Sedative premedication if required	Avoid anticholinergic medication
Avoid pain on injection	Topical anaesthesia	
	Use thiopental sodium	
Avoid coughing or straining on intubation	Use a short-acting non-depolarising muscle relaxant	
	Give remifentanil before intubation	0.5–1 µg/kg over 1 min.
	Use topical laryngeal anaesthesia	
Keep the venous pressure low		
Patient positioning	Head-up tilt of 15–20°	
	Avoid excessive head turning	May obstruct the contralateral internal jugular
IPPV	Normocapnia	
	Slow respiratory rate	Long expiratory time
	No PEEP	
Aim for a systolic blood pressure of 80 mmHg		
Analgesia	Infiltration with lidocaine and adrenaline 1:200 000	
	Remifentanil infusion	0.1–0.5 µg/kg/min
Anaesthesia	Air/oxygen and volatile agent	Titrate to desired blood pressure

IPPV, intermittent positive pressure ventilation; PEEP, positive end-expiratory pressure.

of systolic blood pressure to 80–90 mmHg, a reduction of mean arterial pressure (MAP) to 50–65 mmHg or a 30 per cent reduction of baseline MAP [14]. Previously, labetolol (bolus 0.2 mg/kg maximum 1 mg/kg) was used, largely to control the heart rate. The advent of remifentanil has revolutionised the approach to anaesthesia for this type of surgery [15], blocking any response to stimulation, thereby allowing titration to the desired blood pressure by adjustment of the end-tidal concentration of volatile agent. The blood pressure cuff should be sited on the arm opposite to the operation to avoid interference with readings by surgical activity. The remifentanil infusion should be stopped 10 minutes before the start of closure and the end-tidal concentration of volatile agent reduced, thereby allowing the blood pressure to rise, revealing bleeding points for haemostasis.

PRESERVATION OF THE FACIAL NERVE

The tympanic segment of the facial nerve is at risk during middle-ear surgery and may be difficult to identify in the diseased ear. The facial nerve monitoring used in middle-ear surgery is based upon electromyography and requires neuromuscular function. Neuromuscular block is needed only to facilitate smooth intubation and a short-acting drug should be chosen, allowing return of function before surgery is significantly advanced.

AVOIDING GRAFT DISPLACEMENT

Nitrous oxide (N_2O), being more soluble than nitrogen, diffuses in and out of body cavities more quickly than nitrogen. When the middle ear has been closed by a myringoplasty, termination of N_2O will result in a negative pressure being applied to the graft. Avoiding N_2O throughout the operation is probably the easiest solution, but where this is not possible it should be discontinued 20 minutes before the ear is closed.

An opioid, paracetamol and NSAID analgesia may be given towards the end of surgery for postoperative pain relief. An antiemetic (e.g. cyclizine 1 mg/kg, maximum 25 mg) should be prescribed as PONV can be problematic after middle-ear surgery.

SURGERY FOR CONGENITAL EAR DEFECTS

Children with congenital defects of the external ear present for the insertion of osseo-integrated temporal screws to enable attachment of an artificial pinna- or bone-anchored hearing aid. Reconstructive surgery to form an external ear is also undertaken. These defects are associated with Treacher Collins and Goldenhar syndromes (see Chapter 28), both of which present difficulty for tracheal intubation.

Anaesthesia for these operations can usually be managed using an LMA, which obviates the need for tracheal intubation. It is essential to be satisfied with the performance of the LMA with the head in the position for operation before surgery commences.

NASAL, NASOPHARYNGEAL AND PHARYNGEAL SURGERY

Adenotonsillectomy

Adenoidectomy and tonsillectomy are the most common operations performed in children, often undertaken outside specialist units [16]. Indications for adenoidectomy include chronic obstructive adenoid hypertrophy (mouth breathing, snoring and hyponasal voice) and chronic middle-ear effusion secondary to eustachian tube dysfunction. Indications for tonsillectomy include recurrent infection, acute infection (quinsy), unilateral enlargement and upper airway obstruction (UAO) with OSA.

Adenotonsillar hypertrophy is the most common cause of UAO in children. Children with craniofacial abnormalities (e.g. syndromes with lower- and mid-face hypoplasia, Down syndrome, achondroplasia, mucopolysaccharidoses) and those with neuromuscular disease (hypotonia or spasticity) are predisposed to UAO with lesser degrees of hypertrophy [17]. Upper airway obstruction, when severe, gives rise to OSA characterised by restless sleep and snoring with apnoeic pauses. Polysomnography allows calculation of a respiratory disturbance index (apnoeas per hour) and a sleep disturbance index (arousals per hour). Sleep disturbance often gives rise to behavioural problems and daytime somnolence [18].

Chronic upper airway obstruction can lead to disordered central control of respiration with hypoxia and hypercapnia. If severe, this can result in pulmonary vasoconstriction, right ventricular hypertrophy and right heart failure [19]. Children with sickle cell disease and OSA are at risk of pulmonary complications and cerebrovascular accidents as a result of nocturnal hypoxia [20].

PREOPERATIVE ASSESSMENT

Preoperative identification of patients with OSA is vital and those with severe symptoms require an electrocardiogram (ECG) and echocardiography to assess right heart function. Polysomnography is expensive and time-consuming and is seldom required, though overnight admission for continuous pulse oximetry is sometimes used to support the clinical diagnosis and may be useful in planning postoperative management. Rarely, preoperative treatment with diuretics and continuous positive airway pressure (CPAP) is needed in those with severe right heart failure. Preoperative sedation is contraindicated in patients with UAO and OSA. Patients with sickle cell disease (SCD) should be prepared as described in Chapter 7. Preoperative exchange transfusion exposes patients with SCD to the hazards of transfusion and the development of alloantibodies. There is insufficient evidence to support this approach in all SCD patients and

paediatricians are increasingly recommending a more conservative approach. Nevertheless, patients <5 years of age with SCD and OSA undergoing adenotonsillectomy are at high risk of complications following surgery. When OSA is severe or if there is a significant past medical history (stroke, chest crisis or frequent painful crises) patients should be prepared by exchange transfusion to achieve haemoglobin (Hb) of 9–11 g/dL with an HbS level of <30 per cent. Further guidelines are available in the Addendum to Chapter 7.

ANAESTHESIA

Induction of anaesthesia may be either by inhalation or intravenous. In children with UAO the airway may be difficult to maintain and obstruction will occur at light planes of anaesthesia. Application of CPAP, keeping the mouth slightly open, will help to maintain the airway, until anaesthesia is sufficiently deep to permit insertion of an oral airway.

Children without OSA may be managed using IPPV or spontaneous respiration. A preformed RAE (Ring, Adair and Elwyn) tracheal tube or flexible LMA may be used. Careful insertion of the operative mouth gag is vital in either technique. The gag may be too long or too short, causing compression of either the tracheal tube or the LMA. After gag insertion a manual check for ease of lung inflation is mandatory to ensure unobstructed ventilation, before the operation is allowed to proceed. A major advantage of the LMA is that it can be left in place to secure and protect the airway during recovery until the patient's reflexes return; this circumvents the need to choose between tracheal extubation at a deep plane of anaesthesia (leaving the airway unprotected) and awake extubation (with a risk of coughing or laryngeal spasm) [21]. Postoperatively patients should be left undisturbed in the recovery, with a bite block *in situ* and the cuff inflated, until they remove the LMA themselves. Alternatively, the LMA may be removed before there is any biting and an oropharyngeal airway inserted instead.

In contrast, patients with OSA should be managed using a muscle relaxant, tracheal intubation, IPPV at a light plane of anaesthesia and minimal opioids, so that they can be wide awake at the end of surgery. A pattern of ventilation using permissive hypercapnia (end-tidal carbon dioxide concentration [$ETCO_2$] 6–7 kPa) will facilitate recovery. Laryngeal mask airway anaesthesia should be avoided in these children, as the upper airway is small and the mask may impede the surgical view.

Prophylaxis for PONV is essential [22]. An opioid, paracetamol and NSAIDs [10] should be given intraoperatively. Infiltration of the tonsil bed with 0.25 per cent L-bupivacaine has been advocated, but a systematic review failed to find evidence of efficacy in the postoperative period [23]. Intracapsular tonsillectomy may be associated with significantly less postoperative pain [24].

Blood volume should be calculated (75 mL/kg) and losses should be monitored. Direct vision unipolar suction diathermy for adenoidectomy and low-energy bipolar diathermy dissection for tonsillectomy minimise blood loss [16]. Perioperative fluids should be given and intravenous access must be left *in situ* in case of immediate postoperative bleeding. Patients undergoing adenotonsillectomy should be recovered in a head-down position and on their side until awake.

POSTOPERATIVE CARE

An NSAID and paracetamol are given regularly for postoperative analgesia combined with codeine as required. There are concerns that NSAIDs may increase the incidence of post-tonsillectomy haemorrhage. Meta-analyses [25] suggest that 2 patients out of 100 may require re-operation for bleeding if they receive an NSAID, but at a price of more PONV in those not given an NSAID [10]. However, post-tonsillectomy bleeding is multifactorial, the incidence varying significantly with surgical technique (blunt dissection and ties lowest risk, unipolar dissection highest risk) [16]. Further studies are needed, but, in the absence of contraindications, NSAIDs can be given [26].

Non-steroidal anti-inflammatory drugs are contraindicated in patients with reduced platelet function or those in whom postoperative bleeding may be hazardous [27]. They should be avoided in children with brittle asthma, especially where there is a history of hospital admission, and in children with severe eczema, multiple allergies and nasal polyps [10]. Many mild asthmatics can take NSAIDs with no ill effect [27] or change in lung function [28].

Tonsillectomy is often performed on a day-care basis, with patients remaining in hospital for 5–12 hours of observation. In contrast, children with UAO and OSA are at risk of apnoea and hypoxaemia in the postoperative period and require careful observation using continuous pulse oximetry. Overnight observation is mandatory for the young (<2 years), and those with severe UAO, cor pulmonale, craniofacial hypoplasia, hypotonia or morbid obesity. In those with severe OSA, a nasopharyngeal airway should be placed, under direct vision, at the end of surgery and kept for 12–24 h. On occasion admission to a paediatric intensive care unit (PICU) for CPAP or even intubation may be needed. Hypoxaemic respiratory drive may be important in patients with severe OSA and oxygen should be administered judiciously after discharge from the PICU.

POSTOPERATIVE BLEEDING

Bleeding following tonsillectomy may occur within a few hours of surgery (primary) or at 7–10 days postoperatively (secondary). The incidence is 0.5–2 per cent depending upon the surgical technique [16] and the principles of management are identical for both.

Early signs of blood loss include pallor, slow capillary refill (>1 second) and tachycardia. Restlessness, confusion and hypotension are late signs and suggest significant loss. Large amounts of blood may be swallowed, leading to an underestimate of losses. A full blood count, clotting screen

Table 33.3 Preparation of the operating theatre for a child with post-tonsillectomy haemorrhage

Two suction devices with wide bore tubing, turned on and available for immediate use
Three folding laryngoscopes with the correct size of blade, all open and ready for use
Age-appropriate tracheal tube, half size smaller and larger – two of each size
Wide-bore nasogastric tubes
Surgical assistant scrubbed and ready with all instruments
Surgeon scrubbed and ready

and blood crossmatch should be performed. Although a return to theatre must not be delayed, resuscitation using crystalloid, colloid or blood must be achieved before induction of anaesthesia, as cardiovascular collapse will occur with the onset of anaesthesia in a hypovolaemic child.

Aside from hypovolaemia, anaesthesia is problematic because the child may have a stomach full of blood; moreover active bleeding may make laryngoscopy and intubation difficult. Preparation of the theatre is outlined in Table 33.3.

There is little agreement on the safest technique of anaesthesia for a bleeding tonsil; the anaesthetist should adopt an approach with which they are comfortable, cognisant of the potential hazards. Induction in a head-down, lateral position on the operating table is considered ideal. A rapid sequence induction with pre-oxygenation and cricoid pressure is advocated by some, while others prefer an inhalational induction with sevoflurane in oxygen. If using inhalation, when the child is anaesthetised a laryngoscope blade can be gently introduced to check for bleeding, after which suxamethonium may be given and cricoid pressure applied until the trachea is intubated. Facemask ventilation should be avoided as it may precipitate regurgitation of blood from the stomach.

During the operation further fluid and blood should be given as required; near-patient testing can help guide transfusion requirements. Before termination of anaesthesia, a wide-bore orogastric tube should be passed in an attempt to empty the stomach. Extubation should be in a lateral, head-down position with the child wide awake.

Choanal atresia

Choanal atresia is a membranous or bony occlusion of the posterior nares with an incidence of 1:8000 births [29]. It may be unilateral, when presentation is often delayed. Bilateral obstruction may cause acute respiratory distress in neonates as they are obligate nasal breathers. An oral airway and an orogastric tube should be inserted and taped to the face (Fig. 33.1). Surgery is undertaken within 1–2 days. Other anomalies are common (e.g. CHARGE syndrome)

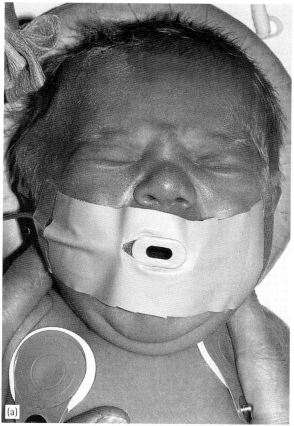

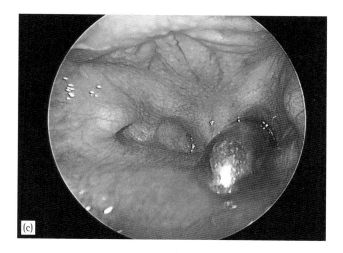

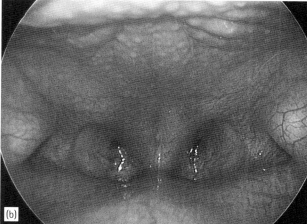

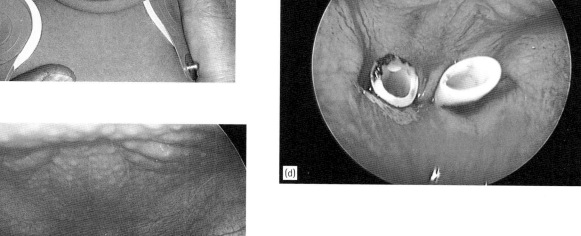

Figure 33.1 (a) Infant with choanal atresia: a Guedel airway is strapped into the oropharynx through which the baby breathes. Surgery is undertaken on the next available routine list and involves an examination of the nasopharynx, (b) confirmation of the diagnosis, (c) perforation of the membrane, and (d) drilling and insertion of stents through which the baby breathes. (Images courtesy of D M Albert FRCS.)

and thorough preoperative assessment including echocardiography is needed.

Surgery involves dividing the membrane; where there is bony occlusion a passageway is drilled. In the latter case, bleeding can be significant despite intraoperative use of topical adrenaline and a preoperative request for group and save serum should be made. Standard techniques for neonatal anaesthesia should be employed, using a muscle relaxant, tracheal intubation (RAE tracheal tube), IPPV and analgesia (paracetamol with codeine). A throat pack is not used, as it obstructs the surgical view. Patency of the new nasal passageway is ensured by the insertion of nasopharyngeal stents fashioned from standard tracheal tubes. These require regular suctioning and are left *in situ* for 8 weeks. Re-stenosis is common (20 per cent) and patients may return for further surgical correction.

Multilocular lymphangioma

Multilocular lymphangioma (cystic hygroma) is a malformation resulting in the development of multiple cystic swellings in the neck, which commonly involve the tongue and oropharynx. Intraoral involvement may lead to respiratory embarrassment and OSA. Laryngoscopy and intubation may be difficult, severe cases requiring tracheostomy. Intraoral disease may be treated with the CO_2 laser, the scler-osant OK-432 can be injected into macrocystic disease [30], while surgical excision may be needed. Requirements for anaesthesia include the management of a potentially difficult intubation and blood loss during surgical excision.

DIAGNOSTIC AND THERAPEUTIC ENDOSCOPY

Diagnostic and therapeutic microlaryngoscopy and bronchoscopy (MLB) is central to paediatric ENT surgery.

Diagnostic endoscopy

Microlaryngoscopy and bronchoscopy is performed in children with mild-to-moderate airway obstruction (see Table 33.1). Most obstructed children present with stridor and the history and examination will direct appropriate preoperative investigations (e.g. chest X-ray, lateral neck X-ray, barium swallow and echocardiography). Previous tracheal intubation may have given rise to airway pathology (e.g. cricoarytenoid fixation, subglottic stenosis, tracheal stenosis), while surgery may have resulted in injury (e.g. recurrent laryngeal nerve palsy during ligation of a patent ductus arteriosus); where possible, a full medical summary should be obtained. Optimal anaesthesia for MLB requires an understanding of the likely pathology and the under-lying medical condition.

SURGICAL REQUIREMENTS

Many common abnormalities of the paediatric airway are dynamic (e.g. laryngomalacia, tracheomalacia and vocal cord palsy). In order to make a diagnosis the surgeon needs a still larynx, unobstructed by a tracheal tube, with preservation of spontaneous respiration. The depth of anaes-thesia may need to be varied rapidly, as accurate assessments of dynamic pathology need the patient to be almost awake yet not prone to laryngeal spasm. This is normally achieved by spontaneous ventilation using a volatile anaesthetic in oxygen, combined with topical anaesthesia.

Formerly MLB was divided into two separate examinations: first, laryngoscopy using a suspension laryngoscope and operating microscope (Fig. 33.2) and, second, a tracheobronchoscopy using a Stortz ventilating bronchoscope (Fig. 33.3). Increasingly, surgeons prefer a unified examination, simply passing the Hopkins rod (see Fig. 33.2b,c) through the

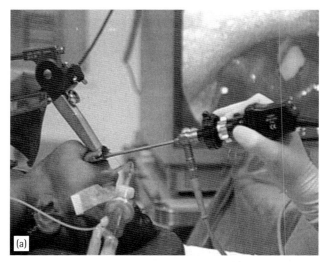

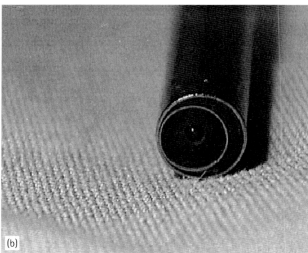

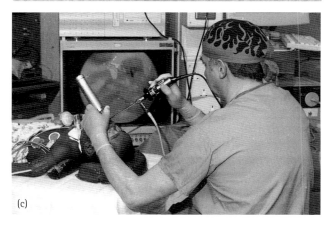

Figure 33.2   (a) Suspension laryngoscope in place for microlaryngoscopy. (b,c) Increasingly surgeons are preferring to undertake microlaryngobronchoscopy using only the Hopkins rod telescope (b) with a folding laryngoscope. (Images courtesy of D M Albert FRCS.)

larynx into the trachea and bronchi. Hopkins rods are available in 0 and 30° view; the latter is preferred for laryngoscopy. Suspension laryngoscopy and use of the bronchoscope are increasingly reserved for therapeutic procedures.

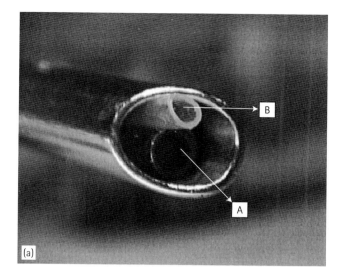

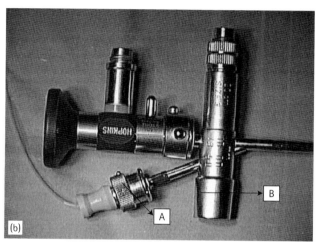

Figure 33.3 Stortz ventilating bronchoscope with Hopkins rod telescope. (a) The bevelled tip with telescope (A) and suction catheter (B). (b) The viewing lens, the body of the instrument and the side arm for instruments or suction (A) and a further side arm (B) for the anaesthesia circuit. (Images courtesy of D M Albert FRCS.)

PREPARATION

Anaesthesia for MLB in a child with upper airway obstruction is hazardous and requires a high level of expertise from all members of the operating team. A wide range of anaesthesia equipment must be available (Table 33.4); items may be needed at very short notice. Bronchoscopes of an age-appropriate size must be ready for use (Table 33.5); because they are available in two lengths (20 and 30 cm) the surgeon must indicate which is required. Both the surgeon and scrub team must be ready, before commencement of anaesthesia.

ANAESTHESIA

Patients should be premedicated with an antimuscarinic (see page 502); by controlling secretions the incidence of coughing, breath-holding and laryngospasm may be reduced. Preservation of spontaneous respiration is an important principle during induction of anaesthesia in children with airway obstruction. Muscle relaxants should be avoided until it is clear that reliable manual inflation of the lungs is possible. Inhalational induction using sevoflurane in 100 per cent O_2 is the method of choice [31]. Once consciousness is lost CPAP is often needed to maintain the airway and improve gas exchange [32]. Where there is significant airway obstruction, minute ventilation will be reduced and induction of anaesthesia will be prolonged. It may take several minutes to achieve a sufficient depth of anaesthesia to permit laryngoscopy; loss of tone in the abdominal musculature is a good clinical sign. While induction is in progress, intravenous access is obtained and a decision on the use of neuromuscular relaxants is made. Short-acting relaxants enable application of topical anaesthesia without causing laryngeal spasm. If mask ventilation is difficult relaxants should not be given; instead anaesthesia should be deepened until it is possible to view the larynx. An alternative approach using a combination of propofol (200–400 µg/kg/min) with remifentanil (0.05–0.1 µg/kg/min) has been described [33]. Where patients have an existing tracheostomy, most elect for induction of anaesthesia by inhalation via the tracheostomy tube.

Lidocaine (3–5 mg/kg, maximum 160 mg) is sprayed onto the glottis and vallecula and into the trachea [34]. A metered dose of 10 per cent lidocaine spray may be used with each spray delivering 10 mg of drug. Accuracy of dosing is difficult to achieve in patients <5 kg and topical lidocaine 1 per cent or 4 per cent may be delivered using a mucosal atomisation device (MADgic; Wolfe Tory Medical, Inc., Salt Lake City, UT, USA). If relaxants are not used the risk of laryngeal spasm is high unless the depth of anaesthesia is assessed carefully.

MICROLARYNGOSCOPY

If a unified examination is proposed, surgical preference is for the trachea not to be intubated as laryngeal trauma can occur even in an apparently effortless and atraumatic intubation [35]. Instead, spontaneous respiration is re-established, a nasopharyngeal airway is passed into the posterior pharyngeal space and anaesthesia is maintained by insufflation of 100 per cent oxygen and a volatile agent.

If a formal suspension laryngoscopy is planned, a naso-tracheal tube may be inserted and anaesthesia is continued in a similar manner with the tracheal tube withdrawn from the larynx once the laryngoscope is in place. Sevoflurane or halothane can be used for maintenance of anaesthesia; both decrease tidal volume in a dose-dependent manner but sevoflurane causes a greater decrease in respiratory rate [36]. If airway obstruction occurs the lower solubility of sevoflurane can lead to unwanted lightening of anaesthesia in the middle of the examination. The cardiovascular profile of sevoflurane is better than that of halothane; it does not sensitise the heart to catecholamines, fewer dysrythmias

Table 33.4 Suggested anaesthetic equipment for microlaryngoscopy and bronchoscopy in children

Item	Equipment	Sizes
Airways	Guedel	0–3
	LMA	1–3
Folding laryngoscopes	Miller	
	Macintosh	Small, medium, large
	McCoy	Paediatric/adult
	Bullard	Paediatric/adult
	Fibre-optic	
Tracheal tubes	Standard	2–9
	Preformed nasotracheal	3–6
	Shouldered neonatal resuscitation (Cole)	1.5–2.5
	Laser tubes	3–6
	Flexo-metallic tracheal tubes (plain and cuffed)	3–8
	Tracheostomy tubes (neonatal and paediatric)	2.5–8
Bougies	Gum elastic (single use)	
Cricothyroidotomy	Cricothyroidotomy needle and cannula with 15 mm connector	18G
Fully equipped difficult intubation trolley		

LMA, laryngeal mask airway.

Table 33.5 Sizes and dimensions of Stortz ventilating bronchoscope and tracheal tubes for microlaryngoscopy and bronchoscopy in smaller children*

Age	Airway diameter at cricoid (mm)	Tracheal tube		Bronchoscope		
		ID (mm)	ED (mm)	size	ID (mm)	ED (mm)
Premature	4.0	2.5–3.0	3.5–4.0	2.5	3.2	4.0
Term neonate	4.5	3.0–3.5	4.0–4.9	3.0	4.2	5.0
6 months	5.0	3.5–4.0	4.9–5.4	3.0	4.2	5.0
1 year	5.5	4.0–4.5	5.4–6.2	3.5	4.9	5.7
2 years	6.0	4.5–5.0	6.2–6.9	3.5	4.9	5.7
3 years	7.0	5.0–5.5	6.9–7.4	4.0	5.9	6.7
5 years	8.0	5.5–6.0	7.4–7.9	5.0	7.0	7.8

*The bronchoscope size refers to the nominal internal diameter (ID), between the Hopkins rod and the outer telescope, the actual ID, is greater. ED, external diameter.

are seen, bradycardia is observed much less often and depression of myocardial contractility is less (see Chapter 10). Lack of sensitisation to catecholamines is advantageous as topical adrenaline is frequently used by surgeons to limit bleeding and reduce oedema in the airway. An alternative approach is to use an infusion of propofol and remifentanil, which has the advantage of avoiding atmospheric pollution. The surgeon can be exposed to undesirably high concentrations of volatile drug when an insufflation technique is used.

The use of 100 per cent oxygen ensures that the oxygen reserves are as high as possible in all patients, even in the premature infant where the risks of hypoxia during the examination are more significant than the risk of retinopathy of prematurity. Close monitoring is essential to detect hypoxia and hypoventilation or excessively light anaesthesia. At the end of the examination anaesthesia is stopped, 100 per cent oxygen is continued and the larynx is observed until the patient is virtually awake. This dynamic examination will reveal vocal cord palsy and laryngomalacia (Fig. 33.4).

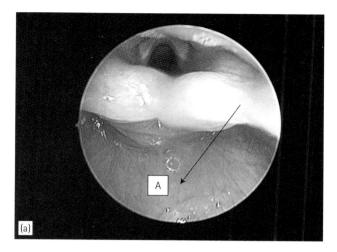

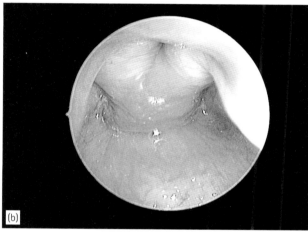

Figure 33.4 (a) Laryngomalacia is a common finding in infants with inspiratory stridor; the aryepiglottic folds are short (A), so the arytenoids are relatively anterior on expiration. (b) On inspiration the arytenoids are drawn into the glottis by the inspiratory airflow, giving rise to turbulence, from which stridor originates. The diagnostic importance of using an anaesthetic technique that maintains spontaneous respiration can be understood. (Images courtesy of D M Albert FRCS.)

BRONCHOSCOPY

The majority of diagnostic ENT bronchoscopies are now undertaken using just the Hopkins rod and anaesthesia continues as described above. On occasion, a full bronchoscopic examination is needed. The inhalational method of anaesthesia is ideal for infants and small children but alternative techniques may be better for prolonged endoscopy in older children (see below).

The correct size and length of a Stortz ventilating bronchoscope will be determined by the size of the patient (Table 33.5). A side arm allows attachment of an anaesthetic T-piece (for use in infants and small child) (see Fig. 33.3). Once the Hopkins rod is in place a closed system exists, allowing ventilation to occur in the annular space between the telescope and the surrounding bronchoscope. A 'spaghetti' suction catheter can also be passed through another side arm on the instrument. Resistance is high in the smaller bronchoscopes, significantly increasing the work of breathing (particularly for infants). Furthermore, resistance increases with the length of the instrument: at a 3 L/min flow rate the resistance of a 30 cm 3.5 bronchoscope is four times that of a 20 cm model [37].

Anaesthesia is continued using oxygen and a volatile agent delivered through a T-piece connected to the side arm or by total intravenous anaesthesia (TIVA) [38]. Assisted ventilation may be needed, especially for infants. Resistance to expiration is high and air trapping can occur unless a long expiratory phase is allowed. It may be necessary to remove the telescope temporarily and allow unobstructed ventilation through the empty bronchoscope.

Fibre-optic endoscopy can be used in the diagnosis of upper airway obstruction, more commonly by respiratory physicians or interventional radiologists. Anaesthesia is best conducted with an LMA or facemask using bronchoscopic swivel mount [39].

Therapeutic endoscopy

A wide range of therapeutic operations are performed on the airway, often in patients with significant airway obstruction. Some procedures can be lengthy and different approaches to anaesthesia may be needed.

OPTIONS FOR ANAESTHESIA

Short therapeutic operations can be performed by continuation of the insufflation technique described above or TIVA (propofol 10–20 mg/kg/h and alfentanil 20–30 μg/kg/h) with spontaneous respiration of oxygen enriched air [40]. Alternatively, an apnoeic oxygenation technique can be employed in which muscle relaxants are given, anaesthesia is maintained by TIVA and a small tracheal tube is passed for ventilation with oxygen. When the surgeon is ready, the tracheal tube is withdrawn and surgery proceeds until ventilation is needed. Repeated interruptions to surgery and trauma from repeated intubations are disadvantages of this approach.

Venturi jet ventilation delivers gas intermittently using an 18 G or 16 G needle attached to the suspension laryngoscope or placed in the trachea [41]. With each delivery, surrounding air is entrained, increasing the volume and reducing the pressure of gas reaching the patient's lungs. Inflation pressures of approximately 120 kPa at the needle tip are reduced to 30 cmH$_2$O in the mid-trachea, which results in visible chest movement. Both TIVA and muscle relaxants are given. The cannula must be aligned with the larynx and the glottis must be unobstructed at all times. Barotrauma and gastric distension are recognised complications. High-frequency positive pressure ventilation using a transglottic or percutaneous transtracheal catheter driven by specific jet ventilation can be used in children [42]. Total

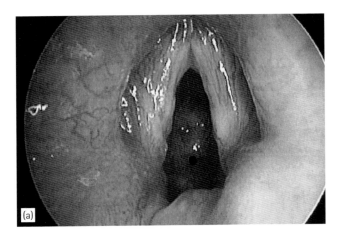

Classification	From	To
Grade I	No obstruction	50% obstruction
Grade II	51% obstruction	70% obstruction
Grade III	71% obstruction	99% obstruction
Grade IV	No detectable lumen	

(b)

Figure 33.5   (a) Organised subglottic stenosis in an ex-premature infant who received respiratory support for 4 weeks after birth. (b) This would be graded as III in the Meyer–Cotton classification [43] of subglottic stenosis, redrawn with permission from Lippincott Williams & Williams. (Image courtesy of D M Albert FRCS.)

intravenous anaesthesia with muscle paralysis is required to ensure a clear glottis.

OPERATIONS ON THE LARYNX

Laryngomalacia may cause infantile failure to thrive as feeding is difficult because of airway obstruction. In an aryepiglottoplasty, redundant mucosa is trimmed from the arytenoids and the aryepiglottic folds with the aim of stopping the arytenoids being drawn into the glottic opening on inspiration. Surgery can usually be performed using insufflation anaesthesia with the tracheal tube withdrawn into the pharynx.

Supraglottic cysts arise from the vallecula and are normally single. Classically, children present with symptoms of intermittent obstruction and treatment involves deroofing and marsupialisation of the cyst base. Relaxants are avoided as the cyst may act as a ball valve, making controlled ventilation impossible. The laryngeal inlet is usually posterior to the cyst, but the glottic opening may be hard to visualise in patients with large cysts, where bubbling associated with air movement may be the only clue. Needle aspiration of the cyst may assist visualisation and permit intubation. Patients should be wide awake before extubation.

Subglottic stenosis (SGS) usually presents with stridor and may be 'soft' with multiple small cysts apparent just below the vocal cords or 'organised' when fibrosis results in concentric narrowing. The degree of narrowing is classified according to the Meyer–Cotton system (Fig. 33.5) [43]. Endoscopic repair may be attempted in grade I and II lesions. In 'soft' deroofing of the cysts with cupped forceps is performed to relieve the obstruction, while radial cuts supplemented by balloon dilatation are used for 'organised' SGS.

The airway may be difficult to maintain as the subglottis tends to close in the absence of CPAP. These patients are often well served by intubation using a fine (1.5 or 2.0 mm) Cole neonatal resuscitation tube, which allows a suitable plane of anaesthesia to be achieved. Thereafter, the tube may be withdrawn to permit surgery; intermittent reintubation may be needed.

Insufflation anaesthesia with a volatile agent, spontaneous respiration and a pharyngeal airway is indicated. Inflation of the balloon in the subglottis results in complete airway obstruction and the maximal inflation time should be 30–45 seconds, allowing ample time for recovery before repetition. Open surgical repair will be required for grade III and IV SGS (see page 513).

Squamous papillomatosis caused by the human papilloma virus (HPV) types 6 and 11 gives rise to cauliflower-like lesions, normally arising from the vocal folds but which may be present throughout the tracheobronchial tree. Children present with voice change and/or inspiratory stridor; treatment is aimed at removing the lesions and maintaining the airway while awaiting the development of immunity. Recently, the microdebrider has been used for their removal but standard treatment involves the use of the CO_2 or potassium titanyl phosphate (KTP) laser [44]. For laryngeal lesions the CO_2 laser is used with the aid of an operating microscope. Tracheobronchial lesions are treated with the KTP laser, using a fibre-optic cable inserted through the side arm of the ventilating bronchoscope. Laser therapy allows precise tissue vaporisation and coagulation with minimal damage to surrounding tissues. Precautions to protect the patient and theatre team are outlined in Table 33.6.

Fire in the airway during laser therapy is a particular risk and practitioners must be aware of this hazard [45,46]. Should this occur the tracheal tube (if present) should be removed, the anaesthetic circuit disconnected and ventilation

Table 33.6 Standard precautions for the use of lasers in the operating theatre

	Hazard	Action
Patient	Inadvertent burn	Lubricant in eyes
		Cover eyes with moist gauze
		Cover head with moist gauze swabs
	Airway fire	Use air–minimal O_2 mixture consistent with adequate oxygenation
		Use laser metal tracheal and tracheostomy tubes
		Fill tracheal tube cuffs with 0.9% saline
		Ensure that surgical pledglets are moist
		Remove all charred material from the airway
Theatre team	Direct beam impact	Use matt instruments to avoid reflection
		Laser-specific eye protection
		Theatre doors shut and windows covered
	Viral particles in laser smoke	Use high-volume filtered smoke extractor
		Wear laser surgical masks

stopped. Saline or water is used to extinguish the fire, after which ventilation can be resumed. The degree of injury should be assessed and supportive care given as indicated, which may include tracheostomy or intubation and IPPV in a PICU.

The choice of anaesthesia technique will depend upon the clinical status of the patient, and local surgical and anaesthetic preferences. Good topical anaesthesia is essential and analgesia is provided by paracetamol and NSAIDs. Codeine (1 mg/kg) may be prescribed as rescue analgesia.

Subglottic haemangioma may on first inspection appear similar to SGS, with significant airway narrowing. The haemangioma is usually soft and compressible, distinguishing it from SGS. Systemic steroid therapy is often given. Endoscopic treatment includes direct steroid injection with elective postoperative intubation and CO_2 laser therapy. Anaesthesia should follow standard lines for therapeutic endoscopy. Open surgical excision by anterior cricolaryngotomy is managed in a similar manner to single-stage laryngotracheal reconstruction (see below).

Laryngeal cleft is a deficiency of the posterior wall of the larynx which prevents competent glottic closure when swallowing; children present with a history suggestive of recurrent aspiration [47]. The cleft may extend a variable length

into the trachea, but interarytenoid or partial cricoid clefts can be repaired endoscopically. A flexo-metallic orotracheal tube is used with muscle relaxants, IPPV and a volatile agent. The suspension laryngoscope allows surgical access to the posterior larynx. When the cleft extends below the level of the cricoid open repair is indicated (see page 515).

OPERATIONS IN THE TRACHEA

Therapeutic procedures in the trachea will be undertaken using the ventilating bronchoscope, employing any of the anaesthetic techniques outlined above.

Removal of an inhaled foreign body merits special consideration as it is common. Inhalation of a foreign body usually occurs between the age of 1 and 3 years; it is more common in boys [48]. The episode is often witnessed; an episode of choking is usually followed by a bout of coughing. Hoaresness and/or stridor suggest that the foreign body is impacted in the larynx; passage into the trachea or main bronchi may cause wheeze or unilaterally reduced breath sounds. Misdiagnosis and treatment for asthma are not uncommon [49]. However, many children may exhibit no obvious signs immediately after the inhalation and if the diagnosis is not to be missed a high index of suspicion is essential, based upon the history [48]. In the UK, peanuts are the most common objects to be inhaled; the nut oil causes mucosal irritation with oedema and pneumonitis distal to the obstruction.

If radio-opaque the foreign body may be seen on chest X-ray (CXR), but the majority are radiolucent. Inspiration and expiration films are required as hyperinflation may be seen on the affected side [50] but a normal CXR does not exclude the diagnosis [51]. In later presentations, collapse and consolidation may be seen distal to the obstruction.

The approach to anaesthesia is the same as diagnostic bronchoscopy. Atropine pre-medication, gaseous induction using oxygen and an inhalational agent, with topical anaesthesia, are satisfactory. If there is respiratory distress urgent bronchoscopy is indicated, otherwise the procedure should wait for an appropriate fasting period. A smooth technique using deep anaesthesia and avoidance of coughing is essential; intubation should be avoided if the foreign body is in or near the larynx, while IPPV is best avoided if the foreign body is in the trachea or creating a ball–valve obstruction [31].

A 30 cm ventilating bronchoscope with Hopkins rod and grasping forceps is used. Application of topical adrenaline (1:10 000) to the area of impaction is useful to reduce oedema and facilitate removal. Ventilation may need to be gently assisted if the bronchoscope is in a main bronchus for a prolonged period. Side holes in the Storz bronchoscope assist proximal ventilation.

Once the object has been firmly grasped in the forceps, the whole instrument is slowly removed from the airway under vision, ensuring that the foreign body does not fall out of the forceps. Once the bronchoscope has been removed anaesthesia is maintained by mask, while awaiting reinsertion to confirm full removal. When withdrawing the bronchoscope with the foreign body, there is a danger of losing the object either in the trachea or in the larynx, causing total obstruction to ventilation. Should this occur the bronchoscope should be passed, pushing the object into the trachea until satisfactory ventilation can be re-established.

A nasogastric tube may be passed if it is considered that the stomach is full; moreover, a tracheal tube can be inserted and the patient extubated once fully awake.

Insertion of tracheal or bronchial stents may be required in children who have stenosis of the trachea or the main bronchi. Patients may have severe airway obstruction and may have already undergone complex surgery (e.g. slide tracheoplasty or lung transplantation). Fibre-optic bronchoscopes are used and inhalational anaesthesia is managed with an LMA or facemask using a bronchoscopic swivel mount.

POST-ANAESTHESIA CARE

Meticulous observation in the PACU is essential following diagnostic or therapeutic endoscopy. Airway oedema as a result of intervention or instrumentation is common and children may develop respiratory distress with stridor. All patients undergoing therapeutic endoscopy and those in whom instrumentation may have been difficult should receive dexamethasone (0.25 mg/kg initial dose, thereafter 0.1 µg/kg every 6 hours). Stridor in the PICU may also require nebulised adrenaline (1:1000, 5 mL); the ECG should be monitored during administration, which should temporarily cease if the heart rate is >190 beats/minute. Patients with a tracheostomy should receive humidified oxygen following the examination.

TRACHEOSTOMY

Tracheostomy is indicated for congenital or acquired airway obstruction, to facilitate long-term respiratory support or in the presence of a neurological abnormality [52]. Children with UAO should receive antimuscarinic premedication and receive an inhalational induction with sevoflurane or halothane in oxygen. Intravenous access is obtained and full monitoring applied. Relaxants should be avoided unless reliable manual IPPV can be achieved. Patients with SGS may be difficult to intubate and a full range of equipment and tracheal tubes must be available. Cole pattern, shouldered, neonatal tracheal tubes are more rigid than the smallest 2.0 tracheal tube and are easier to pass in patients with grade II and III SGS. Some patients (e.g. those with Pierre Robin syndrome) are impossible to intubate; anaesthesia is maintained using oxygen, a volatile agent and spontaneous respiration, while the airway is maintained using an LMA or facemask. On rare occasions it is impossible to maintain the airway, the patient is awoken and the tracheostomy performed under local anaesthesia.

A secure airway allows the use of muscle relaxants, IPPV and a volatile agent. Respiratory obstruction may occur during surgery and hand ventilation permits early detection. The patient is positioned with the head extended

Table 33.7 Potential complications of tracheostomy in children. A complication can occur at any time, but is usually seen at the time indicated

Time	Complication
Immediate (first few hours)	Bleeding
	Surgical emphysema
	Pneumothorax
	Pneumomediatsinum
	Oesophageal injury
	Damage to recurrent laryngeal nerve
Intermediate (first 10 days)	Tube dislodgement
	Obstruction with crusted secretions
	Bleeding
	Local infection
Longer term	Granuloma formation (often tube tip)
	Vascular erosion
	Tracheo-oesophageal fistula
	Suprastomal collapse
	Tracheal stenosis

using a sandbag under the shoulders; strapping is passed around the chin and secured to the operating table, thereby stretching the neck skin and stabilising the head. Infiltration with lidocaine 1 per cent and 1:200 000 adrenaline is made and the trachea identified by dissection. The second and third tracheal rings are identified and two-stay sutures are inserted on either side of the planned tracheal incision. These sutures are taped to the chest at the end of the operation and are not removed until the first tube change 1 week later. They are vital for the patient's postoperative safety: if the tracheostomy tube falls out these sutures are used to pull the trachea to the surface permitting tube reinsertion.

Before the tracheal incision is made 100 per cent oxygen is given and the proposed tracheostomy tube and connector is checked. Standard tracheostomy tubes (Portex, Shiley or Bivona) with 15 mm connectors are used. Once the trachea has been incised, the tracheal tube is withdrawn into the upper trachea and the tracheostomy tube is placed. The anaesthesia circuit is connected to the tracheostomy tube and ventilation is checked (auscultation of the chest, end-tidal CO_2) to confirm correct placement. At the end of surgery the head is taken out of extension and tracheostomy tapes are passed around the neck to secure the tube.

Postoperatively a CXR is taken to confirm correct tube placement and to exclude a pneumothorax. Warmed humidified air/oxygen, using elephant tubing and tracheostomy mask, is given to neonates and infants; cold humidity is used for older children. This is combined with regular sterile suctioning with saline irrigation (1–2 mL) to ensure that crusting and blockage do not occur. A spare tracheostomy tube, tapes and dilators are kept near the patient. Humidification can usually stop after the first tube change and a Swedish nose is used instead.

Tracheostomy can be fatal and must never be underestimated [52]; potential complications are given in Table 33.7.

OPEN OPERATIONS ON THE LARYNX AND TRACHEA

Endoscopic treatment of SGS is appropriate for Meyer and Cotton grade I or II; more severe lesions require open surgery.

Anterior cricoid split

This operation is used in children with SGS, often those unable to be extubated in the PICU, but who are otherwise well with no pulmonary disease [53]. Positioning of the head is the same as for a tracheostomy; the trachea is dissected, after which the cricoid cartilage, and first and second tracheal rings are divided in the midline anteriorly. Anaesthesia with tracheal intubation, a muscle relaxant, an opioid and IPPV by hand is appropriate. Following the split a nasotracheal tube of a larger size is passed with the tube tip position just distal to the lowest divided ring; this acts as a tracheal stent for 5–10 days. A nasogastric tube is passed. Patients are cared for in the PICU where meticulous attention to the tracheal tube is needed. Blockage or accidental extubation is hazardous, as attempts at reintubation can result in the bevel being pushed through the anterior tracheal wall, creating a false passage. Should extubation occur, nasotracheal reintubation should not be attempted in the PICU as the angle of tracheal tube passing through the larynx from the nose encourages anterior perforation through the surgical division. The airway should be supported with a mask, oxygenation ensured and orotracheal intubation attempted. Afterwards, the patient can be returned to theatre for nasotracheal intubation in controlled circumstances. At 5–10 days extubation can be attempted using steroid cover.

Laryngotracheal reconstruction

This involves a similar approach to the cricoid split, but instead opens the larynx anteriorly and posteriorly if required. Harvested rib cartilage is interposed into the anterior and posterior split, thereby increasing the diameter of the airway [54] (Fig. 33.6). If performed as a single-stage procedure, with no covering tracheostomy, the anaesthetic and PICU considerations are the same as those for the cricoid split, including the caveat regarding reintubation. If a posterior graft is needed a sterile, cuffed, flexo-metallic tracheal tube is placed by the surgeon in the trachea distal to the graft site; ventilation is continued in this manner until just before the anterior graft is ready to be placed. At this point a larger nasotracheal tube is passed with the tip positioned just

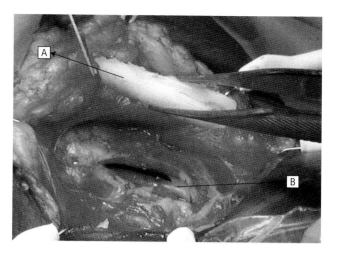

Figure 33.6 Laryngotracheal reconstruction is undertaken for severe subglottic stenosis; insertion of a cartilage graft (A) into a laryngofissure increases the diameter of the subglottis. The operation may be performed as a two-stage procedure (in children with a tracheostomy) or as a single-stage operation involving a postoperative stay in a paediatric intensive care unit as seen here. An age-appropriate nasotracheal tube is placed under direct vision for postoperative care (B). (Image courtesy of D M Albert FRCS.)

below the graft site by the surgeon under direct vision. Wet neurosurgical patties can be packed around this tube to create a seal for IPPV. Once the grafts are in place the patient is returned to the PICU for care, as described above. Patients tolerate nasotracheal tubes well and after the first 24–48 hours only minimal sedation is needed.

Laryngotracheal reconstruction is also performed as a two-stage procedure. The child will have a tracheostomy through which anaesthesia is induced; maintenance is with an opioid, muscle relaxant and volatile agent. Intravenous fluids are given and continued postoperatively.

To manage the airway, a cuffed flexo-metallic tracheal tube is inserted through the tracheostoma, after which the anaesthetist should check for equal ventilation. The tube is secured by surgical suture just below the tracheostoma and fixed to the chest away from the side of rib harvesting using a sterile clear dressing. Care is needed during the operation as surgical manipulation can move the tube resulting in extubation or bronchial intubation; the cuff can also be pierced by suturing. Should this happen the surgeon will need to assist with tube positioning and wet neurosurgical patties will create a seal if the cuff ruptures.

A stent is placed in the trachea to support the grafts, after which the anterior larynx is closed. The flexo-metallic tube is removed after careful tracheal suctioning, a tracheo-stomy tube is reinserted and the patient is awoken to be returned to the ordinary ward. Humidified oxygen is given via a tracheostomy mask. A CXR is required to exclude a pneumothorax which may occur as a result of the rib harvest. Analgesia is with paracetamol, an NSAID and morphine by patient- or nurse-controlled analgesia (PCA

Table 33.8   Clinical croup score*

Clinical sign	Score		
	1	2	3
Inspiratory breath sounds	Normal	Harsh with ronchi	Delayed
Stridor	None	Inspiratory	Inspiratory and expiratory
Cough	None	Hoarse cry	Bark
Inspiratory retractions and flaring	None	Flaring and suprasternal retractions	As 2 with subcostal and intercostal retractions
Cyanosis	None	In air	In 40% O_2

*After Downes and Raphaely [58].

or NCA, respectively). A local anaesthetic infusion (approximately 72 h) through an epidural catheter placed in the site of rib harvest can afford useful relief.

Cricotracheal resection

Short segment tracheal resection can be performed for grade III and IV subglottic stenosis [55]. The patient will already have a tracheostomy and the approach to anaesthesia is the same as the two-stage laryngotracheal reconstruction. A segment of trachea is excised and a new cricotracheal anastomosis is made. Difficulties with the temporary, cuffed, flexo-metallic tube are even more likely in this operation.

Long segment tracheal stenosis demands a different approach as the narrowing may extend throughout the trachea and even into the main bronchi [56]. A combined surgical approach (cardiothoracic and ENT) is therefore needed; a slide tracheoplasty is commonly undertaken to treat this rare disease. General anaesthesia with a muscle relaxant and opioid is used; the patient is intubated with an age-appropriate tracheal tube positioned just above the commencement of the stenosis. Total airway obstruction may occur with tracheal tube movement or airway secretions, humidity and suction may be required and careful tube fixation is needed. The operation is performed using cardiopulmonary bypass; central venous access and an arterial line are needed. The internal jugular veins should be avoided for central venous access as the neck may be dissected during surgery; access via the femoral vein is preferred. When the patient is on cardiopulmonary bypass and the trachea is open, the tracheal tube is advanced under direct vision to support the repair. Supportive care in the PICU is needed following surgery.

AIRWAY EMERGENCIES

The management of paediatric airway emergencies is part of the role of the paediatric anaesthetist. The most common conditions are foreign body inhalation (see earlier), acute

viral laryngotracheobronchitis, acute epiglottitis and bacterial tracheitis. There have been substantial changes in the incidence of these illnesses [57]; consequentially experience in their anaesthetic management has declined.

Viral laryngotracheobronchitis (croup) (VLTB), commonly caused by a parainfluenza virus infection, is diagnosed when a URTI gives rise to a barking cough and inspiratory stridor. The degree of respiratory distress can be assessed using a croup score (Table 33.8) [58]. Traditional therapies (humidified air/oxygen, nebulised adrenaline and dexamethasone 0.6 mg/kg), combined with nebulised budesonide [59], have dramatically reduced the severity of this illness. Less than 0.5 per cent of patients with viral croup admitted to hospital require intubation. Respiratory distress in VLTB develops slowly; serial croup scores will reveal the progressive nature of the illness.

Acute epiglottitis (AE) as a result of *Haemophilus influenzae* infection has all but disappeared following immunisation. Recent experience in Northern Ireland suggests that the incidence may be rising, possibly owing to reduced immunisation after safety concerns over the MMR vaccination in the UK [57]. Occasionally, AE is caused by other bacterial infection. Children present with pyrexia and symptoms of a URTI, which progress over a few hours to difficulty in swallowing and talking. Clinical signs include tachycardia, tachypnoea, dyspnoea, drooling and aphonia. They adopt a classic posture, sitting, leaning forward with facial distress. Inspiratory stridor is a late symptom and a portent of total airway obstruction. If the symptoms are not classic and foreign body inhalation is suspected a lateral X-ray of the neck may assist diagnosis, but the child must be accompanied by experienced medical staff as potentially fatal obstruction may occur at any time with little warning.

Bacterial tracheitis (BT) is now the most frequent acute airway emergency requiring intubation and respiratory support in the PICU [57,60]. It may follow an episode of viral croup; the organisms most commonly implicated are *Staphylococcus aureus*, *H. influenzae* and anaerobes [61]. Children present with pyrexia, copious mucopurulent secretions and signs of endotoxinaemia. Secretions can thicken and fibrin casts of the trachea can form, precipitating respiratory failure from airway obstruction.

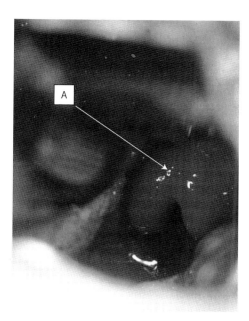

Figure 33.7   Acute epiglottitis: the cherry-red, inflamed epiglottis (A) causes severe airway obstruction, which becomes total with no warning.

Anaesthesia

The principles of airway management outlined above apply in these emergency settings. There is usually no time for atropine premedication; furthermore it is contraindicated in acute epiglottitis as any distress to the child may precipitate total airway obstruction. An ENT surgeon must always be present and the theatre prepared for both MLB and emergency tracheostomy.

Inhalation induction using oxygen and halothane or sevoflurane is the method of choice. Patients with AE will want to remain sitting forward during induction. Intravenous access is obtained after induction, especially in AE after which anaesthesia is slowly deepened using gentle CPAP to maintain airway patency. When deep anaesthesia is achieved, a laryngoscopy is performed. In AE the diagnosis is immediately clear; the whole supraglottic region is inflamed, the epiglottis being cherry red (Fig. 33.7). Indeed, it may be difficult to identify the laryngeal inlet – a clue being the respiratory movements of glottic secretions during respiration. Acute epiglottitis patients should be immed-iately intubated with a smaller nasotracheal tube than would be normal for their age, sedated and moved to the PICU. In VLTB and BT an initial bronchoscopy is performed, using only the Hopkins rod. If the diagnosis is confirmed as VLTB a small-for-age nasotracheal tube is passed, sedation is given and the patient moved to the PICU. In BT a formal bronchoscopy may be needed to clear the trachea of the thick secretions and fibrin casts, after which intubation is undertaken. Muscle relaxants may be used to assist intubation if bag–mask ventilation can be reliably achieved.

Post-anaesthesia care

Antibiotics and supportive care (ventilation, sedation, fluid resuscitation and inotropes) are given in the PICU. Accidental extubation can be fatal in any of these conditions, especially AE; good tube fixation and reliable sedation are important. Humidification of inspired gasses, frequent suctioning and saline irrigation of the tracheal tube are mandatory, especially in BT. As the tracheal tube is smaller than age appropriate it will block easily.

In AE most patients can be extubated after 48 hours if the toxicity has settled and there is a leak around the tube. In VLTB and BT recovery is slower, taking 7–10 days.

REFERENCES

Key references

Anderson BJ. Comparing the efficacy of NASIDs and paracetamol in children. *Paediatr Anaesth* 2004; **14**: 201–17.

Brown K, Aun C, Stocks J, Jackson E, Mackersie A, Hatch D. A comparison of the respiratory effects of sevoflurane and halothane in infants and young children. *Anesthesiology* 1998; **89**: 86–92.

Moiniche S, Romsing J, Dahl JB, Tramer MR. Nonsteroidal antiinflammatory drugs and the risk of operative site bleeding after tonsillectomy: a quantitative systematic review. *Anesth Analg* 2003; **96**: 68–77.

National Prospective Tonsillectomy Audit 2003. London: The Royal College of Surgeons of England, 2005 (http://www.rcseng.ac.uk).

References

1. Mamie C, Habre W, Delhumeau C *et al.* Incidence and risk factors of perioperative respiratory adverse events in children undergoing elective surgery. *Paediatr Anaesth* 2004; **14**: 218–24.

2. Tait AR, Malviya S. Anesthesia for the child with an upper respiratory infection: still a dilemma? *Anesth Analg* 2005; **100**: 59–65.

3. Friesen R, Wurl J, Charlton G. Haemodynamic depression by halothane is age-related in paediatric patients. *Paediatr Anaesth* 2000; **10**: 267–72.

4   Whittet HB, Hayward AW, Battersby E. Plasma lignocaine levels during paediatric endoscopy of the upper respiratory tract. Relatioship with mucosal moistness. *Anaesthesia* 1988; **43**: 439–42.

5. McAuliffe G, Bissonnette B, Cavalle-Garrido T, Boutin C. Heart rate and cardiac output after atropine in anaesthetised infants and children. *Can J Anaesth* 1997; **44**: 154–9.

6. Jöhr M. Is it time to question the routine use of anti-cholinergic agents in paediatric anaesthesia. *Paediatr Anaesth* 1999; **9**: 99–101.

7. Litman RS, Wu CL, Catanzaro FA. Ondansetron decreases emesis after tonsillectomy in children. *Anesth Analg* 1994; **78**: 478–81.

8   Steward DL, Wedge JA, Meyer CM. Steroids for improving recovery following tonsillectomy in children. *Cochrane Database Syst Rev* 2003; (1): CD003997.

9. Anderson BJ. Comparing the efficacy of NASIDs and paracetamol in children. *Paediatr Anaesth* 2004; **14**: 201–17.

10. Lönnqvist PA, Morton NS. Postoperative analgesia in infants and children. *Br J Anaesth* 2005; **95**: 59–68.

11. Kenna MA. Diagnosis and management of otitis media with effusions. In: Cotton RT, Meyer CM III, eds. *Practical pediatric otolaryngology*. Philadelphia: Lippincott-Raven, 1999: 229–46.

12. Paradise JL, Bluestone CD, Rogers KD *et al*. Efficacy of adenoidectomy for recurrent otitis media in children previously treated with tympanostomy tube placement: results of parallel randomised and non-randomised trials. *JAMA* 1990; **263**: 2066.

13. Miyamoto RT, Kirk KI. Controversies in cochlear implantation: technical and surgical considerations. In: Cotton RT, Meyer CM III, eds. *Practical pediatric otolaryngology*. Philadelphia: Lippincott-Raven, 1999: 329–40.

14. Tobias JD. Controlled hypotension in children: a critical review of available agents. *Pediatr Drugs* 2002; **4**: 439–53.

15. Absalom A, Strys MMRF. An overview of TCI and TIVA. Ghent: Academic Press, 2005.

16. National Prospective Tonsillectomy Audit 2003. London: The Royal College of Surgeons of England, 2005 (http://www.rcseng.ac.uk).

17. Rothschild MA. Central and obstructive apnea. In: Cotton RT, Meyer CM III, eds. *Practical pediatric otolaryngology*. Philadelphia: Lippincott-Raven, 1999: 41–58.

18. Clinical Practice Guideline. Diagnosis and management of childhood obstructive sleep apnea syndrome. *Pediatrics* 2002; **109**: 704–12.

19. Brouillette RT, Fernbach J. Obstructive sleep apnea in infants and children. J Pediatr 1982; **100**: 31–40.

20. Siddiqui AK, Ahmed S. Pulmonary manifestations of sickle cell disease. *Postgrad Med J* 2003; **79**: 384–90.

21. Parry M, Glaisyer HR, Bailey PM. Removal of the LMA in children. *Br J Anaesth* 1997; **78**: 337–8.

22. Bolton CM, Myles PS, Nolam T, Sterne JA. Prophylaxis of post-operative vomiting in children undergoing tonsillectomy: a systematic review and meta-analysis. *Br J Anaesth* 2006; **97**: 593–604.

23. Hollis LJ, Burton MJ, Millar JM. Perioperative local anaesthesia for reducing pain following tonsillectomy, 1999 (http://www.cochrane.org/reviews/en/ab001874.html).

24. Isaacson G. Pediatric intracapsular tonsillectomy with bipolar electrosurgical scissors. *ENT J* 2004; **83**: 702–6.

25. Moiniche S, Romsing J, Dahl JB, Tramer MR. Nonsteroidal antiinflammatory drugs and the risk of operative site bleeding after tonsillectomy: a quantitative systematic review. *Anesth Analg* 2003; **96**: 68–77.

26. Cardwell M, Siviter G, Smith A. Non-steroidal anti-inflammatory drugs and perioperative bleeding in paediatric tonsillectomy. *Cochrane Database Syst Rev* 2005; CD003591.

27. Royal College of Anaesthetists. *Guidelines for the use of non-steroidal anti-inflammatory drugs in the perioperative period*. London: Royal College of Anaesthetists, 1998.

28. Short JA, Barr CA, Palmer CD *et al*. Use of diclofenac in children with asthma. *Anaesthesia* 2000; **55**: 334–7.

29. Coates HL. Nasal obstruction in infancy. In: Cotton RT, Meyer CM III, eds. Practical pediatric otolaryngology. Philadelphia: Lippincott-Raven, **1999**: 449–68.

30. Luzzatto C, Midrio P, Tchaprassian Z, Guglielmi M. Sclerosing treatment of lymphangiomas with OK-432. *Arch Dis Child* 2000; **82**: 316–18.

31. Farrell PT. Rigid bronchoscopy for foreign body removal: anaesthesia and ventilation. *Paediatr Anaesth* 2004; **14**: 84–9.

32. Keidan I, Fine GF, Kagawa T *et al*. Work of breathing during spontaneous ventilation in anesthetized children: a comparative study among the face mask, laryngeal mask airway and endotracheal tube. *Anesth Analg* 2000; **91**: 1381–8.

33. Reichert C. Beyond halothane: an update on *Paediatr Anaesth* pharmacology. *Can J Anaesth* 2003; **50**: R1–4.

34. Byers RL, Kidd J, Oppenheim R, Brown TC. Local anaesthetic plasma levels in children. *Anaesth Intensive Care* 1978; **6**: 243–7.

35. Smith OD, Callanan V, Lloyd-Thomas AR, Albert DM. Pseudopolyp of the right laryngeal ventricle following atraumatic intubation: a diagnostic dilemma. *Paediatr Anaesth* 2000; **10**: 559–62.

36. Brown K, Aun C, Stocks J *et al*. A comparison of the respiratory effects of sevoflurane and halothane in infants and young children. *Anesthesiology* 1998; **89**: 86–92.

37. Roberts S, Thornington RE. Paediatric bronchoscopy. *Cont Educ Anaesth Crit Care Pain* 2005; **5**: 41–4.

38. Thaung MK, Balakrishnan A. A modified technique of tubeless anaesthesia for microlaryngoscopy and bronchoscopy in young children with stridor. *Paediatr Anaesth* 1998; **8**: 201–4.

39. Nussbaum E, Zagnoev M. Pediatric fibreoptic bronchoscopy with a laryngeal mask. *Chest* 2001; **120**: 341–2.

40. Kailey J, Cranston A, Moriarty A. Intravenous anaesthesia for laser surgery of the airway in children with recurrent laryngeal papillomatosis. *Paediatr Anaesth* 2002; **12**: 819–20.

41. Grasl MC, Donner A, Schragl E, Aloy A. Tubeless laryngotracheal surgery in infants and children. *Laryngoscope* 1997; **107**: 277–81.

42. Koomen E, Poortmans G, Anderson BJ, Janssens MML. Jet ventilation for laryngotracheal surgery in an ex-premature infant. *Paediatr Anaesth* 2005; **15**: 786–9.

43. Walner DL, Cotton RT. Acquired anomalies of the larynx and trachea. In: Cotton RT, Meyer CM III, eds. *Practical pediatric otolaryngology*. Philadelphia: Lippincott-Raven, **1999**: 515–37.

44. Derkay CS. Recurrent respiratory papillomatosis. In: Cotton RT, Meyer CM III, eds. *Practical pediatric otolaryngology*. Philadelphia: Lippincott-Raven, **1999**: 637–59.

45. Macdonald AG. A brief historical review of non-anaesthetic causes of fires and explosions in the operating room. *Br J Anaesth* 1994; **73**: 847–56.

46. Bruley ME. Surgical fires: perioperative communication is essential to prevent this rare but devastating complication. *Qual Safety Health Care* 2004; **13**: 467–71.

47. Cotton RT, Prescott CAJ. Congenital anomalies of the larynx. In: Cotton RT, Meyer CM III, eds. *Practical pediatric otolaryngology.* Philadelphia: Lippincott-Raven, **1999**: 497–513.

48. Kumar P, Srakar P, Athanasiou T. Inhaled foreign bodies in children. *Diagn Treat Hosp Med* 2003; **64**: 218–22.

49. Lloyd-Thomas AR, Bush GH. All that wheezes is not asthma. *Anaesthesia* 1986; **41**:181–5.

50. Williams H. Inhaled foreign bodies. *Arch Dis Child Educ Pract* 2005; **90**: 31–33.

51. Tokar B, Ozken R, Ilhan H. Tracheobronchial foreign bodies in children: importance of accurate history and plain chest radiography in delayed presentation. *Clin Radiol* 2004; **59**: 609–15.

52. Shinkwin CA, Gibbin KP. Tracheostomy in children. *J R Soc Med* 1996; **89**: 188–92.

53. Eze NN, Wyatt ME, Hartley BE. The role of the anterior cricoid split in facilitating extubation in infants. *Int J Pediatr Otorhinolaryngol* 2005; **69**: 843–46.

54. Wyatt ME, Hartley BE. Laryngotracheal reconstruction in congenital laryngeal webs and atresias. *Otolaryngol Head Neck Surg* 2005; **132**: 232–8.

55. White DR, Cotton RT, Bean JA, Rutter MJ. Pediatric cricotracheal resection: surgical outcomes and risk factor analysis. *Arch Otolaryngol Head Neck Surg* 2005; **131**: 896–9.

56. Kocyildirim E, Kanani M, Roebuck D *et al.* Long segment tracheal stenosis. slide tracheoplasty and a multidisciplinary approach improve outcomes and reduce costs. *J Thorac Cardiovasc Surg* 2004; **128**: 876–82.

57. Devlin B, Golchin K, Adair R. Paediatric airway emergencies in Northern Ireland, 1990–2003. *J Laryngol Otol* 2007; **2**: 1–5.

58. Downes JJ, Raphaely RC. Pediatric intensive care. *Anesthesiology* 1975; **43**: 238–50.

59. Godden CWMJ, Campbell M, Hussey JJ. Cogswell Double blind placebo controlled trial of nebulised budesonide for croup. *Arch Dis Child* 1997; **76**: 155–8.

60. Hopkins A, Lahiri T, Salerno R, Heath B. Changing epidemiology of life-threatening upper airway infections: the re-emergence of bacterial tracheitis. *Pediatrics* 2006; **118**: 1418–21.

61. Brook I. Aerobic and anaerobic microbiology of bacterial tracheitis in children. *Pediatr Emerg Care* 1997; **13**: 16–18.

Eye and dental surgery

IAN JAMES

KEY LEARNING POINTS

- Most ophthalmic anaesthesia is undertaken on a day-care basis.
- Careful anaesthesia and administration of antiemetics are key to avoiding postoperative nausea and vomiting, especially in strabismus surgery.
- Consistent, reproducible anaesthesia is needed for sequential measurement of the intraocular pressure.

OPHTHALMIC SURGERY

Introduction

Surgical procedures on the eye in adults can frequently be performed using local anaesthesia. This is not the case in children for whom general anaesthesia will always be required. Procedures necessitating general anaesthesia are listed in Table 34.1, and encompass the entire paediatric age range, including newborn infants. The most common ophthalmic surgical procedure in children is strabismus surgery, while many infants will require general anaesthesia simply to permit a full eye examination.

Most children undergoing eye surgery are ASA (American Society of Anesthesiology Physical Status) 1 or 2 and will be day cases, and anaesthesia is straightforward. However, many of the eye problems encountered in children are associated with other anomalies, which may have implications for the conduct of general anaesthesia, and it is necessary to be aware of these.

Associated anomalies

Children requiring eye surgery may have other problems, often as part of an associated chromosomal defect, or a metabolic or other congenital disorder. In many cases the associated anomaly is limited to developmental delay, learning disability and behavioural problems and the challenge lies in managing these patients in a sympathetic manner.

In some patients, the association may be of more direct anaesthetic relevance. For example, in several syndromes in which there can be major difficulties with intubation, there may also be cataracts, glaucoma or squints. These include the mucopolysaccharidoses, the craniosynostosis disorders such as Crouzon, Apert and Pfeiffer syndromes, and the craniofacial syndromes such as Goldenhar, Treacher Collins, and Smith–Lemli–Opitz. The Hallerman–Strieff syndrome [1], although rare, may present for cataract surgery in the neonatal period and invariably has a particularly difficult airway to manage. Stickler syndrome, which is associated with early retinal detachment and glaucoma, is a progressive connective tissue disorder that has some of the features of the Pierre Robin anomalad and can also present intubation problems. Appropriate precautions and techniques for patients with potential intubation difficulties should be adopted in all these patients.

The congenital phakomatoses [2], a group of neuro-oculocutaneous disorders that include the Sturge–Weber syndrome, neurofibromatosis, tuberous sclerosis and von Hippel–Lindau disease, all have ocular lesions that may require surgery. These disorders are associated with seizures

Table 34.1 General anaesthesia may be required for the following procedures

Examination of the eye	General examination; fundoscopy
	Measurement of intraocular pressure
	Retinoblastoma follow-up
Extraocular procedures	
On the lids and orbit	Excision of orbital dermoids
	Excision of meibomian cysts
	Steroid injection of haemangiomas
	Tarsorrhaphy
	Ptosis surgery
On the nasolacrimal apparatus	Syringing and probing of ducts
	Dacryocystorhinostomy
On the eye	Strabismus surgery
	Laser surgery/cryotherapy
	Episcleral dermoid excision
	Corneal surgery
	Enucleation
	Evisceration
Intraocular procedures	To reduce intraocular pressure:
	Goniotomy
	Trabeculectomy/trabeculotomy
	Cataract aspiration ± artificial lens insertion
	Lensectomy
	Vitrectomy
	Vitreoretinal surgery

and other intracranial lesions, cardiac lesions and occasionally with phaeochromocytoma, and these patients will require careful preoperative assessment and management.

Patients with homocystinuria, a metabolic disorder in which hypoglycaemia and thromboembolic episodes are common, frequently have dislocated lenses that will require extraction. Adequate perioperative hydration in these children is important and an intravenous glucose infusion should be started preoperatively. Patients with homocystinuria should also be given aspirin over the perioperative period to minimise the risk of thromboembolic episodes. It is important to ensure that these patients are metabolically stable before proceeding with anaesthesia. Dislocated lenses are also common in patients with Marfan syndrome, in whom there may also be aortic root or valve problems. Congenital comorbidity and the significance for anaesthesia is further discussed in Chapter 28.

Infants with congenital cataracts frequently present for surgery in the first few days of life, with all the attendant complications of neonatal anaesthesia (see Chapter 32). These cataracts may be part of a metabolic disorder, or may occur following intrauterine infection. In particular they are common in the congenital rubellar syndrome, though this is now fortunately rare, in which there is frequently a cardiac anomaly. Many of these neonates will be at risk of postoperative apnoeic episodes and will need to be nursed and monitored following surgery in an appropriate environment.

Bacterial endocarditis prophylaxis

Although some patients, such as those with congenital rubellar syndrome or Marfan syndrome, may have an associated cardiac anomaly, the vast majority of ophthalmic procedures do not produce a bacteraemia, and antibiotic prophylaxis for endocarditis is unnecessary. The exceptions are those children undergoing a procedure on the nasolacrimal ducts, in which there is a significant incidence of bacteraemia [3]. These patients should receive appropriate antibiotic prophylaxis if they have a structural cardiac lesion (see Chapter 17).

General principles

Most children undergoing eye surgery are otherwise fit, healthy day-case patients, and for the majority of procedures general anaesthesia is routine. However, particular care should be taken in approaching and handling children who have very poor vision who may not be able to see or be fully aware of what is happening around them.

Some children with glaucoma will be taking regular eyedrops containing β blockers, such as timolol or betaxolol. Some of the administered drug drains through the nasolacrimal canal and is absorbed systemically by the nasal mucosa. It is unusual for there to be side-effects from systemic absorption of these agents in children, but adverse haemodynamic events have been reported in the elderly [4], and it is important to be aware of this possibility in children with cardiovascular comorbidity.

Premedication and induction are a matter of personal preference. Spontaneous ventilation via a facemask will frequently suffice for simple eye examinations, although it is often more convenient to use a laryngeal mask airway (LMA) to allow the ophthalmologist unrestricted access to the eyes. Spontaneous ventilation using an LMA is also satisfactory for the shorter surgical procedures where a sterile operating field is not required, such as laser surgery, and in most of the extraocular cases in older children.

For intraocular procedures, the surgeon will require a still, 'quiet' eye and this is most satisfactorily achieved using paralysis and controlled ventilation. Because of the inaccessibility of the airway when the face is covered in sterile drapes, a secure airway is essential. A preformed RAE (Ring–Adair–Elwyn) tracheal tube is generally used to ensure that bulky connectors are away from the surgical field. However, the use of preformed oral tracheal tubes in neonates can pose a problem as the fixed length of the tracheal portion of these tubes is frequently too long, potentially resulting in bronchial intubation. While it is possible to pack out these tubes at the mouth to prevent this, this results in a cumbersome mass at the mouth that may easily be displaced by the surgical assistant's hands. It is more convenient to use a reinforced, flexible, tracheal tube in infants under 6 months old; this results in a secure airway that does not conflict with the surgical field.

For many surgical procedures a dilated pupil is necessary, and ophthalmologists frequently use mydriatic agents perioperatively. The most commonly used agents are the parasympatholytic drug cyclopentolate 0.5 per cent or 1 per cent, or phenylephrine 2.5 per cent which is a sympathomimetic. These are normally administered topically in the preoperative period but if adequate pupillary dilatation has not been achieved further drops may be applied once the child is asleep. These are generally well tolerated, but serious systemic side-effects consequent upon systemic absorption of these agents have been reported, including hypertension and pulmonary oedema [5]. On occasion, the surgeon may wish to inject subconjunctival mydricaine, a mixture of procaine, atropine and adrenaline, to obtain better pupillary dilatation. It is prudent to avoid an anaesthetic technique utilising a high concentration of volatile agent, particularly halothane, in these cases and to avoid hypercapnia in order to minimise the risk of dysrythmias should there be systemic absorption of these agents.

Most surgical procedures involving the eye and orbit result in only mild-to-moderate pain and discomfort, and are well managed with topical anaesthetic agents and simple analgesics such as paracetamol and the non-steroidal analgesics. These can be given orally preoperatively or rectally at induction. Squint surgery, evisceration of the eye and vitreoretinal surgery are generally associated with more severe postoperative pain, and stronger analgesia may be necessary such as codeine or, in older children, tramadol. However, as squint surgery is associated with a high incidence of postoperative vomiting intraoperative opiate analgesia should be avoided in these patients if possible.

SPECIFIC PROCEDURES

Examination of the eyes (EUA)

Anaesthesia may be required in some children simply because they are too young or uncooperative to allow an adequate examination when awake. Normally this can be carried out satisfactorily using an inhalational technique and a facemask. On occasion it is easier for the surgeon if an LMA is inserted, particularly where it is necessary to use the operating microscope. Many of these children will require regular follow-up examinations and repeated anaesthetics, so it is essential that induction is managed in as gentle a manner as possible.

Measurement of intraocular pressure

Special consideration is required if the primary purpose of the EUA is to measure intraocular pressure (IOP). Most anaesthetic agents reduce IOP and there is a risk that injudicious anaesthesia will lower the IOP to such an extent that a high IOP will be masked, potentially compromising treatment. For this reason some anaesthetists use ketamine,

which does not reduce IOP. Where feasible this should be administered intravenously in a dose of 1–2 mg/kg, but it is not always possible to secure venous access in children before they are asleep. On these occasions, a dose of 5–10 mg/kg ketamine intramuscularly will produce within a few minutes a child who is quiet and still enough to permit a thorough eye examination. It is essential to ensure that the airway is maintained. There may be a slight increase in IOP using ketamine although there are conflicting reports about this [6,7]. However, it is felt that it is safer to have a falsely high IOP than a falsely low one that might result in IOP treatment being delayed.

Many anaesthetists prefer not to use ketamine because of a reluctance to administer intramuscular injections to small children, particularly as these children often require frequent examinations. Ketamine may also be associated with increased pharyngeal and tracheobronchial secretions. An alternative, equally effective technique is to undertake an inhalation induction using sevoflurane, which rapidly induces anaesthesia. The ophthalmologist should be present or close by during induction and available to measure the IOP the instant the child stops moving, and while the eyes are still central. It is important to limit the sevoflurane to 5 per cent, if possible, to minimise the fall in IOP and to ensure that the facemask does not encroach upon and compress the eye, as this will erroneously elevate IOP.

Both anaesthetic techniques are acceptable, and perhaps the more important issue is to ensure that account is taken of the technique used when comparing IOP measurements over a period of time. Whichever method of induction is used, IOP measurements should be taken before laryngoscopy or the use of suxamethonium (although this is now rarely used) as both of these will increase IOP [8–10]. Although insertion of a laryngeal mask does not appear to raise IOP [8,11], it is preferable to measure IOP before LMA insertion.

Syringing and probing of nasolacrimal ducts

Children with blocked nasolacrimal ducts usually present within the first year of life. These can frequently be cleared by probing the duct with a small blunt needle via the punctae at the medial side of the lids, and irrigation with 1–2 mL of saline. This is a short procedure and can safely be managed with an LMA. A very small amount of saline may appear in the nose or nasopharynx, which should be suctioned before removal of the LMA.

On occasion, it is necessary for the surgeon to manipulate or 'fracture' the inferior turbinate to relieve any obstruction at the lower end of the duct. Rarely, where a simple probing has failed, it may be necessary to pass a fine silicone catheter through the duct into the nose and secure it in place for a few weeks. Either procedure may result in a small amount of blood trickling into the nasopharynx. A tracheal tube and throat pack may be more satisfactory, although an LMA is also acceptable in this situation.

Sometimes it is necessary to proceed to a dacryocystorhinostomy (DCR). This is a more extensive procedure involving surgical exposure of the duct and creating a new opening from it into the nasal cavity through the bony upper lateral aspect of the nose. This can produce bleeding which, to assist the surgeon, can be limited by a modest degree of induced hypotension. Application of a topical vasoconstrictor to the nasal mucosa may also be beneficial. Airway protection with a tracheal tube and throat pack is necessary and opiate analgesia should be provided.

All procedures on the nasolacrimal ducts can cause a bacteraemia, and antibiotic prophylaxis should be given to children with structural heart defects [3].

Strabismus surgery

This is the most common ophthalmic surgical procedure in children, a squint occurring in up to 5 per cent of non-premature infants. Surgery is usually performed on a day-stay basis, but the high incidence of postoperative nausea and vomiting (PONV) associated with this procedure occasionally results in unplanned overnight admission. Strabismus surgery is also associated with the oculocardiac reflex, a bradycardic response to extraocular muscle traction, and it has been postulated that these two events might be associated. Although very rare, there is reportedly an increased incidence of malignant hyperpyrexia (MH) in patients with a squint and vigilance should be maintained for this. Suxamethonium should be avoided in these patients, and the temperature monitored. Chapter 29 gives further information in the aetiology and management of MH. In a few older children, the surgeon may elect to place an adjustable suture as part of the technique. This allows the surgeon to make fine adjustments to the repair, using topical anaesthesia, when the patient is awake. In some patients with small degrees of strabismus a minute quantity of botulinum toxin, a paralytic, is injected directly into the extraocular muscles to affect eye movement. This may be done using electromyographic control so muscle relaxants should be avoided.

THE OCULOCARDIAC REFLEX

The oculocardiac reflex (OCR), which was described in 1908 independently by Aschner and Dagnini, is common during squint surgery, occurring in approximately 60 per cent of cases. It is evoked by traction on the extrinsic eye muscles or pressure on the globe, causing a sinus bradycardia [12]. The OCR is a trigemino-vagal reflex, the afferent pathway being the ophthalmic branch of the trigeminal nerve. The bradycardia reverts almost immediately once the stimulus is removed and it is unusual to see a more serious rhythm disturbance. On occasion, however, it can produce major dysrythmias or sinus arrest. Traction on any of the extraocular muscles can evoke the reflex but it is generally felt that it occurs most commonly when the medial rectus muscle is manipulated, though this was not confirmed in a detailed study [12]. The OCR can be successfully blocked by the prior administration of atropine or glycopyrrolate [13], but the resultant tachycardia and the frequently benign nature of the reflex have led many anaesthetists to administer atropine only if the reflex occurs.

As the OCR and the vomiting associated with squint surgery (see below) may share the same afferent pathway, it has been suggested that preventing the OCR may reduce the incidence of vomiting. Anticholinergic prophylaxis is effective at preventing the OCR, but it does not reliably prevent vomiting [13]. However, it has been reported that children with a positive OCR are 2.6 times more likely to develop PONV than those with no measurable reflex [14]. It would seem sensible therefore to prevent the OCR if possible. Blocking the afferent limb of the reflex using a peribulbar block is one way of achieving this [15], but this carries a risk of perforating the globe and is inadvisable in children. It is preferable to administer atropine 20 μg/kg at induction and to accept the resultant modest tachycardia. The administration of atropine is especially necessary if propofol, which has a bradycardic effect, is used for induction or maintenance of anaesthesia.

It is acceptable to allow spontaneous ventilation during squint surgery, although some surgeons prefer a completely immobile eye. Sevoflurane is more suitable than halothane as it is associated with significantly less OCR [16]. Hypercapnia has been shown to double the incidence of significant bradycardia [12], though this has not been confirmed in other studies, and controlled ventilation to ensure normocapnia may be more suitable than spontaneous ventilation during strabismus surgery. If a muscle relaxant is used, consideration should be given to the choice of drug as some, such as rocuronium, appear to attenuate the OCR [17]. Atracurium is associated with a greater incidence of OCR than pancuronium [18] but the shorter duration of action of atracurium makes this a more appropriate relaxant. Cisatracurium, with less histamine release, is equally satisfactory.

VOMITING FOLLOWING STRABISMUS SURGERY

Nausea alone is a difficult entity to quantify in children, who generally have a higher incidence of postoperative vomiting (POV) than adults. This is a well-recognised complication following strabismus surgery, particularly in children over the age of 2 years, and experience suggests that about two-thirds of children undergoing strabismus surgery vomit if no preventive measures are taken. In some studies over 80 per cent of children who received no antiemetic suffered POV [19]. There appear to be two distinct time periods for vomiting, some children vomiting immediately or within the first few hours following surgery, and another group in whom POV does not occur until several hours later, usually within 24 hours but occasionally up to 40 hours postoperatively. A systematic review of publications between 1981 and 1994 on vomiting in children following squint surgery established a mean incidence of 54 per cent POV within 6 hours of operation in children receiving no prophylactic antiemetic, and of 59 per cent within 48 hours [20].

The reason for an increased incidence of vomiting following squint surgery and its precise mechanism remain unknown but it is postulated to be part of an oculoemetic reflex, involving the ophthalmic division of the trigeminal nerve and the vomiting centre in the medulla [21]. Blocking the afferent nerves by way of a retrobulbar or peribulbar block reduces the incidence. It is probable that there are local anatomical reasons for the reflex, as different surgical techniques have been shown to affect the incidence of vomiting. In particular, squint repair using the Faden myopexy technique has a significantly higher incidence of POV than the simpler muscle recession–resection technique [22].

There have been numerous publications on the management of POV in children in general and following squint surgery in particular. Many different strategies have been proposed in an attempt to reduce the incidence, with varying success, including the use of anticholinergic agents, dimenhydrinate, dexamethasone, clonidine, prophylactic antiemetics such as metoclopramide, droperidol or ondansetron, or utilising the putative antiemetic properties of propofol either as induction agent or as part of a total intravenous anaesthesia (TIVA) technique. Studies have also examined the role of nitrous oxide and the use of neostigmine to reverse the muscle relaxants. These publications have been comprehensively reviewed [23].

It is not possible to compare satisfactorily the studies relating specifically to strabismus surgery because they involve very different underlying anaesthetic techniques, in particular in the use or otherwise of premedicants, anticholinergic agents, nitrous oxide, neuromuscular reversal agents and opiates. Furthermore studies have often not taken into account different surgical techniques that may have a significant effect on the incidence of vomiting. There is no doubt, however, that the introduction of the $5HT_3$ (serotonin) antagonists such as ondansetron has led to a significant reduction in the incidence of POV [24], and it should be administered intraoperatively. Ondansetron 0.1 mg/kg is effective, although it has been shown also that smaller doses may be equally effective [19]. Combination therapy, for example using ondansetron with dexamethasone or droperidol, is better than ondansetron alone [25], although droperidol is no longer available in some countries. Concerns about the high cost of ondansetron have prompted others to try cheaper $5HT_3$ antagonists such as dolasetron [26]. Dolasetron 0.35 mg/kg has been shown to be as effective as ondansetron 0.1 mg/kg [27] but is not currently universally available.

Propofol may have antiemetic properties, and it has been demonstrated that anaesthesia induced and maintained by propofol is as effective as ondansetron 150 μg/kg at reducing POV following strabismus surgery [28]. It is possible to reduce the incidence of vomiting to less than 10 per cent using a multimodal approach adopting several of these methods.

Although squint surgery is one of the most painful ophthalmic procedures, opiates should be avoided if possible.

They undoubtedly increase the incidence of vomiting [29] and are usually unnecessary for adequate analgesia, which can usually be achieved satisfactorily using paracetamol and a non-steroidal analgesic such as diclofenac or ibuprofen. Ketorolac 0.75–0.9 mg/kg has been shown to be as effective as morphine or pethidine [29–31]. Where analgesia is inadequate, as it may be for the more painful myopexy repair or repeat surgery, it may be necessary to administer codeine phosphate or tramadol.

Peribulbar block has been shown to be effective in producing good analgesia in children undergoing ophthalmic surgery, as well as reducing the incidence of OCR [15], but most paediatric anaesthetists remain cautious about using this technique because of the significant risks of globe perforation and retrobulbar haemorrhage [32].

As an alternative, pain relief can be enhanced significantly if a sub-Tenon block is administered by the surgeon at the end of the procedure. Tenon's capsule is the fascial layer that extends from the limbus, fusing posteriorly to the optic nerve, separating the globe from orbital fat. Sensation of the eye is provide by ciliary nerves that cross the episcleral space after emerging from the globe. Strabismus surgery on the extraocular muscles is carried out within this space and instilling local anaesthetic here can be effective. Alternatively, Morton et al. have shown that satisfactory postoperative analgesia following squint surgery can be obtained using either diclofenac 0.1 per cent or oxybuprocaine 0.4 per cent eye drops alone [33]. If these are administered selectively to the operative site by the surgeon before suturing the conjunctiva, the problems of an anaesthetic cornea can be minimised.

A suggested anaesthetic technique for strabismus surgery is as follows:

- Premedication can be left to individual preference but is not generally necessary for cooperative patients. Where intravenous induction is planned a topical local anaesthetic cream should be applied.
- Either an intravenous induction with propofol 3–4 μg/kg or gaseous induction is appropriate.
- Following induction atropine 20 μg/kg and a relaxant of choice, depending on the speed of the surgeon, are given along with 100 μg/kg ondansetron and 150 μg/kg dexamethasone to minimise POV.
- Analgesia is provided using diclofenac and paracetamol suppositories.
- Anaesthesia is maintained with oxygen in nitrous oxide or air and a volatile agent via a tracheal tube or LMA, with controlled ventilation to normocapnia.
- One to two drops of topical adrenaline 0.1 per cent can help to reduce conjunctival bleeding.
- A sub-Tenon block or topical anaesthesia drops such as amethocaine should be administered by the surgeon at the end of the procedure.

Patients are often discharged home at around 3–4 hours postoperatively. It is important to warn the parents or other carers that vomiting may start around this time. Restricting oral fluids prior to discharge has been shown to reduce vomiting [34], and limiting activity may also be helpful. If vomiting does occur it is usually self-limiting but additional antiemetics may be necessary. Rarely, overnight admission and intravenous fluids may be required.

Enucleation

Removal of the whole eye may be required because of retinoblastoma, or for cosmetic reasons when there is an unsightly blind eye. As the surgical technique involves dissection of each of the extraocular muscles from the globe, the OCR may readily be evoked. Anaesthetic management should be as for strabismus surgery, although the risks of POV are much reduced.

Evisceration

In this procedure the contents of the globe are removed rather than the whole eye, leaving the sclera behind. There are no specific anaesthetic problems but the procedure can be painful and appropriate analgesia, including an intraoperative opiate such as fentanyl, may be necessary.

Intraocular surgery

Intraocular surgery in children is predominantly for the management of glaucoma, or for cataract extraction with or without an artificial lens implant. Intraocular lens implants are being inserted now even in infants.

Normal IOP is between 10 and 22 mmHg and depends on the balance between the production of aqueous humour, mainly from the ciliary body in the posterior chamber, and its drainage via a trabecular meshwork to the canal of Schlemm in the anterior chamber. Most paediatric glaucoma is a result of an intrinsic disorder of aqueous outflow, and medical therapy is of limited value. The principal surgical procedures to treat glaucoma include goniotomy, trabeculotomy and trabeculectomy. Where surgical procedures are unsuccessful, cyclocryotherapy to ablate the aqueous producing ciliary body is performed. This involves the application of a cryoprobe at $-60°C$ to $-80°C$ behind the corneoscleral limbus, and is painful. Opiate analgesia will be necessary.

It is essential that the eye is motionless during intraocular procedures, and to avoid rises in IOP during the procedure to prevent the extrusion of intraocular contents through the incisions. This is particularly important during corneal grafting (penetrating keratoplasty) when a large defect is created over the cornea. Controlled ventilation should be used, and neuromuscular blockade should be monitored with a peripheral nerve stimulator.

Venous drainage from the eye is valveless and any rise in venous pressure leads to an immediate rise in IOP by altering the volume of the choroid, and by impeding aqueous drainage via the canal of Schlemm. Coughing, straining or vomiting causes acutely increased venous pressure and increased IOP and must be avoided. Generally, arterial pressure has little effect on IOP.

Acetazolamide, which reduces aqueous production, or mannitol may be administered intravenously during these procedures to lower the IOP. It is important in penetrating keratoplasty also to avoid the IOP falling too low as the eye can collapse inwards. The surgeon may suture a ring around the cornea to support the eye during the procedure.

It is good practice to try to prevent as far as possible rises in IOP at the end of the procedure which can be produced, for example, by coughing on the tracheal tube at extubation [35], although with the advent of very fine suture materials allowing complete closure of the ocular wounds this is less important than it used to be. Anaesthesia should be maintained until neuromuscular blockade has been reversed, the patient is breathing spontaneously and extubation has been performed. Some recommend intravenous administration of 1 mg/kg lidocaine prior to extubation. Another useful technique to obtain a smooth extubation is to give a small dose of propofol (0.5–1.0 mg/kg) immediately prior to extubation. In older children topical anaesthesia to the airway can be helpful. This should be avoided in infants, as the simplest way to avoid the elevated IOP associated with crying in the immediate postoperative period is to allow them an early feed.

After initial concerns about possible gastric insufflation and reflux, it has now been shown that pressure-controlled ventilation in children using an LMA is safe and effective [36], and can be used for intraocular surgery, even in small children. This has the advantage of smoother extubation with less coughing and reduced likelihood of acute IOP elevation than with a conventional tracheal tube [37]. However, if an LMA is used, it is imperative to ensure that it is perfectly positioned and secured before proceeding with surgery. If there is any doubt, a tracheal tube should be used.

Intraocular surgery is not particularly painful, and a combination of paracetamol and diclofenac is usually satisfactory. In order to limit the child rubbing the eye postoperatively, some advocate the intraoperative administration of an opiate, intramuscularly or intravenously, during the procedure to obtain some mild sedation postoperatively.

Vitreoretinal surgery

Repair of retinal detachment may be necessary in children, and generally takes place in specialised centres. This usually involves the creation of a chorioretinal scar using cryotherapy and the placement of a scleral buckle towards the back of the eye to obtain apposition of the neuroretina and the retinal pigment epithelium. Sometimes, an intraocular gas bubble containing sulphur hexafluoride (SF_6) or perfluoropropane (C_3F_8) may be injected into the eye to tamponade the detached surfaces together while adhesions develop. It is imperative that nitrous oxide is not administered when these gases are used as it will rapidly diffuse into the gas bubble and alter its size. This is crucially important if subsequent anaesthesia is required, as these gases may remain in the eye for several weeks. Diffusion of nitrous oxide into an existing intraocular gas bubble can result in rapid expansion of the bubble and an acute rise in pressure within the globe, and can cause irreversible ischaemic damage to the retina and optic nerve [38]. Patients and their carers should be given clear instructions about passing this information on to other anaesthetists, should they require further surgery.

Vitreoretinal surgery is painful and appropriate analgesia should be administered perioperatively. In adults a sub-Tenon block has been shown to be effective in providing analgesia [39], and is likely to be equally effective in children.

Emergency eye surgery

Penetrating eye injury may require removal of any foreign bodies and early wound closure and sometimes cannot be delayed to ensure an empty stomach. This has become one of the most contentious areas of anaesthesia because of two conflicting arguments. On the one hand, the possibility of a full stomach demands prompt intubation for airway protection that is conventionally achieved by the rapid induction–intubation sequence using suxamethonium. On the other hand, it has been traditionally taught that there is the need to protect the eye from any acute rise in IOP that may cause extrusion of ocular contents through even very small wounds, leading to total loss of vision. Suxamethonium, it has been argued, causes a transient but definite rise in IOP, even in the absence of fasciculation, which cannot be reliably prevented, and therefore, theoretically, should not be used. Many have therefore recommended that intubation in these cases should be performed using a large dose of a non-depolarising relaxant while cricoid pressure is maintained.

The balance of opinion has fluctuated in recent years and the use of suxamethonium to provide optimal intubation conditions in a rapid sequence induction is now accepted again. In part this stems from the fact that there have been no well-documented reports describing vitreous extrusion following the administration of suxamethonium [40]. One of the causes of this controversy arose from the desire to establish a rigid protocol for the management of patients with a penetrating eye injury but this may not be in the best interests of the patients. Some patients may already have lost most of the vitreous, or have sealed the wound with lens or iris tissue and, if so, a rise in IOP is of much less importance. Unfortunately, this cannot always be assessed until the eye has been examined under anaesthesia. Equally, some patients may not be at risk of a full stomach or can be deferred for sufficient time to reduce the

risks of aspiration, and intubation can be carried out with more confidence using a non-depolarising relaxant. It should not be forgotten that gastric emptying may be considerably delayed following trauma and full consultation with the surgeons is required in making a decision about the timing of surgery.

There are other factors that raise IOP and these must be taken into account. Crying, struggling or vomiting can raise IOP by as much as 40 mmHg, and there should be no attempt at passing a nasogastric tube prior to anaesthesia to empty the stomach. Prior to induction, attempts at securing venous access may not be tolerated and gaseous induction may be more appropriate. This is an acceptable alternative in experienced hands.

Laryngoscopy and intubation themselves produce a significant rise in IOP which can be attenuated by lidocaine 1.5 mg/kg intravenously [41]. Alfentanil 20 µg/kg attenuates the hypertensive response and may limit the IOP rise [42], and the other short-acting opiates can be expected to have a similar effect. However, it is likely that changes in IOP are affected primarily by venous pressure and changes in arterial pressure probably have little effect.

In difficult situations where the eye is at risk and regurgitation is a concern, suxamethonium should be used as part of a conventional rapid sequence induction, particularly if there are any concerns about the airway. If suxamethonium is contraindicated, or if there is less concern about risk of regurgitation, the following technique has been shown to provide good early intubating conditions without raising IOP. A secure intravenous line is established and fentanyl 2 µg/kg is given, followed by vecuronium 0.15 mg/kg. At the first sign of muscle weakness, thiopental 5 mg/kg is given and cricoid pressure applied. Intubation can be performed 80–90 seconds after the vecuronium, which is approximately 60 seconds after loss of consciousness. Premature attempts at intubation provoke coughing, which significantly raises IOP and should be avoided. A nerve stimulator is helpful in indicating when full relaxation has occurred.

Maintenance of anaesthesia is a matter of personal preference since most general anaesthetic agents produce a modest decrease in IOP. The stomach should be emptied as much as possible before the end of anaesthesia. In order to prevent coughing on the tracheal tube it is helpful to maintain anaesthesia until relaxation has been reversed and the patient is breathing satisfactorily, and to extubate while the patient is still asleep. Because of the risk of regurgitation this should be performed with the patient on their side.

Retinopathy of prematurity

Despite meticulous neonatal care severe retinopathy of prematurity (ROP) still occurs and can lead to total blindness. Babies at risk for severe ROP are those of birth weight <1500 g and/or <31 weeks' gestational age. Retinopathy of prematurity, which is characterised by abnormal blood vessel growth in the retina, is classified in five stages, ranging from mild (stage 1) to severe (stage 5). Infants who develop the more severe ROP (stage 3 and above) are at risk of retinal detachment and blindness. It has been shown that the outcome of the disease process can be significantly improved by cryotherapy or laser therapy to ablate the peripheral retina and remove the stimulus to new growth. This needs to be done early in the disease, so early identification is essential and eye examinations in all at-risk infants should take place between 6 and 7 weeks' postnatal age and continued 2-weekly until the risk has passed [43]. Although the examinations, and in some centres the cryotherapy or laser therapy, will usually take place within the neonatal unit some premature infants may be transferred to theatre for their treatment. Cryotherapy is a painful procedure and warrants administration of opiate analgesia such as fentanyl. This has implications for the postoperative care of the patients who, because of their gestational age, will already be at risk of apnoeic episodes following anaesthesia. Provision should be made to provide postoperative ventilation with appropriate support for these babies. Many of these infants will have other systemic disorders consequent upon their extreme prematurity, such as bronchopulmonary dysplasia, which may influence both the conduct of anaesthesia and the need for postoperative support [44], They will need careful preoperative assessment.

DENTAL ANAESTHESIA

Wherever possible dental extractions or conservations in children should be performed using local anaesthesia outside the hospital setting, and this is successful in the majority of children [45]. In some anxious or uncooperative patients in whom behaviour management techniques have been unsuccessful it may be necessary to provide some sedation. There are established clinical guidelines for the use of conscious (or moderate) sedation in paediatric dentistry in the UK [46] and in the USA [47], and inhalational sedation using nitrous oxide remains the mainstay of conscious sedation. Nitrous oxide may, however, be inadequate in some very anxious patients, and the addition of low-dose (0.1–0.3 per cent) sevoflurane has been reported to improve compliance [48]. Intravenous midazolam [49] and propofol [50] are also used, but there are significant concerns about the use of these intravenous agents in children in dental clinics. A recent Cochrane Review was unable to reach any definitive conclusion on which was the most effective method of sedation in these children [51]. If used, it is imperative that these agents are given in doses sufficient only to achieve anxiolysis and cooperation rather than sleep, by staff trained in their use, and with facilities and equipment for resuscitation available.

Some children are unable to cooperate with dental procedures being undertaken under local anaesthesia or sedation and they will require general anaesthesia. Such patients may have a learning disability or behavioural disorder and need to be treated sympathetically. Others will require general anaesthesia because of the extent or nature of the dental work. It is unacceptable for these procedures to be performed by a sole operator/anaesthetist, and a trained anaesthetist must be present with all the appropriate monitoring, recovery and resuscitation facilities. Since 2002 it has been mandatory in the UK that this must take place in a hospital.

Many of these children will be outpatients without other significant health problems and anaesthesia is generally straightforward. Unless there is clear clinical indication to do so there is little value in undertaking any preoperative haematological screening for patients requiring dental treatment [52]. Some patients may have an additional disease process, such as epidermolysis bullosa, in which dental caries is common, or a cardiac disorder, and appropriate precautions and techniques are necessary. Most procedures involved during conservative dentistry cause a significant bacteraemia, most commonly with *Streptococcus viridans* [53,54]. All patients at risk of bacterial endocarditis should therefore be given prophylactic antibiotics.

The procedure may be undertaken in the dental chair or on an operating table. Patient preference and degree of cooperation will usually determine whether induction is intravenous or inhalational. Maintenance of anaesthesia is best achieved using sevoflurane which has a significantly lower incidence of dysrhythmias than halothane, though it has a slightly slower recovery [55,56]. There does not appear to be any benefit in reducing PONV by excluding nitrous oxide [57]. For procedures lasting only a few minutes, usually involving extractions of a few anterior teeth, a nasal mask may be used, but a nasopharyngeal airway provides better operating conditions and fewer episodes of airway obstruction [58].

For longer procedures the airway is best provided with a nasotracheal tube. If this is difficult to insert, an orotracheal tube or an LMA will usually suffice, though this may make the procedure slightly more difficult for the surgeon. If a laryngeal mask is used, this should be removed when the patient has woken and fully regained airway reflexes [59].

Some paediatric patients presenting for dental treatment can be difficult to intubate. In this situation full consultation with the dental surgeon is required to establish whether local anaesthesia may be more appropriate; if not, difficult intubation techniques may be necessary. A throat pack will always be necessary, although it should be recognised that some aspiration can still occur [60]. Thorough examination and suction of the pharynx at the end of the procedure are essential.

Adequate analgesia can usually be provided using paracetamol [61] and diclofenac [62], even for extraction of molar teeth, and dexamethasone can reduce the swelling and the associated pain following extraction of the molars.

REFERENCES

Key references

Blanc VF, Hardy J-F, Milot J *et al*. The oculocardiac reflex: a graphic and statistical analysis in infants and children. *Can Anaesth Soc J* 1983; **30**: 360–9.

Olutoye O, Watcha MF. Management of postoperative vomiting in pediatric patients. *Int Anesthesiol Clin* 2003; **41**(4): 99–117.

Vachon CA, Warner DO, Bacon DR. Succinylcholine and the open globe: tracing the teaching. *Anesthesiology* 2003; **99**: 220–3.

References

1. Cheong KF, Tham SL. Anaesthetic management of a child with Hallermann-Streiff Francois syndrome. *Paediatr Anaesth* 2003; **13**(3): 274–5.
2. Diaz, JH. Perioperative management of children with congenital phakomatoses. *Paediatr Anaesth* 2000; **10**(2): 121–8.
3. Eppert GA, Burnstine RA, Bates JH. Lacrimal-duct-probing-induced bacteremia: should children with congenital heart defects receive antibiotic prophylaxis? *J Pediatr Ophthalmol Strabismus* 1998; **35**: 38–40.
4. Muller ME, van der Velde N, Krulder JWM, van der Cammen TJM. Syncope and falls due to timolol eye drops. *BMJ* 2006; **332**: 960–1.
5. Greher M, Hartmann T, Winkler M *et al*. Hypertension and pulmonary edema associated with subconjunctival phenylephrine in a 2-month old child during cataract extraction. *Anesthesiology* 1998; **88**: 1394–6.
6. Yoshikawa K, Murai Y. The effect of ketamine on intraocular pressure in children. *Anesth Analg* 1971; **50**: 199–202.
7. Ausinsch B, Rayburn RL, Munson ES *et al*. Ketamine and intraocular pressure in children. *Anesth Analg* 1976; **55**: 773–5.
8. Watcha MF, White PF, Tychsen L Stevens JL. Comparative effects of laryngeal mask airway and endotracheal tube insertion on intraocular pressure in children. *Anesth Analg* 1992; **75**: 355–60.
9. Joshi C, Bruce DL. Thiopental and succinylcholine: action on intraocular pressure. *Anesth Analg* 1975; **54**: 471–5.
10. Dear GL, Hammerton M, Hatch DJ *et al*. Anaesthesia and intraocular pressure in young children. A study of three different techniques of anaesthesia. *Anaesthesia* 1987; **42**: 259–65.
11. Duman A, Ogun CO, Okelsi S. The effect on intraocular pressure of tracheal intubation or laryngeal mask insertion during sevoflurane amaesthesia in children without the use of muscle relaxants. *Paediatr Anaesth* 2001; **11**: 421–4.
12. Blanc VF, Hardy J-F, Milot J *et al*. The oculocardiac reflex: a graphic and statistical analysis in infants and children. *Can Anaesth Soc J* 1983; **30**: 360–9.
13. Chisakuta AM, Mirakhur RK. Anticholinergic prophylaxis does not prevent emesis following strabismus surgery in children. *Paediatr Anaesth* 1995; **5**: 97–100.
14. Allen LE, Sudesh S, Sandramouli S *et al*. The association between the oculocardiac reflex and post-operative vomiting in children undergoing strabismus surgery. *Eye* 1998; **12**: 193–6.
15. Deb K, Subramanian R, Dehran M *et al*. Safety and efficacy of peribulbar block as adjunct to general anaesthesia for paediatric ophthalmic surgery. *Paediatr Anaesth* 2001; **11**: 161–7.
16. Allison CE, De Lange JJ, Koole FD *et al*. A comparison of the incidence of the oculocardiac and oculorespiratory reflexes during sevoflurane or halothane anesthesia for strabismus surgery in children. *Anesth Analg* 2000; **90**: 306–10.
17. Karanovic N, Jukic M, Carev M *et al*. Rocuronium attenuates oculocardiac reflex during squint surgery in children anaesthetized with halothane and nitrous oxide. *Acta Anaesthesiol Scand* 2004; **48**: 1301–5.
18. Loewinger J, Friedmann-Neiger I, Cohen M, Levi E. Effects of atracurium and pancuronium on the oculocardiac reflex in children. *Anesth Analg* 1991; **73**: 25–8.
19. Sadhasivam S, Shende D, Madan R. Prophylactic ondansetron in prevention of postoperative nausea and vomiting following pediatric strabismus surgery: a dose–response study. *Anesthesiology* 2000; **92**: 1035–42.
20. Tramèr M, Moore A, McQuay H. Prevention of vomiting after paediatric strabismus surgery: a systematic review using the numbers-needed-to-treat method. *Br J Anaesth* 1995; **75**: 556–61.
21. Van den Berg AA, Lambourne A, Clyburn PA. The oculo-emetic reflex: a rationalisation of postophthalmic anaesthesia vomiting. *Anaesthesia* 1989; **44**: 110–17.
22. Saiah M, Borgeat A, Ruetsch YA *et al*. Myopexy (Faden) results in more postoperative vomiting after strabismus surgery in children. *Acta Anaesthesiol Scand* 2001; **45**: 59–64.
23. Olutoye O, Watcha MF. Management of postoperative vomiting in pediatric patients. *Int Anesthesiol Clin* 2003; **41**(4): 99–117.
24. Sennaraj B, Shende D, Sadhasivam S *et al*. Management of post-strabismus nausea and vomiting in children using ondansetron: a value-based comparison of outcomes. *Br J Anaesth* 2002; **89**(3): 473–8.
25. Splinter WM, Rhine EJ. Low-dose ondansetron with dexamethasone more effectively decreases vomiting after strabismus surgery in children than does high-dose ondansetron. *Anesthesiology* 1998; **88**: 72–5.
26. Meyer T, Roberson CR, Rajab MH *et al*. Dolasetron versus ondansetron for the treatment of postoperative nausea and vomiting. *Anesth Analg* 2005; **100**: 373–377.
27. Olutoye O, Jantzen EC, Alexis R *et al*. A Comparison of the costs and efficacy of ondansetron and dolasetron in the prophylaxis of postoperative vomiting in pediatric patients undergoing ambulatory surgery. *Anesth Analg* 2003; **97**: 390–6.
28. Splinter WM, Rhine EJ, Roberts DJ. Vomiting after strabismus surgery in children: ondansetron vs propofol. *Can J Anaesth* 1997; **44**: 825–9.
29. Mendel HG, Guarnieri KM, Sundt LM Torjman MC. The effects of ketorolac and fentanyl on postoperative vomiting and analgesic requirements in children undergoing strabismus surgery. *Anesth Analg* 1995; **80**: 1129–33.
30. Munro HM, Riegger LQ, Reynolds PI *et al*. Comparison of the analgesic and emetic properties of ketorolac and morphine

for paediatric outpatient strabismus surgery. *Br J Anaesth* 1994; **72**: 624–8.

31. Shende D, Das K. Comparative effects of intravenous ketorolac and pethidine on perioperative analgesia and postoperative nausea and vomiting (PONV) for paediatric strabismus surgery. *Acta Anaesthesiol Scand* 1998; **42**: 1–5.

32. Paruleker MV, Berg S, Elston JS. Adjunctive peribulbar anaesthesia for paediatric ophthalmic surgery: are the risks justified? *Paediatr Anaesth* 2002; **12**: 85.

33. Morton NS, Benham SW, Lawson RA *et al*. Diclofenac vs oxybuprocaine eyedrops for analgesia in paediatric strabismus surgery. *Paediatr Anaesth* 1997; **7**: 221–226.

34. Kearney R, Mack C, Entwistle L. Withholding oral fluids from children undergoing day surgery reduces vomiting. *Paediatr Anaesth* 1998; **8**: 331–6.

35. Madan R, Tamilselvan P, Sadhasivam S *et al*. Intra-ocular pressure and haemodynamic changes after tracheal intubation and extubation: a comparative study in glaucomatous and nonglaucomatous children. *Anaesthesia* 2000; **55**: 380–4.

36. Engelhardt T, Johnston G, Kumar MM. Comparison of cuffed, uncuffed tracheal tubes and laryngeal mask airways in low flow pressure controlled ventilation in children. *Paediatr Anaesth* 2006; **16**: 140–3.

37. Gulati M, Mohta M, Ahuja S, Gupta VP. Comparison of laryngeal mask airway with tracheal tube for ophthalmic surgery in paediatric patients. *Anaesth Intensive Care* 2004; **32**: 383–9.

38. Lee EJ. Use of nitrous oxide causing severe retinal loss 37 days after retinal surgery. *Br J Anaesth* 2004; **93**: 464–6.

39. Farmery AD, Shlugman D, Rahman R, Rosen P. Sub-Tenon's block reduces both intraoperative and postoperative analgesia requirement in vitreo-retinal surgery under general anaesthesia. *Eur J Anaesthesiol* 2003; **20**: 973–8.

40. Vachon CA, Warner DO, Bacon DR. Succinylcholine and the open globe: tracing the teaching. *Anesthesiology* 2003; **99**: 220–3.

41. Lerman J, Kiskis AA. Lidocaine attenuates the intraocular pressure response to rapid intubation in children. *Can Anaesth Soc J* 1985; **32**: 339–45.

42. Morton NS, Hamilton MB. Alfentanil in an anaesthetic technique for penetrating eye injuries. *Anaesthesia* 1986; **41**: 1148–51.

43. The Royal College of Ophthalmologists; British Association of Perinatal Medicine. Report of a joint Working Party. *Retinopathy of prematurity: guidelines for screening and treatment*. London: The Royal College of Ophthalmologists, British Association of Perinatal Medicine, 1995.

44. Allegaert K, Van de Velde M, Casteels I *et al*. Cryotherapy for threshold retinopathy: perioperative management in a single centre. *Am J Perinatol* 2003; **20**: 219–26.

45. Blain KM, Hill FJ. The use of inhalational sedation and a local anaesthesia as an alternative to general anaesthesia for dental extractions in children. *Br Dent J* 1998; **184**: 608–11.

46. Hosey MT. UK National Clinical Guidelines in Paediatric Dentistry. Managing anxious children: the use of conscious sedation in paediatric dentistry. *Int J Paediatr Dent* 1988; **184**: 608–11.

47. American Academy of Paediatric Dentistry Council on Clinical Affairs. Guideline on appropriate use of nitrous oxide for pediatric dental patients. *Pediatr Dent* 2005; **27**: 107–9.

48. Lahoud GY, Averley PA. Comparison of sevoflurane and nitrous oxide mixture with nitrous oxide alone for inhalational conscious sedation in children having dental treatment: a randomised controlled trial. *Anaesthesia* 2002; **57**: 446–50.

49. Averley PA, Girdler NM, Bond S *et al*. A randomised controlled trial of paediatric conscious sedation for dental treatment using intravenous midazolam combined with inhaled nitrous oxide or nitrous oxide/sevoflurane. *Anaesthesia* 2004; **59**: 844–52.

50. Hosey MT, Makin A, Jones RM *et al*. Propofol intravenous conscious sedation for anxious children in a specialist paediatric dentistry unit. *Int J Paediatr Dent* 2004; **14**: 2–8.

51. Matharu LM, Ashley PF. Sedation of anxious children undergoing dental treatment. *Cochrane Database System Rev* 2006(1); CD 003877.

52. Mason C, Porter SR, Mee A *et al*. The prevalence of clinically significant anaemia and haemoglobinopathy in children requiring dental treatment under general anaesthesia: a retrospective study of 1000 patients. *Int J Paediatr Dent* 1995; **5**: 163–7.

53. Roberts GJ, Holzel H, Sury MRJ *et al*. Dental bacteraemia in children. *Pediatr Cardiol* 1997; **18**: 24–7.

54. Roberts GJ, Gardner P, Longhurst P *et al*. Intensity of bacteraemia associated with conservative dental procedures in children. *Br Dent J* 2000; **188**: 95–8.

55. Ariffin SA, Whyte JA, Malins AF *et al*. Comparison of induction and recovery between sevoflurane and halothane supplementation of anaesthesia in children undergoing outpatient dental extractions. *Br J Anaesth* 1997; **78**: 157–9.

56. Paris ST, Cafferkey M, Tarling M *et al*. Comparison of sevoflurane and halothane for outpatient dental anaesthesia in children. *Br J Anaesth* 1997; **79**: 280–4.

57. Splinter WM, Komocar L. Nitrous oxide does not increase vomiting after dental restorations in children. *Anesth Analg* 1997; **84**: 506–8.

58. Bagshaw ON, Southee R, Ruiz K. A comparison of the nasal mask and the nasopharyngeal airway in paediatric chair dental anaesthesia. *Anaesthesia* 1997; **52**: 786–789.

59. Dolling S, Anders NRK, Rolfe SE. A comparison of deep vs awake removal of the laryngeal mask airway in paediatric dental daycase surgery. A randomised controlled trial. *Anaesthesia* 2003; **58**: 1224–8.

60. Davis J, Alton H, Butler J. Aspiration of foreign materials in children while under general anaesthesia for dental extractions. *Anesth Pain Control Dentistry* 1993; **2**: 17–21.

61. Chelliah S, Fell D, Brooks H. Pain and analgesia requirement after day case exodontias in children. *Paediatr Anaesth* 2002; **12**: 834.

62. Littlejohn IH, Tarling MM, Flynn PJ *et al*. Post-operative pain relief in children following extraction of carious deciduous teeth under general anaesthesia: a comparison of nalbuphine and diclofenac. *Eur J Anaesthesiol* 1996; **13**: 359–63.

Plastic surgery

MARK ANSERMINO, MICHAEL RJ SURY

KEY LEARNING POINTS

- In infants, under anaesthesia:
  - cleft lip alone should not cause an airway problem;
  - cleft palate may cause difficulty with laryngoscopy if there is micrognathia – a straight blade placed lateral and almost underneath the tongue should gain a much better view.
- Opioid analgesia is usually necessary after cleft palate repair.

- After palate repair, acute airway obstruction can occur soon after extubation and is caused by a combination of factors, including nasopharyngeal obstruction, blood, secretions, oedema, pharyngeal incoordination and residual effects of anaesthesia.
- Nasopharyngeal airways and nasal tracheal tubes cannot be inserted after a pharyngoplasty.

INTRODUCTION

Plastic surgery in children can improve both appearance and function. This chapter covers surgery for cleft lip and palate, external ear reconstruction and syndactyly. Other common plastic operations are discussed in Chapters 32 and 43.

CLEFT LIP AND PALATE

Background

EPIDEMIOLOGY

Cleft lip and palate are common congenital abnormalities. Cleft lip, with or without a cleft palate, occurs in 1 in 600 live births and the prevalence is higher in Orientals and Native Americans. Isolated cleft palate occurs in about 1 in 2000 births. The risk of having a baby with a cleft rises to between 1 in 20 and 1 in 40 if either one parent or one sibling has a cleft [1,2]. Approximately 1000 cleft lip and palate babies are born per year in England and Wales.

EMBRYOLOGY

Clefts arise because of defects in nasal or maxillary fusion in the first trimester. The palate grows inwards and fuses in the midline in two parts. The primary palate, which is anterior to the incisive foramen, fuses by 5–6 weeks to form the alveolar process (which contains the anterior hard palate, teeth buds and upper lip). The secondary palate, which is posterior to the incisive foramen, fuses later at 7–8 weeks. Cleft lip or palate can be either incomplete or complete, and unilateral or bilateral. A submucous cleft palate occurs when the soft palate mucosa has fused without continuity of the palatal muscles.

NATURAL HISTORY

Unrepaired cleft lip, on its own, does not prevent feeding but by its appearance causes social exclusion. A cleft palate generally prevents suckling and breast-feeding. Swallowing, however, should be unaffected and milk can be trickled into the pharynx by a spoon, a syringe or a squeezable bottle with a very soft nipple. Both the mother and the infant need patience and practice but most infants will thrive. Other feeding problems may result from reflux or pharyngeal incoordination, particularly in isolated cleft palates. If the mandible is small, the pharynx is compressed and it may be difficult to coordinate breathing during feeding. Speech is abnormal due to the escape of air into the nose (velopharyngeal incompetence) and due to poor tongue articulation. Hearing deficits (mainly glue ear) are common with cleft palate and hinder speech development and learning. In many parts of the world resources for surgical correction do not exist and cleft children may suffer from ridicule and bullying at school. Consequently education, employment and marriage are unlikely.

THE EFFECT OF SURGERY

Surgical correction of the lip transforms lives – and revision operations, if necessary, can be achieved in later life. Cleft palate closure is crucial for normal speech development but, unfortunately, it can cause delayed complications of impaired facial growth and unsatisfactory speech. Complications occur because scar tissue forms at important growth sites that may result in maxillary retrusion and contraction of the upper dental arch. Correction of maxillary retrusion is possible with maxillary osteotomy, and dental arch contraction can be modified by prolonged orthodontic care. Surgery can compromise speech either because the soft palate does not seal the nasopharynx or there is a breakdown in the repair leaving an oronasal fistula. The rate of these complications depends upon surgical skill or the type of operation (or both). In the best centres over 90 per cent of primary surgery results in both normal speech and maxillary growth whereas other centres may have only a 30 per cent success rate. There are several recommended surgical techniques and it remains controversial as to which has the best outcome. It is generally accepted that some operations are more damaging than others and, in particular, that the Wardill–Kilner operation tends to cause more scar formation and larger fistulae than the Langenbeck palatoplasty (Fig. 35.1).

Improved results can be expected by concentrating services in dedicated centres, allowing fewer surgeons to operate on a larger number of cases [3]; in the UK, each cleft surgeon should operate on approximately 50 new cases per year. By regular follow-up of patients (until facial growth is complete) surgeons can assess and perfect their technique.

ASSOCIATED ABNORMALITIES

In a review of 1000 cases, over 50 per cent had one or more major anomalies, 22 per cent were syndromic and of these approximately half were unknown and presumed unique (these infants are often labelled dysmorphic) [4]. Major

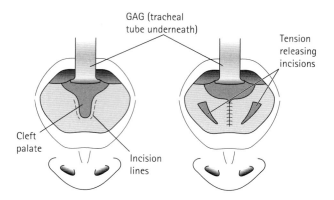

Figure 35.1 Oral views of repair of cleft palate (simplified Langenbeck palatoplasty).

Table 35.1 Important features of velocardiofacial syndrome

Defect	Features
Cleft palate	Very common (75%) – may be submucous
Airway	Pharyngeal hypotonia, retrognathia, laryngomalacia, laryngeal web, vascular ring
Pharynx	Medially placed common carotid arteries – vulnerable during surgical dissection for pharyngoplasty
Cardiovascular	Cardiac anomalies (interrupted aortic arch, pulmonary atresia, aortic coarctation)
	Sensitive to catecholamines (abnormal COMT) [7,8]
Immune and metabolic	Hypoplasia or aplasia of thymus and parathyroids
Other	Developmental delay, behavioural and psychological problems

COMT, catechol-O-methyltransferase.

anomalies are much more common in patients with isolated cleft palate.

Cleft lip and palate has been associated with around 150 different syndromes and the most common is the velocardiofacial syndrome (VCFS). It was first described by Robert Shprintzen in 1978 [5] and its common features are listed in Table 35.1 [6–8]. It has an autosomal dominant inheritance although many cases arise spontaneously.

Important syndromes, listed in Table 35.2, are associated with difficult airways. The Pierre Robin sequence is a combination of a cleft palate, small mandible (micrognathia) and posterior displacement of the tongue (glossoptosis). There may be significant airway obstruction, especially during sleep, which can often be relieved by the prone position. If the mandible is very small there can be life-threatening airway obstruction soon after birth. A nasopharyngeal airway, positioned behind the tongue or just above the epiglottis, usually clears the airway, but in severe cases tracheal intubation is indicated leading to tracheostomy. A laryngeal mask airway (LMA) may provide a temporary clear airway.

Table 35.2 Important cleft syndromes associated with difficult airways

Syndrome	Features
Pierre Robin	Micrognathia, glossoptosis (airway problems resolve with age)
Treacher Collins	Micrognathia (airway problems increase with age)
	Malar hypoplasia, abnormal ears (deafness) and eyelids
Stickler	Micrognathia, retinal and vitreous changes, hearing loss, osteoarthritis, retinal detachment
Goldenhar	Hemifacial microsomia, vertebral dysplasia, cardiac defects
Van der Woude	Lower lip pits, hypodontia
Down	Learning disability, large tongue, atlantoaxial instability, cardiac defects, hypotonia, hypothyroidism, hyperextensible joints
Nager	Micrognathia, malar hypoplasia, limb hypoplasia, ear defects, vertebral anomalies, hearing loss, cardiac defects

Laryngoscopy can be difficult in these babies. In time, the mandible should grow and airway obstruction usually resolves by about 12 weeks. Babies with Stickler and Nager syndromes can have similar airway problems. Airway obstruction makes feeding difficult and a nasogastric tube may be needed to ensure that the baby thrives.

HISTORY OF CLEFT LIP AND PALATE REPAIR

Cleft lip repair was described in the *Leechbook of Bald* in about AD 920 and in China many centuries before that [9], but few palates were repaired before the advent of general anaesthesia in 1846. Before then, the palate was numbed with gargled iced water and few could endure the pain.

John Snow pioneered the use of chloroform and ether for cleft surgery. In 1847, he reported their use in three 6-week-old infants undergoing cleft lip repair [10]. Anaesthetic was administered intermittently either by drip onto an open gauze mask or by a sponge applied to the nostril. The airway was unprotected and blood had to drain away by gravity. Initially, palate repair was considered too hazardous but by the 1860s Collis and Smith published their experience of using chloroform for palate repair [11]. Pharyngeal insufflation of vapour was being used by 1900, and tracheal insufflation by the 1920s. Vapour was insufflated via a small-bore tracheal catheter and the airway was maintained by a larger-bore catheter either in the trachea or above the glottis [12]. The pharynx was packed with gauze to prevent aspiration of blood.

During the 1930s, single-lumen, large-bore, tracheal tubes were in general use and, scaled down, applied to infants.

They were inserted, with skill, under deep anaesthesia without the use of muscle relaxants. In 1937 Ayres introduced the T-piece, specifically for infants undergoing cleft surgery, in order to minimise rebreathing and resistance during spontaneous respiration [13]. Jackson Rees then added an open-ended rebreathing bag to the end of the T-piece to enable assisted ventilation by hand [14]. Finally, controlled ventilation became common practice with the introduction of muscle relaxant drugs.

Since these pioneering days, advances in the understanding of infant physiology and anaesthesia, better drugs, training, equipment and monitoring have all improved the safety and quality of anaesthesia for cleft surgery [15,16].

General issues of surgical management

MULTIDISCIPLINARY CARE

Optimal results are obtained by experienced and integrated teams based in dedicated centres. Families need support and specialist opinion from the time of diagnosis (frequently during pregnancy) to help with feeding, hearing and associated congenital abnormalities. Treatment by speech therapists, orthodontists and psychologists is important later, and parents frequently need genetic advice [17]. Parent support groups are extremely valuable (http://www.clapa.com).

TIMING OF SURGERY

Repair of the cleft lip is done at 2–3 months but can be undertaken at any age. In 1966 a retrospective review [18] showed that there was a fivefold increase in the complication rate of cleft surgery if infants weighed <10 lb (4.54 kg), had a haemoglobin <10 g/dL and a white cell count >10 000/mm³. These 'rules of 10' were later modified to include an age of at least 10 weeks. Understandably, parents want the cleft repaired as soon as possible, yet no psychological disadvantage (to parents) of a delay has been demonstrated [19]. Published complications of neonatal anaesthesia [20–22] and the other disadvantages (and advantages) of neonatal repair are summarised in Table 35.3. In some cultures of the developing world a mother can be socially excluded by giving birth to a cleft baby and this may persuade surgeons to operate early.

Lip or palate surgery should be undertaken only when a baby is thriving; there are exceptions to this rule but the risks must be understood.

A cleft palate should be repaired before speech starts so that speech develops normally. Speech results are best if the palate is repaired before the age of 12 months [23]. It has been suggested that an earlier repair or even a combined repair of the lip and palate in the neonatal period [24,25] is best, but the long-term surgical results (upon maxillary growth and speech) have not been assessed.

Table 35.3 Considerations of cleft lip repair in neonates versus older infants

Consideration	Neonatal repair	Repair at 3 months
Aesthetic result	Improved healing (not proven)	easier repair (not proven)
Blood loss	Higher haemoglobin	Larger blood volume
Physiology	Neonatal physiology (vulnerable to complications of anaesthesia)	Infant physiology
	Undiagnosed abnormalities	Safer use of opioid analgesia
Psychological	Improved parental bonding (not proven)	More support for family may be required
Social	Developing world: cleft mothers can be excluded – early operations may prevent infanticide	Maternal depression (not proven)
Feeding	No advantage	

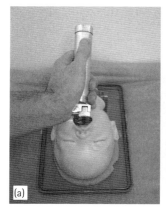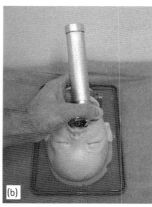

Figure 35.2 Oral views of two methods of laryngoscopy. (a) Midline approach – lifting the tongue with a curved blade; (b) lateral approach – sliding past and underneath the tongue with a straight blade.

Management of cleft lip repair in infants

The challenge for the surgeon is to produce a symmetrical reconstruction of the lip and the nose. Perioral muscles need to be rearranged to ensure a functioning lip. If there is a cleft palate, a flap of mucoperiosteum from the vomer can be raised (a 'vomerine' flap) to close the anterior cleft hard palate.

PREOPERATIVE ASSESSMENT

Special care should be taken to detect associated congenital abnormalities – cardiac anomalies occur in 5–10 per cent of cleft babies. Preoperative haemoglobin measurement is unnecessary in most healthy infants but may be warranted because some infants will have physiological anaemia and others will have significant blood loss, especially during bilateral lip repair [26]. In the premature infant, surgery may reasonably be delayed until 50 or 60 weeks' postconceptual age, but it is more important that the infant is feeding, gaining weight and well.

ANAESTHESIA

The choice of anaesthesia drug or technique depends upon the child and the experience of the anaesthetist. Cleft lip alone does not cause an airway problem. Laryngoscopy should be with a straight-bladed scope and using a lateral approach (Fig. 35.2) [27]. If a midline approach is used the laryngoscope can become caught in a cleft, especially if this is on the right side. A gauze roll placed in the cleft may prevent this happening. A protruding premaxilla can also hinder a midline laparoscopy [27,28]. A south-facing, preformed, oral tracheal tube is secured in the midline on the chin. A throat pack is usual.

Spontaneous ventilation, rather than controlled, is associated with a minor reduction in blood loss [29] but is unlikely to be clinically significant. Blood loss should be carefully measured and intravenous clear fluids infused. At the end of surgery, packs or stents may be inserted into the nose to maintain its shape. These block the nose and can cause respiratory distress in infants – a hollow stent can be used instead.

ANALGESIA

Wound infiltration with local anaesthesia (LA) provides analgesia for a few hours. Longer and more effective analgesia can be obtained by an infraorbital nerve block [30,31] (see also Chapter 26). This nerve innervates the upper lip, lower eyelid, malar skin and side of the nose (but not a vomerine flap). It can be blocked percutaneously either at the infraorbital notch or midway between the palpebral fissure and angle of the mouth [30]. Alternatively, it can be blocked under direct vision during dissection. Paracetamol and non-steroidal anti-inflammatory drugs (NSAIDs) with or without morphine or codeine will be required in some cases, especially if there is a vomerine flap. Older children may need more potent opioid analgesia [32].

SUTURE REMOVAL

Non-absorbable sutures are removed at 5–7 days. In infants this can be achieved under sedation using chloral hydrate, although brief general anaesthesia produces more reliable and steady conditions with a shorter recovery.

Management of primary cleft palate repair in infants

The surgical objectives are both to produce a palate that closes the nasopharynx during speech and to cause minimal scarring. Dissection of palatal muscles is aided by the use of an operating microscope. Surgery should last 60–90 minutes and access is achieved by the use of a gag to depress the tongue. Prolonged pressure from the mouth gag (approximately 3 hours in the literature – seen after 2 hours by MA) can cause significant ischaemia or infarction of the tongue and, when the gag is released, it can swell and obstruct the airway [33–35]. It is prudent to release the gag for a few minutes after 1 hour and then every half hour to ensure that the tongue becomes pink each time. Infants with tongue swelling have been managed with nasopharyngeal airway or tracheal intubation for several days until the swelling has receded. There may be long-term dysfunction.

PREOPERATIVE ASSESSMENT

Surgery must be delayed until the infant is thriving. Appreciable pharyngeal airway obstruction is a contraindication to surgery because it will be exacerbated by palatal closure. If airway obstruction or apnoea is suspected during sleep this should be assessed by overnight oxygen saturation monitoring. Appreciable desaturation may need to be investigated by polysomnography to determine the contribution of central apnoea that could be a feature of cerebral disease. Associated reflux problems are common and need to be controlled beforehand. Rhinorrhoea, caused by reflux of milk into the nose, should not be confused with an upper respiratory tract infection. Cardiac abnormalities must be identified and the timing of palate surgery discussed with cardiologists. Mouth opening should be estimated because cleft palate infants are frequently syndromic and have a small mandible, and laryngoscopy may be difficult. Postoperative airway management should be also planned. Haemoglobin estimation is indicated, especially if significant blood loss occurred with repair of the cleft lip.

LARYNGOSCOPY AND INTUBATION

In a large audit of children with cleft lip and palate in Sri Lanka, the risk of difficult laryngoscopy was 8 per cent when using a curved blade. Most of the difficulty was caused by micrognathia, and protruding premaxilla, and found in infants less than 6 months of age [28]. These observations have been confirmed by a recent survey by Xue *et al.* [36]. A straight blade placed lateral to and almost underneath the tongue should gain a much better view (Fig. 35.3 and see Fig. 35.2). This is because the curved blade tends to compress the tongue and push the larynx further away.

If the mouth opening is severely restricted it may not be possible to perform the operation itself. Once the infant is anaesthetised, the surgeon should be consulted and, before time-consuming laryngoscopy techniques are used, it may

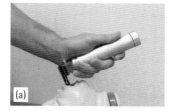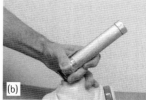

Figure 35.3 Lateral views of two methods of holding a laryngoscope. (a) The standard method used for large children and adults; (b) an alternative method useful in small infants (note the position of the thumb and little finger).

be appropriate to abandon the procedure until the child has grown.

Techniques for difficult laryngoscopy are covered in detail in Chapter 21 but the following have been applied to infants with cleft palate. Often, with conventional laryngoscopy, the larynx can be seen if cricoid pressure is firm and a flexible bougie is used to guide intubation. A tracheal tube can be guided also by the anaesthetist's fingers by 'feel' [37] and one of us (MA) has achieved this in an infant with severe micrognathia.

Fibre-optic laryngoscopy is relatively easy under anaesthesia and via an LMA but intubation itself can be much more difficult in infants than adults for several reasons. A thin scope will easily pass through a size 1 LMA but it will occlude the trachea, so that oxygen desaturation is likely while a tracheal tube (already loaded onto the scope) is advanced. A second tracheal tube has to be loaded onto the scope so that it can push the first through the LMA and into the trachea. Larger endoscopes have a suction port to enable the passage of a guidewire into the trachea [38] but, unfortunately, there may be insufficient space within the LMA for the infant to breathe. Despite these problems fibre-optic intubation via an LMA has been successful in infants with Pierre Robin sequence [39,40], and Treacher Collins [41] and Goldenhar syndromes [42].

Other special laryngoscopes such as the Bullard have been used [43]. This hook-like scope is inserted into the pharynx and pulls the tongue forward without compression. It has a suction port though which a respiratory exchange catheter can be passed into the trachea. The technique may take a little practice but, if successful, is much quicker than flexible fibre-optic laryngoscopy.

If laryngoscopy is difficult, the airway can be managed by LMA alone, although this is not ideal because it can easily be displaced during surgery. A tracheostomy may be necessary especially if the airway is precarious beforehand [15]. Surgery should perhaps be delayed in these circumstances.

Preformed plastic tracheal tubes are satisfactory in most cleft infants but they have thin walls and are occasionally compressed by the gag. This is most likely with the smallest tubes used in retrognathic infants in whom the gag exerts a high pressure. Other more robust preformed tubes are no longer manufactured.

A wire-reinforced tracheal tube is unlikely to be compressed but its correct length is difficult to judge. If it is slightly too long, the gag may push it into a bronchus; if too short it may spring out of the trachea when the gag is removed.

ANAESTHESIA

After induction, care should be taken to ensure that the lungs can be inflated before a muscle relaxant is administered. An inhalational technique has the theoretical advantage that a high inspired concentration of oxygen is inhaled throughout induction. Significant blood loss is unusual but should be estimated. Secure venous access is crucial. Bleeding is reduced by infiltration with a dilute adrenaline solution (1 in 250 000 with 0.5 per cent lidocaine, approximately 4–7 mL). If there is persistent bleeding from raw surfaces the authors recommend intravenous tranexamic acid (10 mg/kg) – a rapid reduction is usually observed. A pharyngeal pack is inserted by the surgeon.

ANALGESIA

Infiltration with local anaesthetic is ineffective for postoperative analgesia. The nerve supply to the palate is more difficult to block than the lip, requiring anaesthesia of the greater and lesser palatine, nasal palatine and glossopharyngeal nerves. Prolonged distraction of the temporomandibular joint probably adds to postoperative discomfort. Consequently, opioid analgesia is usually required, but must be carefully administered to avoid appreciable sedation that might contribute to postoperative airway obstruction. An intraoperative infusion of remifentanil (0.2–0.3 μg/kg/min) allows better control of blood pressure and heart rate, and a significant reduction in intraoperative anaesthetic requirements. Longer-acting opioids can be titrated following extubation. Intraoperative clonidine (2–3 μg/kg) or ketamine (0.5–1 mg/kg) may reduce anaesthesia and opioid requirements and prevent distress in recovery. Non-steroidal anti-inflammatory agents possibly increase bleeding, but are effective for postoperative pain relief and are used routinely in many centres.

An opioid infusion may be necessary for the first 12–24 hours; however, once effective analgesia has been obtained with intravenous morphine, regular administration of oral opioids combined with paracetamol and diclofenac are usually sufficient. Early resumption of oral feeding may reduce distress.

EXTUBATION AND ACUTE AIRWAY OBSTRUCTION

Acute airway obstruction can occur soon after extubation and is caused by a combination of factors including nasopharyngeal obstruction (caused by the repair – Fig. 35.4), blood, secretions, oedema, pharyngeal incoordination and residual effects of anaesthesia. Postoperative respiratory complications should be anticipated in about 9 per cent of

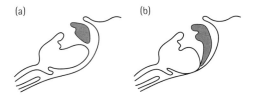

Figure 35.4 Airway obstruction after closure of cleft palate due to small mandible and posterior position of tongue.

normal infants [44] and the risk is significantly increased with pre-existing airway obstruction [45].

Before extubation, it is wise to wait until all bleeding has ceased. After the pack has been removed, the pharynx must be cleared by suction and the infant extubated 'awake'. Venous cannulae must be secured beforehand because they can be pulled or kicked out by the infant.

If the airway is obstructed, a nasopharyngeal airway can be inserted promptly and gently. This is almost always successful and should not disrupt the palatal repair. Some centres leave one in routinely for micrognathic infants. Alternatively, a thick suture can be inserted into the tongue to pull it forward and clear the airway. This may not be as reliable and it can cause haemorrhage and distress. If the airway cannot be cleared, or if there is apnoea, the trachea must be reintubated immediately. After stabilisation, another extubation attempt can be considered when the infant is less sleepy.

POSTOPERATIVE CARE

A nasopharyngeal airway may be needed for the first few hours until the infant can breathe reliably through the mouth. Dexamethasone may reduce obstruction caused by oedema but any definite benefit is unproven. Blood in the nasal airway (or nostril) may coagulate and, with a few drops of saline, gentle suction should clear it. Postoperative analgesics should be titrated to avoid causing sedation and airway obstruction.

Postoperative bleeding is difficult to detect because the blood is usually swallowed. Regular observation by experienced nurses in a high-dependency setting is important. Arm restraints are used by some units to prevent the infant's fingers disrupting the repair; however, a randomised trial showed no benefit and no reduction in the rate of fistulae [46]. Antibiotics (usually penicillin) are recommended to reduce postoperative wound infection and pyrexia [15].

Management of secondary surgery

Many cleft children will require further surgery to improve facial appearance and speech and the following operations require special management.

ABBE FLAP

A pedicle flap can be raised from the lower lip (known as an 'Abbe' flap) and sutured to the upper lip to augment it. The pedicle obviously restricts mouth opening and limits the options for laryngoscopy so that a nasopharyngeal airway may be necessary. Patients should be extubated fully awake. For division of the flap, airway management may need fibre-optic-assisted nasotracheal intubation or, if the flap can be divided easily, ketamine can be used to manage the division and afterwards airway control becomes uncomplicated.

ALVEOLAR BONE GRAFT

A gap in the alveolar margin prevents the normal alignment of teeth. If it is filled with bone 'chips', orthodontic treatment can reposition teeth so that they grow into the new bone. Bone grafting is performed at about 10 years before permanent canines erupt. The bone donor site is usually the iliac crest and it causes prolonged postoperative discomfort. During the first day, pain can be managed by infiltration of local anaesthetic or a continuous infusion of local anaesthetic into the wound [47]. Thereafter non-steroidal drugs are needed for up to 2 weeks. Postoperative nausea and vomiting seems to be a significant problem in these patients.

PHARYNGOPLASTY

Speech defects caused by palatal dysfunction are proven by video-fluoroscopy and nasal endoscopy. Immobile soft palates need surgery to readjust the muscles. If the palate is too short, it cannot reach the posterior pharyngeal wall and it may be necessary to perform a pharyngoplasty. This type of operation lifts flaps of posterior pharyngeal wall and either these can be used to create a pharyngeal ridge that the soft palate can reach (Hynes pharyngoplasty) or a pharyngeal flap (Figs 35.5 and 35.6) is sutured onto the soft palate.

There are two important hazards with pharyngoplasty operations. First there are airway consequences. Nasal airflow, reduced to improve speech, can be so compromised that there is obstructive sleep apnoea. This may last only a few days but can be severe and persist requiring the flap to be taken down [48–50]. Micrognathia and VCFS may increase this problem [51–53]. Death has been reported following pharyngeal flap surgery [54]. Airway obstruction cannot be managed with nasal airways because they will damage the flap. Nasotracheal intubation is contraindicated in future operations unless intraoral surgery cannot be managed otherwise (in these circumstances passing a nasotracheal tube around the pharyngeal obstruction is possible using a nasogastric tube as a guide). Careful postoperative monitoring is recommended for at least 24 h. Opioid analgesia should be used carefully to avoid causing postoperative sedation. There is typically a sore throat for 1–2 weeks and NSAIDs are helpful.

Second, bleeding from the flap donor site may be difficult to control and some children will require overnight intubation while the bleeding is controlled by a pharyngeal pack [48]. Surgeons must be extra careful in children with VCFS because the carotid arteries can be more medial and lie just underneath the pharyngeal flap donor site.

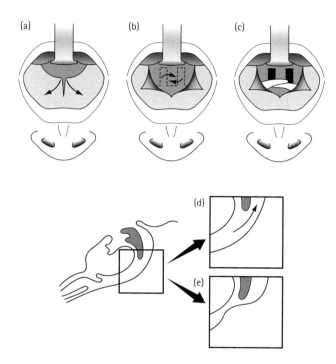

Figure 35.5 Oral and sagittal views of Hynes' pharyngoplasty. The soft palate is incised and flaps are pulled back to expose the posterior pharyngeal wall – as in (a) and (b). Pharyngeal flaps are raised and sutured to create a ridge – as in (c) and (e). Note the raw pharyngeal area of the flap donor sites from which haemorrhage can be difficult to control. Note that after this operation a nasotracheal tube cannot be inserted without causing pharyngeal damage.

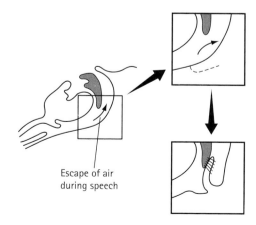

Figure 35.6 Sagittal section of pharyngeal flap. Note that after this operation a nasotracheal tube cannot be inserted without causing pharyngeal damage.

MAXILLARY OSTEOTOMY

This operation is performed in young adults to advance the maxilla to improve facial appearance. Appreciable blood loss should be expected. At the end of surgery, the maxilla and mandible are wired together. Therefore, a nasotracheal tube is needed and must be removed only when the pharynx is clear and the patient is awake.

Cleft anaesthesia in developing countries

Anaesthetists from developed countries frequently travel to underdeveloped parts of the world to participate in cleft surgical programmes [55–58]. Careful selection of patients, attention to technique, drugs and equipment, and thorough intraoperative and postoperative observation (and monitoring if available) should ensure safe anaesthesia delivery. Postoperative nurses are crucial for safety [59].

Children, and adults, may present with unrepaired clefts. Cooperative patients will tolerate lip repair under LA, perhaps with additional sedation. Combined lip and palate repair (in children) is reasonable but will take 3–4 hours to complete and often result in appreciable blood loss. Analgesia should be managed with care because some racial groups may be sensitive to opioids.

EXTERNAL EAR SURGERY

Otoplasty

Prominent ears are a cosmetic deformity present in about 5 per cent of the Caucasian population. Fifty per cent of affected individuals have a family history; inheritance has an autosomal dominant pattern with variable penetrance. Prominent ears can have a severe emotional and behavioural effect on a child once they reach school age. Otoplasty is a common surgical procedure designed to give the auricle a more natural and anatomical appearance. An otoplasty corrects the protrusion, shape and size with a variety of cartilage-splitting or cartilage-sparing procedures.

Surgery may be performed under LA alone in cooperative older children. Good anaesthesia of the ear can be provided by local infiltration and local anaesthetic cream may be used to reduce the initial pain [60]. The lesser occipital and greater auricular nerves can be blocked by injection at the posterior border of the sternocleidomastoid muscle. The auriculotemporal nerve can also be blocked by superficial injection anterior to the tragus. Lidocaine infiltration (with adrenaline to reduce bleeding) has a marginally shorter duration than a regional block using a longer-acting agent [61].

Overall, most children require general anaesthesia and LA techniques can be used as well. There is a high incidence of PONV which is increased with the use of opioid analgesics [62] Ondansetron is a successful prophylactic antiemetic [63]. After surgery, tight dressings may also increase

vomiting [64]. Local anaesthesia alone, without general anaesthesia, may eliminate nausea and vomiting [65].

Significant pain may be encountered when the local anaesthetic effect wears off in 8–10 hours. Regular administration of non-steroidal analgesics is advisable and rescue opioid analgesics (codeine should be sufficient) should be provided on discharge. Pain can be caused by a haematoma or the dressing itself being too tight.

Ear reconstruction

Reconstruction of the ear is required for both congenital microtia and traumatic ear injuries. Microtia is associated with Goldenhar and Treacher Collins syndromes. Surgery is in two stages: first an ear is carved from costal cartilage and inserted under the skin at the ear site; months later, the skin is rearranged around the new ear. Almost all of the pain arises from the cartilage donor site and analgesia by single injections of local bupivacaine and intravenous clonidine lasts 18–24 hours. Some centres use a continuous infusion of local anaesthetic into the wound for the first 24 h. Thereafter, regular NSAIDs should be used.

SYNDACTYLY REPAIR

Syndactyly of the hands arises from defects in differentiation and results in the failure of separation of the fingers into individual appendages. Severity ranges from the mild form where only the soft tissue is fused to the severe forms with bone or cartilage union. Surgical repair may involve various fasciocutaneous flaps, skin grafts (full- or split-thickness from a local or remote sites) or osteotomy. Primary repairs are performed at 6–18 months. A tourniquet is crucial to provide a bloodless surgical field and cuff pressures need to be significantly higher than systolic pressure – 50 mmHg above may be sufficient [66]. Care should be taken with both skin padding and skin preparation solutions to avoid injury under the tourniquet [67].

Syndactyly is associated with Apert syndrome (among other craniofacial syndromes) and caused by amniotic bands and epidermolysis bullosa. Airway management is not usually complicated with craniofacial syndromes except that the mouth needs to remain open during induction because the nostrils are usually obstructed. Insertion of an LMA or tracheal tube is usually straightforward. Venous access cannot be placed in the hands and may therefore be difficult. Axillary brachial plexus block provides excellent postoperative analgesia and significantly reduces the intraoperative anaesthetic requirements. The neurovascular sheath is superficial in children and easily palpated. The block can be performed using single or multiple direct injections [68,69] or cannulation of the sheath guided by palpation, nerve stimulation or ultrasound [70,71] (see Chapter 26). Paracetamol, an NSAID and codeine phosphate (or similar opioid) may be required when the block wears off. Anaesthesia is often required for removal of dressings 1–2 weeks later.

REFERENCES

Key references

Ayres P. Anaesthesia for hare-lip and palate operation. *Br J Surg* 1937; **25**: 796–802.

Bosenberg AT, Kimble FW. Infraorbital nerve block in neonates for cleft lip repair: anatomical study and clinical application. *Br J Anaesth* 1995; **74**(5): 506–8.

Bell C, Oh TH, Loeffler JR. Massive macroglossia and airway obstruction after cleft palate repair. *Anesth Analg* 1988; **67**: 71–4.

Xue FS, Zhang GH, Li P *et al.* The clinical observation of difficult laryngoscopy and difficult intubation in infants with cleft lip and palate. *Paediatr Anaesth* 2006; **16**(3): 283–9.

Xue FS, An S, Tong SY, Liao X, Liu JH, Luo LK. Influence of surgical technique on early post-operative hypoxaemia in children undergoing elective palatoplasty. *Br J Anaesth* 1998; **80**: 447–51.

References

1. Sommerlad BC. Managment of cleft lip and palate. *Curr Paediatr* 1994; **4**: 189–95.
2. Habel A, Sell D, Mars M. Management of cleft lip and palate. *Arch Dis Child* 1996; **74**: 360–6.
3. Clinical Standards Advisory Group. *Cleft lip and palate.* London: Department of Health, 1998.
4. Shprintzen RJ, Siegel-Sadewitz VL, Amato J, Goldberg RB. Retrospective diagnoses of previously missed syndromic disorders among 1,000 patients with cleft lip, cleft palate, or both. *Birth Defects: Orig Artic Ser* 1985; **21**(2): 85–92.
5. Shprintzen RJ, Goldberg RB, Lewin ML *et al.* A new syndrome involving cleft palate, cardiac anomalies, typical facies, and learning disabilities: velo-cardio-facial syndrome. *Cleft Palate* J 1978; **15**(1): 56–62.
6. Driscoll DA, Emanuel BS. DiGeorge and velocardiofacial syndromes: The 22q11 deletion syndrome. *Ment Retard Dev Disabil Res Rev* 1996; **2**(3): 130–8.
7. Graf WD, Unis AS, Yates CM *et al.* Catecholamines in patients with 22q11.2 deletion syndrome and the low-activity COMT polymorphism. *Neurology* 2001; **57**: 410–16.
8. Passariello M, Perkins R. Unexpected postoperative tachycardia in a patient with 22q11 deletion syndrome after multiple dental extractions. *Paediatr Anaesth* 2005; **15**(12): 1145–6.
9. Wallace AF. A history of the repair of cleft lip and palate in Britain before World War II. *Ann Plast Surg* 1987; **19**(3): 266–75.
10. Snow J. Operations without pain. *Lancet* 1847; **i**: 500.
11. Collins MH. Chloroform in cleft palate. *BMJ* 1868; **i**: 131.
12. Magill IW. New inventions: an expiratory attachment for endotracheal catheters. *Lancet* 1924; **i**: 1320.
13. Ayres P. Anaesthesia for hare-lip and palate operation. *Br J Surg* 1937; **25**: 796–802.
14. Rees GJ. Paediatric anaesthesia. *Br J Anaesth* 1960; **32**(3): 132.
15. Doyle E, Hudson I. Anaesthesia for primary repair of cleft lip and palate: a review of 244 procedures. *Paediatr Anaesth* 1992; **2**: 139–45.
16. Jennings FO, Denlaney EJ, Prendiville JB. Ether-cyclopropane anaesthesia for the primary repair of cleft lip and palate (a 20 year experience). *Br J Plast Surg* 1980; **33**: 301–4.
17. Williams AC, Bearn D, Clark JD *et al.* The delivery of surgical cleft care in the United Kingdom. *J R Coll Surg Edin* 2001; **46**(3): 143–9.
18. Wilhelmsen HR, Musgrave RH. Complications of cleft lip surgery. *Cleft Palate* J 1966; **3**: 223–31.
19. Slade P, Emerson DJ, Freedlander E. A longitudinal comparison of the psychological impact on mothers of neonatal and 3 month repair of cleft lip. *Br J Plastic Sur* 1999; **52**(1): 1–5.
20. van Boven MJ, Pendeville PE, Veyckemans F *et al.* Neonatal cleft lip repair: the anesthesiologist's point of view. *Cleft Palate Craniofac J* 1993; **30**(6): 574–7.
21. Stephens P, Saunders P, Bingham R. Neonatal cleft lip repair: a retrospective review of anaesthetic complications. *Paediatr Anaesth* 1997; **7**: 33–6.
22. Ansermino JM, Sommerlad BC. Neonatal cleft lip repair. *Paediatr Anaesth* 1998; **8**(1): 94–6.
23. Sommerlad BC. Surgical management of cleft palate: a review. *J R Soc Med* 1989; **82**(11): 677–8.
24. Lehman Jr JA, Douglas BK, Ho WC, Husami TW. One-stage closure of the entire primary palate. *Plast Reconstr Surg* 1990; **86**(4): 675–81.
25. Sandberg DJ, Magee WP Jr, Denk MJ. Neonatal cleft lip and cleft palate repair. *AORN J* 1997; **75**(3): 490–8.
26. Ansermino JM, Than M, Swallow PD. Pre-operative blood tests in children undergoing plastic surgery. *Ann R Coll Surg Engl* 1999; **81**(3): 175–8.
27. Hatch DJ. Airway management in cleft lip and palate surgery. *Br J Anaesth* 1996; **76**: 755–6.
28. Gunawardana RH. Difficulty laryngoscopy in cleft lip and palate surgery. *Br J Anaesth* 1996; **76**: 757–9.
29. Law RC, Clark C. Anaesthesia for cleft lip and palate surgery. *Update Anaesth* 2002; **14**: 27–9.
30. Bosenberg AT, Kimble FW. Infraorbital nerve block in neonates for cleft lip repair: anatomical study and clinical application. *Br J Anaesth* 1995; **74**(5): 506–8.
31. Ahuja S, Datta A, Krishna A, Bhattacharya A. Infra-orbital nerve block for relief of postoperative pain following cleft lip surgery in infants. *Anaesthesia* 1994; **49**: 441–4.
32. Gunawardena RH. Anaesthesia in cleft lip and cleft palate surgery of children. *Ceylon Med J* 1990; **35**(2): 63–6.
33. Patane PS, White SE. Macroglossia causing airway obstruction following cleft palate repair. *Anesthesiology* 1988; **71**: 995–6.
34. Bell C, Oh TH, Loeffler JR. Massive macroglossia and airway obstruction after cleft palate repair. *Anesth Analg* 1988; **67**: 71–4.

35. Lee JT, Kingston HG. Airways obstruction due to oedema following cleft palate surgery. *J Anaesth* 1985; **32**: 265–7.

36. Xue FS, Zhang GH, Li P *et al.* The clinical observation of difficult laryngoscopy and difficult intubation in infants with cleft lip and palate. *Paediatr Anaesth 2006;* **16**(3): 283–9.

37. Sutera PT, Gordon GJ. Digitally assisted tracheal intubation in a neonate with Pierre Robin syndrome. *Anesthesiology* 1993; **78**: 983–5.

38. Hasan MA, Black AE. A new technique for fibreoptic intubation in children. *Anaesthesia* 1994; **49**: 1031–3.

39. Chadd GD, Crane DL, Phillips RM, Tunell WP. Extubation and reintubation guided by the laryngeal mask airway in a child with Pierre Robin syndrome. *Anaesthesia* 1992; **76**: 640–1.

40. Beveridge ME. Laryngeal mask anaesthesia for repair of cleft palate. *Anaesthesia* 1989; **44**: 656–7.

41. Inada T, Fujise K, Tachibana K, Shingu K. Orotracheal intubation through the laryngeal mask airway in paediatric patients with Treacher Collins syndrome. *Paediatr Anaesth* 1995; **5**: 129–32.

42. Johnson CM, Sims C. Awake fibreoptic intubation via a laryngeal mask in an infant with Goldenhar's syndrome. *Anaesth Intensive Care* 1994; **22**(2): 194–7.

43. Borland LM, Casselbrant M. The Bullard laryngoscope. A new indirect oral laryngoscope (pediatric version). *Anesth Analg* 1990; **70**(1): 105–8.

44. Takemura H, Yasumoto K, Toi T, Hosoyamada A. Correlation of cleft type with incidence of perioperative respiratory complications in infants with cleft lip and palate. *Paediatr Anaesth* 2002; **12**(7): 585–8.

45. Henriksson TG, Skoog VT. Identification of children at high anaesthetic risk at the time of primary palatoplasty. *Scand J Plast Reconstr Surg Hand Surg* 2001; **35**(2): 177–82.

46. Jigjinni V, Kangesu T, Sommerlad BC. Do babies require arm splints after cleft palate repair? *Br J Plast Surg* 1993; **46**(8): 681–5.

47. Lonnqvist PA, Morton NS. Postoperative analgesia in infants and children. *Br J Anaesth* 2005; **95**(1): 59–68.

48. Valnicek SM, Zuker RM, Halpern LM, Roy WL. Perioperative complications of superior pharyngeal flap surgery in children. *Plast Reconstr Surg* 1994; **93**(5): 954–8.

49. Orr WC, Levine NS, Buchanan RT. Effect of cleft palate repair and pharyngeal flap surgery on upper airway obstruction during sleep. *Plast Reconstr Surg* 1987; **80**: 226–30.

50. Sirois M, Caouette-Laberge L, Laocque Y, Egerszegi P. Sleep apnea following a pharyngeal flap: a feared complication. *Plast Reconstr Surg* 1994; **93**: 943–7.

51. Abramson DL, Marrinan EM, Mulliken JB. Robin sequence: obstructive sleep apnea following pharyngeal flap. *Cleft Palate Craniofac J* 1997; **34**(3): 256–60.

52. Shprintzen RJ. Pharyngeal flap surgery and the pediatric upper airway. *Int Anesthesiol Clin* 1988; **26**(1): 79–88.

53. Xue FS, An S, Tong SY *et al.* Influence of surgical technique on early post-operative hypoxaemia in childern undergoing elective palatopsty. *Br J Anaesth* 1998; **80**: 447–51.

54. Kravath RE, Pollak CP, Borowiecki B, Weitzman ED. Obstructive sleep apnea and death associated with surgical correction of velopharyngeal incompetence. *J Pediatr* 1980; **96**(4): 645–8.

55. Fisher QA, Nichols D, Stewart FC *et al.* Assessing pediatric anesthesia practices for volunteer medical services abroad. *Anesthesiology* 2001; **95**(6): 1315–22.

56. Ward CM, James I. Surgery of 346 patients with unoperated cleft lip and palate in Sri Lanka. *Cleft Palate J* 1990; **27**(1): 11–5.

57. Ishizawa Y, Handa Y, Tanaka K, Taki K. General anaesthesia for cleft lip and palate surgery team activities in Cambodia. *Trop Doct* 1997; **27**(3): 153–5.

58. Hodges SC, Hodges AM. A protocol for safe anaesthesia for cleft lip and palate surgery in developing countries. *Anaesthesia* 2000; **55**(5): 436–41.

59. Patterson JF, Belton MK. Anesthesia experiences at a plastic surgery center in Vietnam. Experiences at Children's Medical Relief International surgical facility. *JAMA* 1971; **215**(5): 777–82.

60. Slator R, Goodacre TE. EMLA cream on the ears – is it effective? A prospective, randomised controlled trial of the efficacy of topical anaesthetic cream in reducing the pain of local anaesthetic infiltration for prominent ear correction. *Br J Plast Surg* 1995; **48**(3): 150–3.

61. Cregg N, Conway F, Casey W. Analgesia after otoplasty: regional nerve blockade vs. local anaesthetic infiltration of the ear. *Can J Anaesth* 1996; **43**(2): 141–7.

62. Burtles R. Analgesia for 'bat ear' surgery. *Ann R Coll Surg Engl* 1989; **71**(5): 332.

63. Paxton D, Taylor RH, Gallagher TM, Crean PM. Postoperative emesis following otoplasty in children. *Anaesthesia* 1995; **50**: 1083–5.

64. Ridings P, Gault D, Khan L. Reduction in postoperative vomiting after surgical correction of prominent ears. *Br J Anaesth* 1994; **72**: 592–3.

65. Lancaster JL, Jones TM, Kay AR, McGeorge DD. Paediatric day-case otoplasty: local versus general anaesthetic. *Surg J R Coll Surg Edin* 2003; **1**(2): 96–8.

66. Lieberman JR, Staheli LT, Dales MC. Tourniquet pressures on pediatric patients: a clinical study. *Orthopedics* 1997; **20**(12): 1143–7.

67. Tredwell SJ, Wilmink M, Inkpen K, McEwen JA. Pediatric tourniquets: analysis of cuff and limb interface, current practice, and guidelines for use. *J Pediatr Orthoped* 2001; **21**(5): 671–6.

68. Altintas F, Bozkurt P, Ipek N *et al.* The efficacy of pre- versus postsurgical axillary block on postoperative pain in paediatric patients. *Paediatr Anaesth* 2000; **10**(1): 23–8.

69. Carre P, Joly A, Cluzel FB *et al.* Axillary block in children: single or multiple injection? *Paediatr Anaesth* 2000; **10**(1): 351–9.

70. Fisher WJ, Bingham RM, Hall R. Axillary brachial plexus block for perioperative analgesia in 250 children. *Paediatr Anaesth* 1999; **9**(5): 435–8.

71. Tan TSH, Watcha MF, Safavi F *et al.* Cannulation of the axillary brachial sheath in children. *Anesth Analg* 1995; **80**: 640–1.

Orthopaedic surgery

G R LAUDER

KEY LEARNING POINTS

- Comorbidities are common in orthopaedic patients and may have significant implications for anaesthesia.
- Many patients attend for multiple operations; there may be severe anxiety needing sympathetic care.
- Major blood loss may occur and strategies for blood conservation may be necessary.

- Analgesia should be multimodal employing nerve blocks or regional anaesthesia whenever possible.
- Patients with cerebral palsy have special needs and require careful postoperative management.

INTRODUCTION

In 1741 the Parisian Professor Nicholas Andry coined the term 'orthopaedics' by combing the two Greek words 'orthos', meaning straight, and 'paidios' meaning child. The specialty name therefore literally means 'the straightening of children'. Surgery for orthopaedic procedures in children may be simple or complex. However, many patients have complex medical and/or congenital comorbidities making anaesthesia high risk even for the simplest of interventions. Good communication among the anaesthetist, orthopaedic surgeon, operating room staff, physiotherapist, parents and other relevant personnel is essential for a successful outcome.

GENERAL PRINCIPLES OF ORTHOPAEDIC ANAESTHESIA

Preoperative preparation and assessment

Comorbidity is common in orthopaedic patients (see Chapter 28); a safely conducted anaesthetic and a good

analgesic plan start with preoperative assessment, the general principles of which are outlined in Chapter 17. The history will gauge the degree of restriction from the disease and assess any comorbidities. Physical examination must be comprehensive but also targeted to any associated conditions. Relevant investigations should be guided by the history, examination and type of surgery.

Children often require repeated procedures and past negative experiences cause some to be fearful, anxious and hostile. It is therefore important to 'get it right' in every interaction with the child and parents. The proposed anaesthetic should be discussed in a manner to minimise anxiety but also to include risks (with special reference to analgesic techniques such as epidurals), possible complications, the likelihood of blood transfusion and the use of suppositories. Teenage girls may be taking oral contraceptives or be pregnant. Anaesthesia or radiation from imaging may be teratogenic or cause miscarriage. Pregnancy should be excluded by confidential discussion or urine testing.

Standard approaches to premedication (see Chapter 18) and anaesthesia (see Chapter 19) should be tailored to the individual. Many children will be taking other medication (e.g. anticonvulsants, sedatives, analgesics or antispasmodics) and these must be continued up to and including the day of operation. Before proceeding to surgery the fasting status needs to be ascertained and hospital policy followed [1].

Anaesthesia

The method of anaesthetic induction depends on the patient's previous experiences, their wishes and the underlying medical condition. If the airway is potentially difficult, an inhalational induction and fibre-optic intubation may be indicated (see Chapter 21). Maintenance of anaesthesia must provide good surgical conditions, while allowing recovery to be swift with good analgesia and no postoperative nausea and vomiting (PONV). Local anaesthetic blocks are fundamental to good analgesia, facilitating minimal opioid use and light planes of general anaesthesia by inhalational or total intravenous anaesthesia (TIVA).

Fluid management

In orthopaedic surgery, blood loss may be substantial and it is important to compensate for maintenance fluid deficits before blood loss occurs. The principles of fluid management are discussed in Chapter 4.

Minimising blood loss/blood salvage

Preoperative optimisation of haemoglobin levels can be achieved with oral iron, folate, vitamin B_{12} and erythropoietin. Conservation of blood (see Chapter 24) in paediatric orthopaedic surgery is fundamental to minimise allogeneic blood transfusion. Losses of 10–20 per cent of circulating blood volume can be replaced with crystalloid or colloid if the child remains stable. The haematocrit can be lowered during surgery to minimise red cell loss while operating, so that transfusion can be delayed until haemostasis has been achieved. Serial haematocrit estimations should be made to guide transfusion and postoperative instructions should define the trigger haemoglobin/haematocrit level for further transfusion.

Antimicrobial prophylaxis for orthopaedic surgery

For elective surgery, antibiotics should have good activity against staphylococci and streptococci; the choice is guided by local resistance patterns and given for 24 hours. Salmonella osteomyelitis may occur in those who have sickle cell disease (SCD) or trait. After an open fracture, prevention of infection depends on thorough debridement, wound irrigation and early parenteral antibiotics in high doses.

Tourniquets

Pneumatic tourniquets are applied around the upper or lower extremity to create a bloodless surgical field, in about 40 per cent of paediatric orthopaedic procedures [2] Recommended inflation pressures are determined by the patient's systolic blood pressure and the size of the limb (upper limb 100 mmHg:lower limb 150 mmHg above systolic pressure).

There are complications and risks associated with the use of pneumatic tourniquets. A progressive increase in core temperature can occur during prolonged (90 minutes) use of leg tourniquets (single 0.4–1.6°C, bilateral 1.1–2.3°C) [3]. This is often associated with a progressively increasing tachycardia. Core temperature should be monitored and controlled [3]. Recommendations for application and minimising the systemic and metabolic effects of tourniquet release [2,4,5] are outlined in Table 36.1; they are especially important when tourniquet inflation time exceeds 75 minutes, and when bilateral tourniquets are deflated simultaneously or within 30 minutes of each other.

The use of a tourniquet in patients with SCD is controversial. Tourniquets have been used safely in patients with sickle cell trait [6] and a series of 37 SCD patients has been reported without causing complications from tourniquet use [5]. Even though there are inadequate published clinical data to assess the safety of tourniquets in SCD, the evidence suggests that it is not an absolute contraindication to regional arterial occlusion, provided that patients with SCD have appropriate haematological correction. The benefits of the improved operating conditions achieved using a tourniquet must be carefully balanced against any potential harm in each individual.

Analgesia

Multimodal analgesia is central to an orthopaedic pain management plan which should be tailored to the individual patient and associated support teams [7,8]. Simple analgesics such as paracetamol and/or non-steroidal anti-inflammatory drugs (NSAIDs) in conjunction with local anaesthetic infiltration are effective for minor procedures.

Table 36.1 Recommendations to minimise local, systemic and metabolic effects of tourniquet release in children

- Adequately padding underneath tourniquet
- Prevent skin prep contact with tourniquet
- Use appropriate tourniquet inflation pressure
- Limit inflation times to less than 75 minutes
- Monitor $ETCO_2$ before and after release of the tourniquet
- Increase minute ventilation before tourniquet deflation
- Maintain increased minute ventilation for 5 minutes after tourniquet deflation

$ETCO_2$, end-tidal carbon dioxide concentration in expired air.

Weak opioids or tramadol can be used as rescue analgesia. For major procedures paracetamol and NSAIDs are combined with nurse-controlled analgesia (NCA), patient-controlled analgesia (PCA) and/or regional anaesthesia (nerve blocks, plexus blocks or central neuraxial blocks) (see Chapter 26). Regional techniques should be performed only when there are no contraindications and whenever the potential benefits outweigh the risks.

BONE HEALING AND NSAIDS

Bone healing requires prostaglandins that are synthesised by osteoblasts and stimulate both bone formation and resorption [9] and cyclo-oxygenase-2 (COX-2) function is essential for fracture healing [10,11]. Non-steroidal anti-inflammatory drugs inhibit prostaglandin synthesis and COX-2 function and therefore they may have an adverse effect upon bone healing.

In mice, it is known that COX-2 plays a critical role in mesenchymal cell differentiation during the skeletal reparative process [11] and normal fracture healing fails in mice homozygous for a null mutation in the COX-2 gene [10]. Indometacin inhibits bone formation following femoral reaming in mice [12]. In rabbits the effects of NSAIDs occur both *in vitro* [13] and *in vivo* [14], with both local and systemic NSAIDs [15]. Rat data suggest that fracture healing is significantly poorer in NSAID-treated groups compared with controls [10,16–21] but variations in dosage and study design make it difficult to extrapolate these data to humans.

In adults, heterotopic ossification after hip replacement, acetabular fracture and spinal injury is inhibited by NSAIDs [22–26]. But this may not be of relevance to adult bone healing. Glassman *et al.* demonstrated that ketorolac was associated with a fivefold higher rate of non-union compared with controls following spinal fusion [27]. Subsequently, studies show that NSAID therapy is associated with significant risk of non-union following fracture of the femur [28], long bones [29], tibia [30] and clavicle [31], but none was controlled for confounding variables – e.g. smoking doubles the rate of non-union in adult lumbar spine fusion [32] – and many were not controlled for preoperative bone density, exercise history and diet. In contrast, a number of studies show no effect of NSAIDs on bone healing [33–35]. Until more concrete paediatric evidence is forthcoming, it would be wise to err on the side of caution and limit the use of postoperative NSAIDs to a maximum of 48 hours in operations where bone healing may be impaired.

ANAESTHETIC CONSIDERATIONS FOR SPECIFIC ORTHOPAEDIC CONDITIONS

Trauma

Trauma is the leading cause of death in children less than 14 years of age in the UK [36]. Limb fractures and other extremity injuries are very common in children and are a frequent component of multisystem injury, commonly as a result of road traffic accidents [37]. Severe vascular damage with the potential for critical limb ischaemia as a result of complex or displaced fractures requires urgent surgical repair, but the majority of fractures can be stabilised externally with splints until other serious injuries have been managed. Analgesia is vital to minimise stress, anxiety and pain. Intranasal diamorphine (0.1 mg/kg as a 0.2 mL volume) or inhaled Entonox (50:50 nitrous oxide in oxygen) are safe and accepted methods of immediate analgesia for children [38,39]. Once intravenous access has been achieved, morphine can be administered and titrated to effect using small aliquots (20 µg/kg) to ensure that the patient does not become over-sedated, which may mask a decreased conscious level from other causes. A femoral nerve block is useful for patients with a fractured femur.

The possibility of non-accidental injury (NAI) from physical abuse must be borne in mind for children presenting with orthopaedic fractures. Affected children are usually under 2 years of age [40] and can present with one or multiple bony injuries. Certain fracture patterns are more typical of NAI [41]. Where there is suspicion, local child protection policies should be implemented.

ANAESTHETIC MANAGEMENT

When an immediate operation is needed the patient should be treated as a full-stomach risk and given a rapid sequence induction. Gastric emptying is delayed as a result of the autonomic response to pain and fear, with blood flow being diverted away from the visceral circulation, leading to stasis. Large gastric volumes may remain many hours after injury, [42]. The stomach should be assumed to be full in all emergency patients [43–45]. Delaying the operative procedure may help to reduce the intragastric pressure before anaesthesia is induced [45]. However, children starved for more than 6 hours may still have a large volume of stomach contents [42], especially when the preceding meal was close to the time of injury and when opiate analgesia was given [46]. A safe period between oral intake or injury and induction of anaesthesia cannot be predicted.

For children with multiple trauma, the anaesthetist needs to protect the cervical spine, to continue resuscitation efforts and repeatedly to reassess the child. Compartment syndrome and fat embolism are more likely after trauma.

Compartment syndrome is caused by increased pressure within a myofascial compartment and should be considered whenever there is swelling and pain on passive stretching of the involved muscles. The diagnosis is confirmed by direct pressure measurements within the affected compartment. Epidural analgesia is contraindicated in multiple trauma or trauma to the lower legs, especially tibial trauma, because the sensory block may mask the symptoms. The incidence of fat embolism in paediatric orthopaedic patients is unknown but those with major long-bone fractures, extensive crush injuries and those undergoing surgery with manipulation and/or compression of the intramedullary canal are at risk. The signs of fat embolism include: confusion or sleepiness, desaturation, fever, tachycardia, tachypnoea, hypertension and upper trunk petechiae. The pulmonary shunting leads to hypoxia and haemorrhagic oedema.

Congenital dislocation of the hip

Congenital dislocation of the hip [40] is a displacement of the femoral head out of the acetabular socket. The aetiology is not clear but it is associated with a positive family history, breech presentation and positioning in the neonatal period that keeps the hips adducted and extended. The incidence has been reported as 1–15 per 1000 live births, with girls affected six to eight times more often than boys. Dislocation of the left hip occurs three times more frequently than the right, but in 25 per cent of cases the dislocation is bilateral. Unrecognised congenital dislocation of the hip leads to established dislocation, developmental dysplasia, deformity and eventual osteoarthritis. Prognosis is poor if therapy is begun after 4 years of age. If the diagnosis is made and appropriate treatment begun in the neonatal period then the hip will usually develop normally.

SURGICAL MANAGEMENT

Relocation of the hip can be achieved with skeletal traction. Closed reduction can be achieved with hip spica and/or adductor longus tendon release. If closed reduction is not possible then an open reduction is necessary, secured with a hip spica for the following 4 months. In older children femoral and/or acetabular surgery may be required to give a stable reduction.

ANAESTHETIC MANAGEMENT

Open reduction can be associated with significant blood loss so that crossmatched blood should be available. Analgesia should include a perioperative regional block, postoperative nurse-controlled analgesia (NCA), NSAIDs and paracetamol (see Chapter 27). The immobilisation afforded by a hip spica minimises postoperative pain and intravenous opioids can be stopped after 24 hours. An epidural infusion may be used though catheter management and requires a window to be cut in the hip spica to view the entry site, and urinary catheterisation will be required (Fig. 36.1).

The hip spica

A spica cast is used to maintain position of the hips for congenital dislocation of the hips and following femoral osteotomy. To apply a hip spica the patient is placed with the shoulders and head on a box and the sacrum resting on a horizontal strut attached to the vertical strut between the legs. Great care must be taken in moving to ensure that the

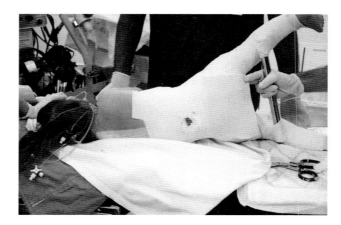

Figure 36.1 Completed hip spica that still requires padding to the edges; epidural catheter inspection window is visible.

surgical repair is not compromised – anaesthesia should be deepened to ensure that this process is smooth. The application of a hip spica can take up to 45 minutes; when undertaken as a sole procedure it may be worthwhile intubating and ventilating the patient. Patient repositioning can lead to accidental extubation.

POSTOPERATIVE CARE

Plaster of Paris (POP) applied immediately next to the operation site can absorb blood so a postoperative haemoglobin check is important. The patient may develop oedematous feet which will then mean that the plaster may have to be split or remoulded. The swelling can be minimised by positioning the patient with the feet up. The capillary refill in the toes and any palpable pulses in the feet should be examined.

Congenital talipes equinovarus

DEFINITION

Congenital talipes equinovarus (CTEV), commonly known as clubfoot, is a congenital idiopathic deformity, of which the salient features are hindfoot equinovarus and midfoot cavus adductus. It occurs in approximately 1 per 1000 live births, is twice as common in boys and is bilateral in 50 per cent. It is usually an isolated deformity but 12 per cent of these children have other anomalies, e.g. spina bifida or arthrogryposis. Recognition of associated neuromuscular problems is essential to avoid the unmasking of these conditions during anaesthesia [47].

SURGICAL MANAGEMENT

The Ponsetti technique involves conservative management using manipulation and cast immobilisation followed by a percutaneous heel cord lengthening. This has been shown to avoid more aggressive posterior medial release (PMR) in 89 per cent of cases and reduces the complications of PMR surgery that include recurrence, over-correction, stiffness and pain [48]. When talipes equinovarus is resistant to conservative measures soft-tissue procedures, such as Achilles' tendon lengthening and capsulotomy, are undertaken. In older children osteotomy may be required to correct and realign CTEV. In resistant cases triple fusion may be required.

ANAESTHETIC MANAGEMENT

Good intraoperative analgesia by regional block should be accompanied by postoperative NCA/patient-controlled analgesia (PCA) with morphine. Muscle spasm may be a significant cause of pain, frequently leading to over treatment with opioids. Diazepam may aid muscle relaxation and minimise use of opioids.

Congenital spinal cord deformities

DEFINITION

Spina bifida occulta is a congenital absence of bony spinous processes and laminae. It occurs in 10 per cent of the general population and is usually of no clinical significance. However, if a sac containing meninges bulges through the defect a meningocele is present; if this also contains neural elements it is called a myelomeningocele. Myelomeningocele is associated with hydrocephalus and the Arnold–Chiari malformation (downward displacement of the cerebellar tonsils and medulla through the foramen magnum). The incidence of these defects is falling owing to maternal folic acid supplementation. The majority of defects occur in the lumbosacral area; 20 per cent are meningocele and 80 per cent are myelomeningocele. Below the defect the nerve roots are abnormal so that bowel, bladder and neuromuscular dysfunction result; the size and location of the myelomeningocele determines the extent of the neurological deficit The open sac is closed in the first few days of life to prevent infection; hydrocephalus may require a ventriculoperitoneal (VP) shunt. Children with myelomeningocele frequently have neuropathic bladders and may require intermittent self-catheterisation. Neuromuscular imbalance occurs when unopposed innervated or spastic muscles work against flaccid muscles and cause joint deformity. Scoliosis is common, especially with higher levels of spinal involvement.

SURGICAL MANAGEMENT

The aim of any surgical intervention is to preserve the ability to stand and walk by releasing soft tissues and realigning bones to produce an extensor posture at the hip and knee, with plantigrade feet [49]. Surgery may also be required for scoliosis correction.

ANAESTHETIC MANAGEMENT

Postoperative drowsiness with nausea and vomiting can easily be dismissed as a consequence of anaesthesia when in fact the problem lies with a blocked shunt. Preoperative VP shunt function should be assessed clinically; raised intracranial pressure is suggested by a history of morning headache, vomiting and/or deterioration in conscious level, mood or schoolwork. Signs include papilloedema or a sixth cranial nerve palsy. If there is a concern the child's neurosurgeon should be consulted. A computed tomography (CT) scan of the head may be required to assess ventricular size. Lung function tests may be helpful to ensure that there is not a life-limiting restrictive lung defect.

Spina bifida patients have a predisposition to latex allergy [50]; 34–67 per cent of children with spina bifida express immunoglobulin E (IgE) antibodies to latex [51,52]. All spina bifida patients should be treated by minimising exposure to latex [53].

Standard anaesthetic techniques can be employed. The sensory level should be identified preoperatively and the analgesia plan amended accordingly. In areas of sensory loss surprisingly little pain relief may be required. It should be remembered that intravenous cannulae can be inserted at sites of decreased sensory innervation. Epidurals and caudals are contraindicated [54] because of the anatomical defect and are often unnecessary because of existing sensory loss.

Cerebral palsy

DEFINITION

Cerebral palsy (CP) is a generic term that describes a spectrum of clinical syndromes where the common feature is the abnormal control of motor function by the brain [55], leading to a progressive disorder of movement and posture, caused by central nervous system (CNS) damage (antenatally or perinatally). It is the commonest cause of childhood motor disability, with an incidence of around 2.5 per 1000 live births in developed countries [56]. The clinical picture evolves over time and the degree and type of disability depend on the extent and site of cerebral pathology. The classification outlined in Table 36.2 is the one most commonly used.

This classification relates only to the motor deficit but the full clinical picture will depend on the part of the brain involved and not all patients have spasticity. Cognitive impairment, intellectual disability, behavioural disturbance and hearing, speech and visual problems are common. Epilepsy occurs in about 35–50 per cent of children with CP; tonic–clonic and complex partial seizures are the most common [57]. Bulbar muscle involvement may lead to feeding difficulties, gastro-oesophageal reflux (GOR), with increased risk of aspiration and recurrent pneumonias (more commonly in those with severe spasticity). These children are often malnourished with poor muscle

Table 36.2 Swedish classification for cerebral palsy (percentage frequency)

Spastic (70%)	Quadriplegia (27%)	Affecting arms and legs
	Diplegia (21%)	Affecting mainly legs
	Hemiplegia (21%)	Affecting one side; arm > leg
Dyskinetic (10%)	Dystonia	
	Athetosis	
	Chorea	
Ataxic (10%)		
Mixed (10%)		

bulk and little subcutaneous fat, hence their weight can be markedly reduced. Conversely, with a feeding gastrostomy *in situ* these patients may be of normal or increased weight. Difficult vascular access is common. Spastic CP results in the development of increasing muscular contractures and secondary bony deformities. Dyskinetic CP is associated with deafness, dysarthria and drooling but often no intellectual impairment. In ataxic CP balance and speech disorders occur with intellectual disability and epilepsy.

SURGICAL MANAGEMENT

Botulinum toxin

Botulinum toxin injections reduce the spasticity of the treated muscles, making them more amenable to stretching, and is a useful adjunct to physiotherapy, splints and surgery [58–61].

Operations

Children with spastic cerebral palsy often present with postural disorders and gait abnormalities resulting from muscle imbalance. Surgical intervention is indicated to:

- improve mobility in the face of contractures
- prevent disability
- arrest the progress of a scoliosis
- reduce or improve pain and aid the carer's ability to manage the child.

Operations commonly performed on the lower limbs include hip surgery, femoral/tibial osteotomies, tendon transfers and tendon releases. Psoas lengthening and adductor release may reduce flexion and internal rotation of the hip and allow muscle balance, so that the femoral head stays in the hip joint. Hypertonic hamstrings cause knee flexion, while spasticity of the calf muscles prevents the child walking or causes a tendency to toe-walk. If physiotherapy and corrective splints cannot produce plantigrade feet, lengthening of Achilles' tendon may improve the position. These may be performed as separate procedures or together in one stage as a 'multilevel' operation to preserve or improve their ability to walk independently [62]. Surgical intervention has little influence on the fine motor control of the hand so surgery to the upper limb is limited to contracture releases of the elbow and shoulder.

ANAESTHETIC MANAGEMENT

Cerebral palsy children are recurrent hospital attendees and require special attention to minimise anxiety. The degree of a child's intellectual impairment cannot be assessed from the first glance [63], and parents will know how their child behaves and how they coped with previous anaesthetics.

The preoperative fluid deficits can be grossly underestimated in patients with CP so that intravenous hydration should be considered the night before. Antiepileptic medication should be prescribed and taken as usual. Sedative premedication is useful for those who have needle or mask phobias. Allergy to latex is reported to be common in cerebral palsy [64,65].

Rapid sequence induction should be performed where there is symptomatic or untreated GOR. Sensitivity to suxamethonium does not occur [66] but resistance to nondepolarising neuromuscular blocking drugs has been reported [67,68]. Thiopental is a useful agent, instead of propofol, for routine induction as it is painless and it reduces the chances of convulsive episodes postoperatively.

How the airway is secured will depend on the extent and duration of the surgical procedure and the individual patient comorbidities. These children are often small and the tracheal tube size may not relate well to the patient's age. Care must be taken after intubation to ensure correct tube length and size. Measurement of the end-tidal concentration of volatile agent is essential; the minimum alveolar concentration (MAC) is reduced in CP children compared with normal controls [69]. A nasogastric tube can be helpful to reduce intraoperative secretions in the mouth, while postoperatively it can be used to give antiepileptics, analgesic drugs and nasogastric feed. A urinary catheter is required for major surgery and always with epidural analgesia.

Temperature regulation is often abnormal in cerebral palsy because of hypothalamic dysfunction; a warming mattress, forced air warmers and intravenous (IV) fluid warmers help to normalise the core temperature. Children must be positioned with care on the operating table because they are at high risk of pressure sores; all pressure areas must be padded.

POSTOPERATIVE CARE

Good analgesia is vitally important in children with cerebral palsy because of the communication problems, intellectual impairment and the need to prevent muscle spasms. Children with cerebral palsy receive less pain assessment and opioids than a normative group of children [70]. Multimodal analgesia is recommended with paracetamol, NSAIDs, infusion epidural analgesia or NCA morphine (1–5 days). The level of insertion of the epidural should take into account the dermatomal levels of skin incision. Where epidural analgesia is used, the risk of compartment syndrome and pressure sores must not be forgotten. Where an epidural is not possible NCA morphine should be given, but this group of patients are at high risk of adverse effects from opioids. Pain from muscle spasms (see below) is poorly responsive to morphine and this may lead to over-treatment; concurrent administration of diazepam will reduce opioid administration.

Children with severe CP can be irritable in the postoperative period, leading to over-treatment with opioids. Irritability can be caused by pain, spasms, disorientation, headache, gastro-oesophageal reflux, hunger, urinary retention, constipation, the unfamiliar environment and/or parental separation. Involvement of carers early in the recovery phase may help reduce the child's anxiety. Facial grimacing and moaning are not uncommon in the child with CP and may be incorrectly thought to be caused by pain. Directing pain control can be difficult and, as self-report is not appropriate, other assessment strategies have to be adopted [71]. Assessment, based on nursing/medical intuition and informal reports from the family, is complex, confusing and problematic [72–75]. Carefully considered behavioural indicators can help improve the management of pain in these children [76] but there is diversity in pain expression which is often in clusters of symptoms (e.g. vocalisation, crying/moaning, change in facial expression, pallor, change in posture or tension, withdrawal, teeth grinding, head banging, increased seizure activity, increased sweating, increase in temperature and tachycardia) [77].

McGrath and colleagues [78] have developed a reliable and sensitive Non-Communicating Children's Checklist for children with neurodevelopmental disorders and severe cognitive impairment. It contains 30 pain behaviours grouped into seven subscales. There are sufficient inconsistencies in pain behavioural indicators in CP children to suggest that reliance on behavioural cues alone can underestimate pain [79,80]. The revised FLACC (face, legs, activity, cry and consolability) tool has recently been shown to improve reliability and validity for acute pain assessment in children with cognitive impairment [81]. It has the advantage of combining observational and behavioural cues to assess pain. Parents develop skill in pain assessment from knowledge of their child's usual behaviours; Hunt and coworkers [82] devised the Paediatric Pain Profile (http://www.ppprofile.org.uk), which is a validated tool that uses these parental skills.

Postoperative muscle spasms are a particular problem in CP children undergoing multilevel lower limb surgery; they occur even in those with no history of spasms. The best treatment is to prevent them occurring. This can be achieved with epidural analgesia or parenteral morphine supplemented by regular diazepam orally, rectally or intravenously, watching for over-sedation. A midazolam infusion, instead of diazepam, can be used for the quadriplegic CP child or the child with athetoid CP as it enables titration to effect when dealing with potentially severe spasms, but needs high-dependency care. Epidural clonidine, when added to bupivacaine, reduces muscle spasms with a reduction in the requirement for diazepam [80]. Increasing doses of baclofen should be avoided because consequent muscle weakness will hinder physiotherapy. Postoperative nausea and vomiting occurs in 52 per cent of CP patients – care in feeding and regular medication are cornerstones of management [83]. It has been reported to be more common in diplegic than quadriplegic patients (68 per cent versus 38 per cent) [84].

The risk of postoperative complications correlates well with the degree of ambulatory function, i.e. a non-ambulatory patient with a gastrostomy or a tracheostomy is at greater risk of complications [85]. Ambulatory cerebral palsy patients having major surgery to the lower limbs are at risk of developing neuropathic chronic pain following surgery [86] (see Chapter 27).

Osteogenesis imperfecta

DEFINITION

Osteogenesis imperfecta (OI) is an inherited rare connective tissue disorder mainly involving bones, making them more fragile. The basic defect appears to be in the maturation of type I collagen. The primary problems are easily fractured, brittle osteoporotic bones and frequent dislocation of joints. Four main groups are described (Table 36.3).

Type I OI often presents with delayed walking. Long-bone fragility is a key symptom and faciocranial disproportion is seen (broad forehead, prominent parietal and temporal bones, and a hanging occiput). Painful, debilitating and deforming fractures occur during infancy and childhood. Fractures have been reported from minimal manipulation, including application of a blood pressure cuff or changing a nappy. After puberty the incidence of fractures decreases with the influence of sex hormones on the bone matrix. Blue sclerae are a distinctive manifestation of this disease; however, the classic triad of multiple fractures, blue sclerae and deafness does not commonly occur [87].

The most severe form (type II) corresponds with OI congenita which is usually lethal and is evident at birth by the occurrence of multiple fractures during delivery, deformity of the limbs, reduced ossification of the cranial vault and facial bones, with a soft skull and vertebrae that are flattened and hypoplastic. Intracranial haemorrhage is the most common cause of death during the neonatal period. If the neonate survives to childhood he or she may develop a small mandible, mid-face hypoplasia, dentinogenesis imperfecta, a raised metabolic rate, severe fragility with deformity of the long bones and chest wall/spinal abnormalities (prominent sternum and scoliosis). Severe thoracic deformity often leads to early respiratory failure and death.

Table 36.3   The characteristics of osteogenesis imperfecta types I–IV

Type	Occurrence	Inheritance	Severity	Characteristic
I	Commonest	Autosomal dominant	Mild	Blue sclerae Bony fragility Dentinogenesis imperfecta
II	1 in 20 000–60 000	Autosomal recessive	Lethal Most severe	Usually lethal Severe porosis Multiple fractures Malformed skeleton
III		Autosomal recessive	Severe	Multiple fractures at birth Progressively deforming Normal sclerae Dentinogenesis imperfecta
IV		Autosomal dominant	Variable severity	White sclerae

Congenital and acquired anomalies associated with OI include: small for age, aortic or mitral valve incompetence from dilatation of the annular rings [88], dentinogenesis imperfecta with brittle, discoloured (often slightly grey–blue) teeth, cleft palate, hydrocephalus, umbilical and inguinal hernias, hyperhidrosis, spina bifida, kyphoscoliosos; premature arteriosclerosis, emphysema, otosclerosis with deafness and lax ligaments with recurrent joint dislocation. Decreased cardiopulmonary reserve may be present in those children with scoliosis; if there is significant chest wall deformity there may be a restrictive lung defect and lung function tests may be of value as a baseline prior to surgery. Odontoid hypoplasia and cervicomedullary compression are rarely seen, even in severe cases. However, if present the base of the skull may collapse onto the cervical vertebrae. Most OI patients dress more lightly and sleep in cooler surroundings then non-OI patients; they are frequently diaphoretic and mildly hyperthermic. An ill-defined platelet dysfunction occurs in OI: the count is often within normal limits but abnormal aggregation [89] may lead to a perioperative bleeding diathesis.

SURGICAL MANAGEMENT

Surgery is indicated for emergency treatment of fractures, or electively for the correction of deformities. Correction of long-bone deformities requires multiple osteotomies, realignment, and insertion/fixation with intramedullary rods. Sofield and Millar have demonstrated that these rods, help prevent recurrent fractures and enable significant mobilisation [90,91].

ANAESTHETIC MANAGEMENT

All known fractures must be documented, while the degree of brittleness must be assessed to determine the risk of further fractures during surgery. These patients may be extremely fragile and can be injured with simple manoeuvres (positioning, blood pressure measurement or airway management). Suxamethonium should be avoided, positioning needs extreme care and it may be necessary to avoid blood pressure measurement. Tracheal intubation needs particular care to avoid damage to the fragile teeth and collapse of the base of the skull on to the cervical vertebrae in susceptible children [92]. If the patient has any of the cardiovascular conditions associated with OI, antibiotic prophylaxis is indicated. If the patient is deaf ensure that they wear their hearing aid to help communication both pre- and postoperatively.

Osteogenesis imperfecta is not associated with malignant hyperpyrexia (MH); however, a non-malignant hyperthermia can occur before and during anaesthesia. Classic MH (see Chapter 29) signs are not seen but tachycardia and metabolic acidosis occur. The mechanism is possibly excess thyroid hormones uncoupling oxidative phosphorylation. Surface cooling, cold intravenous solutions and a decrease in ambient temperature are effective [93,94].

During major surgery coagulopathy related to platelet dysfunction may present and is usually resolved with a platelet transfusion.

Arthrogryposis (amyoplasia congenita)

DEFINITION

Arthrogryposis multiplex congenita (AMC) is a congenital symptom complex characterised by multiple symmetrical non-progressive joint contractures. It results from foetal akinesia due to extrinsic factors (oligohydramnios, amniotic bands, uterine fibroids), or primary neurogenic or myopathic conditions of the fetus [95]. Neurogenic causes account for 94 per cent of these primary cases. These are associated with decreased number and size of anterior horn cells as well as degeneration of nerve roots in the cervical and lumbar spine. The incidence is reported as 1 in 3000 live births. Autosomal recessive and dominant inheritance have been reported [96]. The decreased muscle mass causes the limbs to appear spindly with large, fusiform joints; the skin is featureless with veins that are sparse, small and fragile, making intravenous access difficult. Depending on the primary cause of this symptom complex the extremity contractures may be associated with other anomalies. Rigidity of the temporomandibular joints with limited mouth opening and micrognathia may make mask ventilation and laryngoscopy difficult or impossible [97–100]. About 10–26 per cent of affected patients have associated congenital heart disease, including patent ductus arteriosus, aortic stenosis, coarctation of the aorta and cyanotic congenital heart disease [99,101]. Cleft palate, atlantoaxial subluxations, ribcage deformities with altered pulmonary mechanics, hypoplastic lungs, scoliosis, hip dislocation, gastroschisis, bowel atresias and inguinal hernias have been reported. The majority of AMC patients have normal intellectual function.

SURGICAL MANAGEMENT

Surgery is required to release joint contractures and to improve standing and walking function using a combination of soft tissue releases and realignment osteotomies.

ANAESTHETIC MANAGEMENT

Preoperative assessment must include an inspection of the airway in case of restricted mouth opening and limited neck movement. In the presence of a potentially difficult airway, where intravenous access is a real challenge, an inhalation induction is preferable; difficult airway/intubation equipment should be checked and available [102].

Cervical spine evaluation (flexion/extension films, computed tomography or magnetic resonance imaging) is indicated in patients with clinical symptoms suggestive of cervical spine involvement [97–104].

Arthrogryposis multiplex congenita is not associated with MH [105] but patients with arthrogryposis may be susceptible to a non-malignant hyperthermia related to a hypermetabolic response to anaesthesia and surgery [106]. This manifests as a rise in body temperature that responds to active cooling [105–108].

External fixators

DEFINITION

An external fixator is a device that uses pins or wires attached to bone segments, stabilised by an externally applied frame; they are used to increase limb length in patients with short stature or leg length discrepancies and to correct deformities secondary to trauma or congenital anomalies. Each centimetre of length gained requires the fixator to be in position for a month.

ANAESTHETIC MANAGEMENT

Analgesia is challenging because epidurals are relatively contraindicated as a result of the potential masking of a compartment syndrome, particularly in tibial surgery; moreover, non-steroidal anti-inflammatory agents are restricted because they may impair subsequent bone formation. A 'single-shot' regional technique followed by NCA/PCA morphine works well if supplemented with regular paracetamol. However, if a child has unremitting pain, it may be necessary to introduce a 48-hour course of NSAIDs into the analgesic regimen. If a child has had a previous painful experience with a fixator it may be necessary to place an epidural to ensure adequate analgesia. Entonox is valuable in managing the pain of pin-site cleaning, which usually takes place the day after surgery.

Chronic pain can occur which may be neuropathic or secondary to poorly managed acute pain.

Infections of bones and joints

Infections can occur in both the bones and the joint and they can be acute or chronic. The most common infective organism is *Staphylococcus aureus*. There is an increased incidence of septic arthritis in children who have haemophilia and are human immunodeficiency virus (HIV) positive [109]. The differential diagnosis of septic arthritis from osteomyelitis can be difficult. Acute infection should be considered an emergency because the life-span of infected articular cartilage is approximately 6 hours and there can be significant long-term morbidity if surgery is delayed. Osteomyelitis occurs typically in the metaphyses of the bone, except in the first month of life when it characteristically involves the whole of the bone. It is also seen in the three joints that have intracapsular metaphyses (the hip, shoulder and ankle). The differential diagnosis can be difficult because the osteomyelitis can discharge into the joint, leading to a secondary septic arthritis.

ANAESTHETIC MANAGEMENT

These patients are pyrexial, flushed, irritable, tachycardic and toxic from their sepsis. They are usually emergency cases and anaesthesia requires a rapid sequence induction. Intravenous antibiotics are necessary once samples and blood cultures have been obtained. Long-term venous access may be indicated for chronic infection.

REFERENCES

Key references

Hunt A, Goldman A, Seers K *et al*. Clinical validation of the paediatric pain profile. *Dev Med Child Neurol* 2004; **46**: 9–18.

Lauder GR, White MC. Neuropathic pain following multilevel surgery in children with cerebral palsy: A case series and literature review. *Paediatr Anaesth* 2005; **15**: 412–20.

McGrath PJ, Rosmus C, Canfield C, Campbell MA, Hennigar A. Behaviours caregivers use to determine pain in non-verbal, cognitively impaired individuals. *Dev Med Child Neurol* 1998; **40**: 340–3.

Moriaty T, Ely J. Neuroaxial blockade in children. *Anaesth Intensive Care Med* 2003; **4**: 412–6.

References

1. Splinter WM, Schreiner MS. Preoperative fasting in children. *Anesth Analg* 1999; **89**: 80–9.
2. Lynn AM, Fischer T, Brandford HG, Pendergrass TW. Systemic responses to tourniquet release in children. Anesth Analg 1986; **65**: 865–72.
3. Bloch EC, Ginsberg B, Binner RA Jr *et al.* Limb tourniquets and central temperature in anesthetized children. *Anesth Analg* 1992; **74**: 486.
4. Lee T-L, Tweed WA, Singh B. Oxygen consumption and carbon dioxide elimination after release of unilateral lower limb pneumatic tourniquets. *Anesth Analg* 1992; **75**: 113.
5. Adu-Gyamfi Y, Sankarankutty M, Marwa S. Use of tourniquet in patients with sickle-cell disease. *Can J Anaesth* 1993; **40**: 24.
6. Stein RE, Urbaniak J. Use of the tourniquet during surgery in patients with sickle cell hemoglobinopathies. *Clin Orthop Relat Res* 1980; **(151)**: 231–3.
7. Morton NS. Prevention and control of pain in children. *Pain Rev* 1998; **5**(1): 1–15.
8. American Pain Socity. *The assessment and management of acute pain in infants, children, and adolescents. A Position statement from the American Academy of Pediatrics Committee on Psychosocial Aspects of Child and Family Health and American Pain Society Task Force on Pain in Infants, Children and Adolescents.* The American Pain Society, 2000: http://www.ampainsoc.org/advocacy/pediatric2.htm
9. Kawaguchi H, Pilbeam CC, Harrison JR, Raisz LG. The role of prostaglandins in the regulation of bone metabolism. Clin *Orthop Relat Res* 1995; **313**: 36–46.
10. Simon AM, Manigrasso MB, O'Connor JP. Cyclo-oxygenase 2 function is essential for bone healing. *J Bone Miner Res* 2002; **17**: 963–76.
11. Zhang D, Schwarz EM, Young DA *et al.* COX-2 is critical for mesenchymal cell differentiation during skeletal repair. *J Bone Miner Res* 2001; **16**(suppl 1): S145.
12. Bhandari M, Schemitsch EH. Bone formation following intramedullary femoral reaming is decreased by indomethacin and antibodies to insulin-like growth factors. *J Orthop Trauma* 2002; **16**: 717–22.
13. Martin GJ, Boden SD, Titus L. Recombinant human bone morphogenetix protein-2 overcomes the inhibitory effect of ketorolac, a nonsteroidal anti-inflammatory drug (NSAID), on posterolateral lumbar intertransverse process spine fusion. *Spine* 1999; **24**: 2188–94.
14. Goodman S, Ma T, Trindade *et al.* Cox-2 selective NSAID decreases bone in growth *in vivo. J Orthop Res* 2002; **20**: 1164–9.
15. Engesaeter LB, Sudmann B, Sudmann E. Fracture healing in rats inhibited by locally administered indomethacin. *Acta Orthop Scand* 1992; **63**(3): 330–3.
16. Ro J, Langeland N, Sander J. Effect of indomethacin on fracture healing in rats. *Acta Orthop Scand* 1976; **47**: 588–99.
17. Allen HW, Wase A, Bear WT. Indomethacin and aspirin: effect of non-steroidal anti-inflammatory agents on the rate of fracture repair in the rat. *Acta Orthop Scand* 1980; **51**: 595–600.
18. Endo K, Sairyo K, Komatsubara S *et al.* Cyclooxygenase-2 inhibitor inhibits the fracture healing. *J Physiol Anthropol* 2002; **21**: 235–8.
19. Giordano V, Giordano M, Knackfuss IG *et al.* Effect of tenoxicam on fracture healing in rat tibiae. *Injury Int J Care Injured* 2003; **34**: 85–94.
20. Altman RD, Latta LL, Keer R *et al.* Effect of nonsteroidal anti-inflammatory drugs on fracture healing: A laboratory study in rats. *J Orthop Trauma* 1995; **9**: 392–400.
21. Beck, Krischak G, Sorg T *et al.* Influence of Diclofenac on fracture healing. *Arch Orthop Trauma Surg* 2003; **123**: 327–32.
22. Pritchett JW. Ketorolac prophylaxis against heterotopic ossification after hip replacement. *Clin Orthop* 1995; **314**: 162–5.
23. Burssens A, Thiery J, Kohe P *et al.* Prevention of heterotopic ossification with tenoxicam following total hip arthroplasty: a double blind, placebo-controlled dose finding study. *Acta Orthop Belg* 2005; **61**: 205–11.
24. Moed BR, Letournel E. Low-dose irradiation and indomethacin prevent heterotopic ossification after acetabular fracture surgery. *J Bone Joint Surg [Br]* 1994; **76**: 895–900.
25. Moore KD, Goss K, Angler JO. Indomethacin versus radiation therapy for prophylaxis against heterotopic ossification in acetabular fractures. *J Bone Joint Surg [Br]* 1998; **80**: 259–63.
26. Banovac K, Williams JM, Patrick LD, Haniff YM. Prevention of heterotropic ossification after spinal cord injury with indomethacin. *Spinal Cord* 2001; **39**: 370–4.
27. Glassman SD, Rose SM, Dimar JR *et al.* The effect of postoperative nonsteroidal anti-inflammatory drug administration on spinal fusion. *Spine* 1998; **23**: 834–8.
28. Giannoudis PV, MacDonald DA, Matthews SJ *et al.* Non-union of the femoral diaphysis: the influence of reaming and non-steroidal anti-inflammatory drugs. *J Bone Joint Surg [Br]* 2000; **82**: 655–8.
29. Burd TA, Hughes MS, Anglen JO. Heterotopic ossification prophylaxis with indomethacin increases the risk of long bone non-union. *J Bone Joint Surg [Br]* 2003; **85**: 700–5.
30. Butcher CK, Marsh DR. Nonsteroidal anti-inflammatory drugs delay tibial fracture union. Injury 1996; **27**: 375.
31. Khan IM. Fracture healing: role of NSAIDs. *Am J Orthop* 1997; **26**: 413.
32. Anderson T, Christensen FB, Laursen M *et al.* Smoking as a predictor of negative outcome in lumbar spine fusion. *Spine* 2001; **26**: 2623–8.
33. Adolphson P, Abbaszadegan H, Jonsson U *et al.* No effects of piroxicam on osteopenia and recovery after Colles' fracture. *Arch Orthop Trauma Surg* 1993; **112**: 127–30.

34. Bandolier Extra (March 2004). NSAIDs, coxibs, smoking and bone: http://www.ebandolier.com
35. Van Staa TP, Laufhens HG, Cooper C. Use of NSAID and risk of fractures. *Bone* 2000; **27**: 563–8.
36. Dykes EH. Paediatric trauma. *Br J Anaesth* 1999; **83**: 130–8.
37. Cooper A, Barlow B, DiScala C *et al.* Mortality and truncal injury: The pediatric perspective. *J Pediatr Surg* 1994; **29**: 33–8.
38. Wilson JA, Kendall JM, Cornelius P. Intranasal diamorphine for paediatric anaesthesia: assessment of safety and efficacy. *J Accid Emerg Med* 1997; **14**: 70–2.
39. Kendall JM, Reeves BC, Latter VS. Multicentre randomised controlled trial of nasal diamorphine for analgesia in children and teenagers with clinical fractures. *BMJ* 2001; **322**: 261–5.
40. Tachidijian MO. *Pediatric orthopedics*, 2nd edn. Philadelphia: WB Saunders, 1990.
41. Witherow PJ. Non-accidental injury. In: Benson MKD, Fixen JA, Macnicol MF, eds. *Children's orthopaedics and fractures*. Edinburgh: Churchill Livingstone, **1994**: 749–53.
42. Bricker SRW, McLuckie A, Nightingale DA. Gastric aspirates after trauma in children. *Anaesthesia* 1989; **44**: 721–4.
43. Salem MR, Wong AY, Fizzotti GF. Efficacy of cricoid pressure in preventing aspiration of gastric contents in paediatric patients. *Br J Anaesth* 1972; **44**: 401.
44. Salem MR, Wong AY, Lin YH. The effect of suxamethonium on the intragastric pressure in infants and children. *Br J Anaesth* 1972; **44**: 166.
45. Salem MR, Wong AY, Collins VJ. The pediatric patient with a 'full' stomach. *Anesthesiology* 1973; **39**: 435.
46. Bailey PL, Stanley TH. Intravenous opioid anaesthetics. In: Miller RD, ed. *Anesthesia*, 4th edn. New York: Churchill Livingstone, **1994**: 308–9.
47. Zanette G, Manani G, Pittoni G *et al.* Prevalence of unsuspected myopathy in infants presenting for clubfoot surgery. *Paediatr Anaesth* 1995; **5**: 165–70.
48. Herzenberg JE, Radler C, Bor N. Ponseti versus traditional methods of casting for idiopathic clubfoot. *J Pediatr Orthop* 2002; **22**: 517–21.
49. Sarwark JF. Spina bifida. *Pediatr Clin North Am* 1996; **43**: 1135–57.
50. Szepfalusi Z, Seidl R, Bernert G *et al.* Latex sensitisation in spina bifida appears disease-associated. *J Pediatr* 1999; **134**: 344–8.
51. Pittman T, Kiburz J, Gabriel K *et al.* Latex allergy in children with spina bifida. *Pediatr Neurosurg* 1995; 22: 96–100.
52. Kell KJ, Kurup VP, Reijula KE, Fink JN. The diagnosis of natural rubber latex allergy. *J Allergy Clin Immunol* 1994; **93**: 813–6.
53. Birmingham PK, Dsida RM, Grayhack JJ *et al.* Do latex precautions in children with myelodysplasia reduce intraoperative allergic reactions. *J Pediatr Orthop* 1996; **16**: 799–802.
54. Moriaty T, Ely J. Neuroaxial blockade in children. Anaesth *Intensive Care Med* 2003; **4**: 412–6.
55. Renshaw TS. Cerebral palsy. In: *Lovell and Winter's* pediatric orthopaedics. Philadelphia: Lippincott-Raven, 1996: 469–72.
56. Paneth N, Kiely JL. The frequency of cerebral palsy: A review of population studies in industrialized nations since 1950. *Clinic Dev Med* 1984; **87**: 46–56.
57. Eicher PS, Batshaw ML. Cerebral palsy. *Pediatr Clin North Am* 1993; **40**: 537–51.
58. Corry IS, Cosgrove AP, Duffy CM *et al.* Botulinum toxin A compared with stretching casts in the treatment of spastic equinus: a randomised prospective trial. *J Pediatr Orthop* 1998; **18**: 304–11.
59. Graham HK, Aoki KR, Autti-Ramo I *et al.* Recommendations for the use of botulinum toxin type A in the management of cerebral palsy (Review). *Gait Posture* 2000; **11**: 67–79.
60. Kooman LA, Brashar A, Rosenfeld *et al.* Botulinum toxin type a neuromuscular blockade in the treatment of equinus foot deformity in cerebral palsy: a multicenter, open-label clinical trial. *Pediatrics* 2001; **105**: 1062–71.
61. Boyd RN, Pliatsios V, Starr R *et al.* Biomechanical transformation of the gastroc-soleus muscle with botulinum toxin A in children with cerebral palsy. *Dev Med Child Neurol* 2000; **42**: 32–41.
62. Davids JR, Ounpuu S, DeLuca PA, Davis RB III. Optimization of walking ability of children with cerebral palsy. *J Bone Joint Surg [Am]* 2003; **85**: 2224–34.
63. Kearney PM, Griffin T. Between joy and sorrow: being a parent of a child with developmental disability. *J Adv Nurs* 2001; **34**: 582–92.
64. Delfico AJ, Dormans JP, Craythorne CB, Templeton JJ. Intraoperative anaphylaxis due to allergy to latex in children who have cerebral palsy: a report of six cases. *Dev Med Child Neurol* 1996; **39**: 194–7.
65. Landwehr LP, Boguniewicz M. Current perspectives on latex allergy. *J Pediatr* 1996; **128**: 305–12.
66. Dierdorf SF, McNiece WL, Rao CC *et al.* Effect of succinylcholine on plasma potassium in children with cerebral palsy. *Anesthesiology* 1985; **62**: 88–90.
67. Hepaguslar H, Ozzeybek D, Elar Z. The effect of cerebral palsy on the action of vecuronium with or without anticonvulsants. *Anaesthesia* 1999; **54**: 593–5.
68. Moorthy SS, Krishna G, Dierdorf SF. Resistance to vecuronium in patients with cerebral palsy. *Anesth Analg* 1991; **73**: 275–7.
69. Frei FJ, Haemmerle MH, Brunner R, Kern C. MAC for halothane in children with cerebral palsy and severe mental retardation. *Anaesthesia* 1997; **52**: 1056–60.
70. Hamers JP, Abu-Saad HH, van den Hout MA *et al.* The influence of children's vocal expressions, age, medical diagnosis and information obtained from parents on nurses' pain assessments and decisions regarding interventions. *Pain* 1996; **65**: 53–61.
71. McGrath PA, Seifert CE, Speechley KN *et al.* A new analogue scale for assessing children's pain: an initial validation study. *Pain* 1996; **64**: 435–43.
72. Craig KD. Implications of concepts of consciousness for understanding pain behaviour and the definition of pain. *Pain Res Manage* 1997; **2**: 111–17.
73. Fanurik D, Koh JL, Schmitze ML *et al.* Children with cognitive impairment: parent report of pain and coping. *J Dev Behav Pediatr* 1999; **20**: 228–34.

74. Oberlander TF, O'Donnell ME, Montgomery CJ. Pain in children with significant neurological impairment. *Dev Behav Pediatr* 1999; **20**: 235–43.

75. Lebeer J. Families with a handicapped child: dealing with pain. *WHO Reg Publ Eur Ser* 1992; **44**: 297–301.

76. Anand KJS, Craig KD. New perspectives on the definition of pain. *Pain* 1996; **67**: 3–6; discussion 209–11.

77. Carter B, McArthur E, Cunliffe M. Dealing with uncertainty: parental assessment of pain in their children with profound special needs. *J Adv Nurs* 2002; **38**: 449–57.

78. McGrath PJ, Rosmus C, Canfield C *et al.* Behaviours caregivers use to determine pain in non-verbal, cognitively impaired individuals. *Dev Med Child Neurol* 1998; **40**: 340–3.

79. Beyer JE, McGrath PJ, Berde CB. Discordance between self-report and behavioral pain measures in children aged 3–7 years after surgery. *J Pain Symptom Manage* 1990; **5**: 350–6.

80. Nolan J, Chalkiadis GA, Low J, Olesch CA, Brown TCK. Anaesthesia and pain management in cerebral palsy. *Anaesthesia* 2000; **55**: 32–41.

81. Malviya S, Voepel-Lewis T, Burke C *et al.* The revised FLACC observational pain tool: improved reliability and validity for pain assessment in children with cognitive impairment. *Paediatr Anaesth* 2006; **16**: 258–65.

82. Hunt A, Goldman A, Seers K *et al.* Clinical validation of the paediatric pain profile. *Dev Med Child Neurol* 2004; **46**: 9–18.

83. Tramer MR. *Postoperative nausea and vomiting. Evidence-based resource in anaesthesia and analgesia*, 2nd edn. London: BMJ Books, 2003.

84. Brenn BR, Brislin RP, Rose JB. Epidural analgesia in children with cerebral palsy. *Can J Anaesth* 1998; **45**: 1156A.

85. Stasilkelis PJ, Lee DD, Sullivan CM. Complications of osteotomies in severe cerebral palsy. *J Pediatr Orthop* 1999; **19**: 207–10.

86. Lauder GR, White MC. Neuropathic pain following multilevel surgery in children with cerebral palsy: A case series and literature review. *Paediatr Anaesth* 2005; **15**: 412–20.

87. King JD, Bobechko WP. Osteogenesis imperfecta: an orthopedic description and surgical review. *J Bone Joint Surg* [*Br*] 1971; **53**: 72.

88. White NJ, Winearls CJ, Smith R. Cardiovascular abnormalities in osteogenesis imperfecta. *Am Heart J* 1983; **106**: 1416.

89. Hathaway WE, Solomons CC, Ott J. Abnormalities of platelet function in osteogenesis imperfecta. *Clin Res* 1970; **18**: 209.

90. Sofield HA, Millar EA. Fragmentation, realignment, and intramedullary rod fixation of deformities of the long bones in children (a 10-year appraisal). *J Bone Joint Surg* [*Am*] 1959; **41**: 1371.

91. Millar EA. Observation on the surgical management of osteogenesis imperfecta. *Clin Orthop Relat Res* 1981; **159**: 154–6.

92. Oliverio RM Jr. Anesthetic management of intramedullary nailing in osteogenesis imperfecta: report of one case. *Anesth Analg* 1973; **52**: 232.

93. Solomons CC, Myers DN. Hyperthermia of osteogenesis imperfecta and its relationship to malignant hyperthermia. In: Gordon RA, Britt BA, Kalow W, eds. *International Symposium on Malignant Hyperthermia*. Springfield, IL: Charles C Thomas, **1973**: 319.

94. Stehling LC. Anesthesia for congenital anomalies of the skeletal system. In: Stehling LC, Zauder HL, eds. *Anesthetic implications of congenital anomalies in children*. East Norwalk, CT: Appleton-Century-Crofts, **1980**: 319–30.

95. Thompson GH, Bilenker RM. Comprehensive management of arthrogryposis multiplex congenital. *Clin Orthop Related Res* 1985; **194**: 6–14.

96. Lebenthal E, Shochet SB, Adams A *et al.* Arthrogryposis multiplex congenital: 23 cases in Arab kindred. *Pediatrics* 1970; **46**: 891.

97. Epstein JB, Wittenberg GJ. Maxillofacial manifestations and management of arthrogryposis: literature review and case report. *J Oral Maxillofac Surg* 1987; **45**: 274–9.

98. Steinberg B, Nelson VS, Feinberg SE *et al.* Incidence of maxillofacial involvement in arthrogryposis multiplex congenital. *J Oral Maxillofac Surg* 1996; **54**: 956–9.

99. Oberoi GS, Kaul HL, Gill IS *et al.* Anaesthesia in arthrogryposis multiplex congenital: case report. *Can J Anaesth* 1987; **34**: 288–90.

100. Thomas JA, Chiu-Yeh M, Moriconi ES. Maxillofacial implications and surgical treatment of arthrogryposis multiplex congenital. *Compend Contin Educ Dent* 2001; **22**: 588–92.

101. Friedman WF, Mason DT, Braunwald E. Arthrogryposis multiplex congenital associated with congenital aortic stenosis. *J Pediatr* 1965; **67**: 682–5.

102. Vener DF, Lerman J. The pediatric airway and associated syndromes. *Anesthesiol Clin North Am* 1995; **13**: 585–614.

103. Froster-Iskenius UG, Weterson JR, Hall JG. A recessive form of congenital contractures and torticollis associated with malignant hyperthermia. *J Med Genet* 1988; **25**: 102–12.

104. Leudeman WO, Tatagiba MS, Hussein S, Samii M. Congenital arthrogryposis associated with atlantoaxial subluxation and dysraphic abnormalities. Case report. *J Neurosurg* 2000; **93**(1 suppl): 130–2.

105. Baines DB, Douglas ID, Overton JH. Anaesthesia for patients with arthrogryposis multiplex congenital: what is the risk of malignant hyperthermia? *Anaesth Intensive Care* 1986; **14**: 370–2.

106. Hopkins PM, Ellis FR, Halsall PJ. Hypermetabolism in arthrogryposis multiplex congenital. *Anaesthesia* 1991; **46**: 374–5.

107. Honda N, Konno K, Itohda Y *et al.* Malignant hyperthermia and althesin. *Can Anaesth Soc J* 1977; **24**: 514–21.

108. Ferris PE, Intraoperative convulsions in a child with arthrogryposis. *Anaesth Intensive Care* 1997; **25**: 546–9.

109. Merchan EC, Magallon M, Manso F, Martin-Villar J. Septic arthritis in HIV positive haemophiliacs. Four case reports and a literature review. *Int Orthop* 1992; **16**: 302–6.

Scoliosis surgery

JOHN CURRIE

KEY LEARNING POINTS

- Scoliosis can compromise both respiratory and cardiovascular function. Surgery reduces respiratory postoperative function and the preoperative assessment must determine whether the child will tolerate this.
- Anterior release may be necessary in younger children to control a rapidly accelerating deformity. Most cases can be extubated at the end of the procedure.
- Posterior fusion is usually delayed until adolescence, but may be necessary earlier in severe cases (combined with an anterior release). Many of these children may be thin and undernourished. Blood loss can be considerable. After such a long operation, many children require a period of stabilisation in intensive care.
- Hypotension is at least as potent a cause of poor spinal cord damage as distraction of the spine by the surgeon. Despite spinal cord monitoring, it is reassuring to see good movement of the feet as soon as possible in recovery.

INTRODUCTION

Most scoliosis surgery is performed by orthopaedic surgeons whereas operations for correction of neurological abnormalities are usually dealt with by either paediatric surgeons or neurosurgeons. Anaesthesia for spina bifida surgery and cervical spine stabilisation operations is covered in Chapter 38. Anaesthesia for scoliosis surgery is challenging and, as in many other aspects of paediatric anaesthetic practice, attention to detail is essential. A large team is involved in the preparation and assessment of the child, as well as the operation itself. The children may have associated abnormalities or physiological compromise. Incisions are large and operations can take many hours. There can be major haemorrhage and haemodynamic instability. The operations are also physically demanding and stressful for the surgeon. In all this, the anaesthetist will often act as coordinator and therefore needs to understand the role of each team member.

EMBRYOLOGY AND GROWTH

The vertebral bodies and discs are well developed by the time the foetus is about 13 mm in length. The spine is derived from the sclerotome, which is a group of cells that condense and migrate ventrally around the primitive notochord. Each intervertebral disc is derived from one sclerotome segment, but each vertebra develops from adjoining upper and lower segments. If the sclerotome fails to fuse posteriorly or there is overgrowth of the neural tube a range of spina bifida defects arise.

At birth each vertebra has three parts: a centrum and the right and left sides of the neural arch. The two sides of the arch are united by hyaline cartilage which ossifies during the first year of life. The arches fuse to the vertebral body between the third and sixth years. In prenatal life the spine is uniformly curved and is concave ventrally. In the thoracic and sacrococcygeal regions this ventral concavity persists. The cervical curvature appears when the infant learns to hold the head erect, and look forward, at about the third month. The lumbar curvature appears when the child walks at about 18 months. The cervical and lumbar curves are secondary or 'compensatory' and are concave dorsally.

After birth there is tremendous initial growth and, at periods of rapid growth, any abnormality becomes noticeable. Growth of the spine continues steadily until the pubertal growth acceleration. There is a small increase in growth rate between the ages of 5 and 7 years, called the period of 'middle childhood'. Pressure and traction epiphyses appear about puberty and fuse by year 24. In humans, the epiphyses are rings not the plates found in most other mammals [1,2].

The upper seven ribs are fixed at both ends – the spine and the manubrium sterni. The ribcage is symmetrical with each pair of ribs being of equal length. Any discrepancy in the spine alters this symmetry and leads to rib deformity. Ribs begin to ossify at about prenatal week 9 and full fusion of all epiphyses is complete by year 24.

Scoliosis is a lateral curvature of the spine in the coronal plane as opposed to kyphosis which is curvature in the sagittal plane. Kyphoscoliosis is a combination of these two. Scoliosis may be functional if the curve corrects on sitting or lying and this may be caused by leg length discrepancy, leading to compensatory tilting of the pelvis in an attempt to keep a level gaze and the head central in line over the pelvis. In structural scoliosis there is a fixed deformity and the diagnosis is usually obvious when there is a fixed curve of greater than 10°. The curve may be made more obvious by asking the child to bend forwards (this is called the Adam's forward bending test). A scoliometer is also used and is a device specifically designed to estimate the angle of trunk rotation. The measurements are difficult to standardise but can be used to give a rough assessment of progression of the disease when the child is examined in the clinic.

Ribs will tend to be compressed closer together on the concave side of the scoliosis and splayed on the convex side. The equal length of the ribs also exerts a rotational force [3] so that scoliosis becomes a complex three-dimensional deformity (Figs 37.1 and 37.2). Scoliosis may be congenital, idiopathic or associated with a neuromuscular disease.

CLASSIFICATION

Congenital

Congenital scoliosis presents from birth. Abnormal development of the vertebrae causes a lateral curvature and there

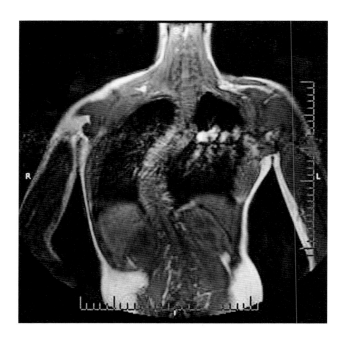

Figure 37.1 Magnetic resonance imaging showing lateral curve in scoliosis.

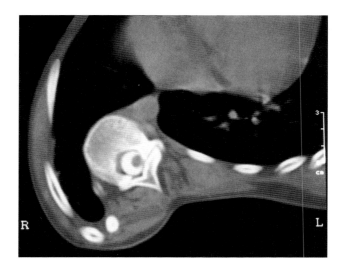

Figure 37.2 Magnetic resonance imaging cross-section showing ribs splayed on the left of the scan, compressed together on the right, with rotation of the vertebrae.

is also lateral longitudinal differential growth. About 30–60 per cent of children with congenital scoliosis have other anomalies in the gastrointestinal tract, the heart or defects of the spinal cord or the cervical spine. The VATER syndrome (**v**ertebral anomalies, imperforate **a**nus, **t**racheo-**o**esophageal fistula, **r**adial or **r**enal anomalies) is associated with vertical abnormalities, an imperforate anus, tracheo-oesophageal fistula and renal dysplasia. Congenital scoliosis is associated with rapid development of deformity in 50 per cent of cases; 25 per cent progress slowly and 25 per cent are static. Seventy-five per cent of patients will require surgery and 10 per cent will require bracing. Braces are applied to most patients because surgery should, ideally, be delayed until after maximum growth.

Idiopathic

This is the most common form of scoliosis. It was first described by Hippocrates and it was Galen (AD 131–201) who first used the term scoliosis [4]. In the past, idiopathic scoliosis has been attributed to poor nutrition, poor posture and genetic predisposition. Attention has been focused on the growth plates of the vertebrae, but no convincing cause has been found. Cases can be divided into the age of presentation: the infantile group presents between birth and 3 years; the juvenile at 3–10 years; and the adolescent group after 10 years of age. Presentation in adolescence is most common. Early-onset scoliosis has a male predominance, whereas females tend to present late [5].

INFANTILE

Children presenting with infantile-type idiopathic scoliosis are carefully monitored and braced as necessary. Progression depends upon skeletal maturity – it is greatest when ossification is least. Skeletal maturity is graded using the Risser method and each grade, from 1 to 4, corresponds to a 25 per cent increment of iliac crest ossification. A low grade indicates that the skeleton still has considerable growth potential. Grade 5 corresponds to skeletal maturity. The lower the Risser grade at the time of curve detection, the greater the risk of progression. The Risser scale is gender specific because of the different timing of skeletal maturity [6–9].

JUVENILE AND ADOLESCENT

Juvenile scoliosis usually presents about the age of 5 or 6 years when the child enters middle childhood. This is usually a period of increased growth when the scoliosis will become more apparent. Children with cerebral palsy often present at about this time because they become more 'wind blown' in their chairs. Adolescent scoliosis is similarly associated with the growth spurt of puberty. This is a time when limiting any further growth may be acceptable and therefore definitive surgery (anterior release, posterior fusion or both) can be performed.

Acquired and other causes

Infection of the vertebrae has long been thought to contribute to scoliosis. Asymmetrical infection causes asymmetrical growth. Tuberculosis is one of the most common spinal infections and it can affect all the vertebrae, which can then collapse – the collapse is also often asymmetrical, leading to wedging of the vertebrae and scoliosis.

Any injury to the spine while it is still growing also leads to asymmetrical growth.

Cerebral palsy causes an imbalance of the muscles as a result of poor neuromuscular function. Children may be unable to sit straight and are often wheelchair bound from an early stage. Poor muscular control leads to falling to one side and this is known as being 'wind blown'. In this position the spine can become fixed and during middle childhood and adolescence the curvature becomes exacerbated. It is often appropriate to fix the spine at an early stage in these children.

Muscular dystrophies also lead to scoliosis because of weakness of the spinal muscles. The most common type of muscular dystrophy presenting for scoliosis surgery is Duchenne muscular dystrophy (DMD) (see page 559). Unlike cerebral palsy children who have fixed scoliosis, children with Duchenne muscular dystrophy have a pronounced scoliosis when sitting yet the spine becomes straighter when they lie down. The usual purpose of scoliosis surgery is merely to arrest any progression of deformity and not to make the spine straight. However, in DMD it is possible to reduce the curve because the deformity lessens when the child is supine. The paradox is that DMD children, unlike cerebral palsy children, have a limited life expectancy but can have surgery to straighten the spine.

Neurofibromatosis is associated with scoliosis but not related to spinal neurofibromas [12]. Friedreich's ataxia (see page 559) is also associated with scoliosis.

INDICATIONS FOR INTERVENTION

The decision to operate depends upon the degree of curvature and its acceleration. Curvature is carefully assessed mainly because of its effect on pulmonary function. As curvature increases, the ribcage becomes more distorted and the lungs become compressed. Distortion restricts rib movement and the thorax is less able to expand during breathing. With kyphosis, diaphragmatic breathing may also be impaired if the spine is bent forward because the abdomen becomes compressed. Standard lung function tests such as forced expiratory volume in 1 second (FEV_1) and forced vital capacity (FVC) [11] are used because indirect tests such as exercise tolerance are not appropriate. Peak flow is a useful indicator of the ability to cough. It will assess the child's ability to tolerate the operation and is particularly useful when there is a degree of muscle weakness. Symptoms tend to occur late in the progression of the deformity.

The curve should be carefully monitored as the child grows and the progression of the curve informs the decision to operate. The Cobb angle is a method of quantifying the radiographic degree of scoliosis [12].

Scoliosis can also compress the mediastinum, especially if there is kyphoscoliosis. This may compromise cardiac function because of restricted ventricular filling. In DMD there may be cardiac hypertrophy which further restricts ventricular filling. Abnormal posture can cause difficulty with feeding and swallowing and may exacerbate any gastro-oesophageal reflux. Weight gain and general well-being of the child are also important.

Surgery reduces the growth of the spine and should be regarded as a last resort. Anterior release affects growth least provided that growth plates are unaffected – sometimes one side of the growth plate will be intentionally damaged so that the other side can grow to reduce the curvature. Spinal fusion completely arrests further growth of the spine [13].

SURGICAL AND ANAESTHETIC MANAGEMENT

Fitting braces and plaster jackets

Braces and plaster jackets try to maintain a normal shape or prevent further curvature prior to surgery. Braces are old-fashioned restraints, composed of leather and metal such as the Milwaukee or Boston braces. They are usually only used in the over-5 age group as they require a degree of cooperation [14,15]. Jackets can be made from modern materials that are lightweight, durable and coloured. Plaster jackets are worn for 4 months followed by a period of not being worn for 2 months. After this period, and reassessment, a new jacket may be fitted and the process repeated. The jacket is known as an EDF cast (EDF: elongation, deformation and flexion).

Fitting a new jacket usually requires anaesthesia. A well-fitting jacket should fix the chest but not restrict diaphragmatic breathing, and it must be tolerable. Preoperative problems of cardiac compression, breathing restriction and gastro-oesophageal reflux must also be evaluated. These children present frequently and will develop their preferences for either intravenous or inhalational induction. It is essential to intubate the trachea because they are placed in a frame, in order to distract the spine before the plaster jacket is applied. Insertion of a Guedel airway protects the tracheal tube from being compressed.

The frame restricts monitoring but electrocardiogram (ECG) leads can be placed on the limbs, a blood pressure cuff on a leg and a pulse oximeter probe on an ear or a suitable digit. It is important to apply positive pressure ventilation because the lungs need to be expanded for best fitting – breathing will be restricted afterwards if the jacket is fixed during the low tidal volume breathing that is typical of spontaneous breathing under anaesthesia. A hole is cut in front of the jacket to allow the diaphragm to descend and for the abdomen to expand.

The trachea should be extubated in the lateral position because it will be too difficult to move the child quickly in case of vomiting, secretions and laryngospasm. Respiratory tract infection is common. In the USA it is usual to cut a hole to allow external cardiac massage. This seems unduly pessimistic and is not our practice.

Waking up with a sensation of being encased in a plaster jacket is frightening and parents can reassure their child during recovery. Assessment of ventilation is essential before discharge to the ward. In the course of a series of jacket applications, the first jacket is usually the most problematic. Thereafter, the child becomes used to the process.

Anterior release

Anterior release reduces the deterioration of scoliosis. It will not correct curvature by itself but may be combined with rib resections to correct deformity of the chest. Anterior release may be necessary in younger children to control a rapidly accelerating curve. Posterior fusion of the spine is usually delayed until adolescence, but may be necessary earlier in severe cases when it may be combined with an anterior release.

Anterior release is usually performed at about the age of 4 or 5 years. It involves a transverse incision between the ribs and only two or three segments are usually released. Sometimes a growth plate is intentionally damaged in order that the spine will grow straighter. The side of incision may not be obvious and must be considered carefully. It may be necessary to disarticulate ribs in order to reduce the curvature. Rib osteoplasty may be performed on the convex side. Surgery reduces respiratory function and the preoperative assessment must determine whether the child will tolerate this.

The anaesthetic is managed with intermittent positive pressure ventilation. Muscle relaxation is used for tracheal intubation but is not necessary for surgery. Anaesthetic agents should be chosen to allow for moderate hypotension without a tachycardia. Epidural analgesia enables cardiovascular stability. A double-lumen tube is unnecessary because the approach is retroplural and the lung can easily be retracted. Our practice is to interrupt surgery every half hour and to re-expand the lungs fully. Re-expansion may limit postoperative atelectasis and reduce the chance of pneumothorax. Increasing inspired oxygen concentration may be necessary during lung retraction.

The operation is usually in the lateral position. Temperature must be monitored and care must be taken with pressure points because surgery can sometimes be prolonged. Appreciable blood loss can be caused by stripping of periosteum but with careful haemostasis it is seldom necessary to transfuse. An arterial line is important to monitor direct blood pressure because lung retraction can compress the mediastinum and great vessels; it will also be necessary for arterial blood gas tension and haemoglobin estimations.

Most patients can be extubated at the end of the procedure and then nursed and monitored in a high-dependency setting. Nasal oxygen is often required. Children are ready, in general, to return to the ward the following day. They are vulnerable to chest lung collapse and chest infection. An epidural will facilitate pain-free respiration and coughing and can be continued for a further 24–36 hours. The jacket, which was made preoperatively, is split into two halves and the child will be nursed on the posterior half. The anterior half can then be applied when the child has recovered from surgery.

Posterior fusion

This is a major and definitive operation for scoliosis. It fixes the spine so preventing further growth. The timing depends upon a balance between needing to arrest the curvature progression and achieving maximal growth. It is therefore usually performed in adolescents. Respiratory function tests should be performed at each clinic visit as these can inform the decision of when to operate. If there is compression of the mediastinum then echocardiography is essential to assess cardiac filling and output.

The patient and parents need to understand that surgery mainly prevents further deterioration and that any reduction in the deformity is 'a bonus'. School will be disrupted for a considerable time. Preparation should include specialist psychological support that will help the child to cope with any teasing and bullying at school. Coping techniques for managing the discomfort and boredom of the postoperative period can be explored. Despite these problems most children are keen to 'have their backs fixed'. A preoperative visit is essential to go through all their questions and explain the procedure and postoperative course. It is important to allow plenty of time to raise any fears that they may have.

Many of these children may be thin and undernourished. Muscle mass may be low and this will be further reduced with the major catabolism of surgery. Treatment of gastro-oesophageal reflux and advice of a dietician at an early stage may be needed.

Until recently, anterior and posterior surgery were separated by 2–3 weeks. This was, apart from the physiological aspects, very debilitating, especially if there had been significant blood loss in the first operation. Modern techniques of limiting blood loss during the posterior fusion operation have now meant that the two operations can be done at the same time, and this has allowed a major improvement in the child's experience. However, combined operations are long.

The deformity may affect the position of the head and neck so that laryngoscopy may be difficult. Large-bore intravenous catheters are inserted. Invasive monitoring with an arterial line and central venous pressure (CVP) are necessary. Monitoring of CVP is helpful to assess cardiac preload but it may be unreliable in the prone position, although it still monitors trend even if absolute values are misleading. Transoesophageal echocardiography may be preferable [16]. The preferred site for CVP catheters is the internal jugular vein. The position of the internal jugular vein is less predictable on the concave side and in this situation ultrasound guidance is most helpful to avoid carotid artery puncture. A urinary catheter should be placed.

Moving into the prone position must be done with great care. Pressure points must be padded and a bed of pillows covered with a layer of cotton-wool padding is adequate. The neck must be slightly flexed and in the midline. Care must be taken to avoid any pressure on the eyes, particularly the edges of the orbits. There may be flexions of the lower limbs and these can be rested upon pillows. The arms are placed on a lateral board; shoulder and elbow extension should be limited to no more than 90° to avoid brachial plexus damage. The knees must be flexed and well padded, the feet dorsiflexed, and no weight taken on the toes. Male genitalia and female breasts should be padded and in a comfortable position. There must be no traction on the catheter and the urine bag must be positioned so that it can be easily seen. Once the child is in position it is wise to conduct a head-to-foot inspection to check all possible pressure points and joint positions. The body weight should rest on the chest and hips to minimise intra-abdominal pressure – this helps to minimise venous haemorrhage during surgery.

Central and peripheral temperature probes are needed and the temperature difference is a guide to peripheral perfusion. Maintaining body temperature at a normal level is important and achieved with a forced-air duvet or blanket placed over the legs and simple insulation over the head. The child may be cool at the beginning but become too warm later. Body temperature often starts to rise once blood transfusion has commenced. Active cooling should start before the pyrexia becomes appreciable. Serial arterial blood gas estimations will confirm adequate ventilation, acid–base status, and lactate and haemoglobin concentrations. Blood loss can be considerable and must be estimated.

Once the spine is prepared by removal of periosteum, rods are fixed to either side of the spine. If the curve is very advanced then it may only be possible to fix a rod to one side, but this is rare. The rods are anchored to the lower spine with strong bolts, and then they are usually attached to the concave side using intralaminar wires. These wires can be tightened to pull the spine onto to the rod. On the convex side hooks are placed under the laminae and then attached to the rod to act as an anchor to push the next hook away from it. Both these manoeuvres tend to straighten the spine. Once the rods, bolts, wires and hooks are in place, small pieces of bone are placed against the raw surface of the spine and this forms the basis of an arthrodesis which fuses the spine. The purpose of the rods is to hold the spine in position until this arthrodesis is complete.

MANAGEMENT OF BLOOD LOSS

Strategies for blood loss are based on controlled hypotension and haemodilution. In addition to standard anaesthesia using isoflurane and analgesia (opioids and epidural local anaesthesia) further control of blood pressure can be achieved using a specific hypotensive drug. Labetalol is a good choice because it combines vasodilatation actions with β-adrenergic receptor blockade which limits reflex tachycardia. Because surgery can be prolonged, hypotension cannot be maintained throughout and should be reserved to help the surgeon during the periosteal stripping phase. After this, while the fixings are being applied, blood loss should not be so severe. Minimum mean blood pressure of 60–65 mmHg is necessary to perfuse the brain and other vital organs. Peripheral perfusion is vital to prevent pressure necrosis during these long operations, and this can be assessed by the temperature difference between central and peripheral probes. Hypotension is at least as potent a cause of poor spinal cord damage as distraction of the spine by the surgeon. Spinal cord perfusion is assessed by electrical monitoring (see below).

Renal perfusion is assessed by urine production. A fall in urine output late in the operation is common and usually increases in the immediate postoperative period. If urine output does not return fluid must be infused to raise the CVP. Occasionally, a diuretic may be necessary.

Blood transfusion can be limited by haemodilution. This can either be normovolaemic or hypervolaemic. The haemoglobin concentration can be reduced to about 80 g/L, so that with haemorrhage less haemoglobin is lost in proportion to volume loss. Later, after haemorrhage has ceased, haemoconcentration allows the haemoglobin concentration to rise again [17,18] Normovolaemic dilution involves blood being taken off and replaced by plasma or crystalloid. In the hypervolaemic method the intravascular space is expanded by vasodilatation, and this method is preferred for good tissue perfusion [18].

In older children a unit of blood can be removed from the circulation at induction of anaesthesia and transfused later in the day [19]. This aids the haemodilution process and provides a unit of 'fresh' blood when most needed. There are rules for the safe handling of donated blood and these must be respected. Alternatively, blood can be taken a few weeks before surgery but this is less attractive because it has administrative implications as well as additional venesection.

An important and effective method of limiting blood loss is to apply gauze packs soaked in 1:500 000 adrenaline in warm saline (1 mg adrenaline in 500 mL saline). There may be an initial increase in heart rate but this settles and the reduction in oozing or blood particularly from the dissected muscles is impressive.

Tranexamic acid (10 mg/kg), an antifibrinolytic, can be given at the commencement of surgery. It is effective and helps with general blood loss including that from the periostium. It has a half-life of about 8 hours and during prolonged surgery a second dose can be given, which has a similar effect [20]. The cell saver is another useful method of reducing blood transfusion, but is not without its problems in orthopaedic surgery (see Chapter 24) [21,22].

All these strategies combine to reduce the need for blood transfusion, and they have been so successful that combined anterior and posterior surgery has become feasible and routine. In larger children it is possible to perform a posterior fusion without autologous blood transfusion.

Postoperatively, a haemoglobin concentration of 80 g/L can be tolerated and treated with diet rather than by exposure to the risks of transfusion [23].

Blood loss can usually be kept to below 40–50 per cent of the circulating volume but occasionally the surgeon may lose control of the haemorrhage. This can lead to coagulopathy and further bleeding and is the main cause of mortality for scoliosis surgery. Clotting tests must be sent at the first sign of increased oozing and the situation may be so severe as to warrant the administration of fresh frozen plasma before the test results are available. Close communication with the haematology and transfusion departments is vital.

SPINAL CORD MONITORING

Ischaemic damage to the spinal cord is a major risk during these operations. This may be produced by either stretching of the cord during distraction of the spine by the surgeon, or hypotension. The anterior spinal artery of Adamkovich is most vulnerable because it has a long course. It is an end-artery with little collateral flow to a large area of the spinal cord (the anterior part of the lower cord). Spinal cord monitoring is used detect damage in this area.

In the past a 'wake-up' test was used and some surgeons may still ask for this. Here the child is woken once distraction is complete and asked to move the toes. It is a sensitive test because foot drop is the commonest problem caused by this type of cord ischaemia. Anaesthesia technique has to be adjusted to allow the child to wake sufficiently in order to move the feet without appreciable discomfort, which would cause excessive movement or hypertension. An opioid-based technique can be successful and, fortunately, the child seldom remembers the event.

There has been debate over whether forewarning the child about the wake-up test was beneficial. This might prepare them to move their feet when asked, or produce alarm and excessive anxiety. Fortunately, the wake-up test is unnecessary with effective spinal cord monitoring.

The monitoring involves measurement of sensory-evoked potentials. A stimulus is applied to the posterior aspect of the upper leg to stimulate the sciatic nerve. The impulse is transmitted through the spinal cord and sensed by electrodes on the back of the neck and head. A characteristic waveform is obtained (Fig. 37.3). Any change in the wave is seen as a possible sign of spinal cord compromise but specifically the reduction in wave amplitude or loss of one of the three peaks. Immediate action must then be taken to restore adequate perfusion by either increasing blood pressure or releasing some of the spinal distraction. A reduction in the latency of the signal is often observed if there is a rise in body temperature (Fig. 37.4). Sensory-evoked potential monitoring is not ideal because it monitors the dorsal columns, which are less likely to be ischaemic. Motor-evoked potential monitoring is being developed and may be more sensitive if it detects ischaemia in the anterior motor tracts. Stimulation of scalp electrodes can cause a motor potential in the sciatic nerve and

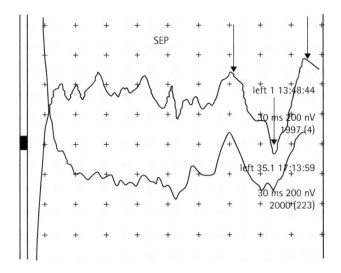

Figure 37.3 Typical triphasic sensory-evoked potential (SEP) trace. Axes: each horizontal line = 3 ms; each vertical division = 200 nV.

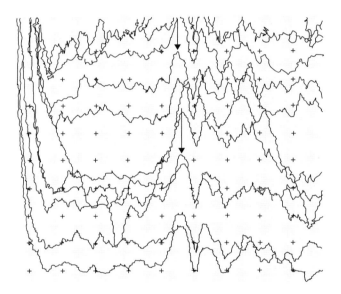

Figure 37.4 Drift of peaks to the left as latency of the signal reduces owing to warming. The lower traces were recorded before the upper ones.

result in a cutaneous signal on the leg, although this may be due to transmission through sensory pathways instead. A motor response needs the absence of muscle relaxation. Despite the monitoring, it is reassuring to see good movement of the feet as soon as possible in recovery.

Other rare complications include air embolism. This is a possibility during any operation on the spine in the prone position [24].

POSTOPERATIVE CARE

Anterior release patients should spend their first night in a high-dependency unit (HDU) for invasive blood pressure monitoring, checking of urine output and close nursing care. The epidural infusion can be adjusted. Posterior spinal fusion

patients should be nursed in an intensive care unit (ICU) because, after such a long operation, they are unlikely to wake up and breathe adequately. These are very painful operations and initial postoperative pain should be first controlled by a morphine infusion while the child is ventilated. About 2–3 hours later the child can be extubated and appropriate patient-controlled analgesia (PCA) or nurse-controlled analgesia (NCA) devices used the following day [25]. Intrathecal morphine can be given by the surgeon during surgery and this may allow for slightly earlier tracheal extubation and better initial pain control. This technique may also reduce the overall morphine consumption in the postoperative period [26].

A nasogastric tube should be inserted because there is usually an ileus for a few days. The child can usually return to the ward the day after surgery. Boredom is then a major problem as they have to lie flat on their back for a week.

DUCHENNE MUSCULAR DYSTROPHY

This pseudo-hypertrophic muscular dystrophy is associated with a high incidence of scoliosis [27]. As these boys grow into their teens their respiratory function deteriorates rapidly because of progressive scoliosis and muscle weakness. There is a 'window of opportunity' to arrest the curvature before the respiratory deterioration makes surgery and anaesthesia unsafe. Pulmonary function tests detect poor function, but the peak flow is a useful indicator and a value of > 150 L/s proves that there is sufficient ventilatory function. Surgery may not lengthen their lives, but it certainly improves quality of life, allowing a more comfortable position in a wheelchair and much easier handling [28].

The weakness is more advanced in the proximal muscles and they may not be able to manage a PCA button. If this is so, a soft, hollow toy can be adapted as a PCA button. Cardiomyopathy develops as they grow into their teens and is the major cause of death. Preoperative echocardiography is essential. The cardiomyopathy is hypertrophic and characterised by poor filling, low ejection fractions and valve leakage [29]; these findings are contraindications to surgery.

Blood loss is increased because the muscular pseudo-hypertrophy affects arterial smooth muscle and, consequently, arteriole muscle contraction is impaired [30]. Blood loss is not usually greater than 60 per cent of the circulating volume provided that all measures previously mentioned are used.

These patients usually have fixed flexed hips which must be carefully positioned for surgery. There is a tenuous association between DMD and malignant hyperthermia which may make total intravenous anaesthesia a safer technique [31]. Pyrexia, late in the procedure, is common and can cause concern. Normal blood gases are reassuring in this situation.

FRIEDREICH'S ATAXIA

The peculiarities in the nervous system in children with Friedreich's ataxia make sensory-evoked potential monitoring impossible because no trace can be obtained [32]. This is perhaps less worrying given that leg function is usually already severely impaired. The wake-up test is not considered necessary and in any case these children do not usually have the temperament to cope with any discus-sion of it.

LATE COMPLICATIONS

Late complications can include infection. Antibiotics are given during and after surgery but there is still a small incidence of infection and it is unusual to be able to identify the organism. If there is infection, the child must return to theatre for drainage of any abscess and, in extreme cases, removal of the rods. The rods may also have to be removed if they protrude through the skin of a cachectic child. This does not usually cause too much blood loss although the procedure may be as extensive and as painful as the original surgery.

REFERENCES

Key references

Almenrader N, Patel D. Spinal fusion surgery in children with non-idiopathic scoliosis: is there a need for routine postoperative ventilation? *Br J Anaesth* 2006; **97**(6): 851–7.

Bunge EM, Juttmann RE, de Koning HJ. Screening for scoliosis: do we have indications for effectiveness? *J Med Screen* 2006; **13**(1): 29–33.

Leong JC, Lu WW, Luk KD, Karlberg EM. Kinematics of the chest cage and spine during breathing in healthy individuals and in patients with adolescent idiopathic scoliosis. *Spine* 1999; **24**(13): 1310–5.

Nigro G, Comi LI, Politano L, Bain RJ. The incidence and evolution of cardiomyopathy in Duchenne muscular dystrophy. *Int J Cardiol* 1990; **26**(3): 271–7.

Sutherland RW, Winter RJ. Two cases of fatal air embolism in children undergoing scoliosis surgery. *Acta Anaesthesiol Scand* 1997; **41**(8): 1073–6.

References

1. Dickson RA, Deacon P. Spinal growth. *J Bone Joint Surg [Br]* 1987; **69**(5): 690–2.
2. Bick EM, Copel JW. The ring apophysis of the human vertebra; contribution to human osteogeny. II. *J Bone Joint Surg [Am]* 1951; **33**(3): 783–7.
3. Dubousset J, Herring JA, Shufflebarger H. The crankshaft phenomenon. *J Pediatr Orthop* 1989; **9**(5): 541–50.
4. Byrd JA III. Current theories on the etiology of idiopathic scoliosis. *Clin Orthop Relat Res* 1988; **229**: 114–19.
5. Calvo IJ. Observations on the growth of the female adolescent spine and its relation to scoliosis. *Clin Orthop* 1957; **10**: 40–7.
6. Risser JC. The iliac apophysis; an invaluable sign in the management of scoliosis. *Clin Orthop* 1958; **11**: 111–19.

7. Noordeen MH, Haddad FS, Edgar MA, Pringle J. Spinal growth and a histologic evaluation of the Risser grade in idiopathic scoliosis. *Spine* 1999; **24**(6): 535–8.
8. Miller NH. Cause and natural history of adolescent idiopathic scoliosis. *Orthop Clin North Am* 1999; **30**(3): 343–52.
9. Hefti FL, McMaster MJ. The effect of the adolescent growth spurt on early posterior spinal fusion in infantile and juvenile idiopathic scoliosis. *J Bone Joint Surg [Br]* 1983; **65**(3): 247–54.
10. Kim HW, Weinstein SL. Spine update. The management of scoliosis in neurofibromatosis. *Spine* 1997; **22**(23): 2770–6.
11. Leong JC, Lu WW, Luk KD, Karlberg EM. Kinematics of the chest cage and spine during breathing in healthy individuals and in patients with adolescent idiopathic scoliosis. *Spine* 1999; **24**(13): 1310–5.
12. Bunge EM, Juttmann RE, de Koning HJ. Screening for scoliosis: do we have indications for effectiveness? *J Med Screen* 2006; **13**(1): 29–33.
13. Sanders JO, Herring JA, Browne RH. Posterior arthrodesis and instrumentation in the immature (Risser-grade-0) spine in idiopathic scoliosis. *J Bone Joint Surg [Am]* 1995; **77**(1): 39–45.
14. Galante J, Schultz A, Dewald RL, Ray RD. Forces acting in the Milwaukee brace on patients undergoing treatment for idiopathic scoliosis. *J Bone Joint Surg [Am]* 1970; **52**(3): 498–506.
15. Perie D, Aubin CE, Petit Y *et al.* Boston brace correction in idiopathic scoliosis: a biomechanical study. *Spine* 2003; **28**(15): 1672–7.
16. Soliman DE, Maslow AD, Bokesch PM *et al.* Transoesophageal echocardiography during scoliosis repair: comparison with CVP monitoring. *Can J Anaesth* 1998; **45**(10): 925–32.
17. Kumar R, Chakraborty I, Sehgal R. A prospective randomized study comparing two techniques of perioperative blood conservation: isovolemic hemodilution and hypervolemic hemodilution. *Anesth Analg* 2002; **95**(5): 1154–61.
18. Copley LA, Richards BS, Safavi FZ, Newton PO. Hemodilution as a method to reduce transfusion requirements in adolescent spine fusion surgery. *Spine* 1999; **24**(3): 219–22.
19. Burbi L, Gregoretti C, Borghi B, Pignotti E. Predeposit, intentional peri-operative haemodilution and erythropoietin level in major orthopaedic surgery. *Anaesthesia* 1998; **53**(suppl 2): 27–8.
20. Neilipovitz DT, Murto K, Hall L *et al.* A randomized trial of tranexamic acid to reduce blood transfusion for scoliosis surgery. *Anesth Analg* 2001; **93**(1): 82–7.
21. Krohn CD, Reikeras O, Bjornsen S, Brosstad F. Fibrinogen, fibrin and its degradation products in drained blood after major orthopaedic surgery. *Blood Coagl Fibrinol* 1999; **10**(4): 167–71.
22. Krohn CD, Reikeras O, Aasen AO. The cytokines IL-1beta and IL-1 receptor antagonist, IL-2 and IL-2 soluble receptor-alpha, IL-6 and IL-6 soluble receptor, TNF-alpha and TNF soluble receptor I, and IL10 in drained and systemic blood after major orthopaedic surgery. *Eur J Surg* 1999; **165**(2): 101–9.

23. Association of Anaesthetists Great Britain and Ireland. *Blood transfusion and the anaesthetist: red cell transfusion.* London: AAGBI, 2001.

24. Sutherland RW, Winter RJ. Two cases of fatal air embolism in children undergoing scoliosis surgery. *Acta Anaesthesiol Scand* 1997; **41**(8): 1073–6.

25. Almenrader N, Patel D. Spinal fusion surgery in children with non-idiopathic scoliosis: is there a need for routine postoperative ventilation? *Br J Anaesth* 2006; **97**(6): 851–7.

26. Gall O, Aubineau JV, Berniere J *et al.* Analgesic effect of low-dose intrathecal morphine after spinal fusion in children. *Anesthesiology* 2001; **94**(3): 447–52.

27. Bridwell KH, Baldus C, Iffrig TM *et al.* Process measures and patient/parent evaluation of surgical management of spinal deformities in patients with progressive flaccid neuromuscular scoliosis (Duchenne's muscular dystrophy and spinal muscular atrophy). *Spine* 1999; **24**(13): 1300–9.

28. Brown JC, Zeller JL, Swank SM *et al.* Surgical and functional results of spine fusion in spinal muscular atrophy. *Spine* 1989; **14**(7): 763–70.

29. Nigro G, Comi LI, Politano L, Bain RJ. The incidence and evolution of cardiomyopathy in Duchenne muscular dystrophy. *Int J Cardiol* 1990; **26**(3): 271–7.

30. Noordeen MH, Haddad FS, Muntoni F *et al.* Blood loss in Duchenne muscular dystrophy: vascular smooth muscle dysfunction? *J Pediatr Orthop B* 1999; **8**(3): 212–5.

31. Takagi A. Malignant hyperthermia of Duchenne muscular dystrophy: application of clinical grading scale and caffeine contracture of skinned muscle fibers. *Rinsho Shinkeigaku* 2000; **40**(5): 423–7.

32. McLeod JG. Electrophysiological and sural nerve biopsy studies in patients with Freidreich's ataxia and Charcot–Marie–Tooth disease. *Proc Aust Assoc Neurol* 1970; **7**: 89–95.

Craniofacial and neurosurgery

SU MALLORY

KEY LEARNING POINTS

- Theoretical neuroanaesthesia principles may not be practical in small uncooperative children.
- Secure tracheal tube fixation and positioning of the patient are crucial.
- Capnography is the best practical monitor for venous air embolism.
- Intensive or high-dependency care is necessary after all craniotomy and craniofacial surgery.
- Blood loss during craniofacial surgery can be massive.

- Analgesia is important but should be adjusted to avoid conscious level effects.
- Electrolyte imbalance may occur and fluid management may be complex.
- Anaesthesia techniques need to adapt to recent advances in imaging, interventional radiology and minimal access surgery.
- Multidisciplinary teamwork is essential in the care of complex patients.

INTRODUCTION

This chapter presents general principles and current practice for both craniofacial and neurosurgery. Where possible, the supporting evidence has been included but given the paucity and difficulties of research in this field some statements represent established practice at the author's hospital. Surgery and imaging have advanced and anaesthesia techniques have had to be adapted and developed to meet new challenges. Problems of major surgery in infants and small children sometimes necessitate compromise on the application of theoretical and ideal neurophysiological principles. In these circumstances the anaesthetist has to be practical and must adapt to the requirements of individual patients.

GENERAL PRINCIPLES

Clinical aspects of central nervous system development and neurophysiology

This is covered comprehensively in Chapter 6; however, some points of particular relevance to clinical practice will be discussed here. In the neonate, the calvarium comprises ossified plates covering the dura. These are separated by fibrous sutures and two fontanelles. The posterior fontanelle closes during the second or third month and the anterior fontanelle usually closes between 10 months and 16 months, fully ossifying in the second decade. High intracranial pressure may be accommodated by separation of fontanelles and non-fused sutures up to early adolescence. While not absorbing acute changes, this separation can provide protection from chronic increase in intracranial volume.

The cerebral metabolic rate is higher in children compared with adults in respect of both glucose (child 6.8, adults 5.5 mg/min/100 g) and oxygen consumption (infant 5.8, adults 3.5 mL/min/100 g) [1]. In the presence of oxygen, the main source of energy for cerebral metabolism is glucose. Storage of glucose or glycogen in cerebral tissue is sparse, allowing only approximately 3 minutes of energy production in the event of anoxia. Cerebral tissue is therefore reliant on its blood supply to provide adequate glucose and oxygen. Children, with their increased metabolic rate, will be less able to maintain normal cerebral metabolism when glucose or oxygen supply is interrupted and, once glycogen stores are depleted, coma and death follow more quickly than in adults.

Cerebral blood flow (CBF) is affected by several factors including carbon dioxide tension, hypoxia, hypothermia, cerebral perfusion pressure (CPP) and a number of anaesthetic agents. These are important because control of intracranial pressure (ICP) relies partly on the ability to manipulate CBF and, in turn, intracranial blood volume. In the neonate CBF is 40–42 mL/min/100 g, infants and children aged 6 months to 3 years have a CBF of 90 mL/min/100 g, 3- to 12-year-olds 100 mL/min/100 g. and adults 50 mL/min/100 g [2]. Regional blood flow also alters with development [3].

Cerebral perfusion pressure is calculated from the formula CPP = MAP − (ICP + CVP), where MAP is mean arterial pressure and CVP is central venous pressure. While MAP remains within a given range, cerebral perfusion is controlled by autoregulatory mechanisms. If excessive hypotension or hypertension, hypoxia, hypercapnia or cerebral ischaemia occurs, then these mechanisms fail. In addition, volatile anaesthetic agents inhibit autoregulation via a dose-dependent cerebral vasodilatation. In children, the lower level of autoregulation is presumed to be related to normal MAP. Sick neonates have impaired autoregulation and CBF in this group follows systemic pressure; this may explain the occurrence of intraventricular haemorrhage [4]. The effects of carbon dioxide on CBF appear, from clinical experience, to be the same as in adults, although in sick neonates there is a linear relationship between arterial partial pressure of carbon dioxide ($PaCO_2$) and CBF [5]. Hyperventilation may restore autoregulation in neonates [6].

Control of intracranial pressure

The ICP in neonates and infants is normally in the range 2–4 mmHg [7] (adult values are 7–17 mmHg). The ICP may be increased by cerebral tissue oedema, or rises in cerebral blood or cerebrospinal fluid (CSF) volumes. Increases in ICP affect CPP. During acute changes, even when the fontanelles are open, the skull is like a rigid box and, once compensatory mechanisms have been exhausted, ICP rises rapidly. Ultimately, there is herniation of the

brain stem through the foramen magnum ('coning'), coma and death. Normally, in adults, an increase in ICP of 10 mmHg can be caused by an increase in intracranial volume of approximately 25 mL, but in infants only 10 mL is required [8]. This explains why a child's neurological status can deteriorate quickly with intracranial haemorrhage.

Intracranial pressure may be affected by surgery but, concomitantly, good operative conditions for neurosurgery are produced by control of ICP (Table 38.1). It is therefore important to minimise or prevent any potentially detrimental effects of anaesthesia. This starts by avoiding excessive sedation with premedication, which may cause respiratory depression and result in hypercapnia. A smooth induction of anaesthesia, avoiding excitation, should be achieved with either propofol, thiopental or sevoflurane and a volatile agent with minimal vasodilatory action, such as isoflurane used for maintenance. Surges in arterial pressure can be reduced with fentanyl, both at laryngoscopy and intraoperatively. Cerebral venous pressure can be minimised by careful patient positioning; head-up tilt and taping (rather than tying) the tracheal tube. Neuromuscular blockade is maintained to prevent rises in intrathoracic pressure or coughing.

Acute rises in ICP are usually managed with hyperventilation and intravenous mannitol. Mild intraoperative hyperventilation (to a minimum $PaCO_2$ of 3.5 kPa) will reduce cerebral blood volume by vasoconstriction but cerebral ischaemia may occur if $PaCO_2$ is allowed to fall too low. Children usually have healthy blood vessels and are less prone to focal ischaemia than adults. Hypotensive agents such as sodium nitroprusside are not generally necessary and they may increase ICP by cerebral vasodilatation. In the past, 20 per cent mannitol (1 g/kg) was used when surgical access to small solid lesions was particularly difficult. The development of modern stereotactic techniques has resulted in improved access to deep-seated lesions. Cerebral dehydration is now reserved for acute life-threatening intracranial crises only. Urine output monitoring is required. A vigorous and rapid response to mannitol can cause a marked reduction in intracerebral volume with tearing of the dural veins. Cerebral dehydration can also be produced with furosemide 0.5 mg/kg, which has the advantage of avoiding

Table 38.1 Methods for control of intracranial pressure during anaesthesia

1. Avoidance of excessively sedative premedication
2. Avoidance of cerebral excitatory/vasodilatory drugs
3. Avoidance of surges in arterial pressure
4. Avoidance of cerebral venous obstruction by careful patient positioning
5. Continuous monitoring of neuromuscular blockade
6. Mild hyperventilation intraoperatively (minimum $PaCO_2$ of 3.5 kPa)
7. Cerebral dehydration (in acute crises)
8. Reduction of cerebral oedema with steroids

$PaCO_2$, partial pressure of arterial CO_2.

an intravascular osmotic load. Hypertonic saline (3 per cent) causes extracellular dehydration by increasing serum osmolality [9]. It has been used to manage ICP in children with head injuries [10]. However, the possibility of rebound phenomenon and concerns about the effect of sodium load in young children means that it should be used cautiously [11]. Steroids can reduce oedema caused by tumours (dexamethasone 0.25 mg/kg as a loading dose followed by 0.1 mg/kg every 6 hours). Concerns about hyperglycaemia and lack of demonstrated efficacy has inhibited the routine use of steroids to treat head injury or acute hypoxia.

Anaesthesia drugs

The effects of anaesthetic drugs in children with central nervous system (CNS) pathology are poorly documented but where studies are available they report similar effects to adults (see Chapter 6). The CBF in normal children increases with 60–70 per cent nitrous oxide compared with an oxygen mixture [12]. Nitrous oxide should not be used if ICP is critically raised or if there is an appreciable risk of venous air embolism. Isoflurane has cerebrovascular stability at 0.5–1.0 MAC (minimum alveolar concentration) [13], and is reliable and predictable for neuroanaesthesia. In animals and children, sevoflurane is similar to isoflurane in its effects on cerebral blood volume, cerebral metabolic rate of oxygen ($CMRO_2$) and ICP [14,15], and it may be useful because its faster elimination allows neurological status to be more reliably assessed during recovery. Desflurane may be less useful as it can increase CBF at concentrations of 1.5 MAC [16].

Total intravenous anaesthesia (TIVA) techniques using propofol supplemented by opiates are common in adult neurosurgical practice but their widespread use in children has been inhibited by fears of complications [17]. It is likely that use of TIVA will increase as the pharmacokinetics are fully delineated (see Chapter 11).

Fentanyl is the standard and commonly used opioid in the management of a ventilated child with raised ICP [18] and, unlike alfentanil and sufentanil, produces no increase in CBF or ICP. Remifentanil is also popular in adult practice and is a good alternative to fentanyl, as its short duration of action means that it can be titrated to surgical stimulus [19]. Establishing effective postoperative analgesia following a remifentanil infusion is crucial.

ANAESTHESIA FOR NEUROSURGERY

Preoperative assessment

Assessment of neurological status is essential and must include a check for signs of raised ICP, depressed conscious level and any focal deficits. Raised ICP frequently presents with vomiting, which may cause dehydration and electrolyte imbalance. If not treated adequately, hypotension and cardiovascular instability may follow induction of anaesthesia. Brain-stem lesions are associated with bulbar palsies that may result in pulmonary aspiration.

Pathology in other systems is rare in children with CNS neoplasia. Other important diseases are found in ex-preterm infants (e.g. lung disease), those with cerebral abscesses (cyanotic heart disease) and children with major spinal defects (renal disease).

At the assessment interview details of anaesthetic induction and postoperative course should be explained to the child and the parents. Parents are likely to be anxious and upset because their child's potentially life-changing or life-threatening illness may have developed recently and rapidly.

Investigations should include a full blood count and electrolytes, especially in those with a history of vomiting or a ventricular drain. Neurosurgery can be associated with large blood loss from disrupted sinuses or dilated veins, especially if ICP is raised. Blood must be crossmatched for craniotomy.

Premedication

If ICP is raised sedative premedication should be avoided because even minor degrees of hypercapnia risks coning. There is a dilemma in children whose high ICP may make them irritable. Children with normal ICP may receive standard sedative premedication, e.g. midazolam 0.5 mg/kg (maximum dose 15 mg) or temazepam 0.5 mg/kg (maximum dose 20 mg).

The use of antisialogogues has decreased with the introduction of modern volatile agents. However, pooling of secretions in the prone or sitting position may wet the tracheal tube tapes and reduce their adhesion. Atropine or glycopyrrolate is useful in this group to reduce secretions and prevent bradycardia and hypotension.

Induction

A compromise may need to be reached between the theoretical advantages of some agents and the difficulty of their administration in uncooperative children. Sevoflurane is currently the standard induction volatile agent and, despite its potential cerebral vasodilator effects, a smooth inhalational induction may have less effect on the ICP than the crying and breath-holding associated with difficult intravenous induction. Following induction, venous access can be achieved, the concentration of volatile agent reduced and a non-depolarising muscle relaxant given. Suxamethonium may be used, despite the theoretical risk of increasing ICP, if rapid paralysis is needed. The airway should be secured with an armoured tracheal tube. The leak around the tube and bilateral lung ventilation must be assessed both with the head in a neutral position and once more in the position for surgery. Any but the smallest leaks may result in hypoventilation. Preformed tubes are often too long and it may be difficult to achieve the correct length without accidental bronchial intubation [20].

Intraoperative anaesthesia

Maintenance of anaesthesia is by a balanced technique with mild-to-moderate hyperventilation ($PaCO_2$ approximately 3.8–4.2 kPa) to control ICP. Isoflurane (0.5–1.0 MAC) in oxygen/air (or N_2O if there is no raised ICP or risk of air embolus) is recommended. Positive end-expiratory pressure (PEEP) increases venous pressures and is not usually necessary. Hyperoxia with a PaO_2 greater than 20 kPa may be beneficial by increasing tissue oxygenation in areas of poor flow following cerebral oedema [21]. High PaO_2 is normal during anaesthesia in patients with healthy lungs and an inspired oxygen concentration (FiO_2) of 0.35.

Blood loss may be reduced by avoiding a hyperdynamic circulation and, provided that there is normovolaemia and brain perfusion is not reduced, both the heart rate and the blood pressure can be reduced by sufficient depth of anaesthesia. Opioids are important in this respect and remifentanil by infusion provides good control. Induced hypotension is used only in specific circumstances where haemorrhage cannot be controlled by other means. Direct arterial pressure monitoring is essential whenever appreciable haemorrhage is expected or when perfusion of the brain is critically dependent on CPP. Occasionally, β blockers or labetalol has been used to control blood pressure. Vasodilator agents such as sodium nitroprusside have also been used but these may result in cerebral vasodilatation and compromise cerebral autoregulation.

Analgesia is usually provided with fentanyl and the maximum dose should not exceed 7–10 μg/kg unless the procedure is prolonged or postoperative ventilation is planned. Remifentanil infusion is an alternative. Reduction of anaesthesia begins once head dressings are complete. When neostigmine is used glycopyrrolate is the preferred antimuscarinic because atropine may have central effects. Ideally, children should be extubated without causing coughing, with good respiratory function, with a normal end-tidal carbon dioxide.

Monitoring

In addition to essential standard monitoring all major cases should have direct arterial pressure measurement. Capnography is a reliable monitor of arterial carbon dioxide tension and is a practical method of detecting venous air embolism (VAE). If necessary, CVP should be measured via a femoral vein catheter because upper body catheters have the potential to obstruct cerebral venous drainage. Intraoperative intravascular volume can be assessed by monitoring CVP and other cardiovascular variables. Urinary catheters are useful in patients who need diuretics, in those with diabetes insipidus or for prolonged surgery. Neuromuscular function should be monitored to prevent increases in intrathoracic pressure caused by raised abdominal tone or coughing.

Monitoring both central and peripheral body temperature is essential. A central temperature of between 36 and 36.5°C is recommended. The large surface area to volume ratio of paediatric neurosurgical patients may make this difficult. Standard warming methods include air mattresses and warming of intravenous fluids. Cooling is usually achieved by cessation of all warming devices. Modest hypothermia has a cerebral protective effect and may reduce the potential for brain damage if cerebral perfusion is low [22]. Temperatures of 34–36°C may provide protection without causing cardiovascular effects [23]. In contrast, hyperthermia, even 1–2°C increases in temperature, is associated with worse neurological function after a period of ischaemia [24]. Postoperative hyperpyrexia exacerbates ischaemia and has a poor outcome if not treated quickly; active cooling methods will be necessary. Hyperpyrexia is more likely after craniopharyngioma resection and hypothalamic, pontine and midbrain manipulations.

Fluid management and blood loss

At least two peripheral cannulae are required in case rapid fluid resuscitation becomes necessary.

In the normal brain it is osmotic forces that are mainly responsible for fluid fluxes. A fall in osmotic pressure of as little as 5–10 mosmol/kg can result in cerebral oedema. Intraoperative maintenance fluid should be isotonic; Hartmann's solution, lactated Ringer's or 0.9 per cent saline are suitable. However, where large volumes of fluid are required Hartmann's solution is mildly hypo-osmolar and may not be ideal. Glucose-containing infusions are usually unnecessary. Hyperglycaemia is associated with adverse outcome in cerebral ischaemia [25] and so blood sugar should be checked regularly during surgery and afterwards.

The relatively large head size of children results in proportionally larger blood loss compared with adults. Blood loss is difficult to measure accurately but can be assessed by measurement of cardiovascular variables and the effect of appropriate volume replacement. Exchange transfusions are not unusual in small children and cause few problems provided that clotting, blood gases and potassium levels are checked regularly. Haemorrhage and rapid transfusion in infants deserve special consideration (see also page 576).

Postoperative management

Patients with respiratory problems should be electively ventilated. Postoperative sedation and ventilatory support are indicated when brain perfusion has been compromised or is unstable.

Most craniotomy patients can be extubated at the end of the procedure but require high-dependency care and direct arterial pressure monitoring for at least 24 hours. Neurological status, cardiorespiratory function and fluid balance must be assessed and monitored. Neurological function can be assessed in children by using a modified Glasgow Coma Scale (GCS) [26]. Analgesia includes regular paracetamol, diclofenac and an opioid. Non-steroidal anti-inflammatory drugs (NSAIDs) are effective in many children although there may be a hazard of reduced platelet function and risk of intracranial haemorrhage (see Chapter 13). Codeine phosphate analgesia [27] may be sufficient and has the advantage of not altering consciousness or pupil size; however, some patients, particularly those who have undergone posterior fossa craniotomy or spinal surgery, will need morphine, either orally or by infusion. Control of postoperative nausea and vomiting (PONV) with ondansetron, is important.

Children who are ventilated postoperatively still require neurological assessment. Low-dose morphine infusion (10 μg/kg/h) usually facilitates this with additional sedation provided by midazolam (2–5 μg/kg/min).

SPECIFIC NEUROSURGICAL PROBLEMS

Acute head injury

Common causes of head injury include road traffic accidents and non-accidental injury [28]. Early intubation and stabilisation may be necessary in a local hospital prior to imaging and transfer to a neurosurgical centre (see Chapter 42). Extradural haemorrhage is rare in children because of the close adherence between the dura and skull but, if it occurs, and there is prompt surgical drainage, it has a good prognosis. In contrast, acute subdural haemorrhage is associated with cerebral trauma and permanent damage. A rare complication is a leptomeningeal cyst or 'growing fracture' that causes scalp swelling and pain. It also requires surgical intervention to prevent brain compression.

Facial injuries may cause airway damage, which will further compromise neurological outcome. Scalp injuries can cause large blood loss and other trauma (limb fractures or abdominal organ damage) may contribute to hypovolaemia. Skull fractures are unusual and because the skull does not fracture easily associated brain injury is more likely than in adults. The impact may cause brain injury by contusion, haemorrhage or diffuse axonal damage. Rapid increase in ICP from secondary cerebral oedema may necessitate urgent surgical intervention. Hyperventilation may assist in the control of ICP while the patient is prepared for operation (see Chapter 42).

Neural tube defects

The majority of these defects are multifactorial in origin but maternal antenatal folic acid supplementation has greatly reduced its incidence [29]. Antenatal diagnosis is usual if the defect is open (anencephaly and meningomyelocele). Maternal serum α-foetoprotein levels (αFP) are used in diagnosis and ultrasound may demonstrate not only the contents of the lesion but also the presence of other congenital abnormalities. Emergency surgery for neural tube lesions is reserved for uncovered defects. Others are investigated with ultrasound, computed tomography (CT) and/or magnetic resonance imaging (MRI). Early surgery is recommended for large lesions or where there is a risk of rupture or meningitis.

These infants may feed poorly owing to neurological deficit, so preoperative intravenous fluids are often required. Induction may be inhalational or intravenous. Intubation in the left lateral position has been recommended in the past, but the supine position is satisfactory if the lesion is surrounded by padding, to remove pressure on the covering layers of the spinal cord; the head and body are supported on foam pads or on a shaped (e.g. Montréal) mattress. This position provides optimal conditions for intubation and ensures an unobstructed airway during induction. The surgery is usually performed in the prone position; inferior vena cava (IVC) compression must be avoided as it causes engorgement of the paraspinal veins. Many neural tube defects have associated haemangiomas in the surrounding tissues, which may increase surgical blood loss. Large lesions may require rotational flaps or tissue expanders to produce skin cover. The base of an encephalocele is frequently associated with a leash of vessels which may cause haemorrhage from the dural veins. Intraoperative opiates are avoided or minimised unless postoperative ventilation is planned, since wound infiltration with local anaesthetic, together with paracetamol, provides effective analgesia. Preterm infants are at an increased risk of postoperative apnoea [30], especially after neurosurgery.

Hydrocephalus

Hydrocephalus occurs in the neonate or infant caused by intrauterine infection, haemorrhage, meningitis or the Arnold–Chiari malformation. The classic clinical picture is of an enlarged head, bulging fontanelles, engorged veins and 'sunsetting' eyes. Ventriculoperitoneal (VP) shunt is the usual treatment. Coexisting inguinal hernias, common in premature babies, have to be repaired to prevent CSF accumulating in the hernia sacs. Peritoneal drainage of CSF is avoided if there is intra-abdominal path-ology, which may require surgical intervention in the future. Atrial shunts are not routinely used because of the potential complications of bacterial endocarditis, pulmonary emboli and pulmonary vascular disease. Alternatively the pleural route can be used but this is usually reserved for cyst or subdural fluid drainage.

Many of these infants will have required intensive care and have a postconceptional age of less than 44 weeks. They may have poor veins and lung function. Exposure of skin surfaces and surgical field preparation may cause appreciable hypothermia. Although blood loss is usually minimal, there is a potential for air embolism during shunt catheter insertion. Excessive drainage of CSF can result in cardiovascular instability. Both cardiovascular and respiratory instability, particularly laryngospasm, have been described during and after anaesthesia in children with the Arnold–Chiari malformation and may warn of brain-stem herniation [31].

Tumours

Central nervous system tumours are the second most common childhood malignancy after leukaemia. Incidence varies worldwide between 15 and 31 per million [32] and appears to be increasing. Treatment varies according to tumour type and patient age. Radiotherapy is not recommended in those less than 3 years because of the detrimental effect on brain development. Chemotherapy may allow infants to reach an age when radiotherapy can be administered. Survival has improved as advances in non-invasive imaging techniques have allowed earlier diagnosis and treatment. Some vascular tumours may be suitable for preoperative embolisation of large feeding vessels, which may reduce operative blood loss. Nevertheless, surgery for vascular lesions has a significant risk of morbidity and mortality.

Posterior fossa tumours

The majority of brain tumours in children occur in the posterior fossa, with a peak incidence between 1 and 8 years. Approximately 30 per cent are astrocytomas, 30 per cent medulloblastomas, 30 per cent brain-stem gliomas and 7 per cent ependymomas.

In some centres the sitting position is considered ideal because it provides excellent conditions for surgical access, improved cerebral venous drainage, decreased blood loss and lowering of ICP, and seems to be associated with improved postoperative recovery including preservation of cranial nerve function [33,34]. Disadvantages of this position include cardiovascular instability, pneumocephalus, spinal cord infarction [35] and an increased risk of VAE [36]. To minimise hypotension, patients are moved gradually to the full sitting position over a period of 3–4 minutes while monitoring the blood pressure and infusing intravenous fluids to compensate for venous pooling; 5 mL/kg of crystalloid is usually sufficient. Appreciable postural hypotension is rare in children unless they are clinically dehydrated. Careful positioning is crucial for both maintaining the venous pressure and minimising the risk of VAE. Head flexion may result in obstruction of the tracheal tube if the bevel abuts against the tracheal wall. Reassessment of tube position in the final position before surgery is essential. Positive end-expiratory pressure is not routine as it increases hypotension, increases the risk of paradoxical air embolus and appears to confer no benefit [37].

The sitting position needs a purpose-built chair and can be used in all ages but is harder to achieve in infants who have no secondary lumbar curve. Small children are stable cross-legged, some sit with flexed legs, and the larger children

have flexed knees with feet supported parallel with the buttocks (Fig. 38.1). Only those approaching adult size are required to have their legs semi-dependent. The legs are strapped with elastic bandages. Antishock trousers are not widely available for infants and children. Blood loss is usually minimal and blood transfusion during surgery is required in less than 10 per cent of our patients.

In a series of 407 consecutive cases from the author's centre, the incidence of VAE in sitting posterior fossa surgery was 9 per cent and this was accompanied by hypotension in 2 per cent. There were only two cases of postoperative morbidity in the VAE group, but neither had permanent injury [38]. There are several methods for detection of VAE. The oesophageal stethoscope detects only large amounts of intracardiac air and is a late warning. Precordial Doppler tends to be oversensitive and the noise interference during diathermy can be problematic [39]. Transoesophageal echocardiography is extremely sensitive and can detect paradoxical emboli [40] but it also detects insignificant emboli and requires operator training. Most hospitals in the UK monitor for VAE using capnography. Significant VAE, causing cardiovascular effects, are thought to be caused by emboli greater than 0.5 mL/kg/min. A patent foramen ovale is associated with a risk of paradoxical embolism [41]. Significant emboli are those that

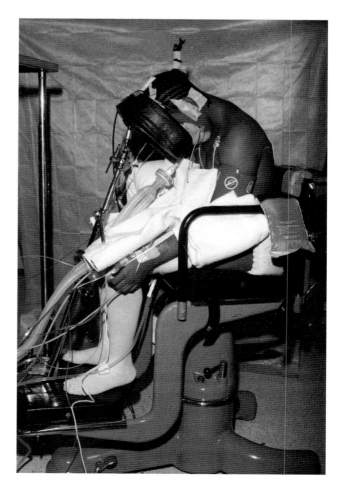

Figure 38.1 The sitting position for posterior fossa surgery.

cause a fall in blood pressure of >10 per cent or changes in heart rate and rhythm. In our experience only emboli associated with a fall in end-tidal carbon dioxide ($P_{ET}CO_2$) to 2.5 kPa or less are likely to be significant. Immediate management should be to limit air entrainment by flooding the surgical site with fluid to seal the veins, applying jugular venous compression (which can be impractical) and increasing the CVP by rapid intravenous volume infusion. The size of the embolus may be reduced by administration of 100 per cent oxygen even though nitrous oxide is not used in these cases. Head-down tilt or even cardiopulmonary resuscitation (CPR) may become necessary and anaesthetic equipment should be set up to anticipate this unlikely event. Although placement of a central venous catheter to allow aspiration of air has been advocated [42], the author has not found this useful.

Postoperative complications specific to the procedure may include posterior fossa syndrome (ataxia, nerve palsies, hemiparesis, irritability and cortical blindness) and cerebellar mutism (loss of speech and, occasionally, the ability to eat or drink). These may become apparent in recovery and complicate postoperative and future anaesthetic management. The cause of these is unclear and recovery is varied [43].

Craniopharyngioma

Craniopharyngioma, although rare, is the most common intracranial tumour of non-glial origin in children. Although histologically benign the clinical effects are progressive, and result in neurological and endocrinological damage due to expansion into the hypothalamus, optic nerves and pituitary stalk. Surgical removal followed by radiotherapy produces major endocrinological defects and therefore some cases are now receiving less aggressive treatment until symptoms warrant further intervention.

Depending on the nature of the pressure effects, these children tend to be either small because of growth failure or obese because of hypothalamic dysfunction. Difficulties in the perioperative period are related to fluid and electrolyte imbalance from diabetes insipidus. This is due to inadequate or inactive arginine vasopressin secretion [44] and later endogenous vasopressin antagonists may be involved [45]. Monitoring of CVP and urinary volumes is important as urine output may increase to up to 25 per cent of the blood volume per hour. An endocrinologist's opinion is essential. Synthetic vasopressin (1-deamino-8-D-arginine vasopressin [DDAVP], known as desmopressin), is usually required [46] and intravenous hydrocortisone is given until normal postoperative adrenal function has been confirmed. There is also an increased incidence of seizures and hyperpyrexia.

Epilepsy surgery

Epilepsy arises from a vast and diverse number of mechanisms. Its incidence has been estimated as 0.5–2 per cent of the world-wide population [47]. A resurgence of surgery for patients with intractable epilepsy has followed encouraging results [48,49]. It is not necessarily curative but may decrease the frequency of seizures and improve psychosocial function. However, it has significant neurological risk. Surgery falls into two types: resection of a specific seizure focus (e.g. temporal lobe resection) and interruption of neural transmission (e.g. corpus callosotomy). Vagus nerve stimulation by an implanted signal generator is an add-itional unusual treatment option in refractory partial-onset seizures, although the mechanism of action is unclear.

Developmental delay, behavioural problems and coexisting disease make anaesthesia challenging. Anaesthesia may be required for diagnostic imaging, electrode/grid insertion or cortical mapping before definitive surgery. Fortunately electrocorticography is not usually affected by anaesthesia; however, anaesthetic drugs may have both pro- and anticonvulsant properties at different doses. Less than 1 MAC isoflurane has minimal effect on the electroencephalogram (EEG) and facilitates mapping of the lesion. Anticonvulsants produce side-effects including sedation, alterations in drug metabolism (both induction and inhibition) and increases in idiosyncratic drug reactions; increased tolerance to neuromuscular blockade and opioid analgesia is of particular importance.

To minimise iatrogenic injury during epilepsy surgery, awake craniotomy techniques have been used in adults. Before awake surgery is contemplated, cognitive level and motivation need to be adequately assessed and patient rapport developed. Awake surgery is not practical in young children but it has been achieved in an older child [50]. Local infiltration with bupivacaine is combined with propofol sedation and remifentanil analgesia. When awake assessment is required, the propofol is discontinued and remifentanil reduced. Low-dose fentanyl has also been used in place of remifentanil. Nausea and vomiting need to be prevented.

Spinal and craniocervical surgery

CONGENITAL SPINAL ABNORMALITIES

Congenital abnormalities of the lumbar region are relatively common and include dermal sinus tracts and thickened filum terminale. They may present with few clinical features, perhaps only dermal pits or hair tuft. Magnetic resonance imaging is used to delineate the lesion. Surgery un-tethers the cord and de-bulks any subcutaneous lesions. These abnormalities are usually avascular and blood transfusion is rare. Spinal monitoring may be used and an anaesthetic technique that does not interfere with neurophysiological studies should be employed, such as low dose (about 1 MAC) isoflurane. The patients are positioned prone with all the potential problems that this may present.

SPINAL TUMOURS

Extramedullary spinal tumours in children tend to arise from abnormal embryogenesis or as metastases rather than the meningiomas or sheath tumours that are more common in adults. Intramedullary tumours are a greater surgical challenge and are likely to be astrocytomas or ependymomas. Spinal tumours are often extremely vascular and, despite optimal positioning and induced hypotension, they cause major haemorrhage. All surgical manipulations of the spinal cord are stimulating and may be associated with arrhythmias and hypotension.

INSTABILITY OF THE CRANIOCERVICAL SPINE

This may be acquired or congenital. Cases with congenital diseases (e.g. Down syndrome, Morquio's disease and pseudo-achondroplasia) often have atlantoaxial subluxation [51,52] and may only present after minor trauma or even surgical positioning for neck surgery [53]. Atlanto-axial subluxation can be posterior but is much more commonly anterior. Subluxation creates a kyphosis over the C2 vertebra so that the spinal cord, tethered by the dentate ligament, is compressed primarily by the dens. Flexion is more hazardous than extension and sudden flexion may cause cord contusion (Fig. 38.2). Traumatic cord compression may cause quadriplegia or sudden death.

Instability of the craniocervical spine presents significant anaesthetic problems. Children with traumatic injury are managed initially with traction. The trachea must be intubated with the neck fixed or held in line by an assistant, who prevents flexion or extension. In cooperative older children securing the airway can be achieved awake or with sedation via fibre-optic intubation (FOI) but in most children, however, asleep FOI is the only method possible. Cricoid pressure is contraindicated [54]. Nevertheless, hypoxia is potentially damaging to a compressed spinal cord and, provided that the head and neck is held still, conventional laryngoscopy may be more practical especially in an emergency. The Bullard laryngoscope can be used to achieve tracheal intubation without moving the head and neck.

Depending on the lesion, the surgical approach will either be posterolateral or transoral. After the latter approach, the child remains intubated for 24–48 hours until all oral swelling has settled.

A halo jacket is fitted and, if laryngoscopy is needed afterwards, it must be appreciated that conventional laryngoscopy can be extremely difficult because the head is fixed and the scope handle impinges on either the lateral rods or the top of the jacket (a polio handle is useful). Fibre-optic intubation should always be available, although many procedures can be performed safely with a laryngeal mask airway (LMA) which may provide both an airway and a pathway for intubation [55].

Imaging and interventional techniques

Sedation is often used for both diagnostic and interventional imaging (see Chapter 44). Anaesthesia may be required or preferred when there are contraindications to sedation, if it has failed previously or if it is inappropriate for the procedure. A simple technique of light anaesthesia using an LMA is usually suitable for most patients.

Embolisation

Intracranial vascular lesions are now routinely treated by embolisation. Arteriovenous malformations (AVMs) in infants present with bruits, cyanosis, murmurs, macrocephaly (from hydrocephalus), seizures due to cerebral ischaemia or cardiac failure. Older children usually present with neurological deficit from the effect of vascular steal. The majority of abnormalities occur in the vein of Galen, or in a midline AV fistula. In those with severe cardiac failure the incidence of pulmonary hypertension is high and nitric oxide may be required for their management [56]. Neonates with these problems have a high mortality (approximately 50 per cent) and morbidity [57,58]. The procedure itself can be hazardous and intracerebral bleeding or migration of embolus material into the lungs can be

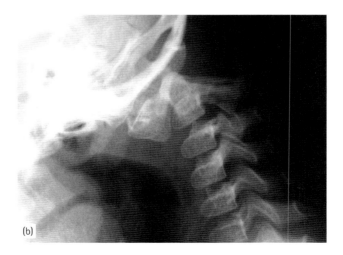

Figure 38.2 Appearance of the unstable C-spine in (a) flexion and (b) extension.

devastating. Iatrogenic cardiac complications and haemorrhage are common Successful embolisation may cause cardiovascular instability and jeopardise cerebral blood flow. Postoperative intensive care is necessary.

Stereotactic surgery

This technique facilitates access to small deep-seated lesions with decreased neurological morbidity. In the past the application of the head frame in small children, which required general anaesthesia, involved moving the anaesthetised patient between CT scanner and operating theatre. These devices have now been superseded by frameless stereotaxy, for which general anaesthesia is still required, but transport from scanner to theatre is not. External markers on the patient's scalp act as reference points for images taken by a pair of cameras above the operating field. These enable accurate positioning of the tip of the surgical tool to a three-dimensional computer-generated image.

Stereotactic procedures can be time-consuming and, usually, there is minimal surgical stimulation.

Neuroendoscopic techniques

Neuroendoscopy is a minimally invasive technique is now being used for treatment of a variety of disorders including hydrocephalus, cyst puncture and periventricular tumour biopsy. This technique is becoming more widely applied as indications and applications expand.

Once the burr hole has been made there is little stimulation The anaesthetic technique is usually dictated by the patient demographics and clinical state rather than the specific procedure. Previously, only the surgeon could view proceedings down the scope, which made effective communication essential [59]. Now, modern video facilities show the progress to the whole operating team. In selected or prolonged cases, invasive monitoring may be indicated [60].

THIRD VENTRICULOSTOMY

This is an alternative to the ventriculoperitoneal (VP) shunt and involves fenestration of the floor of the third ventricle, so that it communicates with the basal cisterns, allowing reabsorption of CSF. It is relatively contraindicated in those with abnormal ventricular anatomy, ventricular haemorrhage or a history of meningitis. However, it eliminates the risk of shunt-related complications and therefore decreases the necessity for repeated VP shunt operations. Complications include haemorrhage, particularly injury to the basilar or perforating arteries (these can be fatal) [61], and transient or permanent consequences of midbrain manipulation (variable cardiovascular instability, bradycardias and asystole). Increases in ICP due to pre-existing disease, irrigation fluid or haemorrhage are also possible. Hypertension and tachycardia may alert to the development of

significantly raised ICP rather than the classic Cushing's reflex of hypertension and bradycardia [62]. Postoperatively, altered mental state, cranial nerve palsies, vomiting and pulmonary aspiration, inappropriate antidiuretic hormone secretion and ventriculitis may all complicate recovery. Hyperkalaemia has been described and may be prevented by using 0.9 per cent saline for intravenous replacement [63].

ENDOSCOPIC TRANSPHENOIDAL SURGERY

This technique can be used to remove a variety of lesions, including pituitary tumours and craniopharyngiomas. Access to the pituitary gland is achieved without brain retraction and morbidity and mortality are reduced [61]. Central venous access is useful for repeated blood tests to monitor endocrine function postoperatively. Nasal instrumentation can cause haemorrhage, which can be prevented by nasal vasoconstrictors but these may cause cardiovascular instability themselves. Emergence and recovery from anaesthesia may be complicated by pharyngeal and gastric blood, and nasal packs. Acute intracranial haematoma may present with sudden blindness, ophthalmoplegia, hypotension and decreased conscious level.

Revascularisation surgery/extracranial–to–intracranial bypass

Children requiring this procedure often have a progressive chronic occlusive cerebrovascular disease called Moyamoya disease. It usually presents with symptoms from stenosis of the arteries of the circle of Willis and the internal carotid arteries. The name Moyamoya is Japanese for 'puff of smoke' and refers to the radiographic appearance of the thin collaterals that develop at the base of the brain. These children may have had transient ischaemic attacks or strokes.

Medical treatment consists of antiplatelet therapy with aspirin in most cases. The anaesthetist's aim is to avoid possible ischaemia and its sequelae. Perioperative management is directed towards balancing cerebral oxygen supply and demand. Preoperative fluids may be advisable to maintain hydration and blood pressure before surgery. Crying and stress need to be minimised and premedication is advised to minimise distress on induction (mild hypercapnia may be beneficial). Normocapnia should be maintained intraoperatively as hyperventilation may reduce CBF and precipitate an ischaemic event and carbon dioxide retention may cause 'steal' from compromised vessels by areas of healthy vasculature. The risk of steal has also led some to advocate the use of TIVA and the avoidance of volatile anaesthesia, although we have experienced no adverse events with isoflurane. Normocapnia is also important after surgery. If analgesia is inadequate, crying can cause hyperventilation. Crying and dehydration appear to be responsible for many of the perioperative complications in this group. Normothermia and normotension are also essential during recovery [64].

ANAESTHESIA FOR CRANIOFACIAL SURGERY

General aspects

The centralisation of expertise into craniofacial units, has facilitated increasingly complex surgical procedures for the repair of craniofacial abnormalities. The development of multidisciplinary teams has been central to the improved management of these patients. In addition, there have been significant advances in imaging, which have allowed detailed surgical planning [65] and assessment of outcome. The care of these, often complex children, requires optimisation of the patient and provision for postoperative care.

Despite its elective nature, the surgical correction of craniofacial abnormality carries a risk of significant perioperative complications, particularly blood loss. Indications for surgery may be functional or cosmetic. Functional indications include raised ICP, compromised respiratory function with central and airway components, feeding difficulties and proptosis causing visual deterioration. Cosmetic correction is important and is usually carried out before school age as craniofacial deformity has wide-ranging effects on a child's behaviour and psychological development. Improved self-image has been demonstrated to decrease behavioural problems for these patients [66]. Surgery is a major undertaking and, in patients with complex problems, may result in morbidity or even mortality [67]. For each individual the risk:benefit ratio needs to be assessed and explained. In a study of 126 children undergoing craniofacial surgery 20 per cent required transfusion in excess of their circulating volume, 3 per cent received CPR or adrenaline (for hypotension) and 29 per cent required postoperative ventilation [68]. Massive haemorrhage and death can occur during craniosynostosis repair [69].

Preoperative assessment

Speech difficulties, optic atrophy, conductive hearing loss and delayed intellectual development can make preoperative communication and assessment difficult. Airway abnormalities are common and are discussed in more detail below. Cervical vertebral abnormalities may restrict neck movement. Venous access may be difficult because of syndactyly and other limb abnormalities (Fig. 38.3). Patient positioning can be restricted by joint contractures. There may be a risk of skeletal fractures (Antley–Bixler syndrome). Protecting proptotic eyes is important, particularly in the prone position. Other abnormalities requiring modification of perioperative care and anaesthesia include raised ICP, renal or urogenital abnormalities (e.g. polycystic kidneys and hydronephrosis), and cardiac anomalies.

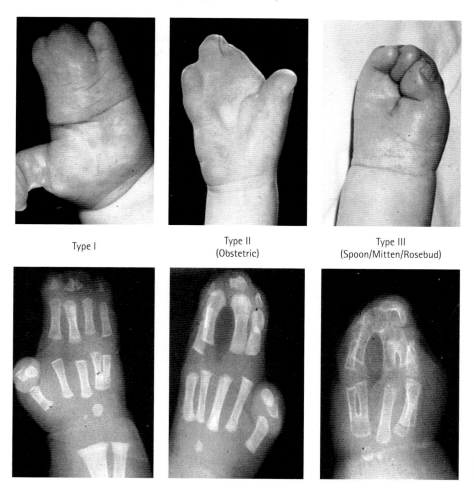

Type I

Type II
(Obstetric)

Type III
(Spoon/Mitten/Rosebud)

Figure 38.3 Limb abnormalities in Apert syndrome.

Airway assessment in craniofacial patients

Craniofacial abnormalities are frequently associated with airway problems. About 20–37 per cent of patients undergoing major craniofacial surgery and 50 per cent of patients with craniofacial synostosis present with some airway compromise [70]. Nasal airway obstruction is common owing to to choanal stenosis or atresia and nasal intubation may be impossible. Maxillary hypoplasia is common in the craniofacial syndromes (Table 38.2) and results in reduced postnasal spaces. There may be shortening of the oropharyngeal and nasopharyngeal airway [71,72], hypoplasia of the mandible [73] and consequent airway obstruction at the pharynx by the tongue. These anatomical abnormalities may be compounded by neurological dysfunction resulting in pharyngeal hypotonia and poor coordination [74]. Fortunately, however, provided that the mouth opening is

Table 38.2 Craniofacial syndromes

Syndrome	Features
Apert	Usually sporadic/autosomal dominant
	Irregular premature fusion of multiple sutures
	Midface hypoplasia/hypertelorism
	Syndactyly
	Possible choanal tracheal stenosis
	Progressive calcification of hands, feet, C-spine
	10% incidence of cardiac defects/genitourinary anomalies
Crouzon	Autosomal dominant
	Premature fusion of multiple sutures, often with brachycephaly (reduced anteroposterior length)
	Maxillary hypoplasia
	Orbital proptosis
	Hypertelorism
Pfeiffer	Usually sporadic/autosomal dominant
	Premature fusion of multiple sutures, patterns seen include brachycephaly (reduced anteroposterior length), turricephaly (cone-shaped head) or *kleebattschaedal* (cloverleaf skull)
	Syndactyly, short broad thumbs and toes
	Multiple abnormalities have been reported including tracheal, cardiovascular and intestinal anomalies
Saethre–Chotzen	Autosomal dominant
	Asymmetrical craniosynostosis including brachycephaly (reduced anteroposterior length) and plagiocephaly
	Deviation of nasal septum and 'beaking' of the nose
	Ptosis/strabismus
	Maxillary hypoplasia
	Syndactyly
	Possible progressive cervical spinal fusion

not restricted, a skilled and experienced anaesthetist is unlikely to find conventional laryngoscopy difficult.

Indications for tracheostomy

A minority of individuals may require a tracheostomy preoperatively. Preoperative tracheostomy is indicated for upper airway obstruction that is deteriorating with age [75,76], and for severe obstructive sleep apnoea in children who are too young for definitive surgery. This improves general health and growth prior to the definitive procedure and may avoid the long-term sequelae of chronic airway obstruction. Elective tracheostomy is needed occasionally if extensive facial osteotomies make reintubation impossible during or after surgery. Tracheostomy itself risks airway complications and death and increases the risk of meningeal infection after cranial reconstruction [77].

Obstructive sleep apnoea

Patients with obstructive sleep apnoea (OSA) may be tired during the day and schoolwork and behaviour may be affected. Severe prolonged OSA can cause right-heart failure and pulmonary hypertension. Sleep studies, using overnight pulse oximetry, may demonstrate profound oxygen desaturation. Airway obstruction during sleep may be produced by abnormal tongue movement against the posterior pharyngeal wall, medial movement of the lateral pharyngeal walls, and pharyngeal constriction [78]. A central component may also be caused by raised ICP, due to herniation of the hindbrain through the foramen magnum. Airway optimisation in children with OSA may involve nasal stenting, nasal continuous positive airway pressure (CPAP), choanal dilatation or adenoidectomy. When these measures fail, tracheostomy is necessary in severe cases [79].

Preoperative investigations

Numerous investigations are required (Table 38.2) and preadmission clinics are helpful and facilitate the multidisciplinary approach. Investigation relevant to anaesthesia include sleep studies, ICP measurement, otorhinolaryngology review, baseline haematological and biochemical parameters, and cardiology review (if indicated). Blood should be crossmatched.

Complex deformities may benefit from cerebral venous imaging to identify anomalous venous drainage [80]. In a small number of cases intracranial venous drainage is dependent on extracranial collaterals and disruption of these during surgery can be fatal [81].

Premedication

Common indications for premedication are to aid pain-free cannulation (an anxiolytic) and to prevent airway secretions (antimuscarinic). Local anaesthetic creams are usually applied to potential cannulation sites preoperatively; however, limb abnormalities and recurrent cannulation can make intravenous induction difficult (see Fig. 38.3). In anxious patients psychological preparation in addition to sedation may make the experience less distressing. Sedative premedication should be used with caution in patients with appreciable airway problems or raised ICP.

Induction and tracheal intubation

Inhalational induction is probably more common than intravenous induction (only 9.5 per cent of patients received intravenous inductions in one series) [68]. This may be due to patient choice, difficulties with venous access due to limb abnormalities and where multiple cannulations have been required in the past. Inhalational induction may also be preferable where a difficult airway is anticipated. A cautious gaseous induction is unlikely to result in apnoea and maintenance of spontaneous ventilation allows confirmation that controlled ventilation is possible before a muscle relaxant is administered. Intravenous induction may be preferred in the older child if the ability to maintain the airway is not in doubt.

In children with craniofacial syndromes, initial problems with induction include ill-fitting facemasks owing to facial abnormality (Fig. 38.4) and exophthalmos. Soft-seal facemasks with highly deformable rims are preferred although leaks around the facemask may still persist, necessitating high gas flows to attain adequate mask ventilation.

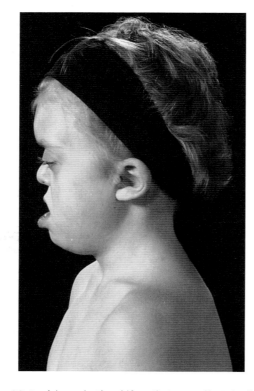

Figure 38.4   A hypoplastic midface that may affect the fit of facemasks.

A common problem in children with midface hypoplasia is upper airway obstruction during light levels of anaesthesia. The obstruction is usually caused by the tongue, as in normal patients, falling into the pharynx. First, it is crucial to open the lips, but an oropharyngeal airway cannot be inserted until anaesthesia is deep enough. Until this can be achieved, distending pressure via a close-fitting facemask together with a jaw thrust manoeuvre is usually effective. An oropharyngeal airway will clear the obstruction.

Alternatively, provided that there is confidence that positive pressure ventilation can be achieved with a facemask, muscle relaxants overcome this problem. Difficulty at laryngoscopy is not usual in children who have midfacial hypoplasia but it may be encountered in those with cervical abnormalities limiting neck movement or restricted mouth opening (e.g. trismus or temporomandibular joint synostosis). The combination of macroglossia with maxillary hypoplasia can cause pharyngeal crowding and may hinder the insertion of the laryngoscope blade. Mandibular hypoplasia (e.g. Treacher Collins or Goldenhaar syndromes) causes much more difficulty (see Chapter 21). Unfortunately, the physical appearance of individuals is not an accurate guide to difficulty with laryngoscopy (Fig. 38.5). Those with maxillary hypoplasia may look abnormal but usually present no problem whereas, conversely, children who have undergone corrective surgery may look more normal but laryngoscopy may be particularly difficult owing to maxillary advancement and restricted mouth opening from temporomandibular joint limitation. Previously uneventful anaesthesia may also be falsely reassuring, particularly for removal of maxillary distraction devices [82].

Difficult laryngoscopy is associated with risks. There may be hypoxia, aspiration, airway oedema and hypertensive responses raising ICP. Where difficulty with tracheal intubation is anticipated provision should include additional airway adjuncts and laryngoscopes (including the Bullard laryngoscope) [83]. Fibre-optic intubation is advocated by some [82,84], but awake FOI is distressing for the child and not usually necessary. An alternative, which is feasible in most craniofacial abnormalities, is introduction of the fibre-optic bronchoscope via an LMA (see Chapter 21).

For intraoral procedures and where intermaxillary fixation (IMF) is to occur the nasal route is preferred although, in most cases, IMF can be achieved with an oral tube posterior to the molar teeth. In major midfacial surgery, reinforced orotracheal tubes resist crushing or kinking during the procedure and can be optimally secured by a circummandibular wire. For cranial vault surgery a preformed south-facing orotracheal tube is a satisfactory option for procedures in the supine position Armoured tubes, with complete facial strapping and protection, are used if the child is to be placed prone. Since the neck is usually fully extended, the optimum tracheal tube position is ensured by initial endobronchial intubation and then withdrawing the tube until breath sounds are heard bilaterally. In children over 6 years old, a cuffed tube is normally preferred.

In conjunction with a throat pack, a cuff helps prevent blood and debris entering the respiratory tract and intra-operative displacement by providing additional tube stability. Potential complications involving the tracheal tube

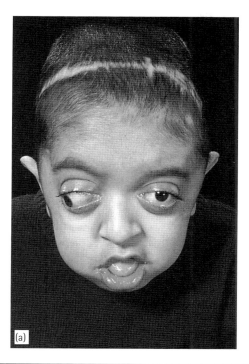

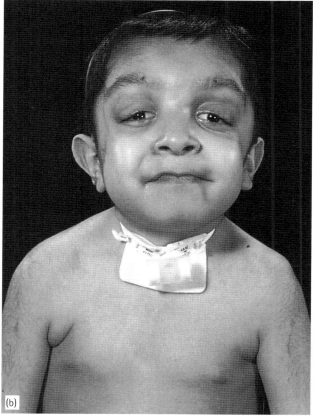

Figure 38.5 Contrary to appearances (a) preoperatively an easy laryngoscopy and (b) postoperatively a difficult laryngoscopy

in craniofacial surgery can occur because the surgical field and airway are shared. Accidental surgical displacement or puncture of the tube or its pilot balloon are common. In the event of tube displacement occurring while facial bones are mobile and access is limited, a laryngeal mask may be lifesaving because it permits continued oxygenation and anaesthesia until reintubation.

Two large-bore venous lines are essential, as massive transfusion is likely. One is a large-bore peripheral line, usually in the long saphenous vein, and the second line may be inserted via the femoral vein, thereby allowing for CVP monitoring. Antibiotic prophylaxis is given on induction and should include cover for anaerobes.

Intraoperative anaesthesia

Anaesthesia is maintained using a balanced technique involving fentanyl (up to 10 μg/kg) and isoflurane, carried in air–oxygen mixture. Alternatives are remifentanil infusion, in place of the fentanyl or TIVA.

Monitoring and patient positioning

Monitoring of oxygen saturation, end-tidal carbon dioxide, ECG, invasive blood pressure, central and core temperatures, and peripheral nerve function is standard for all patients. Monitoring of CVP is useful but not essential. It has been suggested that there may be inaccuracies in monitoring blood loss using invasive monitoring. Suggested alternatives include transoesophageal echocardiography (but availability and experience are limited and its use may be restricted by the surgical access) [85], non-invasive monitoring of aortic blood flow [86] and pulse contour analysis. Patient temperature is controlled by forced air-warming blanket and fluid-warming devices (these are essential).

To protect the airway during surgery extra care must be taken with positioning the patient and the tracheal tube connections. Bony abnormalities, contractures and synostoses need to be padded and may make positioning difficult, especially in the modified prone position. Pressure points are protected and the abdomen must be completely free to allow abdominal movement with ventilation to prevent venous congestion. The chest is auscultated to confirm tracheal tube position and to minimise the risk of bronchial intubation during surgical manipulation of the neck. Cerebral venous congestion is reduced by the 'head-up' position. This may increase the risk of VAE, especially in those who are hypotensive and undergoing extensive vault and sagittal procedures [92]; fortunately, VAE is a rare event (approximately 0.8 per cent of cases) [68]. Acute bradycardia due to the oculocardiac reflex is also recognised in this patient group; sudden falls in heart rate of >30 beats/minute can occur with manipulation around the orbits. It occurs in 10–15 per cent but in the majority of patients it usually responds to cessation of the stimulus or vagolysis with atropine or glycopyrrolate; occasionally adrenaline is required.

Management of blood loss

Strategies to minimise transfusion requirements should be used [87] and are discussed in detail in Chapter 24. Blood loss and major transfusion remain the greatest risk to these infants. A transfusion of more than one circulating volume is frequently required. Over a 5-year period, in one centre, packed red cell transfusion was required in 96 per cent of patients undergoing craniosynostosis repair. About 20–50 per cent of circulating volume can be lost over a 30-minute period in some instances [69]. Common complications of transfusion include coagulopathy, hypocalcaemia, acidosis and hyperkalaemia. Potassium levels were elevated in 10 out of 11 children undergoing craniofacial surgery in one study [88] and, where there is coexisting metabolic acidosis and hypocalcaemia, cardiac arrest has occurred [89]. Other complications of massive transfusion include haemoglobinuria lasting for 24 hours and skin rashes [68]. All of these complications are minimised by careful matching of transfusion volumes to losses, maintaining organ perfusion and avoiding hypovolaemia.

Assessment of blood loss in craniofacial surgery is especially difficult because of the volumes of irrigation fluid used for the surgical power tools and the blood loss onto the surgical drapes. Suction canister volumes and swab weights are grossly inaccurate in this setting, and therefore transfusion has to be based on clinical parameters, which include capillary refill, invasive monitoring parameters (arterial and CVP waveforms) and regular bedside blood gas measurements (base excess, lactate and haemoglobin concentration). Additional information may be obtained from analysis of arterial waveforms, peripheral pulse waves, urinary output [91] and preoperative and postoperative haematocrit measurements [92]. While anaesthetists tend to underestimate blood loss [92] the risks of overtransfusion still remain, and patient age appears to be a strong predictor of this. In a recent series of 20 cases all three patients with excessive haematocrits were less than 14 months old [93]. Younger patients are also more at risk of large volume blood loss [69,93]. One study suggested that the factor most likely to determine the magnitude of any intraoperative transfusion is the anaesthetist [94].

Blood loss may be replaced with various intravenous solutions, each of which are discussed in detail elsewhere. The author uses colloidal gelatin but other centres prefer isotonic salt solutions. Red cells are transfused according to bedside haemoglobin measurement. A concentration of >7 g/dL at the end of surgery is satisfactory if the child is otherwise stable.

Dextrose-containing solutions are not used unless there is hypoglycaemia, as they can lead to hyponatraemia; hyperglycaemia may compound cerebral damage after spells of ischaemia.

Avoidance of transfusion

Preoperative measures to avoid blood transfusion include erythropoietin stimulation and autologous blood donation. Erythropoietin has formed part of protocols in some centres for older Jehovah's Witness children in whom transfusion is unacceptable [95] and reduces the transfusion requirements [96]. Autologous blood donation may be used but the small circulating volume of children and the distress of venesection limits its applicability. During surgery, the need for transfusion is reduced by induced hypotension, scalp infiltration, aprotinin [97], acute normovolaemic haemodilution and intraoperative blood salvage techniques [98] in addition to surgical attention to haemostasis.

Hypotension to limit blood loss is used only in the absence of any contraindications (coexisting raised ICP is an absolute contraindication) because it presents significant risks. Opinion as to its effectiveness varies. In the infant, 'head-up' tilt alone usually provides a satisfactory surgical field. In the older child undergoing major midfacial procedures, moderate hypotension, using a remifentanil infusion, possibly combined with clonidine, may be helpful. Scalp infiltration using a combination of bupivacaine, lidocaine, hyalase and adrenaline [99] can reduce bleeding but its efficacy is limited if the majority of surgical blood loss is from the bone and periosteum.

Acute normovolaemic haemodilution, although successful in some settings [100], has not been demonstrated to reduce blood transfusion in patients undergoing craniosynostosis correction [101]. Intraoperative blood salvage techniques have previously been limited by unfamiliarity with the technique and concerns regarding reinfusing thromboplastic material from brain tissue [102]. Interest in this has recently returned, and this technique may reduce donor exposure, but blood salvage alone is unable to cope with the rapid and massive volume replacement requirements of infants undergoing craniofacial surgery [69,103].

Management of coagulopathy

Massive transfusion is associated with coagulopathy. Varied regimens exist for the administration of clotting factors. Some suggest that blood loss in excess of 40 mL/kg leads to disordered haemostasis and that coagulation profiles should be checked at this point and fresh frozen plasma given according to results [104]. Others suggest that loss of as little as 30 per cent of estimated blood volume should result in the administration of fresh frozen plasma [105] or that empirical transfusion of fresh frozen plasma should follow the loss of a whole blood volume [92]. An audit of the author's practice demonstrated that, provided that tissue perfusion is maintained, coagulopathy is not significant until at least one circulating volume has been lost. Other workers have had similar results [94]. Coagulation profiles are measured after transfusion of one circulating volume and the results guide the administration of clotting factors if there is microvascular bleeding.

POSTOPERATIVE CARE

Indications for intensive care

Improvements in both anaesthetic and surgical techniques have reduced admission rates to intensive care units (ICUs) for many of these procedures [68]. In recent years, the percentage of craniofacial patients being admitted to intensive care postoperatively has been less than 10 per cent. Mechanical ventilation, when required, is usually only for a short period of time [106]. Indications for postoperative ventilation included body temperature <35°C, major intraoperative complications or excessive length of surgery [68], as well as age. Improving expertise and confidence have meant that, despite the increasingly complex procedures being undertaken, the majority of children can be extubated at the end of the procedure and postoperative care can be in a neurosurgical high-dependency unit (HDU), with the continued use of invasive monitoring.

At the end of the procedure tissue swelling may be considerable. Continuing oedema and/or haematoma formation in the initial 48 hours may be reduced by nursing these patients 'head up'. When extensive facial surgery has been performed, it may be necessary temporarily to close the palpebral fissures with 'frost sutures' and to protect the cornea. Bilateral nasopharyngeal airways may be used if there is appreciable facial swelling as these will protect against airway obstruction and avoid the necessity for tracheal intubation. These may remain *in situ* until the oedema has resolved (for up to 7 days in the case of facial bipartition surgery).

Postoperative fluid management

There are continuing losses from surgical drains, haematoma and CSF which need to be carefully monitored postoperatively. Although rare, the risk of developing diabetes insipidus should also be considered [107]. Large fluid losses continue well into the postoperative period. A haemoglobin concentration >7 g/dL is adequate. Problems associated with large volume replacement (e.g. symptomatic hyponatraemia) have been reported [104]. Our protocol (see addendum) has proved effective in minimising postoperative fluid management problems and a recent audit revealed no clinically shocked patients in recovery or on arrival in HDU or ICU.

Clotting screens are repeated postoperatively and coagulopathy corrected if there is abnormal bleeding. At least one clotting index in postoperative blood specimens is outside the normal range [93], with prothrombin time being the most frequently affected.

Pain management

Before emergence from anaesthesia, paracetamol and diclofenac are administered, although diclofenac may be omitted initially if there is excessive bleeding. These drugs, together with oral morphine, provide satisfactory analgesia in most patients as the procedure results in surprisingly little pain. If remifentanil has been used intraoperatively, a bolus of intravenous morphine is given at the end of the procedure. Where older children have undergone major procedures patient-controlled analgesia with morphine may be considered but often nausea limits its use. Iliac crest bone grafts are occasionally required and are painful, a continuous local anaesthetic infusion delivered to the graft site via a fine-bore catheter has proven effective.

SPECIFIC CRANIOFACIAL PROCEDURES

Craniosynostosis repair

The majority of patients requiring craniosynostosis surgery fall into two broad groups: normal children with a single suture craniosynostosis (these simple cases usually have surgery performed in the first 2 years of life) or syndromic individuals with facial abnormalities and multiple suture synostoses (Table 38.3). Over 100 syndromes associated with craniosynostosis have been described; however, many are extremely rare [108]. Crouzon syndrome is the commonest of these but any of these syndromes can present a number of abnormalities, which may challenge the anaesthetist.

Complex cases may require extensive preoperative investigation and evaluation as anomalies are varied. Raised ICP is more common with multiple suture involvement (also in scaphocephaly presenting later than 1 year). Blood losses may be large and oculocardiac reflexes may be triggered with orbital dissection. Sagittal synostosis is usually treated by wide suture excision in the prone position, resulting in blood loss but rarely major complications. Coronal fusion, either single or bilateral, and metopic synostosis (trigonocephaly) are corrected with a 'floating forehead' procedure [109].

Endoscopic strip craniectomy has been developed. Here the bone containing the fused suture is removed endoscopically and claimed advantages are reduced operative times, postoperative ventilatory requirements and blood loss.

Midface advancement and distraction surgery

Traditionally, midface advancement has been achieved by making osteotomies at the points at which the maxilla, zygoma and naso-orbital bones naturally fracture. Thus the Le Fort I corrects hypoplasia of the maxilla by advancing the maxilla inferiorly and buttressing it with bone

Table 38.3   Classification of craniosynostosis

1.	Sagittal craniosynostosis *Scaphocephaly/boat skull*	Elongated and narrow head with increased anteroposterior length Most common form Often seen in preterm infants due to positional moulding
2.	Metopic synostosis *Trigonocephaly/triangle skull*	Broad triangular forehead, hypotelorism and prominent occiput
3.	Unicoronal synostosis *Plagiocephaly/oblique skull*	Unilateral forehead flattening with contralateral bossing
4.	Lamboidal synostosis *Posterior plagiocephaly/ oblique skull*	Unilateral occipital flattening with contralateral bossing Has been confused with positional moulding in infants preferentially sleeping with their heads to one side as appearance is the same
5.	Bicoronal synostosis *Brachycephaly/short skull*	Spherical head shape with recessed forehead and bossing above
6.	Multiple suture synostosis Resulting head shapes include: *Oxycephaly/sharp skull Kleeblattschadel/clover-leaf skull Acrocephaly/tower skull*	May be syndromic or non-syndromic

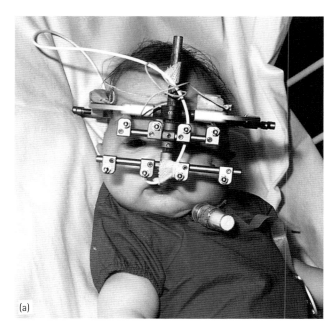

(a)

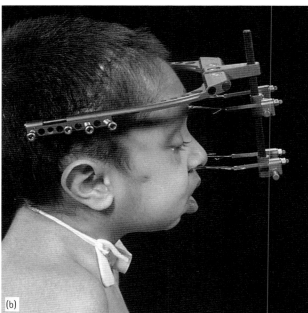

(b)

Figure 38.6 (a,b)   Rigid extraction device frame *in situ*.

grafts, Le Fort II advances the maxilla and nose and Le Fort III corrects midface hypoplasia, allowing advancement of the nose, maxilla and orbits. Distraction osteogenesis, where osteotomy is used to induce bone callus and the two ends of the bone are then distracted, had previously been primarily used for mandibular lengthening. However, this technique has now been successfully applied to other areas in craniofacial surgery including midface advancement. Here application of a rigid extraction device (RED) frame has proved highly successful and is surprisingly well tolerated in even the very young (Fig. 38.6).

The RED frame presents the anaesthetist with some dilemmas, not only at the original surgery but also for procedures in the following months. Certainly, patients will require varying degrees of airway management at induction of anaesthesia but also extubation at the end of the procedure will require forethought and provision for failure (Fig. 38.6). The position of the RED frame's wires makes application of a facemask for ventilation impossible. Moreover, the laryngoscopic view may be inadequate and placement of a tracheal tube may be difficult because of the position of the bars of the halo frame. Fortunately, a laryngeal mask is a useful rescue airway and should be available. Preoperative tracheostomy is advisable in some patients. In an emergency, the device can be removed quickly by cutting the wires and removing the central rod after loosening the Allen screw – equipment for this should stay with the patient throughout their hospital stay.

Facial bipartition surgery

Facial bipartition surgery, although performed rarely, is among the most radical craniofacial surgery undertaken.

It is used to treat conditions such as facial cleft, frontonasal dysplasia and facial dysostosis. The surgical technique of facial bipartition involves the vertical splitting of the facial skeleton into two segments and the use of autogenous bone grafts from the iliac crest to buttress them into the new position. It allows the correction of multiple aspects of craniofacial dysostosis with a single procedure.

Potential airway problems and difficulty with intubation should be anticipated although a survey of our practice found no difficulty in placing an orotracheal tube [93]. This may reflect the fact that all the patients in this series were undergoing primary surgery and it is at subsequent anaesthetic episodes that the problem becomes more apparent [82].

Intraoperative complications encountered include major haemorrhage, bradycardia and airway problems (unintentional extubation). While all patients required transfusion we found that the age of the patient was a strong predictor of over-transfusion of red cells, with patients under 14 months old being most at risk. There is a potential requirement for postoperative ventilatory support, with the risk again significantly greater in younger patients.

ACKNOWLEDGEMENT

We thank Dr Angela Mackersie for her support and invaluable comments.

REFERENCES

Key references

Baykan N, Isbir O, Gercek A et al. Ten years of experience with pediatric neuroendoscopic third ventriculostomy. *J Neurosurg Anesthesiol* 2005; **17**(1): 33–37.

Bissonnette B Leon JE. Cerebrovascular stability during isoflurane anaesthesia in children. *Can J Anaesth* 1992; **39**: 128–34.

Harrison EA, Mackersie A, McEwan A, et al. The sitting position for neurosurgery in children: a review of 16 years experience. *Br J Anaesth* 2002; **88**(1): 12–17.

Kofke WA, Tempelhoff R, Dasheiff RM. Anaesthetic implications of epilepsy, status epilepticus and epilepsy surgery. *J Neurosurg Anesthesiol* 1997; **9**(4): 349–72.

Moylan S, Collee G, Mackersie A, Bingham R. Anaesthetic management in paediatric craniofacial surgery. A review of 126 cases. *Paediatr Anaesth* 1993; **3**: 275–81.

References

1. Sokoloff L. Circulation and energy metabolism of the brain. In: Siegel G et al., eds. *Basic neurochemistry: molecular cellular and chemical aspects*. New York: Raven Press, 1989: 565–91

2. Kennedy C, Sokoloff L. An adaptation of nitrous oxide method to the study of the circulation in children: Normal values for cerebral blood flow and cerebral metabolic rate in childhood. *J Clin Invest* 1957; **36**: 1130–6.

3. Ogawa A, Sakurai Y, Kayama Y. Regional cerebral blood flow with age: Changes in rCBF in childhood. *Neurol Res* 1989; **11**: 173–7.

4. Lou HC, Lassen NA, Friis-Hansen B. Impaired autoregulation of cerebral blood flow in the distressed newborn infant. *J Pediatr* 1979; **94**: 118–21.

5. Wyatt JS, Cope M, Delpy DT et al. Quantification of cerebral oxygenation and haemodynamics in sick newborn infants by near infrared spectrophotometry. *Lancet* 1986; **ii**: 1063–6.

6. Gregory G, Ong B, Tweed W et al. Hyperventilation restores autoregulation in the cerebral circulation in the neonate. *Anesthesiology* 1983; **59**: 427A.

7. Welch K. The intracranial pressure in infants. *J Neurosurg* 1980; **52**: 693–9.

8. Shapiro K, Marmarou A. Mechanism of intracranial hypertension in children. In: McLauren R et al., eds. *Pediatric neurosurgery*. Philadelphia: WB Saunders, 1989; 338–52

9. Smerling A. Hypertonic saline in head trauma. A new recipe for drying and salting. *J Neurosurg Anesthesiol* 1992; **4**: 1–3.

10. Fisher B, Thomas D, Peterson B et al. Hypertonic saline lowers raised ICP in children after head trauma. *J Neurosurg Anesthesiol* 1992; **4**: 4–10.

11. Qureshi AI, Suarez JI, Bhardwaj A. Malignant cerebral edema in patients with hypertensive intracerebral hemorrhage associated with hypertonic saline infusion. *J Neurosurg Anesthesiol* 1998; **10**: 188–92.

12. Leon JE, Bissonnette B. Transcranial Doppler sonography: nitrous oxide and cerebral blood flow velocity in children. *Can J Anaesth* 1991; **38**: 974–9.

13. Bissonnette B, Leon JE. Cerebrovascular stability during isoflurane anaesthesia in children. *Can J Anaesth* 1992; **39**: 128–34.

14. Scheller MS, Tateishi A, Drummond JC et al. The effect of sevoflurane on cerebral blood flow, cerebral metabolic rate for oxygen, intracranial pressure, and the electroencephalogram are similar to those of isoflurane in the rabbit. *Anesthesiology* 1988; **68**: 548–51.

15. Fairgrieve R, Rowney DA, Karsli C, Bissonnette B. The effects of sevoflurane of cerebral blood flow velocity in children. *Acta Anaesthesiol Scand* 2003; **47**: 1226–30.

16. Luginbuehl IA, Fredrickson MJ, Karsli C, Bissonnette B. Cerebral blood flow velocity in children anaesthetized with desflurane. *Paediatr Anaesth* 2003; **13**: 496–500.

17. Hatch DJ. Propofol in paediatric intensive care. *Br J Anaesth* 1997; **79**: 274–5.

18. Moss E, Powell D, Gibson RM et al. Effects of fentanyl on intracranial pressure and cerebral perfusion pressure during hypocapnia. *Br J Anaesth* 1978; **50**: 779–84.

19. Guy J, Hindman BJ, Baker KZ et al. Comparison of remifentanil and fentanyl in patients undergoing craniotomy for supratentorial space occupying lesions. *Anesthesiology* 1997; **86**: 514–24.

20. Black A, Mackersie A. Accidental bronchial intubation with RAE tubes. *Anaesthesia* 1991; **46**: 42–3.

21. Swedlow DB. Anesthesia for neurosurgical procedures. In: Gregory GA, ed. *Pediatric anesthesia*. New York: Churchill Livingstone, 1983: 679–86.

22. Boris-Moller F, Smith M, Siesjo BK. Effects of hypothermia on ischaemic brain damage: a comparison between pre ischaemic and post ischaemic cooling. *Neurosci Res Commun* 1989; **5**: 87–93.

23. Berntman L, Welsh FA, Harp JR *et al*. Cerebral protective effect of low-grade hypothermia. *Anesthesiology* 1981; **55**: 495–8.

24. Wass CT, Lanier WL, Hofer RE *et al*. Temperature changes of >1 C alter functional neurologic outcome and histopathology in a canine model of complete cerebral ischaemia. *Anesthesiology* 1995; **83**: 325–35.

25. Lam AM, Winn RH, Cullen BF *et al*. Hyperglycaemia and neurological outcome in patients with head injury. *J Neurosurg* 1991; **75**: 545–51.

26. Tatman A, Warren A, Williams A *et al*. Development of a modified paediatric coma scale in intensive care clinical practice. *Arch Dis Child* 1997; **77**(6): 519–21.

27. McEwan A, Sigston PE, Andrews KA *et al*. A comparison of rectal and intramuscular codeine phosphate in children following neurosurgery. *Paediatr Anaesth* 2000; **10**(2): 189–93.

28. Loyd B. Subdural haemorrhages in infants. *BMJ* 1998; **317**: 1538–9.

29. MRC Vitamin Research Group. Prevention of neural tube defects: results of the Medical Research Council Vitamin Study. *Lancet* 1991; **338**: 131–5.

30. Steward D. Preterm infants are more prone to complications following minor surgery than are term infants. *Anesthesiology* 1982; **56**: 304–6.

31. Tanaka M, Harvkuni I, Naito H. Intraoperative cardiovascular collapse in an infant with Arnold–Chiari malformation. *Paediatr Anaesth* 1997; **7**: 163–6.

32. Stiller CA, Nectoux J. International incidence of childhood brain and spinal tumours. *Int J Epidemiol* 1994; **23**(3): 458–64.

33. Black S, Ockert DB, Oliver WC *et al*. Outcome following posterior fossa craniectomy in patients in the sitting or horizontal positions. *Anesthesiology* 1988; **69**: 49–56.

34. Orliaguet GA, Hanafi M, Meyer PG *et al*. Is the sitting or the prone position best for surgery for posterior fossa tumours in children? *Paediatr Anaesth* 2001; **11**(5): 541–7.

35. Wilder BL. Hypothesis: the etiology of midcervical quadriplegia after operation with the patient in the sitting position. *Neurosurgery* 1982; **11**(4): 530–1.

36. Bithal PK, Pandia MP, Dash HH *et al*. Comparative incidence of venous air embolism and associated hypotension in adults and children operated for neurosurgery in the sitting position. *Eur J Anaesthesiol* 2004; **21**(7): 517–22.

37. Giebler R, Kollenberg B, Pohlen G *et al*. Effect of positive end-expiratory pressure on the incidence of venous air embolism and on the cardiovascular response to the sitting position during neurosurgery. *Br J Anaesth* 1998; **80**: 30–5.

38. Harrison EA, Mackersie A, McEwan A *et al*. The sitting position for neurosurgery in children: a review of 16 years' experience. *Br J Anaesth* 2002; **88**(1): 12–7.

39. Faberowski LW, Black S, Mickle JP. Incidence of venous air embolism during craniectomy for craniosynostosis repair. *Anesthesiology* 2000; **92**: 20–3.

40. Cucchiara RF, Nugent M, Seward JB *et al*. Air embolism in upright neurosurgical patients: detection and localization by two dimensional tranoesophageal echocardiography. *Anesthesiology* 1984; **60**: 353–5.

41. Fuchs G, Scharz G, Stein J *et al*. Doppler color-flow imaging: screening of a patent foramen ovale in children scheduled for neurosurgery in the sitting position. *J Neurosurg Anesthesiol* 1998; **10**(1): 5–9.

42. Marshall WK, Bedford RF. Use of a pulmonary artery catheter for detection and treatment of venous air embolism: a prospective study in man. *Anesthesiology* 1980; **52**: 131–4.

43. Doxey D, Bruce D, Sklar F *et al*. Posterior fossa syndrome: identifiable risk factors and irreversible complications. *Pediatr Neurosurg* 1999; **31**(3): 131–6.

44. Seckl JR, Dunger DB, Lightman SL *et al*. Neurophypophyseal function during early postoperative diabetes insipidus. *Brain* 1987; **110**: 737–46.

45. Seckl JR, Dunger DB, Bevan JS *et al*. Vasopressin antagonist in early postoperative diabetes insipidus. *Lancet* 1990; **335**: 1353–6.

46. Yasargil MG, Curcic M, Kis M *et al*. Total removal of craniopharyngiomas. *J Neurosurg* 1990; **73**: 3–11.

47. Kofke WA, Tempelhoff R, Dasheiff RM. Anaesthetic implications of epilepsy, status epilepticus and epilepsy surgery. *J Neurosurg Anesthesiol* 1997; **9**(4): 349–72.

48. Sperling MR, O'Connor MJ, Saykin AJ *et al*. Temporal lobectomy for refractory epilepsy. *JAMA* 1996; **276**: 470–5.

49. Kim SK, Wang KC, Hwang YS *et al*. Intractable epilepsy associated with brain tumors in children: surgical modality and outcome. *Child Nerv Syst* 2001; **17**(8): 445–52.

50. Tobias JT, Jimenez DF. Anaesthetic management during awake craniotomy in a 12-year-old boy. *Paediatr Anaesth* 997(7): 341–4.

51. Crockard AH, Stevens JM. Craniovertebral junction anomalies in inherited disorders: part of the syndrome or caused by the disorder? *Eur J Paediatr* 1995; **154**: 504–12.

52. Mitchell V, Howard R, Facer E. Down's syndrome and anaesthesia. *Paediatr Anaesth* 1995; **5**: 379–84.

53. Casey A. TH, O'Brien M, Kumar V *et al*. Don't twist my child's head off: iatrogenic cervical dislocation. *BMJ* 1995; **311**: 1212–13.

54. Landsman I. Cricoid pressure: indications and complications. *Paediatr Anaesth* 2004; **14**: 43–7.

55. Sener E. BS, Sarihasan B, Ustun E *et al*. Awake tracheal intubation through the intubating laryngeal mask airway in a patient with halo traction. *Can J Anaesth* 2002; **49**: 6: 610–13.

56. Ashida Y, Miyahara H, Sawada H *et al*. Anaesthetic management of a neonate with vein of Galen aneuysmal malformations and severe pulmonary hypertension. *Paediatr Anaesth* 2005; **15**: 525–8.

57. Lasjaunias P. Vein of Galen aneurysmal malformation. In: *Vascular diseases in neonates, infants and children*.

Interventional neuroradiology management. Berlin: Springer-Verlag, 1997: 67–202.

58. Friedman DM, Verma R, Madrid M *et al.* Recent improvement in outcome using transcatheter embolisation techniques for neonatal aneurysmal malformation of Galen. *Pediatrics* 1989; **91**: 583–6.

59. Baykan N, Isbir O, Gercek A *et al.* Ten years of experience with pediatric neuroendoscopic third ventriculostomy. *J Neurosurg Anesthesiol* 2005; **17**(1): 33–7.

60. Johnson JO, Jimenez DF, Tobias JD. Anaesthetic care during minimally invasive neurosurgical procedures in infants and children. *Paediatr Anaesth* 2002; **12**: 478–88.

61. Schubert A, Deogaonkar A, Lotto M *et al.* Anesthesia for minimally invasive cranial and spinal surgery. *J Neurosurg Anesthesiol* 2006; **18**(1): 47–56.

62. Kalmar AF, Aken JV, Caemaert J *et al.* Value of Cushing reflex as warning sign for brain ischaemia during neuroendoscopy. *Br J Anaesth* 2005; **94**(6): 791–9.

63. Derbent A, Ersahin Y, Yurtseven T *et al.* Hemodynamic and electrolyte changes in patients undergoing neuroendoscopic procedures. *Child Nerv Syst* 2006; **22**: 253–7.

64. Baykan N, Ozgen S, Serpil Ulstalar Z *et al.* Moyamoya disease and anesthesia. *Paediatr Anaesth* 2005; **15**: 1111–15.

65. Thompson D, Jones B, Hayward R, Harkness W. Assessment and treatment of craniosynostosis. *Br J Hosp Med* 1994; **52**: 17–24.

66. Lefebvre A, Barclay S. Psychosocial impact of craniofacial deformities before and after reconstructive surgery. *Can J Psychiatry* 1982; **27**: 579–84.

67. Whitaker LA, Munro IR, Salyer KE *et al.* Combined report of problems and complications in 793 craniofacial operations. *Plast Reconstr Surg* 1979; **64**: 198–203.

68. Moylan S, Collee G, Mackersie A, Bingham R. Anaesthetic management in paediatric craniofacial surgery. A review of 126 cases. *Paediatr Anaesth* 1993; **3**: 275–81.

69. Meyer P, Renier D, Arnaud E *et al.* Blood loss during repair of craniosynostosis. *Br J Anaesth* 1993; **71**: 854–7.

70. Handler SD, Beaugard ME, Whitaker LA, Potsic WP. Airway management in the repair of craniofacial defects. *Cleft Palate J* 1979; **16**: 16–23.

71. Shprintzen RJ. Palatal and pharyngeal anomalies in craniofacial syndromes. *Birth Defects Orig Artic Ser* 1982; **18**: 53–78.

72. Kreiborg S, Aduss H, Cohen MM Jr. Cephalometric study of the Apert syndrome in adolescence and adulthood. *J Craniofac Genet Dev Biol* 1999; **19**: 1–11.

73. Shprintzen RJ. The implications of the diagnosis of Robin sequence. *Cleft Palate Craniofac J* 1992; **29**: 205–9.

74. Sher AE. Mechanisms of airway obstruction in Robin sequence: implications for treatment. *Cleft Palate Craniofac J* 1992; **29**: 224–31.

75. Mixter RC, David DJ, Perloff WH *et al.* Obstructive sleep apnea in Apert's and Pfeiffer's syndromes: more than a craniofacial abnormality. *Plast Reconstr Surg* 1990; **86**: 457–63.

76. McGill T. Otolaryngologic aspects of Apert syndrome. *Clin Plast Surg* 1991; **18**: 309–13.

77. Jones BM, Jani P, Bingham RM *et al.* Complications in paediatric craniofacial surgery: an initial four year experience. *Br J Plast Surg* 1992; **45**: 225–31.

78. Sher AE, Shprintzen RJ, Thorpy MJ. Endoscopic observations of obstructive sleep apnea in children with anomalous upper airways: predictive and therapeutic value. *Int J Pediatr Otorhinolaryngol* 1986; **11**: 135–46.

79. Moore MH. Upper airway obstruction in the syndromal craniosynostoses. *Br J Plast Surg* 1993; **46**: 355–62.

80. Anderson PJ, Harkness WJ, Taylor W *et al.* Anomalous venous drainage in a case of non-syndromic craniosynostosis. *Child Nerv Syst* 1997; **13**: 97–100.

81. Thompson DN, Hayward RD, Harkness WJ *et al.* Lessons from a case of kleeblattschadel. *J Neurosurg* 1995; **82**: 1071–4.

82. Roche J, Frawley G, Heggie A. Difficult tracheal intubation induced by maxillary distraction devices in craniosynostosis syndromes. *Paediatr Anaesth* 2002; **12**: 227–34.

83. Shulman GB, Conelly NR, Gibson C. The adult Bullard laryngoscope in paediatric patients. *Can J Anaesth* 1997; **44**(9): 969–72.

84. Blanco G, Melman E, Cuairan V *et al.* Fibreoptic nasal intubation in children with anticipated and unanticipated difficult intubation. *Paediatr Anaesth* 2001; **11**: 49–53.

85. Reich DL, Konstadt SN, Nejat M *et al.* Intraoperative transesophageal echocardiography for the detection of cardiac preload changes induced by transfusion and phlebotomy in pediatric patients. *Anesthesiology* 1993; **79**: 10–15.

86. Orliaguet GA, Meyer PG, Blanot S *et al.* Non-invasive aortic blood flow measurement in infants during repair of craniosynostosis. *Br J Anaesth* 1998; **81**: 696–701.

87. Tuncbilek G, Vargel I, Erdem A *et al.* Blood loss and transfusion rates during repair of craniofacial deformities. *J Craniofac Surg* 2005; **16**(1): 59–62.

88. Brown KA, Bissonnette B, McIntyre B. Hyperkalaemia during rapid blood transfusion and hypovolaemic cardiac arrest in children. *Can J Anaesth* 1990; **7**: 747–54.

89. Buntain SG, Pabari M. Massive transfusion and hyperkalaemic cardiac arrest in craniofacial surgery in a child. *Anaesth Intensive Care* 1999; **27**: 530–3.

90. Scholtes JL, Thauvoy C, Moulin D, Gribomont BF. Craniofaciosynostosis: anesthetic and perioperative management. Report of 71 operations. *Acta Anaesthesiol Belg* 1985; **36**: 176–85.

91. Kearney RA, Rosales JK, Howes WJ. Craniosynostosis: an assessment of blood loss and transfusion practices. *Can J Anaesth* 1989; **36**: 473–7.

92. Faberowski LW, Black S, Mickle JP. Blood loss and transfusion practice in the perioperative management of craniosynostosis repair. *J Neurosurg Anesthesiol* 1999; **11**: 167–72.

93. Mallory S, Yap LH, Jones BM, Bingham R. Anaesthetic management in facial bipartition surgery: the experience of one centre. *Anaesthesia* 2004; **59**(1): 44–51.

94. Eaton AC, Marsh JL, Pilgram TK. Transfusion requirements for craniosynostosis surgery in infants. *Plast Reconstr Surg* 1995; **95**: 277–83.

95. Polley JW, Berkowitz RA, McDonald TB *et al.* Craniomaxillofacial surgery in the Jehovah's Witness patient. *Plast Reconstr Surg* 1994; **93**(6): 1258–63.

96. Helfaer MA, Carson BS, James CS *et al.* Increased hematocrit and decreased transfusion requirements in children given erythropoietin before undergoing craniofacial surgery. *J Neurosurg* 1998; **88**: 704–8.

97. D'errico CC, Munro H, Buchman SR *et al.* Efficacy of aprotinin in children undergoing craniofacial surgery. *J Neurosurg* 2003; **99**: 287–90.

98. Tatum SA. Advances in congenital craniofacial surgery. *Facial Plast Surg* 1999; **15**: 33–43.

99. Neil-Dwyer JG, Evans RD, Jones BM, Hayward RD. Tumescent steroid infiltration to reduce post-operative swelling after craniofacial surgery. *Br J Plast Surg* 2001; **54**: 565–9.

100. Schaller RT. Jr, Schaller J, Furman EB. The advantages of hemodilution anesthesia for major liver resection in children. *J Pediatr Surg* 1984; **19**: 705–10.

101. Hans P, Collin V, Bonhomme V *et al.* Evaluation of acute normovolemic hemodilution for surgical repair of craniosynostosis. *J Neurosurg Anesthesiol* 2000; **12**: 33–6.

102. Velardi F, Di Chirico A, Di Rocco C. Blood salvage in craniosynostosis surgery. *Child Nerv Syst* 1999; **15**: 695–710.

103. Fearon JA. Reducing allogenic blood transfusions during pediatric cranial vault surgical procedures: A prospective analysis of blood recycling. *Plast Reconstr Surg* 2004; **113**(4): 1126–30.

104. Wilkinson E, Rieff J, Rekate HL, Beals S. Fluid, blood, and blood product management in the craniofacial patient. *Pediatr Neurosurg* 1992; **18**: 48–52.

105. Imberti R, Locatelli D, Fanzio M *et al.* Intra- and postoperative management of craniosynostosis. *Can J Anaesth* 1990; **37**: 948–50.

106. Hasan RA, Nikolis A, Dutta S, Jackson IT, Clinical outcome of peri-operative airway and ventilatory management in children undergoing craniofacial surgery. *J Craniofac Surg* 2004; **15**(4): 655–61.

107. Poole MD. Complications in craniofacial surgery. *Br J Plast Surg* 1988; **41**: 608–13.

108. Elmslie FV, Reardon W. Craniofacial developmental abnormalities. *Curr Opin Neurol* 1998; **1**: 103–8.

109. Marchac D, Renier D, Jones BM. Experience with the 'floating forehead'. *Br J Plast Surg* 1988; **41**: 1–15.

ADDENDUM: POSTOPERATIVE FLUID REPLACEMENT IN CHILDREN AFTER CRANIOFACIAL SURGERY

Objectives

- Maintain normal circulating blood volume by continuous assessment and reassessment of fluid balance and replacement with appropriate fluids
- Maintain haemoglobin at an appropriate level
- Maintain normal electrolyte balance and normoglycaemia.

Fluid replacement

- Give maintenance fluids
- Replace on-going blood losses (drain losses, haematoma) with Gelofusine and/or packed red cells (see below).

Note that a falling haemoglobin in association with minimal drain losses may indicate an intracranial haematoma, which is a neurosurgical emergency. Please ensure that the craniofacial fellow is called immediately.

Maintenance fluid

- 2.5 per cent dextrose/0.45 per cent saline
- Give 50% of full maintenance for the first 24 hours.

Moderate blood loss ($\leqslant$10 mL/kg/h)

- Measure losses at **half-hourly** intervals and replace at the appropriate **hourly** rate (i.e. if blood loss in first half hour is 25 mL/h, replace at a rate of 50 mL/h). Monitor fluid balance hourly in order to avoid over- or under-transfusion
- Measure Hb after transfusion of each 20 mL/kg blood
- **Replace with blood or colloid in order to maintain Hb >7 g/dL** (4 ml/kg packed cells raises Hb by approximately 1 g/dL. Minimise donor exposure when blood is used by making full use of a unit of blood – transfuse to a Hb of about 12 g/dL and avoid opening a new unit unless necessary).

Massive blood loss (>10 mL/kg/h)

Occasionally, massive postoperative blood loss may occur. It is important to keep up with transfusion to maintain normal circulating blood volume and Hb:

- If Hb 10–12 g/dL give blood:colloid 1:1, i.e. if blood loss 100 mL, give 50 mL blood, 50 mL colloid.
- If Hb >12 g/dL give blood:colloid approximately 1:2, i.e. if blood loss 100 mL, give 30 mL blood, 70 mL colloid.
- If Hb <10 g/dL give blood:colloid approximately 2:1, i.e. if blood losss 100 mL, give 70 mL blood, 30 mL colloid.

Coagulation profile should be checked after each 80 mL/kg infusion (i.e. after infusion of estimated blood volume [EBV]) and repeated serially).

- Fresh frozen plasma (FFP) (10 mL/kg) usually required after rapid transfusion of $1 \times$ EBV.
- Platelets (5 mL/kg) usually required after transfusion of $2 \times$ EBV.

Note that the coagulation results should be taken in the context of the clinical status of the patient and not treated in isolation.

Hypovolaemia is the most common problem after craniofacial surgery

Signs:

- Tachycardia
- Delayed capillary refill ($>$2 seconds)
- Cool, mottled peripheries
- Hypotension – this is a late sign.

Immediate treatment:

- Give an immediate bolus of Gelofusine (10 mL/kg)
- Reassess and repeat as necessary.

Thoracic surgery

PATRICK T FARRELL

KEY LEARNING POINTS

- Understanding the pathophysiology is crucial – beware of air trapping with positive pressure ventilation
- Single-lung ventilation (SLV) is ideal but:
  - technically difficult in infants (surgery can be achieved without it)
  - maintaining oxygenation is the highest priority; if you cannot safely achieve SLV, do not attempt it
  - SLV is better tolerated in the lateral rather than the supine position.

- An anterior mediastinal mass can compress the trachea, bronchi and central veins, and minor postural changes can lead to sudden cardiac arrest. Anaesthesia is dangerous.
- Correction of pectus excavatum causes severe postoperative pain.
- Pulmonary complications after thoracic surgery are common and should be anticipated.

INTRODUCTION

Paediatric non-cardiovascular thoracic anaesthesia requires specific knowledge of pathology, pathophysiology and special techniques. The two major goals are to provide good safe surgical conditions and postoperative analgesia. Surgical access can sometimes be improved by single-lung ventilation (SLV) although this is may be too difficult in small children.

PATHOLOGY OF LUNG LESIONS

Congenital cystic lesions

There are four main types of congenital cystic lung lesions: congenital cystic adenomatoid malformation (CCAM), congenital lobar emphysema, pulmonary sequestration and bronchogenic cysts [1]. The last two are sometimes included in a broader category of bronchopulmonary foregut malformations. For all types of lesions there is a spectrum of disease from a 'threat to life' to an 'asymptomatic finding'. Cystic lesions can be vascular and/or lymphadenomatous and, because they can be connected to the lung or gut, they can be air filled and become infected.

Congenital cystic adenomatoid malformation results from an arrest in the maturation of foetal lung. A disorganised mass of air- and blood-filled cysts forms that does not usually communicate with the normal lung. There are three types depending on the cyst size and structure [2]: 70 per cent are type I with cysts over 2 cm, 15–20 per cent are type II with cysts from 0.5 cm to 2 cm, and type III cysts are less than 0.5 cm and are rarely seen postnatally. Type II cysts are associated with cardiac and renal abnormalities. Diagnosis of CCAM can made on antenatal ultrasound [3] and may resolve spontaneously. Therefore, treatment is based on postnatal clinical evaluation and further imaging including magnetic resonance imaging (MRI) [4]. Congenital cystic adenomatoid malformation is usually unilobar and occurs in the upper and lower lobes with equal frequency. A neonate with a large CCAM presents with severe respiratory distress related to compression of normal lung tissue. Emergency life-saving excision may be required. In older children surgical excision is needed to remove a source of recurrent infection. Congenital cystic adenomatoid malformation may undergo malignant change.

Pulmonary sequestration is a separate bronchopulmonary mass or cyst that is disconnected from the bronchial tree and has a systemic arterial blood supply. Sequestration forms when a supernumerary lung bud arises from the primitive foregut and migrates caudally. It is sometimes classified as a bronchopulmonary foregut malformation. Congenital abnormalities occur in up to 65 per cent of cases. There are two types: extralobar and intralobar.

Extralobar sequestrations are enclosed by a separate pleural membrane with an anomalous blood supply arising from the aorta (this can be a major source of intraoperative haemorrhage). In most cases the sequestration is found between the left lower lobe and the diaphragm but it may occur in the upper abdomen or mediastinum.

Intralobar sequestrations usually lie within the lower lobe and are invested by the pleura of the rest of the lung [5]. In older children they may arise from an inflammatory process following necrotising pneumonia.

Bronchopulmonary foregut malformations include oesophageal duplication, and neurenteric and bronchogenic cysts. Like sequestrations these malformations also develop from abnormal foregut buds but probably later in gestation. They may or may not communicate with the respiratory or digestive tracts and are found most frequently in the mediastinum but can occur anywhere along the foregut from pharynx to duodenum.

Bronchogenic cysts are solitary, unilocular with bronchial-like walls, and contain sterile mucus [6]. They can cause symptoms owing to local compression as they expand, particularly if they become infected. Often, they are an incidental radiographic finding.

Congenital lobar emphysema arises because of collapse of a section of bronchial wall so that a valve-like effect occurs in expiration. The hyper-expanded lung behaves like a pneumothorax [7]. Cartilaginous dysplasia is the commonest cause. Presentation may vary from extreme respiratory distress (requiring rapid surgical decompression) to an incidental finding on chest X-ray.

Tumours

The commonest thoracic tumours in children are mediastinal; the commonest of these is lymphoma [8], and the commonest mediastinal primary is the plasma cell granuloma. Aggressive but less common tumours are pleuropulmonary blastoma and rhabdomyosarcoma. Primary lung and pleural tumours are uncommon [9]. Metastases are usually from osteosarcoma, Ewing's sarcoma and nephroblastoma. Biopsy and resection may require thoracoscopic biopsy or formal thoracotomy.

Infective diseases

Acute pulmonary infections in childhood are common and usually resolve with antibiotic therapy. However, some may progress to abscess formation, empyema or bronchiectasis. Surgery for lung resection or decortication is required if medical treatment fails [10].

Parapneumonic empyema can cause a thick inelastic covering of the lung, which prevents adequate lung expansion. Drainage and minor decortication are indicated for most cases; this can be achieved by thoracoscopy with less pain and shorter intercostal drainage than formal thoracotomy, which is necessary for extensive decortication [11].

Bronchiectasis results from chronic infection and permanent damage to the muscular and elastic components of a medium-sized bronchus. This leads to obstruction, dilatation and poor mucus clearance. It is a common feature of cystic fibrosis (CF). Non-cystic fibrosis bronchiectasis can occur after pneumonia (in association with immunodeficiency or -suppression), and with other underlying congenital lung abnormalities [12]. Bronchiectasis infection uncontrolled by antibiotics and physiotherapy is an indication for resection to try to protect normal lung [13].

Hydatid disease is caused by infection with the larvae of *Echinococcus granulosus*, producing unilocular cystic lesions, usually in the liver or lung. The disease is endemic in Australia and New Zealand, the Middle East, the Mediterranean, and South and Central America. Cyst excision is usually required for pulmonary disease in addition to treatment with ascaricidal agents such as albendazole [14]. Spillage of the contents of a hydatid cyst during surgery can cause a severe anaphylactic reaction.

PREOPERATIVE PREPARATION

The important elements of this task are first to determine the patient's current state of health and then to focus on what can be improved prior to surgery. In cases of chronic infection or large lung cysts, general well-being and lung function may improve only after resection to remove infection and to re-expand viable lung.

History and physical examination

The history of the current illness should focus on cardiopulmonary function, including cough and dyspnoea, recent respiratory tract infections, tachypnoea, chest wall recession, nasal flaring, cyanosis and oxygen requirement. Features of associated defects or syndromes should be sought. In an older child exercise tolerance and the use of medications (e.g. bronchodilators) should be evaluated. Dysphagia, weight loss, failure to thrive and intractable pneumonia are major causes of morbidity [15].

The upper airway should be assessed for difficulty with laryngoscopy. It is particularly important to auscultate the chest because preoperative unilateral signs need to be known not only for checking the position of tubes and blockers for SLV but also to help determine any intra- and postoperative changes. Any chest signs, be they fine crepitations, coarse crackles or rhonchi, are always significant and may indicate the need for further preoperative treatment.

Investigations

Chest X-ray, computed tomography (CT) and magnetic resonance imaging (MRI) all have a place in diagnosis and it is also important to determine the blood supply and other connections of the lesions. Other associated congenital abnormalities may also need investigations (e.g. echocardiography). Pulse oximetry guides the need for further investigations such as arterial blood gases and spirometry. The need for formal lung function tests is arguable and depends on the patient [16]. Blood grouping for cross-match should be performed for any thoracotomy.

Other preoperative issues

Patients with chronic infection, cystic fibrosis and asthma will benefit from preoperative physiotherapy, antibiotics and bronchodilators to reduce the volume and infectivity of their sputum [17]. Atropine may increase the viscosity of secretions and is best avoided [18].

ANAESTHESIA WITHOUT SINGLE-LUNG VENTILATION

The reader must appreciate that there are major technical challenges with bronchial intubation in small infants. Indeed, when SLV is not possible often surgery can still be achieved with the use of a conventional tracheal single-lumen tube. Furthermore, SLV is not always helpful because the surgeon may wish to vary the lung inflation when trying to identify the plane of dissection. In these circumstances the anaesthetist and surgeon have to coordinate their actions. While the surgeon dissects the lung the anaesthetist may inflate it very gently or not at all, and both need to agree the limit of desaturation that will demand lung reinflation. This is not usually hazardous in experienced and skilful hands.

ANAESTHESIA FOR SINGLE-LUNG VENTILATION

The indications and contraindications for SLV are the same as for adults [19,20] and are summarised in Table 39.1.

Table 39.1 Indications and contraindications for single lung ventilation

Strong indications for single lung ventilation or isolation:
  Isolation to avoid ventilating the abnormal lung:
    Major tracheobronchial disruption, i.e. a large air leak
    Giant lung cysts or bullae
  Isolation to avoid contamination of the 'normal' lung:
    Infection
    Massive haemorrhage
    Unilateral bronchopulmonary lavage

Other indications for single lung ventilation:
  Pneumonectomy
  Thoracoscopy
  Lobectomy (especially the upper lobe)
  Mediastinal exposure
  Oesophageal resection
  Procedures on the thoracic spine

Contraindications to single-lung ventilation:
  Severe respiratory impairment such that oxygenation cannot be maintained
  Technical difficulty in bronchial intubation or blockade

Physiology of single-lung ventilation and the lateral decubitus position

Ideally, for the most efficient oxygenation of mixed venous blood, ventilation ($\dot{V}$) and perfusion ($\dot{Q}$) are perfectly matched ($\dot{V}/\dot{Q} = 1$). However, even in the normal upright lung the $\dot{V}/\dot{Q}$ ratio averages 0.85. Any $\dot{V}/\dot{Q}$ mismatches, either low $\dot{V}/\dot{Q}$ (shunt) or high $\dot{V}/\dot{Q}$ (dead space ventilation), cause arterial hypoxaemia and during anaesthesia these may be influenced by gravity, drugs, mode of ventilation and cardiorespiratory pathology. During thoracic anaesthesia both the lateral decubitus position and SLV are major causes of $\dot{V}/\dot{Q}$ mismatch and hypoxaemia.

LATERAL DECUBITUS POSITION

In the lateral decubitus position gravity increases perfusion to the dependent lung and this effect is less in infants because of their smaller size. In the awake state ventilation is also greatest in the dependent lung in adults but not in infants. During anaesthesia ventilation of the dependent lung is decreased because of compression by abdominal and mediastinal organs. The non-dependent lung is not compressed and is better ventilated but less well perfused. The combination of these factors means that the least $\dot{V}/\dot{Q}$ mismatch and best oxygenation are achieved for adults if the normal lung is dependent, in contrast to that for infants when it is optimal for the normal lung to be uppermost [21].

When supine, the gravitational effects are less than for the lateral position and consequently perfusion of the non-ventilated lung during SLV is not as reduced and this increases V̇/Q̇ mismatch. It is therefore important to appreciate that adequate oxygenation may not be possible during SLV anaesthesia in the supine position [22]. Pulmonary V̇/Q̇ mismatch is exacerbated by atelectasis (especially in the dependent lung) [23] but this can be reduced by positive end-expiratory pressure (PEEP). This can be applied differentially to each lung by using a double-lumen tube [24].

SINGLE-LUNG VENTILATION

During SLV there is a homogeneous decrease in blood flow throughout the unventilated lung caused by hypoxic pulmonary vasoconstriction (HPV). This occurs when pulmonary arterioles in the non-ventilated lung constrict mainly in response to low alveolar oxygen concentration. Blood is diverted to better ventilated areas and venous admixture is reduced. Hypoxic pulmonary vasoconstriction is a distinguishing feature of pulmonary arteries, unlike systemic arteries that dilate under hypoxic conditions [25]. Mechanical effects of lung collapse and surgical manipulation are also present but are less important than HPV. Hypoxic pulmonary vasoconstriction is active in infants and children and will help overcome the V̇/Q̇ mismatch. Inhalational anaesthetic agents all tend to reduce the effectiveness of HPV and increase perfusion of the unventilated lung. Isoflurane, for example, will increase perfusion of the non-dependent lung by inhibiting HPV but does not overcome the much larger effect of gravity [26].

Hypoxic pulmonary vasoconstriction is also affected by ventilation; hypocapnia reduces HPV [27]. An increased cardiac output will improve oxygenation by decreasing the effect of the shunt [28]. Non-specific vasodilators such as sodium nitroprusside, nitroglycerin, dobutamine, calcium channel blockers and β_2 agonists all oppose HPV. Vasoconstrictors such as adrenaline and phenylephrine tend to decrease HPV by decreasing blood flow through ventilated areas. Two drugs, almitrine and nitric oxide, enhance HPV and both have been used to prevent hypoxia during SLV [29]. Almitrine bismesylate is a chemoreceptor agonist and pulmonary vasoconstrictor that works possibly by inhibiting potassium ion channels [30]. Inhaled nitric oxide dilates pulmonary vessels in ventilated but not unventilated areas.

Anaesthetic technique and monitoring

Spontaneous ventilation is inadequate for any thoracotomy because lung expansion is prevented by the combination of inadequate negative intrathoracic pressure and mediastinal shift. Historically, these problems limited thoracic surgery until the introduction of positive pressure ventilation [31]. Positive pressure ventilation is required for thoracotomy or thoracoscopy.

INDUCTION

Induction of anaesthesia can be intravenous or inhalational. Inhalational induction is preferred for smaller children and infants because there is a smooth transition of airway control in the constant presence of high inspired oxygen concentrations [32]. Usually muscle relaxation and positive pressure ventilation can begin immediately after induction but in theory spontaneous ventilation is safer in some cases until the airway is controlled. For example, positive pressure ventilation can over-expand congenital lobar emphysema or exacerbate a major air leak. Ideally, isolation of the affected lung should be attempted before muscle relaxation but in practice gentle assisted ventilation and good muscle relaxation rarely result in problems. Local anaesthesia spray to the larynx and trachea reduces autonomic stimulation during prolonged airway instrumentation.

If acute hyperexpansion or tension pneumothorax occurs, decompression can be life saving. If this scenario is anticipated the surgical team must be scrubbed and ready before induction so that the pleura can be drained or the emphysematous lung can be compressed and resected with minimal delay.

MAINTENANCE

The inhibition of HPV by anaesthesia drugs accounts for only a small increase in shunt fraction during SLV [33]. Isoflurane, sevoflurane and desflurane all have similar effects on reducing HPV at a concentration of 1 MAC (minimum alveolar concentration). At higher vapour concentrations, there is more inhibition of HPV and therefore supplementary agents such as opioids or ketamine [34] or local anaesthesia techniques should be used. Propofol has minimal effect on HPV.

Nitrous oxide is not used during thoracic anaesthesia. It is contraindicated where there is air trapped in a cavity because nitrogen is 40 times less soluble and cannot equilibrate with blood as fast as nitrous oxide; 70 per cent nitrous oxide can double the size of a pneumothorax within 10 minutes. It also reduces the maximum inspired oxygen concentration and inhibits HPV. In order to reduce atelectasis the inspired oxygen concentration should be minimised by dilution with air.

There is always potential for major haemorrhage during thoracic surgery and therefore at least two routes of intravenous (IV) access are recommended. Occasionally, a central venous line is necessary and should be inserted on the same side as the surgery.

VENTILATION

There are no clear ventilation guidelines established for SLV. It is suggested for adults that a tidal volume of 10 mL/kg be maintained with an I:E (inspiratory phase time to expiratory phase time) ratio of 1:2 and 100 per cent oxygen and that the respiratory rate be adjusted to maintain a normal end-tidal CO_2 [35]. Small children are usually ventilated with pressure-controlled ventilation and therefore, when there is SLV or surgical manipulation, there is a reduction in compliance and this decreases ventilation. Thus ventilation needs to be adjusted to arterial O_2 saturation SaO_2, and end-tidal or arterial CO_2. Positive end-expiratory pressure to the dependent lung ($< 5\,cmH_2O$) may improve oxygenation but higher pressures do not help because perfusion is reduced and blood is shunted to the non-ventilated lung. Slightly high end-tidal CO_2, 6–7 kPa (permissive hypercapnia), may be beneficial and is preferable to alveolar overdistension which may result in lung injury [36].

MONITORING

In addition to standard apparatus, direct arterial blood-pressure monitoring is advisable, especially in small infants, because haemodynamic changes can occur rapidly. While central venous access is necessary for infusion, pressure measurements can be unreliable in the lateral position [37]. Spirometry is useful to indicate early changes in compliance, especially during pressure-controlled ventilation, when there may be no obvious change in the ventilator's performance.

Bronchial intubation or blockade

Equipment must be prepared and checked in advance; in particular, the correct sizes of tubes, blockers and scopes should be confirmed. There are four choices of technique for SLV [38]:

- single-lumen selective bronchial intubation
- bronchial blockers
- Univent tubes
- double-lumen tubes (DLTs).

SINGLE–LUMEN SELECTIVE BRONCHIAL INTUBATION

The use of a normal single-lumen tracheal tube (TT) to intubate a main bronchus selectively is the simplest technique to provide SLV and is possible even in newborns with pulmonary interstitial emphysema [39]. Owing to the angle of the tracheal division at the carina, intubation of the right main bronchus is usually easier than of the left. Intubating the left main bronchus is easier when the head is turned to the right (this reduces the angle between the trachea and left main bronchus) and rotating or using a right-bevelled TT so that the pointed end is on the left [40,41]. Beware of obstruction caused by the TT orifice abutting against the bronchial wall.

Bronchial intubation will generally be achieved when the patient is supine so that after moving to the lateral thoracotomy position SLV must be rechecked, at least by auscultation, because tube displacement is common. Checking with a bronchoscope may be necessary.

There are advantages and disadvantages with cuffed and uncuffed TTs. With right bronchial intubation, obstruction of the right upper lobe is common and made worse with a

cuff. For left bronchial intubation the cuff may encroach onto the carina and fail to seal the bronchus. This is a problem of the design of TTs where the distance between the cuff and the tip of the TT is too great [42]. The problem of an uncuffed TT is that it may be the correct size for the bronchus (i.e. it leaks at about $20\,cmH_2O$) but it may be too small for the trachea, preventing effective expansion of the lungs when it is withdrawn into the trachea. In this situation a smaller cuffed TT [43], even deflated, will seal the bronchus better and, when it is withdrawn into the trachea, the cuff can be inflated to allow lung expansion.

BRONCHIAL BLOCKERS

In 1969, in the same issue of the *British Journal of Anaesthesia*, Vale and Lines separately described the use of bronchial blockers [44,45]. A Fogarty embolectomy catheter was used by both authors to block the distal bronchus and, even though the catheters became displaced, they were thought to have helped. Several different methods of bronchial blockade have been developed since.

Fogarty embolectomy catheters

These catheters are available in sizes 3–7 (Fr). They have a guidewire, but no distal orifice, and there is a small high-pressure balloon at its end. The balloon diameter varies from 8 mm to 12 mm. Size 3 is suitable for infants under 5 kg and size 5 for larger infants and preschool children [46]. The balloon cuff pressure must be limited to prevent mucosal ischaemia or bronchial rupture. Before use, the balloon can be stretched by inflating it several times and then, once positioned, it is inflated very carefully with 0.1-mL increments of air while auscultating the chest to determine the 'just seal' volume (lung sounds cease). Small increments of air cause large changes in balloon size: 0.2 mL in a 5Fr catheter stretches the balloon diameter to 4 mm and this increases to 7.4 mm with 0.6 mL. Care should be taken never to exceed the manufacturer's limits.

The catheter can be passed beside a small TT or through a larger TT and then positioned by either fluoroscopy (Fig. 39.1) or bronchoscopy. A slight bend in the catheter directs it into the bronchus. Fluoroscopy is the quickest method of checking the balloon position and can be performed without moving the TT or changing the ventilation (contrast can be used to inflate the balloon). Flexible bronchoscopes can obstruct small TTs but are standard for adults. Rigid bronchoscopy can place the catheter balloon before the TT is inserted but this requires skill and experience; however, it has been successfully used even in combination with the prone position [47].

There are problems with the Fogarty catheters. Because there is no central lumen, deflation of the lung is slow. The surgeon can compress the lung before the balloon is inflated but only if the risk of contamination is low. The balloon might not seal the bronchus (risk of contamination of the dependent lung) or it could become dislodged (causing

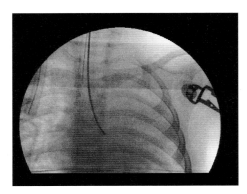

Figure 39.1 An X-ray of a Fogarty catheter placed in the left main bronchus of an infant with congenital cystic adenomatoid malformation. The catheter lies outside the tracheal tube.

tracheal obstruction). Bronchial rupture has been reported where the balloon was inadvertently overinflated [48].

Wire-guided bronchial blockers

The Arndt blocker is a purpose-made bronchial catheter [49,50]. The catheter is available in 5Fr, has a low-pressure high-volume spherical balloon and a central lumen of 0.7 mm, through which a monofilament wire loop can be passed to aid placement. It can be used only within a TT of internal diameter (ID) greater than 4.5 mm because the catheter is 2.5 mm thick and requires the smallest fibrescope (diameter less than 2.0 mm) for positioning. There is a TT adapter that has ports for connection to the anaesthetic circuit and for insertion of both the blocker and the bronchoscope so that ventilation is possible during bronchoscopy. The catheter's central lumen is sufficiently wide to aid lung deflation and the insufflation of oxygen but not for suction of secretions.

Other end-hole catheters

Foley catheters have been adapted for blocking bronchi [51]. They have a central lumen but with a blunt end and side hole. A central lumen is created by cutting off the distal end to allow oxygen delivery and suction (only effective in larger size catheters). Pulmonary artery balloon wedge pressure and atrioseptostomy catheters have also been used, but again the central lumen is so small that suction is not feasible.

UNIVENT TRACHEAL TUBE

The Univent tracheal tube has a second lumen that contains a bronchial blocker [52]. The tube is placed in the mid-trachea and the second lumen is turned towards the bronchus to be blocked so that the blocker can be advanced under fibrescopic control. The smallest size is 3.5 mm (ID) with an outside diameter (OD) of 7.5–8.0 mm (=OD of 5.5–6 mm [ID] conventional TT). There is no cuff or central lumen and it is oval in cross-section. The 4.5 is cuffed

with a central lumen and has an OD of 8.5–9 mm (=OD of 6.5 [ID] conventional TT).The balloons are 'low volume, high pressure' and have a maximum volume of 3 mL, as opposed to the adult versions which take 6 mL. The 3.5 is suitable for children from 6 years to about 10 years of age and the 4.5 for 10 years to about 14 years of age. Larger sizes are available from 6 mm to 9 mm ID for adults. Ventilation can be continued while the blocker is positioned and, in the larger size, the central lumen gives access to the non-ventilated lung for deflation, oxygenation and suction. Again, the central lumen is too narrow to remove major secretions. As with all blockers, lung deflation can be slow, especially during right-sided blockade because the blocker can obstruct the right upper lobe bronchus.

DOUBLE-LUMEN TUBES

Double-lumen tubes (DLTs) are the 'gold standard' for SLV in adults [53] because, in addition to isolating the ventilated lung, they provide access to the non-ventilated lung for deflation, suction, oxygenation, continuous positive airway pressure (CPAP), visualisation and reinflation. The smallest plastic DLTs have low-pressure cuffs and are currently available down to size 26Fr. The OD of a 26Fr is 8.7 mm compared with 28Fr tubes which are at least 9.3 mm. The DLTs are oval in cross-section and there is variation in diameter between tubes from different manufacturers [54]. For example, the Portex 28Fr that the author examined was 9 mm high and 10.2 mm wide with an extra 1.8 mm diameter at the level of the cuff. Since the OD of a size 7 cuffed Portex TT is 9.6 mm, the 28Fr DLT is useful only in larger children. In adults the size of a DLT can be based on gender, weight and height, and the size of both the trachea and the left main bronchus on X-ray [55]. There is no similar work in children. Double-lumen tubes have been used in small infants but these are hand-made from two TTs and they are not readily available [56].

Double-lumen tubes are manufactured in left- and right-sided configurations. A left-sided DLT is recommended as the first choice in most situations because a right-sided DLT is difficult to position without obstructing the right upper lobe orifice. The insertion technique is similar to that used in adults [57]. The stylet is removed once the tip of the tube is past the vocal cords. Then the tube is rotated through 90°, counter-clockwise for a left DLT, and inserted to an appropriate depth. The formula, depth in centimetres = 12.5 + (0.1 × height), has been suggested as a guide for adults [58] but there is no equivalent for children. The position is then checked by a combination of auscultation, resistance to advancement, change in compliance and/or by fibre-optic bronchoscopy [59]. A fibrescope with an OD of less than 3.2 mm is needed for the 28Fr DLT as it has a narrow point at the junction with the connector.

PRACTICAL GUIDE FOR CHOOSING SLV TUBES

A guide to tube selection for SLV in children has been devised by Hammer and colleagues [38]. In children up to age 6 years the only practical techniques are a single-lumen bronchial intubation either with or without a bronchial blocker. Over 6 years of age, the 3.5 uncuffed Univent tube with an OD of 7.5 mm can be used (the OD is equivalent to that of uncuffed TT of 5.5 mm [ID]). The smallest commercial DLTs start from size 26Fr from Rusch and 28Fr from Portex and Broncho-Cath; the 28Fr has an OD of over 10 mm at the cuff and this is equivalent to a 7.5 mm [ID] cuffed oral TT (10.3 mm OD). Consequently the 28Fr DLTs are suitable only for children over 12 years of age.

MANAGEMENT OF HYPOXIA AND HYPERCAPNIA

In practice, the major remediable causes of hypoxia during SLV are under-ventilation, bronchial tube malposition, obstruction from secretions or actions of the surgeon [60]. Table 39.2 shows the steps that may fix the problem. It must be remembered that low cardiac output will exacerbate shunt so that it is important to pay attention to intravascular volume and cardiac function. For lung resection, clamping the pulmonary artery or its branches will instantly decrease shunt.

Hypercapnia is less common and, provided that oxygen saturations remain high, it is of secondary importance. Capnography may indicate hypercapnia but arterial carbon dioxide tension should be measured regularly. High carbon dioxide levels should not be reduced too quickly when the lungs are reinflated. If, after resection, the remaining lung function is borderline the child may need a period of mechanical ventilation support.

Thoracoscopy and video–assisted thoracic surgery

When thoracoscopy was developed, instruments were adapted from other specialties and surgery was limited to biopsy. Now the instruments are purpose-made enabling video-assisted thoracic surgery (VATS) for almost every type of thoracic problem [61] (Table 39.3). The impetus for minimally invasive surgery came from the desire to minimise surgical trauma. Extensive thoracic surgery causes not only immediate pain and morbidity but also other longer-term changes such as scoliosis, muscle girdle weakness and chronic chest wall pain.

Successful surgery needs a high-quality view for the operator. To this end, the major anaesthetic issues relate to providing a relatively still field by using either one-lung ventilation or the insufflation of CO_2 (or both). Once the chest is open, the lung should collapse away from the chest wall to allow surgical view and access – low pulmonary inflation pressures and long expiratory times help to minimise expansion. Thoracoscopy can be achieved with low insufflation pressures or without any inflation pressure at all. Successful SLV makes insufflation of CO_2 unnecessary.

There are risks from CO_2 insufflation. It depresses cardiopulmonary function by increasing intrathoracic pressure,

Table 39.2 Useful steps to treat hypoxia during single lung ventilation

1. Increase inspired oxygen to 100%
2. Check what the surgeon is doing
3. Check the endobronchial/TT position by auscultation or bronchoscopy
4. Suction TT
5. Optimise ventilation to the dependent lung (optimise FRC)
   a. Increase the inspiratory pressure and consequently tidal volume
   b. Alter I:E ratios
   c. Apply 5 cm of PEEP to the dependent lung
6. Oxygenate the operated lung
   a. Insufflating oxygen
   b. Apply 5 cm of CPAP
   c. Intermittently ventilate the operated lung

CPAP, continuous positive airway pressure; FRC, functional residual capacity; I:E ratio, the ratio of inspiratory phase time to expiratory phase time; PEEP, positive end-expiratory pressure; TT, tracheal tube.

Table 39.3 Thoracoscopic procedures performed in children

	Procedure
Pulmonary	Lobectomy
	Decortication
	Cyst excision
Vascular	Aortopexy
	Thoracic duct ligation
	Pericardial window
Oesophageal	Atresia and fistula repair
	Foregut duplication resection
	Myotomy
Spinal	Anterior fusion
Lymphoid	Thymectomy
	Mediastinal mass excision
Other	Sympathectomy
	Diaphragmatic hernia/plication

compressing the central veins and so decreasing venous return. Pulmonary collapse adds to the respiratory acidosis and this can increase pulmonary vascular resistance. To minimise these effects CO_2 should be added slowly, at 1 L/min to a pressure limit of 4–6 mmHg [62]. Cardiovascular changes need to be closely observed and treated with volume loading and occasionally by inotropic support.

Insufflation of CO_2 also risks gas embolism [63], caused by accidental direct insufflation either into a vessel or into a torn pleural vessel. Early detection (usually by capnography, direct arterial blood pressure and pulse oximetry) is the key to a successful outcome. Transoesophageal echocardiography and precordial Doppler are the most sensitive detectors [64] but are not widely available or practical. A 'millwheel' murmur heard on a precordial stethoscope is pathognomonic. If detected, the surgeon must stop insufflation and release the thoracic gas, and the anaesthetist must administer 100 per cent oxygen and support the circulation. The left lateral head-down position [65] is ideal but may not be practical. Fortunately, CO_2 is rapidly absorbed and problems usually resolve quickly. If the foramen ovale is patent paradoxical arterial embolism is possible.

MEDIASTINAL SURGERY

The mediastinum lies between the pleurae, behind the sternum and in front of the vertebra and it contains all of the thoracic viscera except the lungs. It is artificially divided into anterior, middle and posterior compartments based on the lateral chest radiograph (Fig. 39.2). One of the most challenging situations is anaesthesia in a patient with an anterior mediastinal mass.

Mediastinal masses in children can be neoplastic, infectious or congenital. In the anterior mediastinum the common lesions are found in the thymus and lymph glands; the common diseases are infectious adenopathy, lymphoma, leukaemia and germ-cell tumours such as teratoma. In the middle mediastinum adenopathy associated with infection, lymphoma, leukaemia and metastatic disease are commonest; bronchopulmonary foregut malformations are found here also. In the posterior mediastinum ganglion cell tumours such as neuroblastoma, ganglioneuroma and ganglioneuroblastoma are found [66].

Any patient with a large mediastinal mass, especially in the anterior mediastinum, must be managed with great caution. The mass can compress the trachea and bronchi (commonly at the carina) which can be assessed by CT. The central veins may be obstructed – particularly the pulmonary veins, which can be compressed by minor postural changes leading to sudden cardiac arrest. Consequently, inducing anaesthesia in the supine position may lead to complete obstruction of the airway [67] while positive pressure ventilation may cause hypotension by compression of major vessels [68]. Lack of symptoms does not ensure a safe anaesthetic [69] but airway symptoms and superior vena cava syndrome are both associated with the development of acute airway obstruction [70]. The risk of general anaesthesia needs to be balanced against the need for precise tissue diagnosis to guide chemotherapy.

Local anaesthesia and anxiolysis may be adequate to allow a biopsy and avoid the risks of general anaesthesia. Algorithms have been developed in some centres to minimise the risk (Fig. 39.3). The key principle is to use an anaesthetic technique that maintains spontaneous ventilation – muscle relaxation should be used with considerable caution, if at all. The lateral or semi-prone position is recommended and turning the patient to the prone position may be life saving. Overcoming tracheal obstruction may be possible with a rigid bronchoscope and if this fails cardiopulmonary bypass

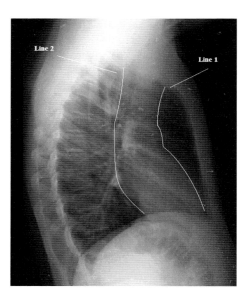

Figure 39.2 Lateral chest X-ray. Line 1 divides the anterior and middle mediastinum and is drawn along the anterior heart border and the brachiocephalic vessels. Line 2 divides the middle from the posterior mediastinum and is along the posterior heart border and trachea.

may be the only option [67]. Postoperative airway obstruction must be anticipated because bronchial or tracheal oedema can be provoked.

CORRECTION OF CHEST WALL DEFORMITY

Pathophysiology of chest wall lesions

Congenital deformities of the anterior chest wall are caused by an overgrowth or aplasia or dysplasia of the rib cartilages. Pectus excavatum is a sunken or funnel chest and accounts for over 80 per cent of cases. Pectus carinatum is a protuberant chest wall, sometimes referred to as a 'pigeon chest', and accounts for 5 per cent; the remainder are mixed deformities. Pectus excavatum occurs in about 1:1000 births and there is often a family history. There is also an association with connective tissue disorders such as Marfan syndrome, Ehlers–Danlos syndrome and scoliosis [71].

There is a spectrum of dysfunction ranging from none through to major respiratory limitation. Patients often have a poor body image and suffer socially [72] even though they have no physical dysfunction. The commonest symptoms are exercise limitation and dyspnoea. Other problems include frequent respiratory tract infections, asthma, cardiac compression or displacement leading to decreased cardiac output, mitral valve prolapse and conduction defects.

The ideal age for surgery is between 7 years and 14 years and a detailed evaluation should be undertaken. Mild cases

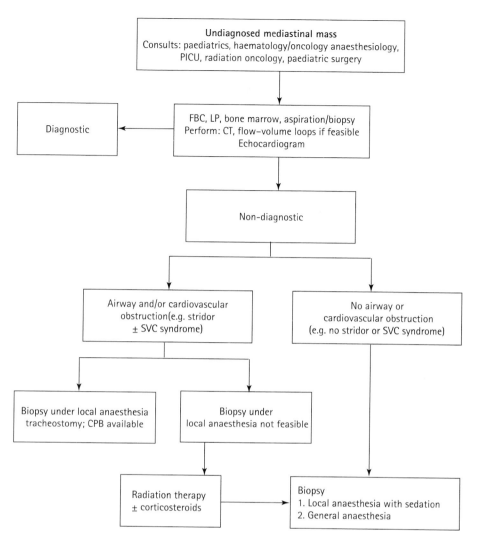

Figure 39.3 Guideline algorithm to manage patients with mediastinal masses in whom the diagnosis is unknown but must be determined before correct treatment can be started. CPB, cardiopulmonary bypass; CT, computed tomography; FBC, full blood count; LP, lumbar puncture; PICU, paediatric intensive care unit; SVC, superior vena cava. Modified with permission from Hammer [67].

are offered an exercise programme. More severe cases undergo extensive investigation including lung function tests and echocardiography. The need for repair is based on several criteria, including the pectus index of Haller [73].

There are two common operations for pectus excavatum: Ravitch (which is often modified) [74] and the more recently introduced minimally invasive procedure of Nuss [75]. In the Nuss procedure, a curved steel bar is inserted beneath the sternum and then rotated to raise and remodel the chest wall. The bar is endoscopically guided via small bilateral incisions in the midaxillary line at the level of T4–5.

Anaesthesia

PECTUS EXCAVATUM

Preoperatively the degree of physiological compromise should be assessed. The anaesthetic requires a conventional cuffed TT and gentle pulmonary inflation to help prevent the surgeon causing pneumothorax, haemothorax and haemomediastinum. Dysrhythmias, and even cardiac puncture, are possible and consequently intra-arterial blood pressure monitoring is essential [76]. Large-bore venous cannulae are necessary. Brachial plexus injuries can be avoided by not extending the arms excessively [77]. Postoperative pain is a major issue and a thoracic epidural with continuous postoperative infusion is recommended [78,79]; epidural or intravenous opioids are usually necessary in addition.

PECTUS CARINATUM

Pectus carinatum is predominately a cosmetic problem. Patients can develop respiratory symptoms but this is uncommon in childhood [80]. Associated conditions include mitral valve prolapse, kyphoscoliosis, Poland syndrome [81], neurofibromatosis, Morquio's disease and vertebral anomalies. Surgical treatment is by costochondral resection with sternotomy [71].

POSTOPERATIVE CARE

Chest tube management

The goal of pleural drainage is to keep the pleural space empty of air, blood or any other fluid. This promotes lung expansion and venous return, and maintains mediastinal position [82]. The drainage system consists of a tube, a unidirectional valve (usually an underwater seal) and a collection container. The tube, usually inserted at the end of surgery, may be either apical or basal. A respiratory swing confirms that the tube is patent and within the pleural space. The smallest tubes that are adequate for the task are best; they cause less pain although they can kink and are less effective at draining thicker effusions [83]. Modern systems have a collection container placed between the tube and the underwater seal drain. The underwater seal bottle must be kept below chest level at all times. The tube in the underwater seal lies 1–2 cm below the water's surface because this creates minimal resistance to air escaping. It is common practice to apply low-level suction of 5–10 cmH$_2$O to the drain. Suction is contraindicated following pneumonectomy because it can cause marked mediastinal shift, which can kink the major vessels leading to cardiovascular collapse. Bubbles indicate that air is escaping from the pleural space and, as the pleural space has negative pressure, bubbles usually escape only during positive pressure from coughing or straining such as a Valsalva manoeuvre. If the child is on positive pressure ventilation the drain must never be clamped because a tension pneumothorax will quickly develop [84].

There are several problems with drain systems. They need constant attention, they can block and be knocked over, are painful and decrease patient mobilisation. There should always be a positive reason to insert the drain and it should be removed sooner rather than later [85]. Serious complications of tube removal are unlikely but include recurrence of pneumothorax and vagal reflex bradycardia [86].

Postoperative analgesia

Acute pain following thoracotomy is acknowledged to be among the worst possible and can develop into chronic pain for 25–67 per cent of adult patients [87]. Chronic pain may be reduced by prolonged effective analgesia. Surgical trauma can also be reduced by using smaller, muscle-sparing incisions and thoracoscopy [88].

Unfortunately, any benefit of pre-emptive analgesia has been disappointing: pain relief does not seem to outlast the expected analgesic effect. This may be due to a wound's ability to generate pain and points to the importance of the duration of treatment and multimodal analgesia. A typical approach would be to combine a regional technique with a low-dose opioid infusion or patient-nurse-controlled analgesia (PCA/NCA, respectively) combined with paracetamol and non-steroidal anti-inflammatory drugs.

The removal of chest drains is very painful and can usually be managed with a combination of opioid and midazolam. Inhaled nitrous oxide alone can be useful in cooperative children. Occasionally, ketamine or anaesthesia is necessary (see Chapter 44 for more details).

REGIONAL ANALGESIA

Several different regional blocks have been recommended for thoracic surgery.

Intrapleural infusion, via a catheter, has a rapid onset [89] but some studies have shown it to be ineffective perhaps because of non-pleural pain (from chest drain sites) and the presence of fluid within the space [90]. Intrapleural infusions also result in higher plasma levels of local anaesthetic [91] than other regional blocks.

Intercostal nerve blocks by 'single shot' may cover a small incision such as a chest tube site but are insufficient for the prolonged pain from more extensive wounds. It has become popular to place a subpleural catheter at the time of surgery and, positioned at the medial aspect of the incision, local anaesthesia may reach the paravertebral space [92]. Plasma levels rise rapidly and by 10 minutes after an injection of 1.5 mg/kg of bupivacaine a blood level can reach 0.87 μg/mL [93]; to delay systemic absorption it has been recommended that bolus injections should be slow and that adrenaline (at least 1:400 000) should be added.

Paravertebral bolus injections and infusions are effective because local anaesthesia will bathe several intercostal nerves. A paravertebral catheter can be inserted percutaneously either before or after surgery [94].

Extradural analgesia has the potential to provide near perfect analgesia. Several series describe its use in infants [95,96]. To be effective, the local anaesthetic must be delivered to the dermatome level of the surgery and appropriate levels can be reached by inserting and passing catheters from the caudal or lumbar routes, or directly at the thoracic level. Radiographs can confirm placement. In a study of 86 caudal catheters in infants less than 6 months old, only 67 per cent of catheter tips where considered to be optimally placed; 12 per cent were too high, 20 per cent were coiled at the lumbosacral level and one was completely outside the epidural space [97]. Ultrasound [98], electrical stimulation [99] and ECG [100] have also been used as a guide to correct placement. Ultrasound is useful in infants less than 6 months of age before the posterior elements of the spine calcify. Electrical stimulation techniques will guide to the desired level but not absolutely confirm placement within the epidural space. The commonest problem is analgesia failure due to either incorrect placement or correct placement but partial block. Extradural additives may be very helpful to intensify and prolong the effects of local anaesthesia [101].

General care

After thoracic surgery pulmonary complications are common and should be anticipated. Continuous positive pressure and other forms of non-invasive ventilation may be necessary. The likelihood of sputum retention, collapse and consolidation with infection can all be reduced by effective analgesia to allow chest expansion and coughing. Appropriate chest physiotherapy, bronchodilators and antibiotics are very important. Oxygen therapy is tolerated best via nasal specula. Pulse oximetry is essential and can be used to monitor the trend in oxygen requirement and respiratory function; capnography via nasal cannulae may also have a useful role.

REFERENCES

Key references

Hammer GB. Anaesthetic management for the child with a mediastinal mass. *Paediatr Anaesth* 2004; **14**: 95–7.

Hammer GB, Fitzmaurice BG, Brodsky JB. Methods for single lung ventilation in pediatric patients. *Anesth Analg* 1999; **89**: 1426–9.

Morrison RR, Kiker MS, Baum VC. What happens when chest tubes are removed in children? *Pediatr Crit Care Med* 2001; **2**(1): 17–19.

Patankar SS. Single lung ventilation in young children: Practical tips on conventional cuffed endotracheal tubes for VATS. *Anesth Analg* 2000; **91**(1): 248.

Wald SH, Mahajan A, Kaplan MB, Atkinson JB. Experience with the Arndt paediatric bronchial blocker. *Br J Anaesth* 2005; **94**(1): 92–94.

References

1. Shanmugam G, MacArthur K, Pollock JC. Congenital lung malformations – antenatal and postnatal evaluation and management. *Eur J Cardiothorac Surg* 2005; **27**: 45–52.
2. Stocker JT, Madewell JE, Drake RM. Congenital cystic adenomatoid malformation of the lung: classification and morphological spectrum. *Hum Pathol* 1977; **8**: 155–71.
3. Davenport M, Warne SA, Cacciaguerra S et al. Current outcome of antenatally diagnosed cystic lung disease. *J Pediatr Surg* 2004; **39**(4): 549–56.
4. Paterson A. Imaging evaluation of congenital lung abnormalities in infants and children. *Radiol Clin North Am* 2005; **43**: 303–23.
5. Corbett HJ, Humphrey GME. Pulmonary sequestration. *Paediatr Respir Rev* 2004; **5**(1): 59–68.
6. Langston C. New concepts in the pathology of congenital lung malformations. *Semin Pediatr Surg* 2003; **12**(1): 17–37.
7. Özçelik U, Göçmen A, Kiper N et al. Congenital lobar emphysema: evaluation and long-term follow up of thirty cases at a single center. *Pediatr Pulmonol* 2003; **35**: 384–91.
8. Strollo DC, Rosado-de-Christenson ML, Jett JR. Primary mediastinal tumors Part II. Tumors of the middle and posterior mediastinum. *Chest* 1997; **112**(5): 1344–57.
9. Cohen MC, Kaschuala RO. Primary pulmonary tumors in childhood: a review of 31 years' experience and the literature. *Pediatr Pulmonol* 1992; **14**(4): 222–32.
10. Cowles RA, Lelli JL, Takayasu J, Coran AG. Lung Resection in infants and children with pulmonary infections refractory to medical therapy. *J Pediatr Surg* 2002; **37**(4): 643–7.
11. Goldschlager T, Frawley G, Crameri J et al. Comparison of open thoracoscopic drainage with open thoracotomy for the treatment of pediatric parapneumonic empyema. *Pediatr Surg Int* 2005; **21**: 599–603.
12. Eastham KM, Fall AJ, Mitchell L, Spencer DA. The need to redefine non-cystic fibrosis bronchiectasis in childhood. *Thorax* 2004; **59**: 324–7.
13. Ötgün İ, Karnak İ, Cahit Tanyel F et al. Surgical treatment of bronchiectasis in children. *J Pediatr Surg* 2004; **39**(10): 1532–6.
14. Durakbasa CU, Sander S, Sehiralti V et al. Pulmonary hydatid disease in children: outcome of surgical treatment combined with perioperative albendazole therapy. *Pediatr Surg Int* 2006; **22**(2): 173–8.
15. Parikh D, Samuel M. Congenital cystic lung lesions: is surgical resection essential? *Pediatr Pulmonol* 2005; **40**: 533–7.
16. Stocks J. Infant respiratory function testing: is it worth all the effort? *Paediatr Anaesth* 2004; **14**(7): 537–40.
17. Gibson RL, Burns JL, Ramsey BW. Pathophysiology and management of pulmonary infections in cystic fibrosis. *Am J Respir Crit Care Med* 2003; **168**: 918–51.
18. Jöhr M. Is it time to question the routine use of anticholinergic agents in paediatric anaesthesia? *Paediatr Anaesth* 1999; **9**: 99–101.
19. Benumof J. *Anaesthesia for thoracic surgery*, 2nd edn. Philadelphia: WB Saunders, 1995.
20. Choudhry, D.K. Single-lung ventilation in pediatric anesthesia. *Anesthesiol Clin North Am* 2005; **23**: 693–708.
21. Heaf DP, Gordon I, Turner HM. Postural effects of gas exchange in infants. *N Engl J Med* 1983; **308**(25): 1505–8.
22. Watanabe S, Noguchi E, Yamada S et al. Sequential changes of arterial oxygen tension in the supine position during one lung ventilation. *Anesth Analg* 2000; **90**: 28–30.
23. Serafini G, Cornara G, Cavalloro F et al. Pulmonary atelectasis during paediatric anaesthesia: CT scan evaluation and effect of positive end expiratory pressure (PEEP). *Paediatr Anaesth* 1999; **9**: 225–8.
24. Brodsky JB. Approaches to hypoxaemia during single-lung ventilation. *Curr Opin Anesthesiol* 2001; **14**: 71–6.
25. Tsai B, Wang M, Turrentine M et al. Hypoxic pulmonary vasoconstriction in cardiothoracic surgery: Basic mechanisms to potential therapies. *Ann Thorac Surg* 2004; **78**: 360–8.
26. Groh J, Kuhnle GEH, Ney L et al. Effects of isoflurane on regional blood flow during one-lung ventilation *Br J Anaesth* 1995; **74**: 209–16.
27. Bindslev L, Jolin-Carlsson A, Santesson J, Gottlieb I. Hypoxic pulmonary vasoconstriction in man: effects of hyperventilation. *Acta Anaesthesiol Scand* 1985; **29**(5): 547–1.
28. Levin AI, Coetzee JF. Arterial oxygenation during one-lung anesthesia. *Anesth Analg* 2005; **100**: 12–14.

29. Silvia-Costa-Gomes T, Gallart L, Vallès J *et al.* Low- vs. high-dose almitrine combined with nitric oxide to prevent hypoxia during open-chest one-lung ventilation. *Br J Anaesth* 2005; **95**(3): 410–16.

30. Lopez-Lopez JR, Perez-Garcia MT, Canet E, Gonzalez C. Effects of almitrine bismesylate on the ionic currents of chemoreceptor cells from the carotid body. *Mol Pharmacol* 1998; **53**(2): 330–9.

31. Brodsky JB. The evolution of thoracic anaesthesia. *Thorac Surg Clin* 2005; **15**: 1–10.

32. Jöhr M, Berger TM. Paediatric anaesthesia and inhalation agents. *Best Pract Res Clin Anaesthesiol* 2005; **19**(3): 501–22.

33. Beck DH, Doepfmer UR, Sinemus C *et al.* Effects of sevoflurane and propofol on pulmonary shunt fraction during one-lung ventilation for thoracic surgery. *Br J Anaesth* 2001; **86**(1): 38–43.

34. Nakayama M, Murray PA. Ketamine preserves and propofol potentiates hypoxic pulmonary vasoconstriction compared with the conscious state in chronically instrumented dogs. *Anesthesiology* 1999; **91**(3): 760–71.

35. Szegedi LL. Pathophysiology of one-lung ventilation. *Anesthesiol Clin North Am* 2001; **19**(3): 435–3.

36. Marraro GA. Innovative practices of ventilatory support with pediatric patients. *Pediatr Crit Care Med* 2003; **4**(1): 8–20.

37. Potger KC, Elliot D. Reproducibility of central venous pressures in supine and lateral positions: a pilot evaluation of the phlebostatic axis in critically ill patients. *Heart Lung* 1994; **23**(4): 285–99.

38. Hammer GB, Fitzmaurice BG, Brodsky JB. Methods for single lung ventilation in pediatric patients. *Anesth Analg* 1999; **89**: 1426–9.

39. Brooks JG, Bustamante SA, Hilton S *et al.* Selective bronchial intubation for the treatment of severe localized pulmonary interstitial emphysema in newborn infants. *J Pediatr* 1977; **91**(4): 648–52.

40. Baraka A. Right-bevelled tube for selective bronchial intubation in a child undergoing right thoracotomy. *Paediatr Anaesth* 1996; **6**: 487–9.

41. Kubota H, Kubota Y, Toshiro T *et al.* Selective blind endobronchial intubation in children and adults. *Anesthesiology* 1987; **67**: 587–9.

42. Lammers CR, Hammer GB, Brodsky JB, Cannon WB. Failure to isolate the lungs with an endobronchial tube positioned in the bronchus. *Anesth Analg* 1997; **85**: 944–5.

43. Patankar SS. Single lung ventilation in young children: practical tips on conventional cuffed endotracheal tubes for VATS. *Anesth Analg* 2000; **91**(1): 248.

44. Vale R. Selective bronchial blocking in a small child. *Br J Anaesth* 1969; **41**: 453–4.

45. Lines V. Selective bronchial blocking in a small child. *Br J Anaesth* 1969; **41**: 893.

46. Tan GM, Tan-Kendrick APA. Bronchial diameters in children – use of the Fogarty catheter for lung isolation in children. *Anaesth Intensive Care* 2002; **30**: 615–18.

47. Turner M, Buchanan C, Brown S. Paediatric one lung ventilation in the prone position. *Paediatr Anaesth* 1997; **7**: 427–9.

48. Borchardt RA, LaQuaglia MP, McDowall RH, Wilson RS. Bronchial injury during lung isolation in a pediatric patient. *Anesth Analg* 1998; **87**: 324–5.

49. Hammer GB, Harrison TK, Vricella LA *et al.* Single lung ventilation in children using a new paediatric bronchial blocker. *Paediatr Anaesth* 2002; **12**: 69–72.

50. Wald SH, Mahajan A, Kaplan MB, Atkinson JB. Experience with the Arndt paediatric bronchial blocker. *Br J Anaesth* 2005; **94**(1): 92–4.

51. Chen KP, Chan HC, Huang SJ. Foley catheter used as bronchial blocker for one lung ventilation in a patient with tracheostomy – a case report. *Acta Anaesthiol Sin* 1995; **33**(1): 41–4.

52. Hammer GB, Brodsky JB, Redpath JH, Cannon WB. The Univent tube for single-lung ventilation in paediatric patients. *Paediatr Anaesth* 1998; **8**: 55–7.

53. Seymour AH, Prasad B, McKenzie RJ. Audit of double-lumen endobronchial intubation. *Br J Anaesth* 2004; **93**(4): 525–7.

54. Russell WJ, Strong TS. Dimensions of double-lumen tracheobronchial tubes. *Anaesth Intensive Care* 2003; **31**: 50–3.

55. Slinger P. Choosing the appropriate double-lumen tube: a glimmer of science comes to the dark art. Editorial. *J Cardiothorac Vasc Anesth* 1995; **9**: 117–18.

56. Pawar D, Marraro GA. One lung ventilation in infants and children: experience with Marraro double lumen tube. *Paediatr Anaesth* 2005; **15**: 204–8.

57. Brodsky JB, Lemmens JML. Left double-lumen tubes: clinical experience with 1,170 patients. *J Cardiothorac Vasc Anesth* 2003; **17**(3): 289–98.

58. Takita K, Morimoto Y, Kemmotsu O. The height based formula for prediction of left-sided double-lumen tracheal tube depth. *J Cardiothorac Vasc Anesth* 2003; **17**(3): 412–13.

59. Cohen E. Double-lumen tube position should be confirmed by fibreoptic bronchoscopy. *Curr Opin Anesthesiol* 2004; **17**: 1–6.

60. Conacher ID. 2000 – Time to apply Occam's razor to failure of hypoxic pulmonary vasoconstriction during one lung ventilation. *Br J Anaesth* 2000; **84**(4): 434–6.

61. Rothenberg SS. Thoracoscopy in infants and children: the state of the art. *J Pediatr Surg* 2005; **40**: 303–6.

62. Tobias JD. Anaesthesia for neonatal thoracic surgery. *Best Pract Res Clin Anaesthesiol* 2004; **18**(2): 303–20.

63. Tobias JD. Anaesthetic implications of thoracoscopic surgery in children. *Paediatr Anaesth* 1999; **9**: 103–10.

64. Jersenius U, Fors D, Rubertsson S, Arvidsson D. The effects of experimental venous carbon dioxide embolization on hemodynamic and respiratory variables. *Acta Anaesthesiol Scand* 2006; **50**: 156–62.

65. Coulter TD, Wiedemann HP. Gas embolism. *N Engl J Med* 2000; **342**(26): 2000.

66. Franco A, Mody NS, Meza MP. Imaging evaluation of pediatric mediastinal masses. *Radiol Clin North Am* 2005; **43**: 325–53.

67. Hammer GB. Anaesthetic management for the child with a mediastinal mass. *Paediatr Anaesth* 2004; **14**: 95–7.

68. Luckhaupt-Koch K. Mediastinal mass syndrome. *Paediatr Anaesth* 2005; **15**: 437–8.

69. Viswanathan S, Campbell CE, Cork RC. Asymptomatic undetected mediastinal mass: a death during ambulatory anaesthesia. *J Clin Anesth* 1995; **7**(2): 151–5.

70. Lam JCM, Chui CH, Jacobsen AS *et al*. When is a mediastinal mass critical in a child? An analysis of 29 patients. *Pediatr Surg Int* 2004; **20**: 180–4.

71. Goretsky MJ, Kelly RE Jr, Croitoru D, Nuss D. Chest wall anomalies: pectus excavatum and pectus carinatum. *Adolesc Med* 2004; **15**: 455–71.

72. Lawson ML, Cash TF, Akers RA *et al*. A pilot study of the impact of surgical repair on disease – specific quality of life among patients with pectus excavatum. *J Pediatr Surg* 2003; **38**: 916–18.

73. Haller JA, Kramer SS, Lietman SA. Use of CT scans in selection of patients for pectus excavatum surgery: a preliminary report. *J Pediatr Surg* 1987; **22**: 904–6.

74. Fonkalsrund EW, Dunn JCY, Atkinson JB. Repair of pectus excavatum deformities: 30 years of experience with 375 patients. *Ann Surg* 2000; **231**(3): 443–8.

75. Nuss D, Kelly RE Jr, Croitoru DP, Katz ME. A 10 year evaluation of a minimally invasive technique for the correction of pectus excavatum. *J Pediatr Surg* 1998; **33**(4): 545–52.

76. Futagawa K, Suwa I, Okuda T *et al*. Anesthetic management for the minimally invasive Nuss procedure in 21 patients with pectus excavatum. *J Anesth* 2006; **20**(1): 48–50.

77. Fox ME, Bemsard DD, Roaten JB, Hendrickson RJ. Positioning for the Nuss procedure: avoiding brachial plexus injury. *Paediatr Anaesth* 2005; **15**: 1067–71.

78. McBride WJ, Dicker R, Abajian JC, Vane DW. Continuous thoracic epidural infusions for postoperative analgesia after pectus deformity repair. *J Pediatr Surg* 1996; **31**(1): 105–7.

79. Barros F. Continuous thoracic epidural analgesia with 0.2 per cent ropivacaine for pectus excavatum repair in children. *Paediatr Anaesth* 2004; **14**: 192–4.

80. Fonkalsrud EW, Beanes S. Surgical management of pectus carinatum 30 years experience. *World J Surg* 2001; **25**(7): 898–903.

81. Fokin A, Robicsek F. Poland's syndrome revisited. *Ann Thorac Surg* 2002; **74**: 2218–25.

82. Kam AC, O'Brien M, Kam PC. Pleural drainage systems. *Anaesthesia* 1993; **48**(2): 154–61.

83. Roberts JS, Bratton SL, Brogan TV. Efficacy and complications of percutaneous pigtail catheters for thoracostomy in pediatric patients. *Chest* 1998; **114**: 1116–21.

84. Laws D, Neville E, Duffy J. British thoracic society guidelines for the insertion of a chest drain. *Thorax* 2003; **58**(suppl II): ii53–9.

85. Waldhausen JH, Cusick RA, Graham DD *et al*. Removal of chest tubes in children without water seal after elective thoracic procedures: a randomized prospective study. *J Am Coll Surg* 2002; **194**(4): 411–15.

86. Morrison RR, Kiker MS, Baum VC. What happens when chest tubes are removed in children? *Pediatr Crit Care Med* 2001; **2**(1): 17–19.

87. Tiippana E, Nilsson E, Kalso E. Post-thoracotomy pain after epidural analgesia: a prospective follow-up study. *Acta Anaesthesiol Scand* 2003; **47**: 433–8.

88. Conacher ID. Post-thoracotomy analgesia. *Anesthesiol Clin North Am* 2001; **19**(3): 611–25.

89. Semsroth M, Plattner O, Horcher E. Effective pain relief with continuous intrapleural bupivacaine after thoracotomy in infants and children. *Paediatr Anaesth* 1996; **6**(4): 303–10.

90. Silomon M, Claus T, Huwer H *et al*. Interpleural analgesia does not influence post-thoracotomy pain. *Anesth Analg* 2000; **91**(1): 44–50.

91. McIlvaine WB, Chang JH, Jones M. The effective use of intrapleural bupivacaine for analgesia after thoracic and subcostal incisions in children. *J Pediatr Surg* 1988; **23**(12): 1184–7.

92. Downs CS, Cooper MG. Continuous extrapleural intercostal nerve block for post-thoracotomy analgesia in children. *Anaesth Intensive Care* 1997; **25**(4): 390–7.

93. Bricker SRW, Telford RJ, Booker PD. Pharmacokinetics of bupivacaine following intraoperative Intercostal nerve block in neonates and in infants aged less than 6 months. *Anesthesiology* 1989; **70**(6): 942–7.

94. Cheung SLW, Booker PD, Franks R, Pozzi M. Serum concentrations of bupivacaine during prolonged continuous paravertebral infusion in young infants. *Br J Anaesth* 1997; **79**: 9–13.

95. Murrell D, Gibson PR, Cohen RC. Continuous epidural analgesia in newborn infants undergoing major surgery. *J Pediatr Surg* 1993; **28**: 548–53.

96. Bösenberg AT. Epidural analgesia for major neonatal surgery. *Paediatr Anaesth* 1998; **8**: 479–83.

97. Valairucha S, Seefelder C, Houck C. Thoracic epidural catheters placed by the caudal route in infants: the importance of radiographic confirmation. *Paediatr Anaesth* 2002; **12**: 424–8.

98. Chawathe MS, Jones RM, Gildersleve CD *et al*. Detection of epidural catheters with ultrasound in children. *Paediatr Anaesth* 2003; **13**: 681–4.

99. Tsui BCH, Wagner A, Cave D, Kearney R. Thoracic and lumbar epidural analgesia via the caudal approach using electrical stimulation guidance in pediatric patients: a review of 289 patients. *Anesthesiology* 2004; **100**: 683–9.

100. Tsui BCH, Seal R, Koller J. Thoracic epidural placement via the caudal approach in infants by using electrocardiographic guidance. *Anesth Analg* 2002; **95**: 326–30.

101. de Beer DA, Thomas ML. Caudal additives in children – solutions or problems? *Br J Anaesth* 2003; **90**(4): 487–9.

40

Cardiac surgery including transplantation

ANGUS McEWAN

KEY LEARNING POINTS

- For children with congenital heart disease, a good understanding of the anatomy and physiology of the lesion is essential for safe anaesthesia.
- Although there are an almost infinite variety of anatomical variations in congenital heart disease, these can be resolved to a small number of physiological correlates.
- Safe anaesthesia depends more on meticulous planning and attention to detail than the specific agent used.

- The site of placement of invasive monitoring catheters will depend on the anatomical lesion and the planned surgery.
- Corrective surgery for congenital heart disease is often staged and the anaesthetic plan for each stage should include consideration of the implications for further stages with particular regard to the preservation of vascular access sites.
- Coagulopathy is common during neonatal cardiac surgery and its treatment requires a multi-modal approach.

INTRODUCTION

Paediatric cardiology and cardiac surgery are a rapidly developing specialty and recently have seen significant advances in both the diagnosis and the treatment of children with congenital heart disease (CHD). Increasingly, diagnostic information is obtained from magnetic resonance imaging (MRI), computed tomography (CT) and echocardiography with less reliance on cardiac angiography. Many patients who would previously have been treated surgically are now treated in the angiography suite with interventional procedures. This has meant that for some patients treatment has been much less invasive, avoiding the need for surgery, cardiopulmonary bypass and long hospital stays, but has resulted in a 'risk transfer' from cardiac theatres to the angiography suite. While more interventional procedures take place in the angiography suite, preoperative diagnosis is primarily with echocardiography and MRI. In addition the advances in foetal echocardiography have led to an increase in antenatal diagnosis of CHD [1]. Furthermore cardiac lesions are corrected earlier in life, many undergoing surgery in the neonatal period [2]. In general, about 50 per cent of those undergoing cardiac surgery are less than 1 year of age and about 25 per cent are less than 1 month.

INCIDENCE OF CONGENITAL HEART DISEASE

The reported incidence of CHD is in the region of 6–8 per 1000 live births. Children with trisomy 21 (Down Syndrome) have a higher incidence of CHD, as do those with other chromosomal abnormalities or congenital syndromes. Having an affected sibling or parent increases the likelihood of CHD, as does the presence of coexisting congenital abnormalities.

As more children with CHD survive into adulthood, a new specialty of 'grown-up congenital heart disease' (GUCH) is emerging. In addition there are children with acquired heart disease or cardiomyopathy, and those who have undergone heart transplantation who require specialist care.

PREOPERATIVE EVALUATION

There are several aims of the preoperative visit, including medical assessment, premedication, formulating an anaesthetic plan, providing information and developing a relationship with the child and family

Medical assessment

Understanding the cardiac diagnosis, the planned surgery and associated pathophysiology is important (see Chapter 30 for further review of this subject). Diagnostic information is obtained from the patient record, including electrocardiogram (ECG), echocardiography, chest X-ray, cardiac catheter and MRI. These data may be summarised in reports from joint planning meetings. Previous operation reports, anaesthetic records or discharge summaries should be reviewed.

A directed history and physical examination should assess the child's general health and any associated conditions such as trisomy 21 or DiGeorge syndrome. Evaluation should include the degree of cardiac failure, the severity of cyanosis, and the presence of, or potential for, pulmonary hypertension or hypercyanotic 'spells'. Invasive monitoring will be needed; suitable routes should be assessed at his stage, as should the need for a re-do sternotomy which has implications for management (see below). Previous aprotinin administration should be noted as re-exposure increases the risk of anaphylaxis [3].

A history of upper respiratory tract infection (URTI) or other febrile illness should be sought, though the decision to proceed with cardiac surgery is difficult if one is identified. Children with cardiac failure are prone to URTIs and may have signs that can mimic a URTI. Moreover, surgery may be relatively urgent; postponement may carry its own risks. One study showed that cardiac surgery in children with a URTI resulted in a longer intensive care unit (ICU) stay and ventilation times, although overall hospital stay was not prolonged [4]. There was an increased incidence of bacterial infections and pulmonary atelectasis. While there was a higher mortality in the URTI group (4.2 per cent)

compared with the non-URTI group (1.6 per cent), it was not statistically significant [4].

Premedication

Sedative premedication can be useful in cardiac anaesthesia but practice varies widely. It is probably unnecessary in infants aged less than 4 weeks but is not contraindicated. The author's preference is to avoid sedative premedication in children with severe heart failure. Crying and struggling during induction can increase cyanosis in patients with tetralogy of Fallot; they often benefit from sedation. Older children are frequently very anxious and premedication may help. Suggested drugs and doses are outlined in Table 40.1.

Topical anaesthetic creams are useful in all patients, even if gaseous induction is planned as intravenous access will be possible at a lighter plane of anaesthesia.

Giving information

Clear information on the perioperative process helps patients and parents deal with anxiety. Details of premedication, fasting times, mode of induction, monitoring, transfusion and ICU stay should be discussed. If a transoesophageal echocardiography probe is to be used this should be explained. Questions about the risk of anaesthesia, surgery or associated procedures often arise and should be answered honestly.

Creating a relationship with the child and family

Instilling confidence and developing a rapport with the child and family will help to alleviate anxiety.

Formulating an anaesthetic plan

Following assessment, it will be possible to formulate a detailed anaesthetic plan, which will also depend on the

Table 40.1 Suggested premedication for cardiac surgery

Age	Weight (kg)	Drug	Dose (mg/kg)	Comments
<4 weeks		No premed		EMLA or Ametop only
From 4 weeks	to 6	Triclofos	50–75	
	6–15	Triclofos	50–75	
	>15	Midazolam	0.5–1.0	Maximum 15 mg
		Temazepam	0.5–1.0	Maximum 20 mg

EMLA, eutectic mixture of local anaesthetics.

Table 40.2 Features of DiGeorge syndrome

- Absent or small thymus
- T-cell abnormality with associated immunodeficiency
- Hypoparathyroidism with associated hypocalcaemia
- Dysmorphic features, particularly small mouth
- Increased surgical morbidity and mortality
- Patients require irradiated blood products to prevent graft-versus-host disease

planned surgery. If there is an associated syndrome, this may influence management. For example, in trisomy 21 a smaller than usual tube may be required and care is needed when manipulating the neck during line insertion. In DiGeorge syndrome (Table 40.2) irradiated blood products should be ordered to prevent transfusion associated graft-versus-host disease.

Repeat sternotomy

Many children return for repeat surgery with reopening of a midline sternotomy. This may result in massive haemorrhage, particularly if there is a retrosternal conduit (e.g. after Rastelli's operation). Should this occur the surgeon will attempt to control the bleeding; simultaneously an assistant will cannulate the femoral or iliac artery which permits rapid transfusion from the bypass machine. Thereafter, when the patient is anticoagulated, pump suckers may be used as an autotransfusion system.

Consequently, before incision, the anaesthetist must ensure that the patient is prepared with the iliofemoral vessels available for immediate arterial cannulation, heparin (300 IU/kg) is drawn up and blood is available immediately. In addition, internal defibrillation will not be possible until the pericardial dissection is complete, so external defibrillator pads should be applied. Antifibrinolytics are often given but aprotinin should not be repeated within 6 months.

ANAESTHETIC TECHNIQUE FOR SURGERY REQUIRING CARDIOPULMONARY BYPASS

Induction

In most conditions, induction of anaesthesia for cardiac surgery may be intravenous or inhalational [5]. In general, older children and those with cyanotic disease have good veins and it is most appropriate to use an intravenous (IV) induction. In small infants without venous access and those on diuretic therapy it is often easier to opt for a gas induction. Practice, however, varies widely between individual anaesthetists and institutions.

Intravenous induction agents

ETOMIDATE

Etomidate has a good cardiovascular safety profile (LD_{50}: ED_{50} of 26). It has little effect on the cardiovascular system whether the patient is healthy or has cardiac disease. Although useful in patients with severe cardiac disease it causes pain on injection and dose-dependent adrenal suppression, and is not available in some countries.

KETAMINE

Ketamine increases blood pressure, heart rate and cardiac output. It is thought to stimulate the release of endogenous catecholamine stores. It is a negative inotrope in the denervated heart [6] so, theoretically, it has limitations in patients in whom endogenous catecholamine stimulation may already be maximal such as those with severe cardiomyopathy. It may also be a poor choice when tachycardia is undesirable (e.g. aortic stenosis). It can be given intramuscularly, which makes it useful in some situations.

FENTANYL

Fentanyl is haemodynamically stable. When given in high doses it may cause bradycardia and/or chest wall rigidity but this is irrelevant when it is used in association with pancuronium. It is not used alone for induction but allows a reduced dose of IV induction agent or sedative.

PROPOFOL

Propofol is frequently used in older children with stable haemodynamics. It causes a dose-dependent decrease in arterial pressure from a reduction in systemic vascular resistance (SVR). In patients with a fixed cardiac output, such as from severe aortic or mitral stenosis, this may result in profound hypotension.

THIOPENTAL

Thiopental also causes a dose-dependent decrease in blood pressure owing to a reduction in SVR, but to a lesser extent than propofol. It may result in prolonged sedation of neonates and small infants, but this is not relevant in long cases or when postoperative intermittent positive pressure ventilation (IPPV) is planned. Absence of pain on injection makes it useful for induction through long-standing peripheral cannulae.

Volatile anaesthetic agents

SEVOFLURANE

Sevoflurane is the volatile agent of choice for induction because it is rapidly acting and non-irritant. Bradycardia, hypotension and respiratory depression will occur with overdose; the minimum concentration required to facilitate vascular access should be used. After intubation a low dose of volatile agent in air/O_2 is given by IPPV. Microbubbles of air are common during bypass and the differential solubility of nitrous oxide and nitrogen increases their size. Accordingly N_2O is generally avoided. Inhalational induction may be prolonged in children with right-to-left shunts but, in practice, this is not clinically relevant.

Muscle relaxants and intubation

A range of muscle relaxants has been used. Pancuronium is popular because its vagolytic and sympathomimetic actions counteract fentanyl-induced bradycardia. If early extubation is planned, atracurium is usual. In neonates and smaller children nasal intubation is common as this is easier to manage in the ICU. In older children, if cuffed tubes are used or in those in whom early extubation is planned oral intubation is more usual.

Monitoring

As far as possible, monitoring should commence prior to induction, including ECG, pulse oximetry and non-invasive blood pressure. Following induction, continuous end-tidal CO_2 monitoring commences, remembering that the measured end-tidal carbon dioxide concentration in expired air ($P_{ET}CO_2$) will be less than the partial pressure of arterial CO_2 ($PaCO_2$) in patients with a right-to-left intracardiac shunt.

ADDITIONAL MONITORING

Central venous pressure (CVP) can be measured from many sites, including the internal jugular, femoral, subclavian or umbilical vein. Where possible, avoid central venous access in veins draining through the superior vena cava in children who will require cavopulmonary connections. The use of ultrasound to guide placement of central lines is becoming routine. Generally multilumen catheters are used. Strict aseptic technique is essential as line sepsis is an important cause of postoperative morbidity [7]. The use of heparin-bonded lines or antibiotic-coated lines reduces the risk of line-related sepsis and heparin-bonded lines may also reduce the risk of line-related thrombosis. Some units avoid percutaneous central access preferring to use surgically placed atrial lines. Pulmonary artery flotation catheters are seldom used in children but other pressure monitoring lines may be inserted by the surgeon (e.g. left atrial or pulmonary arterial).

Direct arterial pressure is usually measured from the radial, femoral or axillary arteries. The brachial artery should be avoided as this is an end-artery. Vessels distal to systemic-to-pulmonary artery shunts should be avoided. In neonates 24Fr cannulae are generally used for the radial artery.

A 22Fr cannulae can be used in other sites. Arterial lines should be flushed with small volumes and slow rates of injection and great care should be taken to avoid air injection.

Nasopharyngeal temperature is commonly used to estimate brain temperature. Skin temperature is also measured. All bypass cases require urinary catheterisation, but this may not be necessary in 'closed' cases such as shunts and pulmonary artery banding.

Other monitors

Transoesophageal echocardiography is increasingly available perioperatively in paediatric cardiac surgery (see page 603).

NEAR-INFRARED SPECTROSCOPY

Near-infrared spectroscopy (NIRS) is an absorption spectrographic method of measuring cerebral oxygenation. It may detect episodes of cerebral deoxygenation, particularly during bypass, but since normal levels of cerebral oxygenation have not been determined in neonates and small infants it is not clear which levels are critical in terms of cerebral damage. In children with CHD, so-called normal values may differ from those of healthy children [8,9].

TRANSCRANIAL DOPPLER

Transcranial Doppler (TCD) measures cerebral blood flow velocity, usually in the middle cerebral artery, and is able to detect microemboli in the cerebral circulation. Like NIRS, interpretation is limited by the lack of normal data but it has the potential to detect inadequate flow during bypass [10,11].

BISPECTRAL INDEX ANALYSIS MONITOR

The Bispectral Index (BIS) analysis monitor is used to determine depth of anaesthesia. It has been advocated for monitoring depth of anaesthesia during cardiopulmonary bypass (CPB) in children [12,13].

MANAGEMENT OF CARDIOPULMONARY BYPASS IN CHILDREN

Before commencement of CPB, antibiotics are given according to local protocols, and a blood sample is taken for baseline activated coagulation time (ACT) and blood gas analysis. Heparinisation is with 3 or 4 mg/kg (300–400 IU/kg) and is usually given at the request of the surgeon. The ACT after heparin should be at least three times baseline or greater than 400 seconds. If aprotinin is used the ACT should be a minimum of 480 seconds. Neonates may be relatively resistant to heparin because of low levels of antithrombin III and usually receive the higher dose. The ACT may also be affected by hypothermia and coagulopathy. Additional anaesthetic drugs are given at this time to allow adequate effect site concentrations before CPB.

Aspects of CPB

The heart is prepared for bypass by dissection, mobilisation and the insertion of cannulation purse strings. The surgeon will divide the bypass sash and following arterial cannulation the arterial limb of the bypass circuit is connected to the cannula. After de-airing, clamps are removed and the perfusionist checks the arterial cannula by measuring the pressure swing with cardiac systole and tests the circuit pressure response to a small transfusion. Venous line(s) are then inserted by the surgeon; the bypass circuit is completed by connection of these to the venous limb of the sash. Bi-caval cannulation (superior vena cava [SVC] and inferior vena cava [IVC]) is required for most paediatric surgery. The CPB commences and the perfusionist increases the flow rate until an average of 2.4–3.2 L/m^2/min is reached ('full flow').

Intermittent positive pressure ventilation is discontinued when full flow is established on CPB. With some lesions, there may be appreciable collateral flow to the pulmonary arteries, which will no longer be oxygenated once ventilation ceases. This is unlikely to be significant with full flow but may cause desaturation at lower flow rates. Anaesthesia can be continued by adding isoflurane into the pump sweep gas and giving bolus doses of fentanyl and midazolam. An alternative is to use a propofol/remifentanil infusion.

Hypotension after the start of bypass may be caused by haemodilution (the haematocrit should be maintained at about 30 per cent by ultrafiltration or the addition of packed cells to the CPB circuit), or the presence of collateral shunts to the lungs (e.g. patent ductus arteriosus [PDA], surgical shunt or pulmonary collateral artery). Such shunts should be ligated as soon as possible after the start of bypass. Once these two causes have been excluded, a vasoconstrictor such as phenylephrine 1–5 μg/kg or metaraminol 1–10 μg/kg is occasionally required to control hypotension resulting from low systemic vascular resistance.

Hypertension may indicate inadequate anaesthesia or analgesia, which should be treated accordingly. If hypertension persists a vasodilator such as phentolamine 1–5 μg/kg may be required.

For some operations surgery is performed on the beating heart but, for repair of most congenital heart disease, it is usually necessary for the heart to be stopped. This is achieved by the infusion of cold blood or (rarely now) crystalloid cardioplegia solution into the aortic root after cross-clamping the aorta. If the aortic valve is competent the coronaries will be effectively perfused but, if there is aortic regurgitation, flow into the coronaries will be inadequate, resulting in poor myocardial preservation. In this situation it is necessary to transect the aorta and selectively catheterise the coronary ostia. Infusion of cardioplegia is repeated every 20–30 minutes.

Activated coagulation time, blood gases and electrolytes are assessed regularly and potassium, calcium, bicarbonate and magnesium are assayed and replaced as necessary.

Hypothermia is used to protect the brain and other vital organs during CPB. For most surgery the core temperature is maintained at 28–32°C. In some centres there is a trend towards bypass at warmer temperatures (32–34°C). For more complex longer operations, or where reduced CPB flow rates may be needed to facilitate the intracardiac repair, lower temperatures are used (25–28°C). Some operations will require deep hypothermic circulatory arrest (DHCA), when the core temperature is lowered to 16–18°C. These may include repair of interrupted aortic arch, neonatal repair of total anomalous venous drainage, the aortic arch repair associated with the Norwood procedure and difficult repairs in very small infants [14]. Generally, DHCA is used sparingly and for as short a period as possible because it is associated with adverse neurological outcomes. Significant neurodevelopmental changes, including lower IQ, may occur after 30 minutes of DHCA [15,16]. This may be ameliorated by maintaining the haematocrit at 30 per cent [17,18] and providing adequate cerebral cooling (perfusion at target temperature for 10–15 minutes before stopping the circulation) and topical cooling of the head. There is no good evidence that steroids improve neurological outcome after DHCA.

PERIOPERATIVE TRANSOESOPHAGEAL ECHOCARDIOGRAPHY

Perioperative transoesophageal echocardiography (TOE) is becoming routine. It has become the standard of care in the USA [19]. Appropriate training and the availability of equipment are key to the successful use of this technology [20]. In some centres the echo examinations are undertaken by anaesthetists but in others these examinations are performed by cardiologists. Perioperative TOE in children is not yet routine in Europe despite evidence of clinical and cost-effectiveness [21,22], yet with adequate training and adherence to published guidelines it may favourably influence surgical and medical management [22,23].

Although the use of TOE in children is generally safe there is an incidence of complications of around 2 per cent [24]. These include damage to the mouth, oropharynx, oesophagus and stomach. Haemodynamic disturbance may result from compression of the left atrium or other structures. Interference with the airway, including inadvertent extubation, right main-stem intubation and compression of the tracheal tube, occurs in a small number of cases.

Transoesophageal echocardiography examination takes place both pre-bypass and post-bypass and falls broadly into two categories: haemodynamic assessment and structural diagnostic information. Haemodynamic assessment evaluates ventricular function and filling [25]. Diagnostic information involves confirmation (or otherwise) of preoperative findings and assessment of the adequacy of the surgical repair.

BLEEDING AFTER CARDIAC SURGERY IN CHILDREN

Bleeding after cardiac surgery contributes to postoperative morbidity including that related to the blood and blood products given. The coagulopathy that occurs during bypass in children is complex, multifactorial and more severe than that seen in adults. The degree of coagulopathy and haemorrhage after surgery is related to the patient's size and weight (Table 40.3) [26]. Severe coagulopathy and haemorrhage can be expected in those weighing <8 kg [27]. The primary defect results from haemodilution, most significantly in neonates and small infants, where a reduction in coagulation factors (fibrinogen 50 per cent and platelets 70 per cent) occurs on initiation of CPB. Antithrombin III is also reduced by about 50 per cent [27]. Coagulation factors and platelets are also consumed by activation of the inflammatory response [28]. Not only are platelets reduced in number but their structure is disrupted and their function impaired [29].

Inadequate heparin levels during CPB in children may also contribute to postoperative bleeding because suboptimal anticoagulation may allow activation of the haemostatic pathways. It has been shown that the ACT shows a poor correlation with heparin levels in children undergoing CPB [28,30] and in one study the use of heparin monitoring and heparin titration resulted in the use of larger doses of heparin but lower doses of protamine. Activation of clotting cascades was also reduced, resulting in less bleeding in the postoperative period [30].

Methods to reduce postoperative bleeding

ANTIFIBRINOLYTIC THERAPY

The antifibrinolytics used in paediatric cardiac surgery include ε-aminocaproic acid (EACA), tranexamic acid (TA) and aprotinin.

Both EACA and TA are lysine analogues that have been shown to reduce bleeding after cardiac surgery in adults and children [31,32]. They do not appear to have any anti-inflammatory activity. Although the optimum dose of TA for use in paediatric cardiac surgery has not been clearly established, a commonly used regimen is 10 mg/kg given at the commencement of surgery, into the pump and after separation from CPB.

Aprotinin is a serine protease inhibitor that is well studied in adults. It has been shown to reduce bleeding significantly, reduce the time taken to extubation, shorten ICU stay and reduce mortality in adults [33]. The same volume

Table 40.3   Features associated with increased risk of postoperative bleeding

- Decreasing age
- Decreasing size (<8 kg thought to be important)
- Preoperative cyanosis
- Preoperative heart failure
- Length of cardiopulmonary bypass
- Degree of hypothermia
- Re-do sternotomy

of evidence has not yet been produced in children although it may reduce bleeding, length of time on the ventilator and ICU stay [3,30,34–36]. It is possible that the doses used in paediatric studies do not take into account the large pump prime to blood volume difference that occurs when children are placed on the bypass circuit [37]. Mossinger has shown that, if a pump dose is given based on the prime volume rather than on the child's weight, plasma aprotinin levels are similar to those seen in adults; postoperative bleeding is reduced and lung function is improved with earlier extubation [37].

Aprotinin is expensive and there is a risk of anaphylaxis particularly with prior exposure and its re-use should probably be avoided within 6 months. There is also a concern that it may be associated with thrombosis and two large studies in adults undergoing coronary revascularisation surgery reported that the use of aprotinin was associated with significantly increased risk of renal failure, stroke and 5-year mortality [38,39]. Although there is no evidence to suggest that this is true in congenital cardiac surgery or in children, it should be used only when there is a clear benefit. More data on the risks and benefits of aprotinin in paediatric cardiac surgery are urgently required.

The topical delivery of the ingredients for clot formation is common in paediatric cardiac surgery. Significant reductions in bleeding have been claimed [40].

Ultrafiltration

Ultrafiltration is a process that removes water and electrolytes from the pump during CPB. Modified ultrafiltration (MUF) is the filtration of the patient's blood after termination of CPB. The latter's benefits include increased haematocrit, concentration of clotting factors and platelets, increased blood pressure for similar or reduced filling pressures, reduced pulmonary vascular resistance, removal of inflammatory mediators and significant reductions in bleeding [41,42].

CLASSIFICATION OF CONGENITAL HEART DISEASE (see also Chapter 30)

Congenital heart disease can be divided according to physiology into simple (left-to-right or right-to-left) shunts,

Table 40.4 Classification of congenital heart disease

'Simple' left-to-right shunt: increased pulmonary blood flow
- atrial septal defect
- ventricular septal defect
- patent ductus arteriosus
- endocardial cushion defect, e.g. atrioventricular septal defect
- aortopulmonary window (AP window)

'Simple' right-to-left shunt: decreased pulmonary blood flow with cyanosis
- tetralogy of Fallot
- pulmonary atresia
- tricuspid atresia
- Ebstein's anomaly

Complex shunts: mixing of pulmonary and systemic blood flow with cyanosis
- transposition of great arteries
- truncus arteriosus
- total anomalous pulmonary venous drainage
- double-outlet right ventricle
- hypoplastic left heart syndrome

Obstructive lesions
- aortic stenosis
- mitral stenosis
- pulmonary stenosis
- coarctation of aorta
- Interrupted aortic arch

Table 40.5 Clinical features of cardiac failure in children

- Failure to thrive
- Difficult feeding
- Breathlessness
- Recurrent chest infection
- Tachycardia
- Cardiac murmur
- Hepatomegaly
- Cardiomegaly
- Pulmonary plethora
- Wheezing

complex shunts or outflow tract obstruction (Table 40.4). This classification is useful as it also guides anaesthetic management.

'SIMPLE' LEFT–TO–RIGHT SHUNTS

These shunts result in increased pulmonary blood flow; Qp:Qs (ratio of pulmonary to systemic flow) can be as much as three to four times normal with volume loading of the right side of the heart. This in turn leads to right atrial enlargement and right ventricular hypertrophy perhaps associated with tricuspid and pulmonary regurgitation. This combination results in cardiac failure, the clinical features of which are listed in Table 40.5. The medical management of these children is primarily with diuretics, sometimes in combination with digoxin.

Untreated high pulmonary blood flow leads to pulmonary vascular disease and ultimately pulmonary hypertension. Early changes are reversible but in time may become irreversible [43,44]. Eisenmenger syndrome refers to severe pulmonary hypertension with suprasystemic pulmonary artery pressures and shunt reversal causing cyanosis – at this point the patient is inoperable. Increasingly, definitive surgery is being performed at a younger age to reduce the risk of pulmonary vascular disease; if this is not possible, a pulmonary

artery band is applied to reduce pulmonary blood flow so that definitive surgery can be postponed without the risk of developing pulmonary hypertension. This is usually performed though a sternotomy incision but without CPB. Significantly increased pulmonary blood flow (Qp:Qs > 2:1) leads to irreversible pulmonary vascular disease by the age of one year; definitive surgery should be performed between 3 months and 6 months to avoid this.

Atrial septal defect

Atrial septal defect is common, occurring in 1:1500 live births. It accounts for up to 10 per cent of all congenital heart disease and has several anatomical variants.

Patent foramen ovale (PFO) is the continuation of the normal foetal communication between the two atria which usually closes functionally soon after birth. In up to 30 per cent of adults the foramen ovale remains probe patent. Patent foramen ovale is usually left untreated in children. A *secundum* ASD is found in the region of the fossa ovalis and results from a deficiency in the septum secundum. A *primum* ASD is located in the inferior part of the atrial septum close to the atrioventricular (AV) valve and is a variant of atrioventricular septal defect (AVSD). A *sinus venosus* ASD occurs high in the atrial septum often close to the opening of the SVC and may be associated with partial anomalous pulmonary venous drainage. A *coronary sinus* ASD (unroofed coronary sinus) is a defect in the atrial wall which allows blood to flow from the left atrium to the right atrium through the coronary sinus. Finally, there may be a complete absence of the atrial septum (*common atrium*). The AV valves may be abnormal or unaffected.

Many ASDs can now be closed using a percutaneous, transcatheter device. Patent foramen ovales and secundum ASDs are most commonly closed using this technique. However, some children will still require surgical closure of the ASD.

ANAESTHETIC CONSIDERATIONS

These patients can frequently be 'fast tracked' and extubated on the operating table or early in the ICU and the opioid dose should be tailored accordingly. Alternatively, an infusion of remifentanil, possibly in combination with propofol, can be used.

Postoperative pulmonary hypertension is seldom encountered.

Ventricular septal defects

Ventricular septal defect (VSD) is the most common congenital defect in children, occurring in 1.5–3.5 per 1000 live births and accounts for 20 per cent of CHD in children [45]. Four types are described: subarterial (5 per cent), perimembranous (80 per cent), inlet (5 per cent) and muscular (10 per cent). If flow through the VSD is small it is referred to as 'restrictive' and if flow is large it is termed 'unrestrictive'. It is now possible to close a small number of VSDs using a percutaneous, transcatheter device.

ANAESTHETIC CONSIDERATIONS

These patients may need inotropic support postoperatively and should be observed for pulmonary hypertension, particularly those with unrestrictive VSDs. Complete heart block may occur, especially after repair of perimembranous VSDs as the conduction tissue is close to the surgical site.

Atrioventricular septal defect

Atrioventricular septal defects are also known as AV canal or endocardial cushion defects and result in deficiency of the atrial and ventricular septa and AV valves. They occur in about 0.2 per 1000 live births and account for about 2–3 per cent of CHD. They are commonly associated with trisomy 21 (Down Syndrome) and may be associated with other cardiac lesions such as tetralogy of Fallot and DiGeorge syndrome (see Table 40.2).

An AVSD may be partial (a primum ASD with a cleft in the anterior mitral valve leaflet) or complete (a large septal defect with both atrial and ventricular components and a common AV valve). The haemodynamic effects are primarily shunting at atrial or ventricular level and AV valve regurgitation.

ANAESTHETIC CONSIDERATIONS

These patients are frequently in cardiac failure preoperatively and may have repeated chest infections. If trisomy 21 is associated, the anaesthetic implications of this need to be managed. Good repair of the left AV valve is important and post-bypass echocardiography is helpful to assess this. Postoperatively, inotropes are frequently required and pulmonary hypertension may occur.

Patent ductus arteriosus

The ductus arteriosus is part of the foetal circulation and extends from the descending aorta to the main pulmonary artery and usually closes after birth. It remains patent in about 1 in 2500 live births and accounts for about 10 per cent of all CHD. In the foetus blood from the right ventricle is directed into the pulmonary artery but, because of the high pulmonary vascular resistance, it flows through the duct, into the descending aorta. After birth, the pulmonary vascular resistance falls and blood flows left to right, from the aorta to the lungs. Patent ductus arteriosus is common in premature babies and its presence may prolong the requirement for IPPV. In these small babies a left thoracotomy is required to ligate the PDA. The condition may also occur in older children in whom transvascular closure is usual.

DUCTAL CLOSURE IN THE NEONATAL INTENSIVE CARE UNIT

A PDA closure in small premature neonates may be undertaken in the neonatal intensive care unit (NICU), which avoids the problems of transferring very small infants to the operating theatre (e.g. hypothermia). The main hazards are difficulty with ventilation during lung retraction, major haemorrhage due to tearing of the friable ductal tissue and inadvertent clamping of the descending aorta or main pulmonary artery. Blood should be immediately available and antibiotics and vitamin K should be administered if not already given.

ANAESTHETIC CONSIDERATIONS

In addition to standard monitors two pulse oximeters should be placed, one on the right hand and one on a lower limb. If the pulse is lost from the lower limb during a test clamping of the duct, this might indicate that the aorta has been clamped inadvertently. Arterial access is useful if already established or if it can be placed reasonably quickly, but is not absolutely necessary. There should be a dedicated intravenous line for fluids and drugs with long (100–150 cm) extension. Full muscle relaxation is combined with high-dose opioids. Some use ketamine (2 mg/kg initially + 1 mg/kg as required). The tracheal tube should have only a small air leak, otherwise ventilation will be impaired during lung retraction. Wound infiltration or intercostal nerve block can be performed by the surgeon on completion of surgery. Total parental nutrition (TPN) or glucose-containing fluids should be continued.

'SIMPLE' RIGHT-TO-LEFT SHUNTS

Tetralogy of Fallot

Tetralogy of Fallot (ToF) accounts for approximately 11 per cent of congenital heart lesions. The four features of the tetralogy are: VSD, overriding aorta, right-ventricular outflow tract obstruction (RVOTO) and right-ventricular hypertrophy (see Fig. 30.1, Chapter 30).

The right-to-left shunt and consequent cyanosis result from a combination of the RVOTO and VSD. The degree of hypoxaemia depends on the relationship between the RVOTO and the systemic vascular resistance.

The RVOTO ranges from mild to severe, and the level of the obstruction also varies. Commonly a dynamic subpulmonary infundibular obstruction is present. Dynamic narrowing of the infundibulum is frequently the cause of hypercyanotic 'spells' (also know as 'tet spells') in which there is an increase in the right-to-left shunt. An RVOTO may also be at the level of the pulmonary valve, or main or branch pulmonary arteries; indeed, pulmonary atresia may exist as a variant of ToF. Patients with pulmonary atresia who have well-developed pulmonary arteries derive their pulmonary blood supply from a PDA. In contrast, patients with hypoplastic pulmonary arteries derive their pulmonary blood supple from major aortopulmonary collateral arteries (MAPCAs).

Tetralogy of Fallot may be associated with a large number of other cardiac and extracardiac anomalies. Extracardiac anaomalies include DiGeorge syndrome (see Table 40.2) and trisomy 21.

HYPERCYANOTIC 'SPELLS'

These episodes of cyanosis are common in untreated patients. They may be initiated by crying or feeding or during anaesthesia. The underlying cause of these spells is unclear but metabolic acidosis, increased partial pressure of carbon dioxide (PCO_2), circulating catecholamines and surgical stimulation are implicated. The management of spells is outlined in Table 40.6.

SURGICAL MANAGEMENT

Controversy still exists as to the optimum management of children with ToF. The choice is between early complete repair or initial palliation with a systemic-to-pulmonary shunt followed by a complete repair when the baby is older. There is a trend towards early complete repair [46,47] which involves closure of the VSD and relief of the RVOTO. The relief of the RVOTO most commonly involves a patch across the pulmonary valve (transannular patch), which necessitates a right ventriculotomy. Consequently, right-ventricular dysfunction is common and a degree of pulmonary regurgitation is almost always present. Junctional ectopic tachycardia (JET) is a particular risk after complete correction.

Anaesthetic considerations

SYSTEMIC-TO-PULMONARY SHUNT

Most frequently this will be a modified Blalock–Taussig (BT) shunt in which a GoreTex tube is inserted from a subclavian artery to a branch pulmonary artery. Surgery is

Table 40.6   Management of hypercyanotic 'spells' during anaesthesia

- 100% oxygen
- Hyperventilation
- Intravenous fluid bolus
- Sedation, e.g. fentanyl
- Sodium bicarbonate
- Vasoconstriction
  - noradrenaline 0.5 μg/kg bolus then 0.1–0.5 μg/kg/min
  - phenylephrine 5 μg/kg bolus then 1–5 μg/kg/min
- β Blockers to relax infundibular spasm and reduce heart rate (e.g. propranolol 0.1–0.3 mg/kg bolus)

usually as neonate or small infant. Sedative premedication may be useful to minimise crying during induction and reduce the risk of a hypercyanotic spell. Either inhalational or intravenous induction is appropriate; both arterial and central venous access are required, with the arterial line placed away from the subclavian artery to be clamped during the operation. Surgery is usually involves a thoracotomy (left or right, depending on side of aortic arch) but may be via a sternotomy; it does not usually require CPB. The tracheal tube should be 'snug' with no air leak as lung retraction during surgery may impair ventilation. The surgeon may request heparin (100 IU/kg) to prevent shunt clot formation. The anaesthetist needs to be prepared for the bleeding, which may occur after the clamps are released. Postoperatively pulmonary blood flow depends upon the systemic blood pressure and the size of the shunt. The higher the blood pressure the more blood flows to the lungs and the higher the arterial saturation; but if the shunt is too small the baby will remain with low saturations. Conversely, if the shunt is too large the baby may develop heart failure or pulmonary oedema. Postoperative IPPV is usually needed.

COMPLETE REPAIR

Early complete correction with no systemic pulmonary shunt, is undertaken in neonates or small infants. These children remain at risk of hypercyanotic spells (Table 40.6). Older children with a BT shunt are much less likely to suffer from a hypercyanotic episode. Sedative premedication is more important in those at risk of a hypercyanotic episode. A CPB is used and the child should be prepared as described above. Postoperatively, right-ventricular dysfunction and pulmonary regurgitation may be seen. Even in the repaired RVOT excessive β-sympathomimetic stimulation from inotropes should be avoided as it may worsen RVOTO by dynamic narrowing or precipitate JET. Milrinone may be particularly useful as it promotes diastolic relaxation of the stiff right ventricle. Core temperature should be kept at about 36°C to minimise the risk of JET. Both direct measurement of the right-ventricular pressure and echocardiography are used to assess the quality of the repair.

COMPLEX SHUNTS: MIXING OF PULMONARY AND SYSTEMIC BLOOD FLOW WITH CYANOSIS

Transposition of the great arteries

Transposition of the great arteries (TGA) is common and accounts for about 6 per cent of all congenital heart lesions. It frequently occurs as an isolated lesion and is rarely associated with extracardiac anomalies. The most common repair is the arterial switch operation (ASO), the short- and long-term results of which have improved to such an extent that children with a good repair can expect a normal life.

Transposition of the great arteries refers to an aorta arising from the morphological right ventricle and a pulmonary artery arising from the morphological left ventricle (Figs 40.1 and 40.2). This is known as ventriculoarterial discordance (VA discordance). The atria are related to the ventricles in the normal way (atrioventricular [AV] concordance). This results in two circulations, which run in parallel; without mixing, the systemic circulation would remain completely deoxygenated. Normally, some mixing does occur through the PDA, or through a VSD, which is present in approximately 25 per cent of cases. If there is no VSD and mixing is inadequate a balloon atrial septostomy must be performed urgently in the neonatal period. Prior to this, ductal patency is maintained with intravenous prostaglandin E2 (5–10 ng/kg/min).

In TGA with intact ventricular septum it is important to perform the ASO early in the neonatal period, preferably in the first 2–3 weeks of life, because the left ventricle is exposed to the pressure of the pulmonary circulation, which falls rapidly after birth; after a short period, the ventricle is unprepared for the work required to pump blood at systemic pressure after the repair. If, however, there is an unrestrictive VSD, both the left and right ventricles are exposed to systemic blood pressure and the left ventricle is better conditioned as a systemic ventricle.

Untreated, the majority of babies with TGA will die in the first year of life from hypoxia and heart failure. Pulmonary vascular disease (PVD) develops early in TGA and contributes to this high mortality [48] and the high risk of pulmonary hypertensive crisis in the postoperative period. The mechanism for the development of PVD is complex and not simply related to high pulmonary blood flow. The presence of a VSD accelerates the process.

Surgical options

ARTERIAL SWITCH OPERATION

This is the operation of choice if the intracardiac anatomy allows. It involves transecting the two main arterial trunks distal to their respective valves and 'switching' them to produce VA concordance. It also involves disconnecting the coronary arteries from the 'old' aorta and reconnecting them

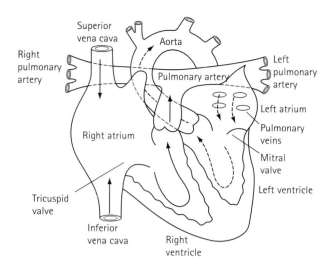

Figure 40.1   Normal heart. From May [83], with permission.

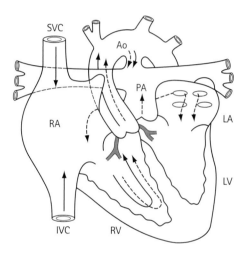

Figure 40.2   Transposition of the great arteries (TGA). The pulmonary artery (PA) arises from the left ventricle (LV) and the aorta (Ao) arises from the right ventricle (RV). Two parallel circuits result. IVC, inferior vena cava; LA, left atrium; RA, right atrium; SVC, superior vena cava. From May [83] with permission.

to the neo-aorta (Fig. 40.3). This restores anatomical and physiological normality. The coronary anatomy varies widely in TGA and must be carefully assessed preoperatively as moving the coronaries to the neo-aorta is the most difficult and important part of the operation. In a proportion of cases the coronaries run in the wall of the aorta (intramural) and this poses particular difficulties for the surgeon. Clearly, ventricular function after surgery depends largely on unrestricted flow in the coronaries.

MUSTARD AND SENNING PROCEDURES

The Mustard or Senning procedures are *atrial* switch procedures. They involve the use of intra-atrial baffles to redirect deoxygenated blood from the vena cava to the left atrium,

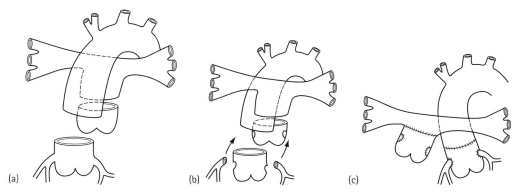

Figure 40.3 The arterial switch procedure. (a) The pulmonary artery and aorta are transected. (b) The coronary arteries are disconnected from the aorta and moved posteriorly. The aorta is also moved posteriorly and the pulmonary artery moved anteriorly. (c) The coronaries are reimplanted into the new aorta. The aorta is attached to what was the pulmonary trunk and the pulmonary arteries are attached to what was the aortic root. From May [83] with permission.

left ventricle and pulmonary artery, and oxygenated pulmonary venous blood to the right atrium, right ventricle and aorta. They create AV discordance, restore physiological but not anatomical normality and leave the morphological right ventricle as the systemic ventricle. These procedures were performed as definitive procedures before the arterial switch became successful and are rarely used as such today. They are still, however, used as palliation in those patients with TGA, VSD and PVD. In these cases the VSD is left open.

THE RASTELLI PROCEDURE

The Rastelli procedure is used in patients with TGA, VSD and left-ventricular outflow tract obstruction (LVOTO). The VSD is closed in a manner that directs blood from the left ventricle to the aorta. The pulmonary artery is ligated just distal to the pulmonary valve and a valved conduit is inserted from the right ventricle to the pulmonary artery. The result of this is continuity between the left ventricle and aorta, and the right ventricle and PA. In addition the LVOTO (subpulmonary area) is bypassed. The Rastelli procedure has traditionally been performed around the age of 2–3 years, following a palliative BT shunt in the neonatal period, but there is a trend towards neonatal Rastelli repair without the need for a shunt.

Anaesthetic implication for the arterial switch procedure

Surgery is performed in the neonate; the immature myocardium requires sensitive management (see Chapter 3). After either inhalational or IV induction arterial and central venous lines are placed. If there is a VSD to close bi-caval cannulation may be needed for CPB and an internal jugular central venous catheter (CVC) may interfere with SVC cannulation – a femoral CVC may be preferable. Otherwise, a single atrial venous cannula is used for CPB and an internal jugular CVC may be inserted.

On release of the aortic cross-clamp, myocardial ischaemia may occur from coronary air emboli or a poor coronary anastomosis: a generous perfusion pressure (>40 mmHg mean arterial pressure [MAP]) assists clearance of air. If ischaemia is thought to be caused by an anatomical problem with the coronaries, they should be redone immediately.

Following weaning from CPB if myocardial dysfunction occurs it is often multifactorial and arises from: (1) an inherently poor left ventricle, (2) poor myocardial protection, (3) poor coronary implantation and (4) coronary air. Inotropes are almost always required, milrinone (0.5 μg/kg/min) and adrenaline (0.02–0.1 μg/kg/min) is a particularly useful combination. Left atrial dilatation should be avoided. After the repair the pulmonary artery is anterior to the aorta and close to the origin of the coronaries. Left-atrial dilatation causes pulmonary venous hypertension and dilatation of the pulmonary artery, which may distort or compress the coronary arteries. Fluid boluses should be given very carefully and a left-atrial monitoring line should be left in place. Pulmonary hypertension may be seen. Cardiopulmonary bypass coagulopathy is common and antifibrinolytics and blood products are frequently used.

Truncus arteriosus

Truncus arteriosus is rare, about 0.7 per 1000 live births and 1 per cent of all CHD. There is a common outlet for the aorta and pulmonary arteries associated with a single (truncal) valve and a VSD. There are three types described depending on how the pulmonary arteries arise from the aorta and on the size of the aorta. There is mixing of blood at the arterial level with a resultant high pulmonary blood flow. This leads to heart failure and the early development of pulmonary hypertension. Surgery should be prompt to prevent pulmonary hypertension from becoming irreversible.

Truncus arteriosus is particularly associated with DiGeorge syndrome (see Table 40.2). Irradiated blood products should be used and calcium levels carefully monitored.

Surgical repair separates the systemic from the pulmonary circulation and closes the VSD. This involves disconnecting the pulmonary artery/arteries from the aorta and repairing the truncal valve. The pulmonary arteries are connected to the right ventricle, usually with a valved conduit. Circulatory arrest may be required. Early postoperative mortality rate is high and varies between 5 and 25 per cent. Factors that influence mortality are truncal valve stenosis, coronary abnormalities and low birth weight.

ANAESTHETIC CONSIDERATIONS

Surgery is in a neonate, with almost certain heart failure that may be of sufficient severity to require preoperative IPPV, diuretics and inotropes. Deep hypothermic circulatory arrest may be needed, requiring ice packs to the head. Cardiopulmonary bypass coagulopathy is likely; antifibrinolytics and blood products are usually necessary. There is a high risk of postoperative pulmonary hypertension; good oxygenation and avoidance of acidosis will minimise the risk.

Anomalous pulmonary venous drainage

Anomalous pulmonary venous drainage comprises about 2 per cent of CHD and may be either total (TAPVD) or partial (PAPVD). Three types of TAPVD exist:

- *Supracardiac* – where the pulmonary veins connect to the SVC via an ascending vertical vein
- *Cardiac* – where the pulmonary veins are connected to the right atrium via the coronary sinus
- *Infracardiac* – where the pulmonary veins connect to the IVC via a common vein, which traverses the diaphragm.

The pulmonary veins may be obstructed.

ANAESTHETIC CONSIDERATIONS

These neonates are usually cyanosed and may be in heart failure. Pulmonary hypertension and pulmonary oedema may be present, particularly if the veins are obstructed. This is one of the few remaining true paediatric cardiac surgical emergencies. The anaesthetic management is similar to that described above for truncus repair. Pulmonary hypertension is even more likely to be seen; nitric oxide (5–20 p.p.m.) may be needed.

Hypoplastic left–heart syndrome

The prognosis of patients with hypoplastic left-heart syndrome (HLHS) has improved in recent years. Previously,

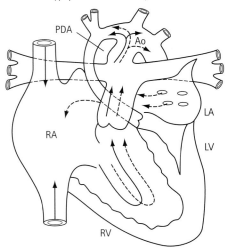

Hypoplastic left heart syndrome

Figure 40.4 Hypoplastic left heart syndrome. Ao, aorta; LA, left atrium; LV, left ventricle; PDA, patent ductus arteriosus; RA, right atrium; RV, right ventricle. From May [83] with permission.

virtually all babies with this condition died, while many children now survive at least into childhood [49]. The longer-term outlook has not been fully determined.

The incidence of HLHS in the USA is about 2 per 10 000 live births. However, in the UK this figure is probably lower as many mothers with a prenatal diagnosis of HLHS opt for termination. The anatomical features of HLHS include: hypoplastic left ventricle, mitral stenosis or atresia, aortic stenosis or atresia, hypoplastic aortic arch and a duct-dependent circulation (Fig. 40.4) The diagnosis is usually prenatal, although it can be difficult and is sometimes missed. Infants present with tachypnoea, tachycardia and cyanosis, and a systolic murmur can be heard.

SURGICAL PALLIATION

The aim of surgical treatment is to establish a single ventricle (Fontan) circulation, in which the right ventricle becomes the systemic ventricle and the pulmonary blood flow is supplied passively from the SVC and IVC. This is done by a series of three operations, termed Norwood stages I, II and III.

Norwood stage I

This is performed in the neonatal period. The aortic arch is reconstructed in such a way that it arises from the pulmonary trunk (Fig. 40.5). The pulmonary valve thus becomes the neo-aortic valve. The branch pulmonary arteries are disconnected from the pulmonary trunk and a new pulmonary blood supply is provided from either a shunt from the subclavian artery (BT shunt) or the right ventricle (Sano modification) [50].

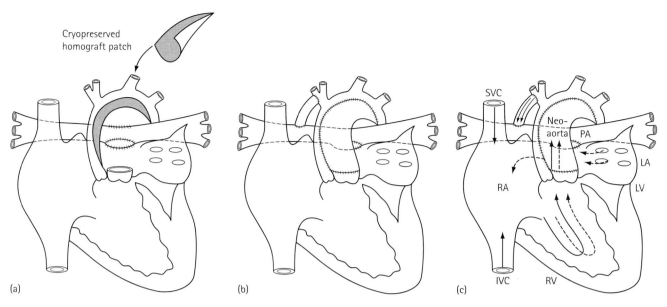

Figure 40.5 (a) The pulmonary arteries are disconnected from the pulmonary root. The hypoplastic aortic arch is laid open. (b) The aorta is reconstructed using a patch and is attached to the pulmonary valve. The systemic circulation is now from the single right ventricle. (c) The final stage is to create the Blalock–Taussig shunt from the subclavian artery to the pulmonary artery to provide the pulmonary blood supply. IVC, inferior vena cava; LA, left atrium; LV, left ventricle; PA, pulmonary artery; RA, right atrium; RV, right ventricle; SVC, superior vena cava. From May [83] with permission.

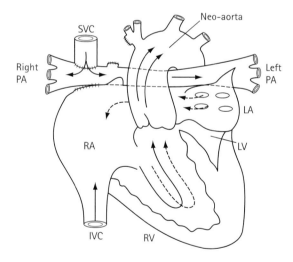

Figure 40.6 Norwood stage II: the Blalock–Taussig shunt is taken down and the superior vena cava (SVC) is connected to the right pulmonary artery. This is called a Glenn shunt. IVC, inferior vena cava; LA, left atrium; LV, left ventricle; PA, pulmonary artery; RA, right atrium; RV, right ventricle. From May [83] with permission.

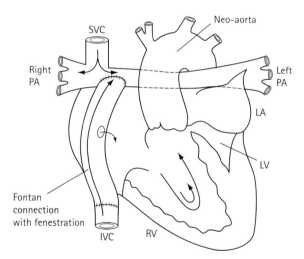

Figure 40.7 Norwood stage III, also called a 'Fontan' circulation. The inferior vena cava (IVC) is now connected to the pulmonary artery via a conduit. LA, left atrium; LV, left ventricle; PA, pulmonary artery; RA, right atrium; RV, right ventricle; SVC, superior vena cava.

Norwood stage II

This surgery takes place at about 6 months of age. The shunt is taken down and the SVC is connected to the right pulmonary artery (Fig. 40.6). The pulmonary blood supply is now provided by systemic venous blood from the SVC. Flow is passive and is therefore dependent on low pulmonary artery pressures. The child remains blue with

arterial saturations in the mid-80s because desaturated blood from the IVC is still draining to the heart and being pumped direct to the systemic circulation.

Norwood stage III

This is the completion of the Fontan circulation (Fig. 40.7). The IVC is connected to the pulmonary artery via an extracardiac or intracardiac conduit. The right ventricle pumps blood to the systemic circulation while the pulmonary blood supply is provided by passive flow of systemic venous blood from the SVC and IVC. It is essential that pulmonary vascular resistance remains low, as any increase in pulmonary vascular resistance (PVR) will reduce pulmonary blood flow. It is common for a small fenestration to be created between the extracardiac conduit and the right atrium so that if the PVR rises blood will be directed to the right atrium and allow cardiac output to be maintained. In this situation the patient will desaturate, but this is much safer than having a low cardiac output and excessive vena caval pressures. Post-operatively, elevated systemic venous pressure may result in pleural effusions, enlarged liver or protein-losing entero-pathy. Later, if PVR remains consistently low, the fenestration can be closed with a transvenous device.

The long-term problem in these patients is that the morphological right ventricle becomes the systemic ventricle and over time is likely to fail. The only recourse, then, is heart transplantation [51,52].

The single-ventricle strategy (Fontan) is used in many different situations other than HLHS. The sequence of events is almost always the same: an initial palliation with a BT shunt, followed later with a Glenn shunt and finally the formation of the Fontan circulation (total cavopulmonary connection [TCPC]).

Anaesthetic considerations

STAGE I NORWOOD

The physiology of HLHS requires maintenance of the balance between the systemic and pulmonary circulation by balancing PVR and SVR. The two circulations are in parallel; if the PVR is reduced blood flow will be directed away from the systemic circulation and the lungs will be flooded. This results in systemic hypotension and hypoperfusion with increasing acidosis. If PVR increases oxygen saturation will fall. Prior to surgery these babies are best managed spontaneously breathing in air with a prostaglandin infusion to maintain ductal patency. If they require IPPV it is important to maintain normal/high arterial CO_2 and low inspired oxygen concentrations (usually 21 per cent).

Surgery is in a neonate with all the implications discussed above. A high-dose opioid-based technique with muscle relaxants is preferred. Central venous access is gained via the femoral or umbilical veins; the internal jugular vein is avoided as narrowing of the SVC would jeopardise the Glenn shunt (stage II). Deep hypothermic circulatory arrest may be required; head ice packs may be needed.

Balancing systemic and pulmonary blood supply is important post-CPB. Some centres use the long-acting α blocker phenoxybenzamine to reduce SVR variability. This allows higher concentrations of oxygen to be used, resulting in an overall increase in oxygen delivery [53]. The alternative approach is to combine a vasodilator such as milrinone with adrenaline (or dopamine) to achieve a similar effect; this also assists myocardial dysfunction which is commonly seen following CPB. The sternum may be left open to avoid cardiac tamponade. Delayed closure in the ICU is usually after several days.

NORWOOD STAGE II

Surgery involves a repeat sternotomy (see page 601), and CPB is used but without aortic cross-clamping, so that the heart remains beating and inotropes are seldom required. Again CVC insertion is via the femoral vein, but a short cannula may be placed in the internal jugular vein to measure pulmonary artery pressure after SVC to pulmonary artery anastomosis. It should be removed early in the postoperative period to avoid any possibility of thrombosis in the SVC. Aprotinin is probably best avoided as it will have been used in the neonatal period and the risk of anaphylaxis is higher on the second exposure, particularly if this is within 6 months. Patients should be nursed 30° head-up after surgery to avoid SVC congestion and should be weaned rapidly from IPPV, as positive intrathoracic pressure reduces flow in the Glenn shunt.

NORWOOD STAGE III

Where possible CVC insertion is via the femoral route but on occasion access for stages I and II causes femoral thrombosis and this site is not available. Surgery involves a repeat sternotomy (see page 601); CPB is required but aortic cross-clamping is not usually necessary unless an intracardiac conduit is formed, so inotropes are not always required. If an inotrope is needed milrinone is a good choice because of its beneficial effects on PVR. The PVR must remain low postoperatively and careful management of ventilation is important to minimise atelectasis; early extubation is recommended. Occasionally, nitric oxide is required [54]. Aprotinin may have a role in preserving lung function in these patients [55] Large amounts of fluid may be required in the early postoperative period.

OBSTRUCTIVE LESIONS

Aortic stenosis

Obstruction to the LVOT can occur at the valvular, subvalvular or supravalvular area or in various combinations and is common, accounting for up to 10 per cent of congenital heart disease [56].

Congenital valvular aortic stenosis (AS) is frequently associated with a bicuspid valve. Severe critical AS in neonates occurs in about 1 in 10 of cases and requires urgent treatment [57]. Supravalvular AS is commonly associated with Williams syndrome [58].

Despite the large number of different anatomical varieties of AS the pathophysiology is essentially the same.

There is an imbalance between myocardial oxygen supply and demand, left-ventricular hypertrophy and the risk of left-ventricular failure. There is always the risk of sudden death. The age of presentation is a risk factor with the younger children being most at risk. Two-thirds of those presenting in the first 3 months of life will require either inotropic or ventilatory support before treatment [59].

TREATMENT OPTIONS

These vary depending on the age, severity and type of lesion. In the neonate with critical AS an urgent valvuloplasty is required. This can be done open using CPB, but it is more usually performed using transluminal balloon angioplasty [60]. In the older child various surgical approaches are used depending on the anatomy. Transluminal balloon valvuloplasty is also commonly performed in the older age group. Valve replacement either with mechanical valves or with bioprosthetic valves is delayed as long as possible because of the long-term problems associated with anticoagulation with a mechanical valve and the inevitable calcification of bioprosthetic valves. The Ross procedure involves moving the pulmonary valve into the aortic valve position, and using a homograft in the pulmonary position. The need for reoperation with the Ross procedure is reduced because the systemic valve (neo-aortic valve) grows with the patient and calcification of the homograft in the pulmonary position is slow. Furthermore, there is no need for anticoagulation [61].

The most common complications of valvuloplasty are aortic incompetence or residual AS.

ANAESTHETIC CONSIDERATIONS

The crucial aim of anaesthesia is to maintain the balance of myocardial oxygen supply and demand. This involves:

- maintaining a normal heart rate (avoiding tachycardia or bradycardia)
- maintaining SVR to preserve coronary perfusion – inhalational induction should be avoided or used with extreme care
- avoiding hypertension
- avoiding myocardial depression.

For surgery with CPB considerations are similar to other neonatal cardiac surgery (see above).

In transluminal balloon valvuloplasty dramatic cardiovascular changes can occur when the catheter crosses the aortic valve and inflation of the balloon occurs: cardiac output falls, myocardial ischaemia occurs and bradycardia is common. The anaesthetist must be prepared to resuscitate the neonate quickly and drugs, particularly adrenaline, should be drawn up beforehand. Occasionally, adenosine is given to slow or stop the heart at the time of balloon inflation to prevent damage to the valve by the inflated balloon being expelled through it. Arterial access will be needed by the cardiologist for the procedure but pressure will not always be displayed. An independent arterial line is very useful. After valvuloplasty, IPPV is commonly needed as as ventricular function can remain poor for some time.

Coarctation of the aorta

Coarctation of the aorta is the discrete narrowing of the aorta and accounts for about 5 per cent of all congenital heart disease. The lesion is often isolated with no other associated abnormalities; it may, however, occur in association with other cardiac abnormalities such as VSD, aortic arch abnormalities or aortic valve abnormalities. The coarctation may be preductal, juxtaductal or postductal depending on the relationship to the ductus arteriosus (DA). The most common form presenting in the neonatal period is the preductal type. Preductal coarctation is associated with minimal collateral circulation below the coarctation and ductal patency should be maintained with prostaglandin E_2 (5–10 ng/kg/min). Both juxtaductal and postductal coarctation are characterised by the development of collateral vessels, which supply the area below the coarctation. This is important, particularly during aortic cross-clamping, as the spinal cord is supplied by these collaterals. In practical terms, coarctation falls into two groups. One group presents in the neonatal period with preductal coarctation, few collaterals and very poor LV function, whereas the second group comprises older children, usually more than 1 year old, who have well-developed collaterals and better LV function.

The neonatal patients have poor LV function and may present in heart failure. Femoral pulses are often weak or absent and there is usually a progressive acidosis.

ANAESTHESIA CONSIDERATIONS

Neonatal repair

These infants are sick and should be treated very carefully: the anaesthetist should not be misled by a baby that looks reasonably well and there should be a low threshold for preoperative IPPV and inotropic support. Those babies who are not so supported need the greatest care at induction.

Intravenous access will often have been established to give prostaglandin. This can be used to administer induction agents. The authors preference is to give incremental doses of fentanyl (up to 5 μg/kg) then muscle relaxant, and supplement this with a very low dose of isoflurane (0.3–0.5 per cent). Ketamine is an alternative. Postoperative IPPV is standard and nasal intubation is preferred. Central venous and arterial access is obtained. The arterial line should be placed in the right arm to allow blood pressure measurement during arterial cross-clamping as the left subclavian will be obstructed during the repair. Some advocate an additional arterial line below the coarctation to measure perfusion pressure during cross-clamping. Alternatively, a blood pressure cuff can be placed on a leg as well as a second pulse oximeter, both of which will indicate the adequacy of the repair after release of the cross-clamps. Inotropes may be required during surgery and these should be available.

Surgery usually takes place through a left thoracotomy without the use of CPB. The lung will be retracted and ventilation may be problematic; for this reason it is important that the tracheal tube is 'snug' fitting and has no leak. Paraplegia may occur in about 1 per cent of cases and is thought to be caused by hypoperfusion during aortic cross-clamping [62]. To reduce the chance of spinal cord damage, babies should be allowed to cool to about 34°C before the cross-clamp is applied, ventilated to normocapnia and upper limb blood pressure maintained. Low-dose anticoagulation may also be administered. A short cross-clamp time is important. As LV function improves in the postoperative period, hypertension may occur and arterial vasodilatation may be necessary.

The older child

These children are not usually as sick as the neonates; induction is with a fentanyl (3 μg/kg) preload and a reduced dose of an IV agent of choice. Arterial and CVC insertion are as described above. Although a collateral blood supply is present the spinal cord remains at risk during the cross-clamping and the same precautions are needed (see above). A brief period of postoperative IPPV is normal, though early extubation is usually possible. Postoperative hypertension is a frequent problem and good analgesia combined with systemic vasodilatation and β blockade is usually required. Many children (up to 30 per cent) will go on to have long-term hypertension that will require therapy.

Increasingly cases are treated with balloon angioplasty with or without stent placement. Splitting or rupture of the aorta is a risk and the institution in which the procedure is undertaken should be in a position to deal with this if it were to occur.

Interrupted aortic arch

Interrupted aortic arch (IAA) is a rare anomaly accounting for less than 1 per cent of CHD. It involves a disruption of the aorta between the ascending aorta and descending aorta. There are three types, depending on where the disruption takes place. A PDA is present and supplies the descending aorta. A VSD is also common. Interrupted aortic arch is frequently associated with a 22q11 deletion which results in the DiGeorge syndrome (see Table 40.2).

These patients, who are often small for dates, are started on a prostaglandin infusion to maintain ductal patency. They are often sick with progressive acidosis and poor cardiac output. There is increasing pulmonary blood flow as the duct closes. Surgical repair depends on the presence of associated lesions, particularly a VSD. In the single-stage repair the arch will be reconstructed and the VSD closed, whilst the two-stage repair involves repair of the aortic arch and banding of the pulmonary artery to limit blood flow to the lungs. The VSD will be closed at a later stage. Either way, deep hypothermic circulatory arrest is likely to be necessary. Topical head cooling should be used and some centres also use selective regional perfusion to try to limit neurological injury [63]. Both early and late mortality are high, and increased with small size, pre-operative acidosis and the presence of associated cardiac lesions[64].

ANAESTHETIC CONSIDERATIONS

Standard care of a sick neonate undergoing CPB with DHCA applies (see above). The frequent association of DiGeorge syndrome requires irradiated blood products and calcium homeostasis. If possible, the blood pressure is monitored above and below interruption, but this is often difficult in practice and either is adequate. Bypass cannulation is usually through a Y-connection with one cannula in the aorta and the other perfusing the lower body through the duct. There is a risk of postoperative pulmonary hypertensive crises.

Recurrent LVOTO may occur at any level and require reoperation. Restenosis of the repaired aortic arch can be dilated with transluminal balloon dilatation.

CARDIAC TRANSPLANTATION

Outcomes in children receiving heart transplants has improved in recent years to such an extent that heart transplantation has become a standard form of treatment [65]. The majority of transplantations take place in children over the age of 1 year but 25 per cent are carried out in infants. The indications for transplantation are primarily untreatable CHD and cardiomyopathy. In those under 1 year the majority are for CHD, usually HLHS, whilst in those over 1 year of age the main indication is cardiomyopathy. Contraindications to heart transplantation are listed in Table 40.7.

Cardiomyopathy

Cardiomyopathy is a rare condition that affects about 1:100 000 children per year [66,67] and may be dilated, hypertrophic (HOCM) or restrictive Many patients with

Table 40.7 Main contraindications to heart transplantation

- Pulmonary hypertension: pulmonary vascular resistance > 6 Wood units/m^2 that is unresponsive to pulmonary vasodilators (oxygen, nitric oxide and intravenous agents)
- Active malignancy
- Multiple-organ failure
- Severe systemic disease
- Severe sepsis

cardiomyopathy will have pulmonary hypertension as a result of increased pulmonary venous congestion secondary to high left atrial pressure.

Anaesthesia in children with cardiomyopathy is challenging. In dilated cardiomyopathy any cardiovascular changes are poorly tolerated and a balanced technique that avoids tachycardia or bradycardia, rises or falls in vascular resistance or depression of contractility must be used. Induction of anaesthesia is particularly hazardous and should be fully monitored. Cautious administration of a small dose (3 μg/kg) of fentanyl followed by a reduced dose of a standard induction agent (e.g. 1–2 mg/kg of thiopental) is usually tolerated; etomidate is a good alternative. For major procedures or the unstable patient, planned postoperative IPPV will allow cardiostable high-dose opiate techniques to be used. In contrast, in HOCM, endogenous or exogenous catecholamine secretion will increase myocardial contractility and worsen LVOTO. Preoperative β blockade should be continued, cardiotonic drugs should be avoided and surgical stimuli should be minimised.

By the time patients with cardiomyopathy come to transplantation they are usually very unwell with little cardiovascular reserve. They may already be on inotropes to support cardiac function. A small number will be on extracorporeal membrane oxygenation (ECMO) or other mechanical support such as a left-ventricular assist device (LVAD). Moving to theatre from the ICU can be challenging.

There remains a critical shortage of donor organs in general and in paediatrics in particular. As a result, the criteria used for selecting donor organs is perhaps less strict than with adult practice. This may lead to difficult decisions about the use of organs and the occasional use of 'marginal donor organs', such as a heart that has required of high-dose inotropic support or suffered a cardiac arrest [68].

Matching a donor to recipient is done according to several criteria, which include:

- blood type (although ABO-mismatched donors are occasionally accepted)
- size of donor compared with recipient (this does not need to be an exact match and frequently the donor organ is large for the recipient; this does not pose major problems)
- condition of the donor heart
- urgency of recipient's need and length of wait, including need for mechanical support which may necessitate the acceptance of marginal organs.

The organisational aspects around the time of transplantation are significant. Most programmes employ a transplant coordinator who is responsible for the logistics. The challenges include coordinating retrieval of the organ, which may be at a considerable distance, timing of admission of the recipient and ensuring that the recipient is in theatre fully prepared to allow the retrieved organ to be implanted without delay.

Tolerable ischaemic times are increasing as better myocardial preservation techniques are used. Four hours was once used as the limit for cold ischaemic time but this has been challenged and times of up to 10 hours have been reported. There is evidence that ischaemic times of up to 8 hours are not associated with adverse outcomes [69].

ANAESTHETIC MANAGEMENT OF HEART TRANSPLANTATION [70,71]

Careful preoperative review is important; understanding the pathophysiology of the recipient is vital as it may vary from complex congenital disease to dilated cardiomyopathy. Close liaison with the transplant coordinator is essential to allow adequate time for anaesthesia and surgical preparation, thereby minimising donor organ ischaemic time.

Induction depends on individual patient pathology, but, in dilated cardiomyopathy, avoidance of myocardial depression is crucial. Muscle relaxants and high-dose opiates are usually given. Monitoring should include central venous and arterial catheters; left atrial and pulmonary arterial catheters are usually sited after bypass by the surgeon.

Re-do sternotomy is common in the congenital group (see page 601) and more time should be allowed for anaesthesia and surgical dissection. The local protocol for immunosuppression and antibiotics should be followed.

Inotropes are very likely to be required post-bypass as ventricular function may be poor. Milrinone is frequently used in combination with a β-adrenergic agonist such as adrenaline or dopamine [72]. The transplanted heart is denervated and will have a relatively slow heart rate; isoprenaline or atrial pacing is used to achieve a desirable rate. Pacing is preferable as the use of isoprenaline may lead to systemic hypotension.

Pulmonary hypertension may occur post-bypass and meticulous ventilation is essential to optimise arterial PCO_2 and PO_2. Despite good ventilation and the use of milrinone, nitric oxide may occasionally be required and can be guided by pulmonary artery pressures. Transoesophageal echocardiography is useful in assessing post-bypass cardiac function and helps to optimise fluid and inotrope management.

Early postoperative problems include bleeding, pulmonary hypertension, poor ventricular function and renal failure. Some renal impairment can be expected in up to 20 per cent of patients post-transplantation [73].

Outcomes after heart transplantation

Early morbidity and mortality are related to the severity of illness before transplantation and to age. Major causes of death after transplantation include acute rejection, graft failure and infection. Later, coronary artery disease becomes a problem along with an increased risk of malignancy. Improvements in immunosuppressive therapy have contributed substantially to increased survival after transplantation.

HEART–LUNG AND LUNG TRANSPLANTATION

Severe CHD sometimes results in irreversible pulmonary vascular disease, which is so severe that the only option is to transplant the heart and lungs as a single block. This procedure is technically easier in small children than double-lung transplantation and so is also sometimes used where there is a primary pulmonary problem.In this circumstance, the recipient's normal heart is available for a further recipient (the 'Domino' procedure). There may even be an advantage for the Domino recipient, who will receive a heart that is conditioned to the high pulmonary artery and right-ventricular pressures that are common to both chronic lung disease and complex congenital disease. Most of the anaesthetic considerations for heart–lung transplantations are the same as those for heart transplantation alone, with the important exception that there will be a tracheal anastomosis and the tracheal tube should be positioned above this.

Lung transplantation, which is usually, but not always, bilateral, is generally performed in children for end-stage irreversible pulmonary hypertension or cystic fibrosis. The transplantation may be performed as a double-lung transplantation with CPB or sequential single lung transplantations without CPB; in both cases there will be two bronchial anastomoses. Surgery is usually performed through a sub-mammary thoracosternotomy (clamshell) incision, which gives good access to both pleurae. Sequential transplantations require lung separation and this limits application in small children (see Chapter 39). In addition, major haemodynamic and respiratory disturbance may occur on clamping and unclamping of the pulmonary arteries and bronchi.

In recipients with cystic fibrosis it is common either to irrigate the tracheal tube in dilute Betadine solution or to change it completely before ventilating the 'new' set of lungs in order to avoid cross-infection. Because the trachea or bronchi distal to the anastomosis are denervated, secretions in this part of the bronchial tree will not stimulate a cough reflex and meticulous physiotherapy is essential.

Outcomes from lung transplantation are not as good as those for heart transplant recipients. The author's institution's current 5-year survival rate is 57 per cent, with early deaths due to acute rejection and infection and late deaths due to obliterative bronchiolitis. Even though it is not considered until life expectancy is thought to be less than 2 years, the main justification for lung transplantation remains a significant improvement in quality of life.

CARDIAC CATHETERISATION

Cardiac catheterisation is used to acquire diagnostic data. It was for a long time the mainstay of cardiological imaging [74] but advances in echocardiography and, more recently, in MRI have reduced the numbers of patients having diagnostic cardiac catheterisations [1].

Diagnostic cardiac catheterisation has traditionally been used to acquire anatomical images, pressures and pressure gradients, and to measure oxygen saturation in the cardiac chambers to calculate shunts and cardiac output. Most commonly, catheters are inserted from the femoral artery and vein although occasionally the internal jugular vein is used. Increasingly, however, cardiac catheterisation is performed for interventional procedures.

Interventional cardiac catheterisation

The first reported interventional cardiac catheterisation (ICC) was the atrial balloon septostomy in 1966 [75]. Since then the repertoire of the interventional cardiologists has increased dramatically.

BALLOON ATRIAL SEPTOSOMY

This is most commonly performed in neonates with transposition of the great arteries and is carried out as an emergency. A balloon-tipped catheter is passed across the atrial septum, and the balloon inflated and then pulled back. This creates an ASD, which allows better mixing of the circulations and improves arterial saturation.

OCCLUSION PROCEDURES

These include the closure of PDAs, ASDs and some VSDs. A variety of different devices can be used for these closures.

BALLOON DILATATION OF VALVES

The pulmonary and aortic valves are most commonly dilated using a balloon, although mitral stenosis can also be treated in this way [76]. During inflation of the balloon the cardiac output drops considerably and ischaemic changes may occur on the ECG. After balloon deflation, cardiac output usually returns to normal but the anaesthetist should be ready to resuscitate the child if necessary. One of the most challenging balloon procedures is the dilatation of the aortic valve in neonates with critical aortic stenosis (see page 612). These babies are frequently very ill and already ventilated and on inotropic support. Surgical treatment of these neonates has poor results and balloon valvotomy is the treatment of choice [76].

BALLOON DILATATION OF ARTERIES WITH AND WITHOUT STENTS

Balloon dilatation of native aortic coarctation is controversial because of the high incidence of recurrence and because of the risk of rupture during dilatation [77,78]. The ballooning of re-coarctation of the aorta is more successful. The indication for stent placement in these patients is still debated.

The ballooning and/or stenting of pulmonary arteries is much more common and well established. This is partly because distal stenoses are difficult to treat surgically.

EMBOLISATION PROCEDURES

These procedures are carried out to occlude unwanted vascular connections such as aortopulmonary collaterals or previously placed BT shunts. Coils are delivered from the end of catheters to occlude the target vessel.

COMPLICATIONS

The overall complication rate is in the order of 8–10 per cent [79,80]. In a study of 4454 patients, the overall incidence of events was 9.3 per cent. Closure of a PDA or ASD had the lowest event rate (4.2 per cent) with an event rate of 11.6 per cent in other interventional procedures. Diagnostic cardiac catheters had a rate of 9.3 per cent. The complication rate for infants was 13.9 per cent compared with 6.7 per cent for those over a year [80].

Many of the complications are related to the catheters themselves. Arrhythmias are common but usually self-limiting and include ventricular ectopic beats, atrial dysrhythmias and short bursts of ventricular tachycardia. Hypotension is common and has a large number of different causes, including perforation of the myocardium resulting in cardiac tamponade, concealed bleeding from the catheter or catheter site, stenting open of valves by stiff catheters, air embolism, reactions to contrast or other drugs, and occlusion of valves or arteries by large catheters or balloons.

Anaesthesia for cardiac catheterisation

In the UK the majority of children undergoing cardiac catheterisation receive a general anaesthetic. In some countries, however, it is more common for children to be sedated for a wide range of procedures and it is possible that an anaesthetist is not involved. In the USA, for example, sedation is often managed by the cardiologist following guidelines from the American Academy of Pediatrics and the American Society of Anesthesiologists [81,82].

Cardiac catheterisation suites are frequently located in remote sites but the same standard of anaesthetic equipment and monitoring that exists in theatres must be provided. Anaesthesia in the catheter suite is relatively high risk and an experienced anaesthetist should be present [80]. Recovery facilities should be of a high standard.

ANAESTHETIC TECHNIQUE

An understanding of the pathophysiology will assist assessment and guide the induction technique. Intermittent positive pressure ventilation is usual and may need to be interrupted for image capture. Small infants will require active warming as the suite is cooled; temperature should be monitored in all patients. The arms are frequently positioned above the head but excessive stretch, which may cause brachial plexus injury, should be avoided.

All standard monitors should be applied. End-tidal CO_2 is particularly useful because it quickly reflects changes in cardiac output and pulmonary blood flow. Some patients may benefit from invasive monitoring.

Cardiac MRI

Cardiac MRI is increasingly used in the evaluation of children with CHD [1]. It has the advantage that it is non-invasive, does not use ionising radiation and is able to provide detailed three-dimensional images, but it is currently unable to provide information about pressure or oxygen saturation. To obtain good-quality images breathing needs to be stopped for some acquisition sequences and this requires the child to be either cooperative or anaesthetised, so there is little place for sedation. Anaesthesia usually involves paralysis and positive pressure ventilation and the anaesthetist must be able to interrupt ventilation. This can be achieved by an anaesthetist inside the MRI scanner or, preferably, from the control room with the use of an extended circuit that can be disconnected and reconnected. Monitoring needs to be of a high standard and MRI-compatible monitors are available.

REFERENCES

Key references

Bettex DA, Pretre R, Jenni R, Schmid ER. Cost-effectiveness of routine intraoperative transesophageal echocardiography in pediatric cardiac surgery: a 10-year experience. *Anesth Analg* 2005; **100**(5): 1271–5.

Chauhan S, Kumar BA, Rao BH *et al.* Efficacy of aprotinin, epsilon aminocaproic acid, or combination in cyanotic heart disease. *Ann Thorac Surg* 2000; **70**(4): 1308–12.

Hoffman TM, Wernovsky G, Atz AM *et al.* Prophylactic intravenous use of milrinone after cardiac operation in pediatrics (PRIMACORP) study. Prophylactic intravenous use of milrinone after cardiac operation in pediatrics. *Am Heart J* 2002; **143**(1): 15–21.

Jonas RA. Deep hypothermic circulatory arrest: current status and indications. *Semin Thorac Cardiovasc Surg* 2006; **5**: 76–88.

Miller BE, Mochizuki T, Levy JH *et al.* Predicting and treating coagulopathies after cardiopulmonary bypass in children. *Anesth Analg* 1997; **85**(6): 1196–202.

Sahn DJ, Vick GW. Review of new techniques in echocardiography and magnetic resonance imaging as applied to patients with congenital heart disease. *Heart* 2001; **86**(suppl 2): 41–53.

References

1. Sahn DJ, Vick GW. Review of new techniques in echocardiography and magnetic resonance imaging as applied to patients with congenital heart disease. *Heart* 2001; **86**(suppl 2): 41–53.

2. Di Donato RM, Jonas RA, Lang P et al. Neonatal repair of tetralogy of Fallot with and without pulmonary atresia. *J Thorac Cardiovasc Surg* 1991; **101**(1): 126–37.

3. Jaquiss RD, Ghanayem NS, Zacharisen MC et al. Safety of aprotinin use and re-use in pediatric cardiothoracic surgery. *Circulation* 2002; **106**(12 suppl 1): 90–4.

4. Malviya S, Voepel-Lewis T, Siewert M et al. Risk factors for adverse postoperative outcomes in children presenting for cardiac surgery with upper respiratory tract infections. *Anesthesiology* 2003; **98**(3): 628–32.

5. Laishley RS, Burrows FA, Lerman J, Roy WL. Effect of anesthetic induction regimens on oxygen saturation in cyanotic congenital heart disease. *Anesthesiology* 1986; **65**: 673–7.

6. Morray JP, Lynn AM, Stamm SJ et al. Hemodynamic effects of ketamine in children with congenital heart disease. *Anesth Analg* 1984; **63**(10): 895–9.

7. Bhutta A, Gilliam C, Honeycutt M et al. Reduction of bloodstream infections associated with catheters in paediatric intensive care unit: stepwise approach. *BMJ* 2007; **334**: 362–5.

8. Kurth CD, Uher B. Cerebral hemoglobin and optical pathlength influence near-infrared spectroscopy measurement of cerebral oxygen saturation. *Anesth Analg* 1997; **84**(6): 1297–305.

9. Kurth CD, Steven JL, Montenegro LM et al. Cerebral oxygen saturation before congenital heart surgery. *Ann Thorac Surg* 2001; **72**(1): 187–92.

10. Abdul-Khaliq H, Uhlig R, Bottcher W et al. Factors influencing the change in cerebral hemodynamics in pediatric patients during and after corrective cardiac surgery of congenital heart diseases by means of full-flow cardiopulmonary bypass. *Perfusion* 2002; **17**(3): 179–85.

11. Zimmerman AA, Burrows FA, Jonas RA, Hickey PR. The limits of detectable cerebral perfusion by transcranial Doppler sonography in neonates undergoing deep hypothermic low-flow cardiopulmonary bypass. *J Thorac Cardiovasc Surg* 1997; **114**(4): 594–600.

12. Mathew JP, Weatherwax KJ, East CJ et al. Bispectral analysis during cardiopulmonary bypass: the effect of hypothermia on the hypnotic state. *J Clin Anesth* 2001; **13**(4): 301–5.

13. Schmidlin D, Hager P, Schmid ER. Monitoring level of sedation with bispectral EEG analysis: comparison between hypothermic and normothermic cardiopulmonary bypass. *Br J Anaesth* 2001; **86**(6): 769–76.

14. Jonas RA. Deep hypothermic circulatory arrest: current status and indications. *Semin Thorac Cardiovasc Surg* 2006; **5**: 76–88.

15. Forbess JM, Visconti KJ, Hancock-Friesen C et al. Neurodevelopmental outcome after congenital heart surgery: results from an institutional registry. *Circulation* 2002; **106**(12 suppl 1): 95–102.

16. Forbess JM, Visconti KJ, Bellinger DC et al. Neurodevelopmental outcomes after biventricular repair of congenital heart defects. *J Thorac Cardiovasc Surg* 2002; **123**(4): 631–9.

17. Shin'oka T, Shum-Tim D, Jonas RA et al. Higher hematocrit improves cerebral outcome after deep hypothermic circulatory arrest. *J Thorac Cardiovasc Surg* 1996; **112**(6): 1610–20, 1620–1.

18. Shin'oka T, Shum-Tim D, Laussen PC et al. Effects of oncotic pressure and hematocrit on outcome after hypothermic circulatory arrest. *Ann Thorac Surg* 1998; **65**(1): 155–64.

19. Stevenson JG. Utilization of intraoperative transesophageal echocardiography during repair of congenital cardiac defects: a survey of North American centers. *Clin Cardiol* 2003; **26**(3): 132–4.

20. Quinones MA, Douglas PS, Foster E et al. American College of Cardiology/American Heart Association clinical competence statement on echocardiography: a report of the American College of Cardiology/American Heart Association/American College of Physicians – American Society of Internal Medicine Task Force on Clinical Competence. *Circulation* 2003; **107**(7): 1068–89.

21. Bettex DA, Pretre R, Jenni R, Schmid ER. Cost-effectiveness of routine intraoperative transesophageal echocardiography in pediatric cardiac surgery: a 10-year experience. *Anesth Analg* 2005; **100**(5): 1271–5.

22. Bettex DA, Schmidlin D, Bernath MA et al. Intraoperative transesophageal echocardiography in pediatric congenital cardiac surgery: a two-center observational study. *Anesth Analg* 2003; **97**(5): 1275–82.

23. Randolph GR, Hagler DJ, Connolly HM et al. Intraoperative transesophageal echocardiography during surgery for congenital heart defects. *J Thorac Cardiovasc Surg* 2002; **124**(6): 1176–82.

24. Stevenson JG. Incidence of complications in pediatric transesophageal echocardiography: experience in 1650 cases. *J Am Soc Echocardiogr* 1999; **12**(6): 527–32.

25. Schiller NB. Hemodynamics derived from transesophageal echocardiography (TEE). *Cardiol Clin* 2000; **18**(4): 699–709.

26. Williams GD, Bratton SL, Riley EC, Ramamoorthy C. Association between age and blood loss in children undergoing open heart operations. *Ann Thorac Surg* **66**(3): 870–5; discussion 875–6.

27. Miller BE, Mochizuki T, Levy JH et al. Predicting and treating coagulopathies after cardiopulmonary bypass in children. *Anesth Analg* 1997; **85**(6): 1196–202.

28. Chan AK, Leaker M, Burrows FA et al. Coagulation and fibrinolytic profile of paediatric patients undergoing cardiopulmonary bypass. *Thromb Haemost* 1997; **77**(2): 270–7 (erratum Thromb Haemost 1997; **77**(5): 1047).

29. Ichinose F, Uezono S, Muto R et al. Platelet hyporeactivity in young infants during cardiopulmonary bypass. *Anesth Analg* **88**(2): 258–62, 1999.

30. Codispoti M, Ludlam CA, Simpson D, Mankad PS. Individualized heparin and protamine management in infants and children undergoing cardiac operations. *Ann Thorac Surg* 2001; **71**(3): 922–7; discussion 927–8.

31. Chauhan S, Kumar BA, Rao BH et al. Efficacy of aprotinin, epsilon aminocaproic acid, or combination in cyanotic heart disease. *Ann Thorac Surg* 2000; **70**(4): 1308–12.

32. Reid RW, Zimmerman AA, Laussen PC et al. The efficacy of tranexamic acid versus placebo increasing blood loss in

pediatric patients undergoing repeat cardiac surgery. *Anesth Analg* 1997; **84**(5): 990–6.

33. Levi M, Cromheecke ME de JE, Prins MH *et al.* Pharmacological strategies to decrease excessive blood loss in cardiac surgery: a meta-analysis of clinically relevant endpoints. *Lancet* 1999; **354**(9194): 1940–7.

34. Boldt J, Knothe C, Zickmann B *et al.* Comparison of two aprotinin dosage regimens in pediatric patients having cardiac operations. Influence on platelet function and blood loss. J Thorac *Cardiovasc Surg* 1993; **105**(4): 705–11.

35. D'Errico CC, Shayevitz JR, Tindale SJ *et al.* The efficacy and cost of aprotinin in children undergoing reoperative open heart surgery. *Anesth Analg* 1996; **83**(6): 1193–9.

36. Dietrich W, Mossinger H, Spannagl M *et al.* Hemostatic activation during cardiopulmonary bypass with different aprotinin dosages in pediatric patients having cardiac operations. *J Thorac Cardiovasc Surg* 1993; **105**(4): 712–20.

37. Mossinger H, Dietrich W, Braun SL *et al.* High-dose aprotinin reduces activation of hemostasis, allogeneic blood requirement, and duration of postoperative ventilation in pediatric cardiac surgery. *Ann Thorac Surg* 2003; **75**(2): 430–7.

38. Mangano DT, Tudor IC, Dietzel C. The risk associated withotinin in cardiac surgery. *N Engl J Med* 2006 26; **354**(4): 353–65.

39. Mangano DT, Miao Y, Vuylsteke A *et al.* Investigators of The Multicenter Study of Perioperative Ischemia Research Group; Ischemia Research and Education Foundation. Mortality associated with aprotinin during 5 years following coronary artery bypass graft surgery. *JAMA* 2007; **297**: 471–9.

40. Codispoti M, Mankad PS. Significant merits of a fibrin sealant in the presence of coagulopathy following paediatric cardiac surgery: randomised controlled trial. *Eur J Cardiothorac Surg* 2002; **22**(2): 200–5.

41. Naik SK, Knight A, Elliott MJ. A successful modification of ultrafiltration for cardiopulmonary bypass in children. *Perfusion* 1991; **6**(1): 41–50.

42. Naik SK, Knight A, Elliott M. A prospective randomized study of a modified technique of ultrafiltration during pediatric open-heart surgery. *Circulation* 1991; **84**(suppl 5): 422–31.

43. Celermajer DS, Cullen S, Deanfield JE. Impairment of endothelium-dependent pulmonary artery relaxation in children with congenital heart disease and abnormal pulmonary hemodynamics. *Circulation* 1993; **87**(2): 440–6.

44. Yamaki S, Abe A, Tabayashi K *et al.* Inoperable pulmonary vascular disease in infants with congenital heart disease. *Ann Thorac Surg* 1998; **66**(5): 1565–70.

45. Mavroudis CBC. Ventriculartal defect. In: Mavroudis CBC, ed. *Pediatric cardiac surgery.* Philadephia, CV: Mosby, 2003: 298–338.

46. Reddy VM, Hanley FL. Cardiac surgery in infants with very low birth weight. *Semin Pediatr Surg* 2000; **9**(2): 91–5.

47. Reddy VM, McElhinney DB, Sagrado T *et al.* Results of 102 cases of complete repair of congenital heart defects in patients weighing 700–2500 g. *J Thorac Cardiovasc Surg* 1999; **117**(2): 324–31.

48. Kumar A, Taylor GP, Sandor GG, Patterson MW. Pulmonary vascular disease in neonates with transposition of the great arteries and intact ventriculartum. *Br Heart J* 1993; **69**(5): 442–5.

49. Pearl JM, Nelson DP, Schwartz SM, Manning PB. First-stage palliation for hypoplastic left heart syndrome in the twenty-first century. *Ann Thorac Surg* 2002; **73**(1): 331–9; discussion 339–40.

50. Mahle WT, Cuadrado AR, Tam VK. Early experience with a modified Norwood procedure using right ventricle to pulmonary artery conduit. *Ann Thorac Surg* 2003; **76**(4): 1084–8.

51. Tanoue Y, Kado H, Shiokawa Y *et al.* Midterm ventricular performance after Norwood procedure with right ventricular-pulmonary artery conduit. *Ann Thorac Surg* 2004; **78**(6): 1965–71.

52. Fraser CD Jr, Mee RB. Modified Norwood procedure for hypoplastic left heart syndrome. *Ann Thorac Surg* 1995; **60**(suppl 6): S546–9.

53. Tweddell JS, Hoffman GM, Fedderly RT *et al.* Phenoxybenzamine improves systemic oxygen delivery after the Norwood procedure. *Ann Thorac Surg* 1991; **67**(1): 161–7; discussion 167–8.

54. Gamillscheg A, Zobel G, Urlesberger B *et al.* Inhaled nitric oxide in patients with critical pulmonary perfusion after Fontan-type procedures and bidirectional Glenn anastomosis. *J Thorac Cardiovasc Surg* 1997; **113**(3): 435–42.

55. Tweddell JS, Berger S, Frommelt PC *et al.* Aprotinin improves outcome of single-ventricle palliation. *Ann Thorac Surg* 1996; **62**(5): 1329–35; discussion 1335–6.

56. Botto LD, Correa A, Erickson JD. Racial and temporal variations in the prevalence of heart defects. *Pediatrics* 2001; **107**(3): E32.

57. Maizza AF, Ho SY, Anderson RH. Obstruction of the left ventricular outflow tract: anatomical observations and surgical implications. *J Heart Valve Dis* 1993; **2**(1): 66–79.

58. Medley J, Russo P, Tobias JD. Perioperative care of the patient with Williams syndrome. *Paediatr Anaesth* 2005; **15**(3): 243–7.

59. Bauer EP, Schmidli J, Vogt PR *et al.* Valvotomy for isolated congenital aortic stenosis in children: prognostic factors for outcome. *Thorac Cardiovasc Surg* 1992; **40**(6): 334–9.

60. Rao PS, Thapar MK, Galal O, Wilson AD. Follow-up results of balloon angioplasty of native coarctation in neonates and infants. *Am Heart J* 1990; **120**(6 Pt 1): 1310–4.

61. Elkins RC, Lane MM, McCue C. Ross operation in children: late results. *J Heart Valve Dis* 2001; **10**(6): 736–41.

62. Park SC, Neches WH. The neurologic complications of congenital heart disease. *Neurol Clin* 1993; **11**(2): 441–62.

63. Lim C, Kim WH, Kim SC *et al.* Aortic arch reconstruction using regional perfusion without circulatory arrest. *Eur J Cardiothorac Surg* 2003; **23**(2): 149–55.

64. Tlaskal T, Hucin B, Hruda J *et al.* Results of primary and two-stage repair of interrupted aortic arch. *Eur J Cardiothorac Surg* 1998; **14**(3): 235–42.

65. Boucek MM, Edwards LB, Keck BM *et al.* The Registry of the International Society for Heart and Lung Transplantation: Sixth

Official Pediatric Report – 2003. *J Heart Lung Transplant* 2003; **22**(6): 636–52.

66. Maron BJ. Hypertrophic cardiomyopathy in childhood. *Pediatr Clin North Am* 2004; **51**(5): 1305–46.

67. Morrow WR. Cardiomyopathy and heart transplantation in children. *Curr Opin Cardiol* 2000; **15**(4): 216–23.

68. Doroshow RW, Ashwal S, Saukel GW. Availability and selection of donors for pediatric heart transplantation. *J Heart Lung Transplant* 1995; **14**(1 Pt 1): 52–8.

69. Scheule AM, Zimmerman GJ, Johnston JK *et al.* Duration of graft cold ischemia does not affect outcomes in pediatric heart transplant recipients. *Circulation* 2002; **106**(12 suppl 1): 163–7.

70. Williams GD, Ramamoorthy C. Anesthesia considerations for pediatric thoracic solid organ transplant. *Anesthesiol Clin North Am* 2005; **23**(4): 709–31.

71. Schindler E, Muller M, Akinturk H *et al.* Perioperative management in pediatric heart transplantation from 1988 to 2001: anesthetic experience in a single center. *Pediatr Transplant* 2004; **8**(3): 237–42.

72. Hoffman TM, Wernovsky G, Atz AM *et al.* Prophylactic intravenous use of milrinone after cardiac operation in pediatrics (PRIMACORP) study. Prophylactic intravenous use of milrinone after cardiac operation in pediatrics. *Am Heart J* **143**(1): 15–21, 2002.

73. Phan V, West LJ, Stephens D, Hebert D. Renal complications following heart transplantation in children: a single-center study. *Am J Transplant* 2003; **3**(2): 214–8.

74. Bing RJ VLGF. Physiological studies in congenital heart disease. *Bull Johns Hopkins Hosp* 1947; **80**: 107–20.

75. Rashkind WJ, Miller WW. Creation of an atrial septal defect without thoracotomy. A palliative approach to complete transposition of the great arteries. *JAMA* 1966; **196**(11): 991–2.

76. Pass RH, Hellenbrand WE. Catheter intervention for critical aortic stenosis in the neonate. *Catheter Cardiovasc Interv* 2002; **55**(1): 88–92.

77. Hernandez-Gonzalez M, Solorio S, Conde-Carmona I *et al.* Intraluminal aortoplasty vs. surgical aortic resection in congenital aortic coarctation. A clinical random study in pediatric patients. *Arch Med Res* 2003; **34**(4): 305–10.

78. Koch A, Buheitel G, Gerling S *et al.* Balloon dilatation of critical left heart stenoses in low birthweight infants. *Acta Paediatr* 2000; **89**(8): 979–82.

79. Rhodes JF, Asnes JD, Blaufox AD, Sommer RJ. Impact of low body weight on frequency of pediatric cardiac catheterization complications. *Am J Cardiol* 2000 1; **86**(11): 1275–8, A9.

80. Bennett D, Marcus R, Stokes M. Incidents and complications during pediatric cardiac catheterization. *Paediatr Anaesth* 2005; **15**(12): 1083–8.

81. American Academy of Pediatrics Committee on Drugs: guidelines for monitoring and management of pediatric patients during and after sedation for diagnostic and therapeutic procedures. *Pediatrics* 1992; **89**(6 Pt 1): 1110–15.

82. Practice guidelines for sedation and analgesia by non-anesthesiologists. A report by the American Society of Anesthesiologists Task Force on Sedation and Analgesia by Non-Anesthesiologists. *Anesthesiology* 1996; **84**(2): 459–71.

83. May L Eliot. *Paediatric heart surgery: a ready reference for professionals.* Milwaukee, TN: Maxishare, 2005.

41

Liver, intestine and renal transplantation

JAMES BENNETT, PETER BROMLEY

KEY LEARNING POINTS

Liver transplantation

- Portal hypertension is a debilitating and life-threatening condition.
- Chronic liver disease is associated with a variety of extra-hepatic manifestations.
- Timing of transplantation is crucial before severe decompensation occurs.
- Acute liver failure is a multisystem disorder with high mortality.
- Coagulopathy and reperfusion syndrome are intraoperative challenges.
- Outcome is excellent, with survivors showing good growth and development.

Intestinal transplantation

- Intestinal transplantation shares many features with liver transplantation.

- Difficulties with venous access should not be underestimated.
- Patients with dysmotility disorders are at risk of aspiration of gastric contents.
- Combined liver–bowel transplantation involves major intraoperative haemodynamic changes.
- Sepsis is a common early complication.
- Results are poor compared with liver transplantation.
- Lymphoproliferative disorder is a major challenge.

Renal transplantation

- End-stage renal failure is rare in children.
- Dialysis is associated with a variety of complications.
- Hypertension and anaemia are common preoperatively.
- Outcome is excellent.
- Most cases are extubated at end of surgery.
- Epidural analgesia is commonly used.

INTRODUCTION

Liver, small bowel and renal transplantations have evolved from experimental procedures to accepted treatments for debilitating end-stage disease. Children undergoing such transplant procedures pose complex challenges to the anaesthetist, from not only their presenting condition, but also the effects of medical therapy such as immunosuppression and dialysis.

Timing of transplantation must balance the progression towards end-stage disease while allowing growth and development of the child. Children who have received transplants often require anaesthesia for unrelated procedures outside of transplant units.

LIVER TRANSPLANTATION

The first successful liver transplantation was performed in 1967 by Starzl on an 18-month-old child who survived for 1 year [1]. Mortality remained very high until the introduction of ciclosporin in 1979. This led to an expansion of transplant centres worldwide [2]. Improved immunosuppressive drugs as well as surgical and anaesthetic techniques have led to survival rates higher than 90 per cent. Children who have received liver transplants are now entering adult life [3].

Indications

Liver disease affects children of all ages and may present chronically or acutely. Disease patterns vary according to age; there are conditions specific to the neonatal period such as neonatal haemochromatosis and conditions affecting infants such as biliary atresia. With increasing age a more heterogeneous disease pattern emerges, with α_1-antitrypsin deficiency and autoimmune hepatitis becoming prevalent until adolescence, when diseases associated with adulthood assume prominence.

There are many classifications of liver disease; however, it is useful to divide the indications into chronic and acute. New indications are being added as practice changes (Fig. 41.1).

Biliary atresia is the commonest indication for paediatric liver transplantation world-wide and is representative of chronic liver disease in infants and children. Infants with biliary atresia undergo a Kasai portoenterostomy to re-establish bile flow; in many, however, progressive liver disease often ensues.

Assessment for liver transplantation

Children with liver disease have complex medical histories requiring a multidisciplinary assessment over a period of days. This admission gives the anaesthetist an excellent opportunity to assess comorbidity and medication, order further investigations and plan the transplant anaesthetic. It is also a valuable time to give information about premedication, anaesthetic induction, venous access and postoperative analgesia.

Children with chronic liver disease develop cirrhosis and portal hypertension with ascites and oesophageal varices.

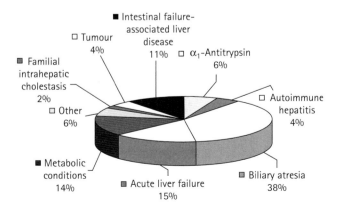

Figure 41.1   Indications for paediatric liver transplantation at the Birmingham Children's Hospital, 1983–2005, $n = 506$.

They are often malnourished with poor growth; progressive jaundice causes troublesome itching and they are prone to infections (recurrent cholangitis, spontaneous bacterial peritonitis or chest infections). The skin becomes fragile with easy bruising from coagulopathy and thrombocytopenia. Metabolic bone disease is common. The clinical implications for the anaesthetist depend on the progression of the liver disease and the presence of extrahepatic manifestations.

Cardiovascular function

Decompensated liver disease is associated with increased cardiac output and low systemic vascular resistance; the mechanism for this remains obscure, but is likely to be a combination of fluid retention and accumulation of vasoactive compounds. Careful cardiac assessment is essential; electrocardiogram (ECG) and transthoracic echocardiograph are reviewed prior to listing to exclude significant cardiac pathology. This is particularly important with biliary atresia where situs inversus and atrial septal defect are relatively common.

Cardiomyopathy is rare in children with liver disease, but it may become apparent in children presenting for retransplantation as a consequence of immunosuppression with tacrolimus [4]. Hypertension is also common in the retransplantation group and requires treatment, which should be continued perioperatively.

Portopulmonary hypertension is very rare in children. Presentation is often late as the symptoms are subtle and may follow the discovery of a new heart murmur, syncope or dyspnoea. Echocardiography and careful cardiological assessment are essential; chest X-ray and ECG are poor screening investigations [5].

Pulmonary hypertension is associated with Alagille syndrome, an autosomal dominant condition characterised by bile duct paucity with cholestasis and itch, in association with cardiac, skeletal and facial abnormalities. The cardiac defect is most commonly a distal pulmonary artery stenosis. Children with Alagille syndrome undergoing liver transplantation have a high mortality rate because of cardiac decompensation [6].

It is not unusual to come across children with minor congenital cardiac abnormalities and for most this proves to be a coincidental finding; reassurance, perioperative prophylactic antibiotic cover and careful attention to avoid air in intravenous infusions and surgical anastomoses are all that are necessary. In more complicated cases the timing of cardiac intervention or surgery must be balanced by the progression of their liver disease.

Respiratory function in liver disease

Impaired respiratory function and arterial hypoxaemia are features of children with advanced liver disease. The most common cause is mechanical, with reduced lung volumes and basal collapse from ascites and hepatosplenomegaly. Pleural effusions may also occur; these further decrease lung volumes and increase the work of breathing. Chest infections are common, particularly in children with encephalopathy and poor gastric emptying as well as those who are debilitated and malnourished.

The hepatopulmonary syndrome (HPS) is arterial hypoxaemia from right-to-left shunting due to vasodilatation of the pulmonary vasculature in patients with liver disease [7]. It is commoner in children and associated with biliary atresia and polysplenia syndrome [8].

The diagnosis of HPS is made clinically by a fall in arterial oxygen levels on standing, dyspnoea and clubbing. A ^{99m}Tc-radiolabelled albumin scan is diagnostic. In normal subjects 95 per cent of the microaggregated albumin is taken up by the lungs; however, in HPS, take-up is in the systemic circulation because of intrapulmonary shunting [9]. Agitated saline contrast echocardiography may also be used; the appearance of 'bubbles' in the left atrium after five beats in the absence of a direct intra-atrial communication is considered diagnostic.

Since the degree of hypoxia may be more advanced than the liver disease, HPS is an indication for early liver transplantation (Table 41.1). Oxygen saturations return to normal following transplantation. Van Obbergh et al. [10] reported a series of seven children with HPS undergoing liver transplantation, all of whom reversed their HPS postoperatively after a mean period of 24 weeks. Most were extubated while still hypoxic with no sequelae. It is essential that the response to oxygen administration is measured and that saturation levels are closely monitored at night or during procedures.

Children with cystic fibrosis and symptoms of portal hypertension are also candidates for liver transplantation. They tend to be older and have well-assessed lung function; respiratory decompensation and chest sepsis are the major postoperative complications [11].

Renal function in liver disease

Renal dysfunction is common in chronic liver disease and is associated with drug toxicity, sepsis and hypovolaemia. Children undergoing retransplantation are particularly prone to perioperative renal failure from immunosuppressive drugs. Children with organic acidaemias and primary oxalosis may be in established renal failure and on renal replacement therapy prior to combined liver and kidney transplantation [12].

The hepatorenal syndrome is less common in children than adults. It is characterised by impaired renal blood flow, low glomerular filtration rate (GFR) and poor urine output. It probably represents an imbalance between vasoconstriction in the renal circulation and splanchnic vasodilatation. It is usually seen in the setting of acute liver failure. There is some evidence to support the use of intravascular filling with albumin and the administration of terlipressin (a nonselective agonist of V1 vasopressin receptors) [13].

Neurological function

Impaired neurological function is a worrying sign in end-stage liver disease. There are many causes: hyponatraemia and hypoglycaemia are easily identified and treated. Hepatic encephalopathy is poorly understood. The aetiology is multifactorial including alterations in cardiac output, and cerebral metabolism with the accumulation of ammonia and neuroactive peptides acting as false neurotransmitters. It is often rapidly progressive in acute liver failure and can be graded clinically (Table 41.2). Patients with grade III or IV coma require intubation and ventilation to protect the airway; all patients with milder grades of encephalopathy require monitoring and review. These patients tolerate sedative drugs poorly and any procedure involving general anaesthesia or sedation must be carefully considered.

Haematological function

Coagulopathy is common and may be severe. Levels of the vitamin K-dependent factors II, VII, IX and X are reduced owing to poor absorption of the fat-soluble vitamins secondary to reduced bile acid secretion in addition to poor liver synthetic activity. Indeed, the prothrombin time is used as a guide to liver synthetic activity. Recombinant factor VIIa is a promising agent to control excessive bleeding associated with liver disease. There are, as yet, few paediatric data although early adult studies show promise [14]. Levels of antithrombin III, and proteins C and S are also reduced in liver disease predisposing to intravascular thrombosis.

Splenomegaly, secondary to portal hypertension, results in sequestration of erythrocytes and platelets causing

Table 41.1 Common causes of hypoxia in children with liver disease

Ascites, hepatosplenomegaly and diaphragmatic splinting
Pleural effusion
Infection
Fluid overload
Cystic fibrosis
Hepatopulmonary syndrome
Cardiac anomalies

Table 41.2 Grading of hepatic encephalopathy

Grade 0	Normal
Grade I	Drowsy but orientated
Grade II	Drowsy but disorientated
Grade III	Agitated and aggressive
Grade IV	Unrousable to deep pain

anaemia and thrombocytopenia. Platelet counts may be further reduced as a result of sepsis, particularly from indwelling central venous lines. Recurrent gastrointestinal haemorrhage and malabsorption may also lead to anaemia.

Metabolic function

The liver is the main store of glycogen in the body. Glycogen synthesis is impaired in liver disease as is gluconeogenesis and children with end-stage liver disease are prone to hypoglycaemia. Blood sugar monitoring is essential particularly during anaesthesia.

Ammonia is produced by amino acid metabolism and converted to urea by the liver. In liver disease, hyperammonaemia may occur and serum urea is low. Enteric bacteria break down amines from blood in the intestinal tract following gastrointestinal (GI) haemorrhage; treatment with lactulose and neomycin to eradicate bacterial overgrowth helps to reduce ammonia production.

Acute liver failure

Acute liver failure in children is an emergency and carries a high mortality. The features are of a multisystem disorder associated with severe impairment of liver function, with or without encephalopathy, associated with hepatic necrosis in the absence of chronic liver disease [15]. The aetiology varies according to age. In the neonate, haemochromatosis is the commonest aetiology, whereas in children viral hepatitis, metabolic conditions and drug toxicity predominate (Fig. 41.2)[16].

These children are best managed in a specialised centre with access to liver transplantation. They should be nursed in a quiet environment and, if encephalopathic, admitted to the intensive care unit for early intubation and ventilation to prevent aspiration, ensure oxygenation and control intracranial hypertension. Invasive lines are placed to allow regular sampling (glucose, electrolytes, international normalised ratio [INR]) and close fluid management. Hypoglycaemia is common and should be treated promptly; enteral nutrition is

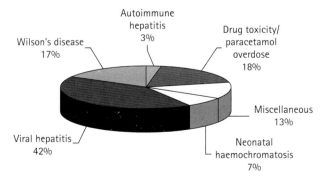

Figure 41.2   Indications for liver transplantation in acute liver failure, at the Birmingham Children's Hospital, 1983–2005, n = 76.

often well tolerated. Broad-spectrum antibiotics and antifungals are given as sepsis is common.

Hypotension is common secondary to vasodilatation with a high cardiac output; intravenous filling and a noradrenaline (norepinephrine) infusion are often required. Renal dysfunction is usually managed with haemofiltration.

Neurological deterioration can be rapid from mild confusion and irritability, to coma and death from intracranial hypertension. At present, most care is supportive and extrapolated from adult practice. Intubation and ventilation with careful sedation are employed to maintain adequate oxygenation and partial pressure of arterial carbon dioxide ($PaCO_2$) in the low normal range. Sedation may be increased to obtund reflexes at the time of invasive procedures. The children are nursed with a 10° head-up tilt, and tube ties are kept loose around the neck to prevent obstruction of venous drainage.

Pupillary changes or evidence of intracranial hypetension are treated with boluses of sedation, ensuring appropriate ventilation and the administration of 20 per cent mannitol 0.5 g/kg. Hypertonic saline [17] and mild hypothermia are promising treatments in adult practice [18].

Intracranial pressure (ICP) monitoring remains controversial; some consider that it guides clinicians in maintaining a cerebral perfusion pressure of 50 mmHg during times of circulatory disturbance or surges of ICP. The risk of intracranial haemorrhage in a child with coagulopathy is high, however. Others suggest that the only proven treatment for acute liver failure is liver transplantation, and the only use for ICP monitoring is to select those children with severe intracranial hypertension who will no longer benefit from transplantation.

The mortality rate in liver transplantation for acute liver failure is significantly greater than for patients with chronic disease as a result of cardiovascular collapse or neurological complications.

Anaesthesia for liver transplantation

The benefits of anaesthetic assessment prior to listing are that most difficulties have been anticipated and an anaesthetic plan has been made for each child.

Preoperatively, full blood count, clotting profile, urea and electrolytes, glucose and liver function tests are scrutinised. Transfusion of platelets and clotting factors is started as indicated prior to theatre. Hyponatraemia is occasionally noted preoperatively, secondary to spironolactone or hypoaldosteronism; the serum sodium must be greater than 125 mmol/L. During liver transplantation serum sodium often rises because of fluid shifts and transfusion, putting the child at risk of central pontine myelinolysis [19].

The parents and child are re-interviewed to explain the anaesthetic procedures, check fasting times and offer premedication. Sedative premedication is not prescribed routinely as it appears to have an unpredictable action in end-stage liver disease and is difficult to time. We ensure that an intravenous dextrose infusion is running in all but the fittest of children and encourage clear, sugar-containing oral fluids up to 2 hours before induction of anaesthesia.

The presence of parents is encouraged at induction of anaesthesia, full monitoring is attached and the children are placed in the semi-recumbent position or in the carer's arms. Usually, an intravenous induction using propofol 2–3 mg/kg, with fentanyl 2 μg/kg, is used. Alternatively, a gaseous induction with sevoflurane in a mixture of nitrous oxide and oxygen is used, but may be slow owing to intra-pulmonary shunting.

Muscle relaxation is achieved with non-depolarising muscle relaxants, usually rocuronium or atracurium. We use a dose of 1–2 mg/kg of rocuronium to achieve rapid conditions for intubation; higher doses than usual are required because of increased volume of distribution, as well as greater binding to acute phase proteins. Rocuronium and vecuronium are metabolised in the liver and thus cleared slowly. We do not routinely employ a rapid sequence induction with cricoid pressure [20] and avoid the use of suxamethonium [21]. Plasma pseudocholinesterase levels are reduced in liver disease and may lead to prolonged action of suxamethonium and mivacurium.

Following adequate muscle relaxation a tracheal tube is placed. In infants, nasal intubation is the route of choice to ensure safe fixation. However, in the presence of coagulopathy and thrombocytopenia the oral route is preferred, thus avoiding the risk of nasal haemorrhage. Tense ascites and hepatosplenomegaly may lead to restriction of diaphragmatic movement during ventilation and a snug-fitting tracheal tube is selected. Moderate hypoxia may occur and relatively high airway pressures with positive end-expiratory pressure (PEEP) are often necessary to maintain adequate gas exchange. Drainage of ascites on opening of the peritoneum often leads to a marked improvement in ventilation.

Children with liver disease are prone to intraoperative hypothermia because of their small size, vasodilatation and malnourished state. Additionally, they are exposed during placement of cannulae, monitoring lines and catheters, and receive cold blood and a cold donor liver graft. Normothermia is important for the metabolic function of the graft as well as other organ systems. The ambient temperature in theatre is raised and the children covered in blankets immediately following induction of anaesthesia. During placement of monitoring lines and catheters they are positioned on a pressure-relieving warming mattress. After anaesthetic preparation, a convective warming system is placed over the body and they are draped with clear PVC drapes, which prevent ascites and blood pooling. They are then surgically prepared and draped. All fluids and blood products are also warmed with devices that allow for rapid infusion such as the Hotline (SIMS Level 1, Inc., Rockland, MA, USA). Temperature monitoring is mandatory using nasopharyngeal and cutaneous probes.

The size and site of intravenous catheters depend on the size of the child and anticipated surgical blood loss. There can be few rules as there is such a range; generally one or two large peripheral cannulae and a multilumen central venous catheter are adequate. All cannulae and central venous catheters are sited in the distribution of the superior vena cava, as manipulation of the inferior vena cava during surgery makes access from the lower part of the body unreliable. High-risk cases may require the placement of large-bore intravenous sheaths in a great vein for rapid infusion. Coagulopathy and previous central access make insertion of central venous catheters a dangerous procedure and there is increasing use of real-time ultrasound guidance [22] (see Chapter 22). Usually, a single arterial catheter for sampling and pressure monitoring is placed in a radial artery. The femoral approach is not recommended because of damping during aortic cross-clamping if an aortic conduit is constructed.

During liver transplantation rapid changes in haemodynamics occur owing to fluctuations in cardiac output, as well as decreased venous return secondary to bleeding and caval manipulation. Cardiac output monitoring is advisable, if not essential. Pulmonary artery catheters are seldom used in children due to complications and size. Less invasive devices are increasingly being used although to date without good comparison. The PiCCO (Pulsion Medical Systems AG, Munich, Germany) is a continuous monitor of cardiac output, which uses a thermodilution catheter inserted via the femoral artery. Saline injections are given via the central venous catheter; stroke volume and cardiac output are calculated using an algorithm derived from pulse contour analysis. The device is also able to calculate other parameters such as extravascular lung water. The LiDCO (LiDCO Ltd, Cambridge, UK) is a similar monitor, which does not require a thermodilution catheter and relies upon the arterial waveform contour to derive cardiac output with lithium dilution calibration.

Transoesophageal echocardiography shows promise as a diagnostic tool and monitor of cardiac output during liver transplantation [23]. A small paediatric probe is gently advanced following induction of anaesthesia. The four-chamber view provides excellent assessment of cardiac structure and function. Sequential measurements of the left ventricle allow calculation of left-ventricular end-diastolic volume, stroke volume and cardiac output. There are concerns over trauma to oesophageal varices.

A urethral catheter and nasogastric tube are also passed. Great care is taken to position the child in order to ensure access to the endotracheal tube and lines, allow good surgical access and avoid pressure damage.

We maintain anaesthesia using isoflurane in a mixture of oxygen and air, supplemented by an opioid infusion. Fentanyl tends to accumulate with repeated doses; alfentanil is highly bound to α_1-acid glycoprotein, levels of which are reduced in liver disease. Remifentanil is broken down by tissue and red cell esterase and is a useful agent at a rate of 0.25–0.5 μg/kg/min. Remifentanil has a tendency to cause bradycardia and has a short half-life requiring the addition of a longer-acting opiate towards the end of surgery.

Atracurium provides good muscle relaxation and is metabolised by non-hepatic mechanisms.

Intravenous maintenance fluid is with 4 per cent dextrose in 0.18 per cent saline initially, and is changed according to serial measurements of blood glucose and serum electrolytes. There is increasing evidence to support tight blood glucose control. During the liver transplantation regular measurement of blood gases and electrolytes, especially ionised calcium, sodium, potassium, lactate and glucose, is essential. The authors monitor coagulation with thromboelastography, prothrombin time and activated partial thromboplastin time in theatre.

Thromboelastography

The thromboelastograph (Figs 41.3 and 41.4) was first developed in the 1940s. It consists of a rotating cup into which is placed the blood sample. A plunger is advanced into the sample and, as clot forms, strain from the rotating cup is transmitted to the plunger. The strain is quantified and displayed on a graph plotted against time. Unlike the standard tests of coagulation, the device provides near-patient analysis of thrombosis and fibrinolysis occurring in whole blood. Classically, during liver transplantation coagulopathy is identified, with fibrinolysis during the anhepatic phase and normalisation of the trace following

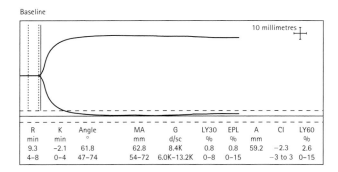

Baseline

R	K	Angle	MA	G	LY30	EPL	A	CI	LY60
min	min	°	mm	d/sc	%	%	mm		%
9.3	−2.1	61.8	62.8	8.4K	0.8	0.8	59.2	−2.3	2.6
4–8	0–4	47–74	54–72	6.0K–13.2K	0–8	0–15		−3 to 3	0–15

Figure 41.3 Baseline thromboelastograph tracing from a patient undergoing liver transplantation.

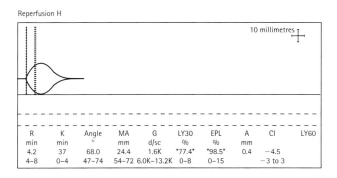

Reperfusion H

R	K	Angle	MA	G	LY30	EPL	A	CI	LY60
min	min	°	mm	d/sc	%	%	mm		
4.2	37	68.0	24.4	1.6K	*77.4*	*98.5*	0.4	−4.5	
4–8	0–4	47–74	54–72	6.0K–13.2K	0–8	0–15		−3 to 3	

Figure 41.4 Thromboelastograph trace demonstrating fibrinolysis following reperfusion.

transfusion of clotting products and function of the grafted liver. The addition of heparinase thromboelastography and accelerators has further refined measurements to target therapy [24].

Types of surgical graft

Short supply of size-matched donor livers means that the majority of paediatric liver grafts are either reduced or split-liver grafts. In the latter technique the left lateral lobe is transplanted into a child and the right lateral lobe is transplanted into an adult recipient. Excellent results may be achieved with such grafts, with 1-year survival rate >90 per cent [25]. Such surgical procedures are technically challenging and carry the risk of vascular complications (hepatic artery and portal vein thrombosis), as well as bleeding from the cut surface of the graft.

Living related transplantation was developed to provide grafts without having an impact on the cadaveric donor pool. First performed in 1989 and now quite commonly world-wide, it involves resection of the left lateral lobe with its vascular supply from a healthy relative and transplantation into a child. The child receives an excellent graft in a planned procedure.

Phases of liver transplantation

The transplant operation is divided into three phases: dissection, anhepatic and reperfusion. The dissection phase lasts from incision to occlusion of the hepatic artery and portal vein; the anhepatic phase is from this point until re-establishment of portal vein inflow to the liver, which is the start of the reperfusion phase, and ends with abdominal closure.

DISSECTION PHASE

This phase may be prolonged in children with previous upper abdominal surgery because of adhesions; loss of blood and ascites may be rapid. Transfusion is guided by haemodynamics and filling pressures, as well as haematocrit, thromboelastogram and other coagulation tests. Ideally, the haematocrit is around 25 per cent to minimise risks of vascular thrombosis. For the same reason only partial correction of coagulation is aimed for, especially if bleeding is from surgical factors. Transplantation operations without any blood product transfusion are not uncommon. Ionised calcium may fall precipitously with infusion of fresh frozen plasma, and calcium chloride infusion is targeted to maintain ionised calcium of 1.2 mmol/L. Improvements in microprocessor technology have allowed manufacture of intraoperative cell salvage devices suitable for children able to process volumes of collected blood as low as 75 mL, and return this to the patient following washing. It is to be expected that in the absence of contraindications transfusion requirements will fall further.

Debate still rages about which fluid to use for intravenous filling: albumin, synthetic colloid or crystalloid? In the absence of good studies this situation is likely to remain contentious. Most units avoid the use of human albumin solutions for intravascular volume expansion, instead opting for a synthetic colloid and transfusing fresh frozen plasma only when indicated by thromboelastogram and clotting studies.

Surgical retraction blades under the diaphragm may lead to movement of small patients and the position and pressure points should be reassessed regularly. Dissection around the porta hepatis and manipulation of the liver may interfere with venous return causing hypotension, which usually responds quickly to fluid administration and pressor support.

ANHEPATIC PHASE

The two major physiological events that occur during the anhepatic phase are decreased venous return to the heart and progressive metabolic abnormalities.

Depending on surgical technique the inferior vena cava is either totally or partially clamped. Despite a compensatory tachycardia, administration of fluid and inotropes may be necessary to correct hypotension. Portal vein clamping similarly reduces venous return, although chronic portal hypertension often results in collateral vessels, allowing blood to return to the heart. Splanchnic and renal circulations may be adversely affected. Excessive fluid administration may lead to high right-atrial pressures at reperfusion when portal and vena cava clamps are released, which may congest the graft and cause significant bleeding.

During the anhepatic phase blood glucose levels fall further and increasing concentrations of intravenous dextrose may be necessary. Despite an often profound metabolic acidosis, buffers are generally avoided unless there is haemodynamic instability or hyperkalaemia. Progressive hyperkalaemia during the anhepatic phase requires control with sodium bicarbonate, dextrose/insulin, furosemide or calcium chloride to avoid dangerous hyperkalaemia on reperfusion.

Core temperature falls during the anhepatic phase and warming equipment is adjusted accordingly.

REPERFUSION

The reperfusion phase is associated with major and sudden changes in haemodynamics. The inferior vena cava and portal vein are unclamped, increasing venous return to the heart. However, systemic hypotension is common as part of the reperfusion syndrome, comprising increased cardiac output, decreased systemic vascular resistance, raised pulmonary vascular resistance and release of endogenous mediators [26]. Although transient, this syndrome may be profound, and is particularly associated with grafts from older donors, higher serum lactate, and liver graft and renal dysfunction. The use of N-acetylcysteine is common to improve reperfusion and early graft function although data regarding its efficacy are limited. N-Acetylcysteine combined with prostaglandin E_1 given at reperfusion and during the postoperative phase has been shown to reduce peak post-transplantation serum alanine transferase, but had little effect on outcome [27]. Conditions should be optimised before reperfusion by tight control of serum potassium and ionised calcium and stable haemodynamics. The surgical team flushes the liver with crystalloid solution or the patient's blood to avoid high levels of potassium, other metabolites and mediators, air and cell debris reaching the recipient's circulation. The portal vein is unclamped slowly and intravenous fluid infused and inotropes given as appropriate. Haemodynamic stability is usually achieved quickly, but may require noradrenaline or adrenaline infusion. Following inspection of the graft for bleeding points the surgical team proceeds to arterialise the graft; good arterial perfusion is required at this stage.

Reperfusion coagulopathy is common and is corrected carefully to prevent bleeding without fluid overload. Heparinase thromboelastography is particularly useful in treating fibrinolysis, which may require treatment with fresh clotting factors and aprotinin. Following arterial and portal revascularisation, acidosis and hyperkalaemia tend to correct spontaneously and serum glucose levels rise due to release from the graft.

Following re-establishment of biliary drainage, drains are placed and surgical closure started. Small infants and those with large grafts are at risk of tight abdominal closure and graft compression; a staged abdominal closure with prosthesis may be employed [28].

If graft function appears to be good preparations for end of surgery are made. Morphine replaces the intraoperative opiate, providing a superior analgesic strategy for the postoperative phase, and a suitable sedative infusion, such as midazolam, is commenced. Most cases are transferred to the intensive care unit; however, good risk candidates are suitable for fast tracking with early extubation. Morphine infusion or patient-controlled analgesia (PCA)/nurse-controlled analgesia (NCA) is widely used for postoperative analgesia.

EARLY POSTOPERATIVE PHASE

The early postoperative phase is associated with ongoing formation of ascites and occasionally significant bleeding requiring aggressive transfusion to maintain good graft perfusion. Haematocrit is maintained at no higher than 25 per cent to lessen chances of hepatic artery thrombosis. The patient is usually weaned off inotropic support, but poor graft function may delay this.

Urine output often falls from the desired 1–2 mL/kg/h secondary to hypovolaemia. Sepsis, poor liver graft function and poor preoperative renal function are risk factors for early renal dysfunction, which often requires haemofiltration.

Respiratory function may be compromised by pleural effusions, fluid overload and a large graft compromising

Table 41.3　Early postoperative complications

Vascular complications
Bleeding
Graft dysfunction
Renal dysfunction
Sepsis
Rejection
Pleural effusion
Pain
Gastrointestinal bleeding and perforation

Table 41.4　Common causes of intestinal failure in children

Gastroschisis
Necrotising enterocolitis
Volvulus
Intestinal atresia
Hirschsprung's disease
Pseudo-obstruction

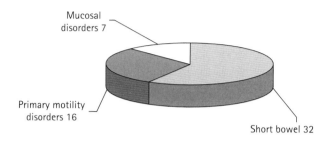

Mucosal disorders 7

Primary motility disorders 16

Short bowel 32

Figure 41.5　Indications for intestinal transplantation at the Birmingham Children's Hospital.

respiratory mechanics. Most children undergoing an elective transplant with good graft function are extubated within 24 hours.

Surgical complications include hepatic artery and portal vein thrombosis, intestinal perforation and bleeding, and usually require early exploration (Table 41.3).

INTESTINAL TRANSPLANTATION

Intestinal transplantation offers the potential for improved quality of life and longevity to those suffering from intestinal failure and life-threatening complications of long-term parenteral nutrition. Unlike renal and liver transplantation the recipients are predominantly children. Intestinal transplantation is relatively new; the first successful small bowel transplantation was performed as part of a multivisceral graft including stomach, duodenum, pancreas and colon in a 3-year-old child in 1987 [29]. However, success rates do not match those of other organ grafts.

Intestinal failure

Children are prone to a diverse range of conditions, which conspire to cause malnutrition at a time when requirements for growth and development are maximal (Table 41.4). This has led to the development of nutritional support both in hospital and at home [30]. One aspect of this is long-term parenteral nutrition (PN), which in many cases is a life-saving therapy. Despite technical advances in long-term central venous catheters and refinements in nutrition, the complications of PN are the main indication for intestinal transplantation.

Some of these complications can be reduced by supplementation with enteral feeding, although this may not be feasible in those who have undergone extensive bowel resection, developed portal hypertension or suffer recurrent episodes of sepsis. The majority of children with intestinal failure have short bowel syndrome; about 20 cm of small intestine with an ileocaecal valve are required, and roughly twice this length without an intact valve. In short gut syndrome poor absorption occurs with ensuing malnutrition,

and dysmotility leads to changes in enteric bacteria, and salt and water losses. Sufferers are prone to episodes of sepsis, diarrhoea and dehydration.

Indications for intestinal transplantation

Children account for around two-thirds of patients undergoing intestinal transplantation world-wide [31]. There are many indications for intestinal transplantation (Fig. 41.5), the majority being postsurgical (often described as short bowel), gastroschisis, necrotising enterocolitis and intestinal atresia. The non-surgical indications are motility disorders such as pseudo-obstruction and aganglionosis, and malabsorption disorders such as microvillus inclusion disease.

Short bowel syndrome is the commonest group of indications and tends to affect infants and small children. Retrospective studies suggest that infants who have undergone intestinal resection and received long-term PN are prone to develop cholestasis with sepsis as a conspicuous feature [32]. Many of these infants develop liver failure and require combined liver and small intestinal transplantation.

Children presenting for intestinal transplantation are typically malnourished and usually have evidence of nutritional therapy such as a nasoenteric tube and/or central venous line. They may have a scarred abdomen and neck from repeated laparotomies, stomas and line insertions. The skin is often fragile with bruising, scars from extravasation and possibly areas of breakdown. Dentition may be poor because of vomiting and the perianal area may be inflamed as a result of persistent diarrhoea. Jaundice and signs of portal hypertension may be apparent.

Timely referral is recommended before the disease progresses to affect other organ systems or loss of central venous access occurs [33].

Assessment

The assessment process is similar to that for children referred for liver transplantation and similarities will be omitted. The complexity of their disease, associated conditions, nutritional therapy and psychological aspects require prolonged and careful assessment. During this admission the children will have a thorough examination and be fully investigated with standard blood tests to study renal and liver function, coagulation and haematological profiles. Careful cardiac assessment is important to exclude valve lesions, pulmonary hypertension or thrombosed veins secondary to central venous catheters. Respiratory review is essential in those cases with a history of prematurity or at risk of aspiration.

One of the key factors in the assessment phase is the extent of their intestinal failure and degree of liver involvement. Radiological assessment of the gut is performed to assess length and motility. Ultrasound scanning of the liver in addition to liver biopsy and endoscopy may be required to identify liver fibrosis or cirrhosis and portal hypertension. A judgement may then be made as to which transplant is necessary: isolated intestinal graft or liver/small bowel graft. In complex cases a decision to proceed to multivisceral transplantation may be made (Fig. 41.6).

A central venous line history is crucial, including previous insertion sites, reasons for removal, infectious agents and complications at insertion. Scars on the neck and chest wall are common, and prominent superficial veins might suggest venous thrombosis and/or superior vena caval syndrome. In one reported series 22 per cent of patients had one thrombosed great vessel, 25 per cent had multiple thrombosed vessels and 2 per cent had all major veins thrombosed [34]. In the authors' unit we perform Doppler ultrasound scans of the great veins. Ultrasound is useful for assessing the internal jugular veins and femoral veins [35]. If imaging of the subclavian veins is inconclusive venography is performed. It is important to exclude thrombosis of the superior vena cava (SVC) as it may be a contraindication to transplantation. If two or more great veins are thrombosed, or there is clinical suspicion, venography or magnetic resonance venography (MRV) is performed to assess patency of the SVC. This provides planning for central venous catheter insertion at the time of transplantation and an indication of the urgency for transplantation.

Surgical aspects

The abdominal incision is usually bilateral subcostal with a midline extension and proposed stoma sites are chosen. It is not unusual for extensive collateral vessels to be present and significant bleeding to occur.

Isolated intestinal transplantation usually involves anastomosis of the donor superior mesenteric artery to recipient aorta via a conduit; the donor portal vein is anastomosed to the recipient portal vein or inferior vena cava. Intestinal

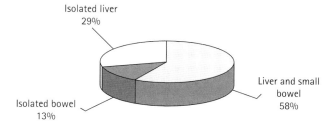

Figure 41.6   Transplantation for intestinal failure by type of graft at the Birmingham Children's Hospital, 1993–2005, $n = 54$.

anastomoses are complex depending on recipient anatomy; a temporary stoma is fashioned to facilitate easy visual and endoscopic surveillance of the graft to identify rejection. The surgical aspects of the combined liver and intestinal grafts are complicated but essentially involve an arterial anastomosis from the infrarenal aorta of the recipient to the liver and intestinal graft via a patch of the coeliac axis and the superior mesenteric artery. Biliary drainage is usually via a roux-en-Y choledochojejunostomy to the donor jejunum.

The availability of size-matched donors is critically limited for infants and small children awaiting combined liver–small bowel grafts. In recent years refinement of surgical technique has led to the successful use of intestine combined with a reduced liver graft. Living related isolated intestinal transplantation programmes are being established and show promise.

Anaesthesia

Anaesthesia for intestinal transplantation is similar to liver transplantation (see above).

Many of these children have received numerous anaesthetics and may be understandably agitated. The presence of parents at induction is usually helpful, and cautious premedication with midazolam may be of use.

Induction is essentially similar to that for liver transplantation, and is usually intravenous using propofol 2–3 mg/kg, fentanyl 2 μg/kg and rocuronium 1 mg/kg via an indwelling central line, and full asepsis. The authors do not routinely perform a rapid sequence induction; however, many of these children will have impaired gastric emptying due to dysmotility conditions and are at risk of aspiration of gastric contents. Intubation often requires a tracheal tube smaller than expected, owing to previous prolonged intubation as a neonate. Anaesthesia is maintained with isoflurane in a mixture of oxygen in air; nitrous oxide is not used to avoid gaseous distension of the bowel. Infusions of atracurium and short-acting opioid are usual. Warming devices and other monitors are the same as for liver transplantation.

Sepsis is a major complication and previous culture reports are scrutinised to identify potential pathogens. If there has been a recent line infection we opt to remove the indwelling tunnelled line and replace it with a temporary multiple lumen line. It is important not to underestimate the difficulty of central line placement in this group of patients. We consult previous radiology reports and place such lines using real-time vascular ultrasound and radiological screening with intravenous contrast if necessary. Strict attention to asepsis is crucial. A full range of catheters and Seldinger wires should be available; occasionally recourse to direct SVC puncture or other advanced method of central venous access is necessary.

Adhesions caused by previous laparotomies make major intraoperative bleeding likely and preparation should be made for rapid transfusion. Children undergoing isolated intestinal transplantation are less likely to suffer dramatic haemodynamic instability compared with liver/small bowel or multivisceral graft recipients as reperfusion syndrome is less profound without the liver graft, and the inferior cava is not clamped.

Children undergoing combined liver/small bowel transplantation may suffer profound haemodynamic changes. Portal hypertension and coagulopathy make surgical dissection difficult and bleeding and ascitic losses are often massive. Reperfusion is somewhat more complicated than the liver-only graft; the reperfusion syndrome still occurs but, additionally, the greater mass of the combined graft necessitates infusion of large volumes of intravenous fluid. Noradrenaline or adrenaline infusions are used as necessary to maintain good arterial perfusion. Profound hypothermia may occur because of the greater mass of the combined graft.

Following completion of surgery a nasojejunal feeding tube is passed to allow early postoperative feeding, and the abdomen is closed. Abdominal closure with a prosthetic patch is often used to avoid compression of the graft, and definitive closure performed later. Sedation with morphine and midazolam is started before transfer to the intensive care unit. Epidural analgesia, which is avoided in liver transplantation because of coagulopathy and intraoperative fibrinolysis, has been used for isolated intestinal transplantation [36].

Postoperative care

The postoperative course of these children is often protracted and complicated. Ventilatory support is continued until acid–base status corrects. Initial fluid requirements remain high owing to ongoing losses and the need to maintain perfusion of the graft. Inotropic support is usually weaned relatively quickly. Nasojejunal feeding commenced when intestinal motility commences. Postoperative haemorrhage or vascular complications usually require early surgical exploration.

Stoma perfusion can easily be observed and biopsy of the graft performed to exclude rejection, vascular injury or infection. Immunosuppression is based on methylprednisolone and tacrolimus, the latter having improved the outcome in intestinal transplantation in recent years.

Recently daclizumab and sirolimus have been introduced. Episodes of rejection can greatly increase stoma output making fluid management very difficult. Sepsis is common and antimicrobial and antifungal agents given according to the results of microbiological surveillance.

Outcomes

Survival for children undergoing intestinal transplantation is not as good as for liver transplantation. Poor prognostic factors appear to be infancy and necrotising enterocolitis, and in general children with short gut fare worse than those with motility disorders. Progression to liver disease is the most important factor associated with poor survival [37]. Results are encouraging for older children undergoing isolated intestinal transplantation for malabsorption [38]; however 1-year patient survival rate for children undergoing combined liver/small bowel transplantation is around 66 per cent [31]. In most series around 70 per cent of children are weaned from total parental nutrition (TPN) to enteral feeding. Long-term complications are sepsis, rejection and post-transplantation lymphoproliferative disorder.

Isolated liver transplantation for intestinal failure

The development of liver disease has an adverse effect on outcome of intestinal transplantation. Some infants referred for intestinal transplantation have established liver disease despite an apparently adequate length of small bowel, which may be capable of adapting to enteral feeding. Such children may be candidates for isolated liver transplantation, and encouraging reports have been published [39].

The complex nature of intestinal failure and transplantation suggests a multidisciplinary approach to the management of these children [40]. Surgical strategies are evolving and include gut lengthening procedures, restoration of intestinal continuity and resection of dysmotile intestine. It is hoped that similar improvements in nutritional care and transplantation will offer children with intestinal failure a brighter future.

RENAL TRANSPLANTATION

Despite advances in the management of renal failure and dialysis, renal transplantation is regarded as the best treatment for children with end-stage renal failure (ESRF).

Renal failure in children

In the UK the incidence of established renal failure requiring renal replacement therapy in children is 10.4 per million population [41]. Renal failure may present at any age

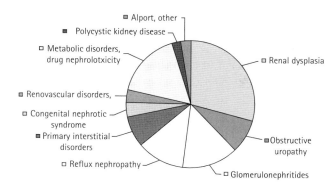

Figure 41.7   Indications for paediatric renal transplantation at the Birmingham Children's Hospital, 1993–2004, $n = 127$.

in childhood but its incidence increases with age, with boys outnumbering girls in a ratio of 1.5:1.

Renal dysplasia and obstructive uropathy are the predominant cause of renal failure in the first 5 years of life; with increasing age, glomerular disorders (glomerular nephritis and nephrotic syndrome) become more common. Renal dysplasia and focal segmental glomerulonephritis are the most common indications for renal transplantation (Fig. 41.7).

Management of end-stage renal failure

Improved medical management has meant that many children with renal failure can remain reasonably well without dialysis; however, dialysis is indicated if there are major problems with fluid overload, electrolyte abnormality or hypertension.

Dialysis is the major treatment modality prior to transplantation in children. The choice of peritoneal dialysis or haemodialysis depends on age and size, the maintenance of vascular access and local experience. Both modalities are associated with complications. Peritoneal dialysis is classically associated with peritonitis, pain, basal atelectasis, pneumonia and pleural effusion. Strict asepsis is essential to minimise the risk of peritonitis; the other complications are secondary to a volume effect and retention of dialysate in the peritoneal cavity. Haemodialysis is associated with haemorrhage due to platelet damage and heparinisation, infection, hypovolaemia and hypotension. Prolonged haemodialysis can lead to metabolic acidosis owing to bicarbonate loss and metabolic bone disease. In children maintenance of vascular access is a major issue; increasingly large-bore (8–12Fr) tunnelled dual-lumen catheters are used for continuous venovenous haemodialysis. Strict asepsis must be observed when using these lines. Thrombosis of the vessels is not unusual and should be excluded before transplantation. Surgically created arteriovenous fistulae may be used for older children for long-term dialysis.

Both modalities may lead to major fluid shifts, and haemodialysis in particular can render the child hypovolaemic; clinical signs and the child's weight chart should be studied carefully. It is essential to document the timing of the last dialysis treatment before anaesthetic induction so that appropriate treatment can be instituted rapidly if hypotension occurs. Renal osteodystrophy is common and explains much of the poor growth displayed by children with ESRF. Most children receive calcium supplementation.

Assessment for renal transplantation

Established renal failure is a multisystem disease and careful preoperative review is essential.

Cardiovascular assessment

Hypertension is common in children on renal replacement therapy, and antihypertensive therapy and blood pressure monitoring must be continued in the perioperative period. Hypertension may worsen and require more vigorous treatment following treatment with steroids and immunosuppressive agents. Left-ventricular hypertrophy and impaired diastolic function have been identified in children and young adults with ESRF [42]. It may be severe and worsen following transplantation [43]. Interestingly, the increase in left-ventricular mass correlates more closely with anaemia and serum creatinine than with systolic blood pressure. Preoperative echocardiography, ECG and cardiology review are clearly important.

Respiratory assessment

This group of patients is prone to chest infections because of their chronic disease state. Basal atelectasis and pleural effusions may be associated with peritoneal dialysis.

Haematological assessment

Significant anaemia is tolerated remarkably well, and compensated by an increase in cardiac output. The combination of preoperative anaemia and intraoperative bleeding can be problematic, but a haemoglobin level of 8 g/dL is generally considered acceptable. Erythropoietin and iron supplements are often necessary and appear to be reducing the incidence of anaemia. Defective platelet function may be present with ESRF and this should be checked preoperatively. Heparinisation secondary to line flush and haemodialysis usually lasts for about 2 hours; scrutiny of coagulation studies is necessary prior to anaesthesia, particularly if epidural anaesthesia is considered.

Surgical aspects

Increasingly, living related transplantation is performed and has the benefit of providing good functioning grafts, which are transplanted in an elective manner. Thus the transplantation may be performed when the child is in optimal condition or pre-emptively before requiring dialysis. Cadaveric grafts remain the most popular option in the UK; however, graft survival is inferior to that of living related grafts.

In older children the donor renal vessels are anastomosed to the iliac artery and vein whereas in small children the anastomoses are made to the aorta and inferior vena cava so the skin incision is either in the iliac fossa or midline.

Conduct of anaesthesia

Premedication with midazolam 0.5 mg/kg may be of use in the anxious child. It is important to ensure that long-term medication, particularly antihypertensive drugs, are given preoperatively. Adult data suggest a more stable intraoperative haemodynamic course when hypertension is controlled preoperatively. Recent haemodialysis in particular may make the child hypovolaemic and at risk of hypotension following induction of anaesthesia. Electrolyte imbalances should be looked for and treated accordingly.

Full monitoring, with ECG, non-invasive blood pressure and oxygen saturation, is important; the blood pressure cuff should be placed away from any arteriovenous fistulae. Induction agents are administered cautiously and intravenous fluid and pressor agents used to correct hypotension.

Gaseous induction with sevoflurane in nitrous oxide and oxygen may be used; otherwise propofol or sodium thiopental with fentanyl is a popular intravenous agent. The choice of muscle relaxant has been made easier since the advent of atracurium. Cisatracurium has the benefit of less histamine release and no accumulation of laudanosine, which may occur with atracurium. Laudanosine is a cerebral stimulant, but is likely to accumulate only with long exposure to atracurium. Suxamethonium is associated with a transient mild rise in serum potassium and is generally avoided in renal failure. A rapid-sequence induction is rarely required in paediatric renal transplantation. There should be no need to proceed without adequate fasting.

In our unit we employ the cautious use of epidural analgesia, ensuring appropriate coagulation profile, platelet count and strict asepsis. We site the epidural catheter via the lumbar vertebral route and advance the catheter according to the height of the block required. The benefits would appear to be superior analgesia and stable haemodynamic profile [44]. Good postoperative analgesia is particularly important in these debilitated children undergoing prolonged surgery, with large incisions, who are extubated at the end of surgery. If an epidural technique is not used, analgesia may be achieved with intravenous morphine; however, the hepatic metabolite morphine-6-glucuronide readily accumulates in renal failure, and may be a cause of postoperative respiratory depression.

Following tracheal intubation, invasive monitoring is placed. Arterial lines are generally not sited in order to avoid damage to future sites of arteriovenous fistulae. Non-invasive blood pressure monitoring is usually adequate and

the cuff is placed on an arm with no fistula. The insertion of a multiple-lumen central venous catheter allows assessment of intravascular volume as well as providing good intravenous access. Previous venous haemodialysis catheters and subsequent thrombosis of the great veins, however, are a potential limiting factor.

Maintenance of anaesthesia is typically with isoflurane in a mixture of oxygen and air, supplemented by a short-acting opiate such as fentanyl or remifentanil. Nitrous oxide is generally avoided because of its potential for bowel distension, which may be important if a relatively large graft is placed, causing tight abdominal closure. Perioperative hypothermia is likely and so the use of fluid warmers and convective heating devices is essential. The presence of renal osteodystrophy and poor tissue cover makes careful positioning equally important to avoid pressure damage.

Reperfusion is tolerated well in children with only mild systemic effects, although it can be a time when significant bleeding occurs and the need for transfusion and pressor support should be anticipated. Usually, careful fluid administration, guided by filling pressures prior to unclamping of the renal vessels, is adequate.

Delayed graft function is common, particularly for cadaveric grafts, and associated with poor graft survival [45]. Early poor graft function has a number of aetiologies: ischaemic–reperfusion injury, donor issues, preservation injury, rejection and unfavourable recipient haemodynamics. It is common practice to improve perfusion of the engrafted kidney by intravascular filling with colloid/crystalloid to a high central venous pressure and maintain high normal arterial blood pressure. Many units use a dose of mannitol and furosemide prior to reperfusion to minimise acute tubular necrosis. The use of dopamine would appear contentious but is still popular. Future developments are likely to be the administration of antioxidant agents to modify ischaemic–reperfusion injury.

In the early postoperative phase the initial diuresis may lead to hypovolaemia and careful fluid management is essential. Similarly, electrolyte disturbances, particularly of sodium, calcium and potassium, may occur rapidly.

Following revascularisation of the graft the ureteric anastomosis is completed, haemostasis achieved and the incision closed. Extubation is usual, particularly if good analgesia and normothermia are achieved. Atelectasis and pulmonary oedema are the commonest reasons for postoperative ventilation. Pulmonary oedema secondary to aggressive fluid administration soon resolves with good graft function. The insertion of a relatively large graft may cause tight abdominal closure, atelectasis and diaphragmatic splinting. Myopathy and poor reversal of muscle relaxation may also necessitate intensive care support postoperatively.

Outcome in renal transplantation

The outcome in paediatric renal transplantation is excellent with 1-year graft and patient survival rates reported at 91 per cent and 99 per cent respectively [46], and results in older children are superior to those in adults because of the higher prevalence of diabetes and cardiovascular disease in adult recipients. The 1-year survival for living related grafts is superior to that of cadaveric grafts, and pre-emptive transplantation before dialysis is needed would appear to be beneficial. Children exhibit catch-up growth following transplantation. The long-term problems remain rejection, disease recurrence and post-transplantation lymphoproliferative disorder.

Future trends in transplantation

In the future xenotransplantation offers hope to children awaiting transplantation, potentially providing size-matched organs free from the problems of rejection and transplanted in an elective fashion. Hepatocyte transplantation may benefit children with metabolic conditions with a normal liver architecture. Similarly bioartificial livers, in which hepatocyte cell lines are incorporated into a dialysis-type membranes would benefit children with acute liver failure, either as a bridge to transplantation or allowing stabilisation and regeneration of their liver.

However, in the shorter term better understanding of disease process should allow improved management of children with organ failure, to allow continuing growth and development, and to minimise complications. Improvements are being seen in the introduction of new immunosuppressant drugs, and the hope is that new agents will reduce the problems of chronic rejection and lymphoproliferative disorder.

The immediate problem remains that there are an increasing number of children who could benefit from transplantation while the number of donors remain static. The remedies to this have to be as much political as medical.

REFERENCES

Key references

Atkinson P, Joubert G, Barron A *et al.* Hypertrophic cardiomyopathy associated with tacrolimus in paediatric transplant patients. *Lancet* 1995; **345**: 894–6.

Atkinson PR, Ross CB, Williams S *et al.* Long-term results of pediatric liver transplantation in a combined pediatric and adult transplant program. *Can Med Assoc J* 2002; **166**(13): 1663–71.

Coupe N, O'Brien M, Gibson P, de Lima J. Anaesthesia for paediatric renal transplantation with and without epidural analgesia – a review of 7 years experience. *Paediatr Anaesth* 2005; **15**: 220–8.

Dhawan A. Acute liver failure in childhood. *J Gastroenterol Hepatol* 2004; **19**: 382–5.

Selvaggi G, Gyamfi A, Kato T *et al.* Analysis of vascular access in intestinal transplant recipients using the Miami classification from the VIIIth International Small Bowel Transplant Symposium. *Transplantation* 2005; **79**: 1639–43.

van Obbergh LJ, Carlier M, DeKock M *et al.* Hepatopulmonary syndrome and liver transplantation: a review of the preoperative management of seven paediatric cases. *Paediatr Anaesth* 1998; **8**: 59–64.

References

1. Starzl TE. History of Liver and other Splanchnic Organ Transplantation. In: Busutil RW, Klintmalm GB, eds. *Transplantation of the liver*. Philadelphia: WB Saunders, 1996: 3–22.

2. Otte JB. History of paediatric liver transplantation. Where are we coming from? Where do we stand? *Pediatr Transplant* 2002; **6**: 378–87.

3. Atkinson PR, Ross CB, Williams S *et al.* Long-term results of pediatric liver transplantation in a combined pediatric and adult transplant program. *Can Med Assoc J* 2002; **166**(13): 1663–71.

4. Atkinson P, Joubert G, Barron A *et al.* Hypertrophic cardiomyopathy associated with tacrolimus in paediatric transplant patients. *Lancet* 1995; **345**: 894–6.

5. Condino AA, Ivy DD, O'Connor JA *et al.* Portopulmonary hypertension in pediatric patients. *J Pediatr* 2005; **147**(1): 20–6.

6. Emerick KM, Rand EB, Goldmuntz E *et al.* Features of Alagille syndrome in 92 patients: Frequency and relation to prognosis. *Hepatology* 1999; **29**: 822–9.

7. Krowka MJ, Cortese DA. Hepatopulmonary syndrome: current concepts in diagnostic and therapeutic considerations. *Chest* 1994; **105**: 1528–37.

8. Fewtrell MS, Noble JG, Revell S *et al.* Intrapulmonary shunting in the biliary atresia/polysplenia syndrome: reversal after liver transplantation. *Arch Dis Child* 1994; **70**: 501–4.

9. Bank ER, Thrall JH, Dartzher DR. Radionuclide demonstration of intrapulmonary shunting in cirrhosis. *Am J Roentgenol* 1993; **140**: 967–9.

10. van Obbergh LJ, Carlier M, DeKock M *et al.* Hepatopulmonary syndrome and liver transplantation: a review of the preoperative management of seven paediatric cases. *Paediatr Anaesth* 1998; **8**: 59–64.

11. Fridell JA, Bond GJ, Mazaregos GV *et al.* Liver transplantation in children with cystic fibrosis: a long term longitudinal review of a single center's experience. *J Pediatr Surg* 2003; **38**(8): 1152–6.

12. Ellis SR, Hulton S, McKiernan PJ *et al.* Combined liver-kidney transplantation for primary hyperoxaluria type 1 in young children. *Nephrol Dial Transplant* 2001; **16**: 348–54.

13. Gines P, Guevara M, Arroy V, Rodes J. Hepatorenal syndrome. *Lancet* 2003; **362**(9398): 1819–27.

14. Lodge JP, Jonas S, Jones RM *et al.* Efficacy and safety of repeated perioperative doses of recombinant factor VIIa in liver transplantation. *Liver Transpl* 2005; **11**(8): 973–9.

15. Bhaduri BR, Mieli-Vergani G. Fulminant hepatic failure: paediatric aspects. *Semin Liver Dis* 1996; **16**: 349–55.

16. Dhawan A. Acute liver failure in childhood. *J Gastroenterol Hepatol* 2004; **19**: 382–5.

17. Murphy N. The effect of hypertonic sodium chloride on intracranial pressure in patients with acute liver failure. *Hepatology* 2004; **39**: 464–70.

18. Jalan R, Olde Damink SW, Deutz NE et al. Moderate hypothermia prevents cerebral hyperemia and increase in intracranial pressure in patients undergoing liver transplantation for acute liver failure. Transplantation 2003; **75**: 2034–9.

19. Hall WA, Martinez AJ. Neuropathology of paediatric liver transplantation. Paediatr Neurosci 1989; **15**: 269–75.

20. Brock-Utne JG. Is cricoid pressure necessary? Paediatr Anaesth 2002; **12**: 1–4.

21. Cheng CAY, Aun CST, Gin T. Comparison of rocuronium and suxamethonium for rapid intubation in children. Paediatr Anaesth 2002; **12**: 140–5.

22. National Institute for Clinical Excellence. Guidance on the use of ultrasound locating devices for placement of central venous catheters. National Institute for Clinical Excellence technology appraisal guide 49. London: NICE, 2002 (http://www.nice.org.uk).

23. Suriani RJ, Cutrone A, Feierman D, Konstadt S. Intraoperative transesophageal echocardiography during liver transplantation. J Cardiothorac Vasc Anaesth 1996; **10**: 699–707.

24. Rudolph F, Ramsay KJ, Ramsay MAE et al. Accelerators in thromboelastograph analysis: effects of tissue factors and heparinase on the thromboelastogram during liver transplantation. Anesth Analg 1998; **86**: S228.

25. Deshpande RR, Bowles MJ, Vilca-Melendez H et al. Results of split liver transplantation in children. Ann Surg 2002; **236**: 248–53.

26. Nanashima A, Pillay P, Crawford M et al. Analysis of post revascularization syndrome after orthotopic liver transplantation: the experience of an Australian liver transplantation center. J Hepatobiliary Pancreat Surg 2001; **8**: 557–63.

27. Bucuvalas JC, Ryckman FC, Krug S et al. Effect of treatment with prostaglandin E1 and N-acetylcysteine on paediatric liver transplant recipients: a single-center study. Pediatr Transplant 2001; **5**: 274–8.

28. Seaman DS, Newell KA, Piper JB et al. Use of polytetrafluoroethylene patch for temporary wound closure after paediatric liver transplantation. Transplantation 1996; **62**: 1034–6.

29. Starzl TE, Rowe MI, Todo S et al. Transplantation of multiple abdominal viscera. JAMA 1989; **261**: 1449–57.

30. Puntis JWL. Nutritional support at home and in the community. Arch Dis Child 2001; **84**: 295–8.

31. Grant D. Intestinal transplantation: 1997 report of the international registry. International Transplant Registry. Transplantation 1999; **67**: 1061–4.

32. Sodheimer JM, Asturias E, Cadnapaphornchai M. Infection and cholestasis in neonates with intestinal resection and long-term parenteral nutrition. J Pediatr Gastroenterol Nutr 1998; **27**: 131–7.

33. Mittal NK, Kato T, Thompson JF. Current indications for intestinal transplantation. Curr Opin Organ Transplant 2000; **5**: 279–83.

34. Selvaggi G, Gyamfi A, Kato T et al. Analysis of vascular access in intestinal transplant recipients using the Miami classification from the VIIIth International Small Bowel Transplant Symposium. Transplantation 2005; **79**: 1639–43.

35. Povoski SP, Zaman SA. Selective use of preoperative venous duplex ultrasound and intraoperative venography for central venous access device placement in cancer patients. Ann Surg Oncol 2002; **9**: 493–9.

36. Goldman LJ, Santamaria ML, Gomez M. Anaesthetic management of a patient with microvillous inclusion disease for intestinal transplantation. Paediatr Anaesth 2002; **12**: 278–80.

37. Bueno J, Ohwada S, Kochoshis S et al. Factors influencing the survival of children with intestinal failure referred for intestinal transplantation. J Paediatr Surg 1999; **34**: 27–32.

38. Ruemele FM, Jan D, Lacaille F et al. New perspectives for children with microvillus inclusion disease: early small bowel transplantation. Transplantation 2004; **77**: 1024–8.

39. Horslen SP, Sudan DL, Iyer KR et al. Isolated liver transplantation in infants with end-stage liver disease associated with short bowel syndrome. Ann Surg 2002; **235**: 435–9.

40. Sudan D, DiBaise J, Torres C et al. A multidisciplinary approach to the treatment of intestinal failure. J Gastrointest Surg 2005; **9**: 165–76.

41. UK Renal Registry. Report from the Paediatric Renal Registry. The seventh annual report from the UK renal registry. Bristol: UK Renal Registry (http://www.renalreg.com).

42. Johnstone LM, Jones CL, Grigg LE et al. Left ventricular abnormalities in children, adolescents and young adults with renal disease. Kidney Int 1996; **50**: 998–1006.

43. Mitsnefes MM, Kimball TR, Border WL et al. Abnormal cardiac function in children after renal transplantation. Am J Kidney Dis 2004; **43**: 721–6.

44. Coupe N, O'Brien M, Gibson P, de Lima J. Anaesthesia for paediatric renal transplantation with and without epidural analgesia – a review of 7 years experience. Paediatr Anaesth 2005; **15**: 220–8.

45. Perico, N. Cattaneo, D. Sayegh, M.H, Remuzzi, G. Delayed graft function in kidney transplantation. Lancet 2004; **364**: 1814–27.

46. Lashley DB, Barry JM, Dermattos AM et al. Kidney transplantation in children: a single centre experience. J Urol 1999; **161**: 1920–5.

42

Trauma and transport

DANIEL LUTMAN, MARK J PETERS

KEY LEARNING POINTS

- Trauma is a major cause of morbidity and mortality in children.
- Early simple intervention – 'airway, breathing, circulation' – can do much to reduce both morbidity and mortality.

- Paediatric retrieval services can support patient stabilisation at the primary receiving facility.
- Early admission to a specialist paediatric intensive care unit (PICU) after stabilisation is essential.

TRAUMA

Trauma has been claimed to be the main cause of death and disability world-wide. Studies in north east England in the late 1980s showed that traumatic brain injury (TBI) accounted for 15 per cent of deaths in children aged 1–15 years [1]. Better pre-hospital (20 per cent) or early inpatient (42 per cent) care could have avoided a high proportion of these fatalities [1]. Airway management, recognition of intracranial haemorrhage and lack of efficient transfers between hospitals were the main deficiencies.

These data predate the modern era of Advanced Paediatric Life Support (APLS), paediatric retrieval services and the centralisation of paediatric intensive care. Encouragingly, more recent data indicate a reduction in the proportion of fatalities attributable to TBI to 2 per cent of deaths in the 0- to 14-year-old group [2]. While this may be due to improvement in emergency medical care, it may also reflect concurrent public health measures such as control of traffic speed and rear seat seatbelt laws. Nevertheless, even now there are still fatalities due to omissions in early basic care.

Paediatric trauma is associated with a high risk of medical errors because of the combination of an unpredictable acute severe illness, urgent time pressures, the involvement of multiple teams, an incomplete history and often out-of-hours presentation to busy emergency departments. Analysis of 44 000 adult trauma cases in the USA suggested that, even in experienced level 1 trauma units, avoidable deaths occur, most commonly as result of failures in the earliest steps of stabilisation [3]. This study identified that of the 2594 trauma deaths the most common avoidable errors were easily remediable (Table 42.1) [3]. The importance of simple high-quality immediate management cannot be overstated.

The ideal structure for paediatric trauma services is unclear; however, outcomes are better if there is specific paediatric provision at the admitting trauma centre. In-hospital mortality and length of stay were significantly higher in adult hospitals managing 0 to 10 year olds with an injury severity score (ISS) of >15 [4].

Paediatric head injury

In the UK the prevalence of TBI in 0 to 14 year olds admitted to the intensive care unit (ICU) is 5.6/100 000 population per year; most cases were pedestrians in a road traffic

Table 42.1 Avoidable errors in the initial management of trauma (adult data) [3]

Avoidable error	Incidence (%)
Failure to intubate, secure or protect the airway successfully	16
Delayed operative or angiographic control of acute abdominal or pelvic haemorrhage	16
Delayed intervention for ongoing intrathoracic haemorrhage	9
Inadequate deep venous thrombosis or gastrointestinal prophylaxis	9
Undertaking lengthy initial operative procedures rather than damage control surgery in unstable patients	8
Over-resuscitation with fluids	5
Complications of feeding tubes	5

Table 42.2 The Glasgow Coma Scale (GCS)

Best motor response	
Obeys	M6
Localises	5
Withdraws	4
Abnormal flexion	3
Extensor response	2
Nil	1
Verbal response	
Oriented	V5
Confused conversation	5
Inappropriate words	3
Incomprehensible sounds	2
Nil	1
Eye opening	
Spontaneous	E4
To speech	3
To pain	2
Nil	1

The score should reflect the best response obtainable. In younger children especially (<4 years of age), scoring can be difficult and subjective based on the observer's knowledge of the child's level of development. Use the AVPU (A = alert; V = responding to voice; P = responding to pain; U = unconscious) score in these patients; recent data suggest that the majority of the predictive capacity of the GCS is contained in the motor component of the score. Any child with a reduction in motor score below 'localising pain' should be treated as a severe head injury equivalent to a total GCS $\leq$ 8.

accidents (RTAs) [2]. Overall 9.2 per cent of children died of their injuries, but children who had suffered TBI as a result of RTAs had the highest mortality rates – the worst mortality was among motor vehicle occupants (23 per cent).

Direct admission of a severely head-injured child to a paediatric trauma centre with paediatric neurosurgical services is the ideal model of care provided that this does not require too long a primary transfer. Since these services are few and far between, and direct admission is often not possible, clear referral pathways and protocols are essential to avoid unnecessary delays and to optimise early care at the initial receiving unit [5].

IMMEDIATE CARE

Advanced Paediatric Life Support underpins the initial management of the critically injured child [6]. The principle that underlies the approach to the severe head injury patient is to 'maintain blood and oxygen going to the brain', remembering that brain injuries are rarely complete at the moment of impact and that secondary damage can occur later and may be avoidable.

Primary brain injury

At the time of impact, damage occurs by tearing of axonal tissue, contusion, disruption of blood supply and bone fractures.

Secondary brain injury

Secondary damage from hypoxia and/or ischaemia are the greatest threats, but cerebral oedema, excitatory neurotoxicity, acute inflammation, osmolar injury and dysregulation of neuronal cell death pathways may all contribute. At present no proven therapies exist other than minimising hypoxia and ischaemia.

STABILISATION OF AIRWAY, BREATHING AND CIRCULATION (ABC)

Optimal management of ABC is the first step in immediate care and takes priority over all other injuries. The Glasgow Coma Scale (GCS) score should be assessed concurrently, as low scores may suggest the need for immediate intervention (Table 42.2).

Airway and breathing

Table 42.3 gives indications for immediate tracheal intubation and mechanical ventilation. Where the receiving unit does not have specialist paediatric intensive care, anaesthesia and neurosurgery, it may be appropriate, if possible, to protect the airway if the coma is less profound (GCS > 8). The trend in the GCS should be observed because a deterioration in score suggests the need for early respiratory support.

The drugs used for intubation and airway control by the North Thames Paediatric Intensive Care Transport team – or Children's Acute Transport Service (CATS) – guideline is shown in Fig. 42.1.

An intubated patient should be ventilated, and given muscle relaxation and appropriate sedation and analgesia, aiming for a partial pressure of arterial oxygen (PaO_2) > 13 kPa and an arterial partial pressure of carbon dioxide

Table 42.3 Immediate intubation and ventilation are required in children with these clinical signs and findings

System	Finding	Comment
Neurological	GCS ≤ 8	There should be early involvement of an anaesthetist or intensivist to provide appropriate airway management
		A depressed conscious level should be ascribed to intoxication only after a significant brain injury has been excluded
		Patients with head injury should not receive systemic analgesia until fully assessed so that an accurate measure of consciousness and other neurological signs can be made
Airway	Ventilatory insufficiency or disturbance	Hypoxaemia ($PaO_2 < 9$ kPa on air or <13 kPa on supplemental oxygen)
		Hypercapnia ($PaCO_2 > 6$ kPa).
		Spontaneous hyperventilation (causing $PaCO_2 < 3.5$ kPa)
		Respiratory arrhythmia, including when seizures occur
	Loss of protective laryngeal reflexes	This should be assessed separately from the GCS
Trauma	Significant facial or neck injury	Burns or smoke inhalation in which oedema may compromise the airway
		Bilateral fractured mandible
		Copious bleeding into the mouth from skull base fracture

GCS, Glasgow Coma Scale; $PaCO_2$, partial pressure of arterial CO_2; PaO_2, partial pressure of arterial oxygen.

($PaCO_2$) of 4.5–5.3 kPa. Hyperventilation can reduce elevated intracranial pressure (ICP) in the short term by diminishing cerebral blood volume. However, hypocapnic cerebral vasoconstriction worsens secondary brain injury owing to ischaemia, thereby negating the benefit of the reduced ICP. Hyperventilation is unsuitable as the primary method of reducing ICP except immediately prior to craniotomy to prevent acute cerebral herniation.

Circulation

An adequate circulation is essential to provide perfusion to the injured brain. In the acute resuscitation phase (before invasive arterial and intracranial pressure monitoring have been established) this means that hypotension must be avoided and that the target blood pressure should be at the higher end of the normal range. Randomised trial data suggest that in this setting intravenous volume loading with crystalloid is better than human albumin solution (HAS) [7].

Thus, in early management, priority should be given to establishing reliable basic monitoring and achieving the targets of oxygenation, avoidance of hypotension and normal carbon dioxide clearance as rapidly as possible. Effective prevention of secondary brain injury in the acute phase does not rely upon invasive monitoring.

COMPUTED TOMOGRAPHY BRAIN SCANNING

Obtaining a scan must not obstruct effective resuscitation; rushing the patient to scan before stabilisation is a common mistake. At this stage the computed tomography (CT) scan is *only* to determine if there is an acute neurosurgical emergency Indications for obtaining a CT scan are given in Table 42.4. Interpretation of a paediatric CT scan is crucial and yet can

be difficult even for radiologists. Sending images, electronically, for a specialist opinion is invaluable (Fig. 42.2).

PAEDIATRIC INTENSIVE CARE OR NEUROSURGICAL REFERRAL

Having controlled the airway and ventilation and stabilised the circulation, referral to a specialist centre should be considered. Indications for referral are outlined in Table 42.5. Continuing careful clinical observation is vital, looking for signs that might suggest the need for other interventions, (e.g. craniotomy, laparotomy, major transfusion or commencing vasoactive drugs). Bradycardia and low GCS are well-recognised indicators, but hypothermia, tachycardia and low respiratory rate are also markers of brain damage that may need further intervention [8].

Other injuries

The smaller physical size of children means that the force applied per unit volume is greater; consequently, more body compartments may be injured than might be suggested from adult experience. As part of the APLS framework for trauma management, primary and secondary surveys should be performed.

Children and infants may have severe circulatory shock despite a normal blood pressure (see Resuscitation, page 641) because the increase in peripheral vascular resistance preserves blood pressure despite a falling cardiac output. Hypotension is a late and dangerous sign of cardiovascular decompensation. An accurate history is the key to anticipating and ruling out injury in advance of physiological

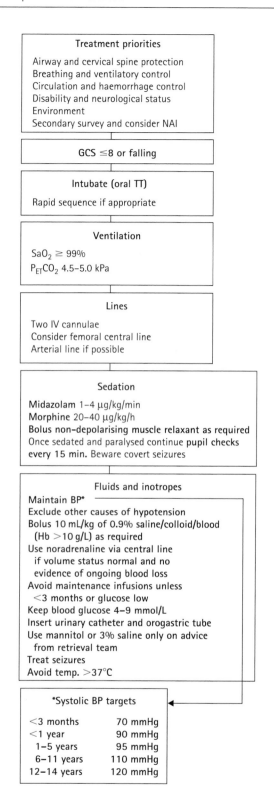

Figure 42.1   Treatment priorities in patients with traumatic brain injury (TBI). A low or falling Glasgow Coma Scale (GCS) score is not the only indication for airway support (see Table 42.3). BP, blood pressure; NAI, non-accidental injury; $P_{ET}CO_2$, end-tidal CO_2 tension; SaO_2, arterial oxygen saturation; TT, tracheal tube.

Table 42.4   Indications for obtaining a computed tomography scan in children with traumatic brain injury once early resuscitation has been completed

Clinical observation	Comment
All patients with any of these risk factors	
GCS < 13	At any time since injury
GCS 13–14	2 hours after injury
Open or depressed skull fracture	
Evidence of basal skull fracture	Haemotympanum 'Panda/Raccoon' eyes CSF otorrhoea Battle's sign (post-auricular ecchymosis)
Post-traumatic seizure	
Focal neurological deficit	
Vomits more than once	Use clinical judgement in those >12 years
Amnesia for >30 minutes prior to injury	Only useful in >5–6 years of age
In patients where there is any loss of consciousness or amnesia since the injury and where the mechanism of injury is dangerous	Pedestrian Ejected from motor vehicle Fall from greater than 1 metre if >5 years of age Any fall if <5 years of age There is a coagulopathy

GCS, Glasgow Coma Scale; CSF, cerebrospinal fluid.

decompensation. However, direct communication is often impossible in children and injuries can remain hidden.

Children are likely to have a good outcome from trauma if they respond well to initial resuscitation. Good signs include reduction in tachycardia (heart rate <130 beats/min) return of usual skin colour and warmth to extremities, improved sensorium and a urine output of 1–2 mL/kg/h. Extensive trauma usually has a poor outcome [9]. Acid–base balance and lactate measured at the end of initial resuscitation are also a useful outcome predictor [10] (Table 42.6). It is important not to confuse a metabolic acidosis with hyperchloraemic acidosis caused by the use of chloride-containing intravenous fluids.

AIRWAY TRAUMA

Thermal injuries and caustic ingestion can compromise the airway. Carbonaceous secretions or a change in cry or voice suggests the possibility of thermal damage to the airway. Early intubation, before significant oedema develops, is recommended and an uncut tracheal tube is favoured as insidious facial swelling can cause accidental extubation if the tube is cut to length [11].

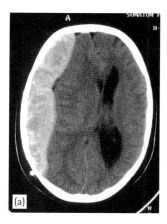

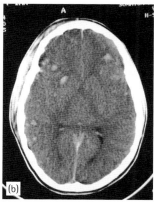

Figure 42.2 (a) Acute extradural haemorrhage with midline shift. This is an arterial bleed, under greater pressure than a venous subdural bleed, hence causing more compression of brain tissue. The variable densities in the haemorrhage reflect the ongoing bleeding. (b) Diffuse axonal injury. Small haemorrhages and contusions are seen throughout brain, with marked early cerebral oedema.

FOREIGN BODY

The aspiration of a foreign body is a leading cause of traumatic death in children under 5 years old and the patient may be brought to the receiving unit *in extremis*. There are two distinct clinical presentations: (1) the foreign body is above the carina or caught in the larynx which can result in subtotal or complete obstruction and a severe risk of death; and (2) the foreign body impacts in a more distal airway causing slower but progressive respiratory distress.

Rigid bronchoscopy is needed for both categories; both the anaesthetic and the bronchoscopy can be highly challenging (see Chapter 33). Ideally, these cases should only be managed by those with considerable expertise and experience in managing the difficult paediatric airway. Consequently, children often have to be moved to a regional centre and this presents a dilemma for the referring hospital: should they attempt to secure the airway? If the foreign body is in the larynx or trachea, intubation may be hazardous and result in total obstruction. Careful clinical judgement by senior doctors is needed.

Table 42.5 Once stabilised referral should be made to a paediatric intensive care unit or paediatric neurosurgical centre if any or some of these clinical signs are present

A CT scan shows intracranial haemorrhage causing midline shift or obstructive hydrocephalus (see Fig. 42.2)
Coma (GCS >8) persists after initial resuscitation
Confusion persisting for more than 4 hours
A deterioration in GCS score after admission (the motor component of the GCS is a sensitive indicator)
Any progressive focal neurological signs detected on repeat examination
Any seizure occurring without full recovery
The presence of a definite or suspected penetrating injury
Any cerebrospinal fluid leak

CT, computed tomography; GCS, Glasgow Coma Scale.

Table 42.6 Metabolic endpoints following initial resuscitation; good outcome is suggested in those with mild acidosis and a low lactate

	Mild	Moderate	Severe
Base excess	2 to −5	−6 to −14	<−15
Lactate (mmol/L)	<2	2–4	>4

SPINE AND CERVICAL SPINE

In paediatric trauma, spinal immobilisation is important. The NEXUS group concluded that cervical spine injuries occur in almost 1 per cent of all head injuries, that most of the injuries were low cervical spine (CS) and that injury was rare in children below the age of 8 years [12]. Immobilising a child is difficult and therefore the need for hard collar and tapes in an uncooperative or confused child should be assessed by an experienced clinician. Paralysed and ventilated patients should receive full spinal immobilisation. 'Scoop' stretchers should be used to move patients between stretcher and bed. Spinal boards are for extrication only and do not provide good cervical immobilisation in children who have larger occiputs.

Current CS imaging recommendations vary. If a head CT is being performed, the neck should be included. Without a neck CT two plain radiological views of the spine are taken in patients <5 years and an odontoid peg view is added in those older than 5 years (S Walsh, Royal London Hospital, personal communication, 2006). Despite the fact that the NEXUS group did not identify CS injury in the absence of radiographic abnormality, normal radiography alone is not usually considered sufficient to discontinue spinal immobilisation. Reliable criteria for ruling out spinal injury in the unconscious patient have yet to be established.

PELVIS

Pelvic fractures are difficult to identify and require expert understanding of the normal radiological appearances of pelvic epiphyses. In the haemodynamically unstable patient CT is often used to rule out pelvic fractures. The pelvis is a site that should be considered in occult haemorrhage; treatment options include external fixation, angiographic embolisation and correction of coagulation abnormalities.

CHEST

Lung contusions can often develop despite the absence of rib fractures, due to the relative elasticity of the paediatric thorax. In major trauma a larger tracheal tube (leak detected at a higher than usual pressure) or a cuffed tracheal tube may be needed to cope with evolving reductions in lung compliance and to deliver positive pressure ventilation by ventilators that provide intermittent flow.

There has been renewed interest in cuffed tracheal tubes in all ages of children [13] and some have recommend cuffed tubes for certain conditions, such as burns [14]. There is a potential for cuffs to cause tracheal or laryngeal mucosal damage especially in small children and infants. However, data from paediatric intensive care are encouraging [15] – meticulous attention to cuff pressure is important.

Pneumothorax is easily missed on supine films. Respiratory or cardiovascular compromise will occur suddenly if a tension pneumothorax develops; moreover, the diagnosis is often difficult to make with certainty in infants and younger children. The authors currently favour drainage of a traumatic pneumothorax in patients receiving intermittent positive pressure ventilation (IPPV), especially if the patient will be transferred to an isolated site (such as the CT scanner) or to another hospital.

ABDOMINAL TRAUMA

Blunt injury

Intra-abdominal injuries in children are usually the result of blunt trauma [16]. Regular observations and assessment for clinical signs suggestive of injury are needed. In the haemodynamically stable child CT is considered the best method of identifying and excluding injury. Focused abdominal sonography for trauma (FAST, an ultrasound scan) is often used during initial assessment and resuscitation [17]. In children, the majority of blunt trauma injuries can be managed conservatively [18].

Hollow viscus trauma

Hollow visceral injuries are often the result of blunt trauma, most commonly motor vehicle accidents. The diagnosis of blunt intestinal injury is difficult to make and often delayed, which contributes to its morbidity and mortality [19].

Solid organ injury

Non-operative management is the accepted treatment of most paediatric solid organ injuries. The indications for operative intervention may include cardiovascular compromise despite 40 mL/kg of fluid, free peritoneal gas on chest or abdominal X-ray and diaphragmatic rupture. In a study of almost 1800 paediatric patients managed conservatively only 5 per cent needed surgical intervention and the median time to intervention was 3 hours [18]. Of those who needed surgery 14 per cent required operation after 12 hours. Laparotomy was more commonly required if more than one organ was injured. Where an isolated organ was damaged, conservative management failed in 3 per cent of kidney injuries, 3 per cent of liver injuries, 4 per cent of spleen injuries and 18 per cent of pancreas injuries.

In terms of mechanism of injury, only bicycle crashes were associated with a significantly increased risk of requiring operative management.

NON-ACCIDENTAL INJURY

Very young infants and children rarely suffer severe accidental head injury because they lack the motor skills to climb onto, or walk into, danger. Non-accidental injury is possible and any clinician involved has a responsibility to consider whether the suggested mechanism of injury has a credible explanation [20]. If there is a significant doubt, the doctor's duty is to inform Social Services according to local arrangements, and make sure that the child remains protected. In the setting of an acutely injured child, protection is effectively provided by the staff attending.

A characteristic 'triad' of acute encephalopathy, subdural haemorrhages and multiple retinal haemorrhages occurs after head injury ascribed to 'shaking' or 'shaking and impact'. A non-traumatic explanation for this triad is, at best, extremely rare. Such findings must prompt a careful and thorough search for infectious, metabolic and haematological causes of each component of the triad as well as for injuries elsewhere. In the acute management phase the treatment priorities remain unchanged by the cause of the injuries.

TRANSPORTING CRITICALLY ILL CHILDREN

Introduction

In the UK paediatric intensive care (PIC) is now provided predominantly in regional referral centres. The report *Paediatric Intensive Care: A Framework for the Future* (1997 see http://www.dh.gov.uk/en/Publicationsandstatistics/ Publications/PublicationsPolicyAndGuidance/DH_40057 60) outlined the benefits of this approach in achieving a critical mass of expertise in the care of severely ill children. One consequence of this centralisation of PIC is the need for paediatric intensive care transport teams (PIC unit of PICU retrieval) with the capacity to move critically ill children long distances safely [21]. In the UK and elsewhere there are two main models of provision: (1) retrieval by the destination PICU team and (2) retrieval by a dedicated regional PIC transport service. Occasionally, the referring hospital may be asked to perform the retrieval, especially when time-critical specialist interventions are anticipated.

Why transfer?

Triage at the primary (ambulance) retrieval level is less common in the UK than in many other countries. The scarcity of paediatric trauma centres in the UK mean that the best option is resuscitation and triage at a local non-specialist hospital, followed by secondary transport to a trauma centre. Early intervention in critical illness improves outcome [22,23]. Moreover, centralisation of PIC improves mortality, hence the initial resuscitation and timely transfer of these patients is crucial. Although the theory of PIC would be familiar to anyone with experience of adult intensive care, non-specialist hospital teams may rarely encounter critically ill children and there are often practical problems in performing interventions.

Who transfers?

RESUSCITATION AND STABILISATION TEAMS

Paediatric intensive care needs a multidisciplinary approach. Many non-specialist hospitals have arranged 'paediatric crash call teams' comprising paediatricians, paediatric nurses, neonatologists, adult anaesthetists and accident and emergency (A&E) staff. The benefits of a team leader or coordinator in resuscitation are clear and the paediatric or A&E consultant will often be the logical choice for this role while the anaesthetist performs necessary interventions. Specialist retrieval teams often use 'dynamic leadership' where the team leader role is swapped between nurse and physician depending on the tasks that they are undertaking at the time. Ideally, this is anticipated and practised in training scenarios or simulators.

Neonatologists may be willing to offer assistance in the emergency management of smaller patients even if they do not fulfil criteria for admission to the neonatal intensive care unit (NICU). Many hospitals have NICUs that may lend expertise or equipment in an emergency.

There is evidence that specialist transport teams provide a higher standard of care during transport than inexperienced or 'ad hoc' teams [24]. This is probably not just because the team has experience in the PICU but because they have experience of the transport environment and can adjust strategies accordingly. However, circumstances occasionally dictate that transport is provided by the referring hospital. This is usually when the risks of delay to the patient are likely to be greater than the benefit of waiting for a specialist team – for example, an expanding extradural haematoma requiring neurosurgical intervention that is not available locally. The most senior clinician possible should be involved in the decision to transport incorporating advice from the PIC provider or regional transport service.

PATIENTS

In the emergency setting patients fall into three broad categories: first, those requiring transfer from a referring hospital by retrieval teams for intensive care; second, those who do not meet criteria for transfer either because they will not benefit from intensive care or because they are not considered sick enough for PICU, yet they need a high-dependency unit (HDU); and third, those who can be cared for within the local non-specialist hospital. The middle group present special difficulties; if a PICU retrieval team is involved in their care intervention is often escalated in order to avoid having to manage a deterioration while in an ambulance. This necessitates an assessment of risk and benefit. While interventions might increase the safety of an interfacility transport, they would not necessarily have been undertaken if the child had remained within an HDU, where any deterioration could be managed more easily.

The management of patients in whom intensive care will be futile is controversial. Some want the death of a child managed in the non-specialist hospital and others believe that the PICU is best. Many clinicians are unsure when withdrawal of care or discontinuation of resuscitation is appropriate. It can be difficult to manage the expectations of the family when there is no hope of survival.

In children who are in cardiac arrest on arrival in A&E, current data suggest that there will be no survivors if more than 20 minutes of in-hospital CPR is needed. Furthermore, there are only a few brain-damaged survivors if spontaneous circulation does not return after more than two doses of adrenaline [25]. If cardiac output returns intermittently or the patient has been cooled the outcome is less clear-cut.

Guidance on the withdrawal of care can be found in a publication produced by the Royal College of Paediatrics and Child Heath [26].

In the acute setting most consultants will either seek the advice of their colleagues locally or contact the PIC provider to help make these decisions.

How to transfer

IDENTIFICATION AND ASSESSMENT

Table 42.7 offers a structured approach to assessing the critically ill child or infant. The development of intrahospital 'early warning scores' designed to identify a child requiring discussion with the local PICU could be useful.

RESUSCITATION

Paediatric Advanced Life Support (PALS), APLS or European Paediatric Life Support (EPLS) offers an excellent framework to deal with many common paediatric emergencies but they are limited in scope to resuscitation. High-dependency or successfully resuscitated patients require significant further attention. The referring hospital needs a single point of contact that can give advice, find a PICU with a bed and organise a retrieval team. Within the UK, regional dedicated PIC transport services such as the Children's Acute Transport

Table 42.7   Rapid clinical assessment of an infant or child*

Airway and breathing	Effort
	Respiratory rate and rhythm
	Stridor or wheeze
	Auscultation
	Skin colour
Circulation	Heart rate
	Pulse volume
	Capillary refill
	Skin temperature
Disability	Mental state or conscious level (AVPU)
	Posture
	Pupils

Normal parameters

Respiratory rate by age (years)	(breaths per minute)
<1	30–40
1–2	25–35
2–5	25–30
5–12	20–25
>12	15–20
Heart rate by age (years)	(beats per minute)
<1	110–160
1–2	100–150
2–5	95–140
5–12	80–120
>12	60–100
Mean blood pressure by age (years)	(mmHg)
<1	40–90
1–3	50–100
7	60–90
10	60–90
12–14	65–95

AVPU: A = alert; V = responding to voice; P = responding to pain; U = unconscious.
*After Advanced Paediatric Life Support (APLS).

Service in North Thames answer these needs (http://www.cats.nhs.uk).

STABILISATION AND REFERRAL

Advanced Paediatric Life Support or EPLS courses and manuals provide guidance on the initial management of critically ill children and infants (http://www.alsg.org). The responsibility for the organisation of paediatric resuscitation within a non-specialist hospital falls to that institution (http://www.resus.org.uk/). Regional PIC transport services offer guidelines for stabilisation on their websites and specimen prescription charts for those unfamiliar with drug calculations in children (http://www.cats.nhs.uk/pages/guidelines.asp).

Accurate observations are important when making a referral. Specialist retrieval teams often use a form to guide

referrers (http://www.cats.nhs.uk/pages/guidelines.asp). Although a referral form often takes a few moments to complete, it initiates reassessment of the child's condition and can highlight gaps in observations and clarify the clinical problem that the referrer needs to discuss.

LOGISTICS

While medical management continues, notes and X-rays will need to be prepared and copied for the transfer. Observations must be continuously recorded; many non-specialist hospitals find it convenient to use an anaesthetic record. These records must be transferred with the patient.

Specialist retrieval teams use paperwork designed to prevent errors and omissions. At the children's Acute Transport Service (CATS), we use a checklist before retrieval and a second pre-departure checklist to ensure that the essentials are not forgotten before returning to base (http://www.cats.nhs.uk/pages/guidelines.asp).

Dedicated retrieval services have access to their own ambulances. For other services a call to the local ambulance service will be needed to a secure suitable vehicle.

TRANSFER EQUIPMENT

Airway

A facemask and a self-inflating bag with an oxygen reservoir should be in clear view on the stretcher at all times. Other hand-ventilation circuits (Jackson–Rees modification of Ayre's T-piece, Mapleson E circuit) are useful but require high gas flows. The airway should be secured and a complete set of intubation equipment (with the calculated endotracheal size and a tube size above and below) should be available.

Specialised transport services often have a bag containing this equipment and this sits on the patient stretcher.

Breathing

Ventilated patients will need a suitable transport ventilator that can operate throughout the anticipated journey and for longer if there are delays – hand ventilation consumes valuable human resources. Pneumatic ventilators are favoured by many retrieval teams as they will operate as long as there is a pressurised gas supply. More complex ventilators may offer more sophisticated ventilation but their power requirements, battery lifetimes and oxygen consumption have to be known in advance to use them safely. Positive end-expiratory pressure (PEEP) can transform gas exchange in a critically ill child and transport ventilators can maintain PEEP only if there is minimal leak around a tracheal tube. Heat and moisture exchangers and bacterial/viral filters of appropriate size are mandatory.

Circulation

Most retrieval services use a minimum of two points of vascular access because one may fall out – it can be very difficult to site venous access during transfer. Correctly placed interosseous needles count as a central point of access and can be used to deliver inotropes or fluid boluses. A triple-lumen central line is relatively unsuitable for fluid challenges because of its high resistance – it does not count as more than one. Intravenous access should always be checked for patency prior to departure for the receiving hospital. At least one fluid bolus should be prepared.

Medication

Resuscitation drugs in prefilled syringes for a cardiac arrest are essential. An adequate supply of the medication being used needs to be prepared. The expected battery lifetime of syringe drivers needs to be known unless power will be available in the ambulance. If the patient is already on an inotrope infusion it may be wise to prepare the next syringe and have it connected and ready to run. Sedation and paralysis may be needed (see Fig. 42.1), as will saline flushes.

Monitoring

Minimal monitoring includes non-invasive blood pressure, pulse oximetry and electrocardiogram (ECG). End-tidal carbon dioxide is highly desirable especially when tracheal tube dislodgement can be so difficult to detect and manage. Specialist transport services have access to equipment designed to make transport easier. End-tidal carbon dioxide monitoring, portable blood gas analysis, lactate and blood glucose monitoring are all available. Oesophageal Doppler and Bispectral Index monitoring are being investigated as possible solutions to the difficulties in estimating cardiac output and over-sedation. Appropriate ambulance power supplies are becoming standard but batteries should be fully charged and their life-time known.

Oxygen

It is easy to run out of oxygen. The oxygen volume needed for the journey can be calculated and it is wise to carry twice the calculated volume if not less than two cylinders. All cylinders have the contents (litres), when full, printed on the collar. The volume of oxygen can be calculated from the cylinder pressure but a graphic tool can be found on the CATS website (http://www.cats.nhs.uk/pages/guidelines.asp) in the guidelines section [27]. Transport oxygen should never be used until leaving the building.

AEROMEDICAL EVACUATION

Interhospital aeromedical evacuation of critically ill children is rarely indicated within the UK as the logistical problems of organising an emergency transport often negate any potential time advantage.

Anaesthetists may be famililar with the physililar effects of altitude on a ventilated patient but may be relatively unfamiliar with the logistical, communication and environmental challenges of flight transport. Training and experience in aeromedical transport are needed to achieve an appropriate risk/benefit in all but the most exceptional circumstances.

Courses covering the theoretical aspects are available within the UK, for example the Paediatric and Neonatal Safe Transfer and Retrieval Cource (www.alsg.org). Requests for emergency aeromedical transport should be directed initially to the local ambulance service duty controller.

Repatriation of critically ill children from abroad is normally performed by private companies that specialise in this field.

RELATIVES

Time must be set aside for communication with the parents, to outline the medical and logistical plan. Audit after retrieval has found that parents are stressed during separation from the child if there is poor communication. We do not currently take written consent for transport, but take care to explain its risks and benefits.

Specialist retrieval teams often have the facility to transport a relative with the child and a study by the South Thames Retrieval Service has demonstrated that this meets parental needs and does not diminish the ability of the team to care for the child [28]. If non-accidental injury is suspected the referring consultant is responsible for contacting the Social Services.

MEDICOLEGAL RESPONSIBILITY DURING RETRIEVAL

United Kingdom case-law is limited on this subject. From US legislation the referring hospital has a duty to attempt to stabilise patients in their care before transport. Nevertheless, there is a degree of shared care throughout the process. The question of who has most responsibility for complications arising from interventions by a retrieval team in the referring hospital has not yet arisen in the UK. In the USA the concept of 'Medical Control' is used where, although care is shared, interventions such as intubation can be 'vetoed' by the local consultant while the patient is on their premises.

RISK, HEALTH AND SAFETY

All interfacility transports contain an element of risk not only to the patient but also to those accompanying them. Data from the USA suggest that teams are seven times more likely to be involved in a road traffic incident when in an emergency ambulance driving with 'blue lights'. Many secondary transfers have been done in the past with unsecured people and equipment at speeds unrelated to the clinical circumstances. Specialist retrieval services with access to dedicated ambulances have tackled this by triaging the patients for clinical urgency and translated this into a driving style. Drivers are specifically trained for emergency response driving. Each retrieval is monitored, using staff feedback forms as well as electronic 'black boxes' in each vehicle. Specialist ambulances have been designed and built to contain patients, staff and retrieval equipment safely in crash conditions.

Table 42.8   Emergency medicine in children: useful internet resources

Children's Acute Transport Service	http://www.cats.nhs.uk
Best Evidence Topics	http://www.bestbets.org
EMedicine	http://www.emedicine.com
PubMed	http://www.ncbi.nlm.nih.gov/entrez/query.fcgi
Pediatric Critical Care Medicine	http://www.pedsccm.org
Nice Guidelines June 2003	http://www.nice.org.uk/pdf/cg4niceguideline.pdf
Resuscitation Council UK	http://www.resus.org.uk/

Future developments

Transport medicine is a rapidly advancing field and useful internet resources are listed in Table 42.8.

REFERENCES

Key references

Advanced Life Support Group. *Advanced paediatric life support, the practical approach*, 4th edn. London: BMJ Books, 2004.

Finfer S, Bellomo R, Royce N *et al.* (on behalf on SAFE study investigators). A comparison of albumin and saline for fluid resuscitation in the intensive care unit. *N Engl J Med* 2004; **350**(22): 2247–56.

Parslow RC, Morris KP, Tasker RC *et al.* (on behalf of the UK Paediatric Traumatic Brain Injury Study Steering Group and the Paediatric Intensive Care Society Study Group). Epidemiology of traumatic brain injury in children receiving intensive care in the UK. *Arch Dis Child* 2005; **90**: 1182–7.

Sharples PM, Storey A, Aynsley-Green A, Eyre JA. Causes of fatal childhood accidents involving head injury in northern region, 1979–86. *BMJ* 1990; **301**: 1193–7.

Tasker RC, Morris KP, Forsyth RJ *et al.* (on behalf of the UK Paediatric Brain Injury Study). Severe head injury in children: emergency access to neurosurgery in the United Kingdom. *Emerg Med J* 2006; **23**(7): 519–22.

References

1. Sharples PM, Storey A, Aynsley-Green A, Eyre JA. Causes of fatal childhood accidents involving head injury in northern region, 1979–86. *BMJ* 1990; **301**: 1193–7.
2. Parslow RC, Morris KP, Tasker RC *et al.* (on behalf of the UK Paediatric Traumatic Brain Injury Study Steering Group and the Paediatric Intensive Care Society Study Group). Epidemiology of traumatic brain injury in children receiving intensive care in the UK. *Arch Dis Child* 2005; **90**: 1182–7.
3. Gruen RL, Jurkovich GJ, McIntyre LK *et al.* Patterns of errors contributing to trauma mortality lessons learned from 2594 deaths. *Ann Surg* 2006; **244**: 371–80.
4. Densmore JC, Lim HJ, Oldham KT, Guice KS. Outcomes and delivery of care in pediatric injury. *J Pediatr Surg* 2006; **41**(1): 92–98.
5. Tasker RC, Morris KP, Forsyth RJ *et al.* (on behalf of the UK Paediatric Brain Injury Study). Severe head injury in children: emergency access to neurosurgery in the United Kingdom. *Emerg Med* J 2006; **23**(7): 519–22.
6. Advanced Life Support Group. *Advanced paediatric life support, the practical approach*, 4th edn. London: BMJ Books, 2004.
7. Finfer S, Bellomo R, Royce N *et al.* (on behalf on SAFE study investigators). A comparison of albumin and saline for fluid resuscitation in the intensive care unit. *N Engl J Med* 2004; **350**(22): 2247–56.
8. Newgard CD, Hedges JR, Stone JV *et al.* Derivation of a clinical decision rule to guide the interhospital transfer of patients with blunt traumatic brain injury. *Emerg Med J* 2005; **22**: 855–60.
9. Orliaguet GA, Meyer PG, Blanot S *et al.* Predictive factors of outcome in severely traumatised children. *Anesth Analg* 1998; **87**: 537–42.
10. Browne GL, Cocks AJ, McCaskill ME. Current trends in the management of major paediatric trauma. *Emerg Med J* 2001; **13**: 418–25.
11. Hammer J. Acquired upper airway obstruction. *Paediatr Respir Rev* 2004; **5**(1): 25–33.
12. Viccellio P, Simon H, Pressman BD, *et al.* (on behalf of NEXUS group). A prospective multicenter study of cervical spine injury in children. *Pediatrics* 2001; **108**(2): E20.
13. Fine GF. The future of the cuffed endotracheal tube. *Paediatr Anaesth* 2004; **14**(1): 38–42.
14. Sheridan RL. Uncuffed endotracheal tubes should not be used in seriously burned children. *Pediatr Crit Care Med* 2006; **7**(3): 258–9.
15. Newth CJ. The use of cuffed versus uncuffed endotracheal tubes in pediatric intensive care. *J Pediatr* 2004; **144**(3): 333–7.
16. Rance CH, Singh SJ, Kimble R. Blunt abdominal trauma in children. *J Paediatr Child Health* 2000; **36**(1): 2–6.
17. Soundappan SV. Diagnostic accuracy of surgeon-performed focused abdominal sonography (FAST) in blunt paediatric trauma. *Injury* 2005; **36**(8): 970–5.
18. Holmes JH, Wiebe DJ, Tataria M *et al.* The failure of nonoperative management in pediatric solid organ injury: a multi-institutional experience. *J Trauma-Injury Infect Crit Care* 2005; **59**(6): 1309–13.
19. Bruny JL. Hollow viscous injury in the pediatric patient. *Semin Pediatr Surg* 2004; **13**(2): 112–18.
20. Richard PG, Bertocci GE, Bonshek RE *et al.* Shaken baby syndrome. *Arch Dis Child* 2006; **91**; 205–6.
21. PICS UK. *1996 Standards of practice for the transportation of the critically ill child: framework for the future*. London: Department of Health, 1997.
22. Pearson G, Shann F, Barry P *et al.* Should paediatric intensive care be centralised? Trent versus Victoria. *Lancet* 1997; **349**(9060): 1213–7.

23. Rivers E, Nguyen B, Havstad S *et al.* Early goal-directed therapy collaborative group. *N Engl J Med* 2001; **345**(19): 1368–77.

24. Edge WE, Kanter WE, Weigle CG, Walsh RF. Reduction of morbidity in interhospital transport by specialized pediatric staff. *Crit Care Med* 1994; **22**: 1186–91.

25. Schindler MB, Bohn D, Cox PN. Outcome of out-of-hospital cardiac arrest in children. *N Engl J Med* 1996; **335**: 1473–9.

26. Royal College of Paediatrics and Child Health. *Witholding or withdrawing life sustaining treatment in children: a framework for practice*, 2nd edn. London: Royal College of Paediatrics and Child Health, 2004.

27. Lutman D, Petros AJ. How many oxygen cylinders do you need to take on transport? A nomogram for cylinder size and duration. *Emerg Med J* 2006; **23**(9): 703–4.

28. Davies J, Tibby SM, Murdoch IA. Should parents accompany critically ill children during inter-hospital transport? *Arch Dis Child* 2005; **90**(12): 1270–3.

43

Burns

BRUCE EMERSON, REBECCA MARTIN

KEY LEARNING POINTS

- Burns in children are common and need prompt first aid followed by treatment from experienced staff to minimise lasting effects.
- Burns over 10 per cent of the body surface area need formal fluid resuscitation.
- Anaesthesia is involved in three phases of burn care:
  1. Emergency care: systematic ABC approach avoids errors, hypovolaemia is rarely caused by the burn unless presentation is delayed and avoid hypothermia early referral to burns unit will assist in prompt management and transfer.
  2. Acute care: several procedures are usually required. Close liaison with the burns unit or intensive care unit is essential. The airway, blood loss, monitoring and analgesia need particular attention.
  3. Reconstruction: this can be life-long with problems of airway management, intravenous access and psychosocial issues.
- A burns centre can provide a complete care package for complex or large burns.

INTRODUCTION

Burns are common in children and can cause significant long-term consequences. They require a spectrum of intervention from simple analgesia to complex intensive care. The optimal treatment is prevention. Once a burn has occurred the child requires a large team to treat and follow them from the emergency phase, through recovery and on to rehabilitation at home. Large burns also have a massive impact on hospital facilities, consuming huge resources. Treatment is targeted at replacing the burned skin with normal skin via the normal healing process or skin grafts from donor sites. All the normal skin functions need to be managed during treatment.

Definition

A burn is a coagulative destruction of tissue and it can be described from its site, size and cause. The cause may be heat, chemical or radiation. Burns units also treat non-burn skin loss such as staphylococcal scalded skin syndrome, Stevens–Johnson syndrome, toxic epidermal necrolysis and septicaemic skin necrosis. There are other complex injuries such as respiratory or electrical burns. The current nomenclature is in terms of depth of injury to the dermis or subdermal structures (Table 43.1 and Fig. 43.1) [1]. Children have thinner skin than adults and so are less able to resist heat. For example, 60°C water will burn an infant in 1 second, a child of 5 years in 5 seconds and yet take 20 seconds in an adult.

Table 43.1   Definitions of burn depth [1]

Depth	Subclassification	Skin structures damaged
1. Superficial burn		Epidermis only
2. Partial-thickness burn	Superficial dermal	Part of dermis
	Deep dermal	Most of dermis
3. Full-thickness burn		Dermis and subcutaneous structures

Table 43.2   Number and type of burns admitted to St Andrew's Burns Centre from April 2001 to June 2005 [2]

Age (years)	Scald	Contact	Flame	Miscellaneous	Total
<1	70	26	0	136	232
1–5	225	105	21	574	925
6–16	51	16	47	246	360
Total	346	147	68	956	1517

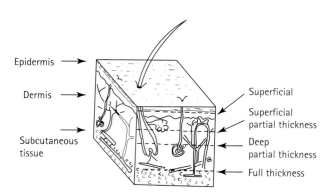

Figure 43.1   Burn depth.

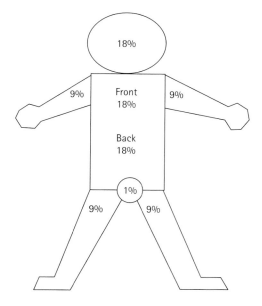

Figure 43.2   Wallace rule of nines [4].

The size and depth give the likely prognosis. Burns heal by keratinocyte proliferation and re-epithelisation. This can be from the surrounding skin or from deeper cells in hair follicles or sweat glands that lie in the deep dermis and upper layers of the subcutaneous tissue. This energy-intense process is one of the reasons for the greatly increased calorie requirement. A superficial or superficial partial-thickness burn will heal within 10–14 days with little or no scarring. Deep burns take 4–6 weeks and full-thickness burns will take up to 3 months with significant scarring that is prone to breakdown. The scar contracts to reduce the area of the wound. Typically, children are burned by scalding and a common story is of a 12- to 18-month-old toddler (approximately 10 kg) who reaches for a cup of tea on a table. This is the commonest type of burn (Table 43.2) and it usually damages approximately 10 per cent of the total body surface area (SA) and is mainly superficial with small, deeper, partial-thickness patches.

Surface area

Paediatric anaesthetists are well aware of the bigger SA to weight ratio in children compared with adults. Children have less area on the legs and more on the head. For each year over one there is a loss of 1 per cent of area from the head and an increase of 0.5 per cent to each leg until the age

of 10 years, when adult proportions are reached. The burn SA is expressed in proportion to total body SA, and it can be estimated by using Lund and Browder charts [3] or the Wallace 'rule of nines' (Figs 43.2 and 43.3) [4]. A useful rule is that the SA of the patient's palm and closed fingers equate to a 1 per cent body SA. The burn SA includes both superficial and deeper areas but excludes simple erythema. A burn SA of 10 per cent is a significant size in children and requires formal fluid resuscitation; 30 per cent to 60 per cent is a major burn and over 60 per cent is known as a massive or extensive burn. Over a 4-year period there have been 1517 children admitted to our burns unit of which 84 per cent had a burn SA less than 10 per cent and 3 per cent greater than 30 per cent.

Epidemiology

Burns occur in accidents or when victims cannot move out of the way of the heat source, e.g. infants or epileptics. A burn in a toddler is usually a scald. Older children experiment with flammable materials and, typically, young teenage boys will be injured more often than girls. In developing countries scalds from hot liquid are common

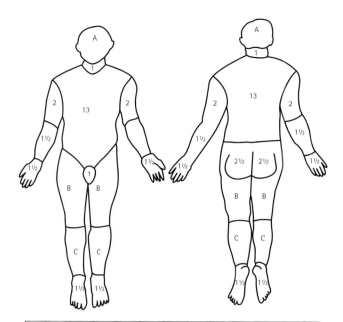

Relative body surface area during growth (%)						
Area	Age 0	1 year	5 years	10 years	15 years	Adult
A – ½ of head	9½	8½	6½	5½	4½	3½
B – ½ of one thigh	2¾	3¼	4	4½	4½	9¾
C – ½ of one leg	2½	2½	2¾	3	3¼	3½

Figure 43.3   Lund and Browder Chart [3]. Redrawn with permission from the Journal of the American College of Surgeons.

because of unprotected cooking apparatus. The incidence increases with overcrowding. Non-accidental injury must be suspected when there is a delayed presentation, an improbable explanation or if there are multiple physical signs of varying ages. Armed conflicts cause tragic civilian burns that will be specific to the weaponry.

Incidence

There are about 100 000 burns treated in hospitals in the UK per year [5]. Approximately 10 per cent need hospital admission and 50 per cent of these are in children <16 years; 10 per cent of these need resuscitation (because the burn SA is >10 per cent), of whom 10 per cent ($n = 50$) need 3–6 months of hospital care. According to the UK census in 2001, the annual incidence of fire childhood casualties was 200 per million. The *UK Fire Statistics 1999–2003* [6] show that the fatality rate in children under 16 years is depressingly static at approximately 50 per year and many die before reaching hospital. Burn care for severely injured children is a low-volume, high-intensity specialty.

Pathophysiology

CUTANEOUS BURNS

Jackson has described a pathological model in which a burn has three zones [7]; there is central coagulative necrosis surrounded by a zone of blood stasis with a peripheral zone of hyperaemia. The treatment of burns is designed to minimise the extension of the burn by maintaining optimal blood flow. There are both local and systemic responses to burn injury. A cascade of proinflammatory molecules causes the basal metabolic rate to rise by up to 50 per cent. Local inflammation is complex and caused by mediators such as histamine, serotonin, prostaglandins, prostacyclin, bradykinin and catecholamines. There is increased microvascular permeability and exudation of protein into tissues.

Large amounts of fluid are sequestered into a burn and when the wound is over 25 per cent SA there is marked generalised oedema formation. This loss causes intravascular volume depletion. Oedema formation starts at about 4 hours and stops at around 30 hours unless there are persisting triggering factors [8]. There is a dilemma about when to limit intravenous (IV) fluid replacement because excess can cause further oedema. Usually there is an initial short period of myocardial suppression followed by a hyperdynamic circulation. The hypermetabolic response can last for up to 18 months in extensive burns.

Infection is a likely major hazard because the skin's ability to control foreign antigens and to present them to the immune system is lost. There is also systemic immunosuppression from protein loss.

AIRWAY BURNS

There are three distinct elements to airway burns: the upper airway, the lower airway and systemic poisoning. The upper airway is occasionally fatally obstructed by burn and subsequent swelling. However, the most common inhalation injury is caused by toxic gases, including carbon monoxide, which can be rapidly fatal. The lower airways may be obstructed by oedema, soot, secretions or bronchoconstriction. The particles in the inhaled smoke dissolve on the mucosal surface causing a chemical pneumonitis. Lower airways do not usually suffer direct thermal injury because of the highly efficient dissipation of heat by the upper airways [9]. If a significant injury is suspected the airway should be examined by laryngoscopy and bronchoscopy [10].

ELECTRICAL INJURY

Three distinct problems occur with electrical injuries: the electrocution itself, the flash burn from an explosion caused by arcing of the current from the source to ground, and tertiary injuries result from being blown away from the explosion. A specific accident in 'oral phase' toddlers is an oral burn from an electrical flex. Electric current will flow through tissues of least resistance, including bones, muscles, blood vessels and nerves. This can produce direct myocardial injury and delayed rhythm disturbances [11]. A patient should be monitored for 24 hours if they have lost consciousness or if there are electrocardiogram (ECG) changes. There may be severe distal limb ischaemia and compartment syndrome should be suspected [12].

CHEMICAL INJURY

About 5 per cent of admissions to the burns unit are because of chemical burns of the skin or ingestion of chemicals. Children are a risk group because of accidental swallowing of either acids, which cause a surface burn, or alkalis which penetrate deeper with more prolonged tissue destruction. The management is to reduce the concentration by dilution with irrigation. The eyes can be damaged by splashing and must be checked. Ingestion of corrosives requires referral to a gastrointestinal surgeon [13].

Pharmacology

There are significant alterations in the effects of drugs on the body in burns [14]. One of the most important is the avoidance of suxamethonium from 24 hours after the burn for up to 18 months later (especially in large burns). Fatal increases in serum potassium have occurred in this period and this is due to extrajunctional proliferation of myoneuronal receptors. Burned children have low albumin and high α_1-acid glycoprotein plasma concentrations. There can be up to a 50 per cent rise in basal metabolic rate and the increased cardiac output translates into an increased renal blood flow and raised glomerular filtration rate but, oddly, a reduced hepatic metabolism [15]. There is a massive rise in volume of distribution because of generalised oedema. There is a decreased sensitivity to non-depolarising muscle relaxants requiring both double dosing and double-frequency boluses [16]. Opioid tolerance develops quickly. Some children develop massive sedation requirements if prolonged intensive care occurs [17]. All these changes are variable and unpredictable.

Outcome and comorbidity

Children can survive massive burns but if there is other significant disease the mortality risk is increased. It is crucial to seek a history of previous medical conditions. Injuries at the time of escape from a fire may also be important. The cause of unexplained acidosis must be sought outside the burn injury. Severity scoring in burns has a poor correlation with outcome.

Burns of all sizes may be fatal. There are very few survivors with 90 per cent burns but children have better outcomes for massive burns than adults. Burns, even as small as 1 per cent, can be fatal if complications such as toxic shock syndrome occur. Most small burns can expect to recover within 2 weeks. Larger burns will need long-term burn wound management; advice to carers is that for each percentage burn their child will need to stay in hospital for 1–2 days.

Children who survive massive burns will inevitably be left with lifelong physical disabilities and they need help from an experienced multidisciplinary team. Strong family support has a positive benefit on recovery. Despite severe injuries their quality of life can be comparable to that of non-burned children [18].

EMERGENCY MANAGEMENT OF BURNS

This section outlines the early management of more serious burns but the principles apply to all burn injuries. The overall aim of emergency care is to identify and treat immediate life-threatening problems and institute appropriate burn management. Burn wounds can be dramatic and distressing; a practical common-sense ABC approach will avoid distraction and so prevent missing other significant injuries.

First aid

First aid should simply stop the burning process, e.g. by extinguishing flames, removing clothing soaked in scalding fluid and cooling the wound. Ideally, the wound should be bathed in lukewarm water for 20 minutes, being careful to avoid causing hypothermia in large SA burns.

ABC approach

All children who have sustained a major burn should be managed by the structured approach outlined in *Advanced Paediatric Life Support* [19] or *Emergency Management of Severe Burns* [20] guidelines. Assessment and treatment should be simultaneous as the problems are encountered.

A: AIRWAY

On arrival in the emergency room there should be a rapid preliminary assessment. Oxygen should be given while airway patency is assessed. Cervical spine protection is mandatory until significant injury can be excluded (potential causes of spinal injury include falling out of windows or from a blast injury). A burnt airway can obstruct owing to oedema, which can form within the first few hours and up to 24–36 hours later. The trachea should be intubated early if there is actual or potential upper airway obstruction, respiratory distress or hypoxia necessitating ventilatory support, reduced level of consciousness or if transport is necessary and there are concerns about airway patency. Figure 43.4 is a useful guide. If there is any doubt, expert advice should be sought; the safest approach is to intubate. Uncut tracheal tubes should be used because the length needs to vary because of facial oedema – a cut tracheal tube can be dislodged.

B: BREATHING

Respiratory effort and adequacy should be assessed. Inhalation of smoke can cause a significant injury to the

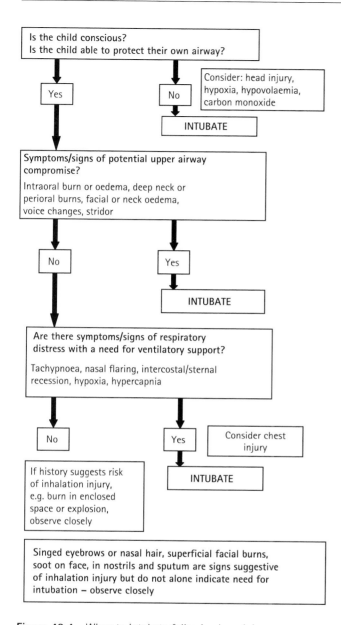

Figure 43.4 When to intubate following burn injury.

C: CIRCULATION

Circulatory shock may be apparent by tachycardia, reduced capillary refill and cool peripheries. Hypotension is a late sign in children because of effective vasoconstriction. Intravenous access should be established in all but the most minor burns and this should be through unburned skin if possible. If venous cannulation cannot be established quickly, intraosseous cannulation may be indicated. In larger burns swelling of the limbs may dislodge cannulae; fixation should be secure. Initial fluid resuscitation in the shocked child following trauma should be by a 10 mL/kg bolus of crystalloid, and repeated if necessary after assessment. In the presence of persistent shock, causes of hypovolaemia other than the burn wound itself should be sought and managed.

Because circumferential limb burns may cause impaired peripheral circulation, the general circulation should be assessed in all limbs. Any affected limb should be elevated and an escharotomy considered. An escharotomy is an incision through inelastic burnt tissue (the eschar). To be effective the incision needs to extend into unburned skin, which is painful and consequently the child will need anaesthesia. Escharotomies may be indicated if transfer to a burns unit is delayed – discussion with the burns unit is recommended.

D: DISABILITY

Rapid assessment of neurological status is important. The AVPU is a simple observational system and involves recording the best responses of the child: they are either alert (A), respond to voice (V), pain (P) or are unresponsive (U). If there is reduced consciousness, the pupillary responses should be recorded.

E: EXPOSURE

The child is vulnerable to hypothermia and should be nursed in a warm environment. All clothes should be removed to ensure that no injury is missed. A soot-covered child may not necessarily have a large burn. Soot can be cleaned off with warm saline to allow the body surface area to be accurately assessed. After the child has been 'rolled' to examine their back they should be wrapped up and kept warm.

Once the burn wound has been examined and carefully documented using a Lund and Browder chart (see Fig. 43.3) fluid resuscitation can be calculated on the basis of the burn SA. Simple erythema is excluded. Formal fluid resuscitation for the burn is required if the burn SA is greater then 10 per cent. The amount of fluid required relates to both the burn SA and the weight of the child. There is no clear consensus on the volume and type of resuscitation fluid needed [21, 22]. We use the Parkland formula [8] (Table 43.3). Children who have delayed resuscitation, significant smoke inhalation or other injuries will

lungs and acute respiratory distress. An inhalation injury should be suspected if there has been a fire in an enclosed space or an explosion. Pulse oximetry can falsely reassure because carboxyhaemoglobin results in high saturations. If suspected, carboxyhaemoglobin levels should be measured and a high oxygen concentration administered. Contamination of the airway by soot is common in house fires but the degree of injury is related to the length of exposure and smoke density. In the conscious child, the need for advanced respiratory support is infrequent but a period of close observation of at least 24 hours will be required.

Full-thickness burns of the chest and abdomen can impair ventilation by reducing chest wall compliance. Chest escharotomy may be required.

Table 43.3　Fluid resuscitation [2]

Fluid resuscitation – Parkland formula

Hartmann's solution: 4 mL/kg per % surface area burned in 24 hours
　　Half given over the first 8 hours from time of burn
　　Half over next 16 hours
PLUS maintenance
　　100 mL/kg/day for first 10 kg body weight
　　50 mL/kg/day for the second 10 kg body weight
　　20 mL/kg/day for each subsequent kilogram of body weight
This is usually given as intravenous Hartmann's solution until oral
　　or nasogastric feeding is started
Glucose-containing solutions are rarely needed
Example
　　12 kg child with 40% flame burn
　　$4 \times 12 \times 40 = 1920$ mL for burn + 1100 mL maintenance over
　　　　24 hours
　　half in first 8 h = 960 mL = 120 mL/h plus 46 mL/h
　　　　maintenance
　　= total 166 mL/h for first 8 h from time of burn (catch
　　　　up will be needed)
　　then 106 mL/h for next 16 h

Table 43.4　Which children to refer to a burns unit?

Factors suggesting a complex burn injury and need for referral	
Age	<5 years
Size	Under 16 years, any burn >5% total body surface area
Site	Face, hands, perineum Flexures, e.g. neck, axilla Circumferential dermal or full thickness
Mechanism	High-tension electrical burn High-pressure steam Suspected non-accidental injury
Inhalation	In the presence of a cutaneous burn – inhalation only to intensive care
Medical conditions	Diabetes Immune suppression Renal failure
Associated injury	Requiring specialist assessment and care

have appreciable extra requirements. Any formula is only a guide and is not a substitute for repeated clinical assessment.

Efficacy of fluid resuscitation should be monitored by clinical parameters and the aim should be to achieve a urine output of 1–2 mL/kg/h. If the urine output is low further fluid boluses should be given and, conversely, excess urine production should prompt a reduction in the hourly fluid rate. Excessive volumes of crystalloid resuscitation are associated with complications such as pulmonary oedema. Myoglobinuria, which can occur in electrical injuries or muscle ischaemia, should be suspected if the urine is pink turning to dirty red in colour. If myoglobinuria is present, intravenous fluids must be increased to achieve a higher urine output in order to minimise renal damage.

Analgesia should be given intravenously in all but the most minor injuries. The analgesic of choice at this stage is morphine 0.1–0.2 mg/kg, titrated to effect. The presence of a parent may help calm the child.

In burns affecting >15 per cent of SA, a nasogastric tube and a urinary catheter should be inserted. Tetanus immunisation status should be checked and a tetanus toxoid booster given if indicated. Prophylactic antibiotics are not required. A full history of events should be documented and any past illnesses and allergies noted. A thorough 'top-to-toe' examination will ensure that other injuries are not missed.

When the child has been assessed and stabilised the most appropriate place for their ongoing care should be chosen. This will usually be a burns unit but will depend on the priorities of any other injuries. The British Burn Association guidelines for referral to a burns unit

should be followed and can be found on their website (http://www.britishburnassociation.org/) (Table 43.4). All complex burns should be referred. If transfer to a burns unit is intended, the wound should be simply cleaned with sterile saline and wrapped in Clingfilm because this reduces pain and allows easy assessment on arrival. Ensure that any dressings used are loose enough to avoid causing constriction as oedema forms. Creams such as silver sulfadiazine (Flamazine) should be avoided as they make wound depth assessment more difficult.

If transfer is not intended, the management of the burn wound itself should be discussed with the local burns unit.

Transfer

The child must be stabilised before transfer. Ideally an experienced paediatric transport or retrieval team should be used. Distance and traffic conditions will dictate the type of transport. If intubation is necessary, we recommend well-fixed straight, and uncut, tracheal tubes. Tube position should be confirmed on chest X-ray to exclude bronchial intubation. There should be continuous monitoring, documentation of fluid balance and vital signs. The child must be wrapped up as they will become cold on transfer; space blankets are useful. Thorough documentation of the initial assessment and treatment should accompany the child.

Ongoing resuscitation

Resuscitation and treatment are a continuous process of re-evaluation of the patient's response to interventions.

The resuscitation formulae are only a guide. An important point in resuscitation is that high fluid requirements may indicate another injury such as occult bleeding. This should be suspected if the fluid requirements approach twice the predicted 4 mL/kg per cent burn SA. High urine output suggests excessive fluid input and this should be reduced as it may be harmful.

ANAESTHESIA AND SURGERY

Optimal care is provided by specialist surgeons and anaesthetists in an operating theatre within a burns unit. The following is a brief description of the treatment and operations to allow non-specialists to plan anaesthetic management. Wound management is either conservative or operative and both may require repeated dressing changes under either general anaesthesia or sedation.

Wound management

Care is designed to restore the skin barrier against water and heat loss, and infection. Covering the burn reduces these problems and will also diminish pain from the exposed pain-and-touch sensory organs. Restoration of appearance, particularly of the face and hands, is also an important consideration. The wound heals best if it is neither wet nor dry and this can be achieved by a combination of exposure to air, special dressings and ointments, and by excision of dead tissue and grafting. The objective is to close the wound by spontaneous epidermal growth or by skin grafting.

Dressings are used to cover the wound to protect it from bacterial contamination and to collect the protein exudates. The classic dressing of paraffin-impregnated gauze covered with a light crepe bandage and then wrapped in bulky cotton wool dressings is not ideal because these dressings need to be changed frequently, resulting in repeated intense procedural pain. Modern dressings aim to make the exchange of dressings and wound inspection as infrequent and as painless as possible. This can be done by using a dressing such as the silicone-based Mepitel®, which replaces the 'old' modern paraffin gauze because it is sufficiently adherent and yet easy to remove. Biobrane® is a biosynthetic non-adherent membrane that is applied closely and stays in place until the burn is healed; it is ideal for superficial partial-thickness burns such as scalds. Any pus can be seen through these dressings but antibiotics are necessary; pressurised pus under Biobrane® can cause septicaemia. Skin grafts are usually split skin (partial thickness). Full-thickness grafts are only occasionally used in cosmetically important areas, e.g. around the eyes and mouth. Most split-skin grafts are shaved from the thigh and then meshed and stretched to maximise surface coverage. Note that the donor site temporarily increases the SA of injured skin.

Preoperative preparation

Identification of potential problems will almost always be found from a careful history, examination and appropriate investigations. Routine 2–4–6 hours fasting times for clear fluids, breast milk and food can be used for small scheduled procedures. In acute burns, or those over 10 per cent, there is a higher risk of pulmonary aspiration and, therefore, ideally, the stomach should be emptied with a nasogastric tube before a rapid sequence induction. Suxamethonium is hazardous beyond 24 hours after a burn. The procedure room must have a high ambient temperature and humidity. Blood loss may be quick, occult and massive, and so preoperative crossmatching is necessary for all but the smallest procedures. Provided that there are no adverse factors, we allow normovolaemic haemodilution down to a haemoglobin concentration of 70 g/L by replacing blood lost with crystalloid.

Operative management falls into three distinct situations:

- acute small burns
- acute large burns
- reconstruction.

Anaesthesia

ACUTE SMALL BURNS (BURN SA < 20 per cent)

Acute small burns can be managed with a standard anaesthetic [23] but always in a fully equipped theatre. The features that may present difficulties are the airway, the hazard of pulmonary aspiration because of gastric stasis, occult blood loss and hypothermia caused by exposure and cleaning fluid. Fortunately, modern dressing techniques may require only a single early general anaesthetic. Subsequent painful dressing changes may not be necessary [24].

Children need a wound inspection and cleaning on admission to determine the burn SA; the areas of smoke discoloration or erythema need to be excluded from the SA estimation. A 'ketamine clean-up' technique has the advantage of potent analgesia and simple anaesthesia, and includes intermittent IV doses of 1 mg/kg titrated until nystagmus occurs. Tracheal intubation is not usually required and supplemental oxygen can be administered by simple face-mask. An empty stomach cannot be guaranteed even though the child will have been fasted for 6 hours; nevertheless aspiration is rare.

Typical burn surgery involves excision of all non-viable tissue and coverage with a skin graft. The burn and the skin of the donor site, plus the surrounding areas, are prepared with an iodine-based aqueous antiseptic solution. Exposure should be minimised to preserve body heat. Monitoring may be lost during skin preparation and should be reinstated promptly. Intravenous access must be securely fixed. The airway often needs to be secured with a tracheal tube. If the surgery is scheduled after overnight fasting, a laryngeal mask may be considered [25]. Bacteraemia occurs with each manipulation of a burn wound and therefore a prophylactic single dose of antibiotics is given. Benzylpenicillin and gentamicin are our first-line choices but the prevalence and sensitivity of local microbiological flora should guide the choice.

Intraoperative opioid analgesia is usually necessary. The use of local anaesthesia may be useful, especially for distal parts of limbs, and a caudal block may cover both operative and skin donor sites. Accurate and reliable regional analgesia is now possible in small children by using high-definition ultrasound probes to guide needle placement. Donor site infiltration or topical local anaesthesia onto dressings are both useful techniques [26]. Common donor sites are the thigh or buttocks. If the donor site is small, blockade of the lateral cutaneous nerve of the thigh is simple and effective. We recommend co-analgesia with intravenous clonidine ($1–2\,\mu g/kg$).

Postoperative analgesia is provided by regular paracetamol, non-steroidal anti-inflammatory drugs and opioids; additional 'rescue' opioid may be necessary for breakthrough pain. Aperients are necessary. Skin grafts need at least two further procedures including dressing changes and removal of staples.

ACUTE LARGE BURNS (BURN SA > 20 per cent)

These challenge even experienced anaesthetists. There will be rapid, massive fluid shifts against a background of multiple organ dysfunction. Patients will be hypermetabolic, with a high temperature and cardiac output. Gastric stasis is likely and surgery should not be delayed on account of fasting times. If a cuffed tracheal tube is used, a feeding tube is placed beyond the pylorus so that enteral feeding may continue during the operation.

Current surgical recommendation is for early and near total burn wound excision because this removes dead tissue, hastens wound healing and reduces mortality [27]. Full-thickness burns may need excision down to fascia whereas partial-thickness wounds need tangential excision or shaving. Paradoxically, tangential excision may bleed more than deep excision. Blood loss is much greater in older and infected burns. Two days after the injury, the wound becomes appreciably more vascular and, consequently, if surgery is delayed operative blood loss may be increased by a factor of three (personal observation by the authors).

Loss of the airway can be fatal in an unstable hypermetabolic state. A full difficult-intubation set of equipment should be available. Emergency tracheostomy can be very difficult if the neck is burnt. In difficult cases airway exchange catheters are useful for tracheal tube changes. Pressure-controlled pulmonary ventilation should aim for a tidal volume of approximately 7 mL/kg.

Large-bore intravenous cannulae are necessary in anticipation of massive blood loss. These lines must be firmly stitched in place with a braided suture such as silk. We recommend a four-point fixation for central lines (a stitch is placed on each of the fixing wings and a further two

sutures to the catheter both proximal and distal to the wings). Adhesive dressings alone are insufficient when the patient is moved for wound cleaning. Arterial lines may be necessary if a limb is unavailable for non-invasive measurement (these must be well secured also). Adhesive ECG electrodes slide off the skin too easily but foetal scalp electrodes can be fixed even into burnt skin and their distal wires attached to standard ECG electrodes on a card base. Special pulse oximetry sensors may be necessary if digits are not available.

It may be difficult to maintain body temperature and therefore important not to begin a procedure if the child is already hypothermic. Active measures include warm air mattress, radiant overhead heating and high ambient theatre temperature (28–30°C). If, during the procedure, the core temperature falls below 35°C, the team should consider either stopping surgery or waiting until the patient is re-warmed. Surgery should also stop if fluid replacement falls behind blood loss or if the lungs become too difficult to ventilate. Blood loss reduction techniques are necessary [28] and these include the use of tourniquets on limbs, subcutaneous infiltration of adrenaline (1 in 100 000 solution) before excision and topical phenylephrine-soaked swabs (20 mg/L saline) after excision. Systemic absorption is rarely of clinical significance. A guide to predicted blood loss during burns surgery is given in Table 43.5 [29].

Maintenance of anaesthesia is usually with volatile agents and morphine infusion. Total IV anaesthesia offers no advantage and a dose algorithm has not been validated in children with burns. After surgery, a period of intensive care with full monitoring is necessary; extreme care is necessary in the transfer from theatre.

RECONSTRUCTION

Common reconstructive procedures include skin resurfacing and the release of contractures. Often these are on the head and neck, and there are potential airway problems. Resurfacing is performed by excising the scar to allow the surrounding skin to spring away from the contracture. The open wound may then be grafted with split skin or covered with an artificial skin substitute such as Integra, which is a bilayer consisting of a basal matrix covered by silicone. The basal layer becomes integrated over 3 weeks and then, at a second-stage operation, the top silicone layer is peeled off and a split-skin graft is placed on top.

Table 43.5 Predicting blood loss during burns surgery for burn surface area (SA) > 30% [29]

Time from burn	Predicted blood loss according to burn SA to be excised (mL/cm²)
<24 hours	0.4
1–2 days	0.6
2–16 days	0.75
>16 days	0.5

A burn can scar and form contractures that may need a lifetime of surgery. If contractures occur across flexible areas such as the joints or the neck there can be severe disability. Normal growth increases tension across burn wounds and corrective operations may be urgent to prevent permanent flexion deformity. Facial and neck contractures cause major airway problems, including limited mouth opening, reduced neck movement and fixation of the anterior neck structures. The nasal cavities may be scarred. Subglottic stenosis is a common complication of a major burn, especially if the burn involved the neck or if there was prolonged intubation. Venous access may still be difficult. Most reconstructive procedures are painful and require local anaesthetic blocks and skin infiltration. Opioids are usually necessary and there may be tolerance because of long-term use.

There are psychological difficulties because of the return to the hospital environment and the need for recurrent anaesthetics to inspect the wound. Each child finds their own level of understanding and coping; their cooperation will vary. Often children and their parents will have their own views about premedication, induction and analgesia and these should be accommodated if possible. Nurses and play specialists have a pivotal role in minimising distress at induction. The anaesthetist needs to work within the team to be most effective.

PAIN AND RECOVERY

Critical care

Specialist critical care aims to attend to the detail of the burn itself and the general problems of the child and family. A team, experienced in all aspects of child burn care, is essential to good quality intensive care [30]. The child should be at the centre of a 'concertina of care' in which staff and facilities are always available but are used or withdrawn as dependency changes.

Severe smoke inhalation can cause acute respiratory distress and require prolonged respiratory support with lung protection ventilation strategies. Tracheal tubes should be securely fixed and this is difficult in the presence of facial burns. We use a combination of Velcro ties and tape, but occasionally in facial burns wire fixation to the teeth is necessary. If the primary reason for intubation is upper airway oedema, extubation may be feasible after a few days if the oedema resolves. Note that pre-existing airway problems such as adenotonsillar hypertrophy, asthma or upper respiratory tract infection are common. Smoke inhalation can lead to bronchial obstruction by casts of soot. Any soot should be sought by early fibre-optic bronchoscopy and then managed with saline lavage and regular chest physiotherapy. Compli-cations of smoke inhalation include bronchoconstriction, microcoagulation and systemic toxicity, and these can be reduced by a combination of nebulised medications including salbutamol (2.5–5 mg), heparin (5000 units) and N-acetylcysteine (3 mL 20 per cent); all are repeated every 4 hours [31].

Secure intravascular access is essential but available sites may be limited. Central venous access may be necessary for drug infusions, antibiotic therapy and blood sampling. Ultrasound can aid line placement. Patients are susceptible to serious line-related complications including infection and vascular compression, and these require prompt line change or re-siting.

Until the burn wound is closed many visits to the operating theatre may be needed. The National Burn Care Review Committee (http://www.britishburnassociation.org/Downloads/2001-nbcr.pdf) recommends that an operating theatre is located within the burns unit. After each skin harvest and grafting procedure there is an inevitable general deterioration but while the burn is unhealed the child is susceptible to sepsis within the wound itself, the lungs or the intravascular lines.

The hypermetabolic response to burn injury should be minimised to aid wound healing and recovery. This means limiting the stressful procedures, effective analgesia, being nursed in a warm environment, infection control and meeting the extra calorie requirements. Enteral feeding via nasogastric or postpyloric tubes should be established early. Calorie intake should be calculated to meet the child's need. Typical requirements are the basal metabolic rate plus additional calories related to age and the burn SA. Infants and toddlers need $1000\,kcal/m^2$ burn SA and children need $1300\,kcal/m^2$ [32]. A fall in body weight may indicate that feeding is ineffective. Antacid prophylaxis is required as burns patients are prone to gastric erosions and stress ulceration (these were first described in burns patients by Curling in 1842 [33]).

Standard pulse oximetry monitoring may be difficult because of lack of digits and so reflectance skin probes may be necessary. The adequacy of circulation volume may be assessed by a combination of core to peripheral temperature gradient, pulse rate, blood pressure and urine output. Daily weight may not be useful because of exudates in dressings. Cardiac output monitoring may be required and oesophageal Doppler or pulse contour analysis technology is sometimes useful. Inotropes are rarely required during the resuscitation phase. If cardiovascular support is needed noradrenaline should be used cautiously because it can reduce skin perfusion. The ongoing fluid and electrolyte loss through the burn wound needs to be replaced and assessed each day; the formulae are a useful guide (see Table 43.3).

Maintaining satisfactory sedation may be extremely difficult because of the changes in the volume of distribution, metabolism and excretion, and the development of gross tolerance. We have found a combination of IV morphine, ketamine and midazolam infusions plus oral clonidine to be effective. Oral rather than intravenous clonidine seems to have fewer cardiovascular side-effects [34]. Additional analgesia is usually required for dressing changes and wound cleaning. As the child is weaned from mechanical ventilation, analgesia and sedation can be changed from IV to oral. Intravenous propofol can be useful to cover the final stages of weaning [35].

Regression of a child's behaviour is inevitable after a burn. There may be serious psychosocial and familial issues. Non-accidental injury and child protection issues need to be considered. This is an emotionally exhausting time for the child, family and staff, and psychological support is imperative.

Pain management [36]

Burn pain has three components: background, break-through and procedural pain. Early effective pain management is vital to gain the confidence, trust and cooperation of the child and their carers. It also has a role in modulating the neuroendocrine response which may help to limit any damaging metabolic consequences. The link between emotional and physical aspects of pain should not be ignored [37].

To allow effective pain management, robust systems must be in place to assess pain and its treatment regularly. Age-related pain-scoring systems should be used. It is important to involve the child and their carers in pain assessment and to listen to and act upon their responses. Staff need to be consistent and realistic and the support of an acute pain team is valuable.

BACKGROUND AND BREAKTHROUGH PAIN

The mainstay of pain control is regular, oral opioid analgesia. Extra doses must be available to treat breakthrough pain. Regular paracetamol should be given to all children unless contraindicated. It is important to remember that adjustments in background analgesia will be required if the child undergoes surgical procedures. Intravenous morphine infusions, controlled by either the nurse or the patient, are often appropriate in both the acute and the postoperative settings. Patient-controlled analgesia is not possible if the hands are burnt.

Children with major burns may develop morphine tolerance and, if doses are too high or side-effects develop, alternatives such as oxycodone or methadone can be used instead [38]. Adjuncts such as clonidine can be added. Regular aperients should be given to prevent constipation and antiemetics may be required. There can be features of neuropathic pain for which gabapentin may be effective. As the burn heals it can be itchy and this, rather than pain, may be the cause of distress in a small child. We find that if chlorphenamine alone is ineffective then a combination of cyproheptadine and hydroxyzine helps. An early report suggests that low-dose gabapentin may be beneficial for itching that is unresponsive to conventional antihistamines [39].

Non-steroidal anti-inflammatory drugs are effective analgesics but their value should be carefully balanced with potential side-effects. They should be avoided during the initial phase in larger burns and used with caution during critical care because of the risk of gastric erosions. They are effective for managing donor-site pain in children with smaller burns.

Local anaesthesia is safe and efficacious in the perioperative period either by topical application or by infiltration into the donor site. Single 'shot' regional or nerve blocks benefit some children. Catheter techniques risk infection.

The recovery from a major burn injury is a long process and even with effective analgesia children are very anxious and distressed. After initial management, probably requiring benzodiazepines, play specialists and psychologists are extremely valuable. The child may be weaned off analgesics as they recover but analgesics should not be withdrawn abruptly. As discharge from hospital approaches the analgesia regimen should be simplified. Weaning from opioids can be achieved at home with the advice of the pain team and primary care support.

PROCEDURAL PAIN

Examples of painful procedures include dressing changes, physiotherapy and simple bed-sheet changes. First, the child should be prepared with an appropriate explanation and discussion about sedation and analgesia. There will be a need for drugs with rapid onset and offset for short procedures, and longer-acting agents for complicated dressing changes. Modern dressings have allowed dressing changes to become less traumatic. The introduction of Biobrane has reduced the number of wound procedures.

The authors' unit uses ward-based sedation. Anaesthetic staff are always involved but the level varies according to the sedation technique. Techniques include, in ascending order of complexity, oral opioids, oral ketamine (8–10 mg/kg) and midazolam (0.5 mg/kg to a maximum of 30 mg), IV ketamine, and then conventional general anaesthesia. The chosen technique may not be sufficient and can be immediately 'stepped up', safely, by the anaesthesia team. Later, as the child progresses, lesser techniques become appropriate. Adjuncts such as fentanyl lozenges and Entonox can be effective in older children for short procedures.

The benefits of behavioural techniques such as play therapy and music are increasingly recognised and also more advanced technology with virtual reality systems are showing promising results.

REFERENCES

Key references

Barret JP, Wolfe SE, Desai MH, Herndon DN. Total burn wound excision of massive paediatric burns in the first 24 hours post-injury. *Ann Burns Fire Disaster* 1999; X11: 25–7.

Benjamin D, Herndon DN. Special considerations of age: the pediatric burned patient. In: Herndon DN, ed. *Total burn care*, 2nd edn. London: WB Saunders, 2000: 427–38.

Hettiaratchy S, Papini R, Dziewulski PD (eds). *ABC of burns*. Oxford: Blackwell Publishing Ltd, 2005.

The Education Committee of the Australia and New Zealand Burn Association Ltd. *Emergency management of severe burns course manual EMSB* (UK edn). Manchester: British Burn Association, 2004.

National Burn Care Review Committee. *Standards and strategy for burn care: a review of burn care in the British Isles*. London: NBCR Committee, 2001.

References

1. Latarjet J. A simple guide to burn treatment. International Society for Burn Injuries in collaboration with the World Health Organization. *Burns* 1995; **21**: 221–5.
2. *St Andrew's Burns Unit Handbook*. Chelmsford: St Andrew's Centre for Burns 2005.
3. Lund CC, Browder NC. The estimation of areas of burns. *Surg Gynecol Obstet* 1944; **79**: 352–8.
4. Wallace AB. The exposure treatment of burns. *Lancet* 1951; **i**: 501–4.
5. National Burn Care Review Committee. *Standards and strategy for burn care: a review of burn care in the British Isles*. London: NBCR Committee, 2001.
6. Office of the Deputy Prime Minister. *Summary fire statistics United Kingdom 1999–2003*. London: The Stationery Office, 2003.
7. Jackson DM. The diagnosis of the depth of burning. *Br J Surg* 1953; **40**: 588–96.
8. Baxter CR. Fluid volume and electrolyte changes of the early post burn period. *Clin Plast Surg* 1974; **1**: 693–703.
9. Rabinowitz PM, Siegel MD. Acute inhalation injury. *Clin Chest Med* 2002; **23**: 707–15.
10. Muehelberger TM, Kunar D, Munster A, Couch M. Efficacy of fiberoptic laryngoscopy in the diagnosis of inhalation injuries. *Arch Otolaryngol Head Neck Surg* 1998; **124**: 1003–7.
11. George EN, Schur K, Muller M *et al*. Management of high voltage electrical injury in children. Burns 2005; **31**: 439–44.
12. Koumbourlis AC. Electrical injuries. *Crit Care Med* 2002; **30**: S424–30.
13. Weigert A, Black A. Caustic ingestion in children. *Contin Educ Anaesth Crit Care Pain* 2005; **5**: 5–8.
14. Martyn JA. Clinical pharmacology and drug therapy in the burned patient. *Anesthesiology* 1986; **63**: 67–75.
15. Mills AK, Martyn JA. Neuromuscular blockade with vecuronium in paediatric patients with burn injury. *Br J Clin Pharmacol* 1989; **28**: 155–9.
16. Uyar M, Hepaguslar H, Ugur G. Balcioglu, T. Resistance to vecuronium in burned children. *Paediatr Anaesth* 1999; **9**: 115–18.
17. Sheridan RL, Stoddard F, Querzoli E. Management of background pain and anxiety in critically burned children requiring protracted mechanical ventilation. *J Burn Care Rehab* 2001; **22**: 150–3.
18. Sheridan RL, Hinson M, Liang MH *et al*. Long-term outcome of children surviving massive burns. *JAMA* 2000; **283**: 69–73.
19. Mackway-Jones K, Molyneux E, Phillips B, Wieteska S. *Advanced paediatric life support: the practical approach,* 4th edn. Oxford: Blackwell Publishing Ltd, 2005.
20. The Education Committee of the Australia and New Zealand Burn Association Ltd. *Emergency management of severe burns course manual EMSB* (UK edn). Manchester: British Burn Association, 2004.
21. Cocks AJ, O'Connell A, Martin H. Crystalloids, colloids and kids: a review of paediatric burns in intensive care. *Burns* 1998; **24**: 717–24.
22. Marinov Z, Kvalteni K, Koller J. Fluid resuscitation in thermally injured paediatric patients. *Acta Chir Plast* 1997; **39**: 28–32.
23. Black RG, Kinsella J. Anaesthetic management for burns patients. *Br J Anaesth/CPD Rev* 2001; **1**: 177–80.
24. Barret JP, Dziewulski P, Ramzy PI *et al*. Biobrane versus 1% silver sulfadiazine in second degree pediatric burns. *Plast Reconstr Surg* 2000; **105**: 62–5.
25. McCall JE, Fischer CG, Schomaker E, Young JM. Laryngeal mask airway use in children with acute burns: intraoperative airway management. *Paediatr Anaesth* 1999; **9**: 515–20.
26. Bussolin L, Busoni P, Giorgi L *et al*. Tumescent local anesthesia for the surgical treatment of burns and postburn sequelae in pediatric patients. *Anesthesiology* 2003; **99**: 1371–5.
27. Barret JP, Wolfe SE, Desai MH, Herndon DN. Total burn wound excision of massive paediatric burns in the first 24 hours post-injury. *Ann Burns Fire Disaster* 1999; **X11**: 25–7.
28. Losee JE, Fox I, Hua LB *et al*. Transfusion-free pediatric burn surgery: techniques and strategies. *Ann Plastic Surg* 2005; **54**: 165–71.
29. Desai MH, Herndon DN, Broemeling L *et al*. Early burn wound excision significantly reduces blood loss. *Ann Surg* 1990; **211**: 753–9.
30. Hettiaratchy S, Papini R, Dziewulski PD (eds). *ABC of burns*. Oxford: Blackwell Publishing Ltd, 2005.
31. Desai MH, Mlcak R, Richardson J *et al*. Reduction in mortality in pediatric patients with inhalation injury with aerosolized heparin/*N*-acetylcystine therapy. *J Burn Care Rehab* 1998; **19**: 210–12.
32. Benjamin D, Herndon DN. Special considerations of age: the pediatric burned patient. In: Herndon DN, ed. *Total burn care*, 2nd edn. London: WB Saunders, 2000: 427–38.
33. Curling TB. On acute ulceration of the duodenum in cases of burn. *Medico-Chir Trans Lond* 1842; **25**: 260–81.
34. Arenas-López S, Riphagen S, Tibby SM *et al*. Use of oral clonidine for sedation in ventilated paediatric intensive care patients. *Intensive Care Med* 2004; **30**: 1625–9.
35. Sheridan RL, Keaney T, Stoddard F *et al*. Short term propofol infusion as an adjunct to extubation in burned children. *J Burn Care Rehab* 2003; **24**: 356–60.
36. Stoddard FJ, Sheridan RL, Saxe GN *et al*. Treatment of pain in acutely burned children. *J Burn Care Rehabil* 2002; **23**: 135–56.
37. Henry DB, Foster RL. Burn pain management in children. *Pediatr Clin North Am* 2000; **47**: 681–98.
38. Williams PI, Sarginson RE, Ratcliffe JM. Use of methadone in a morphine-tolerant burned paediatric patient. *Br J Anaesth* 1998; **80**: 92–5.
39. Mendham JE. Gabapentin for the treatment of itching produced by burns and wound healing in children: a pilot study. *Burns* 2004; **30**: 851–3.

44

Anaesthesia and sedation outside operating theatres

MICHAEL R J SURY

KEY LEARNING POINTS

- Many procedures outside theatres require sedation or anaesthesia.
- Sedation is less reliable than anaesthesia.
- Anaesthesia resources are limited.
- Sedation is dependent upon the procedure.
- Non-anaesthetists must use drugs with a wide margin of safety.
- Non-anaesthetists need training.
- Short, painful procedures need special anaesthesia techniques that allow rapid patient throughput and recovery.

Management of painless imaging

- Most well children can be managed with behavioural and sedation techniques.
- Ill children need anaesthesia.

Management of painful procedures

- Cooperative children may cope with local anaesthesia, behavioural techniques or conscious sedation.
- Cooperation can be improved with careful preparation – reassurance and practice will gain trust and confidence.
- Most procedures are best managed with anaesthesia.
- Without anaesthesia services, subanaesthetic doses of ketamine may be the best option.

INTRODUCTION

This chapter covers the management of procedures outside operating theatres but does not address long-term sedation for intensive care. The second section (Useful drugs and techniques for non-anaesthetists) summarises safe sedation drugs that could be used by trained non-anaesthetists and in the subsequent sections (Management of painless imaging and Management of painful procedures). The range of effective management is discussed but with emphasis on the 'best' and 'fastest' anaesthesia techniques.

GENERAL ISSUES

Demand and range of procedures

Currently, in my hospital, approximately 4000 anaesthetics per year take place outside operating theatres. Together with the number of procedures completed under sedation, and this includes many dental procedures, this amounts to a major workload. Over the past decade five local services have undergone major expansion and each has resulted in strategic changes as well as specific developments in anaesthesia and sedation techniques. They include:

- painless imaging
- insertion of long-term venous access
- intrathecal chemotherapy
- gastroenterological endoscopy
- cardiac angiography.

More recently, the demand for sedation and analgesia for minor injuries within accident and emergency departments has also increased. All these services require special planning to maximise the efficient use of limited anaesthesia resources and, when anaesthesia is not possible, to deliver effective and safe sedation by non-anaesthetists.

Appropriate techniques

Techniques should be appropriate to both the procedure and the child. For example, usually a simple intravenous (IV) cannula can be inserted with a combination of local anaesthesia and distraction, whereas a complex cardiac angiograph in a sick infant needs monitored anaesthesia and controlled ventilation. Table 44.1 shows the range of management techniques available and the appropriateness of them will depend upon the degree of discomfort, the longevity of the procedure and the ability of the child to cooperate. The appropriate management of common procedures will be discussed in detail later.

BEHAVIOURAL TECHNIQUES

It is important to recognise that many procedures can be managed by behavioural methods alone, and the role of play specialists [1] and psychologists should not be underestimated. Standard techniques such as play, distraction and guided imagery are valuable and hypnosis is potentially useful even in small children [2]. All behavioural tools are only helpful with the child's active participation and are not designed to trick the child into false expectations; they enable the child to develop coping strategies and work best in combination with brief informational preparation.

Anaesthesia versus sedation

The crucial difference between anaesthesia and sedation is not related to the drugs, but relies upon the expertise of the user. An anaesthetist can use any drug to its best advantage whereas a non-anaesthetist must avoid drugs that are likely to cause airway and breathing side-effects. Sedation drugs, therefore, tend to be weak or impotent, slow acting, long lasting and unreliable (depending, of course, upon the procedure for which they are used). If anaesthetists are called upon, they can choose anaesthesia drugs because these are potent, short acting, have fast recovery and always succeed.

Table 44.1 Techniques*

Behavioural techniques
Systemic analgesia
Anxiolysis
Conscious sedation
Deep sedation
Dissociative sedation
Minimal anaesthesia
Conventional anaesthesia
Intensive care

*Techniques are arranged in ascending order of complexity (appropriate use of local anaesthesia is assumed).

Subanaesthetic doses can be used initially and increased if necessary and, if there are any major physiological effects, skills are available to overcome them.

There is a perception among anaesthesia professionals that sedation is less safe because non-anaesthetists may not be able to manage airway obstruction or apnoea. The public, however, and non-anaesthetists, tend to believe that sedation is a safer option because they wish to avoid the need for airway and breathing support. There are few data to support either view, and it is likely that safety is dependent upon several factors, including the procedure, the drugs, the practitioner and the patient group. For example, sedation in elderly patients having oesophagoscopy has an appreciable mortality but it is unreasonable to believe that sedation of children for magnetic resonance imaging (MRI) is similar.

The availability of personnel is influential. Even in many 'first-world' hospitals there are insufficient anaesthetists to provide a comprehensive service for all procedures and it follows that 'others' must deliver sedation, and they need training to use safe and effective protocols [3,4].

Definitions

Standard definitions [3,5] (Table 44.2) are often imperfect in common scenarios. Their problems, and other controversial definitions, are discussed below.

CONSCIOUS OR MODERATE SEDATION

Conscious sedation is a safe and useful concept for cooperative adults but not for most children, especially if they are sick. In an uncooperative child, sedation does not change a 'no' to a 'yes'. It is generally accepted that true conscious sedation is unlikely in most clinical scenarios but exceptions will be discussed later. The rousability of the subject depends to some extent upon the stimulus used. Whenever verbal contact is inappropriate, such as in infants or nonverbal children, a non-painful stimulus is useful but if the child rouses the procedure may be more difficult. In the USA the term 'moderate sedation' is preferred.

Table 44.2 Standard definitions*

Minimal sedation (anxiolysis)	Drug-induced state during which patients respond normally to verbal commands. Although cognitive function and coordination may be impaired, ventilatory and cardiovascular functions are unaffected
Moderate sedation/analgesia (conscious sedation)	Drug-induced depression of consciousness during which patients respond purposefully to verbal commands, either alone or accompanied by light tactile stimulation (reflex withdrawal from a painful stimulus is not a purposeful response). No interventions are required to maintain a patent airway and spontaneous ventilation is adequate. Cardiovascular function is usually maintained
Deep sedation/analgesia	Drug-induced depression of consciousness during which patients cannot be easily roused but respond purposefully following repeated or painful stimulation. The ability to maintain ventilatory function independently may be impaired. Patients may require assistance in maintaining a patent airway, and spontaneous ventilation may be inadequate. Cardiovascular function is usually maintained. (In the UK, deep sedation is considered to be part of the spectrum of general anaesthesia.)
General anaesthesia	Drug-induced loss of consciousness during which patients are not rousable, even by painful stimulation. The ability to independently maintain ventilatory function is often impaired. Patients often require assistance in maintaining a patent airway, and positive pressure ventilation may be required because of depressed spontaneous ventilation or drug-induced depression of neuromuscular function. Cardiovascular function may be impaired

*Standard definitions used by American Society of Anesthesiologists [5] and the Scottish Intercollegiate Guidelines Network [3].

DEEP SEDATION

In the USA a state of 'deep sedation' has been accepted in 'which the patient is not easily roused' but that 'it may be accompanied by a partial or complete loss of protective reflexes and includes the inability to maintain a patent airway independently'. Following reports of adverse events, insurance companies forced hospitals to ensure that deep sedation is managed to the same standards as for anaesthesia. Thus standards of care have become similar in the UK and USA, yet there is a difference in the personnel. In the UK, only anaesthetists can use techniques 'deeper' than conscious sedation, whereas this is not so in the USA.

SLEEP SEDATION

Children do not lie still for painless imaging unless they are asleep. While it is true that it should be possible to rouse the sleeping child if necessary, trying to prove rousability during the procedure itself is impractical. Nevertheless, whatever the depth, sleep must be safe. A working definition of deep sedation for children could be:

'. . . a technique in a state of depression of the nervous system such that the patient is not easily roused but which has a safety margin wide enough to render the loss of airway and breathing reflexes unlikely' [6].

This could be called 'sleep sedation' because the depth is uncertain unless the child is tested with a stimulus.

MINIMAL ANAESTHESIA

Low doses of anaesthetics can cause sleep that is unlikely to have appreciable airway effects and from which recovery is rapid. Several authors have called these techniques deep sedation but this is unsatisfactory because unintended anaesthesia occurs, albeit briefly, in a proportion of children. Nevertheless this is different from 'conventional anaesthesia' that needs airway support. 'Light anaesthesia' [7] could be used but, as for sleep sedation, once the child is asleep, it is counterproductive to test their rousability; if they do not need attention, there is no need. Experienced anaesthetists have developed techniques that begin with a brief anaesthetic followed by a sleep, maintained by low doses, from which the child may be easily roused. Such techniques could be called 'minimal anaesthesia' [8].

DISSOCIATIVE SEDATION

Ketamine provides a unique state of 'dissociation' and it is argued that a separate definition is justified. In low doses, ketamine causes a trance-like amnesic state in which the eyes may be open, vital reflexes are present and there is sufficient analgesia to manage minor painful procedures. Surgery can be managed under higher doses that may still preserve protective airway reflexes, spontaneous breathing and cardiovascular stability. It is argued that ketamine has a margin of safety so wide that non-anaesthetists can use it provided that they have the necessary training [9].

Assessment and monitoring of consciousness

OBSERVATIONAL SCALES

Consciousness is an elusive concept and several observational scales have been developed to help describe it. In order to be practical, the number of levels within a scale should be limited so that the observer can make repeated and frequent scores. Scales with five or six points are popular but the descriptors may not be adequate for all situations and therefore validity and reliability may be poor. This is a recognised difference between the detailed scales used by psychologists and the practical scales of clinical medicine. There are many clinical scales and, as a rule, each was designed for a different scenario. Two widely used validated scales are the Observer's Assessment of Alertness/Sedation [10] and the University of Michigan Sedation [11] scales but only the latter was developed for children and specifically for painless imaging. For painful procedures, scales vary from a modified Ramsay scale that has eight levels [12] to much more complicated and time consuming scales that are useful in psychological research [13,14]. Examples of sedation scales used in other scenarios are the COMFORT [15] in intensive care and modified Glasgow Coma Scale [16] in children with coma.

Within a scale there are two descriptors of any level: the stimulus used to challenge consciousness and the response achieved by that stimulus. It is obvious that the stimulus is crucial and that the depth consciousness results from a balance between the arousal stimulus and the sedation. Moreover, in the absence of stimulation sedation can become too deep.

Sedation drugs often have a long and unpredictable recovery profile and it is important to decide when it is safe for close observation to end. This will depend upon the drugs used but it is wise, for most drugs, to wait both for at least 2 hours and until the child is increasingly active. A test of sleepiness has been proposed whereby the child's ability to remain awake is tested by observing them in a quiet, darkened room [17]. The length of time chosen will depend upon the situation, e.g. in infants recovering from chloral hydrate, if they can stay awake for 20 minutes they are highly likely to meet all other discharge criteria.

MONITORS OF CONSCIOUSNESS

Monitors of consciousness are either indirect or direct. Indirect monitors include pulse oximetry and capnography, which indicate respiratory depression associated with sedation. Pulse oximetry is mandatory for all sedated and anaesthetised children. Capnography is extremely useful and a good waveform can be obtained if a soft catheter is placed in a nostril. Tubing systems are available that combine both the delivery of oxygen and the aspiration of tidal gas [18]. Electrocardiogram and non-invasive blood pressure should be applied if possible.

Heart rate variability is related to autonomic activity, and is a potential monitor of anaesthetic depth (in adults). It encompasses several mathematical expressions of the variation of the time difference between successive ECG R waves. If a 'steady-state' RR sequence is analysed over about 5 minutes, underlying autonomic rhythms can be quantified but, as yet, the technique is currently only a research tool [19,20]. Direct measurement of brain function using processed electroencephalogram (EEG) or auditory-evoked

potentials (AEPs) is of limited value because of both theoretical and practical limitations. Processed EEG such as Bispectral Index (BIS) or entropy change in natural sleep as well as sedation and have never been adequately validated in small children. With experience, monitors such as BIS may assist in monitoring conscious level in some techniques [12,21] including propofol [22] but do not seem to help with sevoflurane [23].

None of these monitors should predict, with certainty, whether or not an individual will move in response to a physical stimulus because movement is caused by activity of the spinal cord and does not necessarily involve higher cerebral centres of consciousness [24].

Safety recommendations for sedation

In 1992 the Royal Colleges recommended two very safe principles: if a patient is unable to respond to a verbal command then they should be managed by an anaesthetist and techniques by non-anaesthetists should 'carry a margin of safety wide enough to render unintended loss of consciousness unlikely' [25]. Meanwhile the USA accepted the concept of deep sedation but now, in effect, the safety standards are similar because it requires the same standards of care as for anaesthesia [26].

In 2002 the Scottish Intercollegiate Guidelines Network (SIGN) published a clinical guideline and its updated 2004 version is available on the internet (http://www.sign.ac.uk/) [3]. It contains most of the available evidence but is mainly a statement of opinion and, as such, is a guideline. Unfortunately it does not satisfy the evidence-base standards of the Royal College of Paediatrics and Child Health, although it is referenced on their website.

Sedation of children for dental procedures has long been a problem and clear UK guidelines are available via the internet (SIGN, http://www.sign.ac.uk/; British Society of Paediatric Dentistry, http://www.bspd.co.uk/; and Department of Health, http://www.dh.gov.uk). Any sedation in children under 16 years old, other than nitrous oxide alone, should be undertaken only in a hospital setting.

In 2001 the Academy of Medical Colleges responded to reports of unacceptable mortality in adult patients having oesophagogastroscopy [4] and its report might easily apply to paediatrics. Briefly, the report recommends that:

- safe sedation techniques should be defined for each specialty
- organisations should ensure that staff receive sedation training
- hospitals should appoint two lead consultants (an anaesthetist and non-anaesthetist) to lead and support sedation services.

Sedation protocols for non-anaesthetists

In a report of 95 sedation disasters, in which there were 51 deaths and 9 cases of permanent neurological damage, the most common avoidable factors were an obvious failure to apply basic standards of monitoring and airway management [27]. Protocols aim to improve success and maintain safety. In a recent review of over 30 000 sedation records from centres conforming to safety standards, rates (per 10 000) of other complications were unexpected: apnoea 24, stridor or laryngospasm 4.3 and significant desaturation 157. Since there were no deaths and only one child required cardiopulmonary resuscitation this infers that minor complications can be managed successfully by non-anaesthetsists [28].

PRINCIPLES OF SAFETY AND SUCCESS

The principles of safety and success in sedation are in conflict. For example, a low dose will be safer than a high dose but will not be as successful. Similarly, a hungry child will not sleep easily but a recent meal increases the risk of aspiration. Table 44.3 presents some principles for the design of protocols for non-anaesthetists; the most important factors for both safety and success are the judgement and the skill of the staff. With the exception of nitrous oxide sedation (see later), all sedated and anaesthetised patients must be monitored with pulse oximetry (at least) and have someone assigned to them give undivided care. That person must be trained for all common eventualities and make a contemporaneous record of their observations. Suitable assistance must be available to help prevent or manage complications. Full resuscitation expertise must be available within the hospital or unit.

Many anxious children can be calmed and a procedure may be undertaken either without drugs or with alternative 'easier' techniques such as nitrous oxide sedation. Skills required to calm children are invaluable.

PATIENT ASSESSMENT AND COMMON CONTRAINDICATIONS TO SEDATION

The most important safety factor in any protocol involves the assessment of fitness for sedation. Many children have contraindications to conventional sedation techniques and should be managed by an anaesthetist instead. Table 44.4 presents contraindications published by SIGN and a more

Table 44.3 Principles for design of safe and successful sedation protocols for non-anaesthetists

Success	Experienced staff
	Minimise the distress of the procedure
	Selection of children
	Choose effective drugs/techniques
	Quiet and child-friendly environment
Safety	Experienced staff
	Enforce contraindications to sedation
	Safe drugs – do not exceed maximum doses
	Recovery and discharge criteria
	Good facilities and equipment

detailed list appropriate for painless imaging. Children should be fasted for any sedation technique in which pulmonary aspiration is possible (6 hours for food and milk and 3 hours for clear fluid). In emergency departments these fasting rules may not be appropriate because either stomach emptying cannot be relied upon or the procedure is too urgent. New guidance has been developed for minimising risk in these circumstances so that the risk of using effective sedation and analgesia in unfasted children may be justified [29].

PAINFUL VERSUS PAINLESS PROCEDURES

Sedation for painful procedures is much more difficult than for painless scans and it is reasonable to separate sedation management into these two groups. Painful procedures in uncooperative children are best managed by anaesthetists because potent short-acting drugs are more effective. In contrast, the majority of children will keep still for painless imaging with behavioural or sedation techniques and only if this fails, or if the child is not fit for sedation, is anaesthesia is required.

SEDATION FAILURE

Standard doses may not be effective in some children and, if doses are increased, there should be a limit to prevent accidental anaesthesia. For painful procedures the issue of restraint may arise and guidance is available on the Royal College of Nursing (http://www.rcn.org.uk) and SIGN websites. For these reasons it is wise to accept a failure rate, to delay the procedure and to try again with either a different technique or anaesthesia.

RESPONSIBILITY AND CONSENT

A surgeon takes consent for surgery and bears responsibility for explaining benefit and risk, and this model can be applied for many procedures outside theatres. For imaging, however, both the referring clinician and the radiologist understand the potential benefit but may not appreciate the hazards of sedation or anaesthesia techniques. Similarly, an anaesthetist understands the risks but not the benefits. Ideally, the referring clinician should obtain prior written consent and the sedationist or anaesthetist should then explain the recommended technique. In the unlikely event that the clinician has not appreciated that the risks outweigh the benefits, more communication and reassessment are required. It is important that parents and children are fully informed of the intended procedures and that someone takes responsibility.

Resources and planning

TRAINING OF 'SEDATIONISTS'

People are the most important resource and they should be deployed within a team. It is very common for the

Table 44.4   Scottish Intercollegiate Guidelines Network (SIGN) contraindications to sedation and common contraindications to sedation for painless imaging

SIGN contraindications to sedation in children [3]	
abnormal airway	
raised intracranial pressure	
depressed conscious level	
history of sleep apnoea	
respiratory failure	
cardiac failure	
neuromuscular disease	
bowel obstruction	
active respiratory tract infection	
known allergy or adverse reaction to sedative	
child too distressed despite adequate preparation	
older child with severe behavioural problems	
consent refusal by parent or patient	
Common contraindications to sedation for painless imaging [6]	
1. Airway problems	Any actual or potential airway obstruction (e.g. snoring or stridor, blocked nose, small mandible, large tongue)
2. Apnoeic spells	Related to brain damage or previous drug treatment
3. Respiratory disease	Peripheral haemoglobin oxygen saturation (SpO_2) less than 94% in air
	Respiratory failure (high respiratory rate, oxygen treatment)
	Inability to cough or cry
4. High intracranial pressure	Drowsiness
	Headache
	Vomiting
5. Epilepsy	Generalised convulsions requiring rectal diazepam within the last 24 hours *or* rectal diazepam used more frequently than once in 2 weeks
	Previous adverse reaction to sedation, i.e. exacerbation of seizures
	Children requiring resuscitation during a convulsion within the last month
	Children who not only have convulsions but also have other major neurological or neuromuscular disease such as apnoeic spells or hypotonia as part of global neurological disease, intracranial hypertension due to cerebral tumour or encephalitis
	Generalised convulsions with cyanosis more frequent than once per day
	Children who have had a convulsion less than 4 hours before sedation
	Failure to regain full consciousness and mobility after a recent convulsion
6. Risk of pulmonary aspiration of gastric contents	Abdominal distension
	Appreciable volumes draining from nasogastric tube
	Vomiting
7. Severe metabolic, liver or renal disease	Requiring peritoneal dialysis or haemodialysis

non-anaesthetists to focus on the 'what' or 'how' but it is the 'who' that is most important. Training is often an item missing from protocols. Organisations recommend training but have not specified what is to be taught and, until they do, resuscitation courses can teach relevant skills. Courses that teach how to assess a sick child are important. Qualification and registration also need to be considered.

In our unit we train a team of experienced nurses who have a background of anaesthesia, intensive care or emergency medicine. They undergo tutorials in resuscitation and then practise airway and intravenous skills on anaesthetised children. These skills are revalidated every 3 months, and safety is increased further because they work as a team [6]. Other centres have similar sedation teams [30–32].

Simulation is a tool that could be developed but is limited to the management of complications rather than technique. Three scenarios could be practised; airway obstruction, anaphylaxis and cardiac arrest.

EQUIPMENT AND FACILITIES FOR SEDATION

The equipment and monitoring should be equal to that used for anaesthesia except for the presence of an anaesthesia machine – this may be necessary to manage failed sedation. The facilities will vary according to the procedure. Painless imaging requires a quiet area to induce sleep and it is best sited close to the scanner to minimise disturbing the child during transfer. In other situations sedation is undertaken in the procedure room itself and will need sufficient space for staff involved. A recovery area, of suitable size, needs qualified staff and should not be isolated. Some centres have developed 'mobile' services for the wards [33] and others utilise intensive care units [34]. The Association of Anaesthetists of Great Britain and Ireland website (http://www.aagbi.org/) publishes guidelines that will assist anyone planning a new anaesthesia facility and the principles can be applied to sedation also.

Distressing procedures should be undertaken in a procedure room so that the child can be comforted by returning to their own bedspace (their 'place of safety').

ECONOMICS OF SEDATION VERSUS ANAESTHESIA

There is no doubt that anaesthesia is faster than sedation and therefore more efficient. In terms of cost per session, anaesthesia is probably cheaper per patient but only if a comparison is made with 'like' patients. The cost is related to personnel (equipment should be similar and drug costs are small by comparison) and anaesthesia is cheaper only if the patient throughput is efficient. Fast anaesthesia techniques will be discussed later.

Sometimes anaesthesia resources may not be available or the procedures themselves may not justify the expense. In many situations the need for anaesthesia can be minimised by offering behavioural and sedation techniques to suitable children. Assessment of children several days before the procedure allows planning and preparation.

USEFUL DRUGS AND TECHNIQUES FOR NON-ANAESTHETISTS

The drugs and techniques below are potentially useful because they have a wide margin of safety. Nevertheless, non-anaesthetists need training to manage unexpected loss of consciousness and airway complications. Doses are available in local and national formularies but, in the main, those quoted are from the *British National Formulary for Children* 2005 (website: bnfc.org).

Painless imaging [8]

INFANTS < 5 KG

Infants aged less than 6 months often sleep naturally after food if they are comfortable and warm.

SMALL CHILDREN (<15 KG)

Small oral doses of chloral hydrate or triclofos calm irritable children and are suitable for computed tomography (CT) or echocardiography. Larger doses (50–100 mg/kg, max. dose 1 g) reliably cause sleep lasting 30–60 minutes in 95 per cent of children and are effective for MRI. Chloral hydrate has an unpleasant taste and is a gastric irritant; triclofos is better tolerated but has a slower onset. Several large series demonstrate that chloral hydrate can cause unpredictable and prolonged sedation.

Oral barbiturates are useful for MRI. Secobarbital makes 90 per cent of children younger than 5 years sleep successfully, and pentobarbital (4 mg/kg) is also reliable and may be safer than chloral hydrate for infants (pentobarbital is not available in the UK).

Of all the benzodiazepines, midazolam has the shortest action and when administered by mouth (0.5 mg/kg), via the nose (0.2 mg/kg) or per rectum (0.25–0.5 mg/kg) will begin to calm children within a few minutes. Nasal administration is distressing but made less so by using a simple spray or 'atomising' attachment to the syringe. Excessive sedation is unlikely and can be reversed with flumazenil (intravenously or via the nose, 10 μg/kg, maximum dose 200 μg) but, because of flumazenil's shorter action, resedation can occur. Paradoxical reactions can be troublesome and may also be reversed [35] but flumazenil may provoke seizures and should be used with care [36].

Other benzodiazepines, lorazepam and diazepam, administered orally or by injection, are used infrequently but may be useful for long periods of anxiolysis and sedation (not recommended in neonates).

CHILDREN > 15 KG

It is difficult to sedate safely an uncooperative child of this size. Play specialists can provide invaluable help but children with behavioural problems are especially difficult. Benzodiazepines alone are usually insufficient for scans that need prolonged sleep. Temazepam (orally, 1 mg/kg) combined with droperidol (orally, 0.25 mg/kg) has a 70 per cent success rate in children between 15 kg and 25 kg and the success rate increases to 95 per cent with intravenous diazepam [6]. Droperidol is no longer be available and sufficient data to recommend any alternative are not available. An outdated combination of morphine and alimemazine had a success rate of around 80 per cent.

Dexmedetomidine (intravenously, 1 μg/kg followed by infusion 0.5 μg/kg/h) combined with midazolam is promising [37].

Pentobarbital (up to 5 mg/kg), is regarded as a safe intravenous sedative in North America; however, it is not available in the UK and significant numbers of children have airway obstruction or paradoxical excitement. Secobarbital also causes paradoxical reactions too often to be valuable.

Melatonin may promote natural sleep. In an uncontrolled study 10 mg caused 50–65 per cent of children to sleep through an MR scan and it may also help children to sleep for electroencephalography (EEG) [38]. However, in a randomised controlled trial, melatonin did not improve the reliability of sedation for MRI [39]. Tiredness due to sleep deprivation may be helpful, although some children become more irritable.

Painful procedures [9]

The use of local anaesthesia is assumed.

NITROUS OXIDE

With care and patience, nitrous oxide is effective for many short painful procedures provided that the child is cooperative enough to allow one to apply the facemask firmly to avoid air dilution. In the UK, nitrous oxide (Entonox) is available only in cylinders with a demand valve but, in France it is available as Kalinox and can be delivered via a free-flow apparatus that is more practical for small children [40]. Dentists are expert in using nitrous oxide and their technique is called inhalational sedation – formerly known as relative analgesia (RA) [41,42]. Inspired concentration of nitrous oxide is gradually increased to a maximum of 70 per cent from a custom-built apparatus and via a soft nasal mask (scavenging is inbuilt). Usually around 30 per cent is effective and dysphoria is common at 70 per cent. Up to 90 per cent of children can be managed for dental treatment in this way. If nitrous oxide is limited to children over 1 year, and provided that no other drugs are used, and that the conscious state of the child is not depressed beforehand, up to 50 per cent inspired concentration can be used with little chance of causing an unrousable state [40]. There are a few specific contraindications to nitrous oxide. Neither fasting nor pulse oximetry monitoring is considered necessary, except in the USA [43].

OPIATES

Care must be taken to match the potency and length of action of opiate with the procedure-related pain; in the absence of pain respiratory depression can occur. Incremental intravenous fentanyl (1 µg/kg) is effective for minor injuries [9] and nasal diamorphine (0.1 mg/kg atomised in 0.1 mL) is valuable in children with limb fractures [44]. If naloxone (10 µg/kg) is necessary, pain may return.

OPIATES COMBINED WITH BENZODIAZEPINES

This combination is helpful but its efficacy and safety are unpredictable. A safe incremental dose of midazolam may be between 25 and 50 µg/kg [9]. Usually, the length of action of the sedation is much longer than the pain of the procedure itself. For example, the common combination of midazolam and fentanyl is useful but does have an appreciable adverse

reaction rate (5 per cent) that includes respiratory depression, paradoxical reaction and vomiting; these effects are unpredictable but more common in small children [45].

KETAMINE

The margin of safety for low-dose ketamine may be wide enough for use by non-anaesthetists, although this is controversial [46,47]. Intravenously, 1–2 mg/kg will quieten a child and facilitate a short minor procedure such as wound care. Larger intramuscular (4–5 mg/kg) or oral (5–10 mg/kg) doses are effective and suit some situations. Laryngospasm or apnoea can occur in less than 1 per cent but these are almost always self-limiting or can be managed with basic airway skills [48]. Ketamine can cause vomiting in up to 30 per cent and dysphoria or hallucinations in around 1–5 per cent [49,50]. Midazolam does not prevent ketamine hallucinations [51].

MANAGEMENT OF PAINLESS IMAGING [8]

Behavioural techniques are especially valuable for painless imaging and the success of any sedation technique should be judged on those children in whom behavioural techniques have failed. Computed tomography is fast and quiet and most children lie still enough. For longer CT scans or for children who are too irritable, a calming dose of midazolam may be sufficient and, provided that the dose is limited to 0.5 mg/kg, rigid fasting rules may be relaxed so that sleep is more likely – this is a controversial practice. Calming doses of sedatives are not sufficient for noisy MRI or long uncomfortable nuclear medicine scans. Here, sleep or deep sedation is effective in about 90 per cent of selected cases. Children who are unfit or whose behaviour is too disturbed (usually children older than 8 years or larger than 40 kg) need anaesthesia. A management strategy for painless imaging is suggested in Fig. 44.1. It may be reasonable to

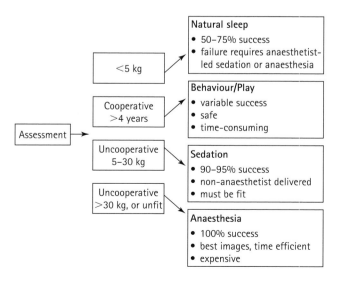

Figure 44.1 General strategy for management of children for painless imaging.

relax fasting rules for some sedation techniques but only if there is confidence that the level of sedation does not depress pharyngeal reflexes.

Anaesthesia involving conventional airway and breathing support can be modified to improve recovery. Almost all infants and children lying supine do not need artificial airway support during anaesthesia; at most, they may need minor extension of the neck. In this situation, once anaesthesia has been achieved, by either intravenous or inhalational means, doses can be reduced because there is no stimulation from any airway device. Recovery may therefore be faster and may be associated with less airway irritation such as laryngospasm or coughing. In a few children this technique fails to either keep them still or maintain unobstructed breathing. Also, the natural movement of breathing can cause movement artefact and, if so, controlled ventilation is necessary. In MRI there are important technical hazards and restrictions (Table 44.5).

If an artificial airway is not considered necessary a single dose of intravenous thiopental or propofol will cause sufficient sleep, and for long scans propofol infusions are used widely (6 mg/kg/h is effective) [52]. Intravenous pentobarbital (maximum dose 5 mg/kg) is a popular technique in the USA. Rectal drugs such as thiopental (25–50 mg/kg) are effective in small children but are not as reliable as intravenous or inhalational methods. Inhalational drugs can be administered with oxygen via simple plastic oxygen masks [53] or nasal catheters [54]. In this technique the inspired concentration cannot be controlled with much precision but the measurement of end-tidal concentration will guide changes to the vaporiser setting or gas flow. Scavenging can be achieved with a plastic canopy to cover the head. Conventional anaesthesia, using a laryngeal mask, is a popular and reliable method but seems to be associated with crying in recovery (author's unpublished observations). There is evidence that there is more distress or delirium during recovery from sevoflurane than from halothane after painless imaging [55]. Finally, ketamine causes secretions that may provoke unwanted swallowing.

Radiotherapy, although not imaging, requires similar anaesthesia, aiming for perfect immobility and fast recovery [56]. Transthoracic echocardiography can be difficult in irritable infants and small children but calming should be sufficient and midazolam or triclofos is usually successful. Transoesophageal echocardiography, as for any oesophagoscopy, is safer under anaesthesia.

MANAGEMENT OF PAINFUL PROCEDURES

Table 44.6 summarises the recommended management of painful procedures and the main areas of expansion of services are discussed in detail. The use of local anaesthesia is assumed.

INTERVENTIONAL RADIOLOGY

Interventional radiology encompasses a variety of procedures that involve a wide range of pain, time taken and difficulty. Overall, the delivery of an efficient service is best achieved by an anaesthetist who can choose a technique to suit the procedure and the child. The most common procedure is the insertion of long-term venous access using ultrasound imaging. This service has probably achieved a major reduction in the suffering of children who have previously required multiple venous cannulations or blood sampling. Whereas some children can be managed without anaesthesia many, if not most, are too ill or have inaccessible veins to make conscious sedation practical. Ketamine can be used if its side-effect profile is accepted. In many cases controlled ventilation is needed to ensure perfect immobility.

Some biopsies can be achieved with nitrous oxide alone but only with full cooperation.

Table 44.5 Technical problems with monitoring and equipment for magnetic resonance imaging (MRI)

Technical problem	Details
Ferromagnetic equipment may be attracted to the strong magnetic field	Special equipment required *or* strict policy with ferromagnetic equipment Steel gas cylinders are dangerous – piped gases only Non-ferromagnetic patient trolleys
Conventional electrical monitoring produces electromagnetic noise which disrupts image acquisition	Powerful MR scanners are screened by a copper shield within the walls, ceiling and floor of the scanning room Conducting cables passing through the screen to the scanning room will transfer electromagnetic interference and disrupt imaging
During scanning, the changing magnetic gradients induce electric current	Conventional electrical monitoring inside the scanning room may not function Coiled wires can burn skin Metallic implants must be checked for compatibility

Note that it is extremely valuable to have an area next to the scanner where patients can be induced, recovered and, if necessary, resuscitated without any magnetic restriction. (Recommendations for MRI are published on the Association of Anaesthetists of Great Britain and Ireland website: http://www.aagbi.org.)

Table 44.6   Recommended management

Painless procedures (whenever behavioural methods are ineffective)

Transthoracic echocardiography/ultrasound	Conscious sedation (calming)
Computed tomography	Conscious sedation/short sleep
Magnetic resonance imaging	Sleep (anaesthesia or sedation)
Radiotherapy	Sleep (anaesthesia or sedation)
Electroencephalography	Sleep (natural or melatonin)
Brain-stem-evoked responses	Sleep (anaesthesia or sedation)
Eye examinations	Sleep (anaesthesia or sedation)

Painful procedures (the use of local anaesthesia is assumed)

Dental procedures	Nitrous oxide (or anaesthesia)
Venepuncture and venous access	Behavioural, nitrous oxide
Wound care, removal of sutures	Analgesia, nitrous oxide, (conscious sedation for short procedures, anaesthesia for remainder)
Minor injuries (accident and emergency)	Ketamine or anaesthesia
Burns dressings	Opiate-based conscious sedation, ketamine or anaesthesia
Removal of chest drains	Opiate-based conscious sedation, or nitrous oxide, or ketamine, or anaesthesia
All other painful minor procedures (includes oncology procedures, renal/hepatic biopsy, muscle and joint injections, interventional radiology and insertion of long-term venous access, cardiac angiography, oesophagogastroscopy and colonoscopy)	Anaesthesia (nitrous oxide or other conscious sedation technique for cooperative children)

This is a quick guide to successful management of various procedures (see text for detailed discussion).

MINOR ONCOLOGY PROCEDURES [57]

Intrathecal chemotherapy and bone marrow aspiration are not comfortable with local anaesthesia alone. Surprisingly, a survey of practice in the USA and Europe found that some centres did not offer any additional analgesia or anaesthesia [58]. Behavioural techniques will benefit a few motivated children and, if anaesthesia is not available, sedation helps. Nevertheless, most centres prefer an anaesthesia service and, because many children have long-term venous access, intravenous techniques are popular. Propofol alone is sufficient, but the dose can be reduced by potent analgesia with a short-acting opiate. Only small doses of fentanyl or alfentanil should be used if spontaneous breathing is desired. Remifentanil is useful and, although apnoea is likely, this can be managed by manual ventilation as one would for a muscle relaxant. Bradycardia or muscle rigidity side-effects are rare provided that the bolus dose is limited to 2 µg/kg. Usually, bolus doses of propofol (3 mg/kg) and remifentanil (1–2 µg/kg) are sufficient for a lumbar puncture, which should take only a few minutes; recovery from these doses is rapid and children are usually eating and drinking within 30 minutes [59]. This technique is likely to be much faster than an inhalational technique using sevoflurane. Etomidate may allow fast recovery but is associated with vomiting in 10 per cent when combined with an opiate [60].

Sedation techniques with combinations of opiates and benzodiazepines have a high failure rate and risk hypoxia.

Nitrous oxide (inspired concentration 50 per cent) is a standard technique in France and, if used with care and skill, is remarkably successful [40]. Success is highest with unhurried preparation in cooperative children. Ketamine is a useful 'standby' drug but should be necessary only when other techniques fail or are unavailable.

Central venous lines must be used with care. Some centres prefer anaesthetists to use a full sterile technique but, because this imposes practical difficulties of combining sterility and rapid attention to the airway, a clean technique may be acceptable in which the central line is used only after cleaning with alcohol and by gloved hands. After anaesthesia, the line must be flushed with sufficient volume of 0.9 per cent (normal) saline, and later flushed again with heparinised saline, before discharge home.

GASTROINTESTINAL ENDOSCOPY

Oesophagoscopy is difficult under conscious sedation in uncooperative children [61]. Deep sedation or anaesthesia is necessary to suppress the gag reflex during insertion of the scope although, after this, stimulation is much less. Also, the scope can compress and obstruct the trachea [62]. In general, sedation is not recommended for oesophagoscopy in children [63], but a recent survey from France shows that sedation is still used widely [64]. Combinations of opiate and benzodiazepines are used but, even with good judgement, there is a risk of hypoxia [65,66].

Anaesthesia managed by tracheal intubation is standard but other techniques have been described. If an anaesthetist is present, an artificial airway device may not be needed, especially if the procedure is short. Most diagnostic gastroscopies can be completed within 10 minutes and, with sufficient endoscopes, four cases per hour could be completed if recovery was also fast. Propofol (2–3 mg/kg) suppresses the gag reflex sufficiently and smaller bolus doses are effective thereafter [67–70]; opiates are not usually necessary. Nasal catheters that combine the delivery of oxygen and aspiration of tidal gas for capnography are very useful. Longer procedures are probably easier with an airway device and laryngeal masks are available that incorporate an additional port to allow insertion of a scope. Longer procedures are best managed with a propofol infusion or an inhalational technique.

Colonoscopies cause pain from bowel distension and a propofol infusion may require opiate supplementation. Pain may warn the gastroenterologist that the colon is at risk of perforation and, if conventional anaesthesia reduces colonic tone, sedation may be safer in this respect. Ketamine is another alternative but has an appreciable rate of laryngospasm during oesphagoscopy, perhaps owing to increased pharyngeal secretions [71].

Achalasia causes an oesophageal liquid residue and is dangerous; it should be drained before any sedation or anaesthesia is given.

CARDIAC ANGIOGRAPHY

The majority of cardiac diagnoses are now achieved by echocardiography and, consequently, angiography is reserved for diagnosis of complex anatomy and physiology or for interventions such as dilatations and insertions of stents, coils and other blocking devices. It is now possible to insert pulmonary valves during angiography. In most cases conventional anaesthesia and controlled ventilation are justified. This allows optimum conditions for prolonged detailed imaging and creates stable respiratory conditions if the cardiovascular status is unstable or destabilised by the procedure itself. Indeed, the cardiac angiography department may have the highest cardiac arrest rate in a paediatric hospital outside intensive care [72].

Sedation techniques are in use in many centres and the rate of respiratory depression will vary according to drug technique and skill [73–75]. The catheters, inserted into the femoral vessels, can be virtually painless with local anaesthesia and, if the child is sufficiently prepared and cooperative, sedation may not be needed or limited to anxiolysis. Deeper sedation levels with combinations of midazolam with either ketamine or opiates can be successful but are probably better described as minimal anaesthesia.

When cardiac anatomy is complex the estimation of cardiac output and shunt fraction may be needed and this involves the measurement of blood oxygen content. The accuracy of these estimations is improved by minimising the oxygen content of venous blood and this is best achieved in the awake state because anaesthesia and muscle relaxation minimise oxygen consumption. This poses a dilemma. Anxiolysis or conscious sedation may provide a 'natural' cardiovascular state, but if the child will not keep still sedation must be deeper with a degree of cardiorespiratory depression [75]. However, the unnatural state of anaesthesia can provide reproducibly steady conditions. Close cooperation and discussion with the cardiology team are important.

Beware of brachial plexus injury due to extreme extension of the arms during prolonged imaging [76].

DENTISTRY

Dentists have been pioneers in sedation and have considerable experience in managing anxious children; there are specific guidelines for the UK [41,42] and the USA [43]. Inhalational sedation with nitrous oxide alone is very successful because dentists have the time to reassure and gain trust; treatment is rarely urgent. The operator usually delivers the nitrous oxide but there must be a trained assistant and resuscitation equipment present. For anxious children the addition of 'subanaesthetic' concentrations of sevoflurane improves the success rate [77] but there are not sufficient data to make this an established or recommended technique. Intravenous benzodiazepine administered alone, carefully titrated, is the only other recommended (in the UK) sedation technique for dentistry, but only in adults. Other drugs have been combined for dentistry but they risk unintentional anaesthesia.

If a patient becomes unconscious their ability to open their mouth is lost. This is a useful sign of deepening sedation and therefore a mouth gag should not be used for conscious sedation.

ACCIDENT AND EMERGENCY; MINOR INJURIES [9]

Children present with minor injuries that cannot be managed with conscious sedation. Large emergency units should have anaesthesia services but others may not, either because of their remote position or because of other organisational issues. Whatever the reasons, accident and emergency departments are developing their own procedural sedation and analgesia (PSA) protocols and these include the use of nitrous oxide, benzodiazepines, opiates and ketamine. Although ketamine has its side-effects, it is very effective and may be safe enough for non-anaesthetists; this is controversial [3,47]. Certainly intravenous benzodiazepine and opiate combinations are not completely safe [45,78] and may not be as effective as ketamine. Ketamine may be safest if fasting is uncertain or if there is hypovolaemia. Whatever the technique, users must be trained to manage airway problems.

CHEST DRAINS – INSERTION AND REMOVAL

Chest drains are usually inserted either as an emergency or during thoracic surgery. In an emergency, analgesia (and sedation, if any) must be used very carefully to avoid causing any additional respiratory dysfunction; ketamine may be the best technique. However, the removal of chest drains is a common and difficult problem in conscious children. There is some published experience of using nitrous oxide or morphine alone in cooperative children but these are not very effective [79]. Careful titration of opiate and midazolam is probably the best (easiest and safest) technique because it modifies the pain and causes amnesia. Ketamine or anaesthesia may be justified in some situations.

REFERENCES

Key references

Bennett D, Marcus R, Stokes M. Incidents and complications during pediatric cardiac catheterization. *Paediatr Anaesth* 2005; **15**(12): 1083–8.

Gall O, Annequin D, Benoit G *et al.* Adverse events of premixed nitrous oxide and oxygen for procedural sedation in children. *Lancet* 2001; **358**(9292): 1514–15.

Green SM, Rothrock SG, Lynch EL et al. Intramuscular ketamine for pediatric sedation in the emergency department: safety profile in 1022 cases. *Ann Emerg Med* 1998; **31**:688–97.

Krauss B, Green SM. Procedural sedation and analgesia in children. Lancet 2006; **367**(9512): 766–80.

Sury MR, Harker H, Begent J, Chong WK. The management of infants and children for painless imaging. *Clin Radiol* 2005; **60**(7):731–41.

References

1. Pressdee D, May L, Eastman E, Grier D. The use of play therapy in the preparation of children undergoing MR imaging. *Clin Radiol* 1997; **52**(12): 945–7.
2. Butler LD, Symons BK, Henderson SL *et al.* Hypnosis reduces distress and duration of an invasive medical procedure for children. *Pediatrics* 2005; **115**(1): e77–85.
3. SIGN. *Safe sedation of children undergoing diagnostic and therapeutic procedures. A national clinical guideline.* Edinburgh: Scottish Intercollegiate Guidelines Network, 2004 (http://www.sign.ac.uk).
4. Academy of Medical Royal Colleges. *Safe sedation practice for healthcare procedures in adults.* Report of an intercollegiate working party chaired by the Royal College of Anaesthetists. 2001. London: Academy of Medical Royal Colleges, 2001.
5. American Society of Anesthesiologists. continuum of depth of sedation – definition of general anesthesia and levels of sedation/analgesia. Park Ridge: American Society of Anesthesiologists, 2001.
6. Sury MRJ, Hatch DJ, Deeley T *et al.* Development of a nurse-led sedation service for paediatric magnetic resonance imaging. *Lancet* 1999; **353**: 1667–71.

7. Vangerven M, van Hemelrijck J, Wouters P *et al.* Light anaesthesia with propofol for paediatric MRI. *Anaesthesia* 1992; **47**: 706–7.
8. Sury MR, Harker H, Begent J, Chong WK. The management of infants and children for painless imaging. *Clin Radiol* 2005; **60**(7): 731–41.
9. Krauss B, Green SM. Procedural sedation and analgesia in children. *Lancet* 2006; **367**(9512): 766–80.
10. Chernik DA, Gillings D, Laine H *et al.* Validity and reliability of the Observer's Assessment of Alertness/Sedation Scale: study with intravenous midazolam. *J Clin Psychopharmacol* 1990; **10**(4): 244–51.
11. Malviya S, Voepel-Lewis T, Tait AR *et al.* Depth of sedation in children undergoing computed tomography: validity and reliability of the University of Michigan Sedation Scale (UMSS). *Br J Anaesth* 2002; **88**(2): 241–5.
12. Gill M, Green SM, Krauss B. A study of the Bispectral Index Monitor during procedural sedation and analgesia in the emergency department. *Ann Emerg Med* 2003; **41**(2): 234–41.
13. Powers SW, Blount RL, Bachanas PJ *et al.* Helping preschool leukemia patients and their parents cope during injections. *J Pediatr Psychol* 1993; **18**(6): 681–95.
14. Tucker CL, Slifer KJ, Dahlquist LM. Reliability and validity of the brief behavioral distress scale: a measure of children's distress during invasive medical procedures. *J Pediatr Psychol* 2001; **26**(8): 513–23.
15. Ambuel B, Hamlett KW, Marx CM, Blumer JL. Assessing distress in pediatric intensive care environments: the COMFORT scale. *J Pediatr Psychol* 1992; **17**(1): 95–109.
16. Tatman A, Warren A, Williams A *et al.* Development of a modified paediatric coma scale in intensive care clinical practice. *Arch Dis Child* 1997; **77**(6): 519–21.
17. Malviya S, Voepel-Lewis T, Ludomirsky A *et al.* Can we improve the assessment of discharge readiness? A comparative study of observational and objective measures of depth of sedation in children. *Anesthesiology* 2004; **100**(2): 218–24.
18. Sury MR, Harker H, Thomas ML. Sevoflurane sedation in infants undergoing MRI: a preliminary report. *Paediatr Anaesth* 2005; **15**(1): 16–22.
19. Blues CM, Pomfrett CJ. Respiratory sinus arrhythmia and clinical signs of anaesthesia in children. *Br J Anaesth* 1998; **81**(3): 333–7.
20. Toweill DLB. Linear and nonlinear analysis of heart rate variability during propofol anesthesia for short-duration procedures in children. *Pediatr Crit Care Med* 2003; **4**(3): 308–314.
21. Agrawal D, Feldman HA, Krauss B, Waltzman ML. Bispectral index monitoring quantifies depth of sedation during emergency department procedural sedation and analgesia in children. *Ann Emerg Med* 2004; **43**(2): 247–55.
22. Powers KS, Nazarian EB, Tapyrik SA *et al.* Bispectral index as a guide for titration of propofol during procedural sedation among children. *Pediatrics* 2005; **115**(6): 1666–74.
23. Rodriguez RA, Hall LE, Duggan S, Splinter WM. The bispectral index does not correlate with clinical signs of inhalational

anesthesia during sevoflurane induction and arousal in children. *Can J Anaesth* 2004; **51**(5): 472–80.

24. Antognini JF, Carstens E. *In vivo* characterization of clinical anaesthesia and its components. *Br J Anaesth* 2002; **89**(1): 156–66.

25. Royal College of Anaesthetists and Royal College of Radiologists. *Sedation and anaesthesia in radiology.* Report of a joint working party. London: Royal College of Anaesthetists and Royal College of Radiologists, 1992.

26. American Academy of Pediatrics, American Academy of Pediatric Dentistry, Cote CJ, Wilson S, the Work Group on Sedation. Guidelines for monitoring and management of pediatric patients during and after sedation for diagnostic and therapeutic procedures: an update. *Pediatrics* 2006; **118**(6): 2587–602.

27. Coté CJ, Notterman DA, Karl HW *et al.* Adverse sedation events in pediatrics: a critical incident analysis of contributing factors. *Pediatrics* 2000; **105**(4 Pt 1): 805–14.

28. Cravero JP, Blike GT, Beach M *et al.* Incidence and nature of adverse events during pediatric sedation/anesthesia for procedures outside the operating room: report from the Pediatric Sedation Research Consortium. *Pediatrics* 2006; **118**(3): 1087–96.

29. Green SM, Roback MG, Miner JR *et al.* Fasting and emergency department procedural sedation and analgesia: a consensus-based clinical practice advisory. *Ann Emerg Med* 2007; **49**(4): 454–61.

30. Egelhoff JC, Ball WS Jr, Koch BL, Parks TD. Safety and efficacy of sedation in children using a structured sedation program. *Am J Roentgenol* 1994;1259–62.

31. Keengwe IN, Hegde S, Dearlove O *et al.* Structured sedation programme for magnetic resonance imaging examination in children. *Anaesthesia* 1999; **54**(11): 1069–72.

32. Beebe DS, Tran P, Bragg M *et al.* Trained nurses can provide safe and effective sedation for MRI in pediatric patients. *Can J Anaesth* 2000; **47**(3): 205–10.

33. Lowrie L, Weiss AH, Lacombe C. The pediatric sedation unit: a mechanism for pediatric sedation. *Pediatrics* 1998; **102**(3): E30.

34. Hertzog JH, Dalton HJ, Anderson BD *et al.* Prospective evaluation of propofol anesthesia in the pediatric intensive care unit for elective oncology procedures in ambulatory and hospitalized children. *Pediatrics* 2000; **106**(4): 742–7.

35. Sanders JC. Flumazenil reverses a paradoxical reaction to intravenous midazolam in a child with uneventful prior exposure to midazolam. *Paediatr Anaesth* 2003; **13**(4): 369–70.

36. Shannon M, Albers G, Burkhart K *et al.* Safety and efficacy of flumazenil in the reversal of benzodiazepine-induced conscious sedation. The Flumazenil Pediatric Study Group. *J Pediatr* 1997; **131**(4): 582–6.

37. Koroglu A, Demirbilek S, Teksan H *et al.* Sedative, haemodynamic and respiratory effects of dexmedetomidine in children undergoing magnetic resonance imaging examination: preliminary results. *Br J Anaesth* 2005; **94**(6): 821–4.

38. Johnson K, Page A, Williams H *et al.* The use of melatonin as an alternative to sedation in uncooperative children

undergoing an MRI examination. *Clin Radiol* 2002; **57**: 502–6.

39. Sury MR, Fairweather K. The effect of melatonin on sedation of children undergoing magnetic resonance imaging. *Br J Anaesth.* 2006; **97**: 220–5.

40. Gall O, Annequin D, Benoit G *et al.* Adverse events of premixed nitrous oxide and oxygen for procedural sedation in children. *Lancet* 2001; **358**(9292): 1514–15.

41. Hosey MT. UK National Clinical Guidelines in paediatric dentistry. Managing anxious children: the use of conscious sedation in paediatric dentistry. *Int J Paediatr Dent* 2002; **12**(5): 359–72.

42. Department of Health U. *Conscious sedation in the provision of dental care.* Report of an Expert Group on Sedation for Dentistry, Standing Dental Advisory Committee, 2003 (15 March accessed 2006). Available from: http://www.doh.gov.uk/dental

43. American Academy of Pediatric Dentistry. Elective use of minimal, moderate, and deep sedation and general anesthesia for pediatric dental patients, 2004. Available from: http://www.aapd.org/media/Policies_Guidelines/G_Sedation.pdf

44. Kendall JM, Reeves BC, Latter VS. Multicentre randomised controlled trial of nasal diamorphine for analgesia in children and teenagers with clinical fractures. *BMJ* 2001; **322**(7281): 261–5.

45. Pena BM, Krauss B. Adverse events of procedural sedation and analgesia in a pediatric emergency department. *Ann Emerg Med* 1999; **34**(4 Pt 1): 483–91.

46. McGlone RG, Howes MC, Joshi M. The Lancaster experience of 2.0–2.5 mg/kg intramuscular ketamine for paediatric sedation: 501 cases and analysis. *Emerg Med J* 2004; **21**(3): 290–95.

47. Morton NS. Ketamine is not a safe, effective, and appropriate technique for emergency department paediatric procedural sedation. *Emerg Med J* 2004; **21**(3): 272–3.

48. Green SM, Rothrock SG, Lynch EL *et al.* Intramuscular ketamine for pediatric sedation in the emergency department: safety profile in 1022 cases. *Ann Emerg Med* 1998; **31**: 688–97.

49. Gingrich BK. Difficulties encountered in a comparative study of orally administered midazolam and ketamine. *Anesthesiology* 1994; **80**: 1414–15.

50. McDowall RH, Scher CS, Barst SM. Total intravenous anesthesia for children undergoing brief diagnostic or therapeutic procedures. *J Clin Anesth* 1995; **7**(4): 273–80.

51. Wathen JE, Roback MG, Mackenzie T, Bothner JP. Does midazolam alter the clinical effects of intravenous ketamine sedation in children? A double-blind, randomized, controlled, emergency department trial. *Ann Emerg Med* 2000; **36**(6): 579–88.

52. Frankville DD, Spear RM, Dyck JB. The dose of propofol required to prevent children from moving during magnetic resonance imaging. *Anesthesiology* 1993; **79**: 953–8.

53. Sury M, Harker H, Thomas M. Sedation for MRI using sevoflurane. *Paediatr Anaesth* 2005; **15**: 1025; author reply 1025.

54. De Sanctis Brigg's V. Magnetic resonance imaging under sedation in newborns and infants: a study of 640 cases using sevoflurane. *Paediatr Anaesth* 2005; **15**: 9–15.

55. Cravero J, Surgenor S, Whalen K. Emergence agitation in paediatric patients after sevoflurane anaesthesia and no surgery: a comparison with halothane. *Paediatr Anaesth* 2000; **10**(4):419–24.

56. Keidan I, Perel A, Shabtai EL, Pfeffer RM. Children undergoing repeated exposures for radiation therapy do not develop tolerance to propofol: clinical and bispectral index data. *Anesthesiology* 2004; **100**(2): 251–54.

57. Culshaw V, Yule M, Lawson R. Considerations for anaesthesia in children with haematological malignancy undergoing short procedures. *Paediatr Anaesth* 2003; **13**(5): 375–83.

58. Hain RD, Campbell C. Invasive procedures carried out in conscious children: contrast between North American and European paediatric oncology centres. *Arch Dis Child* 2001; **85**(1): 12–15.

59. Glaisyer HR, Sury MR. Recovery after anesthesia for short pediatric oncology procedures: propofol and remifentanil compared with propofol, nitrous oxide, and sevoflurane. *Anesth Analg* 2005; **100**(4): 959–63.

60. McDowall RH, Scher CS, Barst SM. Total intravenous anesthesia for children undergoing brief diagnostic or therapeutic procedures. *J Clin Anesth* 1995; **7**: 273–80.

61. Bishop PR, Nowicki MJ, May WL *et al.* Unsedated upper endoscopy in children. *Gastroint Endosc* 2002; **55**(6): 624–30.

62. Casfeel HB, Fiedorek SC, Kiel EA. Arterial blood oxygen desaturation in infants and children during upper gastrointestinal endoscopy. *Gastrointest Endosc* 1992; **36**: 489–493.

63. Stringer MD, McHugh PJM. Paediatric endoscopy should be carried out under general anaesthesia. *BMJ* 1995; **311**: 452–3.

64. Michaud L. Sedation for diagnostic upper gastrointestinal endoscopy: a survey of the Francophone Pediatric Hepatology, Gastroenterology, and Nutrition Group. *Endoscopy* 2005; **37**(2): 167–70.

65. Balsells F, Wyllie R, Kay M, Steffen R. Use of conscious sedation for lower and upper gastrointestinal endoscopic examinations in children, adolescents, and young adults: a twelve-year review. *Gastrointest Endosc* 1997; **45**(5): 375–80.

66. Lamireau T, Dubreuil M, Daconceicao M. Oxygen saturation during esophagogastroduodenoscopy in children: general anesthesia versus intravenous sedation. *J Pediatr Gastroenterol Nutr* 1998; **27**(2): 172–5.

67. Carlsson U, Grattidge P. Sedation for upper gastrointestinal endoscopy: a comparative study of propofol and midazolam. *Endoscopy* 1995; **27**(3): 240–3.

68. Kaddu R, Bhattacharya D, Metriyakool K *et al.* Propofol compared with general anesthesia for pediatric GI endoscopy: is propofol better? *Gastrointest Endosc* 2002; **55**(1): 27–32.

69. Walker JA, McIntyre RD, Schleinitz PF *et al.* Nurse-administered propofol sedation without anesthesia specialists in 9152 endoscopic cases in an ambulatory surgery center. *Am J Gastroenterol* 2003; **98**(8): 1744–50.

70. Barbi E, Petaros P, Badina L *et al.* Deep sedation with propofol for upper gastrointestinal endoscopy in children, administered by specially trained pediatricians: a prospective case series with emphasis on side effects. *Endoscopy* 2006; **38**(4): 368–75.

71. Green SM, Klooster M, Harris T *et al.* Ketamine sedation for pediatric gastroenterology procedures. *J Pediatr Gastroenterol Nutr* 2001; **32**(1): 26–33.

72. Bennett D, Marcus R, Stokes M. Incidents and complications during pediatric cardiac catheterization. *Paediatr Anaesth* 2005; **15**(12): 1083–8.

73. Rautiainen P. Alfentanil infusion for sedation in infants and small children during cardiac catheterization. *Can J Anaesth* 1991; **38**(8): 980–4.

74. Lebovic S, Reich DL, Steinberg LG *et al.* Comparison of propofol versus ketamine for anesthesia in pediatric patients undergoing cardiac catheterization. *Anesth Analg* 1992; **74**(4): 490–4.

75. Friesen RH, Alswang M. Changes in carbon dioxide tension and oxygen saturation during deep sedation for paediatric cardiac catheterization. *Paediatr Anaesth* 1996; **6**: 15–20.

76. Souza NE, Durand PG, Sassolas F *et al.* Brachial plexus injury during cardiac catheterisation in children. Report of two cases. *Acta Anaesthesiol Scand* 1998; **42**(7): 876–79.

77. Averley PA, Girdler NM, Bond S *et al.* A randomised controlled trial of paediatric conscious sedation for dental treatment using intravenous midazolam combined with inhaled nitrous oxide or nitrous oxide/sevoflurane. *Anaesthesia* 2004; **59**(9): 844–52.

78. Kennedy RM, Porter FL, Miller JP, Jaffe DM. Comparison of fentanyl/midazolam with ketamine/midazolam for pediatric orthopedic emergencies. *Pediatrics* 1998; **102**(4 Pt 1): 956–63.

79. Bruce E, Franck L, Howard RF. The efficacy of morphine and Entonox analgesia during chest drain removal in children. *Paediatr Anaesth* 2006; **16**(3): 302–8.

PART **V**

ORGANISATION AND PHILOSOPHY

Risk

JOHAN VAN DER WALT

KEY LEARNING POINTS

- Up to 80 per cent of anaesthesia adverse events may be related to human error, but poor systems are also important.
- Clinical governance and risk management are crucial to safety.
- After a serious adverse event, families will become more distressed unless they are given an early and honest explanation.
- Frequency of deaths is likely to represent only the 'tip of the iceberg' of hazardous practice.

- True risk is difficult to calculate because of the uncertainty of the denominator.
- The 1992 UK National Confidential Enquiry into Perioperative Deaths (NCEPOD) report was concerned with paediatric surgery and anaesthesia and recommended: subspecialty training, avoidance of infrequent practice, concentration of services, appropriate selection and transfer of sick children.

INTRODUCTION

'*primum non nocere*' – above all, do no harm!

This aphorism has been attributed to the French pathologist and clinician Auguste François Chomel (1788–1858) and has been a laudable aim in medical practice for over 150 years. Yet it implies that harm is part of medical practice and this is especially important to anaesthetists because anaesthesia has no inherent therapeutic value. However, doing nothing can also be harmful. If we accept that anaesthesia is risky we should consider risk management and develop a culture of safety [1,2].

Anaesthesia is often likened to aviation. There are similarities, in that anaesthetists have copied the principles of incident reporting and psychology of human error, but there are some important differences. First, the aviation industry is driven by commercial incentives and has huge financial resources available. Second, because an aviation disaster creates massive media attention, there is government regulation and enforcement of standards. Third, the human body is much less predictable than a machine and is

often ailing – often, it cannot be repaired before 'takeoff'. It is reasonable to say that anaesthesia is practised in a highly pressured, tightly coupled and complex physiological system where there is always the potential for error, accidents and harm.

To manage risk effectively it is essential to identify and understand the nature and scope of the risks, the outcomes, and their causes or associated factors. Adverse anaesthesia outcomes and risks have been studied more extensively in adults than in children but both share similar problems and solutions. Nevertheless, paediatric anaesthesia has some unique issues.

RISK MANAGEMENT

Clinical risk management is the systematic identification and management of risks and factors that contribute to clinical error with the aim of minimising harm and improving outcomes. A useful guidance document has been published by the Association of Anaesthetists of Great Britain and Ireland [3] in which four linked stages of risk management

Table 45.1   Commonly used risk management terms [5]

Patient safety	The absence of the potential for, or occurrence of, health care-associated injury to patients. Created by avoiding medical errors as well as taking action to prevent errors from causing injury*
Error	Mistakes made in the process of care that result in, or have the potential to result in, harm to patients. Mistakes include the failure of a planned action to be completed as intended or the use of a wrong plan to achieve an aim. These can be the result of an action that is taken (error of commission) or an action that is not taken (error of omission).* Errors can include problems in practice, products, procedures and systems[†]
Incident	Unexpected or unanticipated events or circumstances not consistent with the routine care of a particular patient, which could have, or did, lead to an unintended or unnecessary harm to a person, or a complaint, loss or damage[†]
Near miss	An occurrence of an error that did not result in harm [14]
Adverse event	An injury resulting from a medical intervention [14]
Preventable adverse event	Harm that could be avoided through reasonable planning or proper execution of an action*

*Patient Safety Initiative: building foundations, reducing risk. Interim report to the Senate Committee on Appropriations. Rockville: AHRQ Publications, 2003, 04-RG005).
[†]http://www.quic.gov/report/errors6ver6.doc (accessed 8/12/05).
[†]http://www.ashrm.org (accessed 8/12/05).

are recognised. These are: (1) *risk identification* leading to (2) *policies* for (3) *risk control*, which will have implications for (4) *funding*. Clinical governance is regarded as fundamental to safety; it relies upon individuals taking responsibility at all levels of an organisation. Risk management underpins everything anaesthetists do to deliver a competent or good quality service, and most anaesthetists already apply risk reduction; it is part of the practice of anaesthesia [4]. However, patient safety is still evolving and individuals may need to be more formal in their approach. Important defin-itions are summarised in Table 45.1 [5].

Medical practice, in general, is associated with an alarming incidence of harm caused by errors and mistakes. The rate of iatrogenic harm in patients of all ages has been shown to be consistent and running between 10 per cent and 12 per cent in the USA [6], Australia [7], UK [8], New Zealand [9], Canada [10] and Denmark [11]. In Australia, with a population of 20.4 million, preventable clinical adverse events (AEs) are associated with 50 000 permanent disabilities and 14 000 deaths per year and this is estimated to cost about 8 per cent of the national health budget [12]. Almost 50 per cent of these AEs were found to result from surgery. Anaesthesia accounted for only 2 per cent and was associated with less liability and deaths – such statistics have made anaesthesia a leader in patient safety [13,14]. Similar findings have been found in 5.7 million hospitalised children in the USA where as many as 4500 children die from medical errors each year (excluding errors associated with medication) [15]. Deaths occurred more frequently in infants and those in lower socioeconomic groups. There were significant increases in length of stay that resulted in more than $ US1 billion in excess costs. The analysis also found that the rate of 'anaesthesia complications' was 6 per 10 000 discharges, which amounted to 245 cases out of a pool of 384 295.

Human factors and error

It has often been stated that 80 per cent of AEs are caused by human error but it is clear that there are two elements to human fallibility: the person and the system [16]. The person approach focuses on the variability and error in individuals and considers forgetfulness, ignorance, inattention, carelessness, negligence and recklessness. These human characteristics suggest that there is blame, and it is understandable, although unfortunate, that a culture of 'name, blame and shame' has sometimes developed. The system approach concentrates on the background conditions that create the situations and conditions under which individuals work. Often poor human performance results from faults in system design, planning or administration. Rectifying these problems can improve the performance of individuals.

Errors [16] have been categorised as:

- latent – i.e. occurring 'upstream' in management, personnel processes and the design of equipment
- active – i.e. occurring 'downstream' at the site of care delivery (Fig. 45.1).

Active errors are subcategorised as skill based (slips, lapses in the performance of familiar tasks that take place without much conscious thought), mistakes (performance of an incorrect task believing it to be correct) and violations (deliberate deviations from rules, policies, standards, procedures, instructions and regulations). Mistakes are further divided into rule based (actions based on acquired rules and procedures) and knowledge based (practitioner relies on judgement not based on rules or procedures).

The enhancement of patient safety encompasses three complementary activities: preventing errors, making errors visible and mitigating the effects of errors

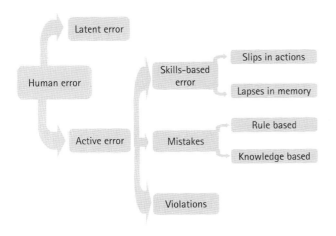

Figure 45.1   Categories of human error [16].

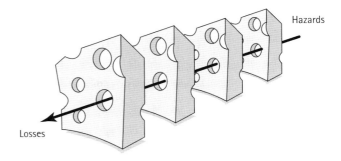

Figure 45.2   Swiss cheese layers of defensive barriers.
(Reproduced from Reason [16] with permission.)

(http://www.quic.gov/report/errors6ver6.doc, accessed 8/12/2006). These activities require organisations to recognise and to expect human fallibility and therefore to develop appropriate defences – such organisations are said to have a good 'risk culture'. Outside medicine, examples of good risk cultures can be seen in nuclear power plants and air traffic control centres, and they have been called 'high reliability organisations' because they expect to make errors and they prepare to recognise and recover from them. They rehearse scenarios to look for new and unexpected problems in order to reform and improve systems [16]. Reason has described a systems approach as being multilayered with defences, barriers and safeguards, each with its own weaknesses that will be breached given a certain set of circumstances [16]. He has likened these defensive layers to having multiple holes (like a Swiss cheese) that protect the patient most times but when the holes line up at some stage in a dynamic system there is patient harm (Fig. 45.2). It is possible to engineer alarms or phys-ical barriers (e.g. pin yoke index for connecting breathing gases) but there will always be a reliance on clinical staff, procedures and administrative controls. Mostly they do this very effectively, but there are always weaknesses.

These principles are being incorporated into anaesthesia research. For example, Biboulet and colleagues found that human error occurred in 91 per cent of anaesthesia-related cardiac arrests [17] and that the causes were multifactorial and associated with inadequate preoperative assessment (and risk estimation), intraoperative errors or misjudgements and poor patient health. Marcus has studied human factors in paediatric anaesthesia [18] and out of 28 023 anaesthetics at a single institution there were 668 incidents (2.4 per cent), of which airway incidents were most common (52.2 per cent). Of 284 human factors that could be identified 43 per cent were errors of judgement, 18 per cent were failure to check, 9 per cent were skill failure, 8 per cent resulted from inexperience, 6 per cent resulted from inattention or distraction and 6 per cent were problems with communication. Common errors of

judgement included 'inadequate depth of anaesthesia', 'inadvisable anaesthetic technique', 'anaesthetising a child with an upper respiratory tract infection (URTI)', and 'trachea extubated at wrong time'. The most common cognitive mechanisms involved were rule-based mistakes (28 per cent) and latent system errors (25 per cent); there were also knowledge-based mistakes, rule violations and skill-based error slips (each contributed 13–15 per cent).

In a major review of anaesthesia-related mortality Aitkenhead found that that the pattern of human error has not changed much over 40 years [19]. Inadequate preparation of patients, wrong choice of agent or technique, overdose, inadequate crisis management, inadequate resuscitation, inadequate postoperative care, failure to check, lack of vigilance and carelessness remained the commonest errors. Even with improved monitoring and anaesthesia techniques, high-risk patients can survive the operative phase but die later from avoidable causes. A review of perioperative adult deaths in South Australia found that the postoperative period accounted for 50 per cent of all anaesthesia associated deaths [20].

Recording and analysis of adverse events

Clinical governance requires organisations to have quality improvement procedures that respond to incidents, AEs and sentinel events. Sentinel events are speci-fied subsets of AEs and are of such significance that they are often defined and sometimes even legislated by regional governments to be reported. Well-known examples of sentinel events are death due to drug error, procedure error (wrong operation or wrong patient), gas embolism, blood transfusion error resulting from ABO incompatibility, retained instrument or other material after surgery, and maternal death or serious disability associated with labour. These serious events happen rarely but require formal and rapid investigation using a process called root cause analysis (RCA). This identifies organisational deficiencies that may not be immediately obvious but which may have caused or contributed to the event [21]. The RCA report also includes risk reduction strategies to decrease the chance of a similar event occurring again.

Risk mitigation

Risk management must have a plan for risk mitigation. This is important not only for the staff involved but also for the institution in order to promote good public relations and prevent bad publicity. This is why complaints management is vital. Staff need training and a process to manage complaints successfully. Legal formalities must be attended to in case of litigation. It is the author's experience that these principles are often neglected in stressful situ-ations and that this adds to the misery for everyone involved. With proactive, timely and sensible processes many problems are avoided. A prepared protocol is essential and an example can be found in the Australian Patient Safety Foundation (APSF) crisis management manual [22].

A common mistake of medical and industrial accidents is to fail to communicate. Families are distressed and become angry unless they are given an early and honest explanation. Risk management consultants know that the less competent practitioner with a good 'bedside manner' is less likely to be sued than the highly competent expert doctor who has an offhand autocratic attitude to his or her patients.

Adverse events may result if key clinical information is not available. Clinicians have a duty to advise colleagues of known hazards but a system-based automatic warning system can be developed that ensures that important information is presented during preoperative assessment [23,24].

Crisis management

The Australian and New Zealand College of Anaesthetists has recommended that training in crisis resource management should be mandatory for medical personnel undertaking anaesthesia or sedation for interventional medical or surgical procedures [25]. The APSF has recently published a crisis management manual that has been validated on an analysis of 4000 reports to the Australian Incident Monitoring Study (AIMS) [26]. Although approximately only 10 per cent of these reports were in children [27] the flow charts within the manual are useful to paediatric practice. The crisis management of laryngospasm is a good example [28]. The complete list of 25 subjects covered can be accessed on the internet at http://qhc.bmjjournals. com/cgi/content/full/14/3/156 [26]. Simulation is now available in many institutions to ensure that staff of all disciplines are trained and maintain good standards and competencies; it can provide the opportunity to rehearse scenarios and to look for new and unexpected problems so that systems and practice can be improved [16].

ANAESTHESIA MORTALITY AND MORBIDITY

Safety in anaesthesia is conventionally measured by the frequency of deaths but this is likely to represent only the 'tip of the iceberg'. To address this problem incident monitoring,

AE reporting and clinical audit have been developed (prospectively or retrospectively) to provide different, but complementary, information. Retrospective medical record review provides information on the frequency of specific adverse drug events. Prospective incident monitoring is much better because it is more reliable and it records the contributing factors. With reliable information, preventive strategies can be developed with confidence [29]. It is interesting to note that minor AEs consume about 60 per cent of resources spent on medical negligence and should therefore be monitored in addition to serious AEs [30,31].

Risk is multifactorial. It can be difficult to compare the risks found in different studies because of variations in the populations studied [32]. Age is a crucial factor, e.g. differing maximum ages have been used for inclusion in paediatric studies ranging from 10 years to 18 years. For infants, there has been insufficient age differentiation, and it is important to distinguish premature babies, neonates, and 6- to 12-month-old infants; gestational age and postconceptional age (PCA) are also important.

The lack of a denominator in most mortality and morbidity studies is another problem that places considerable limitations on the conclusions of individual studies. However, over time, enough data accumulate from multiple studies to identify patterns and clusters of events. Trends can be identified so that resources can be directed to improve systems. Common themes emerge from comparison of all data collected from mortality [20,25,33] and morbidity reviews, incident reporting [34] and closed claims studies [31,35]. The medical profession must perform data collection and analysis to give confidence to the public and authorities who need reassurance that doctors are to be trusted to maintain and improve standards of medical practice.

Mortality in patients of all ages

It is promising that outcomes from anaesthesia in both adult and paediatric populations have improved dramatically over the last 50 years. Beecher and Todd produced figures from the 1950s showing that anaesthesia was the principal cause of death in 3.7 per 10 000 patients of all ages [36]. In his classic studies, at Cape Town's Groote Schuur hospital in South Africa, Harrison showed that anaesthesia-related mortality decreased sixfold over three decades from 4.3 per 10 000 in the 1950s to 0.7 per 10 000 in the 1980s [37]. The UK National Confidential Enquiry into Perioperative Deaths (NCEPOD) estimated a frequency of 1 in 185 000 deaths due to anaesthesia [38]. The mortality rate for anaesthetic deaths of all ages in Australia for the triennium 1988–90 was estimated to be 'not less than 1.8 per 100 000' (0.18 per 10 000) [33]. A Canadian report in 2001 of 24 000 anaesthetised patients revealed that mortality was 0.6 per 10 000 [17] and children (aged <20 years) accounted for 6.5 per cent of the deaths. Figures of one death per 200 000–300 000 have been published for the USA [14]. The most recent Australian national study analysed 130 deaths over the triennium during which an estimated 10.336 million anaesthetics were administered which yielded a rate of 1 death per 79 509 [25] and this is a significant reduction of approximately 26 per cent over the two previous reports. In Japan a total of 2 363 038 anaesthesia cases were analysed over 5 years [39] and the mortality (within seven postoperative days) totally attributable to anesthesia was 0.21 per 10 000 cases. The two principal causes of cardiac arrest attributable to anesthesia were drug error (15.3 per cent) and serious arrhythmia (13.9 per cent). Preventable errors caused 53.2 per cent of cardiac arrest. Only a minority (22 per cent) of deaths were totally attributable to anesthesia [39]. These statistics demonstrate a steady improvement and it is possible that eventually we may reach the point of an 'irreducible minimum' risk. However, a recent report from South Australia, analysing 290 perioperative deaths, found that the number of anaesthetic and surgical deaths had reduced by 73 and 33 per cent, respectively, compared with the previous triennium [20]. It is worth reiterating that despite these improvements there are recurring errors common to all these studies [19]. A salutatory lesson comes from Biboulet *et al.* who concluded that cardiac arrests, totally related to anaesthesia, were all avoidable [17]. In a review of all published mortality studies Lagasse found that the anaesthesia-related mortality rate, as determined by peer review, has been stable during the 1990s decade at about 1 death per 13 000 anaesthetics [40]. Certainly, anaesthetists should not be complacent.

Paediatric anaesthesia mortality

In 1964 Graff provided an estimate of the paediatric anaesthetic mortality rate of 3.3 per 10 000 [41]. At about the same time another report quoted an incidence of cardiac arrest in children in association with anaesthesia as high as 1 in 525 and an operative mortality and morbidity greatest in the first year of life [42]. At the Boston Children's Hospital the mortality rate was 1.8 per 10 000 for children aged 0–10 years for the period 1954–66 with a reduction to 0.8 per 10 000 over the next decade to 1978 [43]. In France, a multicentre survey of 40 240 children demonstrated a further improvement

with an anaesthetic mortality rate of 0.25 per 10 000 [44]. Morray and colleagues reported on 289 cases of cardiac arrest from the Pediatric Perioperative Cardiac Arrest (POCA) registry involving 63 institutions in the USA and Canada and, of these, 150 were considered to be related to anaesthesia. They stated that the incidence of cardiac arrest related to anaesthesia was 1.4 per 10 000 anaesthetics and the mortality rate was 0.05 per 10 000 [45]. In Canada, the anaesthesia mortality in 23 832 children was reported as 0.8 per 10 000 [17]. There are recent reports from single institutions where no anaesthesia-related deaths have been reported [46–48].

RISK FACTORS

Both the USA closed claims study [49] and the AIMS [27] have found that 10 per cent of all AEs occur in children; the common major factors are summarised in Fig. 45.3. These multicentre reports do not have denominator data but have now been validated by studies from single institutions [46–48]. A common finding in these studies is that mortality and morbidity are highest in infants [48,50,51]. Many incidents and AEs may be avoidable because up to 80 per cent occur in healthy children (Table 45.2) and we know that

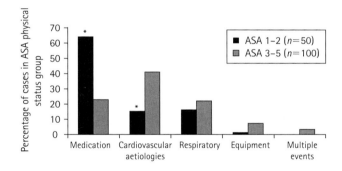

Figure 45.3 Primary cause of anaesthesia-related cardiac arrest in relation to American Society of Anesthesiologists' (ASA) status (comparison of ASA 1–2 versus 3–5; * $P < 0.05$) [45]. CV, cardiovascular.

Table 45.2 Comparison of types of incidents and adverse outcomes in paediatric studies

Source	Respiratory (%)	Cardiac (%)	Medication (%)	ASA 1–2 (%)	ASA 3–5 (%)	Anaesthesia mortality rate (%)
Morray *et al.* 1993 [49]	43	13	3	49*	10*	50
Van der Walt *et al.* 1993 [27]	43	13		80	20	NA
Morray *et al.* 2000 [45]	20	32	37	33	66	26
Tay *et al.* 2001 [46]	77	11	4	80	20	0
Murat *et al.* 2004 [47]	53†	12.5†		NA	NA	0
Marcus 2006 [18]	52	15	4	NA	NA	0

ASA, American Society of Anesthesiologists; NA, not available.
*Out of 238 patients 40 did not have an ASA score.
†Intraoperative figures.

drug errors are often responsible for cardiac arrests [45,48]. Respiratory disease frequently affects children whereas cardiovascular disease is common in adults [27,49]. The period of anaesthesia most commonly associated with AEs is the maintenance phase of anaesthesia, especially in the younger age groups [44]; AEs are more likely during emergency procedures [44,48]. Other risk factors have been identified such as anaesthetic technique and experience and training.

In respect of morbidity, postoperative vomiting is a frequent problem in the 8- to 16-year group [47,51].

The anaesthetist as risk factor

Competence of staff caring for children has been the subject of government enquiries in the UK [52] and Australia [53]. These have had major implications for all doctors, especially clinical directors, because they have introduced and reinforced clinical accountability and governance.

Questions have been raised regarding the relationship between the competency of anaesthetists and major morbidity and mortality. A number of publications have demonstrated the benefit of a trained paediatric anaesthetist in decreasing the incidence of perioperative events [45,54].

A French survey found that anaesthetists with small annual paediatric caseloads had significantly more complications [55] (per 1000 cases, there were 7–24.8 complications in the 1–100 patients per year group, 2.8–10.1 complications in the 100–200 group and 1.3–4.3 complications in the >200 patient group). Similar volume to outcome relationships have also been shown for congenital heart surgery [56,57].

However, not all children can be transferred into the care of high case-load anaesthetists and therefore guidelines are needed to place the children in institutions with appropriate resources. This will require the accreditation of institutions as well as the staff. Leaders in paediatric anaesthesia should project a vision for the ideal yet realistic delivery of paediatric anaesthesia services in both cities and rural areas. Guidelines and protocols are needed that delineate clinical skills and resources appropriate to patients. These should be agreed with service providers and subjected to continuous outcome audit and review.

It may be difficult to provide necessary skills and competencies outside specialist hospitals and even regional centres may have staff deficiencies. In these circumstances children may need to travel to a suitable hospital and therefore early recognition of illnesses becomes important. Neonatal and paediatric retrieval is now very sophisticated and even the most critically ill children can successfully be transferred.

The 1992 UK NCEPOD report had four major recommendations (Table 45.3):

- subspecialty training for surgeons and anaesthetists
- avoidance of infrequent paediatric practice

Table 45.3 National Confidential Enquiry into Perioperative Deaths (NCEPOD) recommendations

NCEPOD recommendations for paediatric anaesthesia [58]	NCEPOD recommendations for children 1999 [59]
No occasional paediatric surgeons and anaesthetists	Concentration of children's surgical services
Appropriate selection and transfer of infants	Regional perspective for acute referrals
Named consultant	Subspecialty training for surgeons and anaesthetists
Maintaining skills for 'children's' anaesthetists in major hospitals	Surgical illness severity scoring system
Specific designated paediatric operating lists	Guidelines for trainees to consult with consultants
Adequate supervision of trainees	Adequate supervision of trainees
	PICU and HDU (2000) issues
	Audit of perioperative deaths

HDU, high-dependency unit; PICU, paediatric intensive care unit.

- concentration of paediatric surgical services
- appropriate selection and transfer of sick children [58,59].

Other countries have also published guidelines for the management of elective surgery and the Australian and New Zealand College of Anaesthetists has provided some basic guidelines on appropriate facilities outside specialist hospitals [60]. In order to promote and test good practice, interdepartmental peer review has commenced in the UK [61].

American Society of Anesthesiologists' classification

The American Society of Anesthesiologists' (ASA) physical status classification system has been in wide use for over 50 years and there have been many reports that demonstrate a close relationship with severe adverse outcomes [45]. Nevertheless data show that even healthy children are at risk [27,46,49] – one-third of paediatric cardiac arrests were seen in otherwise healthy children [45].

The ASA system is imperfect because its application is variable in both adults [62] and children [63]. For example, the ASA system does not adequately describe the status of neonates and small infants – a system is needed that encompasses paediatric-specific factors [20].

Patient age

Every study of anaesthesia-related AEs, morbidity and mortality has demonstrated that risks are more serious and frequent in infants and neonates. Intraoperative respiratory

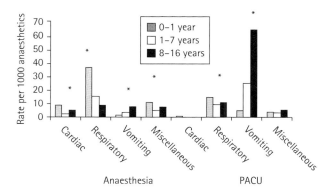

Figure 45.4 Rate and type of adverse events during anesthesia and in the postanaesthesia care unit (PACU) in the different age groups. Rate is expressed as rate per 1000 anaesthetics. Stars indicate significant differences within age groups calculated on actual numbers (χ^2, $P < 0.05$) [47].

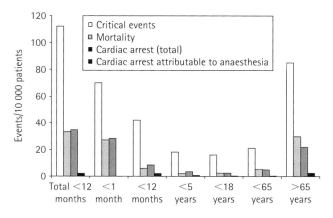

Figure 45.5 Relationship between age and complications associated with anaesthesia. The values in the first set of columns are a combination of all infants below the age of 12 months to demonstrate the high incidence of complications in infancy [50].

events are most frequent in infants and postoperative vomiting is the major problem in older children (Fig. 45.4) [47,51]. A study by Morita and colleagues shows clearly how complications in the neonatal age group far outstrip those in other age groups (Fig. 45.5) [50]. Tay *et al.* also found that critical incidents in infants (8.6 per cent) were four times more common than in older children (2.1 per cent) [46].

Prematurity

The risk of postoperative apnoea in former preterm infants less than 60 weeks' PCA was identified in the 1980s. Risks were higher if infants had required significant respiratory support and required oxygen or were anaemic at the time of their surgery. Many of these infants subsequently develop intraventricular haemorrhage, retinopathy and chronic lung disease. However, studies have been based on small numbers and a clearer picture emerged only when the results from several studies were combined [64]. This led to the

conclusion that the risk of significant postoperative apnoea was 1 per cent in ex-preterm infants 55 weeks (PCA) old. Coté has recommended that all infants aged below 60 weeks' PCA should be admitted after routine anaesthesia for observation with pulse oximetry and apnoea monitoring for not less than 12 apnoea-free hours [64].

Respiratory factors

Respiratory AEs are more common in children than in adults and the effects are even more frequent and severe in infants. Murat found that 53 per cent of AEs were from respiratory events versus 12.5 per cent were from cardiac events [47]. Braz and colleagues noted that 71.5 per cent of anaesthesia-attributable cardiac arrests were caused by respiratory events [48]. General anaesthesia is associated with impaired oxygenation due to atelectasis that occurs in the dependent parts of the lung within 5 minutes of the onset of general anaesthesia [65–67]. Infants are most susceptible because they have unstable alveolar architecture, although atelectasis can be reduced by volume-recruitment manoeuvres [68]. If there is a respiratory AE, high oxygen consumption promotes rapid hypoxaemia and bradycardia.

UPPER RESPIRATORY TRACT INFECTION

One of the most common dilemmas is how to manage children presenting with a current or a recent upper respiratory tract infection URTI, otherwise known as the common cold. Upper respiratory tract infections vary in their severity but can affect the whole respiratory tract with secretions, mucosal inflammation, oedema and congestion, leading to possible airway obstruction, airway irritability, coughing, laryngospasm, bronchospasm and atelectasis. There are also concerns about the systemic effects of pyrexia causing increased oxygen demand, ventilation and cardiac output. Viraemia may cause a myocarditis that has been implicated but not substantiated in perioperative deaths [69–71]. Because of these concerns the usual practice has been to avoid anaesthesia in these children, although this causes frequent 'last minute' cancellations with the attendant social and economic issues.

Two similar risk stratification studies in 2001 have provided results leading to a more rational evidence-based approach [72,73]. The outcome from these two studies has been an acceptance that AEs associated with URTI are both minor and manageable. Tait *et al.* have proposed that risk is related to the airway device; children with mild URTI can be managed with minimal risk without tracheal intubation and others (mainly infants) with moderate-to-severe symptoms who require tracheal intubation should ideally be postponed for at least 4–6 weeks until URTI symptoms resolve [73]. However, there will be many pertinent factors to consider for each case that may provide justification for proceeding. This has been eloquently discussed by Coté who describes this approach and comments that the use of a suitable technique usually results in an uneventful outcome [74].

A more recent finding from Mamie and colleagues suggests that the risk from URTI is less important than the age of the child and the experience of the anaesthetist [75].

Another study of risk factors in children with URTI having open heart surgery found an increased incidence of respiratory complications both intraoperatively and post-operatively. Fortunately, there were no long-term effects or increase overall length of hospital admission [76].

Laryngospasm is a frequent and feared event in paediatric anaesthesia. An AIMS report [28] comments that bradycardia was a frequent complication of laryngospasm causing hypoxaemia in 20 per cent of infants.

Cardiovascular factors

The most recent comprehensive study of cardiac events has been the POCA registry [45] and it has reported on 150 arrests from 63 institutions. The estimated frequency of arrests was 1.4 per 10 000 anaesthetics, of which 26 per cent died. Infants accounted for 55 per cent of the total and the most common causes were medication related (37 per cent) and cardiovascular (32 per cent). Two-thirds of the drug-related arrests were caused by cardiovascular depression from halothane, alone or in combination with other drugs. Children with severe disease having emergency procedures were more likely to have a fatal outcome. Although the incidence of respiratory-related cardiac arrests accounted for only 20 per cent of the total, it is well known that cardiac arrest following respiratory failure in children is associated with significant hypoxaemia and permanent neurological damage. In this series, cardiac arrests occurred during induction of anaesthesia in 37 per cent and maintenance in 45 per cent. There were warning signs of bradycardia (54 per cent), hypotension (49 per cent), abnormality of oxygen saturation (46 per cent), inability to measure blood pressure (25 per cent), abnormality of end-tidal carbon dioxide (21 per cent), cyanosis (21 per cent) and arrhythmia (16 per cent) [45]. A study in a tertiary care hospital in Brazil reported on 15 253 anaesthetics over a 9-year period [48]. There were 35 cardiac arrests (22.9:10 000) and 15 deaths (9.8:10 000). They found an incidence of anaesthesia-related cardiac arrests in children of 4.58 per 10 000 with no anaesthesia-attributable deaths. Major risk factors for cardiac arrest were neonates and children under 1 year of age with ASA 3, 4 or 5 physical status and those having emergency surgery. The main causes of anaesthesia-attributable cardiac arrest were respiratory events (71.5 per cent) and medication-related events (28.5 per cent). Based largely on the POCA registry Mason has classified anaesthesia-related cardiac arrests according to the causes: cardiac disease, airway problems, problems with intravascular volume and medication (inhalational agents, suxamethonium and intravascular local anaesthetic injection) and allergic reactions [77]. Mason reviewed the aetiology and prevention of anaesthesia-related cardiac arrest and commented on the preoperative approach to these patients.

Children who present with a previously undiagnosed heart murmur do not usually have significant pathology, but some have an anatomical defect. Any child with a murmur should be assessed by a paediatrician and, if necessary, referred to a cardiologist for their opinion (with or without echocardiography). Cardiac anomalies that may have problems during anaesthesia include cardiomyopathy, pulmonary hypertension and other causes of severe limitation to cardiac output such as valve disease. Further discussion of cardiac risk can be found in Chapter 30.

The view that cardiac pathology must be clearly elucidated is reinforced by a study from Baum and colleagues showing that a diagnosis of congenital heart disease (CHD) adds significant risk of mortality in children having routine non-cardiac surgery [78]. Mortality was 3.8 per cent without CHD and 6.0 per cent with CHD, and was twice as high in infants than in other children.

Although sudden death in children is not common it is important to know the likely causes at various ages [70] as it is relevant for proper preoperative assessment and subsequent management.

Cardiac catheterisations, especially interventional rather than diagnostic procedures, have a high risk of major AEs. Bennet and colleagues reported that AEs occurred in 9.3 per cent of catheters: the AE rate was highest in infants (13.9 per cent) compared with 6.7 per cent for older children [79].

Drug errors

Drug error is a recurring problem in both adult and paediatric anaesthesia [39,45]. Braz and colleagues have reported that 28.5 per cent of AEs were drug related [48]. A New Zealand-based study of the 'wrong drug' problem have suggested recommendations to reduce this problem that focus on human factors [80].

Sedation

Sedation has not been well managed in many institutions, often with inappropriate techniques leading to significant adverse outcomes including death. In keeping with trends in general anaesthesia in children, most AEs are avoidable and the respiratory system is most commonly involved (obstruction, hypoventilation, hypoxaemia and apnoea) [81]. Healthy children less than 6 years of age are at greatest risk and all classes of drugs are associated with complications [82]. Anaesthetists should be involved either to provide sedation or to advise on safe practice.

Intravenous fluids

Perioperative hypoglycaemia is uncommon in infants and children and glucose-containing solutions may cause intraoperative hyperglycaemia [83]. Tight control of blood glucose in neonates with necrotising enterocolitis is associated with increased survival rates (mortality rate of 29 per cent is reduced to 2 per cent in those neonates with blood glucose <11 mmol/L) [84], but in other intensive-care scenarios insulin infusions may risk hypoglycaemia.

During surgery, the current recommended practice is to use a balanced salt solution for both fluid replacement and maintenance. If hypoglycaemia is suspected, blood glucose should be measured and extra intravenous glucose provided if necessary. Children are more at risk than adults from dilutional hyponatremia which can easily be caused by fluids that contain glucose, which, when metabolised, become hypotonic; the secretion of antidiuretic hormone reduces excretion of water and exacerbates the problem [85]. Hyponatraemia has caused fatal cerebral oedema. Blood transfusion in infants also has the significant risk of hyperkalaemia and hypocalcaemia if the blood has been stored for a long time [86].

Anaphylaxis

The estimated incidence of life-threatening anaphylaxis in the anaesthesia population of all ages is 5 per 10 000 anaesthetics with a mortality rate of 3–6 per cent [87]. Allergy to latex became evident in the 1980s and became the main cause of intraoperative anaphylactic reactions in children (allergy to muscle relaxants drugs was the main cause in adults) [88]. It is therefore important to reduce latex expos-ure of neonates and small children and manufacturers are now producing latex-free equipment. However, possibly the most practical and cost-effective strategy is to ban the use of powdered latex gloves.

The recognition and management of an anaphylactic crisis in children and adults is similar and a crisis management plan should be developed and practised [87]. Anaphylactic and anaphylactoid reactions should be considered with any unexpected, dramatic and severe hypotension. Bronchospasm is present in less than 50 per cent of anaphylaxis under general anaesthesia. Skin reactions may be seen late because the patient is covered. The early use of IV adrenaline is critically important.

Other diseases

There are many situations and conditions that impose additional risks beyond the scope of this chapter. The anaesthetist must be prepared to consult an expert or other resources such as textbooks or the internet. One invaluable source of information is the textbook *Anesthesia for Genetic, Metabolic and Dysmorphic Syndromes of Childhood* and it should be available to all who anaesthetise children on a regular basis [89].

There are other more obscure risks that are currently being discussed such as the potential risk of the effects of combining immunisation with anaesthesia [90]. Guidelines have recently been suggested although the advantages of protection from infectious diseases must be considered [91].

CONFLICTING AGENDAS IN RISK MANAGEMENT

Anaesthetists aim to deliver a high standard to minimise risk and eliminate side-effects. Parents demand assurances for a safe and high-quality anaesthesia service and return of their child unharmed. Health-care administrators require a standard that will deliver anaesthesia at minimal cost with maximal patient throughput, and with minimal complaints and litigation. Obviously, these issues are conflicting and a balanced outcome of quality of care is difficult to achieve. Informed consent now imposes a professional as well as a legal obligation to be able to articulate the risks in a way that allows a parent to understand the risks. 'Cast iron' assurances are not possible but safety should improve as our knowledge of pharmacology, technology and risk management progresses. Communication reassures parents because it indicates expertise and professional insight (Table 45.4). It is also important that surgeons, paediatricians, radiologists or other professionals involved in health care (administrators, lawyers and politicians) understand that paediatric anaesthesia has specific risks. For example, a general anaesthetic for a hernia repair in a preterm infant is radically different from that in an adult. Major medicolegal problems have occurred when clinicians do not fully disclose material risks that the court may view as negligent. The UK Department of Health have provided some guidelines of what should be discussed with parents and the children (Table 45.5) [92].

Risk must also be put into perspective for professional and lay people with everyday examples to enable meaningful discussion. Smith has some good advice (Table 45.6) and explains the use of a variety of visual tools to illustrate and keep risks in perspective, such as the risk ladder [93].

Table 45.4   What do you tell parents?

'From my examination I do not expect any surprises. BUT, nothing in life is truly safe! In the same way that there are risks with most everyday activities that you as a parent accept, for example, car travel, there are risks with every anaesthetic.
From my assessment the special (additional) risks for your child are ...'

(mention those risks that have been identified during the preoperative consultation)

'Because I have identified the specific risks for your child and I understand the nature of these risks, as a specialist anaesthetist, I will take all necessary precautions to prevent and manage them and bring your child safely back to you. I never take any chances and will always act in the best interests of your child.'

One can then discuss the specific issues and risk factors and involve the parent in the decision-making and make an appropriate entry in the patient's case notes.

Table 45.5 Seeking consent: what information do children and their parents need?

Children and their parents clearly need enough information before they can decide whether to consent to, or refuse, treatment. In particular, they need information about:

- the benefits and the risks of the proposed treatment
- what the treatment will involve
- what the implications of not having the treatment are
- what alternatives may be available
- what the practical effects on their lives will be of having, or not having, the treatment

Table 45.6 How to communicate risk to patients

1. Remember that communicating any message depends critically on trust
2. Assume that all patients should be told as much as possible about risks and side-effects. This may not always be possible, or even desirable, but we should avoid deciding on the patient's behalf what they should be told
3. Be aware that words can convey feelings as well as facts. How do you want patients to feel about their anaesthetist and about themselves as they start to think about undergoing anaesthesia and surgery? Much of the preparation that patients need to make is emotional and psychological and we can help with this – and it's not just about reducing anxiety
4. When communicating risks, we need to consider not only the patient's educational background but also their attitudes to risk. Attitudes to risk depend critically on perceived benefits. We should not try to 'second guess' other people's values
5. Face-to-face risk communication allows for more personal tailoring of risks and, in fact, including individual risk estimates tends to make risk communication interventions more effective. The best way is probably to use a combination of words and numbers, supplemented by visual methods

REFERENCES

Key references

Marcus R. Human factors in pediatric anesthesia incidents. *Paediatr Anaesth* 2006; **16**: 242–50.

Morray JP, Geiduschek, JM, Ramamoorthy C *et al*. Anesthesia-related cardiac arrest in children: initial findings of the Pediatric Perioperative Cardiac Arrest (POCA) Registry. *Anesthesiology* 2000; **93**: 6–14.

National Confidential Enquiry into Perioperative Deaths. '*Extremes of Age: The 1999 report of the National Confidential Enquiry into Perioperative Deaths*. London: NCEPOD, 1999: http://www.ncepod.org.uk (accessed 9/12/06).

Reason J. Human error: models and management. *BMJ* 2000; **320**: 768–70.

Visvanathan T, Kluger MT, Webb RK, Westhorpe RN. Crisis management during anaesthesia: laryngospasm. *Qual Safety Health Care* 2005; **14**: e3.

References

1. Frei FJ. Anaesthetists and perioperative risk. *Paediatr Aanesth* 2000; **10**: 349–51.
2. Heine MF, Lake CL. Nature and prevention of errors in anesthesiology. *J Surg Oncol* 2004; **88**: 143–52.
3. Association of Anaesthetists of Great Britain and Ireland. *Risk management*. London: AAGBI, 1998.
4. Fleisher LA. Risk indices. What is their value to the clinician and patient? *Anesthesiology* 2001; **94**: 191–3.
5. Pronovost PJ, Thompson DA, Holzmueller CG *et al*. Defining and measuring patient safety. *Crit Care Clin* 2005; **21**: 1–19.
6. Thomas EJ, Studdert DM, Runciman WB *et al*. A comparison of iatrogenic injury studies in Australia and the USA. I: Context, methods, casemix, population, patient and hospital characteristics. *Int J Qual Health Care* 2000; **12**: 371–8.
7. Runciman WB, Webb RK, Helps SC *et al*. A comparison of iatrogenic injury studies in Australia and the USA. II: Reviewer behaviour and quality of care. *Int J Qual Health Care* 2000; **12**: 379–88.
8. Vincent C, Neale G, Woloshynowych M. Adverse events in British hospitals: preliminary retrospective record review. *BMJ* 2001; **322**: 517–19.
9. Davis P, Lay-Yee R, Briant R *et al*. AEs in New Zealand public hospitals: principal findings from a national survey. Wellington: Ministry of Health, 2001.
10. Baker GR, Norton PG, Flintoft V *et al*. The Canadian Adverse Events Study: the incidence of adverse events among hospital patients in Canada. *Can Med Assoc J* 2004; **170**: 1678–86.
11. Schioler T, Lipczak H, Pedersen BL *et al*. Incidence of AEs in hospitals. A retrospective study of medical records. *Ugeskr Laeger* 2001; **163**: 5370–8.
12. Wilson R McL, Runciman WB, Gibberd RW *et al*. The Quality in Australian Healthcare Study. *Med J Aust* 1995; **163**: 458–71.
13. Gaba DM. Anaesthesiology as a model for patient safety in health care. *BMJ* 2000; **320**: 785–8.
14. Kohn L, Corrigan J, Donaldson M, eds. *To err is human: building a safer health system*. Washington, DC: National Academy Press, 1999.
15. Miller MR, Zhan C. Pediatric patient safety in hospitals: a national picture in 2000. *Pediatrics* 2004; **113**: 1741–6.
16. Reason J. Human error: models and management. *BMJ* 2000; **320**: 768–70.
17. Biboulet P, Aubas P, Dubourdieu J *et al*. Fatal and non-fatal cardiac arrests related to anesthesia. *Can J Anaesth* 2001; **48**: 326–32.
18. Marcus R. Human factors in pediatric anesthesia incidents. *Paediatr Anaesth* 2006; **16**: 242–50.

19. Aitkenhead AR. Injuries associated with anaesthesia. A global perspective. *Br J Anaesth* 2005; **95**: 95–109.

20. van der Walt JH, ed. Report on perioperative deaths in South Australia and Northern Territory 1998–2000 by the South Australian Perioperative Mortality Committee under the auspices of the Department of Human Services. Adelaide: Department of Human Services, 2004.

21. Rooney JJ, Vanden Heuvel LN. Root cause analysis for beginners: 2004, http://www.asq.org/pub/qualityprogress/past/0704/qp0704rooney.pdf (accessed 19/6/06).

22. Bacon AK, Morris RW, Runciman WB, Currie M. Crisis management during anaesthesia: recovering from a crisis. *Qual Safety Health Care* 2005; **14**: e25.

23. Kerridge RK, Crittenden MB, Vutukuri VLSP. A multiple-hospital anaesthetic Problem Register: establishment of a regionally organized system for facilitated reporting of potentially recurring anaesthetic-related problems. *Anaesth Intensive Care* 2001; **29**: 106–112.

24. van der Walt JH, Sainsbury DA, Pettifer R. Anaesthesia alert: an integrated, networked, register of paediatric anaesthetic problems. *Anaesth Intensive Care* 2001; **29**: 113–16.

25. Gibbs N, ed. *Safety of anaesthesia in Australia. A review of anesthesia related mortality 2000–2002*. Melbourne: Australian and New Zealand College of Anaesthetists 2002.

26. Runciman WB, Merry AF. Crises in clinical care: an approach to management. *Qual Safety Health Care* 2005; **14**: 156–163.

27. van der Walt JH, Sweeney DB, Runciman WB *et al.* Paediatric incidents in anaesthesia: an analysis of 2000 incident reports. *Anaesth Intensive Care* 1993; **21**: 655–8.

28. Visvanathan T, Kluger MT, Webb RK, Westhorpe RN. Crisis management during anaesthesia: laryngospasm. *Qual Safety Health Care* 2005; **14**: e3.

29. Malpass A, Helps SC, Runciman WB. An analysis of Australian adverse drug events. *J Qual Clin Pract* 1999; **19**: 27–30.

30. Runciman WB, Edmonds MJ, Pradhan M. Setting priorities for patient safety. *Qual Safety Health Care* 2002; **11**: 224–9.

31. Cohen MM, Duncan PG, William DB *et al.* The Canadian four-centre study of anaesthetic outcomes: II. Can outcomes be used to assess the quality of anaesthesia care? *Can J Anaesth* 1992; **39**: 430–9.

32. van der Walt JH. Searching for the Holy Grail: measuring risk in paediatric anaesthesia. *Paediatr Anaesth* 2001; **11**: 637–41.

33. National Health and Medical Research Council. Working Party on Anaesthetic Mortality. *Report on deaths associated with anaesthesia in Australia 1988–1990.* Canberra: NHMRC, 1992.

34. Webb RK, Currie M, Morgan CA *et al.* The Australian Incident Monitoring Study: an analysis of 2000 incident reports. *Anaesth Intensive Care* 1993; **21**: 520–8.

35. Cheney FW, Posner K, Caplan RA, Ward RJ. Standard of care and anesthesia liability. *JAMA* 1989; **261**: 1599–603.

36. Beecher HK, Todd DP. A study of the deaths associated with anesthesia and surgery. *Ann Surg* 1954; **140**: 2–34.

37. Harrison GG. Death due to anaesthesia at Groote Schuur Hospital, Cape Town: 1956–1987. Part I. Incidence. *S Afr Med J* 1990; **77**: 412–15.

38. Lunn JN, Devlin HB. Lessons from the confidential enquiry into perioperative deaths in three NHS regions. *Lancet* 1987; **ii**: 1384–6.

39. Kawashima Y, Takahashi S, Suzuki M *et al.* Anesthesia-related mortality and morbidity over a 5-year period in 2,363,038 patients in Japan. *Acta Anaesthesiol Scand* 2003; **47**: 809–17.

40. Lagasse RS. Anesthesia safety: model or myth? *Anesthesiology* 2002; **97**: 1609–17.

41. Graff TD, Phillips OC, Benson DW *et al.* Baltimore Anesthesia Study Committee: factors in pediatric anesthesia mortality. *Anesth Analg* 1964; **43**: 407–14.

42. Rackow H, Salanitre E, Green LT. Frequency of cardiac arrest associated with anesthesia in infants and children. *Pediatrics* 1961; **28**: 697–704.

43. Holzman R. Morbidity and mortality in pediatric anesthesia. *Pediatr Clin North Am* 1994; **41**: 239–56.

44. Tiret L, Nivoche Y, Hatton F *et al.* Complications related to anaesthesia in infants and children. *Br J Anaesth* 1988; **61**: 263–9.

45. Morray JP, Geiduschek, JM, Ramamoorthy C *et al.* Anesthesia-related cardiac arrest in children: initial findings of the Pediatric Perioperative Cardiac Arrest (POCA) Registry. *Anesthesiology* 2000; **93**: 6–14.

46. Tay CLM, Tan GM, Ng SBA. Critical incidents in paediatric anaesthesia: an audit of 10 000 anaesthetics in Singapore. *Paediatr Anaesth* 2001; **11**: 711–18.

47. Murat I, Constant I, Huy HM. Perioperative anaesthetic morbidity in children: a database of 24 165 anaesthetics over a 30-month period. *Paediatr Anaesth* 2004; **14**: 158–66.

48. Braz LG, Braz JRC, Modolo NSP *et al.* Perioperative cardiac arrest and its mortality in children. A 9-year survey in a Brazilian tertiary teaching hospital. *Paediatr Anaesth* 2006; **16**: 860–6.

49. Morray JP, Geiduschek JM, Caplan RA *et al.* A comparison of pediatric and adult anesthesia closed malpractice claims. *Anesthesiology* 1993; **78**: 461–7.

50. Morita K, Kawashima Y, Irita K *et al.* Perioperative mortality and morbidity in the year 2000 in 520 certified training hospitals of Japanese Society of Anesthesiologists: with a special reference to age – report of Japanese Society of Anesthesiologists Committee on Operating Room Safety. *Masui* 2002; **51**: 1285–96.

51. Cohen MM, Cameron, Duncan PG. Pediatric anesthesia morbidity and mortality in the perioperative period. *Anesth Analg* 1990; **70**: 160–7.

52. Bristol Royal Infirmary. Bristol Royal Infirmary Inquiry 2001: http://www.bristol-inquiry.org.uk (accessed 9/12/06).

53. Douglas N, Robinson J, Fahy K. Inquiry into obstetric and gynaecological services at King Edward Memorial Hospital 1990–2000, 2001: http://www.health.wa.gov.au/kemhinquiry (accessed 9/12/06).

54. Keenan RL, Shapiro JH, Kane FR *et al.* Bradycardia during anesthesia in infants. *Anesthesiology* 1994; **80**: 976–82.

55. Auroy Y, Ecoffey C. Relationship between complications of pediatric anesthesia and volume of pediatric anesthetics. *Anesth Analg* 1997; **84**: 234.

56. Jenkins KJ, Newburger JW, Lock JE *et al*. In-hospital mortality for surgical repair of congenital heart defects: preliminary observations by hospital caseload. *Pediatrics* 1995; **95**: 323-30.

57. Hannan EL, Racz M, Kavey R-E *et al*. Pediatric cardiac surgery: The effect of hospital and surgeon volume on in-hospital mortality. *Pediatrics* 1998; **101**: 963-9.

58. National Confidential Enquiry into Perioperative Deaths. 'Extremes of age' the 1999 report of the National Confidential Enquiry into Perioperative Deaths. London: NCEPOD, 1999: http://www.ncepod.org.uk (accessed 9/12/06).

59. Lunn JN. Implications of the National Confidential Enquiry into Perioperative Deaths for paediatric anaesthesia. *Paediatr Anaesth* 1992; **2**: 69-72.

60. Australian and New Zealand College of Anaesthetists. *Statement on anaesthesia care of children in healthcare facilities without dedicated paediatric facilities.* ANZCA PS 29. Melbourne: ANZCA, 2002: http://www.anzca.edu.au/ publications/profdocs/profstandards/ps29_2002.htm (accessed 9/12/06).

61. Crean PM. Stokes MA, Williamson C, Hatch DJ. Quality in paediatric anaesthesia: a pilot study of interdepartmental peer review. *Anaesthesia* 2003; **58**: 543-8.

62. Haynes SR, Lawler PGP. An assessment of the consistency of ASA physical status classification allocation. *Anaesthesia* 1995; **50**: 195-9.

63. Ragheb J, Malviya S, Burke C, Reynolds P. An assessment of interrater reliability of the ASA physical status classification in pediatric surgical patients. *Paediatr Anaesth* 2006; **16**: 928-931.

64. Coté CJ, Zaslavsky A, Downes J *et al*. Postoperative apnea in former preterm infants after inguinal hernorrhaphy: a combined analysis. *Anesthesiology* 1995; **82**: 809-22.

65. Hedenstierna G. Gas exchange during anaesthesia. *Br J Anaesth* 1990; **64**: 507-14.

66. Coté CJ, Goldstein EA, Cote MA *et al*. A single blind study of pulse oximetry in children. *Anesthesiology* 1988; **68**: 184-8.

67. Hatch D, Fletcher M. Anaesthesia and the ventilatory system in infants and young children. *Br J Anaesth* 1992; **68**: 398-410.

68. Marcus RJ, van der Walt JH, Pettifer RJA. Pulmonary volume recruitment restores pulmonary compliance and resistance in anaesthetised young children. *Paediatr Anaesth* 2002; **12**: 579-84.

69. Critchley LA. Yet another report of anesthetic death due to unsuspected myocarditis. *J Clin Anesth* 1997; **9**: 676-7.

70. Liberthson RR. Sudden death from cardiac causes in children and young adults. *N Engl J Med* 1996; **334**: 1039-44.

71. Tabib A, Loire R, Miras A *et al*. Unsuspected cardiac lesions associated with sudden unexpected perioperative death. *Eur J Anaesthesiol* 2000; **17**: 230-5.

72. Parnis S, Barker D, van der Walt JH. Clinical predictors of anaesthetic complications in children with respiratory tract infections. *Paediatr Anaesth* 2001; **11**: 29-40.

73. Tait AR, Malviya S, Voepel-Lewis T *et al*. Risk factors for perioperative adverse respiratory events in children with upper respiratory tract infections. *Anesthesiology* 2001; **95**: 299-306.

74. Coté CJ. The upper respiratory tract infection (URI) dilemma. Fear of a complication or litigation? *Anesthesiology* 2001; **95**: 283-5.

75. Mamie C, Habre W, Delhumeau C *et al*. Incidence and risk factors of perioperative respiratory adverse events in children undergoing elective surgery. *Paediatr Anaesth* 2004; **14**: 218-24.

76. Malviya S, Voepel-Lewis T, Siewert M *et al*. Risk factors for adverse outcomes in children presenting for cardiac surgery with upper respiratory tract infections. *Anesthesiology* 2003; **98**: 628-32.

77. Mason LJ. An update on the etiology and prevention of anesthesia-related cardiac arrest in children. *Paediatr Anaesth* 2004; **14**: 412-16.

78. Baum VC, Barton DM, Gutgesell HP. Influence of congenital heart disease on mortality after noncardiac surgery in hospitalized children. *Pediatrics* 2000; **105**: 332-5.

79. Bennett D, Marcus R, Stokes M. Incidents and complications during pediatric cardiac catheterization. *Paediatr Anaesth* 2005; **15**: 1083-8.

80. Jensen LS, Merry AF, Webster CS *et al*. Evidence-based strategies for preventing drug administration errors during anaesthesia. *Anaesthesia* 2004; **59**: 493-504.

81. Malviya S, Voepel-Lewis T, Tait AR. Adverse events and risk factors associated with the sedation of children by nonanesthesiologists. *Anesth Analg* 1997; **85**: 1207-13.

82. Kaplan RF, Yaster M, Strafford MA, Cote CJ. Pediatric sedation for diagnostic and therapeutic procedures outside the operating room. In: Cote CJ, Todres ID, Ryan JF, Goudsouzian NG, eds. *A practice of anesthesia for infants and children.* Philadelphia: WB Saunders Co., 2001: 584-609.

83. Leelanukrom R, Cunliffe M. Intraoperative fluid and glucose management in children. *Paediatr Anaesth* 2000; **10**: 353-9.

84. Hall NJ, Peters N, Eaton S, Pierro A. Hyperglycemia is associated with increased morbidity and mortality rates in neonates with necrotizing enterocolitis. *J Pedatr Surg* 2004; **39**: 898-901.

85. Arieff AI, Ayus JC, Fraser CL. Hyponatraemia and death or permanent brain damage in healthy children. *BMJ* 1992; **304**: 1218-22.

86. Brown KA, Bisonette B, McIntyre B. Hyperkalemia during rapid blood transfusion and hypovolaemic cardiac arrest in children. *Can J Anaesth* 1990; **37**: 747-54.

87. Currie M, Kerridge RK, Bacon AK, Williamson JA. Crisis management during anaesthesia: anaphylaxis and allergy. *Qual Safety Health Care* 2005; **14**: e19.

88. Murat I. Anaphylactic reactions during paediatric anaesthesia; results of the survey of the French Society of

Paediatric Anaesthetists (ADARPEF) 1991–1992. *Paediatr Anaesth* 1993; **3**: 339–43.

89. Baum VC, O'Flaherty JE. *Anesthesia for genetic, metabolic and dysmorphic syndromes of childhood*. Philadelphia: Lippincott, Williams & Wilkins, 1999.

90. van der Walt JH, Roberton DM. Anaesthesia and recently vaccinated children. *Paediatr Anaesth* 1996; **6**: 135–41.

91. Short JA, van der Walt JH, Zoanetti DC. Immunization and anaesthesia – an international survey. *Paediatr Anaesth* 2006; **16**: 514–22.

92. Department of Health. *Seeking consent: working with children*. London: Department of Health, 2001: http://www.dh.gov.uk/assetRoot/04/06/72/ 04/04067204.pdf (accessed 9/12/2006).

93. Smith A. European Society of Anaesthesiologists. *Risk perception and communication in anaesthesia*. Brussels: European Society of Anaesthesiologists, 2003: http://www.euroanesthesia.org/education/rc2003glasgow/ 1rc1.pdf (accessed 9/12/06).

Ethics

DUNCAN MACRAE

KEY LEARNING POINTS

- Effective communication of doctors, parents and children is the key to obtaining valid consent and to taking forward challenging decisions on withdrawing or withholding treatment.
- For consent to be valid, the person making the decision must be competent, have received sufficient information on what is proposed and give consent voluntarily.
- There is no ethical difference between withholding and withdrawing life-sustaining treatment.

- When life-sustaining treatment offers no realistic possibility of benefit, doctors have a duty to consider whether starting or continuing the treatment is in the best interests of the child.
- A palliative care treatment plan must always be in place when curative treatment is withheld or withdrawn.
- Doctors must respect reasonable decisions made by parents on behalf of their children even if those decisions do not accord with the doctor's view.

INTRODUCTION

Ethical judgements are an inevitable part of everyday life for all members of civilised societies. In paediatric medical practice ethical considerations are especially prominent in the area of withholding or withdrawing life-saving treatment and in obtaining consent. The basis of ethical decision-making in these areas is discussed in this chapter, which also outlines the legal context in which such decisions are made. Readers should, however, note that, while the ethical principles outlined may transcend regional or national boundaries, the legal framework pertaining to medical decisions differs between legal jurisdictions and practitioners should familiarise themselves with laws and regulations relevant to their own legal system.

PRINCIPLES OF ETHICS IN CLINICAL PRACTICE

In recent years, healthcare professionals, particularly in acute hospital specialities, have become more aware of the ethical problems created by caring for other people. Whenever we struggle with 'value questions' we are, *de facto*, making a moral or ethical judgement, whether we explicitly acknowledge this or not. Ethics is an ambiguous term and may refer to the theoretical study of so-called 'moral philosophy'. It is usually taken to have a more practical meaning, i.e. pertaining to the whole area of value judgements as they relate to life or, in the case of medical ethics, to the practice of medicine and delivery of health care. Finally, the term 'ethics' may be applied to narrowly defined codes that set out the principles underpinning professional activity. If we accept that we frequently make value judgements, whether at a medical scientific, technical or social level, it is clear that we must understand the principles and practicalities of ethical decision-making.

There a number of theoretical traditions within ethics. These deserve brief mention, as they underpin the approaches taken by those teaching medical ethics and, even unconsciously, our day-to-day value judgements. Consequentialism views an action according to its likely consequences in the real world. 'Utilitarian' philosophers such as Jeremy Bentham were consequentionalists, asserting that we should act to seek the greatest good for the greatest number of individuals. Such philosophers emphasise that we need to determine the consequences of an action not just on individuals closely involved, but also on society as a whole, before being able judge it ethical. Deontologists take a different approach to the development of moral theory. Their philosophy holds that some actions have singular moral worth. Religious and legal codes often contain examples of duties required of the follower or subject which are based on their supposed intrinsic moral value. The imperative not to kill is one such example. The professional duties of a doctor, enshrined by Hippocrates and carried forward to this day in codes of conduct for doctors, are an example of deontological thinking. Moral codes such as the 'Ten Commandments' exist in many religions.

Despite the variations in moral theory over the ages, a number of guiding principles currently underpin our understanding of ethics in medicine: beneficence, non-malificence, autonomy and justice.

Beneficence, the first principle, demands that doctors provide care that benefits patients. This may seem to be a fairly straightforward duty to fulfil but conflicts can arise in relation to, for example, financial interests of a doctor in a particular treatment. Families may have difficult judgements to make when faced with choices of supporting a critically child who may not survive but whose survival may severely impact on the general well-being of the rest of the family – the judgement being whether to frame the decision narrowly and concentrate on benefiting the sick child or to frame it more widely and consider the whole family.

Non-malficence contrasts with beneficence. According to this principle, doctors have a duty to avoid harming patients. Decisions in the critically ill often relate to the potential of 'heroic' interventions to benefit a patient weighed against the considerable harm that they may also cause. This principle reminds us starkly that pain and suffering must be weighed carefully when considering medical interventions.

The principle of *autonomy* suggests that we must respect the right of individuals to decide for themselves, to the fullest extent possible, what is in their best interests. In paediatrics the exercise of autonomy is, at least in the case of very young children, devolved to parents or those with parental responsibility. Rules vary between legal jurisdictions as to the circumstances under which an older child who is still legally a 'minor' may be judged to have developed sufficient capacity to decide for themselves. Ensuring autonomy in practice requires doctors to establish that the patient or parent deciding for a child is able to do so without undue influence of others, including doctors, parents, siblings or peers. In summary, the principle of autonomy tells us that individuals, families or communities may have different moral perspectives, values and aims that, while discordant with our own, we should respect.

The fourth principle underpinning thinking in ethics is *justice*. In simple terms, the principle of justice requires us to use medical interventions and resources fairly so as to avoid treatment based on factors other than medical need. In the UK, the National Health Service aims to ensure that health care is available to all, 'free to all at the point of care', and goes a long way to ensure that justice prevails. However, it is all too easy to cause injustice by unknowingly designing inequality into the delivery of health care by, for example, making it more difficult for some groups or individuals to gain access to care [1].

Justice, however, is not simply delivered by ensuring that all individuals have equal access to care. In fact, as the popular media constantly remind us, society as a whole has difficulty in agreeing what is fair in the allocation of medical resources, and how the medical system should deal with this. There is clearly a limit to how much money a country and individuals within a society can spend on health care. So, if resources are limited, how should they be allocated? Should we spend huge sums on expensive intensive care which, in the case of adults, has been shown to most commonly be a very costly intervention late in life, or concentrate resources instead on interventions that prevent disease (immunisation, nutrition, abolishing deprivation). Is it more just to refuse an individual with ischaemic heart disease who might benefit from an expensive drug-eluting stent the benefit of that intervention on the basis that the money would be better spent on primary prevention? A recent paper reported that deaths from injury fell by 63 per cent in the 20-year period to 2001. Below the surface, a worrying picture emerged – that there were steep social class gradients and that the gains had failed to benefit children from poorest families. Therefore, a 'macroeconomic' argument might be made to divert resources away from acute care towards injury prevention and social care, and therefore redress the balance.

Another example of ethical dilemmas in health care is the enforcement of evidence-based care and in particular the interpretation of evidence when incorporated into policy by health-funders. An insurance organisation may adopt a policy of limiting the availability of an expensive drug or intervention. This may seem just to most people if reasonable alternatives exist, but is it then just to deny an individual patient access to the intervention which, in their particular case, doctors caring for them have judged that there may be exceptional benefit?

In the paediatric intensive care unit and the operating department we are constantly making value judgements related to the allocation of resources. Should a theatre case requiring postoperative intensive care be cancelled if no intensive care unit (ICU) nurse can be found? The case may be urgent. There is some risk of a poorer outcome if surgery is delayed, but admission to an overstretched ICU might put the child and others at risk from substandard nursing care. We all make similar ethical judgements on an almost daily basis within our medical practice.

WITHHOLDING OR WITHDRAWING LIFE–SUSTAINING TREATMENT

All involved in providing health care, together with parents, have a common purpose in acting together to restore a sick child to health. Advances in medicine, and particularly technological advances in surgery, anaesthesia and intensive care, have extended the boundaries of what is possible. However, it is sometimes clear either before treatment begins or during treatment that, while life might be temporarily sustained, to attempt to do so would confer no benefit and would be against the child's best interests.

In the UK, the Royal College of Paediatrics and Child Health have identified five situations where it may be ethical and legal to consider withholding or withdrawing life sustaining treatments [2]. Other authors have described similar approaches from different countries [3,4].

- **The brain dead child** – in the older child where absence of brain-stem function can be assessed according to standard criteria [5], it is widely agreed that recovery cannot occur and that technical survival is made possible only by continued mechanical ventilation and intensive care. It is widely accepted that in such circumstances continuing care is futile and that withdrawal of treatment is appropriate.
- **The permanent vegetative state** – a child may develop a permanent vegetative state following major global cerebral insults to the extent that they are totally reliant on others for all aspects of care and do not relate to the outside world in any way.
- **The 'no chance' situation** – describes situations where a child has such severe disease that life-sustaining treatment simply delays death without any significant improvement in quality of life or reduction of suffering.
- **The 'no purpose' situation** – describes a situation where a child may be able to survive with treatment but the resulting degree of physical or mental impairment would be so great that it would be unreasonable to expect them to bear it.
- **The 'unbearable' situation** – where the child or family feel that, in the face of progressive and irreversible illness, further treatment is more than can be borne, irrespective of the medical opinion that it may be of some benefit.

There are clear legal and ethical frameworks that underpin decisions to withdraw or withhold treatment. In the UK, the law pertaining to the care of children and decisions on their health care is formed of statutes such as the Children Act (England and Wales, 1989, Scotland, 1995) and court-defined judgements making up the 'common law'. The United Nations Convention on the Rights of the Child, the Children Act in the UK and similar legislation in other countries support the rights of children to have fair access to health care, to receive information and have their opinions valued, and to have decisions made in their 'best interests'. Although the healthcare team have a legal and ethical duty to provide care to a sick child, and must always act to cherish and support the child, there is no obligation in law to give treatment that is futile or burdensome, and to do so in some circumstances may be regarded as an assault.

Axioms on which to base practice in withdrawing or withholding life sustaining treatment, based on the ethical principles outlined, can be enumerated:

1. It is held to be both legal and ethical to withdraw or withhold treatments where the healthcare team, parents and, where appropriate, the child are in agreement that this is in the child's best interests.
2. There is held to be no significant difference between withdrawing and withholding treatments, as the ethical intention is the same. There may, however, be a perception that withdrawal of treatment is more 'difficult' than not to start treatment. It is therefore necessary that all parties clearly understand the clinical and ethical circumstances of the specific case and are able to contextualise the decision in the ethical spectrum.
3. A doctor's duty of care is not an absolute duty to preserve life by all means. There can be no sanction against doctors who reasonably decide that a particular treatment is not consistent with the current treatment plan, or where the burden to the patient outweighs the possible benefits of treatment.
4. The way in which decisions are reached is important. There should be wide-ranging open discussion within the healthcare team, the family and, where appropriate, the child [6]. Within the healthcare team, a high level of consensual agreement is required with individual opinions balanced according to expertise and depth of knowledge of the individual child and family. Individuals within the healthcare team may on occasions disagree with decisions by reason of their personal moral stance; such disagreements should be respected but should not deter the team from acting on their openly achieved consensus decisions. It is important that the professionally agreed consensus is communicated with authority by a lead consultant, as information from multiple sources, however well intentioned, can lead to a perception by parents of there being 'disagreement' over actions where none actually exists.
5. Parents may ethically and legally decide on behalf of children who are unable to decide for themselves. Parental decisions should be respected if they are reasonable, even if they do not accord absolutely with the views of the healthcare team. If parents' views are clearly aberrant, and are judged to be against the best interests of the child, additional steps are required in an attempt to reach an acceptable position. One of the most challenging aspects of decision-making is the

judgement of 'best interests'. Many children and adults with severe disabilities report that they are happy with their circumstances, which to many able-bodied observers may seem to be impossibly burdensome. Families may wish to care for and cherish their child in such circumstances and should be encouraged to do so, provided that they make that decision based on the fullest possible explanation of what the future holds. While courts have upheld the rights of children who are of sufficient maturity to consent to treatment themselves, a child's refusal of treatment may be overruled by parents (a course of action supported by court decisions in the UK and elsewhere).

6. Where disagreements arise between parents and the healthcare team, a number of options can be considered that may lead to resolution. The most important element contributing to resolution of disagreements in this situation is to maintain confidence of the parents in the healthcare team. Ongoing discussion is vital, even if views expressed are opposed. Parents may find the opinion of another doctor (second opinion), clinical psychologist, counsellors, extended family or religious advisors helpful. The healthcare team may negotiate a limit to treatment or time-limited extension of intensive therapy. If, after an extended dialogue and appropriate supportive inputs, agreement is not reached, parents may wish to explore the possibility of transferring their child to another hospital where treatment will be offered or, as a last resort, a hospital may seek assistance from the courts in deciding the matter.

7. A move away from curative care does not imply withdrawal of care. It is never permissible to withdraw drugs or interventions designed to alleviate pain or suffering. When curative care is no longer the objective, a care plan based on comfort and symptom relief must be implemented. Parents' wishes for their child's end-of-life care must be respected to the fullest extent, and may include a delay in withdrawing treatment to facilitate family or religious observances, and a request to take a child home from hospital.

8. To ensure comfort, analgesic, sedative and muscle relaxant drugs necessarily administered during therapy can be continued when treatment including ventilation is withdrawn. Sedative and analgesic drugs should be administered to ensure that children are comfortable and pain free. Occasionally administration of such drugs hastens death but their administration is justified if their primary aim is to relieve suffering. The cause of death remains the underlying disease, not the sedative or analgesic drug. Muscle relaxant drugs that have not been an ongoing part of therapy should not be introduced at the time of withdrawal of ventilation simply to facilitate an outwardly quiet death. Muscle relaxants do not have sedative or analgesic properties and there can be no 'best interest' argument for their new use at the time of ventilation withdrawal.

9. In euthanasia, the intended action is to cause death. Euthanasia is illegal in the UK but not in all countries [7–9]. Thus, in the UK any act specifically aimed at causing death is illegal.

10. Where withdrawal of supportive or curative care does not lead to death, even if death was expected, palliative care must be offered. The lives of unexpected survivors must be respected and they should be cared for appropriately.

11. Feeding and other medical treatments may be withdrawn from patients in whom the vegetative state is thought to be permanent. However, it is strongly advised that this be done only after legal advice has been taken.

CONSENT

Consent is another area of everyday medical practice with important legal and ethical considerations.

From the time of Hippocrates, the practice of medicine has been largely authoritarian. Doctors relied on the notion of beneficence or 'doing good' to justify a paternalistic view that it was often unnecessary to obtain what, in the current era, we would term 'valid consent'. It is now clear that consent, which should be sought before any healthcare intervention, is necessary for two reasons. First it provides clinicians with a defence to subsequent charges of battery under criminal law or trespass to the person under common law tort. More importantly, obtaining consent is part of the process of establishing trust between the doctor and patient by sharing of information and invokes the ethical principle of ensuring the autonomy of the individual [10,11].

Consent is a patient's agreement for a health professional to provide care. For consent to be valid, the patient must be competent to make their own decision, have received sufficient information on what is proposed and to act under their own volition. Twenty-first century health care is complex and there are often many treatment options. Seeking consent should be considered to be a process of joint decision-making between doctor (or other healthcare professional) and the patient during which information exchange occurs in both directions. Patients need to hear about therapeutic options. Doctors need to understand the patient's individual needs and priorities which in turn may be influenced by cultural, religious or occupational factors. Although the conclusion of the consenting process is usually the event of 'taking consent', consent for a complex procedure is often the culmination of a process with many inputs including those of GPs, nurses, consultant physicians, surgeons and anaesthetists, which may take place over an extended period of time. The signing of a consent form is simply a formal conclusion or acknowledgement of this process. Consent may be expressed in many ways and need not always be written. This is of particular relevance to anaesthesia and intensive care, when the generality of what will happen is explained but the minutiae of care delivery (e.g. how many cannulation attempts or how many arterial blood gas samples) are not specifically consented and are held to be implied by the general agreement to proceed.

For consent to be valid, a person giving consent must have 'capacity' to do so. This means that they must be able to understand information relevant to the decision-making process. This does not mean that the person needs to have PhD-level intellect, but simply the ability to process information relevant to the decision before them. A child may be judged to have capacity and therefore able to make their own decisions about healthcare interventions (see below). The capacity of a child or adult to understand may be temporarily affected by factors such as panic, fatigue, injury, pain or medication. Parents or those with parental responsibility consenting on behalf of their children must meet the same standards.

A structure for assessing capacity has been laid out in UK law in the Mental Capacity Act 2005. This states that an adult is able to make a decision for themselves if they can understand the information relevant to the decision, can retain the information to use or weigh as part of the process of making the decision and are able to communicate their decision by verbal or non-verbal means. These principles provide a helpful structure to practitioners faced with assessing a patient's (or parent's) capacity to consent to healthcare treatment.

Consent must be given voluntarily and not under any form of duress or undue influence of other health professionals, family or friends. These considerations also apply in the case of parents asked to consent to a healthcare intervention in their child. For example, a young parent may be unduly influenced by the opinions of a (grand)parent and it is important that their own wishes are ascertained. Particular care must be taken if a child is consenting for themselves to ensure that their decision is made voluntarily and not under the influence of others, including family members or peers.

Parents or children deciding for themselves can make a valid judgement to consent to a treatment or procedure only if they are provided with sufficient information. The main domains that must be covered when providing information are listed in Table 46.1.

The standard of practice required of a medical practitioner by law in the UK in relation to the area of consent, as in other areas of professional practice, is the standard first elucidated in the cases of *Hunter v Hanley* 1955 in Scotland and *Bolam v Friern Hospital Management Committee* 1957 in England [12]. According to these judgements, a doctor is not guilty of negligence if he or she acted in accordance with a practice accepted as proper by a responsible body of medical men and women skilled in that particular art. In simpler terms, doctors are judged against standards of their peers. Applying this test to consent obtained from a patient, a doctor would have to warn of all risks that 'a responsible body of medical opinion' would consider a patient should

Table 46.1 Information that patients may want or ought to know before consenting to treatment or investigation

- Details of the diagnosis and likely prognosis if left untreated
- Uncertainties about the diagnosis and how treatment will be handled if more information becomes available
- The purpose, nature and extent of the proposed treatment
- Likely benefits of treatment
- Possible risks or disadvantages of treatment
- The nature of any follow-up treatment (intensive care, analgesia, prolonged drug therapy, likely supplementary procedures)
- Right to withdraw from treatment at any time
- Right to a second opinion
- A patient should always know the name of the consultant in charge of their care

be warned of, rather than every conceivable risk. The landmark case *Sidaway v Bethlem Royal Hospital Governors and Others* 1985 [13] illustrates this point. A patient underwent surgery to decompress a cervical nerve root and developed serious lasting spinal cord damage. She sued the hospital and surgeon. At trial medical witnesses stated that it was common practice of neurosurgeons at the time not to warn patients of the less than 1 per cent risk of paralysis or death in order not to frighten the patient. The trial judge dismissed the case. Lord Browne-Wilkinson has added to this area of law, by stating that the court would 'not stand idly by if the profession, by an excess of paternalism, denies their patient a real choice', and stressed that the practice held by the body of responsible practitioners had to be one that is 'rightly and properly held'.

Information must be provided to patients in a language in which they are fluent. It is good practice to use medical interpreters who are independent of the patient's family so that the consenting doctor knows that information is accurately conveyed. Interpreters should be asked to co-sign the consent form.

The clinician providing the treatment or investigation is responsible for ensuring that the patient has given valid consent before treatment begins. The UK General Medical Council guidance states that the task of seeking consent may be delegated to another health professional. This professional must be suitably trained and qualified and have sufficient knowledge of what is proposed to satisfy the patient's need for information (Table 46.1) and to undertake any discussion of that information.

When an anaesthetist is involved in a patient's care, it is their responsibility to ensure that relevant information about the conduct of anaesthesia has been given and valid consent for anaesthesia obtained. For elective surgery, it is good practice to provide information about anaesthesia at the same time that surgery is first discussed, perhaps in the form of a leaflet or at a preoperative assessment clinic. The anaesthetist who will administer the anaesthetic should ensure that discussion with the patient and their consent is documented. Guidance on consent for anaesthesia has been published by the Association of Anaesthetists of Great Britain and Ireland [14].

Valid consent may be given orally, verbally or non-verbally. A signed consent form is a record of the consenting process but it does not in itself make consent valid if the process by which the signature was obtained did not meet the required standards in relation to voluntariness, information and capacity.

There is no temporal limit to the validity of consent provided that the circumstances prevailing at the time consent was agreed still prevail. Thus, a consent agreed at an outpatient appointment months before elective surgery may be valid on admission to hospital for the proposed elective procedure provided that the patient has not withdrawn their consent, and that the patient's circumstances are unchanged.

Patients with capacity may withdraw consent to healthcare interventions at any time. It is good practice to encourage the patient to discuss their reasons for withdrawing consent since this may be the result of a misunderstanding or anxiety that can easily be allayed. Legally, a child lacking capacity whose parents or guardian have consented to a healthcare intervention cannot withdraw that consent but, if a child shows substantial resistance to what is proposed, most practitioners will, acting in the child's best interests, choose to delay all but an emergency procedure.

The legal framework relating to consent [15] of or on behalf of children varies between legal jurisdictions. However, it can be stated that, in general, people with parental responsibility are entitled to give consent on behalf of their child. A child's mother will invariably have parental responsibility unless removed by a court, as will a father married to a child's mother at the time of conception or birth. An unmarried father may have or acquire parental responsibility but laws between jurisdictions differ widely. Others (e.g. local authority, other relatives) may also have acquired parental responsibility through the courts or by parental nomination.

Under common law, any young person in the UK can consent to medical, surgical or nursing treatment without involvement of their parents if they are considered sufficiently mature to understand the issues at stake. Similar laws apply in other countries and legal jurisdictions. This concept of minors having capacity to consent, often termed 'Gillick competence' in the UK (*Gillick v West Norfolk and Wisbech AHA* 1986 [16]) is perhaps best summarised by the guideline enumerated by Lord Fraser in his 'Gillick' judgement (Table 46.2).

In cases where parents disagree about proposed treatment and it is a clinical priority to proceed, clinicians are authorised to proceed provided that they have consent from one of the child's parents. Courts may intervene to limit the power of one parent to consent to (or refuse) treatment if it is shown that they are acting against the best interests of the child.

Table 46.2   Fraser guidelines

1. The young person understands the advice that is being given
2. The young person cannot be persuaded to inform or seek support from their parents, and will not allow the healthcare worker to inform the parents of advice being given
3. The young person's physical or mental health is likely to suffer unless they receive advice or treatment
4. It is in the young person's best interest to receive advice or treatment without parental consent

In cases where the person with parental responsibility is judged incompetent (e.g. as a result of a road traffic collision in which the child was also injured) the clinician should seek legal advice, although in an emergency the clinician should act in the best interests of the child.

When babies or young children are being cared for in hospital, it is not usually practicable to seek their parents' consent on every occasion an intervention is required (e.g. blood gases, urine tests, cannula insertion), especially in the ICU. It is therefore important that parents are made aware of routine procedures that will be necessary and ensure that they consent in advance to these forms of care. Parents will, however, quite reasonably wish to be reassured that they will be consulted and their permission sought before any non-routine intervention. If a parent cannot be contacted and there is an urgent clinical need to proceed, doctors should act in the child's best interests while recording clearly in the clinical record why treatment was required urgently and what attempts were made to contact the child's parents to seek prior consent.

If parents refuse to consent doctors must decide if it is in the child's best interests to proceed. If so, where time permits, legal advice should be sought and, if the matter is not resolved, redress to the courts may be required. In an emergency situation, after consulting widely with appropriate colleagues to ensure consensus on the way forward, treatment should proceed but be limited to that which is reasonably necessary. Good documentation of all discussions with colleagues and parents is necessary in such situations.

Some situations of this type – such as in the care of children of Jehovah's Witness parents – can be predicted and avoided. This is discussed further in Chapters 17 and 36.

Treatment of many conditions is imperfect and parents may be asked to allow their child to participate in clinical trials of new treatments or investigations, which lead ultimately to the development of new treatments. Ethically, such research activities on human subjects must be conducted after prior approval of the proposed research by a research ethics committee. A competent patient, including a competent child, may consent on their own behalf to take part in clinical research but should do so only after the potential risks, benefits and alternatives have been fully delineated. In practice, however, it is advisable always to ensure that parents support a child's wish to participate in clinical research. Where children lack capacity to consent, parents may give consent for their child to take part in therapeutic research that is at least as likely to benefit their child as standard therapy and to non-therapeutic research provided that it is minimally invasive. If a child shows unwillingness to participate in a research procedure their wish should be respected. Research should be conducted in children only if the research question can be answered by the involvement of these groups rather than the ethically preferable option of competent adults. Similar considerations apply to adults lacking competence. The Royal College of Paediatrics and Child Health publish guidance relating to the conduct of research involving children [17]. In the UK a recent piece of legislation, the Mental Capacity Act 2005, sets out clear parameters for the conduct of research involving or in relation to persons lacking capacity. It states that such research may be lawfully carried out if an 'appropriate body' (normally a research ethics committee) agrees that the research is safe, relates to the person's condition and cannot be done as effectively using people who have full mental capacity. The situation where research is required into a new approach to cardiopulmonary resuscitation may well fall within the remit of this part of the Act.

REFERENCES

Key references

Association of Anaesthetists of Great Britain and Ireland. *Information and consent for anaesthesia*. London: AAGBI, 1999.

Department of Health. *Reference guide to consent for examination and treatment*. London: Department of Health, 2005.

Edgar J, Morton NS, Pace NA. Review of ethics in paediatric anaesthesia. *Paediatr Anaesth* 2001; **11**: 355–9.

General Medical Council. *Seeking patient's consent: ethical considerations*. London: GMC, 1998.

Royal College of Paediatrics and Child Health Guidelines for the ethical conduct of medical research involving children. *Arch Dis Child* 2000; **82**: 177–82.

References

1. Sinuff T, Kahnamoui K, Cook DJ *et al.* Rationing critical care beds: a systematic review. *Crit Care Med* 2004; **32**(7): 1588–97.

2. Royal College of Paediatrics and Child Health. *Withholding and withdrawing life sustaining treatment*, 2nd edn. London: Royal College of Paediatrics and Child Health, 2004.

3. Burns JP, Rushton CH. End-of-life care in the pediatric intensive care unit: research review and recommendations. *Crit Care Clin* 2004; **20**(3): 467–85.

4. Hubert P, Canoui P, Cremer R, Leclerc F; GFRUP. Withholding or withdrawing life saving treatment in pediatric intensive care unit: GFRUP guidelines. *Arch Pédiatr* 2005; **12**(10): 1501–8.

5. Task Force for the Determination of Brain Death In Children. Guidelines for the determination of brain death in children. *Ann Neurol* 1987; **80**: 298–9.

6. Vince T, Petros A. Should children's autonomy be respected by telling them of their imminent death? *J Med Ethics* 2006; **32**(1): 21–3.

7. Hendin H, Foley K, White M. Physician-assisted suicide: reflections on Oregon's first case. *Iss Law Med* 1998; **14**(3): 243–70.

8. Jochemsen H. Dutch court decisions on non-voluntary euthanasia critically reviewed. *Iss Law Med* 1998; **13**(4): 447–58.

9. Quirk P. Euthanasia in the Commonwealth of Australia. *Iss Law Med* 1998; **13**(4): 425–6.

10. General Medical Council. *Seeking patient's consent: ethical considerations*. London: GMC, 1998.

11. Department of Health. *Reference guide to consent for examination and treatment*. London: Department of Health, 2005.

12. Bolam v Friern Hospital Management Committee 2 ALL ER 18 [1957].

13. Sidaway v Bethlem Royal Hospital Governors and others [1985] 1 All ER 6.

14. Association of Anaesthetists of Great Britain and Ireland. *Information and consent for anaesthesia*. London: AAGBI, 1999.

15. Edgar J, Morton NS, Pace NA. Review of ethics in paediatric anaesthesia. *Paediatr Anaesth* 2001; **11**: 355–9.

16. Gillick v West Norfolk and Wisbech AHA [1986] AC 112.

17. Royal College of Paediatrics and Child Health. Guidelines for the ethical conduct of medical research involving children. *Arch Dis Child* 2000; **82**: 177–82.

47

Research

ANDREW R WOLF

KEY LEARNING POINTS

- Success in medical research requires commitment over several years.
- Medical treatments should rely on research to provide an 'evidence base' in order to optimise individual treatment.
- Before undertaking a project, it is wise to read relevant reviews and to search reference databases thoroughly.
- To be successful in winning a grant, the research question should be strong enough to compete with other projects, as

well as to advance the knowledge in the specialty – collaboration of clinical and basic sciences is important.
- Early statistical advice is essential in designing the trial.
- Any drug trial involving safety or efficacy must conform to the standards of the International Conference on Harmonisation Good Practice Guideline (ICH GCP).

INTRODUCTION

Medical research covers a very wide span of activities from genomic and proteonomic science through integrated cellular and animal studies to single-centre, multicentre and epidemiological trials. In addition, with the rise of evidence-based medicine, and as a platform from which established views of medical practice are challenged, our routine management and use of drugs (often applied from adult to paediatric practice without testing) has come under scrutiny. The sheer bulk of medical literature that bombards the practitioner is enormous but cannot be ignored. Understanding the relevance, quality and importance of published research is essential to both the trainee and the established practitioner who is required to maintain lifelong learning and development of their chosen discipline. The paediatric anaesthetist must therefore have a reasonable knowledge of research methods and have learned data interpretation skills that allow critical assessment of published or presented work.

These will form the basis from which they will modify their techniques and incorporate new drugs into their practice.

Medical research is undergoing significant change at present as a result of pressures from financial, ethical and societal expectations. Funding has gravitated to areas that are likely to make the greatest impact on health economics such as diabetes, obesity and cardiovascular disease. Furthermore, universities and funding bodies tend to focus on research that will result in high-impact journal publications and favourable publicity. Success at this level in medical research requires full-time commitment and dedication over several years and is not always compatible with *craft* specialties, such as paediatric anaesthesia, that require lengthy training. Nevertheless, the application of developments in basic science and pharmaceutical research require individuals within the specialised disciplines who can interpret and apply these advances outside the laboratory and into everyday practice. The process of clinical trials has also been under review in recent years. Regulations governing research such as ethical review, the use of medicines outside product licence, the costs of research borne by the medical facility and issues of responsibility and indemnity for adverse events have made even the most simple piece of clinical research into a challenging undertaking. These constraints are particularly cumbersome in paediatric practice where establishing a research sponsor (the body that will accept legal responsibility and liability for the study) and securing additional indemnity insurance may have additional funding implications.

Despite these difficulties it is imperative that clinical research in paediatric anaesthesia is nurtured to allow rigorous evaluation of new techniques and sustained development of the specialty. In addition, as a profession we need to have the knowledge and abilities to work with science groups, and to support translational research that lifts basic science developments into practical benefits. The philosophy and methods of research are complex and of considerable relevance to contemporary healthcare science [1], but they are outside the scope of this chapter, which concentrates on the practical aspects of trial design and data interpretation that are relevant to 'everyday' paediatric anaesthetic research. Specific issues of paediatric research will be discussed and include consent, ethics and some guidelines on how to set up a clinical trial.

WHAT IS RESEARCH?

Research is a systematic and rigorous method of enquiry by which a process can be described, leading to explanation in terms of concepts, theories and advancement of knowledge. Medical treatments should rely on research to provide an 'evidence base' in order to optimise individual treatment. In the past, and still to a lesser extent today, our management was influenced by empiricism, anecdote and tradition. An early example of the linkage of enquiry, evidence and medical practice, was the work of James Lind, a Royal Navy surgeon, who, in 1747, undertook a clinical trial, based on 6 treatment groups of 12 sailors with scurvy. He was able to show that sailors given citrus fruit as part of their diet recovered from their disease, while the others did not. This then led to the provision of limes on British ships and the prevention of scurvy at sea.

In general terms research methods can be *deductive* or *inductive*. The deductive approach begins with a general idea that leads to a hypothesis or theory that can then be tested by gathering data (a 'top-down' approach). In contrast, in inductive methods, the investigator starts with observations from which the ideas are generated (a 'bottom-up' approach). These in turn can be tested from further observations. An example of this can be found in the cholera outbreak in London in the 1850s when the anaesthetist Dr John Snow made the observation that families taking their water from the Broad Street pump appeared to get the disease while those using another water supply did

not. Removal of the pump head prevented residents from drawing the water and brought an end to the epidemic. Snow's observation, hypothesis and subsequent intervention produced a relatively clear-cut result, but in medical science absolute associations cannot be made. This has led to the evolution of statistics applied to biomedical research to underpin data and to attach relative weight to subsequent results. John Snow effectively applied *probabilistic inductive logic* on which to base his conclusions before the mathematics of biomedical statistics had been conceived. Nowadays, using the same data from 1854, the relative risk of contracting cholera from the Broad Street pump can be calculated as 14, indicating a strong association or high probability that the water supply was the underlying cause [2].

TYPES OF RESEARCH

Research has moved from case study and case series approaches to more sophisticated trial designs using appropriate sample sizes and statistical analyses in order to make conclusions more robust. Clinical studies can be complicated by endpoints that are difficult to measure in study populations with large individual variation (e.g. pain measurement in children). The difficulty of trying to separate a chance finding from a robust and clinically important result has given rise to calls for a more standardised approach with rigorous trial design, avoidance of bias and involvement, from start to finish, of a medical statistician. The gold standard for research investigation is the prospective randomised clinical trial, overseen by an independent clinical trials unit. Ascribing the value and weighting of a finding from one or more clinical trials has been formalised by the Oxford Centre for Evidence Based Medicine to allow a reader to interpret the 'level of evidence' (Table 47.1). Systematic reviews of the literature use this system to base conclusions that make recommendations varying from A (strongest – consistent findings from level 1 studies) to D (weakest – inconsistent or no conclusions at any level).

Prospective versus retrospective studies

Most studies in paediatric anaesthesia are longitudinal (i.e. they investigate a process over a period of time). This can be prospective, in which the patients are followed forward in time after an intervention to look at outcome, or retrospective, which examines outcomes backwards from exposure. Prospective trials in general allow a more definitive answer to a research question because there is less bias and confounding. They need sufficient numbers of patients in order to make robust conclusions. The study population should be defined and the outcomes compared with those from a control group. Observer bias can be reduced by randomisation and blinding. Results should be reproducible by other workers following the same methods.

Table 47.1 Simplified grading of recommendations and importance of medical research evidence*

Grade of recommendation	Level of evidence	Description of study design
A	1a	Systematic review (with homogeneity) of randomised clinical trials
	1b	Individual randomised clinical trials (with narrow confidence interval)
	1c	A trial where all patients died before the drug became available, but now some survive with the drug, or before the drug was available some patients died, but none now die on it
B	2a	Systematic review (with homogeneity) of cohort studies
	2b	Individual cohort study (including low-quality randomised clinical trial)
	2c	'Outcomes' research
	3a	Systematic review (with homogeneity) of case–control studies
	3b	Individual case–control
C	4	Case series (and poor quality cohort and case–control studies)
D	5	Expert opinion without explicit critical appraisal, or based on physiology or bench research
Z	6	Abstracts

*From the Centre for Evidence Based Medicine, Oxford (http://www.cebm.net/levels_of_evidence.asp).

Observational studies

When it is not possible to have a control group, or to randomise patients, it may be necessary to undertake this type of study. An example would be the effects of cardiopulmonary bypass on different organ systems; it can be seen as an exploratory analysis that may lead to the formation of a hypothesis.

Cohort studies

These are longitudinal studies in which patients in a group (or cohort) have been subject to a particular event and are followed to determine outcome. A typical example would be the identification of impaired neurological development in young infants exposed to general anaesthesia (animal data suggest that exposure to general anaesthetic agents results in cerebral apoptosis, but there are no human data).

Sequential studies

Data are often accumulated over time with some patients having completed the study before others start. If the results of the study have major implications, such as survival from a new technique or drug, then it may be unethical to continue after a clear difference has emerged from an interim analysis.

Multicentre studies

In a single paediatric centre, it may be impossible to recruit sufficient numbers of patients to achieve adequate statistical power (see below) within a reasonable period. Involving more than one centre is often needed to get adequate recruitment rates for relatively rare conditions, e.g. evaluating a new treatment in sepsis [3].

Meta-analyses

This technique pools data from several randomised trials. It effectively increases the sample size in order to quantify a clinical effect with greater confidence and is particularly valuable when single studies have conflicting conclusions. A useful example has been the comparison of regional analgesia with general anaesthetic techniques on postoperative outcome [4].

OTHER METHODS OF ENQUIRY

While research is the cornerstone of evidence-based medicine, there are other approaches based on data collection or opinion that can result in improved care at both a global and a local level. These include audit and the formation of consensus guidelines. Audit is not strictly research in the sense of acquiring scientific knowledge and it is not as rigorous in terms of qualitative/quantitative method. However, it can be effective in achieving quality, improving outcome, increasing efficiency and enhancing a culture of education and reflection. The audit cycle has several phases: observation of current practice, identifying issues that can be improved, setting standards of care, implementing change and comparing new and old practices. It is complementary to research in that audit concentrates on the mechanistic and practical features of clinical care while research addresses principles and core knowledge.

Evidence and consensus guidelines can be developed to establish what is considered best practice and to try to achieve recommendations. The process requires an initial systematic review of objective literature with predefined goals for a specific clinical question. This then leads to key recommendations that are then refined by consensus. The Delphi Process [5] is achieved through a panel of experts (and consumers if appropriate) who are presented with statements that are graded in terms of strength of agreement/disagreement. The responses are sequentially modified by several rounds of discussion, feedback and modification leading to a final consensus from the expert panel that can then advocate guidelines and recommendations. In the UK several organisations and institutions have been formed to try to improve consistency and evidence basis for clinical practice. The Scottish Intercollegiate Guideline Network (SIGN) [6] has over 100 published guidelines and many of them relate to paediatric practice. The Royal College of Paediatricrics and Child Health (RCPCH) has reviewed evidence-based practice for many key issues (http://www.rcpch.ac.uk).

ETHICS AND CONSENT

The issues surrounding the ethics of research in children and obtaining consent have become increasingly complex in recent years. Societal views on rights of the individual, particularly those of a child, have shifted towards an increased emphasis on informed choice and protection of the individual. At the same time, there is strong pressure to discover, develop and deploy new techniques and drugs with comprehensive safety and efficacy data. There is clearly a dilemma, in that drugs and techniques need to be evaluated in children to obtain data before safety and efficacy profiles can be properly established. Several recent reviews are available that consider ethics of paediatric research and consent of the child in detail [7,8].

The ethical dilemmas of undertaking research in children bring into focus issues such as therapeutic versus non-therapeutic research, risks versus benefit of a trial, and clinical equipoise. A 'therapeutic trial' usually involves evaluation of a technique or drug that may convey benefit to that individual patient within the trial, e.g. the evaluation of a new drug for postoperative pain relief. A randomised controlled trial (RCT) is appropriate to determine the efficacy and safety of that drug. In contrast, 'non-therapeutic research' conveys no direct potential benefit to the subject although the results of the study may change practice and improve clinical care for others in the future (e.g. a pharmacokinetic study that improves prescribing or dosing regimens). The division between 'therapeutic' and 'non-therapeutic' research is secondary to the overriding issue of risk versus benefit. Clearly, high-risk low-benefit research is not ethical, and a study that has no benefit or worth should not be undertaken even if there are no associated risks. However, evaluation and agreement of what constitutes an acceptable risk within the context of potential benefits either to an individual or to others are hard to define. These issues are best discussed by independent ethical committees, although in the past there has been wide variation in opinion from local paediatric research ethics committees about what constitutes an acceptable risk–benefit ratio. Recently, in the UK, committees have become more centralised in an attempt to set consistent standards of practice although many of the issues still remain unresolved (see http://www.corec. org.uk, the Central Office for Research Ethics Committees [COREC], National Patient Safety Agency, UK).

A comparative trial must attempt to answer a clinical dilemma in terms of the relative benefits for the different treatments [9]. Therefore, the concept of clinical equipoise requires that before a trial can be approved there must be genuine uncertainty within the expert medical community about which treatment is better. An excellent example was the lack of data available to determine if extracorporeal membrane oxygenation (ECMO) was better than conventional ventilatory strategies for the treatment of life-threatening neonatal respiratory illness [10]. It was rapidly adopted in the USA without such a trial and because it was expensive it provoked questions of efficacy. A UK multicentre trial was designed that acknowledged clinical equipoise but recognised that it would be unethical to continue the trial if it could be demonstrated that one treatment was significantly better. Data were therefore monitored objectively by a clinical trials group and the trial was terminated once a clear benefit in terms of long-term quality survival of infants in the ECMO group had been demonstrated.

Human research is expected to be carried out using the principles set out in the Declaration of Helsinki of 1964 and updated in the International Code of Ethical Guidelines and Practices for Research Involving Human Subjects [11]. Some of the key principles that underpin human research are presented in Table 47.2.

Before data collection begins a study will be reviewed by several committees that consider different aspects of safety. National committees include the Food and Drug Administration (FDA) in the USA or the Medicines and Healthcare products Regulatory Agency (MHRA) in the UK. Local committees include the research ethics and hospital development committees. Funding bodies assess the project by peer review and will also provide a check to maximise safety.

Ethical issues need to be considered by local, regional or national ethical committees before a trial is sanctioned. The committee will include lay people as well as medical practitioners or scientists who will independently judge the merits of the study using the principles in Table 47.2. Paediatric research should be carried out only when the research question cannot be effectively answered in adults and the committee will want to know why the research is necessary; in anaesthesia projects common reasons include age-related pharmacological and physiological variation or the need to test different and specialised equipment.

Table 47.2 Seven of the key principles from the International Code of Ethical Guidelines and Practices for Research Involving Human Subjects (11)

1. The science underlying the research must be valid and the trial is limited to expose the minimum number of patients calculated with statistical input to answer the research question effectively
2. The risk–benefit ratio must be acceptable both for the overall research question and for the individual taking part
3. There should be no conflict of interest between the researchers and patient
4. There must be gain or potential future gains to patients
5. Taking part should be completely voluntary
6. Patients should be able to withdraw from the study at any time without the need for discussion and withdrawal from the trial will not affect future care
7. The recruitment process must be fully open, and all aspects have been discussed fully before taking formal written consent

In addition they will also consider the practical aspects of making sure that the study will be successful:

- Does the statistical input optimise the goals and effectiveness and minimise the number of subjects needed to answer the research question?
- How and when will consent be obtained?
- What are the risks or hazards? These will need to have been fully considered before the study starts. Independent procedures must monitor for adverse reactions and intervene if necessary (data monitoring committee).
- How will the data be managed? A comprehensive plan is needed before starting the study to ensure confidentiality, accuracy and objectivity.
- Who is responsible or liable?
- What will be the duration of study? The feasibility of recruitment within the study period must be stated.

Once approved the study must be carried out strictly according to the research proposal in terms of recruitment, time-frame and procedures. Increasingly, research trials are overseen by an independent clinical trials unit that collates the data, monitors recruitment and screens the data for adverse events. This ensures independent and unbiased data collection and avoids potential ethical conflicts. Any serious adverse events need to be reported immediately to the ethical committee and if necessary the study needs to be interrupted while necessary investigations take place. The rigorous nature of ethical review, driven in part by the necessity to protect children, has made the process of obtaining ethical approval time-consuming and sometimes complex. Small studies that used to be undertaken by clinical staff (managed within clinical services) may no longer

be practical because of the paperwork and regulation of data processing. Most research needs to be managed by staff with sufficient time dedicated to the project and, consequently, this brings a financial burden. In respect of the pharmaceutical companies, there have been concerns that they may choose not to test or develop new drugs in paediatrics because the costs of research are unlikely to be offset by profits. Some companies may choose not to undertake paediatric testing at all or test their new drugs in counties with more lenient policies on paediatric research. This has led to initiatives in both the USA and the UK to support pharmaceutical research. In the USA, the Orphan Drug Act (Federal law passed in 1983) encourages the testing and development of drugs for the treatment of rare diseases – drug companies are given tax concessions and allowed 7 years' monopoly. A similar approach exists in the European Union administered by the Committee on Orphan Medicinal Products within the European Medicines Agency.

Consent

Consent for paediatric research can be difficult. For competent adult patients undergoing an elective procedure the researcher can approach the potential trial subject, to give them all the information with which they can make a fully informed choice. Usually, this involves an initial interview and presenting a written information sheet, followed by formal written consent after a period of reflection. Subjecting children to research who are unable to understand its implications completely means that another individual (a parent or guardian) is required to make decisions on their behalf. Ideally, there should be no risk or additional discomfort associated with the research, but there are exceptions to this rule. *High gain* research may be deemed so important (*high impact*) that significant risk or discomfort may be justified. An example is the first insertion of an implantable intracardiac device in a child which has potentially a large gain to the patient but the risk is unknown and potentially high.

Often children cannot be expected to understand fully the nature of consent or the implications of a research study. The researcher is therefore required to provide, to the parent or guardian, detailed information of what is proposed, why it is being done and how it will be done, together with an explanation of risk, benefit and legal rights. Older children will need appropriate explanations depending on their maturity and understanding. Clearly, infants and toddlers cannot take part in the consent process and there are special considerations and implications for studies that involve resuscitation techniques, studies of the critically ill and studies of child abuse when informed consent cannot be obtained. Although children as young as 7 years of age have been included in the process of consent, it has been questioned whether children less than 10 years old are reliably able to provide assent (agreement to the proposal) for a research procedure let alone consent (accept to undertake a proposal from another person with full understanding) [12]. Children tend to acquiesce to the wishes of an adult without regard to the implications. Increasingly ethics committees will ask for an age-appropriate information sheet in addition to the full parental information sheet and consent forms. The rules pertaining to ethics and consent are constantly changing and are not yet fully consistent either nationally or internationally. It is essential to be fully aware of local legislation and guidelines during the planning of research.

UNDERTAKING A CLINICAL STUDY

Even the simplest of clinical studies requires considerable planning to ensure that the research question is answered effectively and to avoid errors that may devalue the study or make the answer invalid. The key steps are outlined below.

Evaluation of published research

In the quest for lifelong learning and development it is essential to continue to read and evaluate published research. This requires critical appraisal to determine the quality, validity of conclusions and importance of the study findings. A research question may develop from many sources. It may come from individual observation, from reading previously published work or from discussion with a colleague within or outside clinical medicine. Irrespective of the source of the hypothesis it is essential to have a wide and detailed understanding of the subject before embarking on the project.

It is wise to read the reviews of topical or important subjects that are readily available (see Cochrane, Bandolier, SIGN or RCPCH websites) in which usually the authors have achieved relatively robust conclusions made by considering all the relevant evidence. However, there is a large body of published evidence that the reader must assess themselves in order to judge whether it is important enough for them either to change their practice or to consider undertaking a trial.

Much published literature has little clinical impact: the work may be a repetition or a minor variation of previous work. This does not break new ground but it is still valuable because it confirms that results are not due to chance and that conclusions are more certain. Some research may not prove anything and therefore may seem inconsequential but the data can be used to qualify future research findings and make progress to prove or disprove hypotheses. Finally, occasionally, there will be novel research that stimulates considerable debate and may alter future practice. A recent example of this is observation that the developing rat brain is damaged by anaesthesia and this has provoked calls for prospective human trials to determine its clinical relevance [13].

The quality of a manuscript should be judged in terms of its hypothesis, study design, statistics, data handling, results and conclusions. The hypothesis question should be based on the gap between the known and unknown facts and then the study should be designed to answer it. Publications in peer-reviewed journals are cited in the major bibliographic electronic databases such as MEDLINE, EMBASE and PubMed and will have been read and appraised by at least two other specialists. Peer review is important to screen out unsuitable articles.

There is pressure for authors to publish in high prestige journals such as *Nature*, the *New England Journal of Medicine* or *The Lancet* because this is regarded as academic achievement and it leads to promotion and successful grant applications. In these 'high-impact factor' journals, only the most highly scrutinised and most significant articles are published and the reader can then be reassured about their quality. Despite this process there are still instances (fortunately rare) of fabrication of data or fraud and these not only destroy the reputation of the authors but also damage the wider public image of medical research.

In reading a manuscript each section should be checked:

- Introduction: what is the hypothesis or question and is it relevant or important?
- Methods: can the trial design answer the question and what is the primary outcome measure? Are the method and measurement rigorous? Is the study biased (could observers be influenced)? Is their an appropriate control group?
- Statistics: are sufficient patients enrolled (is the sample size large enough) to determine a difference if it exists (to disprove the null hypothesis)? Are data monitoring, handling and statistical tests appropriate?
- Results: are the control data similar to previously published data? Have all the necessary information and results been presented? If there is a statistical difference between the groups, is it appreciable or important?
- Discussion: what is the relevance of the study findings in the context of previous published data? What were its potential pitfalls? Are the conclusions justified?

The research question

Having absorbed the information surrounding the area of interest it is now essential to form a robust hypothesis that will withstand careful scrutiny. The effort required to undertake and complete a research project has become considerably more difficult in recent years because of the competitive nature of grant and funding applications, the increasing standards required for ethics and other institutional approvals (including full economic costing), and the exacting prerequisites of statistical planning, trial surveillance, communication and publication. This makes it mandatory for the research question to be strong enough to achieve grant funding and institutional support, and to advance the knowledge in the specialty. Many research projects in the past have been simple repetitions or minor variations from previous work, mostly with minimal impact. Developing a novel hypothesis with potential large impact is difficult, but achievable. Research questions are increasingly generated by collaboration with other specialties in both clinical and basic sciences. Good questions do not need to be complex to be important. An example is the recent extensive work on establishing the effective dosing and efficacy of paracetamol in infants and children [14,15].

Pilot studies

It is sometimes important to undertake a small pilot study before a larger, definitive study. This can serve several purposes. If a new treatment could be potentially harmful it is important to limit the exposure of patients to that treatment. A careful pilot study allows evaluation of benefit and risk. The measurement process and data collection methods can be tested; staff can test and practise observations. Assuming that there is some evidence of benefit from the pilot study, these data can then be used to determine how many patients will be required in a larger study to provide a statistically robust conclusion (power analysis).

Writing a research proposal

The exact format of a research proposal will vary according to the funding body. Table 47.3 lists the usual sections in a written proposal and summarises the content.

Statistical advice

The effective resolution of a research hypothesis requires a robust trial design with reliable and accurate data collection. Early statistical advice is essential in designing the trial and is now a prerequisite of ethical approval. Larger trials should be organised through a clinical trials unit which must be involved at an early stage. They can advise on how best to construct the trial to answer the research question as well as take a central role in obtaining, monitoring and analysing high-quality data. The following summarises the common and important statistical considerations and approaches in paediatric research.

The variation of a characteristic (a measurement or outcome) within a population can be estimated from a sample of individuals, and the confidence of such estimations can be calculated and used to make predictions. For example, determining the dose of anaesthetic required to prevent movement to a standard skin incision can be estimated by testing a range of doses in several sample groups of patients. A dose–response curve can be generated and used to predict the probability of movement or non-movement. Effective doses causing immobility in 50 per cent or 95 per cent are interpolated (or sometimes extrapolated). Although the effect upon an individual cannot be predicted with certainty the probability estimation is still useful.

The size of a sample group is important and this should be the minimum number of subjects needed to provide a statistically acceptable conclusion. In a single hypothesis project with two groups (a control group and a treatment group) there are likely to be two outcomes: there is or is not

Table 47.3 Checklist of the requirements for a research proposal

1. Title	Concise to allow the reader to grasp rapidly what is being proposed
2. Abstract	Précis of the main proposal including the research question, how it will be answered and the implications of the study
3. Lay summary	A non-technical summary to allow a lay person to understand the basic elements of the proposal
4. Background	A detailed review of the literature that sets out what is known, what is unknown and what forms the basis of the hypothesis. The articles cited in this literature review will need to be referenced, usually at the end of the proposal
5. Hypothesis	In terms of obtaining funding this is the key to being successful. The hypothesis will be short and should demonstrate a clear question that needs to be resolved by a research study. The hypothesis may have several components but should not be vague. While the hypothesis must be focused, the wider issues can be incorporated into the section on aims of the study
6. Study design	This sets out how the trial will be carried out. It will include where the study is to be undertaken, the patient age group and numbers, specifics on how and what will be done, exclusion and inclusion criteria for recruitment, and what happens if the procedure does not go according to the proposed plan
7. Data handling/ statistics	Usually planned in conjunction with a clinical trial unit to ensure that the research question is answered effectively in terms of statistics recording and processing of trial data
8. Costing and resource implications	A detailed financial plan is necessary for the funding body to assess the requested grant
9. Timelines	The study needs to be completed within the ethical and funding window requested. Therefore the proposal should set out a timing plan. This becomes of key relevance if several individual experiments are planned Care must be taken to match the data collection with speed of recruitment. Poor time planning can result in failure of the study

a difference between the groups. Two errors are therefore possible. Type 1 (or α) error occurs when the null hypothesis is erroneously rejected. The possibility of this occurring is usually set at 5 per cent (corresponding to a P value of 0.05). A type 2 (or β) error occurs when the null hypothesis is erroneously accepted and is usually set at around 10–20 per cent. The power is 100 per cent minus the type 2 error (i.e. if the error is 10 per cent the power is 90 per cent) and is defined as the chance of determining a difference between the groups if such a difference truly exists. It is important to appreciate that, if the variation in the variable is large and the treatment itself has only a small effect, a small sample is unlikely to demonstrate a difference between the groups. The variation in the variable and the effect size can be estimated either from previous research or from a pilot study. Sample sizes can be estimated by standard formulae or published nomograms.

Trial design

The sample population needs to represent the wider population and, in a trial with two or more sample groups, these should be selected at random using random number allocation (tables or a similar technique) to avoid bias. Occasionally, parents ask that their child be allocated to one arm of the study. This is a source of bias and cannot be allowed. The parent's wishes may be accepted but the child must be withdrawn from the study. In heterogeneous groups a stratified randomisation helps to ensure that different types of patient are allotted equally within the treatment groups.

The best way to assess a treatment effect is to compare it with a placebo. Everyone, including the child, their family, the nurses and the researchers, needs to remain 'blind' or unaware of whether the child received the drug or the placebo. Any effect is therefore unlikely to be due to bias and all procedures are carried out similarly to all patients. Procedures must be in place, however, so that, if there is a complication, adverse event or similar problem, someone in responsibility can decide whether to stop the trial or not.

Some trial designs can allow for individual subjects to receive the two treatments (a crossover trial). For example, in chronic pain therapy, two pain-relieving drugs could be administered, in random order, to the same patient provided that there a suitable period of time separating them to prevent any interaction. This is of considerable value because it means that each patient acts as their own control. Different drug doses can be compared within the same patient and any effect is more likely to be caused by the drug (or dose) rather than any other patient characteristic. The numbers of patients required for within-patient comparison is usually half that required for between-patient comparisons.

Based on the numbers needed to achieve a robust conclusion the trial may need to be reconfigured. If patient recruitment is likely to be outside the scope of a single centre, then several centres need to be recruited and the study becomes multicentre. If the study is potentially dangerous then the design must incorporate independent monitoring with interim analysis using either a sequential trial design or a fixed sample analysis.

Project registration and ethical approval

The administrative procedures necessary to undertake human research are now considerable and involve significant administrative efforts, particularly those that involve assessment of drugs or medical devices. The legislation is evolving at a rapid rate and has become more complex year after year. Most studies now require significant funds not only to carry out the study itself but also to provide the infrastructure for administration and data monitoring that complies with current legislation. Therefore, obtaining adequate funding to cover the costs of the study itself and the administrative burden associated with it is now essential before proceeding to the approvals to study. Some of the steps now required include national and international registration and ethical committee approval in addition to local hospital approval.

Drug research regulations

Recent attempts have been made to lay down an international standard for designing, conducting, recording and reporting of research trials that involve participation of human subjects. Counties including the European Union, Japan, the USA, Australia, Canada and the Nordic countries have developed guidelines (The International Conference on Harmonisation Good Practice Guideline – ICH GCP) which aims to protect the rights of human subjects participating in clinical trials, and to ensure the scientific validity and credibility of the data collected (see http://www.mhra.gov.uk). Compliance with the ICH GCP is a mandatory step in the authorisation to undertake clinical research trials that involve drugs, but within a few years the GCP principles may be a requirement for all clinical research. Completing this documentation and obtaining approval are labour intensive and can be daunting to an individual planning a research project. It has made it almost essential for a clinician wishing to engage in clinical research to undertake the necessary consents and administrative steps via a professional clinical trials unit that has the experience necessary to undertake this time-consuming work. Applying these directives into paediatrics has been complex. On the one hand, there are many drugs that are used without adequate paediatric testing but, on the other, there is a need to protect the best interests of the child in any research undertaken. The Ethics Working Group of the Confederation of European Specialists in Paediatrics (CESP) has addressed these issues in trying to interpret the principles of ICP GCP into paediatric research [16].

Hospital approval and indemnity

Undertaking a study has financial and service implications. A study may take extra time in the operating theatre, use additional hospital equipment and even have hidden costs such as space, paper, electricity and telephone charges. This is the basis of full economic costing for research, and is now expected to be accounted for within a research proposal. In addition, before the study can be sanctioned, it must be determined who accepts the overall responsibility for the study and who indemnifies the study. It is the duty of sponsor and the holder of the indemnity to address any problems of the study. In a commercial trial of a new medication or device, the company setting up the trial will be required to provide this indemnity. In the UK, paediatric studies are often not covered by existing indemnity agreements from universities or medical schools, and these institutions may insist on independent insurance to be covered by the grant. In respect of running costs, UK hospitals have central funding set aside for research and development and therefore want an assessment and agreement on all the cost implications before the study is approved.

Funding

Commercial drug trials are usually independently funded and should meet all costs. Potential sources of grants for non-commercial projects consist of national research institutions (such as, in the UK, the Wellcome Trust or the Medical Research Council), government-based initiatives, large charitable organisations (such as Action Research and the British Heart Foundation) and local charities (often associated with a hospital). Occasionally, commercial bodies such as drug companies will provide unrestricted grants. Specialist clinicians, including paediatric anaesthetists, are often unsuccessful in obtaining large independent peer-reviewed grants because their research impact cannot compete with the major clinical priorities of cancer and ischaemic heart disease. However, important research questions with high impact will be considered and the chance of success of an application can be improved by linking basic science questions to clinical practice in groups that have a high reputation and a strong record in obtaining grant funding. Funding bodies usually require a detailed research proposal which they send for independent peer review. Even if the application is unsuccessful, the comments presented by the reviewers can be helpful in improving the proposal to increase the chance of success on subsequent attempts. Assistance with grant applications should be available from research and development departments. The internet is another interesting and valuable source of information.

Data acquisition, storage and analysis

Research data are confidential and must be collected and stored to prevent identification of participants. Anonymity

can be achieved by assigning trial numbers to the patients that are kept separate from the data. Particular care must be taken with data stored on computer from both data loss and loss of confidentiality. Meticulous records need to be kept with every conceivable piece of information, even if this may not seem relevant at the time. It can be impossible to obtain data retrospectively once the study has finished and secondary hypotheses are often generated by unforeseen analysis of all the data. In large or multicentre trials a clinical trials unit should coordinate the collection and storage of the data as well as provide surveillance monitoring to ensure that protocols and procedures are being adhered to.

It is a legal requirement to store research data for many years after the trial has been completed because late adverse events can occur and it may be necessary to review the data. Also, the raw data may be of considerable value to other research groups who may wish to use it in a meta-analysis.

A detailed account of data analysis is outside the scope of this chapter and the reader should refer to one of the many specialised books and articles on biomedical statistics [17]. However, in basic terms, the data from two or more groups are likely to be in one of three forms: normally distributed, non-normally distributed or nominal (i.e. something has or has not happened). Normal (gaussian) distribution data are described by mean and standard deviation, and differences between groups are analysed using parametric statistical tests (e.g. t- and F-tests). Both the means themselves and the differences between the means can be described by confidence intervals. Small data-sets, and those that are not normally distributed (i.e. skewed), are usually described by medians and ranges, and comparisons are made using non-parametric tests such as the Wilcoxon signed rank (for paired data) and Mann–Whitney tests (for non-paired data). Skewed data can sometimes be log-transformed into a normal distribution so that parametric tests, which are more robust, can be applied. Nominal data are usually analysed using a χ^2 or Fisher's exact test.

Data may be used to look for association and correlation of two observations such as the fall in blood pressure, after a spinal local anaesthetic technique, with age. Statistical evaluation techniques include linear or multiple regression analysis. The Kaplan–Meier survival curve is a useful technique for analysing the time of outcome of a drug effect because it allows for some patients to 'drop out' of the study or for some not having an effect at all. Comparison between two groups can then be achieved using a logrank test [17].

WRITING UP THE STUDY

Having obtained and processed the data it is hoped that the results will answer the primary research question. Further analysis of the data may also reveal secondary outcomes which may be of interest, but must be regarded as provisional. It is tempting to trawl through the data disregarding negative associations and ascribe unwarranted importance to differences that achieve a statistical significance. This approach to data analysis is usually regarded with scepticism by statisticians and manuscript reviewers. However, they can be presented as *post hoc* analysis and can form a pilot set of data for a subsequent definitive study. Journals have individual styles and these should be checked beforehand. Word counts are almost always limited and in general it is harder but better to use fewer words. Brevity is usually associated with clarity. The following offers guidance to inexperienced writers on writing up studies.

Title, authors and introduction

The title of the research article should be brief yet give as much information to the reader as possible. When researchers are searching databases of publications they rely upon titles as well as key words. Examples of good titles are 'Pharmocokinetics and pharmacokinetic interactions of morphine in neonates, infants and children' and 'Evidence of neurodevelopmental delay after exposure to inhaled anaesthetics in preterm human infants' because these give the reader a fair idea of what is about to be discussed. Cryptic titles are unhelpful.

The principal investigator, who has usually collected the data and written the majority of the manuscript, should be the first author. Other individuals can be added but only if they have made appreciable contributions (their contributions should be stated). These may include those who have provided help with study design, statistical advice or laboratory investigations. There is a tradition that the last name on the authorship is reserved for the senior researcher who has supervised the study. All authors share responsibility for the probity of the project. There have been instances of fraudulent work being given credibility by senior researchers who have failed to check its authenticity. Research fraud is equivalent to medical misconduct and can result in disciplinary procedures including erasure from the medical register.

The introduction should then set the scene for the paper and is one of the most important sections, especially for an assessor of the manuscript. It should be concise (not a full review of the literature) and explain what is known in the area of study and what is unknown. The last sentence is a simple statement of the research question or hypothesis.

Methods and results

The methods describe what was done and include details of ethical approval, patient recruitment, group allocation, individual research management and analysis techniques including a statistics section. They should allow the reader to have enough information to repeat the experiment. New procedures or analyses must be described in detail. Previously used methods need only be mentioned, or summarised, and referenced. The sample size (α error and power) should be justified.

Results and discussion

The results should describe, in the simplest form possible, what was found and its relationship to the primary question or hypothesis. The demographic details of the sample of patients and any deviations from protocol should be described first to introduce the data-set. It is possible that patients who have been recruited for a study may not have produced complete data. This could be due to withdrawal of consent, protocol violation or withdrawal of the patient from the study by the researchers (e.g. a patient develops an unexpected and unrelated complication). It should have been predetermined how such data are treated and analysed. 'Intention to treat' means that all patients are included in the data-set once randomisation has been made whereas in 'per protocol' design only those who complete the study protocol are included in the analysis.

The primary outcome should be described first before any secondary analysis is presented. It is also important to include non-significant findings, which may not be as exciting to the reader but may be clinically important. Figures, tables or photographs should be included only if they add clarity. A well-designed figure can replace many words and conveys the key findings to the reader in a direct fashion. Data description should always include measures of central tendency and dispersion where possible. Adverse outcomes, critical incidents and complications must be described.

The discussion allows the results to be put in the context of previous data. It should not include further results but should begin by stating what was found. The strengths and then the limitations of the research method need to be explored fully. Data from other studies should be discussed, particularly if it is in conflict with the current results of the study, and the current state of knowledge needs to be assessed in the light of the new information. Finally, there should be a conclusion and a proposal for any further research questions posed by the study. Suggestions for further research are often a useful way to close the discussion.

PRESENTATION AND PUBLICATION

Presenting original work can take several forms: informal presentation (work in progress), formal presentation at regional, national or international meetings, or definitive publication in a peer-reviewed journal. Presentations of work in progress to a department can be very useful to clarify laboratory methods, to discuss results and their interpretation and to gain new directions for the project. Work in progress is less suitable for clinical studies because interim analysis (unless that is part of that design) could introduce bias into subsequent data and alter the final outcome. This applies to both the presentation of interim clinical results at meetings and the subsequent publication of abstracts. Pilot data, planned interim analysis that has been collected independently and final data from a definitive clinical trial submitted before peer-reviewed publication are appropriate for abstract presentation. Larger national and international meetings will publish an abstract of the work that is presented and these will usually be peer reviewed for scientific content prior to publication. Multiple presentations of the same work is not considered good practice, and generally the definitive publication should follow the abstract presentation.

In order for the research to reach the most appropriate and largest readership possible, it is necessary to be realistic at the outset of the quality, specialisation and impact of the work. There are currently just under 5000 biomedical journals indexed on MEDLINE and the articles within them are easily accessed world-wide. It is therefore important to publish within this domain for maximum impact. *Paediatric Anaesthesia* is the only subspecialty journal but other mainstream journals regularly have important paediatric research and review articles. All have a careful process of peer review by which only acceptable quality manuscripts are accepted. Often the reviewers will require modification of the work to improve its quality even after provisional acceptance. Occasionally, important work will be deferred pending further research data that can provide more definitive proof of the hypothesis.

Journals are rated in terms of quality and importance by 'impact factor' and this is calculated from the number of citations of the journal over a 2-year period divided by the total number of articles appearing in the same time. Journals such as *The Lancet* or *New England Journal of Medicine* have impact factors of 15–25, whilst anaesthesia journals, at best, have impact factors of 1–5. This may reflect importance of research but may also simply demonstrate that specialist issues are not often quoted in research dealing with large general issues. It must be reiterated, however, that only research of the highest quality can achieve publication in high-impact journals. The journal *Paediatric Anesthesia* is read world-wide by specialist anaesthetists and will have significant influence in the specialty irrespective of assessments of impact factors.

Publishers of medical journals are obliged to be profitable, yet in doing so their output may be too expensive for individuals or even for organisations with financial restrictions. Indeed, some high-impact publications are so expensive that the information – even valuable information – is restricted to the few who can afford it. This can be counterproductive to researchers and the public. An alternative approach is being promoted whereby research outputs are made available by free-access journals [18]. The quality of these publications can be maintained by peer review and an editorial board, which should be the same process for all journals. Inevitably there are costs involved and these could be paid by the researchers or their sponsors or the 'free-access publisher', although this will add to the cost of the research. Abandoning paper in favour of electronic publication should save money for the publishers.

REFERENCES

Key references

British Medical Association. Consent, rights and choices in health care for children and young people. Boulder: NetLibrary, 2001.

Freedman B. Equipoise and the ethics of clinical research. *N Engl J Med* 1987; **317**(3): 141–5.

Gill D. Ethical principles and operational guidelines for good clinical practice in paediatric research. Recommendations of the Ethics Working Group of the Confederation of European Specialists in Paediatrics (CESP). *Eur J Pediatr* 2004; **163**(2): 53–7.

Mayer D. *Essential evidence-based medicine*. Cambridge: Cambridge University Press, 2004.

McIntosh N, Bates P, Brykczynska G *et al*. Guidelines for the ethical conduct of medical research involving children. Royal College of Paediatrics, Child Health: Ethics Advisory Committee. *Arch Dis Child* 2000; **82**(2): 177–82.

References

1. Bowling A. *Research methods in health: investigating health and health services*, 2nd edn. Buckingham: Open University Press, 2002.
2. Mayer D. *Essential evidence-based medicine*. Cambridge: Cambridge University Press, 2004.
3. Bernard GR, Margolis BD, Shanies HM *et al*. Extended evaluation of recombinant human activated protein C United States Trial (ENHANCE US): a single-arm, phase 3B, multicenter study of drotrecogin alfa (activated) in severe sepsis. *Chest* 2004; **125**(6): 2206–16.
4. Block BM, Liu SS, Rowlingson AJ *et al*. Efficacy of postoperative epidural analgesia: a meta-analysis. *JAMA* 200312; **290**(18): 2455–63.
5. Jones J, Hunter D. Consensus methods for medical and health services research. *BMJ* 1995; **311**(7001): 376–80.
6. Scottish Intercollegiate Guideline Network. *A guideline developers' handbook*. Edinburgh: SIGN, 2002.
7. McIntosh N, Bates P, Brykczynska G *et al*. Guidelines for the ethical conduct of medical research involving children. Royal College of Paediatrics, Child Health: Ethics Advisory Committee. *Arch Dis Child* 2000; **82**(2): 177–82.
8. British Medical Association. *Consent, rights and choices in health care for children and young people*. London: BMJ Books, 2001.
9. Freedman B. Equipoise and the ethics of clinical research. *N Engl J Med* 1987; **317**(3): 141–5.
10. UK collaborative randomised trial of neonatal extracorporeal membrane oxygenation. UK Collaborative ECMO Trial Group. *Lancet* 1996; **348**(9020): 75–82.
11. Council for International Organizations of Medical Sciences, World Health Organization. *International ethical guidelines for biomedical research involving human subjects*. Geneva: CIOMS; 2002.

12. Ondrusek N, Abramovitch R, Pencharz P, Koren G. Empirical examination of the ability of children to consent to clinical research. *J Med Ethics* 1998; **24**(3): 158–65.

13. Jevtovic-Todorovic V, Hartman RE, Izumi Y *et al.* Early exposure to common anesthetic agents causes widespread neurodegeneration in the developing rat brain and persistent learning deficits. *J Neurosci* 2003; **23**(3): 876–82.

14. Anderson BJ, van Lingen RA, Hansen TG *et al.* Acetaminophen developmental pharmacokinetics in premature neonates and infants: a pooled population analysis. *Anesthesiology* 2002; **96**(6): 1336–45.

15. Anderson BJ, Holford NH, Woollard GA *et al.* Perioperative pharmacodynamics of acetaminophen analgesia in children. *Anesthesiology* 1999; **90**(2): 411–21.

16. Gill D. Ethical principles and operational guidelines for good clinical practice in paediatric research. Recommendations of the Ethics Working Group of the Confederation of European Specialists in Paediatrics (CESP). *Eur J Paediatr* 2004; **163**(2): 53–7.

17. Bland M. *An introduction to medical statistics*, 3rd edn. Oxford: Oxford University Press, 2000.

18. Frank M. Access to the scientific literature – a difficult balance. *N Engl J Med* 2006; **354**(15): 1552–5.

48

Organisation of services

KATHY WILKINSON

KEY LEARNING POINTS

- Paediatric anaesthetic services have developed in parallel to general paediatric and surgical services for children, enabling advances in all areas.
- Since the publication of the first National Confidential Enquiry into Perioperative Deaths (NCEPOD) report in 1989, marked organisational changes have occurred in UK systems of care. Occasional practice has been discouraged and this has resulted in large numbers of infants and children being transferred to tertiary centres.

- All UK anaesthetists are specifically trained in the care of children; they should be able to participate in the resuscitation of acutely ill infants and children and provide anaesthesia for a fit child aged 5 years and over undergoing minor surgery.
- The responsibilities of paediatric anaesthetists extend (as in adult services) to the provision of acute pain relief and intensive care.
- Important parallels and differences exist in the delivery of paediatric anaesthetic services in other healthcare systems.

INTRODUCTION

The chapter outlines the evolution of paediatric services in the UK over the last 150 years and is intended to provide a context for the development of surgical and anaesthetic services for children generally. The current recommendations for organisation of services will be discussed, in relation to the UK paediatric anaesthetic service, together with a brief description of that in other healthcare systems.

ORGANISATION OF ALL PAEDIATRIC SERVICES IN THE UK

Before the foundation of the UK children's hospitals and dispensaries in the late eighteenth and early nineteenth centuries, secondary care for children was delivered in a very piecemeal fashion in hospitals all over the country. Children were treated mainly as outpatients and usually not in separate facilities. Indeed, in 1843, of the 2643 patients treated in all the London hospitals, only 136 were children under 10 [1]. Yet half of the 50 000 people who died in London each year at that time were children. Even within the new children's hospitals the physicians who delivered the care would have had no real training in paediatric medicine, but did this work alongside their adult, mainly fee-paying practice. There was little medical literature to guide and inform care. Thomas Phaire's *The Boke of Chyldren* [2], was the first text on paediatrics ever written in English, while Walter Harris's *Acute Diseases of Infancy* (1689) apparently remained the standard source of reference for more than a century. Dedicated children's doctors became a reality only in the mid-twentieth century. In 1900, The Society for the Study of Children's Diseases was founded in London, with more than 800 members from all over the UK. This preceded the formation of the British Paediatric Association (BPA) in 1928, which became the main organisation representing paediatricians. At about the same time UK medical schools were founding the first departments for the management of diseases of children; Edinburgh in particular started to train paediatric doctors and nurses in 1931. The inception of the National Health Service (NHS) in 1948 gave rise to a structure of remuneration that enabled specialists to work exclusively with children and consultant paediatricians were appointed. The BPA was dissolved in 1996, when children's medicine finally separated from the Royal College of Physicians, to form the Royal College of Paediatrics and Child Health (RCPCH).

The Platt report [3] was one of the first to give recognition to the special requirements of children in hospital. It focused on the need to improve the emotional welfare of the child and responded to the representations of many professional and voluntary groups, concerned about restrictions that limited parental visits. The National Association for the Welfare of Children in Hospital (NAWCH), now 'Action for Sick Children', drew attention to the lack of facilities for parents in hospitals, and continued to press for unrestricted parental access. By 1976 when the Court Report *The Welfare of Children in Hospital* was published [4], there had been only minor improvement in services for children. It is interesting to note that the report emphasised the need to balance the desire to treat a child near to home with the need to concentrate services into a reasonable-sized unit, advocating: 'A child and family centred service in which skilled help is readily available and accessible: which is integrated in as much as it sees the child as a whole and as a continuously developing person'. The Department of Health report *Welfare of Children and Young People in Hospital, 1991* [5] formed a further attempt to set standards that should be achieved by providers of health care and expected by those purchasing it. The cardinal principles are outlined in Table 48.1. Until the recent publication of the National Service Framework (NSF) for Children [6] this report formed the basis for contracting of children's services.

In 1993 the Audit Commission published an independent survey of in-patient care for children in England and Wales [7]. The data are useful in quantifying current paediatric surgical activity at that time. Approximately half of the inpatient paediatric workload was surgical, with a peak of activity at around 5 years of age, which is probably accounted for by the increase in ear, nose and throat (ENT) problems in this age group. In the early 1990s, children and adolescents up to age of 18 years constituted 28 per cent of the population and consumed about 5 per cent of the hospital service budget. Many of the recommendations within the report reappeared in the recent Children's NSF [6].

Today there are 10 dedicated children's hospitals in the British Isles. Most coexist alongside larger (adult) trusts, and many are physically sited adjacent to or within the

Table 48.1   Basic principles of contracting for hospital services for children

- Children are admitted to hospital only if the care they that require cannot be provided as well at home, in a day clinic or on a day-stay basis
- Children requiring admission to hospital are provided with a high standard of medical, nursing and therapeutic care to facilitate a speedy recovery and minimise complications and mortality
- Families with children have easy access to hospital facilities for children without needing to travel significantly further than to other similar amenities
- Children are discharged from hospital as soon as socially and clinically appropriate and full support provided for subsequent home or day care
- Good child health is shared with parents and carers and they are closely involved in the care of their child at all times unless, exceptionally, this is not in the best interests of the child. Accommodation is provided for them to remain with their children overnight
- Accommodation, facilities and staffing are appropriate to the needs of children and adolescents and separate from those provided for adults. Where possible separate accommodation is provided for adolescents
- Like all other patients, children have a right for their privacy to be respected and to be treated with tact and understanding. They have an equal right to information appropriate to their age, understanding and specific circumstances

From *Welfare of Children and Young People in Hospital*, Department of Health, 1991 [5].

adult centre. This may be advantageous administratively. Clinically, there are potential gains with smoother transition from child to adolescent and then adult facilities. Developmentally, larger organisations may attract better opportunities for research, more advanced information technology and other vital support systems.

In comparison, many other children's facilities are integrated within university and district hospitals. Within these units there is less scope to keep services separate and specifically designed for children and their families. Children's units of all sizes now have stronger and established links to community services.

The spectrum of illnesses suffered by children changed in the latter part of the last century. In particular the profile of infectious disease has been altered by immunisation (e.g. against measles, pertussus, *Haemophilus influenzae* and meningoccus type C) and antimicrobials. There has also been an increase in other acute conditions such as allergy and trauma. The development of improved chemotherapy has allowed malignancy to be treated with increasing success. Moreover, complex supportive care and transplantation have saved many children who would otherwise have died.

The availability of information through the internet has altered the perception and attitude towards disease, and there is a greater expectation of treatment and cure.

The reported rate of chronic disease in childhood more than doubled between 1972 and 1991, and this trend is continuing [8]. This can be partly explained by a greater recognition and diagnosis of disease (e.g. asthma), and to improved survival in many chronic conditions. Some chronic diseases (e.g. asthma and diabetes) would appear to be becoming more common. There has been the appearance of new diseases such as human immunodeficiency virus (HIV)/ acquired immune deficiency syndrome (AIDS), which has added an extra burden of care in some groups, more so in metropolitan areas.

Delivery of care has radically changed over the last 20 years, with an increasing emphasis on supporting the child and family in the home whenever possible. This has resulted in markedly reduced inpatient length of stay (LOS); as a result bed capacity has been reduced. The reasons for shortened LOS are multifactorial. They include improvements in clinical care with speedier recovery, a recognition that prolonged admission is not needed for many conditions and an understanding that families and children prefer a limited hospital stay. Generally, only the sickest and most complex cases now receive overnight care. In the UK providers will henceforth be remunerated for treatments delivered ('payment by results'). Consequently, cost of care is an issue and departments are now challenged to deliver surgical care in a timely and predictable fashion, e.g. by providing preassessment in an outpatient environment to facilitate admission on the day of surgery, and reduce the possibility of cancellation. Paediatrics in the UK, as well as the care of children in society, has been under recent scrutiny by the combined impact of the results of the Bristol Children's Cardiac Surgery enquiry by Lord Kennedy [9] and Lord Laming's report [10] on the events surrounding the death of a child in the care of social workers. The reports revealed the apparent failings in the systems of care for children, both in hospitals and in the community. This led to an overhaul of health and social care arrangements, with the appointment of the first National Clinical Director for Children in 2001 and subsequently the first Children's Commissioner in 2005. Alongside this legislation there was the publication of the first National Service Framework for Children [6]. This huge document covers all aspects of care for children in both hospital and the community, and is presented as a series of 10 standards. Throughout it reiterates the need for separate and high-quality systems of care in all settings, whatever a child's particular needs. Child protection training emerges as a clear priority for all who work with children. There is little specific mention of the role of the children's anaesthetist. However, of particular relevance to paediatric surgery and anaesthesia is the Hospital Standard (Standard 7) [11], which outlines three key areas for standard setting in hospital (Table 48.2). These comprise 'Child centred services', 'Quality and safety of care' and 'Quality of environment'.

Table 48.2 Key hospital standards

- Children and young people should receive care that is integrated and coordinated around their particular needs, and the needs of their family. They, and their parents, should be treated with respect, and should be given support and information to enable them to understand and cope with the illness or injury, and the treatment needed. They should be encouraged to be active partners in decisions about their health and care and, where possible, be able to exercise choice
- Children, young people and their parents will participate in designing NHS and social care services that are readily accessible, respectful, empowering, follow best practice in obtaining consent and provide effective response to their needs
- Children and young people should receive appropriate high-quality, evidence-based hospital care, developed through clinical governance and delivered by staff who have the right set of skills
- Care will be provided in an appropriate location and in an environment that is safe and well suited to the age and stage of development of the child or young person

From *Getting the Right Start – National Service Framework for Children, Young People and Maternity Services. Standard for Hospital Services,* Department of Health, 2003 [11].

The means by which these standards will be implemented calls for a 'shift in culture' to gear services to the needs of the individual child and family. The Hospital Standard, as with the other elements of the NSF, forms part of a 10-year plan. It was recognised at the outset that the framework described the desired destination but did not outline the means by which these changes would be made. In late 2005 the Health Care Commission (an independent inspectorate of healthcare standards in UK) commenced a process of reviewing all acute hospitals in England against standards, which have evolved from the NSF. Questionnaires were sent to all acute hospitals, in which children aged 0–16 years constituted about 4 per cent of their total workload. The recent results of this pilot review of children's services showed that a large majority were rated as poor or 'fair', with only a minority in the good range [12]. The Health Care Commission [12a] have subsequently published a final summary report. The review focused on the provision of care by trusts in five areas:

1. Life support
2. Child protection
3. Pain relief
4. Communication skills
5. Child-friendly environment.

It found that there were particular problems in relation to both the training and ongoing experience of anaesthetists and surgeons working with children in life support and child protection. In relation to the overall surgical and anaesthetic services for children, it found that in 8 per cent of trusts surgeons carrying out planned cases did not work enough with children to maintain their skills with very young children, and it recommended that the service should be supported by a clinical network of local regional providers of children's surgery. This has also been suggested by a number of other publications.

ORGANISATION OF PAEDIATRIC SURGICAL SERVICES IN THE UK

UK paediatric surgical services

As with paediatric medicine, the early surgeons who operated on children had a primary commitment to their adult fee-paying patients. However, their work features very early on in the activities of the emerging children's hospitals, with initially no attempt at subspecialisation. The British Association of Paediatric Surgeons was founded in 1953, at the same time as many other surgical subspecialty groups. However, the vast majority of general surgery in children continued to be performed outside specialist hospitals and was done primarily by adult surgeons and anaesthetists, albeit with a paediatric interest. As with medical paediatrics the formation of the NHS in 1948 was helpful in the development of paediatric surgery as a subspecialty with the appointment of further dedicated posts, largely in the children's hospitals where the bulk of the more complex cases were managed.

National Confidential Enquiries

The Confidential Enquiry into Perioperative deaths (CEPOD) was founded in 1982 as a joint venture between the Association of Anaesthetists and the Association of Surgeons. The first enquiry looked at surgical and anaesthetic practice in three UK regions [13]. After publication of the report on this preliminary work, national funding was awarded and it was decided that the first comprehensive project would concentrate on children under the age of 10 years. This was for two reasons:

1. Children provided a small identifiable sample for the first national survey
2. It was felt to be timely in view of the increasing specialisation of children's and neonatal surgery.

By extrapolation from the preliminary report it was suggested that there would be about 400 perioperative deaths annually in this age group. In the event just less than 300 deaths were reviewed, approximately two-thirds of which were after cardiac surgery [14]. The general conclusions of the report, which has proved so influential in shaping paediatric anaesthetic and surgical practice in the UK in the last 25 years, are given in Table 48.3.

The lack of universal reliable data in the NHS, and in particular the lack of numerators, did not allow meaningful

Table 48.3   General conclusions of the National Confidential Enquiry into Perioperative Deaths (NCEPOD), 1989 [14]

1. The overall surgical and anaesthetic care of children as revealed in this enquiry is excellent
2. Few children die following surgery. Those who do have multiple congenital anomalies often not compatible with life or malignant tumours, or suffer severe multiple trauma
3. Much surgery and anaesthesia for children are given by clinicians with a regular paediatric practice. However, this is not always so
4. While most children's surgery and anaesthesia is undertaken by, or under the supervision of, consultants, on some occasions this supervision was lacking
5. The clinical competence of some locum appointments to care for the special needs of children must be questioned
6. The needs of children in single-specialty units are not always fully met. While the natural dominance of surgical requirements (for neurosurgery and burns in particular) are paramount, an absence of facilities in intensive care for children and a lack of skilled paediatric anaesthetists, paediatricians and paediatric nurses were found in some units
7. Local audit meetings to review the management of children occur in 83% of cases. This is a considerable improvement on the situation reported in the report of the Confidential Enquiry into Perioperative Deaths (1987) [13]
8. The system established by NCEPOD for the collection of data worked well. Its success was ensured by the enthusiasm of the consultants who participated. NCEPOD has again demonstrated that consultant anaesthetists and surgeons are willing to review their performance (only 0.2% of consultants refused to participate)
9. The data systems in the NHS are inadequate. Rates of events (admissions, operations and deaths) cannot be calculated because contemporary data are not available. Thus valid comparisons between hospitals, districts or regions cannot be made promptly enough to influence clinical practice

conclusions about whether deaths were indeed more common with 'occasional' paediatric practice. This was one of the main criticisms of this very important piece of epidemiological research. However, the survey did highlight the extent of occasional practice. It also revealed, in the details of several case summaries in the report, the difficulties encountered by some general surgeons and anaesthetists, particularly in out-of-hours and emergency work in the very young. The impact of the first National Confidential Enquiry into Perioperative Deaths (NCEPOD) report has been enormous, partly because of the way that it was interpreted. During the last 15 years, there have also been coincident generic changes in healthcare, and advances in surgical and anaesthetic training, that have contributed. In the early 1990s a series of reports, reviews and editorials broadly reinforced and expanded on the NCEPOD recommendations [15–17]. They attempted to define 'occasional' practice, and discuss the reasons why it was detrimental to patient care. An influential summary was produced by the BPA in 1994 *The Transfer of Infants and Children for Surgery* [18]. This included details of what had become known as the Lunn criteria, defining occasional practice in terms of the suggested number of cases that might maintain expertise. A further report by the RCPCH in 1996 re-examined workload, and stated that to maintain competence anaesthetists and surgeons required 'ideally the equivalent of one operating session per week on children' [19]. It was this latter recommendation that has tended to be regarded as the minimum necessary.

The British Association of Paediatric Surgeons was the first to define their role in a series of guidance documents to purchasers [20–22]. However, there was a continued dilemma as to where this care should be delivered. A controversial review, in 1998, called for more debate about the provision of paediatric surgical care, with respect to both the role of the specialist centre, and the majority non-specialist practice delivered in the district hospital [23].

Some answers emerged in 1999, when, 10 years after its original publication, NCEPOD presented the results of a further survey on perioperative death in childhood (Fig. 48.1) [24]. This time cardiac surgical deaths were excluded, and the sample was extended to include children under the age of 16 years. Of the 139 deaths the largest number now occurred in children's and university hospitals, and a minority in the district general hospital (DGH). Occasional practice would appear to have been considerably reduced.

Most deaths were associated with congenital abnormalities, nectrotising enterocolitis, tumours or trauma. There were no reported deaths after the common childhood operations of appendicectomy and tonsillectomy. However, these had not been noted in the 1989 report either. Deaths of babies with hernias in the DGH had disappeared, but still occurred, albeit outside the DGH. The authors commented, 'In the management of acute children's surgical cases a

regional organisational perspective is required'. This particularly applies to the organisation of patient transfer between units. Paediatric units have a responsibility to lead this process. 'Concerns were raised about a recurrent problem of poor or absent data on children's surgery' – this had been previously noted in 1989. Local discussion of perioperative deaths was sometimes also still lacking. However, the first recommendation was that further concentration of children's surgical services (whether at local or regional level) 'would increase expertise and further reduce occasional practice'. In summary the 1997–98 NCEPOD report [24] reflected the change in practice since 1989 with the sickest children now being transferred to regional centres in advance of, or during, their final illness. It represented the start of a continuing trend.

In an attempt to address the many ongoing issues in paediatric surgery, in 2000 the Royal College of Surgeons of England assembled a paediatric forum. This comprised nominated representatives of the 10 surgical specialist associations, the Royal College of Anaesthetists (RCoA), College of Ophthalmologists, the RCPCH and the Royal College of Nursing. The aims of the forum at its inception were to:

- define a set of national standards for the management of children requiring surgery
- ensure that children receive treatment in an appropriate environment
- outline the special provisions that must be made within education and training programmes for surgeons involved in the care of children
- recommend an appropriate assessment relating specifically to children in the intercollegiate examinations
- promote the provision of and encourage participation in audit and appropriate continuing professional development (CPD) activities for all surgeons involved in the care of children.

There was broad recognition that an integrated, high-quality surgical service was dependent on the collaboration of a wide group of professionals, and this group was particularly large in paediatric surgery. In addition, with the exception of ENT, it was pointed out that children comprise a relatively small proportion of the total workload of each speciality. Although altogether surgery for children constituted a larger grouping, individually each subspecialty was relatively insignificant. In creating a forum, it was the totality of paediatric surgical provision that would be represented. The first report of the forum was published in May 2000 [25] and provided an opportunity for all members to give a summary of current provision, scope of practice, training and education, and suggest future recommendations. It was broadly supportive to the DGH providing surgical care for children, assuming that facilities were adequate. It also promoted the idea of 'hub and spoke' arrangements to integrate the tertiary centres more closely with the DGHs that they served. This had first been discussed in an important joint editorial by Rollin in 1997 [26]

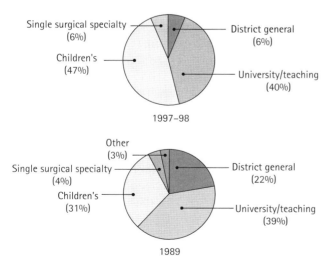

Figure 48.1 Comparison of the type of hospitals in which surgery took place in 1997–98 and 1989 (percentage of final operations) [24]. Reused with permission from NCEPOD.

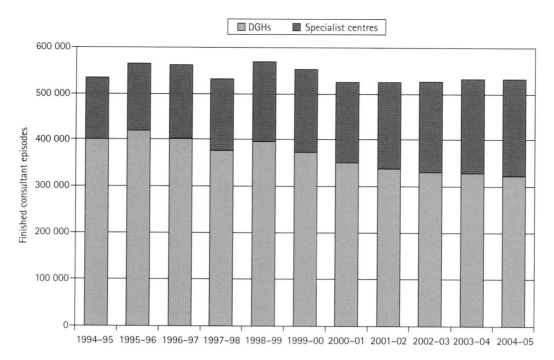

Figure 48.2　Finished consultant episodes for children with an operation, 1994–95 to 2004–05. Reused with permission from NCEPOD.

and been widely accepted as an example of good practice. A revision of the 2000 surgical forum recommendations has been very recently published [26a], and is presented with generic recommendations ('Standards of Care') in the areas of consent, child protection, resuscitation, pain management and transition to adult services. There is also a strong recommendation that lead clinicians in general surgery for children be identified. Specific recommendations in all sub-specialty areas are again presented. As an appendix to this publication an important 'Statement on the future provision of General Paediatric Surgery in the DGH' was made. There is agreement within this statement that general paediatric surgery in the DGH in the UK is facing a crisis with many general surgeons with an interest in paediatrics approaching retirement and a huge shortage of those trained and prepared to take their place. In summary it strongly suggests (as in many previous recommendations) the urgent need for networks of care for children's surgical services within regions, with local provision of care whenever possible. The reference statistics that support this statement were provided by a paper commissioned by the forum and published in February 2007 [26b], and which describe trends in children's surgery over a 10-year period 1994–2004.

In this period there was a reduction in overall children's surgical activity of the order of 20 per cent in DGHs (from about 450 000 finished consultant episodes (FCEs) to 350 000 FCEs (Fig. 48.2). This is mirrored by an increase of about 90 per cent in the tertiary centres from 100 000 to just under 200 000 FCEs. The reasons around these changes are complex, and reflect changes in surgical management as well as the changes in the 'confidence' of DGH teams to deal with

surgical problems in children. Of note is the fact that the largest reduction of workload in the DGH has been in the 0–4 age range. Of interest, in Scotland most general surgery in children has been carried out in the three children's hospitals, with around 80 per cent of children's surgery taking place in these specialist centres. It is likely that this will become greater in the future, with only 13 per cent of current general surgical consultants in Scotland in a recent survey expecting their successors to perform general paediatric surgery [27]. Therefore, we are currently at a point in the UK where the last 15 years has seen a real reduction in the amount of surgical work carried out in children in the DGH. This has been particularly the case in general surgery. Operating on children has become less popular for several reasons. These include:

- The increasing tendency of general surgery training programmes to promote subspecialisation in one area (e.g. vascular, colorectal). Although it has been possible for some years for a training module within paediatrics to be undertaken, it is unlikely that a DGH can provide the ongoing work to sustain more than one surgeon with these skills. This is because the volume of paediatric general surgery work is relatively low. The result has been that there are very few applicants for the current training programme for the 'general surgeon with an interest in children'. Indeed a postal survey of 1044 DGH general surgeons in England and Wales in 2004 indicated that only 18 (<2 per cent) indicated general paediatric surgeon as a special interest [28].

- The combined effects of the recent reorganisation of UK medical training [29] and the European Working Time Directive (EWTD) [30].
- The lack of paediatric independent practice.
- The combined effect of recommendations for both surgeons and anaesthetists to avoid 'occasional' practice (and the possible risk of litigation).
- The increasing strength and prominence of specialist paediatric surgeons within the UK and the lack of clear definition in their role.
- Paediatric practice often results in antisocial patterns of work, and is more likely, especially in the smaller unit, to be consultant delivered (this relates to point 1).

This problem has been recently recognised by the Royal College of Surgeons of England (RCSEng). The Intercollegiate Surgical Curriculum Project [31] states, in its most recent training objectives for general surgeons of the future, the following with respect to children's surgery:

'Specialist paediatric surgical practice aspires to provide care for children and teenagers. . . . Much of the elective work comprises day case surgery and the emergency work is usually that of common emergency abdominal conditions such as appendicitis and urogenital tract such as torsion of the testicle. Conditions of greater complexity should be the preserve of Specialist Paediatric Surgery and it is felt inappropriate to train general surgeons in this area. The volume and complexity of the work involved does not merit designation as a stand-alone sub-specialty.'

This would tend to indicate an admission that, like anaesthetists, all *general* surgeons must undertake a minimum amount of training in order to care for children.

The British Association of Paediatric Surgeons with the Association of Paediatric Anaesthetists (APA), the RCPCH, the Senate of Surgery and Association of Surgeons have recently addressed this problem, producing a statement on the future organisation of general surgical services for children (Table 48.4) [32]. This envisages a system of managed clinical networks for children's surgery, such as those described for many aspects of specialist care [33]. These have already been explored in many areas within paediatrics [34] and there are examples of good practice already in existence [35]. It promotes the idea of two distinct varieties of paediatric surgeon: the specialist and the generalist. The latter will offer an improved service to the DGH, performing, for example, day-care lists on site and outpatient clinics. Out-of-hours small DGHs will need to decide on their capabilities with respect to the competencies of their general surgeons and children below a certain age will require transfer to a regional centre. It is likely that, if this is accepted, it will have similar effects on other surgical services for children, which might be organised on a three-centre model. It remains to be seen how much of these very different recommendations will be embraced and implemented.

Table 48.4 Model of service provision for general paediatric surgery*

1. The small district general hospital (DGH)
   These hospitals should be able to provide resuscitation and stabilisation of all infants and children with surgical pathology. They should also be capable of providing elective surgery for ages down to 1 year by visiting general paediatric surgeons. Most urgent and emergency surgery under 5–8 years (dependent on skills of resident general surgeons) will need to be transferred to intermediate or tertiary regional centres
2. The intermediate centre (large DGH or university hospital)
   These hospitals may be large enough to employ general paediatric surgeons (as defined above) who will provide on-site emergency and elective care for non-specialist paediatric surgery (including babies generally outside the neonatal period, trauma, intussusception) and elective outreach services for neighbouring DGHs. They will require the support of trained paediatric anaesthetists, radiologists, pathologists, etc., and on-site paediatric high-dependency unit facilities
3. The specialist or tertiary regional centre
   This centre should provide the full range of paediatric surgical care including neonatal, urological and cancer surgery, supported by neonatal and paediatric intensive care on site and full retrieval facilities. This care will be delivered by a complement of specialist paediatric surgeons and anaesthetists. Dependent on the geography/population distribution of the regional network, general paediatric surgeons may also work from the same site (e.g. in large conurbations)

*From BAPS/APA/RCoA, *Joint Statement on General Paediatric Surgical Service Provision in District General Hospitals in Great Britain and Ireland*, 2006 [32].

DEVELOPMENT OF UK PAEDIATRIC ANAESTHETIC SERVICES

Although there was anecdotal evidence that some departments had taken the recommendations of NCEPOD 1989 very seriously [36], this was not borne out by a national survey of UK anaesthetists published in 1994 [37]. The results were based on a postal survey to all Fellows of the Royal College of Anaesthetists in 1993. Only those involved with anaesthesia in children aged under 3 years were asked to respond (which may explain why only 32 per cent did so). The majority of responders were in DGH practice and just under half of these had received 6 months of training in a specialist centre. However, UK anaesthetists would have received at least 3 months of paediatric anaesthetic training before accreditation. Perhaps the most worrying fact that emerged was that two-thirds were still anaesthetising babies for pyloromyotomy, with most caring for only one or two annually. This tended to suggest that occasional practice in this vulnerable group was still common. More recent statistics support the fact that changes have occurred, not least

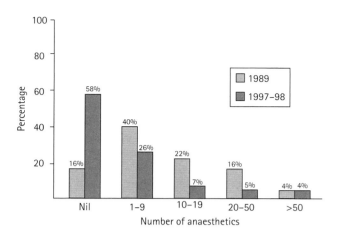

Figure 48.3 Percentage of consultant anaesthetists anaesthetising infants aged less than 6 months, grouped by number of cases anaesthetised [24]. Reused with permission from NCEPOD.

those supplied by NCEPOD in 1999 [24], which gave considerable detail about anaesthetists working with children, 58 per cent of whom said that they no longer worked with babies less than 6 months of age (compared with 16 per cent in 1989) (Fig. 48.3). The proportion anaesthetising only small number of infants had also fallen (from 40 per cent in 1989 to 26 per cent in 1997–98).

More recently a survey conducted by the Association of Paediatric Anaesthetists in Great Britain and Ireland (APAGBI) was able to identify a lead for paediatric anaesthesia within most UK departments – this was slightly more likely in the DGH and major acute general hospitals than in the university hospital [38]. This would tend to indicate a good level of compliance with both the NCEPOD and RCoA recommendations on an organisational framework for paediatric anaesthesia.

ORGANISATION OF PAEDIATRIC ANAESTHETIC SERVICES AT DEPARTMENTAL LEVEL

In 1994 the RCoA produced a detailed compendium of recommendations for all departments which was to be used to set standards, and could in turn be passed on to purchasers of health care and hospital management teams. There were separate chapters for all subspecialty areas of anaesthesia, pain and intensive care. This document has subsequently undergone two revisions and the current version (2005) will be discussed in more detail [39]. It can be used as a template around which the organisation of paediatric anaesthetic services is designed (Table 48.5).

Studies have shown that anaesthesia workload in general has been subject to major growth in the last 10–20 years [40,41]. This is because increased safety has permitted anaesthesia in a larger and sicker population. There has also in many countries been an increased use of regional anaesthesia. In many large departments of paediatric

Table 48.5 Summary of the Royal College of Anaesthetists' (RCoA) guidance on the provision of paediatric anaesthetic services, 2005*

- Anaesthesia services for children require specially trained clinical staff together with equipment, facilities and an environment appropriate for the needs of a child
- The service should be led at all times by consultants who regularly anaesthetise children
- At all times there must be adequate trained assistance; skilled assistance for paediatric anaesthesia should be provided by staff specifically trained for the task
- In a life-threatening emergency where transfer is not feasible, the most senior appropriately experienced anaesthetist should undertake anaesthesia
- Paediatric resuscitation equipment must be available wherever and whenever children are treated and staff must receive regular re-training in paediatric life support
- There should be a properly staffed and funded acute pain service that covers the needs of children
- Paediatric high-dependency and intensive care services should be available as appropriate for the type of surgery performed
- Parents (or carers) should, wherever possible, be involved in all aspects of care and decisions regarding the management of their children

*From *Guidance on the Provision of Paediatric Anaesthetic Services*, RCoA, 2005 [39]. Reused with permission from RCoA.

anaesthesia the profile of work has also changed, with an increased involvement in interventional radiological and cardiology procedures [42]. In theatres there has been a marked increase in laparoscopic general surgical and urological work performed.

Staffing

Much has been made of the need for children to be cared for by anaesthetists and surgeons who have ongoing paediatric experience, and what constitutes occasional practice. However, it may be unrealistic in many DGH departments to create separate on-call rotas for paediatric anaesthesia. Infants present special anaesthetic risk [42], and arrangements need to be made for this group to be cared for by those with additional training and ongoing experience in a regional centre. Perioperative morbidity also relates to ASA status [42]. This needs to be prioritised when making decisions on where surgery is performed, with consideration being made to transfer to a regional centre. However, all anaesthetic departments will need to provide a level of on-site competence, which allows them to cover resuscitation of the sick infant and child out of hours. In addition there may be an age guideline (e.g. 5 years) at which they would be expected to provide anaesthesia confidently, assuming that the child is otherwise well and undergoing minor surgery, such as manipulation under anaesthesia (MUA) or appendicectomy. For those who regularly cover children's lists this should be straightforward, and this group may also be confident to look after children to a lower age limit (e.g. 1–3 years), particularly in the elect-ive setting. However, others will need to have their skills refreshed on a regular basis, by undertaking a list on an occasional basis with or without a colleague who does it regularly, either in their own hospital or on secondment to a regional centre. The RCoA is quite clear that supervision of other grades (SAS grades and trainees) in paediatric practice should be by a consultant with appropriate experience [43–45]. Most departments have clear local rules on this subject, which are dictated by the level of competence of resident staff and their other responsibilities when on call. Generally, and as a minimum standard, care of infants is under the direct supervision of a consultant. Comorbidity and type of surgery may also influence this decision and guidelines should be suitably broad so that care is never compromised (e.g. suggesting telephone discussion between trainee and consultant if any doubt exists). Assistance for the anaesthetist is extremely important in paediatrics; at present operating department practitioners, and anaesthetic and recovery nurses undertake a variable amount of specific paediatric training. There is a need for generic paediatric training for all theatre staff that includes a regular resuscitation elem-ent. The recommendation is that the organisation of recovery facilities is under the supervision of a registered children's nurse, and it is advantageous if they have current advanced life support training in paediatrics [46,47]. Children's surgery and anaesthesia should generally be delivered in units with on-site paediatric (medical) staff, who are available when necessary to give advice and support for the child with comorbidity. On occasion, there will not be a paediatric ward on site (e.g. when day-case surgery is undertaken). Nevertheless a senior paediatrician must be available to assist if the child unexpectedly requires postoperative high dependency care or if a child protection matter arises. Wherever children are nursed in the preoperative and postoperative period there is a recommendation that two registered children's nurses are available. This may be particularly difficult in certain circumstances, such as the (mixed) day procedure and outpatient dental facilities, and in single speciality surgical units, such as neurosurgery and burns units.

REMOTE AND RURAL LOCATIONS

Several parts of the UK are relatively isolated from secondary care and those facilities that do exist may be limited in size. Models of care within these locations may necessarily be very different [47a]. Anaesthetists play a very important role in these facilities, providing resuscitation and assisting in management not only for sick adults, but also for newborns and children. Numbers of (surgical) cases are often very small, so special arrangements need to be made for ongoing maintenance of skills. The further use of telemedicine is also being explored, e.g. during the resuscitation and early intensive care management of the sick child.

Equipment

In the intervening 10 years between the two NCEPOD reports that related to paediatric anaesthesia (1989–99), there were major changes in the UK with respect to the quality and availability of monitoring equipment. In 1989 more than one-third of children were not managed with oximetry (which had become available from the early 1980s) and more than 80 per cent had no capnography. With the advent of 'minimal monitoring' standards, both modalities were used virtually 100 per cent of the time by 1997–98, when the second survey was carried out. However, the full range of equipment that is required for babies and children of all ages and sizes is large. It is important to have a member of the consultant team who takes a particular interest in paediatric equipment, and that checking of all essential equipment is part of established and routine anaesthetic practice.

Support services

Support services will include the provision of on-site high-dependency or intensive care for children which should be matched to the profile of surgery undertaken. However, in all units where children undergo surgery, there should be the ability to resuscitate and initiate intensive care, and systems in place for urgent transfers. Transfers may be required within the hospital as well as to other centres and portable equipment should be ready for this eventuality, as well as a bag containing a small supply of essential additional transfer items. An acute pain service for children is increasingly important, particularly if the volume of major surgery is large and complex analgesic techniques are undertaken. In smaller centres these will need very close supervision by attending anaesthetists, a system that may fall short of the ideal, particularly out of hours. Clear agreed guidelines and staff training are a prerequisite for the smooth running of such a service. It is helpful if drug doses used are compatible with those described in nationally recognised references [48]. In the UK the newly published UK *British National Formulary for Children* [49] has provided a valuable resource, and includes simple information about epidural and intravenous opiate regimens. A generic formulary such as this should be used in all parts of the hospital where children are treated.

Suitable pain assessment tools for children of all ages are also an essential means by which recovery and ward staff are enabled to provide analgesia for children, and should be employed in areas where children are usually admitted (e.g. accident and emergency department and assessment units). Pharmacy support should allow for suitable doses/preparations to be available, to provide advice and to assist in the provision of special regimens for children. Sophisticated epidural and parenteral opiate techniques cannot function without the aid of appropriate infusion devices. On-site pathology and blood transfusion services should be able to process small samples when required in infants, and provide blood and blood products for babies and children in an appropriate manner and according to national guidelines [50]. Many theatre suites employ point-of-care testing – these are particularly useful when dealing with major haemorrhage when transfusion triggers may be breached, and can provide important dynamic information on the coagulation cascade.

Facilities

Separate facilities for children can be provided by either physical or temporal separation from adults. The former, as well as representing a more ideal environment for the child, can achieve greater throughput, particularly if staffed by trained paediatric anaesthetic personnel [51]. There are recommendations for the facilities which should be available in the paediatric operating theatre [52]. These list the environment, equipment and personnel needs but rarely mention location. If the operating theatre is relatively isolated from the ward then a holding area is useful and should be suitably decorated and provide occupation for the waiting parent and child. If isolated from the main theatre suite, consideration should be given as to whether it is appropriate to carry on emergency work in such a location out of hours. The ability of parents to accompany their child at induction and recovery is greatly enhanced by the provision of a waiting area very close to the theatre suite and with intercom or telephone communication links [53]. In smaller DGHs and/or low-volume surgical subspecialties, consideration needs to be given to separate children's lists, which might occur at, for example, 2-weekly intervals. This is preferable to a mixed list. However, when this is impossible because there is a need for a regular weekly throughput (e.g. to accommodate plaster changes in orthopaedics or plastic surgery), then children should be scheduled early in the day so that fasting times can be minimised and theatres prepared in advance.

Areas of special requirement

INTENSIVE CARE

A relatively small group of babies and children undergoing surgery have serious comorbidity and/or require major surgery likely to require postoperative ventilation. The biggest groups are those undergoing cardiac surgery and neurosurgery. In paediatric general surgical practice, the neonate forms the largest single group requiring intensive care postoperatively. This relates to the incidence of congenital abnormalities, the association of these abnormalities with prematurity and the requirement for relatively major corrective surgery, commonly involving thoracolumbar incisions. In the elective situ-ation, when the need for postoperative ventilation is planned, or there is a significant chance that it will be required, it should be available on site (i.e. the child

should undergo surgery in a hospital with the appropriate intensive care facilities readily available) [54]. Anaesthetists also have a major role in the resuscitation and stabilisation of sick infants and children, be they medical or surgical. This is particularly the case where there are no on-site paediatric intensive care (PIC) facilities. With a move to subspecialisation in paediatric anaesthesia in the UK, there have been concerns about the ability of all anaesthetists to deliver such a service. The UK Department of Health has recently reported on this subject, producing recommendations that extend to pre-hospital care [55].

DAY SURGERY AND ANAESTHESIA

Children's surgery is particularly suited to the day-care setting and it has been estimated that up to 75 per cent of all types of surgery in children may be performed on a day-stay basis. Day care for children may be organised around several models, the ideal being a mixed medical/surgical facility with a nearby, dedicated theatre. This is rarely possible outside the specialist centre. An alternative is to have 'children's days' within a mixed adult/child facility. Staff with specific expertise in day care and in paediatrics should be employed. Comorbidity should be an unusual reason to deny children surgery on a day-stay basis. However, this might include the very immature (e.g. less than 60 weeks' postconceptional age if born prematurely), children with unstable metabolic disease and those at risk from postoperative airway/respiratory compromise, particularly if there has been a history suggestive of sleep apnoea or hypoventilation. Children should not be discharged if they have actual or predicted unmet analgesia needs, or persistent vomiting. The organisation of day surgery for children has been specifically discussed [56].

SEDATION

An increasing number of children are referred for procedures that, in the past, might have been carried out with restraint and/or oral sedatives (e.g. lumbar puncture or joint injection). Still more are being referred for newer investigations or procedures that require sedation, such as magnetic resonance imaging (MRI) and interventional radiology. Anaesthetists have been at the forefront of making recommendations in this area [57]. Unfortunately, funding of many of these additional services, particularly in smaller centres, where numbers may be low, is often problematic. In relation to the administration of chemotherapy, new UK regulations apply [58]. In all areas, systems of care need to be strictly regulated, with senior members of staff involved and clear guidelines developed.

Training and education

The RCoA has produced guidance for training anaesthetists at all levels and aims to provide, even those whose career aim is to be in general (adult) practice, the necessary competencies to provide safe anaesthesia and analgesia for the fit 5 year old undergoing minor surgery [44,45]. Those who wish to specialise need to undertake 6–12 months of additional training in a tertiary setting, the latter being the minimum necessary to practise as a specialist paediatric anaesthetist. In order to specialise in paediatric practice in a DGH it is recommended that a minimum of 6 months of additional paediatric anaesthesia training be undertaken. Ongoing experience is important, and this might be gained through a regular paediatric list. Although this will provide some of the skills to equip the individual to undertake the early management of the sick baby or child, the additional competencies for the early intensive care may need to be gained by other means and be regularly refreshed. Various ways of maintaining skills and knowledge have been recommended and include simulation training, clinical attachments and attendance at the large number of 'core topics' sessions organised locally and nationally. Teaching on the advanced life support courses for children may also be helpful. It is clear that, in the DGH or university setting, anaesthetists are likely to need to maintain a range of additional competencies, which may not be necessary if there is a PIC unit (PICU) on site. In the UK the impact of the shorter working hours for anaesthetists in training, embodied in the EWTD, is currently being realised and assessed. One recent paper from a large national children's hospital demonstrated that the reduction of hours worked by anaesthetic trainees had led to changes in training opportunities, which may be detrimental [59]. The study demonstrated a 13 per cent decrease in the number of operating lists undertaken by each specialist registrar after the change in working hours. The greatest impact was on exposure to general lists and those in remote locations. They concluded that the EWTD had had a measurable impact on the training of paediatric anaesthetists, and that the significance of this change for clinical practice had not yet been measured. In the UK anaesthetic training is currently competency based. Sufficient time must be spent if these competencies are to become embedded in an individual's skill base and the number of cases is probably still important. More difficult to ensure are the competencies of support staff in theatres as these are less well defined. This is an important area for future development. There are many areas of commonality in other developed countries in their organisation of paediatric anaesthesia services. In the USA there have been similar discussions about the difficulties associated with subspecialisation [60], albeit 10 years ago.

GUIDELINE DEVELOPMENT

A well-functioning anaesthetic department will have mechanisms in place for local guideline development and promotion [61]. In the UK there is a minimum list of guidelines that should be available in all locations where anaesthetics are administered [62]. Specific to paediatric anaesthesia there will usually also be local guidelines on

when to call for senior assistance, the management of the child with stridor, and on child protection. Policies in many general areas need to have sections pertinent to the child (e.g. fluid administration, acute pain, latex policy, major blood loss, preoperative starvation and sedation). It is helpful to have a nominated individual whose responsibility it is to develop and update these guidelines.

Research and audit

Clinical research in children may be more difficult to perform for various reasons:

- There are separate and specific guidelines for research in children [63].
- Consent may be more difficult to obtain [64].
- To date drug companies have had little incentive to fund research for all but high-volume use drugs. Children, who remain relatively low users of drugs can thus be deemed 'therapeutic orphans', and there is widespread use of off-label and unlicensed medicines [65]. This may be a particular problem in PIC [66]. Recent work in the UK has stimulated progress in this area [67].
- Assessment of endpoints may be more difficult and must allow for developmental level.

Nevertheless, research in paediatric anaesthesia is important if the specialty is to move forwards with the rest of medicine. Within the UK and Europe there is a current initiative to improve and facilitate multidisciplinary drug research in children and it is hoped that anaesthesia and intensive care will both benefit from this process. Audit of practice is also important against agreed standards [68]. It has been suggested that all deaths in children in the perioperative period should be discussed in a multidisciplinary forum and this might be one of the functions of a hospital's children's surgical committee (see Organisation and administration below). Regular review of morbidity is also essential.

Organisation and administration

Increasingly children are admitted on the day of surgery. For the majority of ASA 1 and 2 children this is acceptable, provided that they have been screened for comorbidity, surgery is minor and sufficient information has been delivered to both parent and child at preassessment. This must include very clear instructions about fasting. Even if children are scheduled for more major surgery, they and their parents may be accommodated in 'hotel'-type facilities the night before surgery. This should not prevent the anaesthetist from having important discussions with the child and family. As in adult practice the concept of preoperative evaluation is increasingly being discussed for children; the advantages are related to a decrease in wasted operating time due to inadequate patient preparation [69]. This has major resource implications, as sessions are specifically allocated to outpatient duties, and additional staff and space are required. This may be difficult to arrange if the family have to travel long distances and the social disruption incurred may be too high a price to pay for 'admission on the day'. It is the recommendation of the RCoA that there is a multidisciplinary committee consisting of a paediatrician, anaesthetist, surgeon, pharmacist and registered children's nurse, which should be responsible for 'the overall management, improvement, integration and audit of anaesthetic and surgical services for children'. Other useful individuals within this group are a senior member of theatre staff and a play therapist. Just as with the national forum, there is a need for multidisciplinary representation. The function of the group is to regulate all aspects of the surgical and anaesthetic care of children, including deciding admission and transfer criteria, and maintaining and improving the perioperative environment. Such a committee must be recognised within the hospital administrative structure, and consulted when appropriate; ideally it should operate across directorates. Since the publication of the Children's National Service Framework in England in 2003 [11], there has been a statutory recommendation that there is a representative for children on the board all UK trusts. It would be logical if that person also participated in the children's surgical committee. It is recommended that specialised paediatric care in the UK is increasingly part of a 'managed clinical network', in which there are clear and well-established links with regional centres. The organisation of children's surgical and anaesthetic services have been shown to fit well within this model of care.

Patient information and consent

Good communication with parents and children is essential at all stages of the perioperative course and begins with information imparted before admission. Many departments have produced generic leaflets, which cover the surgical admission and may also supply information about anaesthesia and analgesia. In the UK the joint RCoA–AAGBI information project included two specific information leaflets for parents and older children [70]. There have also been many attempts to provide information specifically for children, and these include illustrated booklets, videos and web-based programmes. Preoperative discussion should involve the child whenever possible at a level appropriate to their development and degree of understanding. Discussion of risk may be particularly difficult. It is incumbent upon anaesthetists to attempt to provide this whenever possible and particularly for invasive procedures. Ideally, when risks are substantial these discussions should take place some time in advance of surgery and anaesthesia, which makes the possibility of preassessment attractive in terms of best practice. In cases where parents and/or children refuse treatment it is important that there are local mechanisms to support clinicians, such as a clinical ethics committee, to offer help and advice. Anaesthetists should be well informed about consent issues in children [64] and need to be confident in dealing with refusal to treatment in the competent child.

Child protection

Legislation with respect to the child is changing [71] and anaesthetists should be aware of the implications of this. In particular, there have been recent changes in the recommendations with respect to suspected child abuse [72]. It is important that all professionals working with children have some training in this area so that appropriate local mechanisms can be activated and there is good interdisciplinary cooperation. In the UK a joint guideline has recently been produced by the APA, RCoA and RCPCH [73]. All UK anaesthetists are now aware of the need to refer suspected cases of child abuse, and will undergo basic child protection training.

PAEDIATRIC ANAESTHESIA IN OTHER HEALTHCARE SYSTEMS

Organisation

Paediatric anaesthesia has emerged in many developed countries in a similar fashion to the UK, and in parallel with specialist medical and surgical services [74,75]. However, there are important and useful comparisons to be made in the way in which the service is delivered, with similar issues for discussion, e.g. maintenance of skills in paediatric anaesthesia and training.

In the USA, as in the UK, there is a range of centres caring for children, with the possibility of 'occasional' practice. There is perhaps more potential for this, given that the system of care delivery is to a greater extent privatised. This has led to discussions about the need to introduce more widespread 'credentialling' in paediatric anaesthesia training and practice.

A survey of paediatric regional anaesthesia from the French Language Society of Pediatric Anesthesiologists also revealed large variations in the size of institution where care was delivered [76]. Data were collected prospectively on >85 000 anaesthetics. Most participating hospitals were in France itself, with a range in size of 100–300 beds. In a small number of these it was stated that there was no on-site department of paediatrics. A similar survey of analgesia more recently from Germany [77] shows that, of the 383 hospitals analysed, 8.4 per cent had an annual workload of <2500 anaesthetics in children. A further 63 departments responded that their paediatric workload was too small to partake in the survey.

In Australia the perception is that most children having elective surgery will be anaesthetised in a regional setting.

This is backed by a recent survey from Western Australia, in which the majority of children received care in a tertiary hospital or a private (metropolitan) hospital [78]. Of the 28 522 anaesthetics given over the year, only 14 per cent received it in a rural setting, with 8 per cent in a public metropolitan (non-specialised) hospital. In particular, infants were most commonly cared for in a tertiary public hospital (62 per cent). However, the authors note that 6 per cent of infants were cared for in non-specialist units.

In a recent survey of practice from Japan, there were not enough specialist paediatric anaesthetists in the children's hospitals, and smaller centres lacked case numbers to maintain a subspecialist rota [79].

Training

In 1997 the Accreditation Council for Graduate Medical Education in the USA recognised fellowship training in paediatric anaesthesia. Paediatric anaesthesia thus joined critical care and pain management in having a formal training requirement at fellowship level. The possible consequences of this were discussed at the time in a survey and editorial in the same year [80,81].

Latterly, there has been an examination of the effects of lengthening all anaesthesiology residency programmes in the USA [82]. There was a general increase in numbers of residents undertaking 1-year programmes. The specific subspecialty distribution of fellows had changed. However, there was little alteration in the numbers undertaking paediatric training.

The Australian and New Zealand College of Anaesthetists has recently published a new learning portfolio for anaesthetic trainees [83]. The recommendation is that all trainees spend a minimum of 50 half-day sessions in module 8 (paediatric anaesthesia). There are no specific recommendations with respect to duration of paediatric anaesthetic training prior to taking up consultant/staff specialist positions in tertiary centres. In practice, a minimum of 12 months is suggested by those in the larger children's hospitals, and overseas experience is encouraged (D Baines, personal communication, 2006).

SUMMARY

In outlining the development of paediatric surgical and anaesthetic services in the latter part of the twentieth century, the evolution alongside recommendations has been discussed. It is striking how much has been achieved, and how many recommendations are repeated in the many different documents from various agencies on the care of children. Providing a high-quality service such as that outlined is an increasingly difficult challenge in both the specialist centre and the DGH. There has been a marked change in the location of care away from the DGH in the last 10 years, which may prompt further reorganisation. Remarkably,

children's services are often not given the priority that they deserve in modern healthcare systems. The challenge is to provide a local service whenever possible, at least for routine surgery in children, and maintain the skills and interest of staff. Very young children, particularly those requiring complex or out-of-hours surgery, may require transfer. The hope is that this can be recognised and organised equitably. There are many areas for development within paediatric anaesthesia [84–86], and anaesthetic research in children must continue if these developments are to be proven and high standards maintained.

REFERENCES

Key references

Department of Health. *The acutely or critically sick or injured child in the district general hospital: a team response.* Department of Health, Gateway ref 4758. London: Department of Health, 2006 (http://www.dh.gov.uk).

National Confidential Enquiry into Perioperative Deaths. *Extremes of age.* The 1999 report of the National Confidential Enquiry into Perioperative Deaths. London: NCEPOD, 1999.

Royal College of Anaesthetists. *Guidance on the provision of paediatric anaesthetic services.* London: Royal College of Anaesthetists, 2005 (http://www.rcoa.ac.uk/publications).

References

1. Kosky J, Lunnon R. *Great Ormond Street and the story of medicine. The hospitals for sick children.* 1991. Cambridge: Granta.
2. Phaire T. *The boke of chyldren* (1545) . Edinburgh: E & S Livingstone, 1955 (reprinted by British Paediatric Association).
3. Platt H. *The welfare of children in hospital.* Report of a Committee of the Central Health Services Council. London: HMSO, 1959.
4. Court Report. *Fit for the future: report of the Committee on Child Health Services* (Cmnd 6684). London: HMSO, 1976.
5. Department of Health. *The welfare of children and young people in hospital.* London: HMSO, 1991.
6. Department of Health. *National service framework for children, young people and maternity services.* London: Department of Health, 2004 (http://www.dh.gov. uk/PolicyAndGuidance/HealthAndSocialCareTopics/ChildrenServices).
7. Audit Commission. *Children first: a study of hospital services.* London: HMSO, 1993.
8. Blair M, Stewart-Brown S, Waterson T, Crowther R. *Child public health.* Oxford: Oxford University Press, 2003.
9. Department of Health. *Learning from Bristol.* The report of the Inquiry into children's heart surgery at The Bristol Royal Infirmary. London: HMSO, 2002 (http://www.bristolinquiry.org.uk).

10. Department of Health and The Home Office. *The Victoria Climbié inquiry – report of an inquiry by Lord Laming.* London: The Stationery Office, 2003 (http://www.victoria-climbie-inquiry.org.uk/finalreport).

11. Department of Health. *Getting the right start – National service framework for children, young people and maternity services.* Standard for hospital services. London: Department of Health, 2003 (http://www.dh.gov.uk).

12. Healthcare Commission. *Improvement review into services for children in hospital.* London: Healthcare Commission, 2006 (http://www.heathcarecommission.org.uk/nationalfindings/nationalthemedreports/childrenswork).

12a. Commission for Health Audit and Inspection. Improving services for children in hospital. London: Health Care Commission (http://www.healthcare commission.org.uk).

13. Buck N, Devlin HB, Lunn JN. *Report of the confidential enquiry into perioperative deaths.* London: Nuffield Provincial Hospitals Trust, 1987.

14. Campling EA, Devlin HB, Lunn JN. *The report of the national confidential enquiry into perioperative deaths.* London: NCEPOD, 1989.

15. Lunn JN. Implications of the national enquiry into perioperative deaths for paediatric anaesthesia. *Paediatr Anaesth* 1992; **2**: 69–72.

16. Atwell J, Spargo P. The provision of safe surgery for children. *Arch Dis Child* 1992; **67**: 345–9.

17. Anonymous. NCEPOD and perioperative deaths in children. *Lancet* 1990: **ii**: 1498–500 (Editorial).

18. British Paediatric Association (RCPCH). *The transfer of infants and children for surgery.* London: Royal College of Paediatrics and Child Health, 1994.

19. Royal College of Paediatrics and Child Health. *Children's surgical services.* London: Royal College of Paediatrics and Child Health, 1996 (http://www.rcpch.ac.uk).

20. British Association of Paediatric Surgeons. *A guide for purchasers and providers of paediatric surgical services.* Edinburgh: Royal College of Surgeons of Edinburgh, 1995.

21. British Association of Paediatric Surgeons and Royal College of Surgeons of England. *Surgical services for the newborn – a joint report.* London: Royal College of Surgeons of England,1999 (http://www.rcseng.ac.uk). London: 1999.

22. Senate of Surgery of Great Britain and Ireland. *The provision of general surgical services for children.* Senate paper 3 July. Glasgow: Senate of Surgery of Great Britain and Ireland, 1998 (http://www.rcseng.ac.uk).

23. Arul GS, Spicer RD. Where should paediatric surgery be performed? *Arch Dis Child* 1998; **79**: 65–72.

24. National Confidential Enquiry into Perioperative Deaths. *Extremes of age.* The 1999 report of the National Confidential Enquiry into Perioperative Deaths. London: NCEPOD, 1999.

25. Royal College of Surgeons of England. *Children's surgery – a first class service.* Report of the paediatric forum of the Royal College of Surgeons of England. London: Royal College of Surgeons of England, 2000 (http://www.rcseng.ac.uk/publications).

26. Rollin AM. Paediatric anaesthesia – who should do it? The view from the district general hospital. *Anaesthesia* 1997; **52**: 515–16.

26a. Children's Surgical Forum of the Royal College of Surgeons, England. *Surgery for children – delivering a first class service.* London: Royal College of Surgeons, 2007: www.rcseng.ac.uk

26b. Cochrahe H, Tanner S. *Trends in Children's surgery 1994-2004 – evidence from Health Episode Statistics data.* London: Department of Health.

27. Craigie RJ, Duncan JL, Youngson GG. Children's surgery performed by adult general surgeons in Scotland: the present and future. *Surgeon* 2005; **6**: 391–4.

28. Association of Surgeons of Great Britain and Ireland. February 2005 newsletter. London: ASGBI, 2005 (http:\\www. asgbi.org.uk).

29. Department of Health. *Modernising medical careers: the next steps. The future shape of foundation, specialist and general practice training programmes.* London: Department of Health, 2004.

30. Council of the European Union. Directive 93/104/EC of 23 November 1993 concerning certain aspects of the organisation of working time. Brussels: Council of the European Union, 1993 (http://europa.eu.int).

31. Royal College of Surgeons of England. Intercollegiate Surgical Curriculum Project. London: Royal College of Surgeons of England, 2005 (http://www.iscp.ac.uk).

32. British Association of Paediatric Surgeons *et al. Joint statement on general paediatric surgical service provision in district general hospitals in Great Britain and Ireland.* London: BAPS, 2006 (http://www.baps.org.uk).

33. Department of Health. *A guide to promote a shared understanding of the benefits of managed clinical networks.* Gateway reference. 4968. London: Department of Health, 2005 (http://www.dh.gov.uk/publications).

34. Cropper S, Hopper A, Spencer SA. Managed clinical networks. *Arch Dis Child* 2002; **87**: 1–4.

35. Partners in Paediatrics. A grouping of child health provides, 2005 (http://www.partnersinpaediatrics. org. uk).

36. Bowhay AR, Morgan Hughes JO. Paediatric anaesthesia in the district hospital. *Anaesthesia* 1989; **4**: 139–42.

37. Stoddart PA, Brennan L, Hatch DJ, Bingham R. Postal survey of paediatric practice and training among UK anaesthetists. *Br J Anaesth* 1994; **73**: 559–63.

38. Peutrell J. *APA survey of UK paediatric anaesthesia.* London: APA, 2005 (http://www. apagbi.org.uk).

39. Royal College of Anaesthetists. *Guidance on the provision of paediatric anaesthetic services.* London: Royal College of Anaesthetists, 2005 (http://www.rcoa.ac.uk/publications).

40. Clergue F, Auroy Y, Pequignot F *et al.* Evolution of anaesthetic workload – the French experience. *Best Pract Res Clin Anesthesiol* 2002; **16**: 459–73.

41. Lalwani K. Demographics and trends in non-operating room anaesthesia. *Curr Opin Anesthesiol* 2006; **19**(4): 430–5.

42. Murat I, Constant I, Maud'Huy H. Perioperative anaesthetic morbidity in children: a database of 24 165 anaesthetics over a 30 month period. *Paediatr Anaesth* 2004; **14**: 158–66.

43. Royal College of Anaesthetists. *CCST in anaesthesia. General principles.* A manual for trainees and trainers. London: Royal College of Anaesthetists, 2003 (http://www.rcoa. ac.uk/docs/ccstptied2.pdf).

44. Royal College of Anaesthetists. *CCST in anaesthesia III: competency based specialist registrar years 1 and 2 training and assessment.* A manual for trainees and trainers. London: Royal College of Anaesthetists, 2003 (http://www.rcoa. ac.uk/publications).

45. Royal College of Anaesthetists. *CCST in anaesthesia IV: competency based specialist registrar years 3, 4 and 5 training and assessment.* A manual for trainees and trainers. London: Royal College of Anaesthetists, 2003 (http://www.rcoa.ac.uk/publications).

46. Resuscitation Council (UK). *European paediatric life support course.* London: Resuscitation Council UK, 2006 (http://www.resus.org.uk).

47. Advanced Life Support Group. *Advanced paediatric life support* (APLS). Manchester: Advanced Life Support Group, 2006 (http://www.alsg.org.uk).

47a. Oates B. The RARI Paediatric Project. Child health services in remote and rural Scotland. Interm report. Remote and rural areas resource initiative. Edinburgh: Scottish Executive, in press.

48. Association of Paediatric Anaesthetists. Good practice in post-operative and procedural pain. *Paediatr Anaesth* 2008; in press.

49. Paediatric Formulary Committee. *British national formulary for children.* London: BMJ Publishing Group and RPS Publishing, 2005 (http://bnfc.org/bnfc).

50. Boulton F. Transfusion guidelines for neonates and older children. *Br J Haematol* 2004; **124**: 433–53.

51. Kain Z, Fasulo A, Rimar S. Establishment of a pediatric surgery center: increasing anesthetic efficiency. *J Clin Anesth* 1999; **11**: 540–4.

52. American Academy of Pediatrics (Section of Anesthesiology). Guidelines for the pediatric perioperative anesthesia environment. *Pediatrics* 1999; **103**: 512–15.

53. Hall PA, Payne JF, Stack CG, Stokes MA. Parents in the recovery room: a survey of parental and staff attitudes. *BMJ* 1995; **31**: 163–4.

54. NHS Executive. *Paediatric intensive care – a framework for the future.* Report from the National Coordinating Group on Paediatric Intensive Care to the Chief Executive of the NHS Executive. Leeds: NHS Executive, 1997 (http://www.dh.gov.uk).

55. Department of Health. *The acutely or critically sick or injured child in the district general hospital: a team response.* Department of Health, Gateway ref 4758. London: Department of Health, 2006 (http://www.dh.gov.uk).

56. Thomas R. *Just for the day – children admitted to hospital for day treatment.* London: Action for Sick Children, 1991.

57. Scottish Intercollegiate Guideline Network. *Safe sedation of children undergoing diagnostic and therapeutic procedures.* Guideline 58. Edinburgh: SIGN, 2004 (http://www. sign.ac.uk/guidelines/fulltext/58/index.html).

58. Department of Health. *HSC 2001/022: national guidance on the safe administration of intrathecal chemotherapy.* London: Department of Health, 2001 (http://www.dh.gov.uk).

59. White MC, Walker IA, Jackson E, Thomas ML. Impact of the European working time directive on the training of paediatric anaesthetists. *Anaesthesia* 2005; **60**(9): 870–4.

60. Morray JP. Implications for subspeciality care of anaesthetised children. *Anesthesiology* 1994; **80**: 969–71.

61. Royal College of Anaesthetists, Association of Anaesthetists. *Good practice guide.* London: Royal College of Anaesthetists, Association of Anaesthetists 2002 (http://www.rcoa.ac.uk/publications).

62. Royal College of Anaesthetists, Association of Anaesthetists. *Departmental portfolio.* London: Royal College of Anaesthetists, Association of Anaesthetists, 2002 (http://www.rcoa.ac.uk/publications).

63. Royal College of Paediatrics and Child Health Ethics Advisory Committee. Guidelines for the ethical conduct of medical research involving children. *Arch Dis Child* 2000; **82**: 177–82.

64. British Medical Association. *Consent, rights and choices in health care for children and young people.* London: BMJ Publications 2001.

65. Conroy, S, Choonara I, Impicciatore P *et al.* Survey of unlicensed and off-label drug use in paediatric wards in European countries. *BMJ* 2000; **320**: 79–82.

66. Turner S, Gill A, Nunn T, Choonara I. Use of 'off label' and unlicensed drugs in paediatric intensive care units. *Lancet* 1996; **347**: 549–50.

67. Royal College of Paediatrics and Child Health. *Safer and better medicines for children – developing the clinical and research base of paediatric pharmacology in the UK.* London: Royal College of Paediatrics and Child Health, 2004 (http:\\www.rcpch.ac.uk/publications).

68. Royal College of Anaesthetists. *'Raising the Standard': a compendium of audit recipes.* London: Royal College of Anaesthetists, 2000 (http://www.rcoa.ac.uk).

69. Ferrari L. Preoperative evaluation of pediatric surgical patients with multisystem considerations. *Anesth Analg* 2004; **99**: 1058–69.

70. Royal College of Anaesthetists, Association of Anaesthetists of Great Britain and Ireland. *Raising the standard: information for patients.* London: RCoA, AAGBI, 2003 (http:\\www.youranaesthetic.info).

71. Department for Education and Skills. The Children Act 2004. London: HMSO, 2004 (http:\\www.opsi.gov.uk/ acts/acts2004/20040031.htm).

72. Department of Health. *What to do if you're worried a child is being abused.* London: Department of Health, 2003 (http://www.dh.gov uk).

73. Royal College of Paediatrics and Child Health. Child protection and the anaesthetist – safeguarding children in the operating theatre. Intercollegiate document. London: Royal College of Paediatrics and Child Health, 2007 (http://www.rcpch.ac.uk).

74. Cass NM, Cooper MG. Paediatric anaesthesia in Australia: origins and developments. *Paediatr Anaesth* 1996; **6**: 69–78.

75. Costorino AT, Downes JJ. Pediatric anesthesia historical perspective. *Anesthesiol Clin North Am* 2005; **23**(4): 573–95.

76. Giaufre E, Dalens B, Gombert A. Epidemiology and morbidity of regional anesthesia in children: a one year prospective survey of the French – Language Society of Pediatric Anesthesiologists. *Anesth Analg* 1996; **83**: 904–12.

77. Stamer UM, Mpasios N, Maier C, Stuber F. Postoperative analgesia in children – current practice in Germany. *Eur J Pain* 2005; **9**: 555–60.

78. Sims C, Stanley B, Milnes E. The frequency of and indications for general anaesthesia in children in western Australia 2002–2003. *Anaesth Intensive Care* 2005; **33**: 623–8.

79. Shimada Y, Nishwaki K, Sato K *et al*. Pediatric anesthesia practice and training in Japan: a survey. *Paediatr Anaesth* 2006; **16**: 543–7.

80. Rockoff M, Hall S. Subspecialty training in pediatric anesthesiology: What does it mean? *Anesth Analg* 1997; **85**: 1185–90.

81. Haberkern C, Geiduschek JM, Sorenson GK *et al*. Multi-institutional survey of Pediatric Anesthesia Fellowship: assessment of training and current professional activities. *Anesth Analg* 1997; **85**: 1191–5.

82. Havidich JE, Haynes GR, Reveres JG. The effect of lengthening anesthesiology residency on subspeciality education. *Anesth Analg* 2004; **99**: 844–56.

83. Australian and New Zealand College of Anaesthetists. Learning portfolio. Melbourne: Australian and New Zealand College of Anaesthetists, 2006 (http://www. anzca.edu.au).

84. Greeley W. Pediatric anesthesia: Where do we go from here? *Anesth Analg* 2000; **90**: 1232–3.

85. Bingham R. Paediatric anaesthesia: past, present, future. *Anaesthesia* 2003; **58**: 1194–6.

86. Costorino AT. Pediatric anesthesia: thoughts on the future. *Anesthesiol Clin North Am* 2005; **23**(4): 857–61.

49

Education and simulation

MARK THOMAS

KEY LEARNING POINTS

- Adult learning demands a different approach.
- New technologies can help us to acquire new skills and knowledge.
- Competency-based training requires a new approach on behalf of both the trainee and the trainer.
- Simulator learning may become a key component of anaesthesia training.

INTRODUCTION

Medical education is changing; reduced working hours [1] and the need to keep up to date [2] demand effective and efficient teaching, supported by new technologies.

ADULT LEARNING

In medical training, teaching methods have to accommodate the autonomous and self-directed strategies that adults use for absorbing and retaining knowledge [3]. Adults learn best with goal-orientated well-defined objectives; they have more interest in problem-centred teaching and are best motivated by internal drives when new knowledge is appreciated as being both relevant and practical in their everyday working lives. Self-esteem varies from person to person and adults need to be shown respect throughout the learning process. One of the main barriers to effective adult teaching is pride: humiliation in front of peers is counterproductive and teachers need to acknowledge all positive aspects of performance.

Thomson O'Brien and co-workers looked at common formats of continuing medical education (CME) in a Cochrane review assessing the impact of teaching upon clinical practice [4]. They found, in six out of ten studies, that interactive workshops were effective in significantly improving clinical practice. Moreover, when workshops were combined with didactic presentations the change was even more marked. Didactic teaching alone had very little effect on clinical practice.

Medical educationalists have adapted their teaching in recognition of these factors. Most resuscitation courses, for example, incorporate small-group interactive sessions as a major part of the teaching curriculum. These allow learners to challenge the perceived wisdom, thrash out ideas and incorporate new knowledge into their current practices – all primary goals in adult learning.

After a learning episode, recall of newly acquired data declines in the subsequent weeks, reaching a plateau beyond which knowledge becomes residual and thereafter retained. This is known as the Ebbinghaus retention curve and has been demonstrated in many areas of medical learning including resuscitation course MCQ (multiple choice questionnaire) scores [5]. The Ebbinghaus effect can be minimised by two strategies. One is to 'over learn' and 'over train' to such a degree that even when the predictable decline in knowledge occurs the retained part is still enough to practise safely and effectively.

Another method is to practise new skills and apply newly acquired knowledge at regular intervals. Unless those intervals are sufficiently close together there is a risk that re-training virtually from scratch will be required in order to regain prior levels of achievement.

Problem-based learning

The challenge in a busy clinical job is how to narrow the gap between good educational theory and the practical acquisition of knowledge and skills. The recent trend, given the theories described above, has been towards problem-based learning (PBL) [6].

Teachers, acting as facilitators, give groups of students an illustrative case or scenario in order for them to define their learning objectives. They undertake self-directed study, then come back to the group to discuss and modify what they have learned. In this way, other generic skills such as problem solving and team working become an integral part of the learning process. Problem-based learning needs to be used in the context of a defined core curriculum in order to avoid gaps in knowledge. It results in better long-term retention of knowledge.

There are drawbacks to PBL: it is demanding of tutor time since it requires close supervision and regular feedback. Moreover, students need simultaneous access to learning resources and may find it hard to distinguish the relevant from the irrelevant.

One can envisage how this approach might work well in the context of a clinical attachment. Illustrative cases such as pyloric stenosis or inguinal hernia repair could be researched and studied before an operating list. A group of trainees could then meet with a facilitator having completed their background reading, to discuss preoperative assessment, the anaesthesia plan, fluid balance and postoperative analgesia for these patients before starting their lists.

One-to-one teaching

Anaesthetic practice often presents a one-to-one learning opportunity for teacher and trainee that should be the envy of our clinic-based colleagues.

In the context of a mutually trusting relationship, one can explore the needs and attitudes of the learner to a greater extent than is possible in a group setting [7]. One-to-one teaching is a powerful tool in influencing the practice of the learner, allowing the incorporation of knowledge and skills tailored to their needs. This setting also allows for frank feedback and honest reflection, which are two key components of the learning process. To maximise the

trainee's gain, the teacher should plan the session guided by some simple questions, for example:

- What are the main learning goals?
- How will you judge how effectively these goals have been achieved?
- How would you like the learner to describe the experience to a peer?

At the end of the operating list, both trainee and trainer should reflect upon their learning experience.

Large-group teaching

This is the most tried and tested form of learning; it is a time-efficient method of delivering core knowledge and allows students to identify areas for further self-directed learning. Lecturers should encourage students to interact rather than adopt a passive learning role. It has been shown that audience involvement during a lecture improves content recall [8]. Lecturers should encourage students to ask questions or ask the audience questions; posing a 1-minute paper or short multiple choice questions at regular intervals can also help to engage students' minds [9]. It should be appreciated that attitudes, skills and analytical thinking are not best taught or modified in this type of forum.

Small-group teaching

Large-group teaching has the disadvantage of being a passive learning environment whereas one-to-one teaching is labour intensive. The strength of small-group teaching lies in its ability to strike a happy medium between these two extremes. The key to this form of learning lies in good planning and skilful group leadership. An effective facilitator avoids answering questions (some teachers count to 10 silently before speaking after having been asked a question), avoids interrupting too often and constantly scans the group to involve reticent participants. Many different forms of small-group format can be used and have been given exotic names such as *buzz groups*, *fishbowl*, *snowball* or *horseshoe*. Each uses different group dynamics and subgroup divisions aimed at enlivening discussion. Whatever the name, the aim is the same. They are all designed to encourage discussion between participants with the group leader interjecting or steering the discussion as appropriate. The interested reader is directed to the *ABC of Learning and Teaching in Medicine*, where this topic is comprehensively covered [10].

Technology-based teaching

The advent of medical simulators and web-based learning resources has led to a plethora of choice for the motivated learner, but caution is required in evaluating these. It is easy to be wooed by the technology and lose sight of key learning points and objectives; furthermore, it is vital that web-based resources are peer reviewed and evaluated by trusted sources.

MEDICAL SIMULATION

The Royal College of Anaesthetists (http://www.rcoa.ac.uk/), along with many other similar educational bodies worldwide, has developed a competency-based curriculum for medical education. The change towards competency-based training has been driven partly by the need for public accountability and partly to improve efficiency in shorter training times. Anaesthesia lends itself well to the interface between computer-based technology and clinical learning, and many competencies can be taught using high-fidelity simulators [11]. The past decade has seen an expansion in the number of simulator centres for anaesthesia and the formation of a specialist society devoted to their development (SESAM: the Society in Europe for Simulation Applied to Medicine, http://www.sesam.ws). Anaesthesia simulation has been the subject of recent reviews [12,13].

In parallel with the development of simulator courses has come the realisation that our understanding of the science of teaching, let alone trainee assessment, in this environment is in its infancy. It would be a major step forward in appraisal and revalidation if simulated scenarios could be developed that reliably correlated with clinical performance. However, performance is more complicated and multi-layered than this simplistic approach allows at present. The aviation industry is famous for successfully adopting simulator training as a major part of training and revalidation of pilots. However, patients are not as predictable in their responses as aeroplanes. It makes sense to train on a machine in order to operate a machine even if that machine is as complicated as a modern jet. Patients are not machines.

Simulators can reproduce, with a high degree of reality, clinically rare yet life-threatening scenarios without any risk to patients. Teaching and rehearsing crisis management in the simulator is highly effective as it exploits the two major simulator strengths, namely, acquiring technical skills and teaching team management. Human error is a major contributory factor in up to 80 per cent of critical incidents in anaesthesia and performance of team-working strategies that help minimise human error can be learned and rehearsed [14,15]. Chopra and coworkers [16] found that anaesthetists' performance in a malignant hyperpyrexia scenario improved significantly, compared with a control group, if they had received prior training on the simulator. This enhanced performance seemed to be independent of any increase in familiarity with the simulator itself, as those trained in an anaphylaxis algorithm acted as controls. Furthermore, the enhanced performance remained significant 4 months after the initial training.

Technical skills such as airway maintenance [17] and venous cannulation [18] can also be taught. Medical interns

in New York, for example, have been easily trained in airway management skills on a simulator [19]. Furthermore their learning was not influenced by the grade of trainer and retesting confirmed good retention of skills and knowledge weeks and even months after the initial training.

WEB–BASED LEARNING

On-line and computer-based modules are increasingly popular ways of enhancing learning [20]. They have the advantage of being able to be completed at a time and place convenient to the student without necessarily taking them away from clinical experience opportunities. Unlike article and textbook reading they engage the participant and allow self-evaluation. They also allow more demonstrable evidence of having read and absorbed the new information and can be linked to a printable certificate of completion.

There are many excellent resources within our specialty (Table 49.1). The website http://www.doctors.net.uk, for example, hosts several on-line anaesthesia learning modules. The management of a child with obstructive sleep apnoea requiring tonsillectomy and the management of pyloric stenosis are two examples and there are excellent modules on basic and advanced paediatric life support. A pre-course multiple choice questionnaire is followed by a series of case scenarios. Once completed these allow the busy practitioner to gain Royal College of Anaesthetists' CME points and add these to an on-line personal development profile.

Web-based assessment has the advantage of being time efficient and immediate. Multiple choice questions are marked and feedback is immediate; these are excellent ways of encouraging and directing progress. However, only factual knowledge can be accurately assessed in this way and it may be difficult to ensure the authenticity of an individual student's work. More complicated cognitive reasoning is not so easily assessed using this simplistic approach and web-based learning is probably most effectively used when combined into more conventional teaching programmes. Clinical skills and attitudes will always be best learned and assessed at the patient's side.

The Higher Education Academy offers online resources to help design web-based assessment courses at http://www.heacademy.ac.uk/.

Web–based resources

There are many excellent websites devoted to paediatric anaesthesia [21]. Table 49.1 cites some of the most popular but there are many others.

As with all e-learning resources the source needs to be trusted. Increasing effort is being made to peer review web-based resources to ensure their accuracy and educational value through schemes such as Health On the Net Foundation (http://www.hon.ch/med_prof.html) and Intute (formerly OMNI) (http://www.intute.ac.uk/healthandlifesciences/medicine/).

Table 49.1   Some useful web-based teaching resources

Subspecialty	Web address	Summary
General	www.doctors.org.uk	A general resource aimed at UK doctors with on-line CME points and modules
Basic paediatric anaesthesia	http://pedsanesthesia.stanford.edu	Practical guidelines and information on most aspects of the specialty, including pain management
	http://www.virtual-anaesthesia-textbook.com/vat/peds.htm	A web-based textbook describing the anaesthetic management of many procedures, with practical background and clinical information
Cardiology	http://www.kumc.edu/kumcpeds/	A superb cardiology site with diagrams and descriptions of all major cardiac defects including echocardiography footage
Cardiac surgery	http://www.cincinnatichildrens.org/health/heart-encyclopedia/anomalies/	Although primarily written for lay people this is a beautifully illustrated site with descriptions of major congenital cardiac defects, their symptoms, signs and management
Neonates	http://www.neonatology.org/neo.clinical.html	An alphabetically indexed electronic textbook with an extensive number of links to other sites concerned with the care of our smallest patients
Syndromes	http://www.ncbi.nlm.nih.gov/entrez/query.fcgi?db=OMIM	This is a highly extensive list of inherited conditions with detailed descriptions. Whilst not specifically aimed at anaesthetists it is a powerful resource
Pain	http://www.ich.ucl.ac.uk/cpap/	A site run by our own hospital and the Institute of Child Health with links to other resources and courses as well as practical guides
	http://painsourcebook.ca/	A collection of useful pain resources including scoring systems and treatment protocols
	http://www.nysora.com/techniques/pediatric/ultrasound/	A useful, well-referenced resource from the New York School of Regional Analgesia with an emphasis on ultrasound-guided blocks

CME, continuing medical education.

Table 49.2   Assessment and training resources

Body	Web address	Summary
The Postgraduate Medical Education and Training Board (PMETB)	http://www.pmetb.com/	UK body overseeing postgraduate medical education in association with the specialty Royal College
NHS Modernising Medical Careers	http://www.mmc.nhs.uk/	NHS agency: useful information on assessment and competency
NHS Healthcare Assessment and Training	http://www.hcat.nhs.uk/	Detailed information on assessment exercises to be used in training
Royal College of Anaesthetists	http://www.rcoa.ac.uk/docs/cctptiv.pdf	Detailed key competencies expected of a trainee in paediatric anaesthesia

COMPETENCY–BASED TRAINING

Using the teaching and learning resources discussed above, the trainee in paediatric anaesthesia will be expected to demonstrate mastery of key competencies. The Royal College of Anaesthetists have provided a list of expected training competencies for both intermediate and higher level subspecialist trainees in paediatric anaesthesia [22]. The Royal College works with the Postgraduate Medical Education and Training Board (PMETB) to oversee competency assessment (Table 49.2).

Trainees in the UK will be taught relevant skills and, after a period of practice, they will undergo formal assessment. For direct clinical care there are three main assessment tools: (1) Mini-Clinical Evaluation Exercise (mini-CEX); (2) Direct Observation of Procedural Skills (DOPS); and (3) Case-based Discussion (CbD). Documentation, presently restricted to Foundation years (general training, before specialist training), can be seen at http://www.hcat.nhs.uk/foundation/assessments.htm.

Mini-CEX is used for the evaluation of an observed clinical encounter. In paediatric anaesthesia, a mini-CEX could be employed in the assessment of an anaesthesia trainee undertaking a preoperative visit. Among areas assessed are history taking, physical examination skills, communication skills, clinical judgement and professionalism. After the assessment the trainer is required to give feedback to the trainee as part of the learning process.

Direct Observation of Procedural Skills is a structured checklist for the assessment of practical procedures. In paediatric anaesthesia, DOPS could be used, for example, for trainees performing central venous access or an epidural block. Detailed aspects of the procedure are scored, e.g. pre-procedure preparation, aseptic technique, technical ability and post-procedure management. Trainees are scored as being above or below the expected performance of a doctor at their stage of training. A successful trainee would be expected to show improvement over a series of DOPS assessments.

Case-based Discussion is a structured discussion of clinical cases managed by the trainee and is used to evaluate clinical reasoning. In paediatric anaesthesia, the trainee would discuss a range of their clinical workload, with their competency being assessed under a number of broad categories, among which are record keeping, clinical assessment, treatment, post-operative plan and follow-up.

It is the responsibility of the trainee to ensure that the assessments are done, and progress in training is halted if assessments are delayed. It is hoped that this more structured approach to training will ensure competency and help to counteract the effect of reduced working hours and experience.

There are clearly many new and exciting methods of teaching at our disposal. While we should embrace and critically appraise them we should not lose sight of the fact that successful practice in our specialty relies as much on intricate manual skills and sensitive communication within and between teams as it does on knowledge. Knowledge is relatively easy to acquire and test but the nuances of team working and highly technical skills are more subtle and will continue to provide rewarding challenges for teacher and learner alike.

REFERENCES

Key reference

Cantillon P, Hutchinson L, Wood D, eds. *The ABC of learning and teaching in medicine*. London: BMJ Publications, 2003.

References

1. Fitzpatrick B, Gotthardt M, Laulom S *et al.*, eds. *Effective enforcement of EC labour law*. Dordrecht: Kluwer Law International, 2003.
2. General Medical Council. Guidance on good practice. London: General Medical Council, UK, 2006: http://www.gmc-uk.org/education/pro_development/pro_development_guidance.asp
3. Brookefield SD. Adult learning: an overview. In: Tuinjman A, ed. *International encyclopaedia of education*, 2nd edn. Oxford: Pergamon Press, 1996: 375–80.
4. Thomson O'Brien MA, Freemantle N, Oxman AD *et al.* Continuing Medical Education meetings and workshops: effects on professional practice and health care outcomes. *Cochrane Database Syst Rev* 2006, Iss 4.
5. Ali J, Howard M, Williams J. Is attrition of advanced trauma life support acquired skills affected by trauma patient volume? *Am J Surg* 2002; **183**:142–5.
6. Wood DF. ABC of learning and teaching in medicine: problem based learning. *BMJ* 2003; **326**: 326–30.
7. Gordon J. ABC of learning and teaching. One to one teaching and feedback. *BMJ* 2003; **326**: 543–5.
8. Bligh DA, ed. *What's the use of lectures?* San Francisco, CA: Jossey-Bass, 2000.
9. Cantillon P. ABC of learning and teaching in medicine: teaching large groups. *BMJ* 2003; **326**: 437.
10. Jaques D. ABC of learning and teaching in medicine: teaching small groups. *BMJ* 2003; **326**: 492–4.
11. Galvin R. Simulation and anaesthetic training. *R Coll Anaesth Bull* 2006; **35**: 1746–8.
12. Wong AK. Full Scale computer simulators in anaesthesia training and evaluation. *Can J Anaesth* 2004; **51**: 455–64.
13. Wantman A, Chin C. Use of simulation in paediatric anaesthesia training. *Paediatr Anaesth* 2003; **13**: 749–53.
14. Fletcher GC, McGeorge P, Flin RH *et al.* The role of non-technical skills in anaesthesia: a review of current literature. *Br J Anaesth* 2002; **88**: 418–29.
15. Cooper JB, Gaba DM. A strategy for preventing anesthesia accidents. *Int Anesthesiol Clin* 1989; **27**: 148–52.
16. Chopra V, Gesink BJ, de Jong J *et al.* Does training on an anaesthesia simulator lead to improvement in performance? *Br J Anaesth* 1994; **73**: 293–7.
17. Mayo PH, Hackney JE, Mueck JT *et al.* Achieving house staff competence in emergency airway management: results of a teaching program using a computerized patient simulator. *Crit Care Med* 2004; **32**: 2549–50.
18. Scerbo MW, Bliss JP, Schmidt EA *et al.* A comparison of the CathSim system and simulated limbs for teaching intravenous cannulation. *Stud Health Technol Inform* 2004; **98**: 340–6.
19. Rosenthal ME, Adachi M, Ribaudo V *et al.* Achieving housestaff competence in emergency airway management using scenario based simulation training: comparison of attending vs housestaff trainers. *Chest* 2006; **129**: 1453–8.
20. McKimm J, Jollie C, Cantillon P. ABC of learning: web based learning. *BMJ* 2003; **326**: 870–3.
21. Tong JL, Thomas ML. World wide web resources and the paediatric anaesthetist: surfs up. *Paediatr Anaesth* 2001; **11**: 19–27.
22. Royal College of Anaesthetists. *IV: competency based higher and advanced level (ST years 5, 6 and 7) training and assessment*. A manual for trainees and trainers. London: Royal College of Anaesthetists, 2007 (http://www.rcoa.ac.uk/docs/cctptiv.pdf).

50

Paediatric anaesthesia in developing countries

ADRIAN BÖSENBERG

KEY LEARNING POINTS

- Paediatric anaesthesia with limited resources is challenging.
- Children often have major complications of the disease process because of delays in presentation.
- The spectrum of pathology is different and comorbid conditions such as human immunodeficiency virus, tuberculosis and malaria are common.
- War, trauma and violence may be part of everyday life for some children.
- Safe blood products are in short supply.
- Basic safe standards of anaesthesia should be a priority.

INTRODUCTION

Paediatric anaesthesia in the developing world is challenging [1,2]. Up to 45 per cent of the population of many developing countries are less than 15 years of age. Malnutrition is widespread, adding to the health burden, while most children live in rural areas with limited access to basic health care [3]. Spending on health is a low priority for many governments in poorly developed countries and paediatric anaesthesia in the developing world has not advanced to the extent that it has in the developed world. Perioperative mortality and morbidity may be considered to be high compared with the developed world; expectations, however, are often commensurate with the facilities and quality of the available care.

This chapter outlines some of the many challenges facing the paediatric anaesthetist in developing countries. The problems faced in the tropics [4] may be completely different to those faced on a tropical island in the South Pacific [5] or the West Indies [6], at altitude in Nepal [7] or in the humidity of sub-Saharan Africa [1,8]. However, the main problems are: lack of trained personnel; the spectrum and nature of the pathology; the facilities and equipment available; and the use of cheap, generic and perhaps outmoded drugs that are also not always available [2,9].

THE CHILD

Children of the developing world are victims of circumstance: natural disasters, war, social unrest [10] and economic crises render their lot an unenviable one. For many, medical care, or timely access thereto, is a remote or even non-existent possibility [2,3,7,11]. Fear, poor understanding and poor education often result in delayed presentation to medical facilities. Frequently, traditional healers will have had prior involvement, with the consequent risk of bowel perforation from enemas [12] or hepatorenal toxicity from potions. Further delays are engendered when patients have to undertake long journeys to hospital and, if initial misdiagnosis occurs, tertiary referral is made only when complications arise [2,7,13]. A typical example is appendicitis, which is relatively uncommon in the developing world, where many other causes for a change in bowel habit are initially suspected. Most present for surgery with generalised peritonitis and perforation is common. In the developing world, the prospect of providing anaesthesia for a toxic, acidotic and dehydrated child is daunting. Another example is infantile hypertrophic pyloric stenosis, a rare condition in developing countries, where symptoms other than the classic triad of bile-free vomiting, visible peristalsis and a palpable tumour are more likely [14]. The unsuspecting anaesthetist, who may have no access to a laboratory [1] and is also limited in the choice of fluid for resuscitation, would be challenged to manage the gross metabolic derangements in these patients. Superstition may also play a role in increasing anaesthetic risk. For example, rural Vietnamese believe that it is not good to die with an empty stomach; parents consider surgery an enormous risk so they feed their children beforehand. Passage of a nasogastric tube prior to induction is routine [15].

Perinatal mortality in some parts of the developing world is 10 times greater than that in developed countries [16]. The majority of babies are born at home or in rural health centres [3], where basic neonatal resuscitation equipment is often deficient. Those requiring surgery may need to be transferred, but specialised transport teams rarely exist. In some hospitals neonates are not operated on because 'they always die' [17], whereas in others they may undergo surgery without anaesthesia [6,18] because 'it is safer' and the belief that neonates do not feel pain persists. When surgery is undertaken there are additional challenges, particularly in emergency situations [6]. Not only is there a lack of appropriately sized equipment, but it may be extremely difficult to maintain normothermia even in relatively warm climates without improvisation. Regional anaesthesia can play a significant role in neonatal anaesthesia [19] and in some centres may be the only choice [3,20]. Apart from providing analgesia without respiratory depression, the need for postoperative ventilatory support for conditions such as oesophageal atresia [21], congenital diaphragmatic hernia [22] and abdominal wall defects is reduced by continuous epidural analgesia. Regrettably, even neonates who have skilful anaesthesia and surgery may die because of inadequate postoperative care [20]. Unfortunately, the development of highly specialised neonatal anaesthetic and surgical services [3,16,17] is a low priority.

Children and war

Children may be victims of all aspects of violence; they face an intense struggle for survival as a consequence of displacement, separation from or loss of parents, poverty, hunger and disease. They are vulnerable to the abuse of abandonment, abduction, rape and enforced soldiering. An estimated 300 000 children are currently being used as child soldiers in over 30 countries [23]. Many sustain physical injuries and permanent disabilities, while a large number acquire sexually transmitted infections including human immunodeficiency virus (HIV)/acquired immune deficiency syndrome (AIDS). These HIV-positive soldiers become disease vectors in communities where they are deployed [24]. For many of these children acts of violence become the only form of normality, and former victims become the perpetrators [10]. Survivors are subjected to the collapse of economic, health, social and educational infrastructures. Lost and abandoned children sleep on the streets and are forced to beg for food while trying to find their families. Many become child labourers or turn to crime or prostitution for survival [25].

Children in war-torn areas sustain bullet, machete and shrapnel wounds, while others are burned – mutilating injuries that are not commonly seen in civilians [26]. Landmines are responsible for killing or maiming an estimated 12 000 civilians per annum. In Angola, a country with the highest rate of amputees in the world, there were an estimated 5.5 landmines for every child. Continuing landmine explosions remain a chronic legacy of this conflict [26]. Blast injuries leave children without feet or lower limbs, with genital injuries, blindness and deafness – a pattern of injury that has become a post-civil war syndrome encountered by surgeons world-wide [26]. The terrible psychological effects of war persist even though the armed conflict may be over. Mental and psychiatric disorders including post-traumatic stress disorder are common among child survivors.

Pain

Children from an impoverished background seem more stoical and indifferent to even severe pain; following cardiac surgery, children appear to need very little pain relief and are easily soothed by lollipops (A Davis, 2005, personal communication) or play therapy [11]. The majority walk from the intensive care unit to the general ward on the first postoperative day (A Davis, R Ing, personal communication, 2005). This may be an indication that pain assessment in children from an impoverished background is difficult. Many children in acute pain do not show facial expression. Is this stoicism or simply a reflection of malnutrition, lack of social stimulation, severity of illness or even cultural attitude? Language difficulties, cultural barriers and outdated attitudes of the caregiver may endorse this quandary. Although there are many pain assessment instruments available, few have been validated in children from the developing world [27].

HUMAN RESOURCES

Anaesthesia does not have a high profile in developing countries and the consequent critical shortage of personnel is a barrier to progress. It is not perceived as an attractive career for many undergraduates [28], who receive little, if any, exposure to the specialty [29]. Indeed, very few developing countries can afford specialist anaesthetists, except possibly in their principal hospitals, and salaries are usually insufficient to attract suitably trained and qualified practitioners for more than short periods. Emigration further depletes scarce resources. In many African [30] and Asian countries [31] the doctor:patient ratio is so low that the ideal of employing a physician specifically to provide routine anaesthesia is usually out of the question. Anaesthesia is generally provided by non-medical staff; in some centres it is provided by nurses [32] and in others by medical assistants with only rudimentary training [1]. Supervision is invariably inadequate [32] and remuneration is poor. Many provide high-quality anaesthesia for a limited range of surgery but few receive formal training in paediatric or neonatal anaesthesia. Inadequately trained anaesthetists tend to shy away from children, particularly neonates and infants, because of the perceived difficulty and fear. This is understandable in view of the lack of supervision, the severity of the patients' conditions and the deficiency in equipment that is more suited for adults. Invariably the 'paediatric anaesthetist' is someone who may have a special interest or affinity for children or has simply been allocated to paediatric anaesthesia for the day because there is no one else. The paediatric anaesthesiologist as such is a luxury.

PATHOLOGY

Many pathological conditions that are seldom seen in industrialised countries are more prevalent in developing countries because of poor health education, malnutrition, the close proximity of livestock to humans, earth-floored homes, poor sanitation and contaminated water supplies. Some conditions that are prevalent world-wide are of particular relevance to the anaesthetist.

HIV/AIDS

An estimated 40 million people are living with HIV, mostly in the developing world (90 per cent) with sub-Saharan Africa (26 million) and south-east Asia (7.5 million) making up more than 75 per cent of the global total, of which about 6 per cent are children (Fig. 50.1a) [33]. More than 25 million have died of AIDS since 1981; as a consequence, there are an estimated 12 million orphans in Africa alone [33].

Although some success has been achieved in slowing down the transmission of HIV in developed countries, [34,35], in developing countries there are numerous barriers to the treatment of HIV-infected children. The treatment of children has lagged behind that of adults, partly because of the expense of antiretrovirals and the lack of paediatric drug formulations, but mainly because of poor human resources and infrastructure for administration of treatment [36].

Children can be infected by vertical transmission from the mother (>90 per cent) or when sexually abused (around 2 per cent) by an infected adult [37]. Transmission via blood products remains a risk, but, with the global trend towards volunteer donors and more sophisticated testing of blood, this risk is expected to diminish.

Vertical transmission can occur either *in utero*, during labour and delivery, or postnatally. Risk factors include maternal plasma viral load and breastfeeding. Current data indicate that mixed feeding (breastfeeding with other oral foods and liquids) is associated with the greatest risk of transmission [38]. Perinatal transmission rates have been dramatically reduced by single-dose nevirapine treatment, but this strategy protects only about 50 per cent of infants, and more than 75 per cent of women receiving nevirapine develop a major nevirapine-resistant viral mutation. In developed areas of the world, antiretroviral therapy has reduced perinatal transmission by more than 90 per cent compared with the 1993 rate [38].

Differentiating those infants who are infected by vertical transmission from those who are not infected presents a difficult dilemma since all children born to HIV-positive mothers will have HIV antibody for the first 6–18 months. Only 30–40 per cent of those infants who are actually infected begin to make their own antibody to HIV and may go on to develop AIDS. The presence of HIV antibody is therefore not a reliable indicator of infection because one cannot easily differentiate between actively or passively acquired antibodies. More sophisticated expensive tests have been developed but are not yet widely available. All children born to HIV-positive mothers should therefore be considered potentially infected; if antibody persists beyond 15 months, infection should be assumed.

Progression of the disease depends on the mode of transmission; vertically acquired infection is more aggressive. Twenty to thirty per cent of HIV-infected children will develop profound immune deficiency and AIDS-defining illnesses within a year, whereas two-thirds will have a slowly progressive disease. The disease course depends on a variety of factors that include timing of infection *in utero*, the viral load and stage of the disease in the mother.

The clinical manifestation of HIV in infants and children is variable. The majority may have asymptomatic infections, and the presentation may be subtle, e.g. failure to thrive, lymphadenopathy, hepatosplenomegaly, interstitial pneumonia, chronic diarrhoea or persistent oral thrush. Some present for the first time with severe life-threatening disease. Chronic diarrhoea, wasting and severe malnutrition predominate in Africa, whereas systemic and pulmonary pathologies are more common in the USA and Europe. Recurrent bacterial infections, chronic parotid swelling, lymphocytic interstitial pneumonitis (LIP) and early onset of progressive neurological deterioration are characteristic of children with AIDS.

Pulmonary disease is the leading cause of morbidity and mortality [39,40] Bacterial pneumonia, viral pneumonia and pulmonary tuberculosis (TB) are common in children

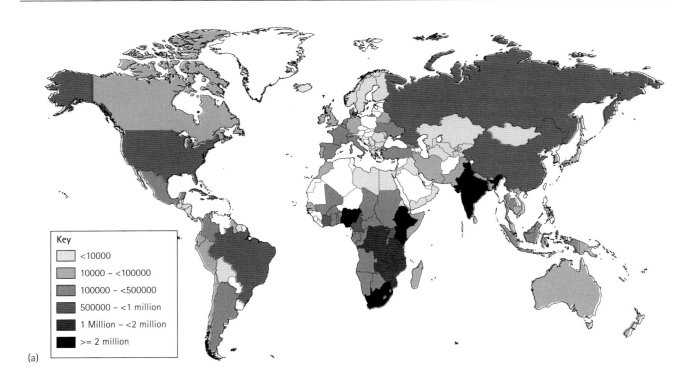

(a)

Key

- <10000
- 10000 – <100000
- 100000 – <500000
- 500000 – <1 million
- 1 Million – <2 million
- >= 2 million

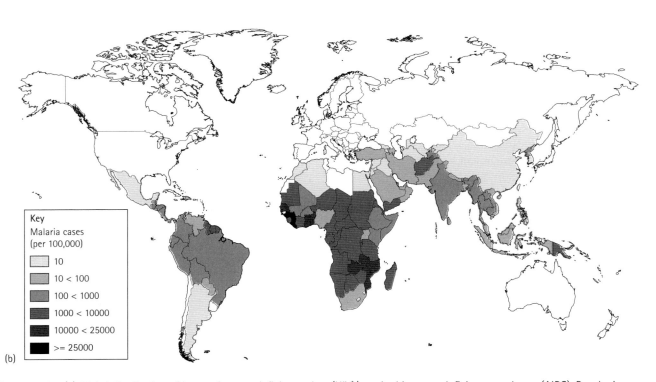

(b)

Key

Malaria cases
(per 100,000)

- 10
- 10 < 100
- 100 < 1000
- 1000 < 10000
- 10000 < 25000
- >= 25000

Figure 50.1   (a) Global distribution of human immunodeficiency virus (HIV)/acquired immune deficiency syndrome (AIDS). Developing countries, particularly sub-Saharan Africa, carry the greatest health burden with the poorest resources. Source: UNAIDS/WHO/UNICEF Epidemiological Fact Sheets on HIV/AIDS and STIs (September 2002). Reproduced with permission from the World Health Organization. (b) Global distribution of malaria. The distribution is remarkably similar to that of HIV/AIDS. Blood products in these regions carry an enormous risk even if family members act as donors. Source: WHO/Malaria Department and Public Health Mapping Group, © World Health Organization, January 2004. Reproduced with permission.

throughout the developing world. The course of these diseases is more fulminant when associated with HIV infection. Acute opportunistic infections occur when the CD4 T-cell count falls, including *Pneumocystis carinii* pneumonia (PCP), *Pneumocystis jirovecii* pneumonia (PJP) and cytomegalovirus, as well as the more typical *Haemophilus influenzae,* streptococcus pneumonia and respiratory syncytial virus infections [39,40]. The classic presentation of PCP is fever, tachypnoea, dyspnoea and marked hypoxaemia, but in some children the presentation is more indolent with hypoxaemia preceding clinical or radiological changes. A slowly progressive chronic form of lung disease, LIP or pulmonary lymphoid hyperplasia, is seen in older children and can lead to an insidious onset of dyspnoea, cough and chronic hypoxia with normal auscultatory findings. In contrast to adults, LIP may cause acute respiratory failure in children and is treated with steroids and bronchodilators. Management of the upper airway may be difficult in the presence of stomatitis and gingival disease. Intubation may be difficult in the presence of acute (*Candida*) or chronic epiglottitis (lymphoid hyperplasia), or necrotising laryngotracheitis or Kaposi's sarcoma.

Cardiac disease is being recognised with increasing frequency in HIV-infected children. The pathogenesis of the cardiomyopathy is multifactorial and includes pulmonary insufficiency, anaemia, nutritional deficiencies, specific viral infections and drug therapy. Left- and right-ventricular dysfunction, arrhythmias and pericardial effusions are seen. Human immunodeficiency virus may directly infect the myocardium itself leading to early electrocardiogram (ECG) changes, or abnormal echocardiograms showing either hyperdynamic left-ventricular dysfunction or evidence of diminished contractility.

The gastrointestinal tract is commonly involved [41], particularly in tropical countries, and affected children show evidence of malabsorption ('slim'), chronic recurrent diarrhoea, dysphagia, failure to thrive or enteric infection. These children may require endoscopy for diagnostic studies. From the anaesthetist's point of view there is an increased risk of reflux secondary to oesophagitis, which may be infective (e.g. *Candida* or cytomegalovirus) or drug induced (e.g. zidovudine), while pseudobulbar palsy or oesophageal strictures also occur. Pseudobulbar palsy may be a manifestation of central neurological involvement.

Nausea and vomiting may have a neurological, infective or drug-related cause. Pancreatitis, lymphomas or smooth muscle tumours may delay gastric emptying. Hepatomegaly is invariably present but severe hepatocellular dysfunction is seldom a major problem unless chronic hepatitis (hepatitis B or C, or cytomegalovirus) is present. Cholestasis and fluctuating transaminase levels may be caused by HIV or poor nutrition, or be drug induced.

Neurological impairment is seen in most symptomatic HIV-infected children – commonly a progressive encephalopathy with developmental delay, progressive motor dysfunction and behavioural changes. Craniofacial dysmorphic features have been described. Haematological abnormalities can reflect depression of all cell lines. Anaemia

may be caused by primary marrow failure, malnutrition or be drug induced, while thrombocytopenia may occur as a result of autoimmunity.

Universal precautions should be strictly applied for all anaesthetic procedures. Extra care should be taken when anaesthetising an HIV-infected patient. Precautions should also be taken to prevent contamination of the anaesthetic circuits. Disposable equipment, bacterial filters and disposable circuits are recommended; however, the prohibitive cost for most institutions in developing countries limits the use of disposables. Reusable equipment should be cleaned, sterilised and decontaminated according to the manufacturer's instructions. Fortunately, HIV is sensitive to a wide range of disinfectants [42].

Tuberculosis

Tuberculosis remains an important cause of morbidity and mortality [43]. The epidemiology of paediatric TB is shaped by risk factors such as age, race, immigration, poverty, overcrowding and HIV/AIDS [43,44]. The emergence of drug-resistant TB adds to the burden and is a constant danger to healthcare workers in general and anaesthetists in particular.

Primary TB infection usually does not produce clinical illness in well-nourished immunised children, whereas reactivated pulmonary TB is a chronic or subacute disease, which may present a variety of challenges for the anaesthetist. These difficulties range from a need to prevent transmission by contamination of the anaesthetic circuits to the risks associated with pleural effusions, pulmonary cavitation and bronchiectasis. Mediastinal and hilar lymphadenopathy may severely compromise the airway.

Primary TB and its complications are more common in children than in adults. Once infected, young children are at increased risk of progression to extrapulmonary disease [43,44]. *Mycobacterium tuberculosis* can cause symptomatic disease in any organ of the body, usually a reactivation of a latent site of infection. The most common sites of reactivation are lymph nodes, bones and joints, and the genitourinary tract. Less frequently the disease involves the gastrointestinal tract, peritoneum, pericardium or skin. Tuberculosis meningitis and miliary TB, more common in children, carry a high mortality [43]. Because of the high prevalence of HIV infection in tuberculous children, HIV testing should be performed on all children with TB; conversely, TB should be sought in all HIV-positive children.

Malaria

Malaria is a febrile flu-like illness caused by one of four species of malaria parasites: *Plasmodium falciparum, Plasmodium vivax, Plasmodium ovale* and *Plasmodium malariae* (Fig. 50.1b). Effective and safe prophylaxis against malaria has become increasingly difficult because the species that causes the most severe illness, *P. falciparum,* has become widely resistant to chloroquine and in some areas to other antimalarial drugs as well [45]. Severe malaria even when optimally treated carries a mortality rate of 10–25 per cent [45].

Prompt diagnosis and early treatment are an important determinant of outcome. Uncomplicated malaria usually presents as fever, headache, dizziness and arthralgia. Gastro-intestinal symptoms may predominate and include anorexia, nausea, vomiting and abdominal discomfort or pain that may mimic appendicitis. Malaria in children can present with an acute life-threatening disease or run a chronic course with acute exacerbations. The acute manifestations include three overlapping syndromes: respiratory distress secondary to a severe underlying metabolic acidosis (pH < 7.3) usually a lactic acidaemia; severe anaemia (haemoglobin < 5 mg) with hypovolaemia [46]; and neurological impairment as a manifestation of cerebral malaria. Seizures are an important presenting feature of cerebral malaria in 60–80 per cent of cases. Prolonged seizures refractory to treatment, and those that occur on antimalarial treatment, are ominous signs and are associated with neurological sequelae or death [46]. Cerebral malaria can also manifest as a prolonged post-ictal state, status epilepticus, severe metabolic derangement (hypoglycaemic and metabolic acidosis) and/or primary neurological syndrome ranging from diffuse cortical involvement to brainstem abnormalities.

Children with chronic malaria adjust physiologically to low haemoglobin levels but may decompensate rapidly when challenged with a febrile illness or surgery. The characteristic physical findings in children with severe anaemia are respiratory distress and a hyperdynamic circulation. Blood transfusion can be administered rapidly in children with metabolic acidosis since most of these children have depleted intravascular volumes.

Although controversial, exchange transfusion has been advocated for severe malaria (i.e. those with cardiorespiratory compromise, hyperparasitaemia and/or cerebral malaria). The rationale is to remove harmful metabolites, toxins and cytokines, to decrease the parasite load and remove deformed red cells, while restoring normal red cell mass, platelets and other clotting factors [45]. Unfortunately, many malaria endemic areas also have a high prevalence of HIV, adding significantly to the risk of blood transfusions.

Chronic recurrent malarial infections may manifest with splenic enlargement. This may cause delayed gastric emptying and pose an aspiration risk on induction of anaesthesia. The spleen may also enlarge acutely, or rupture spontaneously during coughing, vomiting or defecation. Rupture during external cardiac massage has also been described. Malaria may cause bloody diarrhoea with massive fluid loss fluid resembling dysentery in children.

Cardiac disease

Paediatric cardiac services are generally too expensive for most developing countries and the increasing economic divide threatens those services that do exist [47]. In North America each cardiac centre serves 120 000 people; in contrast, one centre serves 16 million people in Asia and 33 million in Africa [48]. Despite the need, few units in the developing world can treat the required volume of cases. Unless families have the financial means to travel to a developed country, the options for diagnostic or therapeutic cardiac procedures are poor [11]. Medical missions may provide immediate help, but their impact on a developing country is short term and potentially disruptive. These visiting teams, ultimately, have little impact on the complex socioeconomic and sociopolitical problems that exist [47].

Rheumatic heart disease is more common than congenital heart disease in many developing countries, reflecting the socioeconomic problems of poverty, overcrowding, malnutrition and lack of antibiotics. Children often present late with life-threatening symptoms secondary to repeated infections and superimposed endocarditis. The acute deterioration precipitated by endocarditis may be the factor that prompts the search for medical attention. Valve replacement may be life saving but long-term follow-up of anticoagulant therapy is often not feasible.

Congenital heart disease is an additional challenge and it is not uncommon to see congenital heart defects in adults in developing countries. Those who have survived without the benefit of palliative or corrective surgery also present with a high incidence of pulmonary hypertension or endocarditis. Total correction of these defects is generally not feasible and palliative surgery may be the more effective alternative. Excellent palliation with reasonable quality of life can be achieved relatively cheaply [47].

Tetanus

Tetanus is a disease characterised by painful tonic muscle spasms, hyperreflexia and autonomic instability. It is caused by the exotoxin of *Clostridium tetani*, an organism that is ever present in the soil and in contaminated wounds. Although rarely seen in developed countries, tetanus is prevalent in countries where children are not immunised routinely. Tetanus neonatorum carries a high mortality and is still encountered in those areas where it is customary to apply faeces to the umbilical cord to stop it bleeding.

The clinical manifestations of the disease are not the result of invasive tissue injury but are secondary to the production of a potent neurotoxin, tetanospasmin, at the site of the injury. The injury may be trivial and may not even be detectable at the time of presentation. The incubation period is inversely proportional to the distance between the site of the injury and the central nervous system. In children this usually occurs within 14 days of the injury.

Trismus is the presenting symptom in the majority of cases, and sustained trismus produces a characteristic sardonic smile (risus sardonicus). Persistent contractions of the chest and back muscles result in opisthotonus.

Restlessness and irritability may be followed by tetanic seizures often precipitated by trivial stimuli (touch, noise). Glottic or laryngeal spasm can cause sudden death. Late deaths may occur as a result of nosocomial infection, renal failure, sudden cardiac arrest or cerebral haemorrhage as a result of the autonomic instability [49].

Treatment consists of surgical debridement of the wound, administration of human tetanus immunoglobulin, antibiotic therapy and intensive supportive medical care. Ventilatory support is invariably necessary because the frequent spasms impair ventilation, which is already compromised by sedative therapy. Benzodiazepines and opiates are the mainstay of treatment but numerous protocols have been tried [49]. Pain management should also be considered and the author has been encouraged by the use of continuous epidural analgesia for these children. Further advantages of epidural analgesia include good control of the autonomic instability, earlier wean from ventilatory support and possibly a reduction in the complication rate [49]. Trismus responds to muscle relaxants and does not pose as significant an intubation problem as the uninitiated might expect.

EQUIPMENT

Essential equipment to provide safe anaesthesia for children and neonates is often lacking [7]. Small intravenous cannulae are a precious resource and butterfly needles are still used (and in some cases reused). Syringe pumps and other control devices are impractical in environments that have an erratic electricity supply. A full range of sizes of tracheal tubes is rarely found and they are always recycled as there is no other option. Intravenous fluids are very expensive if not manufactured locally, and many developing countries do not have any local production facilities [2]. The choice of intravenous fluid is therefore limited and in short supply.

Monitoring is basic: a precordial stethoscope and a finger on the pulse [1]. Appropriately sized blood pressure cuffs are seldom available. Pulse oximetry has been shown to be the most useful monitor and should ideally be made available in all centres where paediatric surgery is performed [1,7].

Anaesthetic machines in developing countries fall into two categories: modern sophisticated machines or simple low-maintenance equipment. Modern electronic machines, provided by well-meaning donors have a poor track record in austere environments. Sophisticated equipment needs to be understood, but this is not aided by operating manuals in a foreign language. Often these machines are discarded at their first fault because maintenance is inadequate or non-existent, guarantees are not likely to be honoured, and faults are too expensive to repair. Poorly maintained equipment is generally unusable but, in untrained hands, becomes hazardous or even life threatening.

Simplicity and safety have long been the key to anaesthetic equipment in developing countries [1,2]. Ideally, a suitable anaesthetic machine should be inexpensive, versatile, robust and able to withstand extreme climatic conditions. It should be able to function even if the supply of cylinders or electricity is interrupted, easy to understand and operate by those with limited training, economical to use and easily maintained by locally available skills [50,51]. The cheapest, most practical, and most widely used anaesthetic is inhalational anaesthesia administered through an EMO (Epstein–Macintosh–Oxford, Penlon Ltd, Abingdon, UK) or OMV (Oxford Miniature Vaporiser, Penlon Ltd) draw-over vaporiser. Oxygen concentrators supplement oxygen delivery and eliminate the need for expensive oxygen cylinders with reducing valves that are often faulty or destroyed in these austere environments. The most appropriate ventilator is the Manley Multivent Ventilator, which essentially functions like a mechanical version of the OIB (Oxford Inflating Bellows) and can be used with a draw-over system [51].

A general scheme for inhalational anaesthesia in developing countries is shown in Fig. 50.2 [52] and was first proposed by Ezi Ashi et al. [53]. Applying this scheme four different modes can used and modified according to the available supplies and services. The basic mode, mode A, is for use when there is no electricity and no supply of compressed gases. The apparatus consists of a low-resistance vaporiser linked by valves to the patient to act as a draw-over system with room air as the carrier gas. The self-inflating bag or hand bellows makes it possible to provide artificial ventilation while the vaporiser remains as a draw-over. The addition of low-flow oxygen to the inspired gas in mode B is dependent on the availability of an oxygen cylinder. The addition of a length of reservoir tubing to the circuit enables oxygen to be stored on expiration, to be used on the next inspiration, substantially improving its economy [54].

When electricity is available (mode C) the operation of the anaesthetic apparatus can be extended by permitting: (1) the use of an air compressor to provide continuous gas flow (which in turn would allow the use of a Boyle apparatus and plenum vaporiser); (2) oxygen concentrator; and (3) ventilators. When nitrous oxide is available (mode D), all types of inhalational anaesthesia currently available in developed countries can be practised. In situations where services and supplies are interrupted, even acutely, it is possible to change from one mode to another without requiring other anaesthetic apparatus. These techniques may be of little interest to the anaesthetist working comfortably in the well-maintained sophisticated environment of developed nations. However, their role is considerable in the field (e.g. war and natural disasters) and today's anaesthetist should be acquainted with their functioning in this unpredictable world.

Draw-over anaesthesia

Draw-over anaesthesia enables inhalational anaesthesia to be administered using atmospheric air as the carrier gas. The essential features of this system consist of a calibrated

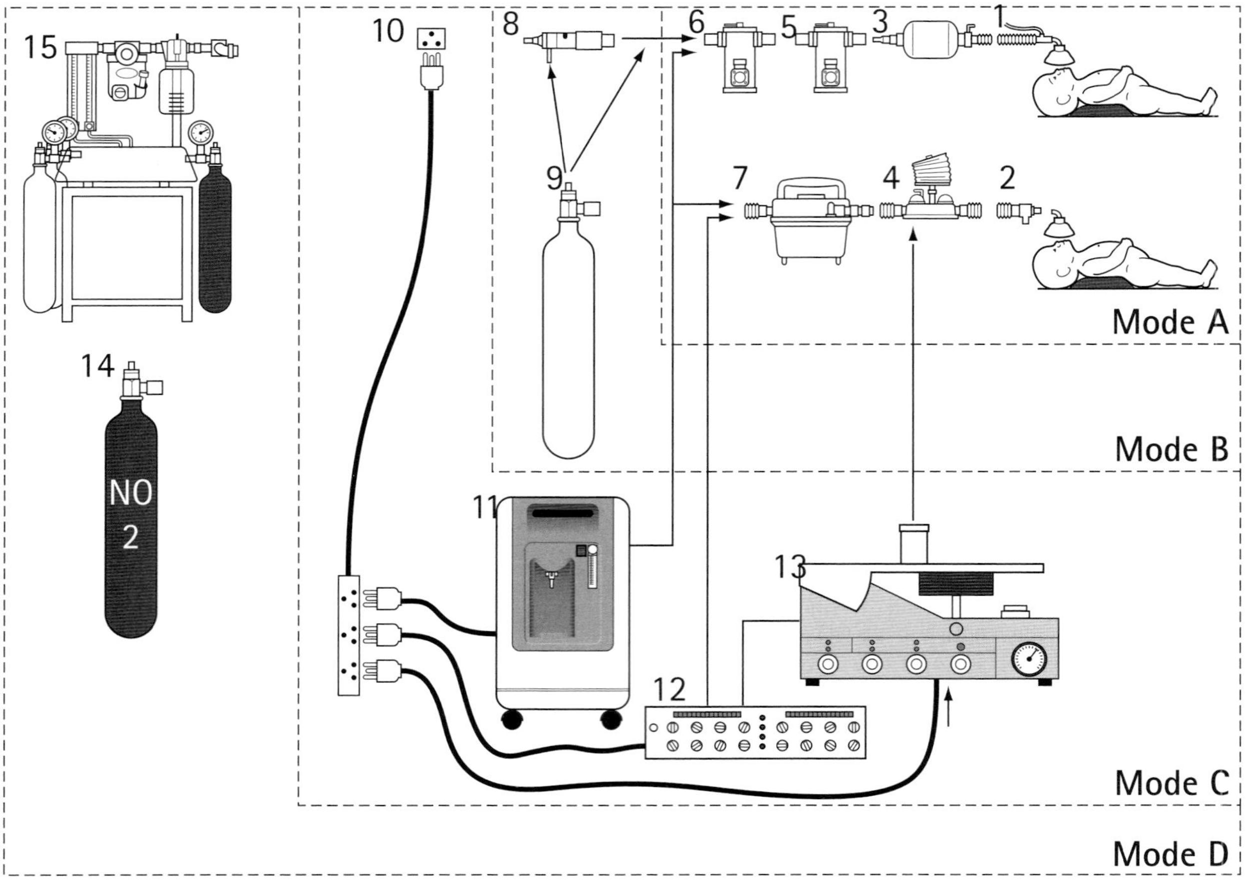

Figure 50.2 A schematic diagram of anaesthetic systems that could be used depending on available resources. Mode A provides basic inhalational anaesthesia with air, spontaneous ventilation or self-inflating bags. Draw-over vaporisers are required. Mode B provides oxygen enrichment but requires the availability of oxygen cylinders. Plenum vaporisers can be used. Mode C requires electricity to power the oxygen concentrator, air compressor and/or ventilator. A mechanical ventilator, e.g. Manley, does not require electrical power. Mode D requires a Boyle machine and nitrous oxide cylinders. 1, T-piece with reservoir tube and face-mask; 2, Ambu Paedi valve; 3, self-inflating (AmBu) bag; 4, Oxford Inflating Bellows (OIB); 5, Oxford Miniature Vaporiser (OMV) with halothane; 6, OMV with trichloroethylene; 7, EMO (Epstein–Macintosh–Oxford) vaporiser with ether. These circuits and manual ventilators are interchangeable and ether, halothane or trichloroethylene can be used on its own or in series. 8, Farman's entrainer with an oxygen cylinder (9) can be used to supplement oxygen, or an electrical power source (10) is available with an oxygen concentrator (11), air compressor (12) or Manley ventilator (13). Nitrous oxide (14) and Boyle apparatus (15) allow anaesthesia practice equivalent to that of developed countries.

vaporiser with sufficiently low resistance (EMO and OMV) to allow the negative pressure created by the patient's inspiratory effort to draw room air through the vaporiser during spontaneous ventilation. Positive pressure ventilation can be provided by means of a self-inflating bag or bellows (OIB), with a valve to prevent the gas mixture re-entering the vaporiser, as well as a unidirectional valve at the patient's airway to direct expired gases to the atmosphere, preventing rebreathing (Fig. 50.2, mode A). In this way an anaesthetic can be administered in the absence of compressed gases. The vaporiser has an inlet for supplementary oxygen that can be attached to the oxygen output tube of an oxygen concentrator, or oxygen cylinder when available (Fig. 50.2, modes B and C).

The EMO and the OMV are the more commonly used low-resistance vaporisers. The EMO is calibrated only for

ether but its performance is linear for other agents. The OMV is calibrated for a variety of agents [17,51], but despite the lack of temperature compensation its performance is stable under most conditions. Both these vaporisers have been used successfully in paediatric anaesthetic practice [11] but it is recommended that they be converted to form a T-piece for greater safety.

The OMV has been evaluated as a simple draw-over system for paediatric anaesthesia. Wilson and Bem [17] showed that, when a self-inflation bag is used in a draw-over mode, more efficient vaporisation occurs despite vaporiser cooling. However, the respiratory efforts of neonates or weak infants are insufficient to operate the valve mechanisms of the self-inflating bag (e.g. AmBu bag), necessitating continuous assisted ventilation even in the presence of ether, which stimulates ventilation.

Oxygen concentrators

Improved oxygen availability, independent of compressed gas and electrical power supply, can be provided by linking oxygen concentrators to a draw-over anaesthetic apparatus as was first described by Fenton [55]. Maintenance requirements are low and servicing is recommended only after about 10 000 hours of usage. The benefits are enormous.

The concentrator functions by having ambient air pumped by a compressor through one of two canisters containing a molecular sieve of zeolite granules that reversibly absorb nitrogen from compressed air [8,51]. The controls are simple and comprise an on/off switch for the compressor and a flow-control knob that is set to deliver up to 5 L/min. The flow of oxygen continues uninterrupted as the canisters are alternated automatically so that oxygen from one canister is available while the other regenerates. A warning light on a built-in oxygen analyser illuminates if the oxygen concentration falls below 85 per cent and the concentrator switches off automatically when the oxygen concentration falls below 70 per cent. This is heralded by visual and audible alarms. Air is then delivered as the emerging gas. Modern machines are relatively silent.

The oxygen output of the concentrator is dependent on the size of the unit, inflow of oxygen, minute volume and pattern of ventilation. The addition of deadspace (or oxygen economiser tube) at the outlet improves the performance, and predictable concentrations of greater than 90 per cent oxygen can be obtained with flows from 1 L/min to 5 L/min independent of the pattern of ventilation. Much lower concentrations and less predictability were noted when the deadspace tubing was omitted [54].

The possible hazards of oxygen concentrators are few provided that they are positioned in the operating room so that the in-draw area is free from pollutants. Failure of power supply or failure of the zeolite canisters will result in the delivery of ambient air. A bacterial filter at the outlet combined with the use of dust-free zeolite should prevent contamination of the delivered gas. Dirty internal air filters may produce lower oxygen concentrations and must be checked. An oxygen storage tank and booster pumps afford protection against the vagaries in electrical supply.

DRUGS

The supply of anaesthetic gases and drugs to rural medical facilities is erratic and unreliable. Furthermore, the cost of many drugs, particularly the modern agents, has risen alarmingly above and beyond the reach of most health budgets. Anaesthetists in developing countries therefore have to resign themselves to using cheaper agents or generics. Ether and halothane remain the mainstay of anaesthesia in many countries [1,2,8,9] but in some trichloroethylene is still available, and is sometimes used in combination with ether or halothane. Ether is cheaper than halothane and is probably safer, although its use is limited by its flammability. Flammability may also limit its transportation and therefore its availability.

Ketamine is probably the most commonly used anaesthetic agent, particularly by the occasional paediatric anaesthetist. It is simple to use, effective and relatively safe when used as a sole agent for short procedures, in combination with muscle relaxants or to supplement general anaesthesia for major surgery. The dosage used ranges from 5 mg/kg to 10 mg/kg when given intramuscularly, 1 mg/kg to 2 mg/kg intravenously and 2 mg/kg to 5 mg/kg/h or by continuous infusion. Ketamine should be used with midazolam 10–20 μg/kg/h to reduce the hallucinatory side-effects. However, benzodiazepines are not always available. Morphine and other opiates may not be permitted in some cultures. The choice of muscle relaxants is also limited in many areas. Suxamethonium, gallamine, curare, alcuronium or pancuronium is the usual option, and the choice is dictated by their availability or the availability of reversal agents.

The cost of nitrous oxide may be prohibitive in terms of storage, erratic delivery and budgetary constraints [53,55]. Closed or semi-closed anaesthetic systems are considered dangerous in an environment where the oxygen supply is erratic [53] and agent monitors are not available [7]. The erratic supply of soda lime and compressed gas cylinders further limits it use. Consequently, the potential benefits and cost saving of low-flow anaesthesia is lost [53].

Regional anaesthesia has many benefits, in terms of safety, cost savings and for postoperative analgesia [3,6,18,19,22,56,57]. Generally, children in developing countries accept this form of analgesia. However, there seems to be a general reluctance to perform regional anaesthesia on children. Possible reasons include lack of training or expertise, fear of failure and the unavailability of drugs, disposables and other ancillary equipment.

Access to the epidural space can be obtained if the appropriate equipment is not available. A catheter can be threaded into the epidural space through an intravenous cannula inserted into the caudal space via the sacral hiatus in neonates and small infants [58]. Cheaper non-insulated needles have also been used successfully for peripheral nerve blocks when more expensive insulated needles are not available [59].

BLOOD SAFETY

Blood transfusion services, if they exist, aim to provide a life-saving service by ensuring an adequate supply of safe blood [60]. Patients, particularly children, in developing countries face the greatest risks from unsafe blood and blood products [61]. An estimated 70 per cent of all blood transfusions in Africa are given to children with severe anaemia caused by malaria.

Fewer than 30 per cent of developing countries have a nationally coordinated blood transfusion service. Many of these do not even perform the most rudimentary tests for diseases such as HIV or hepatitis B and C because of economic constraints. Even limited testing doubles the basic cost of a unit of blood. It is estimated that, annually, some six million tests that should be done globally to check for infections are not done.

Many countries still rely on paid donors or a family member to donate blood prior to surgery. In Argentina, for example, up to 92 per cent of the blood supply is from family members. Although Pakistan, for example, has increased its voluntary unpaid blood donation to 20 per cent in the last 5 years, family donors made up 70 per cent and paid donors 10 per cent in 2004 [61]. Over the past decade, through concerted efforts by the World Health Organization to improve blood safety world-wide, the number of voluntary unpaid donors has increased considerably. In China, voluntary blood donation went from 45 per cent of donations in 2000 to 90 per cent in 2004. In Bolivia the rate of voluntary, unpaid donations increased from 10 per cent in 2002 to 50 per cent in 2005. Malaysia, China and India reached 100 per cent screening of donated blood for HIV by the year 2000 [62].

There are risks in any system. Family and paid donors may hide aspects of their health and lifestyle that could make the blood unsafe (see Chapter 24). Family members may feel pressured to donate whereas paid donors are driven by need and avoid important details about their health status. The commercial plasma industry and blood trade can fuel the transmission of HIV. In 1999, 26 million litres of plasma were fractionated for global use [63]; the major source was paid donors from developing countries. Voluntary, unpaid donors have a greater sense of responsibility towards their community and keep themselves healthy so as to be able to keep giving safe blood. South Africa has had 100 per cent voluntary, unpaid donation since it established a national blood service. With HIV prevalence approaching 30 per cent in the adult population, only 0.02 per cent of its regular blood donors have contracted HIV.

Storage of blood is difficult considering the unreliable and unpredictable electricity supply. To obviate the risk of transmission of malaria, HIV and other infectious diseases, blood should be transfused only when absolutely necessary. In sophisticated units the use of pre-donated autologous blood is an option [64]. In poorer countries this is not practical because malnutrition and chronic anaemia are common in many adults and children. Lack of appropriate equipment and cost are also prohibitive. Similarly, intraoperative blood salvage, let alone cell savers appropriate for use in children, is simply not available. Recombinant factor VII, which is being used more and more to reduce blood usage by those who can afford it [64], is not available in many countries.

THE VISITOR

Personality traits compatible with survival have been suggested as a prerequisite for working in the austere environments of the developing world. These traits include an almost pathological desire for hard work, a willingness to merge or at least sympathise with a different culture, patience to relate to and teach people sometimes far removed educationally, the ability to withstand prolonged periods of cultural isolation but mostly a never-failing ability to improvise and make the best of a bad situation [52,65]. There is no place for risk-taking 'cowboy anaesthetists' [65].

International travel, particularly visits to many parts of the developing world, needs careful preparation and planning whether the anaesthetist is part of a volunteer organisation [11,66,67] or travelling as an individual. Detailed advice [66,67] is beyond the scope of this chapter but some generalisations are made based on personal experience and observations of colleagues. Changing political climates and international health guidelines dictate visa and vaccination requirements. Expert advice should be sought to tailor the traveller's needs according to the individual's medical and immunisation history, the duration of stay and proposed itinerary.

Physical acclimatisation (ranging from jet lag to altitude sickness, heat or sunburn) will be necessary, as well as an adjustment to the local culture and cuisine. Social graces acceptable in a western culture may be deemed offensive in some other cultures. An interpreter is an important ally. However, the inability to understand a language or the local dialect places a visiting anaesthetist at a serious disadvantage, particularly when dealing with children. Children often use subtle ways to describe their feelings that even a skilled interpreter may fail to convey.

The hospital environment may be disconcerting for some. In contrast to the familiar comforts of a clean child-friendly hospital, the visitor may be struck by the relatively shabby, bland appearance of many hospitals in developing countries. The buildings may not have received a coat of paint since they were originally built and broken windowpanes provide the only air conditioning. Children are usually cared for in adult wards.

In the operating room the visitor may be faced with anaesthetic equipment barely recognisable from its original manufacture or in a state of disrepair with non-standard improvisations in an attempt to make it functional. The choice of drugs may be limited; the names of locally manufactured generic drugs and the presentation of intravenous solutions may add to the confusion. Surgical safety may be the next issue. Informed consent, as we know it, and patient identification in the absence of parents may not be obvious to the newcomer. A local or itinerant surgeon may suggest an extensive procedure on a malnourished child without consideration for monitoring, blood transfusion or availability of intensive care or postoperative analgesia in an unmonitored environment. The anaesthetist is obliged to consider the risks and benefits carefully in such circumstances.

Different standards of anaesthetic practice may emerge from different parts of the world. Such standards need not necessarily be considered inferior but may well open the way for the assimilation of new ideas [68]. A safe anaesthetic is not necessarily the most expensive one. After all, it is not the agents that we use but the skill with which we use them that determines outcome. It should never be necessary to depart from the dictum *'primum non nocere'*. Simplicity may be the key, but there is no place for double standards. Guidelines, evolved over time in the UK, the USA and Australia may be untenable in many parts of the world [68], but every attempt should be made to exercise the same standard of care as expected in the developed countries. Children deserve no less!

ACKNOWLEDGEMENTS

The author acknowledges the input provided by Haydn Perndt (Ethiopia), Isabelle Murat (Francophone Africa), Anneke Meursing (Malawi), Carol Parrot (Vietnam), Annette Davis (Mozambique), Richard Ing (Nicaragua), Jeff Morray (Khazakstan), David Baines (East Timor), Narko Tuotuo (Solomon Islands), Zippy Gathuya (Kenya), Felix Namboya (Malawi), Sats Bhagwanjee, Dave Muckart and Larry Hadley (South Africa) – all of whom have worked or are working in a developing country. All tried, as I did, to ensure that important points were not omitted. I would also like to thank my hosts Philemon Amambo (Namibia), Eric Borgstein (Malawi), Ali Salaama (Sudan), Carlos Parsloe (Brazil), Dr Gunnesar (Mauritius), the Indian Society of Paediatric Critical Care, the Malaysian Society of Anaesthetists and the Zimbabwean Society of Anaesthetists, who afforded me the opportunity to visit their respective countries and gain a glimpse of anaesthetic practice in those parts of the world.

REFERENCES

Key references

Bosenberg AT, Bland BA, Schulte-Steinberg O, Downing JW. Thoracic epidural anaesthesia via caudal route in infants. *Anesthesiology* 1988; **69**: 265–9.

Eltringham RJ, Varvinski A. The Oxyvent. *Anaesthesia* 1997; **52**: 668–72.

Ezi Ashi TI, Papworth DP, Nunn JF. Inhalational anaesthesia in developing countries. *Anaesthesia* 1983; **38**: 729–35.

References

1. Hodges SC, Hodges AM. A protocol for safe anasthesia for cleft lip and palate surgery in developing countries *Anaesthesia* 2000; **55**: 436–41.
2. Steward DJ. Anaesthesia care in developing countries. *Paediatr Anaesth* 1998; **8**: 279–82.
3. Ameh EA, Dogo PM, Nmadu PT. Emergency neonatal surgery in a developing country. *Pediatr Surg Int* 2001; **17**: 448–51.
4. Crofts IJ. Trials and tribulations of surgery in rural tropical areas. *Trop Doct* 1980; **10**: 9–14.
5. Hatfield AH. Anaesthesia and anaesthetic training in the Pacific Islands. *Anaesth Intensive Care* 1989; **17**: 56–61.
6. Duncan ND, Brown B, Dundas SE *et al.* 'Minimal intervention management' for gastroschisis: a preliminary report. *West Indian Med J* 2005; **54**: 152–4.
7. Hoffmann E, Duck M, Oberhur A, Paul M. Anaesthesia for repair of cleft lip, maxilla and palate in Nepal. *Eur J Anaesthesiol* 2003; **20**: 677–78.
8. Fenton PM. The cost of Third World anaesthesia: an estimate of consumption of drugs and equipment in anaesthetic practice in Malawi. *Cent Afr J Med* 1994; **40**: 137–9.
9. Brown TCK. Two worlds of anaesthesia. *Anaesth Intensive Care* 1989; **17**: 6–8.
10. Albertyn R, Bickler SW, van As AB *et al.* The effects of war on children in Africa. *Pediatr Surg Int* 2003; **19**: 227–32.
11. Schechter WS, Navedo A, Jordan D *et al.* Paediatric cardiac anaesthesia in a developing country. Guatemala Heart Team. *Paediatr Anaesth* 1998; **8**: 283–92.
12. Grant HW, Buccimazza I, Hadley GP. A comparison of colo-colic and ileo-colic intussusception. *J Pediatr Surg* 1996; **31**: 1607–10.
13. Wiersma R, Hadley GP. Minimizing surgery in complicated intussusceptions in the Third world. *Pediatr Surg* 2004; **20**: 215–17.
14. Emmink B, Hadley GP, Wiersma R. Infantile hypertrophic pyloric stenosis in a Third-world environment. *S Afr Med J* 1992; **82**: 168–70.
15. Scheepstra GL. The Dutch Interplast in Vietnam. *World Anaesth* 1997; **1**: 2.
16. Sola A, Farina D. Neonatal respiratory care and infant mortality in emerging countries. *Pediatr Pulmonol* 1999; **27**: 303–4.
17. Wilson IH, Bem MJ. A view from developing countries. In: Hughes DG, Mather SJ, Wolf AR, eds. *Handbook of neonatal anaesthesia*. London: WB Saunders Co., 1996: 338–50.
18. Kikunga, Sikolo B *et al.* Spinal blocks in paediatric surgery. All Africa Anaesthetic Congress, 1997: 80 (Abstr).
19. Williams RK, Adams DC, Aladjem EV *et al.* The safety and efficacy of spinal anesthesia for surgery in infants: the Vermont Infant Spinal Registry. *Anesth Analg* 2006; **102**: 67–71.
20. Chowdhary SK, Chalapathi G, Narasimhan KL *et al.* An audit of neonatal colostomy for high anorectal malformation: the developing world perspective. *Pediatr Surg Int* 2004; **20**: 111–13.
21. Bosenberg A, Wiersma R, Hadley GP. Oesophageal atresia: caudothoracic epidural anaesthesia reduces the need for postoperative ventilatory support. *Pediatr Surg Int* 1992; **7**: 289–91.
22. Hodgson RE, Bosenberg A, Hadley GP. Congenital diaphragmatic hernia repair – impact of delayed surgery and epidural anaesthesia. *S Afr J Surg* 2000; **38**: 31–4.
23. Uppard S. Child soldiers and children associated with fighting forces. *Med Confl Surviv* 2003; **19**: 121–7.
24. Tripodi P, Patel P. HIV/AIDS peacekeeping and conflict crises in Africa. *Med Confl Surviv* 2004; **20**: 195–208.

25. Spry-Levenson J. Lessons in survival for children of war. *Gemini News* 1996 (http://www.pangaea.org/street_children/Africa/Kigali.htm).

26. Pearn J. Children and war. *J Paediatr Child Health* 2003; **39**: 166–72.

27. Bosenberg A, Thomas J, Lopez T et al. Validation of a six-graded faces scale for evaluation of postoperative pain in children. *Paediatr Anaesth* 2003; **13**: 708–13.

28. Akinyemi OO, Soyannwo AO. The choice of anaesthesia as a career by undergraduates in a developing country. *Anaesthesia* 1980; **35**: 712–15.

29. Soyannwo OA, Elegbe EO. Anaesthetic manpower development in West Africa. *Afr J Med Med Sci* 1999; **28**: 163–5.

30. Harrison GG. Anaesthesia in Africa: difficulties and directions. *World Anaesth* 1997; **1**: 2.

31. Lertakyamanee J, Tritrakern T. Anaesthesia manpower in Asia. *World Anaesth* 1999; **3**: 13–15.

32. Adnet P, Diallo A, Sanou J et al. Anesthesia practice by nurse anesthetists in French speaking Sub-Saharan Africa. *Ann Fr Anesth Reanim* 1999; **18**: 636–41.

33. UNAIDS/WHO. *Epidemic update*: December, 2005. Geneva: UNAIDS/WHO, 2005.

34. Anabwani GM, Woldetsadik EA, Kline MW. Treatment of human immunodeficiency virus (HIV) in children using antiretroviral drugs. *Semin Pediatr Infect Dis* 2005; **16**: 116–24.

35. Asamoah-Odei E, Garcia Calleja JM, Boerma JT. HIV prevalence and trends in sub-Saharan Africa: no decline and large subregional differences. *Lancet* 2004; **364**(9428): 35–40.

36. Vermund SH. Prevention of mother-to-child transmission of HIV in Africa. *Trp HIV Med* 2005; **12**(5): 130–4.

37. Lalor K. Child sexual abuse in sub-Saharan Africa: a literature review. *Child Abuse Negl* 2004; **28**: 439–60.

38. Thorne C, Newell ML. Prevention of mother-to-child transmission of HIV infection. *Curr Opin Infect Dis* 2004; **17**: 247–52.

39. Graham SM. Impact of HIV on childhood respiratory illness: differences between developing and developed countries. *Pediatr Pulmonol* 2003; **36**: 462–8.

40. Graham SM. Non-tuberculosis opportunistic infections and other lung diseases in HIV-infected infants and children. *Int J Tuberc Lung Dis* 2005; **9**: 592–602.

41. Wittenberg D, Benitez CV, Canani RB et al. HIV Infection: Working Group Report of the Second World Congress of Pediatric Gastroenterology, Hepatology, and Nutrition. *J Pediatr Gastroenterol Nutr* 2004; **39**(suppl 2): S640–6.

42. Schwartz D, Schwartz T, Cooper E, Pullerits J. Anaesthesia in the child with HIV disease. *Can J Anaesth* 1991; **38**: 626–33.

43. Wells T, Shingadia D. Global epidemiology of paediatric tuberculosis. *J Infect* 2004; **48**: 13–22.

44. Feja K, Saiman L. Tuberculosis in children. *Clin Chest Med* 2005; **26**: 295–312.

45. Singhai T. Management of severe malaria. *Indian J Pediatr* 2004; **71**: 81–8.

46. Newton CR, Taylor TE, Whitten RO. Pathophysiology of fatal *Falciparum malaria* in African children. *Am J Trop Med Hyg* 1998: **58**: 673–83.

47. Hewitson JH, Brink J, Zilla P. The challenge of pediatric cardiac services in the developing world. *Semin Thorac Cardiovasc Surg* 2002; **14**: 340–5.

48. Neirotti R. Paediatric cardiac surgery in less privileged parts of the world. *Cardiol Young* 2004; **14**: 341–6.

49. Bhagwanjee S, Bosenberg AT, Muckart DJJ. Management of sympathetic overactivity in tetanus with epidural bupivacaine and sufentanil: Experience with 11 patients. *Crit Care Med* 1999; **27**: 1721–5.

50. Eltringham RJ, Varvinski A. The Oxyvent. *Anaesthesia* 1997; **52**: 668–72.

51. Eltringham RJ, Nazal A. The Glostavent: an anesthetic machine for use in developing countries and difficult situations. *World Anaesth* 1999; **3**: 9–10.

52. Bösenberg A. Special problems in developing countries. In: Bissonette B, Dalens BJ, eds. *Pediatric anesthesia: principles and practice*. New York: McGraw-Hill, 2002.

53. Ezi Ashi TI, Papworth DP, Nunn JF. Inhalational anaesthesia in developing countries. *Anaesthesia* 1983; **38**: 729–35.

54. Jarvis DA, Brock-Utne JG. Use of an oxygen concentrator linked to a Draw-Over vaporiser (anaesthetic delivery system for underdeveloped nations). *Anesth Analg* 1991; **72**: 805–10.

55. Fenton PM. The Malawi anaesthetic machine. *Anaesthesia* 1989; **44**: 498–503.

56. Aguemon AR, Terrier G, Lansade A et al. Caudal and spinal anesthesia in sub-umbilical surgery in children. Apropos of 1875 cases. *Cah d'anesthesiol* 1996; **44**: 455–63.

57. Bosenberg A. Pediatric regional anaesthesia: an update. *Paediatr Anaesth* 2004; **14**: 398–402.

58. Bosenberg AT, Bland BA, Schulte-Steinberg O, Downing JW. Thoracic epidural anaesthesia via caudal route in infants. *Anesthesiology* 1988; **69**: 265–9.

59. Bosenberg AT. Lower limb nerve blocks in children using unsheathed needles and a nerve stimulator. *Anaesthesia* 1995; **50**: 206–10.

60. Sullivan P. Developing an administrative plan for transfusion medicine-a global perspective. *Transfusion* 2005; **45**: 224S–40S.

61. Dhingra N, Lloyd SE, Fordham J, Amin NA. Challenges in global blood safety. *World Hosp Health Serv* 2004; **40**: 45–52.

62. World Health Organisation. *Blood safety and donation a global view*. Geneva: WHO, 2005 (http: //www.who.int/mediacentre/factsheets/fs27).

63. Volkow P, Del Rio C. Paid donation and plasma trade: unrecognised forces that drive the AIDS epidemic in developing countries. *Int J STD AIDS* 2005; **16**: 5–8.

64. Barcelona SL, Thompson AA, Cote CJ. Intraoperative pediatric blood transfusion therapy: a review of common issues. Part II: transfusion therapy, special considerations, and reduction of allogenic blood transfusions. *Paediatr Anaesth* 2005; **15**: 814–30.

65. Fisher Q. Anesthesia in the developing world. *Soc Pediatr Anesth Newsl* 1999; **12**(1): 15.

66. Fisher QA, Nichols D, Stewart FC et al. Assessing pediatric anesthesia practices for volunteer medical services abroad. *Anesthesiology* 2001; **95**: 1315–22.

67. Fisher QA, Politis G, Tobias JD et al. Pediatric anesthesia for voluntary services abroad. *Anesth Analg* 2002; **95**: 336–50.

68. Unger F, Ghosh P. International cardiac surgery. *Semin Thorac Cardiovasc Surg* 2002; **14**: 321–3.

Appendix 1

Accepted normal ranges of vital cardiorespiratory variables quoted from the European Paediatric Life Support (EPLS) manual

Respiratory rate (breaths/minute)

Age (years)	Respiratory rate
<1	30–40
1–2	26–34
2–5	24–30
5–12	20–24
<12	12–20

Heart rate (beats/minute)

Age	Mean	Awake	Deep sleep
0–3 months	140	85–205	80–140
3 months–2 years	130	100–180	75–160
2–10 years	80	60–140	60–90
>10 years	75	60–100	50–90

Systolic blood pressure (mmHg)

Age	Normal	Lower limit (95th centile)
0–1 month	>60	50–60
1–12 months	80	70
1–10 years	$90 + 2 \times$ age in years	$70 \times 2 \times$ age in years
>10 years	120	90

Appendix 2

Anaesthesia drugs

Common premedicants

Drug	Dose	Comments
Atropine	*IM:* 20 mcg/kg	45 mins preop **Min dose: 100 mcg** **Max dose: 500 mcg** 90 mins preop
	PO: 20–40 mcg/kg	**Min dose: 100 mcg** **Max dose: 500 mcg**
Midazolam	*PO:* 500 mcg/kg	30–45 minutes preop **Max dose: 15 mg**
Temazepam	*PO:* 0.5–1 mg/kg	90 minutes preop **Max dose: 20 mg** Use in children >20 kg who can take tablets
Triclofos Sodium	*PO:* 50–75 mg/kg	30–40 min preop **Max dose: 1 g in a single dose**
Ametop Gel	Apply 30 minutes prior to surgery. Max application time 1 hour. Effective for 4–6 hours after removal	
EMLA Cream	Must be applied at least 1 hour before surgery, may be left on as long as required.	

Injection induction agents

Drug	Dose	Comments
Propofol	2–3 mg/kg IV	Unpremedicated day cases may require up to 5 mg/kg. Add Lidocaine 1 mg for each 10 mg of propofol to prevent pain on injection.
Thiopental	4–6 mg/kg IV	*Neonates:* 2 mg/kg
Ketamine	*IV: 1–2 mg/kg* *IM: 5–10 mg/kg*	IV increments: 1 mg/kg
Etomidate	*300 mcg/kg IV*	

Muscle relaxants

Drug	Dose	Increments	Comments
Atracurium	500–600 mcg/kg	250 mcg/kg every 30 mins	Infusion: 5–10 mcg/kg/min.
Cis-atracurium	100–400 mcg/kg	50 mcg/kg	Duration of larger dose = 40–50 mins.
Mivacurium	100–200 mcg/kg	100 mcg/kg	Infusion: 10–15 mcg/kg/min
Pancuronium	100 mcg/kg (Neonates: 50 mcg/kg)	20% of loading dose	If used in neonates respiratory support is necessary after surgery
Rocuronium	600 mcg/kg	100–200 mcg/kg	
Suxamethonium	1–2 mg/kg		
Vecuronium	100 mcg/kg (Neonates: 80 mcg/kg)	30–50 mcg/kg	Infusion of 1–10 mcg/kg/min

Intraoperative opioids

Drug	Dose	Details
Alfentanil	30–50 mcg/kg	
Codeine	IM: 1–1.5 mg/kg/dose	Every 6 h Never intravenously
Fentanyl	0.5–10 mcg/kg	Wide does range dependant on pain and duration of surgery Cardiac surgery: up to 50 mcg/kg
Morphine Sulphate	50–200 mcg/kg	Cardiac surgery: Up to 1 mg/kg total dose
Remifentanil	Loading dose: 1–2 mcg/kg Infusion: 0.05–2 mcg/kg/min as clinically indicated	Several dilutions are practical (in 5% glucose): • 300 mcg/kg in 50 ml → 1 ml/h = 0.1 mcg/kg/min • 5 mg in 500 ml → 1 ml/kg/h = 0.13 mcg/kg/min • 2 mg in 500 ml → 1.5 ml/kg/h = 0.1 mcg/kg/min
Bolus dose of Remifentanil when used with Propofol for short painful procedures	Use in separate syringes Remifentanil for each patient dilute 4 mcg/kg in 20 ml so that 5 ml contains 1 mcg/kg. Propofol for each patient dilute 5 mg/kg in 20 ml so that 4 ml contains = 1 mg/kg. Technique For lumbar puncture or bone marrow aspirate the dose of Propofol is typically 12 ml (=3 mg/kg) followed by Remifentanil 5 ml (=1 mcg/kg). Flush IV line with 20 ml of 0.9% sodium chloride when finished.	Dilute 1 mg of Remifentanil in 50 ml 0.9% sodium chloride solution → 20 mcg/ml.

Muscle relaxant reversal agents

Drug	Dose	Comments
Neostigmine	50 mcg/kg	
Atropine	25 mcg/kg	With neostigmine
Glycopyrrolate	10 mcg/kg	With neostigmine

Postoperative analgesia and anti-emetics

Drug	Route	Dose	Comments
Paracetamol	NEONATES:		
	Oral:	Loading dose: 15 mg/kg Then: 10–15 mg/kg	Max dose:
	Rectal:	Loading dose: 20 mg/kg Then: 15 mg/kg	60 mg/kg/day
	OTHERS:		
	Oral:	Loading dose: 20 mg/kg Then: 15 mg/kg	Max dose:
	Rectal:	Loading dose: 30–40 mg/kg Then: 20 mg/kg	90 mg/kg/day
	Intravenous:	Loading dose: 15 mg/kg Then 15/mg/kg 6 hourly	Limit to 5 days duration **Max IV dose 60 mg/kg/day**
Diclofenac	Oral/Rectal:	1 mg/kg every 8 hours **Max single dose:** 50 mg **Max daily dose:** 150 mg	Not in infants <6 months old. Caution in asthma or renal disease
Ibuprofen	Oral:	5 mg/kg every 6 hours **Max single dose:** 200 mg **Max daily dose:** 800 mg	Not in infants <6 months old. Caution in asthma or renal disease
Piroxicam	Sublingual:	20 mg once daily	Not recommended for younger children. Available as melt.
Codeine	Oral/Rectal: IM:	1–1.5 mg/kg every 4 hr 1 mg/kg every 4 hr **Max dose:** 60 mg	Combine with paracetamol. **Never IV**
Morphine	Oral: IV:	≥1 yr 200–400 mcg/kg every 4 h **Loading dose:** 50–100 mcg/kg **Infusion:** 10–30 mcg/kg/hr	Always prescribe NALOXONE For respiratory depression (see below)
Morphine infusion	IV:	Dilute 1.0 mg/kg in 50 ml 5% dextrose **Rate:** 0.5–1.5 ml/hr (1 ml/hr = 20 mcg/kg/hr)	For age ≥6 months with suitable monitoring
Naloxone	IV:	4 micrograms/kg	Use if respiratory rate <20/min in children <5 yrs old, and if rate <10/min for older children
Cyclizine	Oral/IV:	1 mg/kg **Max single dose:** 50 mg **Max daily dose:** 150 mg/day	Every 8 hours
Ondansetron	Oral/IV:	100 mcg/kg **Max single dose:** 4 mg **Max daily dose:** 12 mg	Every 8 hours
Dexamethasone	IV:	100 mcg/kg **Max dose:** 8 mg	Every 8 hours

Appendix 3

Other drugs that may be required either during anaesthesia, intensive care or postoperatively

Preparation	IV Dilution/ reconstitution	Dose	Comments
Adenosine		*Bolus: IV:* 100 mcg/kg (max 6 mg) increasing to 200 mcg/kg (max 12 mg)	Flush cannula with saline immediately
Amiodarone	Dilute in 5% glucose only	5 mg/kg slowly IV	Preferably via central line
Aminophylline	40 mg/kg in 50 ml 5% glucose 1 ml/hr = 0.8 mg/kg/hr	*IV Bolus:* 5 mg/kg *Then infusion:* 0.8 mg/kg/hr	Bolus dose infused over 20–30 minutes Suggested doses are for asthma
Aprotinin		*Loading dose:* 1 ml/kg *Pump:* 2 ml/kg *Infusion:* 1 ml/kg/hr	Test dose required.
Captopril		*Initially PO:* 100 mcg/kg *Then:* 300 mcg-3 mg/kg/day	Increase gradually in 3 divided doses
Chlorphenamine		*Bolus: IV:* 100 mcg/kg every 8 hrs	For opioid induced itching not responsive to naloxone
Chlorpromazine		*IM:* 500 mcg/kg	
Dexamethasone Phospate		*Initially:* *IV:* 250 mcg/kg *Then:* 100 mcg/kg 6 hourly for 3 doses either IV or IM *Anti-emetic dose* 0.1–0.25 mg/kg *Croup:* *Initially:* IV or NG: 150 mcg/kg	Usage: prevention of laryngeal oedema and post-extubation stridor For PONV give after induction prior to opioid adminstration Followed by prednisolone 1 mg/kg every 12 hours (via naso-gastric tube)
Diazepam		*PO/PR:* 0.1–0.2 mg/kg every 6 hours Max dose 2 mg	For muscle spasms
Flumazenil		*Bolus:* 1–2 mcg/kg *Infusion:* 1–5 mcg/kg/hr	Titrate against level of sedation. **NB: Half life shorter than most benzodiazepines**
Furosemide	*Infusion:* 50 mg in 50 ml 0.9% saline given at 100–300 mcg/kg/hr	*Up to:* 1 mg/kg IV	Repeatable every 6 hours

(Continued)

Preparation	IV Dilution/ reconstitution	Dose	Comments
Heparin		*IV:* 300 units/kg 400 units/kg for neonates	Cardio-pulmonary Bbypass anticoagulation.
Hydralazine	In 10 ml 0.9% saline (2 mg/ml)	*IV:* 200 mcg/kg *PO:* 1.5–3.0 mg/kg/day	Bolus titration to clinical effect. In 3 doses.
Indometacin	In 1 ml water for injection (1 mg/ml)	*IV:* 200 mcg/kg for 3 doses at 12 hour intervals	Give over 1 hr for closure of PDA.
Labetalol		*IV bolus:* Increments of 20 mcg/kg *Infusion:* 1–3 mg/kg/hr	Titrate against clinical effect. **Max dose intraop 1 mg/kg.**
Magnesium Sulphate	In 10 ml with 5% glucose (100 mg/ml)	100 mg/kg (1 ml/kg of 10% solution) **Max dose** 10 ml	Give slowly by IV injection, not faster than 10 mg/kg/min.
Mannitol	20%	*Start with:* 200 mg/kg (1 ml/kg) *Up to:* 1 g/kg (5 ml/kg)	Ensure patient is catheterised
Methyl- prednisolone		*IV:* 30 mg/kg	
Milrinone	<30 kg: 10 mg made up to 50 ml in 5% glucose >30 kg: 50 mg in 50 ml (i.e. neat solution)	load over 20 minutes with 50 mcg/kg then dose range 0.375–0.75 mcg/kg/min	Titrate against clinical effect
Naloxone – reversal of opioid induced respiratory depression – treatment of itching or urinary retention		*IV:* 4 mcg/kg *IV:* 0.5 mcg/kg	**Repeatable after 20 minutes.** NB: The half life of naloxone is much shorter than the agonists it is reversing.
Nitric Oxide	5–20 ppm. Take soda lime out of circuit and increase FGF to above minute ventilation. Administration by module automatically senses the ventilator flows and injects appropriate amount of nitric oxide. For manual ventilation the calculation is as follows:		

$$\frac{\text{Oxygen flow rate (ml/min)} \times \text{desired Nitric Oxide (ppm)}}{400} = \text{Nitric Oxide flow (ml/min)}$$

Preparation	IV Dilution/ reconstitution	Dose	Comments
Phenobarbital		*PO:* 3 mg/kg/12 hourly	
Phentolamine	1 mg/ml with 5% glucose	*IV:* Increments of: 50–100 mcg/kg	Titrate to control blood pressure (used during cardiopulmonary bypass)
Phenylephrine	in 500 ml 5% glucose (20 mcg/ml)	*IV:* 1–4 mcg/kg (0.05–0.2 ml/kg) slowly and titrate against effect	Titrate to control blood pressure (used during cardiopulmonary bypass)
Phenytoin		*Loading dose:* *IV:* 15 mg/kg over 30 mins	Check blood levels. Monitor ECG.

(Continued)

Preparation	IV Dilution/ reconstitution	Dose	Comments
Propranolol	100 mcg/ml with 5% glucose	*IV:* 50–100 mcg/kg	Slowly. Titrate to clinical effect in increments of 50 mcg/kg
Prostaglandin E_2	15 mcg/kg in 50 ml 5% glucose 1 ml/hr = 5 nanogram/kg/min	*Infusion:* 3–10 nanogram/kg/min *PO:* 5–10 mcg/kg hrly for 24 hrs	*PO:* Then decrease frequency to every 2–4 hours
Protamine		*IV:* 6 mg/kg	Slow IV to reverse heparinisation
Salbutamol	3 mg/kg in 50 ml 5% glucose 1 ml/hr = 1 mcg/kg/min	*IV:* 0.2–4 mcg/kg/min	Increase slowly by 0.01 mcg/kg/min every 15 mins
Theophylline		*Neonatal apnoea:* PO/NG: 6–9 mg/kg/dose	

Appendix 4

Doses and calculations for commonly used IV infusions

Dilutent normally glucose 5% (Neonates glucose 10%) except those marked**

	Normal dose range	Normal starting dose	Infusion
Adrenaline Isoprenaline Noradrenaline	0.01–0.5 mcg/kg/min	0.1 mcg/kg/min =	300 mcg/kg in 50 ml at 1 ml/hr
Dobutamine Dopamine	2.5–20 mcg/kg/min	5 mcg/kg/min =	3 mg/kg in 50 ml at 5 ml/hr **or** 15 mg/kg in 50 ml at 1 ml/hr
Nitroglycerin* Nitroprusside	0.5–5 mcg/kg/min	1 mcg/kg/min =	3 mg/kg in 50 ml at 1 ml/hr
Midazolam	1–6 mcg/kg/min	2 mcg/kg/min =	3 mg/kg in 50 ml at 2 ml/hr **or** 6 mg/kg in 50 ml at 1 ml/hr
Milrinone	0.375–0.75 mcg/kg/min	0.5 mcg/kg/min	See Appendix 3
Vecuronium	1–10 mcg/kg/min	2 mcg/kg/min =	6 g/kg in 50 ml at 1 ml/hr
Epoprostenol	**5–20 ng/kg/min	5 ng/kg/min =	15 mcg/kg in 50 mls at 1 ml/hr
Prostaglandin E2	3–10 ng/kg/min DUCT Up to 100 ng/kg/min PHT	5 ng/kg/min =	15 mcg mcg/kg in 50 mls at 1 ml/hr
Fentanyl	4–8 mcg/kg/hr	4 mcg/kg/hr =	100 mcg/kg in 50 ml at 2 ml/hr
Morphine (continuous infusion in the PICU. For routine post-operative analgesia see Chapter 27.)	10–40 mcg/kg/hr *Neonates* 5–15 mcg/kg/hr	20 mcg/kg/hr = *Neonates:* 10 mcg/kg/hr =	1 mg/kg in 50 ml at 1 ml/hr 1 mg/kg in 50 ml at 0.5 ml/hr

NOTES

General formulae: 3 mg/kg in 50 ml at 1 ml/hr = 1 mcg/kg/min
300 mcg/kg in 50 ml at 1 ml/hr = 0.1 mcg/kg/min (100 ng/kg/min)
30 mcg/kg in 50 ml at 1 ml/hr = 0.01 mcg/kg/min (10 ng/kg/min)
1 microgram (mcg) = 1000 nanograms (ng) Epoprostenol was formerly known as prostacyclin

* Concentration limit: Nitroglycerin **max dose**: 50 mg in 50 ml
** Dilution recommendations: Epoprostenol **minimum dose**: 70 mcg in 50 ml.
Dilute in 0.9% saline.

Infants below 5 kg

Drug	Solution	Rate
Dobutamine or Dopamine	15 mg/kg made up to 50 ml (5 × strength concentration)	Thus 1 ml/hr = 5 mcg/kg/min
Adrenaline or Noradrenaline	300 mcg/kg made up to 50 ml (1 × strength concentration)	Thus 1 ml/hr = 0.1 mcg/kg/min
Glyceryl Trinitrate (GTN) or Nitroprusside	6 mg/kg made up to 50 ml (2 × strength concentration)	Thus 1 ml/hr = 2 mcg/kg/min

Appendix 5

Basic Life Support and resuscitation algorithms

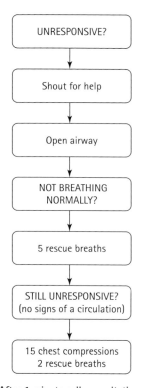

Figure A5.1 Paediatric Basic Life Support algorithm. CPR, cardiopulmonary resuscitation.

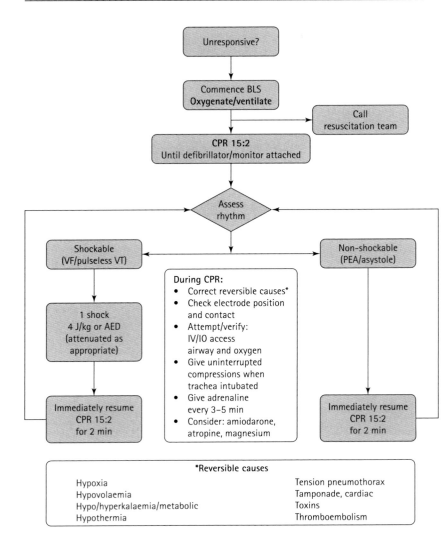

Figure A5.2   Paediatric Advanced Life Support algorithm. AED, automated external defibrillator; BLS Basic Life Support; CPR, cardiopulmonary resuscitation; IO, intraosseous; IV, intravenous; PEA, pulseless electrical activity.

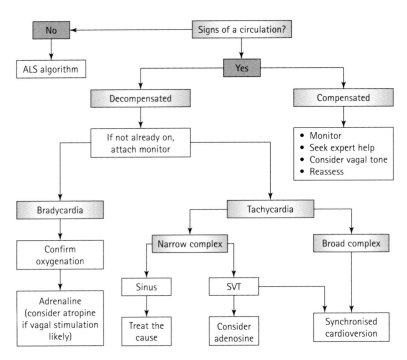

Figure A5.3   Algorithm detailing the approach to arrhythmias in children. ALS, Advanced Life Support; SVT, supraventricular tachycardia.

Index